ANESTHESIA EQUIPMENT

PRINCIPLES AND APPLICATIONS

ANESTHESIA EQUIPMENT

PRINCIPLES AND APPLICATIONS

Jan Ehrenwerth, M.D.

Professor of Anesthesiology
Director, Section of General Anesthesia
Yale University School of Medicine;
Attending Anesthesiologist
Yale New Haven Hospital
New Haven, Connecticut

James B. Eisenkraft, M.D.,
M.R.C.P. (U.K.), F.F.A.R.C.S.

Professor of Anesthesiology
Director of Anesthesia Research
Mount Sinai School of Medicine
of the City University of New York;
Attending Anesthesiologist
The Mount Sinai Medical Center
New York, New York

with 655 illustrations

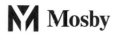 Mosby

St. Louis Baltimore Boston Chicago London Philadelphia Sydney Toronto

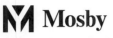

Mosby

Dedicated to Publishing Excellence

Editor: Susan M. Gay
Assistant Editor: Sandra E. Clark
Project Supervisor: Barbara Bowes Merritt
Book Designer: Julie Taugner
Cover Designer: Kathy Barkey
Editing and Production: York Production Services

Printed in the United States of America.

Mosby–Year Book, Inc.
11830 Westline Industrial Drive
St. Louis, MO 63146

Library of Congress Cataloging in Publication Data
Anesthesia equipment : principles and applications / [edited by] Jan
  Ehrenwerth, James B. Eisenkraft.
     p.   cm.
   Includes bibliographical references and index.
   ISBN 0-8016-1556-9
   1. Anesthesiology—Aparatus and instruments.   I. Ehrenwerth,
Jan. II. Eisenkraft, James B.
   [DNLM: 1. Anesthesiology—instrumentation.   WO 240 A579]
   RD78.8.A54   1993
   617.9′6′028--dc20
   DNLM/DLC
   for Library of Congress   92-48755
                                       CIP

93 94 95 96 97 CL/MY 9 8 7 6 5 4 3 2 1

CONTRIBUTORS

Isaac Azar, M.D.
Associate Director of Anesthesiology
Beth Israel Medical Center
Professor of Anesthesiology
Mount Sinai School of Medicine
New York, New York

Steven J. Barker, Ph.D., M.D.
Professor and Chairman
Department of Anesthesiology
University of California, Irvine
Orange, California

Charlotte Bell, M.D.
Assistant Professor
Department of Anesthesiology
Yale University School of Medicine;
Attending Anesthesiologist
Yale New Haven Hospital
New Haven, Connecticut

Sorin J. Brull, M.D.
Assistant Professor of Anesthesiology
Yale University School of Medicine;
Attending Anesthesiologist
Yale New Haven Hospital
New Haven, Connecticut

Enrico M. Camporesi, M.D.
Professor and Chairman
Department of Anesthesia;
Professor of Physiology
SUNY Health Science Center
Syracuse, New York

Hansel de Sousa, M.D.
Department of Anesthesiology
Cortland Memorial Hospital
Cortland, New York

Jan Ehrenwerth, M.D.
Professor of Anesthesiology
Director, Section of General Anesthesia
Yale University School of Medicine;
Attending Anesthesiologist
Yale New Haven Hospital
New Haven, Connecticut

John H. Eichhorn, M.D.
Professor and Chairman
Department of Anesthesiology
University of Mississippi Medical Center
Jackson, Mississippi

James B. Eisenkraft, M.D., M.R.C.P. (U.K.),
F.F.A.R.C.S.
Professor of Anesthesiology;
Director of Anesthesia Research
Mount Sinai School of Medicine
  of the City University of New York;
Attending Anesthesiologist
The Mount Sinai Medical Center
New York, New York

Carl E. Englund, Ph.D.
Head
Information and Decision Management Branch
Naval Ocean Systems Center
San Diego, California

Jeffrey M. Feldman, M.S.E., M.D.
Associate Director of Research and Obstetric Anesthesia
Department of Anesthesiology
Albert Einstein Medical Center
Associate Professor of Anesthesiology
Temple University School of Medicine
Philadelphia, Pennsylvania

Michael L. Good, M.D.
Assistant Professor of Anesthesiology
University of Florida College of Medicine
Gainesville, Florida

Joachim S. Gravenstein, M.D.
Graduate Research Professor in Anesthesiology
University of Florida/Shands Teaching Hospital
Gainesville, Florida

Nikolaus Gravenstein, M.D.
Professor of Anesthesiology and Neurosurgery
Interim Chairman
Department of Anesthesiology
University of Florida College of Medicine
Gainesville, Florida

Alan W. Grogono, M.D., F.F.A.R.C.S.
Chairman and Merryl and Sam Israel, Jr.
Professor of Anesthesiology
Tulane University Medical Center
New Orleans, Louisiana

Simon C. Hillier, M.B., Ch.B., F.F.A.R.C.S.
Assistant Professor of Anesthesia
Indiana University School of Medicine
Indianapolis, Indiana

Cindy W. Hughes, M.D.
Assistant Professor
Department of Anesthesiology
Albany Medical College
Albany, New York

David Eric Lees, M.D.
Professor and Chairman
Department of Anesthesia
Georgetown University School of Medicine
Washington, DC

Robert G. Loeb, M.D.
Assistant Professor
Department of Anesthesiology
University of California, Davis
Davis, California;
Medical Director of Ambulatory Surgery Unit
University of California, Davis Medical Center
Sacramento, California

William L. McNiece, M.D.
Assistant Professor of Anesthesia
Indiana University School of Medicine
Indianapolis, Indiana

Jolie Narang, M.D.
Assistant Professor
Department of Anesthesiology
Mount Sinai School of Medicine
   of the City University of New York
New York, New York

Autry J. Parker, M.D.
Clinical Fellow in Chronic Pain
Johns Hopkins University School of Medicine
Baltimore, Maryland

Annette G. Pashayan, M.D.
Associate Professor of Anesthesiology and Neurosurgery
University of Florida College of Medicine
Gainesville, Florida

James H. Philip, M.E. (E.), M.D.
Anesthesiologist
Director of Bioengineering
Department of Anesthesia
Brigham and Women's Hospital;
Associate Professor of Anaesthesia
Harvard Medical School
Boston, Massachusetts

Timothy J. Quill, M.D.
Associate Professor
Department of Anesthesiology
Dartmouth-Hitchcock Medical Center
Hanover, New Hampshire

Daniel B. Raemer, Ph.D.
Associate Professor of Anaesthesia
Harvard Medical School;
Director of Biomedical Engineering
Brigham and Women's Hospital
Boston, Massachusetts

Sivam Ramanathan, M.D.
Professor of Anesthesiology and Critical Care Medicine
University of Pittsburgh School of Medicine
Magee-Women's Hospital
Pittsburgh, Pennsylvania

Leslie Rendell-Baker, M.D.
Professor of Anesthesiology
Loma Linda University School of Medicine
Loma Linda, California

E.S. Siker, M.D.
Chairman
Department of Anesthesiology
Mercy Hospital
Pittsburgh, Pennsylvania

David G. Silverman, M.D.
Associate Professor of Anesthesiology
Director of Departmental Clinical Research
Yale University School of Medicine
New Haven, Connecticut

Raymond S. Sinatra, M.D., Ph.D.
Associate Professor of Anesthesiology
Director, Pain Management Service
Yale University School of Medicine
New Haven, Connecticut

N. Ty Smith, M.D.
Professor of Anesthesiology
University of California, San Diego
School of Medicine
San Diego Veterans Affairs Medical Center
San Diego, California

Theodore Craig Smith, M.D.
Chief of Anesthesia
E.A. Hines Jr. Veterans Affairs Hospital
Maywood, Illinois;
Professor of Anesthesiology
Loyola University Chicago
Stitch School of Medicine
Chicago, Illinois

Richard M. Sommer, M.D.
Assistant Professor of Anesthesiology
New York University School of Medicine;
Chief of Anesthesiology
Veterans Affairs Medical Center
New York, New York

Joe T. Travis, M.D.
Resident in Anesthesiology
Tulane University Medical Center
New Orleans, Louisiana

Daniel M. Thys, M.D.
Director, Department of Anesthesiology
St. Luke's/Roosevelt Hospital Center
Professor
Department of Anesthesiology
College of Physicians and Surgeons
Columbia University
New York, New York

Kevin K. Tremper, Ph.D., M.D.
Professor and Chairman
Department of Anesthesiology
University of Michigan
Ann Arbor, Michigan

Jan J. van der Aa, Ph.D.
Adjunct Assistant Professor
Department of Anesthesiology
University of Florida College of Medicine
Gainesville, Florida

Matthew B. Weinger, M.D.
Assistant Professor of Anesthesiology
University of California, San Diego
Staff Physician
Veterans Administration Medical Center
San Diego, California

Roxanne F. Zarmsky, M.D.
Assistant Professor
Department of Anesthesiology
Yale University School of Medicine
New Haven, Connecticut

Ross H. Zoll, Ph.D., M.D.
Assistant Professor
Department of Anesthesiology
Yale University School of Medicine
New Haven, Connecticut

To Sally, Corey, and Megan,
and to my parents.

JAN EHRENWERTH

To my mother,
to the memory of my father,
and to Gail, Michelle, and Jonathan.

JAMES B. EISENKRAFT

FOREWORD

The last ten years have seen a great advance in the quality and safety of anesthesia. This is in part due to an enhanced understanding of underlying physiology and the introduction of new drugs of high specificity and low toxicity. These developments have been matched by modest advances in anesthesia equipment, but the quantum leap has been in monitoring of the process and the patient. Meanwhile the challenges to the anesthesiologist have multiplied in the form of more adventurous surgery as well as such novel environments as lithotripsy, laparoscopic procedures, and magnetic resonance imaging. Never before have anesthesiologists been surrounded by equipment of such complexity, and the trend will surely continue. There is an inevitable price to pay for technological advances on this scale, and failure of equipment or its misuse by the anesthesiologist becomes an even more important cause of misadventure.

Textbooks on anesthesiology usually rate a chapter or two on the equipment used in our discipline, while a few books have been devoted entirely to the technicalities of equipment. It might, therefore, appear that the ground was fully covered. In fact the present volume has detected an unfilled niche. The special objective of this book is to present equipment in the context of its physiological and pharmacological relevance and also to explain the physical principles that underlie the way in which the equipment works. The topics are further broadened by an exposition of the rationale of its use and, where appropriate, the risk management and medicolegal significance of its employment. All of this is more important than the pure technology, which changes from year to year. Throughout the book, emphasis is on patients and clinical practice rather than simply on equipment as the name of the book might seem to imply. The whole book has its feet firmly on the ground and dispassionately reviews the pros, cons, and practicalities of new and future technology.

The contents of this book embrace an exceptionally wide range of equipment, dealing with the anesthesia machine, monitors, and the anesthetic environment. Can a single book do justice to this broad field? Drs. Jan Ehrenwerth and James Eisenkraft, the editors, have succeeded in this daunting challenge. They have assembled the expertise in these changing fields and melded it into a logical and consistent exposition of the state of the art. There is obvious merit in the provision of clear and concise answers to questions about the design and function of the entire range of anesthesia equipment in a single volume.

In today's world, particularly valuable sections of the book deal with Hazards and Safety Features (Part IV) and Maintenance and Quality Assurance (Part V). These broadly based sections are not confined to hazards of the equipment itself, but also address the very difficult issues of vigilance, ergonomics of the workspace, record-keeping (both manual and automated), alarms and their interpretation, the role of computers, and integrated "smart" monitoring systems. Regulations of the United States Food and Drug Administration receive detailed consideration.

In Part VI, Special Situations, the reader will discover a miscellany of topics that might otherwise be difficult to locate. This section is especially important because of increasing demands for anesthesia services outside the operating room, in the presence of novel modalities of therapy and investigation, in abnormal physical environments, and in developing countries. The section on low flow techniques may well become highly relevant to the use of more expensive volatile anesthetics. The final chapter (Chapter 33) on future trends portends the transformation of the anesthesia apparatus which now appears overdue.

If ever there was a current need for a single reference text, this one is it. This is not a book to molder on the library shelves but one which should be prominently accessible in the clinical area for instant access and also for the education of the resident.

J.F. Nunn
E.S. Siker

PREFACE

Anesthesia Equipment: Principles and Applications is intended to provide the student and practitioner of anesthesiology with a contemporary review of the equipment used in the delivery and monitoring of a basic anesthetic. Dr. Richard Kitz stated, "Of the three legs of the tripod labelled anesthesiology—pathophysiology, pharmacology, and technology—technology is the least stressed in our educational programs."* Because of the complexity of modern anesthesia equipment, many anesthesia practitioners regard it as somewhat of a "black box" that is little understood, expensive, and not to be tampered with for liability reasons. Meanwhile, studies of complications in relation to anesthesia equipment have shown that while overt failure is rare, user error and failure to recognize spurious data are not uncommon. A basic understanding of the equipment used routinely is therefore essential to the safe practice of anesthesia.

Our fundamental approach to describing equipment is to first define *principles* of operation, including where applicable the physics and technological aspects. Once these are understood the applications and limitations of the equipment will be more readily appreciated.

This volume is organized into six parts. Part I covers the *Design Features* of the basic delivery system for inhalational anesthesia. While the contemporary delivery systems used in North America are emphasized, the principles described will be applicable to other systems used elsewhere in the world. Designs and arrangements that are no longer contemporary in North America and which may be considered unsafe (e.g., in-circuit vaporizers) have been deliberately omitted. Measured flow vaporizing systems (e.g., Copper Kettle) are included, however, since they illustrate important principles; also these systems are still used on modern field anesthesia machines. The clinical relevance and safety aspects of the anatomy of the delivery system are emphasized throughout.

Part II, *System Monitors*, describes the basic monitors of the delivery system that ensure that it is functioning correctly and as intended by the user. Part III, *Patient Monitors*, describes additional equipment used for basic intraoperative monitoring as defined in the standards published by the American Society of Anesthesiologists. More specialized monitors such as the electroencephalogram, evoked potentials, and transesophageal echocardiogram are deliberately omitted since they are not considered basic or routinely used.

Part IV covers *Hazards* as well as *Safety Features* of anesthesia equipment. This section considers the anesthesia workspace as a whole and includes chapters on computer applications in anesthesia practice and automated anesthesia information management systems (record-keepers).

Part V describes *Maintenance and Quality Assurance* aspects of anesthesia equipment. This is clearly an area of extreme importance since equipment requires a large financial investment and any malfunction may have medicolegal implications. Part VI, *Special Situations*, includes chapters on use of equipment for other-than-routine adult anesthesia in the main operating room suite of the hospital, closed circuit anesthesia, and infusion pumps used to deliver intravenous agents. As anesthesia equipment continues to evolve and in preparation for the 21st century, the final chapter considers the future direction of anesthesia delivery systems.

The editors wish to acknowledge the efforts of all those who have made this book possible and in particular the contributors, without whose work and expertise this book would not have been possible. We would also like to thank all of the equipment manufacturers for providing technical information and many of the illustrations used, and especially acknowledge the help of Paul Baumgart and Ross Garland of Ohmeda, and Joseph Condurso and Peter Schreiber of North American Dräger. Our sincere appreciation also goes to our secretaries Jill Fuggi (Yale) and Joanne Delerme (Mount Sinai) for their superb assistance; to Susan Gay, Executive Editor, Mosby–Year Book for her constant encouragement in the formulation and production of this book; to Sandra Clark, Assistant Editor, Mosby–Year Book; and to Sandra Schnetzka, Production Coordinator, York Production Services.

*Kitz RJ: Can technology education during medical school make better doctors? Society for Technology in Anesthesia First Annual Distinguished Lecture, January 1991. *J Clin Monit* 8:243-249, 1992.

We are grateful to all of our own teachers and mentors for stimulating our interest in the science and technology of anesthesia, and in particular to Drs. E.S. Siker and John F. Nunn, who also contributed the Foreword. We also thank our families for their constant patience and support throughout the genesis of this work. Last, but by no means least, we would both like to thank Dr. Paul G. Barash, the *shadchan* whose matchmaking brought us together to compile and edit this book.

Jan Ehrenwerth, M.D.   **James B. Eisenkraft, M.D.**
New Haven, Connecticut   New York, New York

CONTENTS

Part I

DESIGN FEATURES

Structure, function, and rationale

Chapter 1

MEDICAL GASES: STORAGE AND SUPPLY

John H. Eichhorn, M.D.
Jan Ehrenwerth, M.D.

Anesthesia providers were once expected to know a great deal about the storage and supply of medical gases.

In both large and small institutions, anesthesiologists often had to rely on their own knowledge and skill in this area to manage the many aspects of medical gases, from purchasing to troubleshooting.

Today, changes in technology and institutional organization often relieve the anesthesiologist of most of these responsibilities. However, this should not excuse anesthesia providers from understanding the basic facts and safety principles associated with the use of medical gases for anesthesia. Almost without exception, the only medical gases encountered by practicing anesthesiologists today are oxygen, nitrous oxide, and compressed air. For safety reasons, flammable agents are rarely if ever used in operating rooms today. Nitrogen is used almost exclusively to power gas-driven equipment. Helium, carbon dioxide, and particularly premixed combinations of oxygen and helium or carbon dioxide are generally no longer used. The anesthesiologist who finds it necessary to use one of these gases must be fully versed in its characteristics and safe handling. Detailed information and numerous references relating to the handling and use of these and other unusual medical gases, along with a wealth of general information about medical gas cylinders, is presented in two publications from the Compressed Gas Association.*[1,2]

Medical gas manufacturers are subject to more stringent government and industry-based regulations and inspections than in the past. This has helped reduce markedly the number of accidents related to medical gases. For these reasons, anesthesia training programs may not emphasize

---

*Compressed Gas Association, Inc., 1235 Jefferson Davis Highway, Arlington, VA 22202, (703) 979-0900.

instruction in the various aspects of storing and using medical gases.

In addition, the recent increased concern with the safety of anesthetized patients has helped to reduce the number of gas-related injuries. Almost universal use of inspired oxygen monitors (with lower-limit alarms) provides the anesthesia practitioner with an early warning in the event that the oxygen supply becomes inadequate. Should the oxygen monitor fail, pulse oximetry can alert the anesthesiologist to problems with patient oxygenation that are related to inadequate oxygen supply.

MEDICAL GAS CYLINDERS AND THEIR USE

Medical gases are stored either in metal cylinders or in the reservoirs of bulk gas storage and supply systems. The cylinders are almost always attached to the anesthesia gas machine. Bulk supply systems use pipelines and connections to transport medical gases from bulk storage to the anesthesia machine.

Virtually all facilities in which anesthesia is administered are equipped with central gas supply systems. Today, E cylinders are rarely the only source of medical gas for anesthesia machines. If, however, an anesthetic is being administered using only E cylinders, then *both* the anesthesiologist and related support personnel must first ensure that an adequate supply of reserve cylinders is available. In addition, the amount of gas in the cylinders being used must be continually monitored, and the cylinders must be replaced before they are completely empty. The importance of this cannot be overemphasized. Most anesthesia practitioners today have not been confronted with the possibility of running out of oxygen and having to change a tank while administering an anesthetic.

Anesthesia practitioners should be familiar with two sizes of gas cylinders. The E cylinder (approximately 2 feet long and 4 inches in diameter) is the cylinder most often used by anesthesia providers. E cylinders are also routinely used as portable oxygen sources when a patient is transported between the OR and an Intensive Care Unit. H cylinders are larger (approximately 4 feet long and 9 inches in diameter) and are generally used as sources of gas for small or infrequently used pipeline systems. They may be used as intermediate or long-term sources of gas at the patient's bedside. Almost all hospitals store H cylinders of oxygen in bulk as a backup source in case the pipeline oxygen fails or is depleted. H cylinders of nitrogen are often used to power gas-driven medical equipment. Occasionally, H cylinders containing oxygen, nitrous oxide, or air have been used in operating rooms, connected to the anesthesia machine via special reducing valves and hoses. Such unconventional configurations not only can be hazardous but also defeat certain safeguards. Any practitioner using such a system must become thoroughly familiar with it and be certain that it complies with applicable regulations and guidelines.[1-5]

Oxygen tanks*

Oxygen (O_2) has a molecular weight of 32 and a boiling point of $-183°$ C at atmospheric pressure 760 mmHg (14.7 psia).[†] The boiling point of a gas (the temperature at which it changes from liquid phase to gas) is related to ambient pressure in such a way that as pressure increases, so does the boiling point. However, a certain *critical temperature* is reached above which, no matter how much pressure is applied to the liquid phase, a gas boils into its gaseous form. The critical temperature for oxygen is $-118°$ C, and the *critical pressure,* which must be applied at this temperature to keep oxygen liquid, is 737 psia. Because room temperature is usually 20° C and therefore in excess of the critical temperature, oxygen can exist only as a gas at room temperature.

E cylinders of oxygen are filled to a pressure of approximately 1900 psig[‡] at room temperature. When full, they contain a fixed number of gas molecules (fixed mass of gas). These molecules obey Boyle's law, Pressure × Volume = Constant (or $P_1V_1 = P_2V_2$), provided that temperature does not change. A full E cylinder of oxygen with internal volume 5 L (V_1) and pressure 1900 psig (P_1) will, therefore, evolve approximately 660 L (V_2) of gaseous oxygen at atmospheric pressure (V_2) (14.7 psia). Thus Boyle's law, $P_1V_1 = P_2V_2$, gives $V_2 = (P_1 × V_1)/P_2 = (1900 × 5)/14.7 = 660$ L (approximately).

If the oxygen tank's pressure gauge reads 1000 psig, then the tank is (1000/1900) or 52% full and will evolve only (660 × 52%) 340 L of oxygen (Fig. 1-1). If such a tank were being used at an oxygen flow rate of 6 L/min, it would empty in just under an hour (actually 340/6 = 57 minutes). Likewise, a full (2200 psig) H cylinder will evolve 6900 L of oxygen at atmospheric pressure. It is important to understand these principles when oxygen tanks are being used to supply the machine or a ventilator or to transport patients. Thus, because oxygen exists only as a gas at room temperature, the tank's pressure gauge can be used to determine how much gas remains in the cylinder. Clearly, if a machine is equipped with two E cylinders of oxygen, only one should ever be open at any time so that both tanks are not emptied simultaneously.

Nitrous oxide tanks*

Nitrous oxide (N_2O) has a molecular weight of 44 and a boiling point of $-88°$ C at 760 mmHg. Because it has a critical temperature of 36.5° C (and critical pressure of 1054 psig) nitrous oxide can exist as a liquid at room temperature (20° C). E cylinders of nitrous oxide are filled to

---

*Portions of this chapter are reproduced by permission from Eisenkraft J.B.: The anesthesia delivery system, Part I, vol 3, In *Progress in anesthesiology,* San Antonio, Texas, 1989, Dannemiller Memorial Educational Foundation.
†Psia = pounds per square inch absolute pressure.
‡Psig = pounds per square inch gauge pressure. One atmospheric of pressure (760 mmHg) = 0 psig = 14.7 psia.

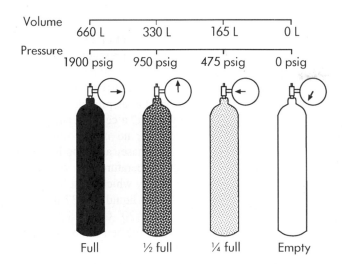

Fig. 1-1. Oxygen remains a gas under high pressure. The pressure falls linearly as the gas flows from the cylinder; thus, in contrast to nitrous oxide, the pressure remaining always reflects the amount of gas remaining in the cylinder. (Redrawn from Bowie E, Huffman LM: *The anesthesia machine: essentials for understanding*. With permission from Ohmeda, a Division of BOC Health Care, Inc.)

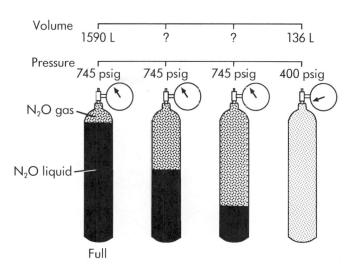

Fig. 1-2. At ambient temperature (20° C), nitrous oxide liquifies under high pressure and the pressure of the gas above the liquid remains constant *independent* of how much liquid remains in the cylinder. Only when all the liquid has evaporated does the pressure start to fall, and then it does so rapidly as the residual gas flows from the cylinder. (Redrawn from Bowie E, Huffman LM: *The anesthesia machine: essentials for understanding*. With permission from Ohmeda, a Division of BOC Health Care, Inc.)

90% to 95% capacity with liquid nitrous oxide. Above the liquid in the tank is nitrous oxide vapor, that is, gaseous nitrous oxide. Because the liquid nitrous oxide is in equilibrium with its vapor phase, the pressure exerted by the nitrous oxide vapor is its saturated vapor pressure (SVP) at the ambient temperature.

A full E cylinder of nitrous oxide will evolve approximately 1590 L of gaseous nitrous oxide at one atmosphere pressure (14.7 psia). As long as some liquid nitrous oxide remains in the tank and temperature remains constant (20° C) the pressure in the tank will be 745 psig, which is the SVP of nitrous oxide at 20° C (Fig. 1-2). It becomes clear that, unlike oxygen, the content of a tank of nitrous oxide cannot be determined from the pressure gauge. It can, however, be determined by removing the tank, weighing it, and subtracting the weight of the empty tank (tare weight), which is stamped on each tank. The difference is the weight of the contained nitrous oxide. By Avogadro's volume, 1 g molecular weight of any gas or vapor occupies 22.4 L at standard temperature and pressure. Thus 44 g of nitrous oxide occupies 22.4 L at 0° C and 760 mmHg pressure. At 20° C this volume increases to $(22.4 \times 293/273 =)$ 24 L. Thus each gram weight of nitrous oxide is equivalent to 0.55 L of gas at 20° C.

Only when all of the liquid nitrous oxide in the tank has been used up and the tank contains only gaseous nitrous oxide can Boyle's law be applied. In this instance, where the tank pressure (P_1) is 745 psig (due to gas only) and the internal volume (V_1) of the E cylinder is approximately 5 L, the volume (V_2) of nitrous oxide gas that will be

evolved at atmospheric pressure (P_2) is

$$V_2 = (P_1 \times V_1)/P_2 \quad \text{or} \quad (745 \times 5)/14.7 = 253 \text{ L}$$

At this point the tank is (253/1590) 16% full. A tank showing a pressure of 400 psig at 20° C will evolve (400/745) × 253 = 136 L of nitrous oxide gas.

While anesthesia is being administered, it is not practical to remove the nitrous oxide cylinder from the anesthesia machine and weigh it accurately enough to determine how much nitrous oxide is left. When the nitrous oxide is being used rapidly, the latent heat of vaporization causes the cylinder itself to become cold. If there is sufficient humidity in the surrounding atmosphere, some moisture or even frost may collect on the outside surface of the cylinder over the portion that is filled with liquid nitrous oxide. The moisture or frost line, which may actually fall as the gas is used, can provide an indication of when the nitrous oxide will run out. A number of tapes and devices are available with which to mark the cylinders for this purpose, but these are apparently unreliable. If the anesthesiologist is going to use only tanks of nitrous oxide for an anesthetic, it is best to begin with a full cylinder. When this is done, the length of time that the cylinder will last can be calculated. For example, a full E cylinder of nitrous oxide used at a flow rate of 3 L/min will last about 9 hours (3 × 60 × 9 = 1620 L). The anesthesiologist must remember that when the pressure in the cylinder begins to fall, there are about 250 L left to be evolved and the tank will need replacement in the near future.

Table 1-1. Typical medical gas cylinders volume and weight of available contents.* All volumes at 70° F (21.1° C)

Cylinder style and dimensions	Nominal volume cu in/liter	Contents	Air	Carbon dioxide	Cyclo-propane	Helium	Nitrogen	Nitrous oxide	Oxygen	Mixtures of oxygen	
										Helium	CO$_2$
B 3½ in. od × 13 in. 8.89 × 33 cm	87/1.43	psig liters lb-oz. kilograms		838 370 1-8 0.68	75 375 1-7¼ 0.66				1900 200 — —		
D 4½ in. od × 17 in. 10.8 × 43 cm	176/2.88	psig liters lb-oz. kilograms	1900 375 — —	838 940 3-13 1.73	75 870 3-5½ 1.51	1600 300 — —	1900 370 — —	745 940 3-13 1.73	1900 400 — —	** 300 ** **	** 400 ** **
E 4¼ in. od × 26 in. 10.8 × 66 cm	293/4.80	psig liters lb-oz. kilograms	1900 625 — —	838 1,590 6-7 2.92		1600 500 — —	1900 610 — —	745 1,590 6-7 2.92	1900 660 — —	** 500 ** **	** 660 ** **
M 7 in. od × 43 in. 17.8 × 109 cm	1337/21.9	psig liters lb-oz. kilograms	1900 2850 — —	838 7,570 30-10 13.9		1600 2260 — —	2200 3200 — —	7.45 7,570 30-10 13.9	2200 3450 122 cu ft —	** 2260 ** **	** 3000 ** **
G 8½ in. od × 51 in. 21.6 × 130 cm	2370/38.8	psig liters lb-oz. kilograms	1900 5050 — —	838 12,300 50-0 22.7		1600 4000 — —		745 13,800 56-0 25.4		** 4000 ** **	** 5330 ** **
H or K 9¼ in. od × 51 in. 23.5 × 130 cm	2660/43.6	psig liters lb-oz. kilograms	2200 6550 — —			2200 6000 — —	2200 6400 — —	745 15,800 64 29.1	2200† 6900 244 cu ft —		
Pin Index Safety System Pin positions (see Fig. 1-6)			1-5	—	3-6	—	1-4	3-5	2-5	4-6 2-4	2-6 1-6

Adapted with permission from Compressed Gas Association: Characteristics and safe handling of medical gases, publication P-2 (ed 7), Arlington, Va, 1989, The Association.

*These are computed contents based on nominal cylinder volumes and rounded to no greater variance than ± 1%.

**The pressure and weight of mixed gases will vary according to the composition of the mixture.

†275 cu ft/7800 L cylinders at 2490 psig are available upon request.

CHARACTERISTICS OF GAS CYLINDERS
Size

Table 1-1 gives a list of the sizes, weights, and volumes of the common cylinders that contain the various medical gases. As noted, the anesthesia provider will most often encounter oxygen and nitrous oxide in E cylinders and a variety of gases in H cylinders. Although other gas cylinders (i.e., those used for gas-powered equipment, laparoscopy equipment, and lasers) are found in the operating room, these are not likely to be in the domain of anesthesia personnel.

Color coding

Table 1-2 lists the color markings used to identify medical gas cylinders. Although the internationally accepted color for oxygen is white, the United States continues to use green, primarily for reasons of tradition. Yellow is used to identify compressed air in the United States, and this represents another exception to international standards. Anesthesiologists working in countries other than the United States should be aware of these differences.

Cylinder markings

Certain codes are stamped near the neck on all medical gas cylinders. The code "DOT" indicates that the cylinder was manufactured according to specifications of the United States Department of Transportation (DOT) (Fig. 1-3). The DOT has extensive regulations of its own concerning the marking and shipping of medical gas cylinders. The service pressure (psig), which is stamped on each cylinder,

Table 1-2. Color marking of compressed gas containers intended for medical use

Gas intended for medical use	United States color	Canada color
Oxygen	Green	White*
Carbon dioxide	Gray	Gray
Nitrous oxide	Blue	Blue
Cyclopropane	Orange	Orange
Helium	Brown	Brown
Nitrogen	Black	Black
Air	Yellow*	Black and white
Gas mixture (other than mixtures of oxygen and nitrogen)	Color marking of mixtures shall be a combination of colors corresponding to each component gas	

Gas mixtures of oxygen and nitrogen

19.5% to 23.5% oxygen	Yellow*	Black and white
All other oxygen concentrations	Black and green	Pink

Adapted with permission from Compressed Gas Association: Standard color marking of compressed gas containers intended for medical use, publication C-9 (ed 3), Arlington, Va, 1988, The Association.
*Historically, white has been used in the United States, and yellow used in Canada, to identify vacuum systems. Therefore, it is recommended that white *not* be used in the United States, and yellow *not* be used in Canada, as a marking to identify containers for use with any medical gas.

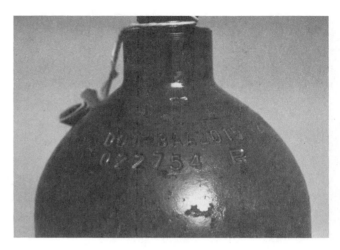

Fig. 1-3. Some of the cylinder markings on an E cylinder. *DOT-3AA* indicates that the cylinder was manufactured according to the specifications of the United States Department of Transportation. *3AA* indicates the type of steel used. *2015* indicates the maximum filling pressure of the cylinder in psig. The number below *DOT* is the cylinder serial number, and the mark beside it is the manufacturer's name.

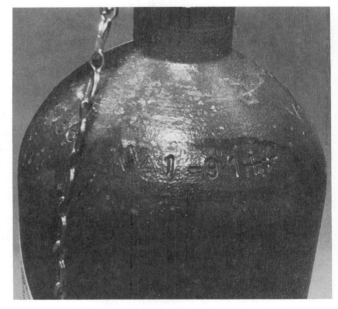

Fig. 1-4. An E cylinder of oxygen. The inspection date, January 1991, has been circled in black marker to indicate the cylinder was checked at the time it was delivered to the facility. All cylinders must be checked for leaks and structural integrity with an overpressure test at least once every 10 years.

should never be exceeded. Each cylinder is also given its own serial number and commercial designation. The final code stamped on the cylinder is usually the date of the last inspection and the inspector's mark. Medical gas cylinders must be inspected at least once every 10 years, at which time they should also be tested for structural integrity. This is done by filling the cylinder to 1.66 times the normal service pressure. The date of this inspection is often circled with a black marker to indicate that the cylinder has been checked by the supplier (Fig. 1-4).

All medical gas cylinders should come from the supplier having a tag with three perforated sections, each designating a different stage of use. These are "empty," "in use," and "full." The portion of the tag marked "full" should be removed when a cylinder is put into service. This is not usually critical, however, as it is generally obvious when a cylinder is in use. Making use of the tag marker does become important when an empty cylinder is removed from the machine. If the tag is not used correctly at the outset, the problem becomes compounded with each successive stage of the cylinder's use, and the final result is storage of an empty cylinder as a full one. Although a discrepancy in weight may well alert a user to an incorrectly labeled cylinder, it may be easily overlooked in an emergency situation and can lead to a serious problem. Thus all anesthesia personnel must recognize the importance of correct labeling.

Pressure relief valves

All medical gas cylinders must incorporate a mechanism to vent the cylinder's contents before it explodes from excessive pressure.[6] Explosion can be a result of exposure to extreme heat (i.e., a fire) or accidental gross overfilling. These mechanisms are of three basic types that are incorporated into the cylinder and cannot be inspected by the user. The fusible plug, made of a metal alloy with a low melting point, will melt in a fire, allowing the gas to escape. With certain gases, such as oxygen or nitrous oxide, this can aggravate the fire. The frangible disc assembly consists of a metal disc that is designed to break when a certain pressure is exceeded and thereby allow the gas to escape through a discharge vent. Finally, the safety relief valve is a spring-loaded mechanism that closes a discharge vent. If the pressure rises, the valve opens until the pressure falls below the valve's opening threshold. Some cylinders have combination devices incorporating a fusible metal plug with one of the other two mechanisms.

Connectors

Figure 1-5 illustrates the tops of typical valves for both small (E) and large (H) cylinders. As previously mentioned, large cylinders such as H cylinders have valve outlets that are coded and unique to the gas content of the cylinder. The coding is based on the threads and diameter of the outlet port orifice.[4] Regulators to reduce and control the pressure of the gas, also specific for each type of gas, are attached to these threaded valve ports. It is highly unsafe to use a regulator for one type of gas on a valve port of a cylinder of another type of gas.

Small cylinders such as E cylinders have cylindrical ports or holes in their valves to receive the yoke (either on an anesthesia machine or freestanding) from which the gas will flow. A washer (usually Teflon) is necessary to make this connection gas-tight. One must be careful not to place the retaining screw that holds the cylinder in the yoke into the safety relief device instead of its intended location in the conical depression opposite the valve port (Fig. 1-5, *A*). The connection between cylinder valve and yoke is made gas-specific by the pin-index system for small-cylinder connections.

GAS CYLINDER SAFETY ISSUES
Prevention of wrong gas cylinder connections

In the past, cylinders containing the wrong gas (for example, nitrous oxide instead of oxygen) were sometimes connected to anesthesia gas delivery systems, with disastrous results. This led to the development of systems designed to help ensure use of the correct cylinder. Most of the gas used for anesthesia comes from E cylinders or other small cylinders, for which the pin-index system was developed in 1952. The Pin Index Safety System[4] has two (5-mm) stainless steel pins on the cylinder yoke connector just below the fitting for the valve outlet port. There are seven different pin positions, depending on the type of gas in the cylinder (Fig. 1-6). The yoke connector for an oxygen cylinder, for example, has pins at positions 2 and 5 (Fig. 1-7). Pin positions for the various gases are listed in Table 1-1. These pins fit exactly into the corresponding holes in the cylinder valve (Fig. 1-8). This system is an additional measure and, along with color coding, is de-

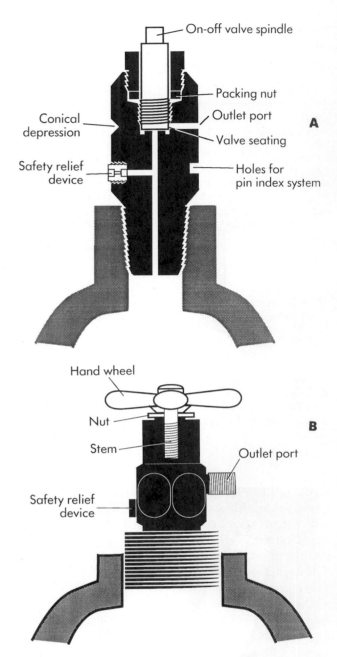

Fig. 1-5. Typical cylinder valves. **A,** A small-cylinder packed valve such as would be found on an E cylinder. Note that the female type of port is not unique to the gas type. **B,** A large-cylinder packed valve such as would be seen on an H cylinder. Note that the male type of outlet port has unique diameter and threads as a safety feature intended to help ensure correct connections. (Redrawn with permission from Parbrook GD, et al: *Basic physics and measurement in anesthesia,* ed 3, Oxford, Butterworth-Heinemann Limited and the author.)

signed to ensure that the correct gas is connected to its corresponding cylinder yoke. Obviously, connectors with either damaged or missing index pins are unsafe and should not be used under any circumstances. Because a pin can easily be lost or damaged when a cylinder is handled

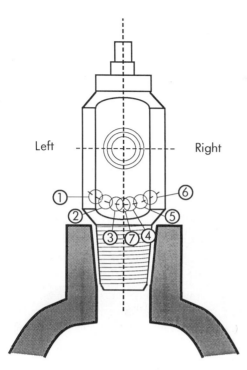

Fig. 1-6. Pin Index Safety System pin location. Perspective shown looking at the placement of holes in the tank. Pins are placed precisely complementary in the tank yoke. Two pins are used to identify each type of gas. Pin configurations are listed in Table 1-1.

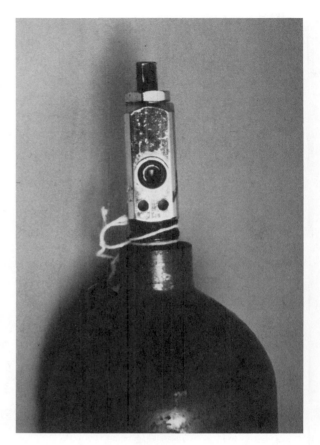

Fig. 1-8. Cylinder valve at the top of an E cylinder showing the two holes for the pin index system and the outlet port with an attached washer.

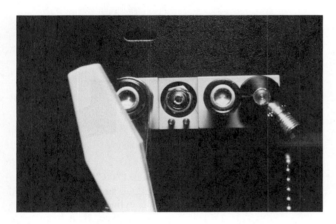

Fig. 1-7. A cylinder yoke on the anesthesia machine. Note the two pins for the pin index system at the bottom of the yoke and the hole (not gas specific) that aligns with the outlet port of the tank. To the right of the yoke is the threaded DISS connection attaching the hose from the central gas supply.

roughly, the person changing a cylinder must make certain that both pins are intact.

Securing cylinders against breakage

Gas cylinders should always be secured when they are placed in an upright position. If left freestanding, a cylinder can easily fall over in such a way that it would fracture at the neck (Fig. 1-9). The cylinder's highly pressurized gas would be suddenly released, and the cylinder would become an unguided missile of tremendous force. The cylinder could generate enough force to penetrate a cinder-block wall several feet thick. The potential danger of such an occurrence is obvious. Therefore, *all gas cylinders must be secured when they are upright*. If that is not possible, the solution may be simply to lay the cylinder on its side. Individual E cylinders can be placed in a broad-based wheeled carriage for support when in use.

Transfilling

Anesthesia personnel should never attempt to refill small cylinders from larger ones. Even if gas-tight connections were possible, the risk of explosion from the heat of compression in the small cylinder would still be serious. In addition, there is always the possibility that the wrong gas would be placed in the cylinder. The practice of transfilling is forbidden, and medical gases must be obtained *only* from a reputable commercial supplier.

Cylinder hazards

A study of 14,500 medical gas cylinders consecutively delivered from supposedly reputable suppliers found 120

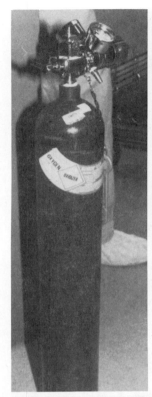
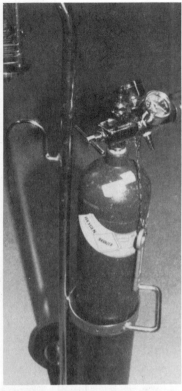
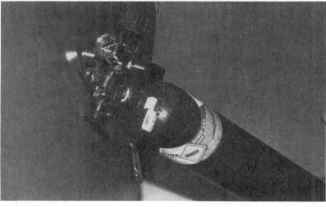

Fig. 1-9. Gas cylinders must never be left standing upright and unsecured. They are vulnerable to being knocked over by such events as a door being opened *(upper left)*. If upright, individual cylinders should be secured in some type of holder, often a rolling stand for E-sized cylinders *(upper right)*. Failure to secure upright cylinders leads to their eventually being knocked over. Cylinders that fall directly to the floor, and especially cylinders that fall so that the top just hits a wall *(lower panel),* are at great risk for breaking at the cylinder neck, creating an incredibly dangerous "unguided missile" as the high-pressure gas escapes out the narrow neck, rocketing the cylinder forward with enough force to penetrate a brick wall.

(0.83%) with potentially dangerous irregularities.[7] Forty cylinders were delivered either empty or partially filled. Three were found dangerously overfilled to near bursting pressures. Six cylinders of compressed air were found to be contaminated with volatile hydrocarbons. Thirty cylinders were unlabeled; and the labels of many others were illegible, having been painted over. Four cylinders were incorrectly color coded. Five large cylinders were fitted with incorrect valve outlet ports. This is especially dangerous because an oxygen valve on an air cylinder enables air to be fed into an oxygen outlet. Valve assemblies were loose on 14 cylinders and were inoperable on 4. On a large number of cylinders, the current inspection date was either absent or painted over and illegible. Numerous examples were cited of cylinders being improperly stored or secured. The results of this study serve to remind anesthesia practitioners of the danger of assuming that their gas supplies are perfectly safe. Rather, it is wise to establish a system to ensure that each cylinder of medical gas is inspected and tested upon delivery to the facility.

GUIDELINES FOR USE OF MEDICAL GAS CYLINDERS

Numerous rules govern the safe handling of cylinders containing medical gas.[1,2] Summarized here are the practical points that anesthesia practitioners must consider on a routine basis.

Supply

As noted, medical gases should be purchased only from a reputable commercial supplier. Outside metropolitan areas, the only supplier of any type of compressed gas may be the local welding company. Purchasing medical gases from such a source can be appropriate once it has been established that this supplier meets all safety requirements and standards for the manufacture and supply of medical gases. Such verification should be incorporated into the system to promote maximum safety.

Storage

Very specific regulations and standards govern the storage of medical gas cylinders.[2,3] For example, full cylinders and empty cylinders must be stored separately, each in their own "tank rooms" if possible. Small cylinders should be placed in nonflammable racks, and large cylinders should be chained to a wall. At least one anesthesiologist in each facility should be aware of these requirements and how they are being implemented. Anesthesia caregivers should also assume responsibility for all aspects of medical gas supplies, on which they depend.

Transport and installation

Medical gas cylinders must be handled with care. The serious damage that a broken cylinder can cause has already been mentioned. Valve assemblies can easily be damaged by rough handling, with unpredictable consequences. Cylinders should undergo a final inspection just before they are used. Should there be any question concerning safety or content, the user should forego using the cylinder (and initiate an investigation before returning it to the supplier). Before a small cylinder (E cylinder) is installed in the hanger yoke, the plastic wrapping surround-

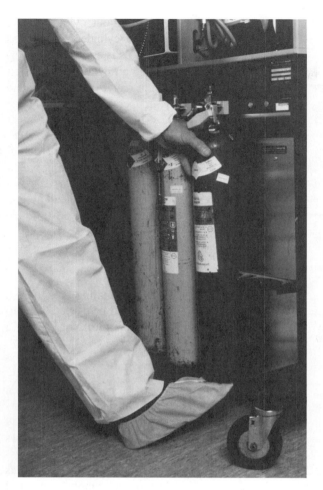

Fig. 1-10. Proper method for attaching an E cylinder to the yoke of an anesthesia machine. The tank is first supported on the anesthesiologist's foot while the holes on the tank are aligned with the pins in the yoke. The tank is then slid into place on the yoke and the T-handle is tightened in order to make a gas-tight seal.

ing the cylinder valve outlet must be completely removed. If this is not done, the plastic wrapper will prevent the gas from entering the gas inlet in the hanger yoke. All cylinders should be opened slightly "cracked" immediately prior to installation. This blows any residual oil, grease, and debris from the valve outlet port that would otherwise be released into the anesthetizing apparatus. Furthermore, cylinders should always be opened *slowly* to prevent dramatic heating of the suddenly pressurized piping. If, when the cylinder is opened, an abnormal odor is detected, gas should be collected from the tank and analyzed by gas chromatography to detect hydrocarbon contamination.[8] If a problem is confirmed, the cylinder in question should be sequestered (not returned to supplier) and the appropriate authorities (both local and federal) should be contacted.

Connections between gas cylinders and anesthesia machines must be tight. Figure 1-10 illustrates the proper method for balancing the tank when securing it to or removing it from the yoke. Washers are necessary for small-

cylinder yokes and must occasionally be replaced. If a hissing noise is heard when a cylinder is opened, there is a leak. The tightness of a connection can always be quickly checked by dripping soapy water onto it and inspecting for bubbles. One should never over-tighten a connection in an attempt to compensate for a leak; this may damage or even crack the cylinder valve. As in all aspects of anesthesia practice, brute force is almost never appropriate.

Once a new cylinder is in place, the pressure must be checked on the applicable gauge. Correct pressures of full cylinders are listed in Table 1-1. Over-pressurized cylinders are dangerous and must be removed at once and reported to the supplier.

MEDICAL GAS PIPELINE SYSTEMS

Medical gas pipeline systems consist of three main components: (1) a central supply of gas, (2) pipelines to transport the gases to the points of use, and (3) connectors at these points, which connect to the equipment utilizing the medical gas. Anesthesia caregivers are primarily concerned with piped oxygen and nitrous oxide. Operating rooms may have two other medical gas supply pipelines— one for compressed air and the other for nitrogen to power gas-driven equipment.

Detailed standards and guidelines exist for the use of medical gas delivery systems. In North America, these are published by the American National Standards Institute (ANSI), the American Society of Mechanical Engineers (ASME), the Compressed Gas Association (CGA), the National Fire Protection Association (NFPA),* the Canadian Standards Association (CSA),† and the American Hospital Association.‡[9] In the United States, a hospital must meet the NFPA standards in order to be accredited by the Joint Commission on Accreditation of Healthcare Organizations (JCAHO) and, often, to obtain insurance coverage. The construction of a medical facility is governed by standards, and the procedures required for operating a medical gas system must be followed by the plant engineering or maintenance departments. Problems in the construction of gas pipelines have led to anesthesia deaths.[10] Anesthesia providers therefore should be aware of these standards and the gas delivery system at their facility.

MEDICAL GAS CENTRAL SUPPLY SYSTEMS

The central supply (bulk storage) system is the source of medical gases that are distributed throughout the pipeline system. For oxygen, the central supply can be a series of standard cylinders connected by a manifold system or, for larger installations, pressure vessels of liquid oxygen with accompanying vaporizers. For medical air, it can be

*1 Batterymarch Park, Quincy, MA 02269-9101.
†178 Rexdale Blvd., Rexdale (Toronto), Ontario Canada M9W 1R3.
‡840 North Lake Shore Dr., Chicago, IL 60611.

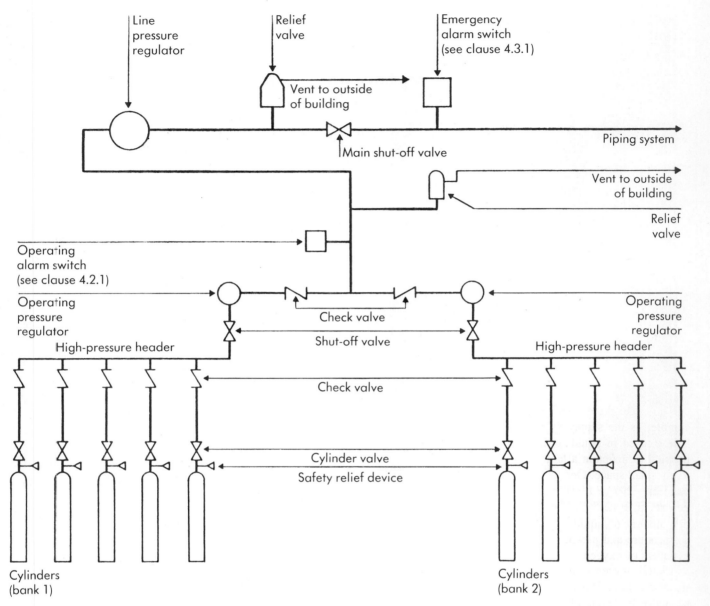

Fig. 1-11. Typical cylinder (H size) supply system, as would be seen in a very small hospital or a free-standing facility. There is no reserve supply. (Reproduced with permission from CSA Standard Z305.1-1975, Nonflammable medical gas piping systems, Rexdale, Ont, 1975, Canadian Standards Association. The notes in the drawing refer to sections of that publication.)

cylinders of compressed air, cylinders of oxygen and nitrogen with the gases mixed by a regulator, or air compressors. Generally, for nitrous oxide or nitrogen, a series of cylinders with a manifold system is used.

Oxygen

Central supply systems carrying oxygen are the most common as well as the most important supply systems, and as such they have received considerable attention. Standards for bulk systems (involving the storage of oxygen as a liquid) are contained in NFPA Publication 50.[11] Oxygen systems are treated extensively in NFPA Publication 99[12] and in the CSA Standard Z305.1.[13]

Very small systems have a total storage capacity of less than 2000 cu ft of gas (a single H cylinder of oxygen contains 244 cu ft or 6900 L) and have additional separate standards when based in nonhospital facilities. Systems in very small hospitals may store oxygen in a series of standard H cylinders connected by a manifold or high-pressure header system. Typically, these systems do not have reserve supplies. (See Figs. 1-11 and 1-12 for diagrams of such a system.) Note that there are two banks of cylinders. All central supply systems for medical gases must be present in duplicate, with two identical sources (often referred to as the primary and secondary supplies and not to be confused with the entirely separate reserve system) able to provide the needed medical gas interchangeably.

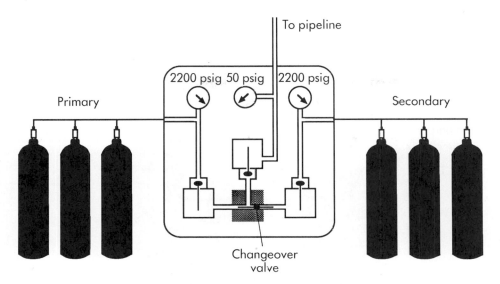

Fig. 1-12. A simplified version of Fig. 1-11. The oxygen is supplied in H tanks from both a primary and a secondary supply. The tanks are connected by a manifold; when the tanks are full the pressure is 2200 psig. A changeover valve automatically switches to the secondary supply once the primary supply has been exhausted. A reducing valve decreases the pressure to 50 psig before the oxygen enters the hospital pipeline. (Adapted with permission from Parbrook GD et al: *Basic physics and measurement in anesthesia,* ed 3, Oxford, Butterworth-Heinemann Limited and the author.)

The larger the oxygen demand of the facility, the more complex is the supply system. Most hospitals store their bulk oxygen in liquid form (Fig. 1-13). This enables the hospital to maintain a large reservoir of oxygen in a relatively small space. One cu ft of oxygen stored at a temperature of $-297°$ F $(-183°$ C) expands to 860 cu ft of oxygen at 70° F (21° C).[14] Since 1 cu ft is equal to 28.3 L, this amount of liquid oxygen provides 24,338 L at room temperature and pressure. That is the equivalent of 3½ H cylinders of oxygen.

Liquid oxygen is stored in a special container and kept under pressure. This container has an inner and outer layer separated by layers of insulation and a near vacuum. This construction is similar to that of a thermos bottle and serves to keep the liquid oxygen cold by inhibiting the entry of external heat (Fig. 1-14).

Liquid oxygen systems must be in constant use in order to be cost-effective. If the system goes unused for a period of time, the pressure increases as some of the liquid oxygen boils. The oxygen is then vented to the atmosphere. The liquid oxygen system contains vaporizers that heat the liquid and convert it to a gas before it is piped into the hospital. Environmental as well as mechanical heat sources can be used to aid in vaporization.

Liquid oxygen can be very hazardous. Fires are an ever-present danger. In addition, personnel can receive severe burns if they come in contact with liquid oxygen or an uninsulated pipe carrying liquid oxygen.

Small hospitals probably require central supply systems that store oxygen in replaceable liquid oxygen cylinders and a reserve of oxygen stored in high-pressure H cylin-

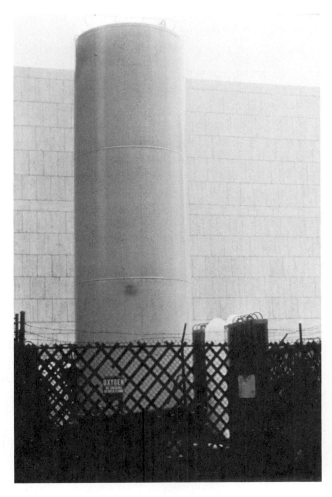

Fig. 1-13. A typical bulk storage vessel for liquid oxygen.

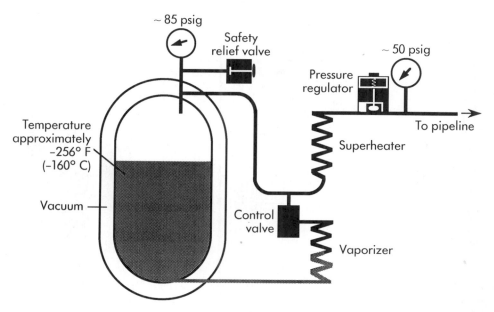

Fig. 1-14. Diagram of a liquid oxygen supply system. The vessel resembles a giant vacuum bottle, and the liquid oxygen is at approximately −256° F (−160° C). Pressure inside the vessel is maintained at approximately 85 psig. When oxygen is used from the top of the vessel, it passes first through a super heater and then through the pressure regulator to keep the pipeline pressure at 50 psig. During times of rapid use, the temperature and therefore the vapor pressure in the tank may fall. The control valve causes liquid oxygen to pass through the vaporizer, which adds heat and thus maintains the pressure in the tank. (Redrawn with permission from Parbrook GD et al: *Basic physics and measurement in anesthesia,* ed 3, Oxford, Butterworth-Heinemann Limited and the author.)

ders. The reserve system is automatically activated when the main supply (with its component primary and secondary storage) fails or is depleted (see Fig. 1-15). Hospitals of average size may store liquid oxygen in single large, or bulk, pressure vessels rather than in liquid oxygen cylinders. The storage vessel is filled through a cryogenic hose (designed to function at extremely low temperatures) from a liquid oxygen supply truck. In such a system, the size of the reserve system depends on the rate of oxygen use, as the reserve must constitute at least one average day's supply. This may be stored in a series of high-pressure H cylinders. However, large hospitals are required to have a second liquid oxygen storage vessel that serves as the reserve system because of the impracticality of storing and connecting enough cylinders to provide an average day's reserve supply of oxygen (Fig. 1-16).

Built into all these central supply systems for oxygen are a variety of mandatory safety devices. Pressure-relief valves are designed to open if pressure in the system exceeds the normal level by 50%. This prevents the rupture of vessels or pipes from the excessive pressure generated by a frozen valve or a malfunctioning pressure regulator. Alarm systems indicate when the supply in the main storage vessel is low and when the reserve supply has been put into use. The sounding of an oxygen alarm should activate a rehearsed protocol within the hospital that results in contact with the oxygen supplier and subsequent verification that an oxygen delivery is on the way.[15] Pressure alarms,

built into the main supply line, sound when the line pressure varies by ±20% from the normal operating pressure of approximately 55 psig. Pressure alarms should also be located in various areas in the pipeline to detect oxygen supply problems beyond the main connection (Fig. 1-17).

All these alarm systems must sound in two different locations, one being the hospital maintenance or plant engineering department and the other in an area occupied 24 hours a day, such as the telephone switchboard. These alarms should be tested periodically as part of a regular maintenance program. Failure of alarms has led to crisis situations. Testing the various alarms can be difficult but is possible if the system is properly designed.

Another critical safety feature is the T fitting located at the point where the central supply system joins the hospital piping system. This fitting allows delivery of an emergency supply of oxygen from a mobile source in the event of extended failure, extensive repair, or modification of the hospital's central supply.

The location and housing of oxygen central supply systems are governed by strict standards.[11] A bulk oxygen storage unit should be located away from public areas and flammable materials.

Medical air

The central supply of medical air can come from three sources: (1) cylinders of compressed air that has been cleaned to medical quality by filtration distillation; (2) a

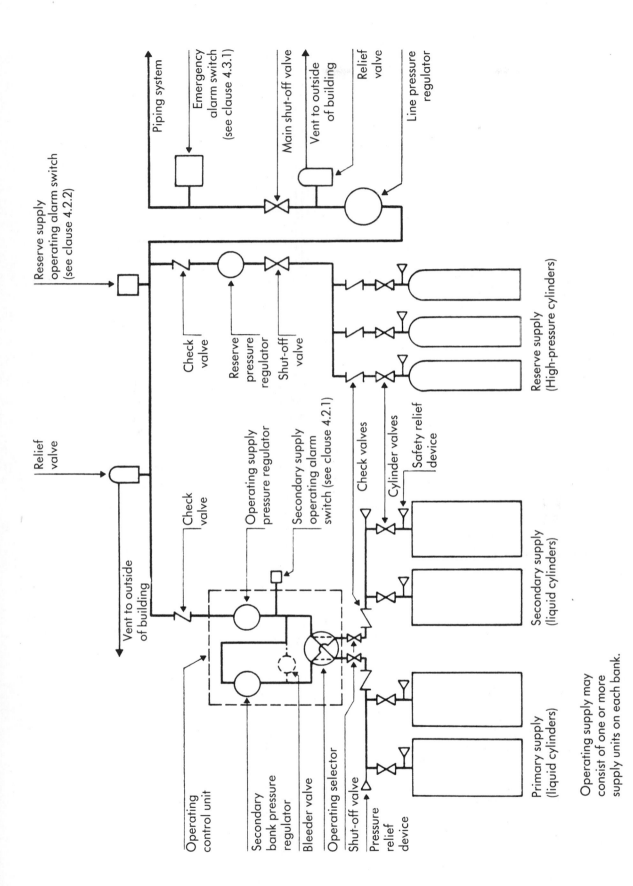

Fig. 1-15. Typical cryogenic cylinder supply system for liquid oxygen with a high-pressure cylinder reserve supply, as would be seen in a small hospital. The redundant primary and secondary liquid cylinders are intended to be the continuous oxygen source; there is an automatic switchover to the other bank when one is depleted (and thus ready for replacement). The reserve supply is activated automatically when both banks of cylinders are depleted or fail. (Reproduced with permission from CSA Standard Z305.1-1975, Nonflammable medical gas piping systems, Rexdale, Ont, 1975, Canadian Standards Association. The notes in the drawing refer to sections of that publication.)

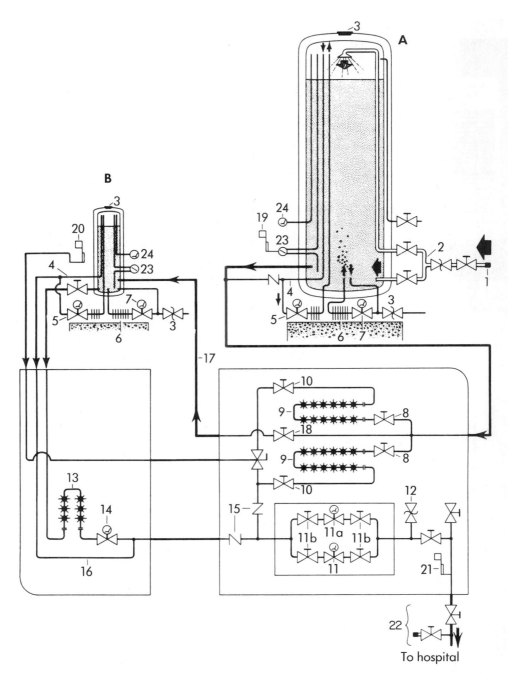

Fig. 1-16. Typical bulk supply system for oxygen, as would be seen in a large hospital. Very large hospitals may require more than one system of this magnitude. **A,** Main liquid oxygen reservoir, **B,** reserve liquid oxygen reservoir. *(1)* Connection to supply vehicle, *(2)* top and bottom fill lines, *(3)* reservoir pressure-relief valves, *(4)* "economizer" circuit, *(5)* gas regulator in pressure building circuit, *(6)* pressure building vaporizer, *(7)* liquid regulator in pressure building circuit, *(8)* cryogenic liquid control valves, *(9)* liquid vaporizers, *(10)* downstream valves for isolation of vaporizers, *(11)* primary line-pressure regulator, *(11a)* secondary line-pressure regulator, *(11b)* valves to isolate regulators for repair, *(12)* pressure-relief valve for main pipeline, *(13)* reserve-system liquid vaporizer, *(14)* reserve-system line pressure regulator, *(15)* gas flow check valves, *(16)* reserve-system "economizer" line, *(17)* reserve-system fill line, *(18)* valve controlling flow to reserve system from main cylinder, *(19)* low-liquid-level alarm, *(20)* reserve-in-use alarm, *(21)* main-line-pressure alarm, *(22)* main shut-off valve and T-fitting, *(23)* liquid-level indicators, *(24)* vapor or "head" pressure gauges. In normal operation, liquid oxygen flows from the lower left of the main vessel, **A,** via a cryogenic pipe through valves, *8* and to the vaporizer *9,* where the liquid becomes gaseous oxygen. It then flows through pressure regulators *11* and hence into the supply pipeline to the hospital. (*Anesthesiology* 52:504-510, 1980. Reproduced with permission of J.B. Lippincott.)

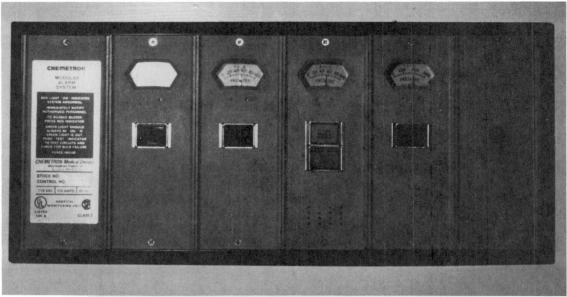

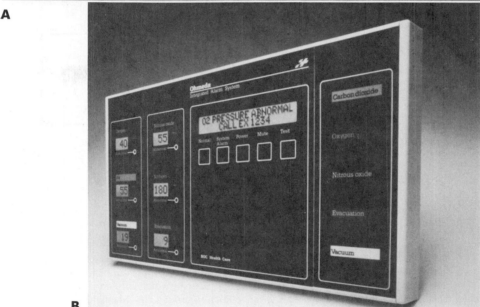

Fig. 1-17. A, A bank of pressure gauges that monitor the gases in one zone of the operating room. These gauges are for nitrous oxide, air, oxygen, and nitrogen. Note that individual gases being monitored are not identified on the panel. **B,** A modern gas monitoring panel that identifies the individual gas being monitored and gives a visual readout of the alarm message. (Photo courtesy of Ohmeda, a Division of BOC Health Care, Inc.)

(relatively uncommon) proportioning system that receives oxygen and nitrogen from central sources, mixes them in a proportion 21% oxygen to 79% nitrogen, and delivers this mixture to the medical air pipeline (these systems usually have compressed air cylinders or an air compressor as a reserve system); and (3) air compressors (Fig. 1-18), which represent the most common source of medical air in hospitals. The compressor works by compressing ambient air and then delivering the pressurized air to a reservoir or holding tank.[14] The medical air is then fed to the pressure regulator and from there to the hospital piping system.

Air compressor systems are subject to rigorous standards.[12,13] As with other systems, two duplicate compressors are necessary—each with the capacity to meet the entire hospital's medical air needs. The system must be used only for the medical air pipeline and not for the purpose of powering equipment. The compression pumps must not add contaminants to the gas, and the air intake must be lo-

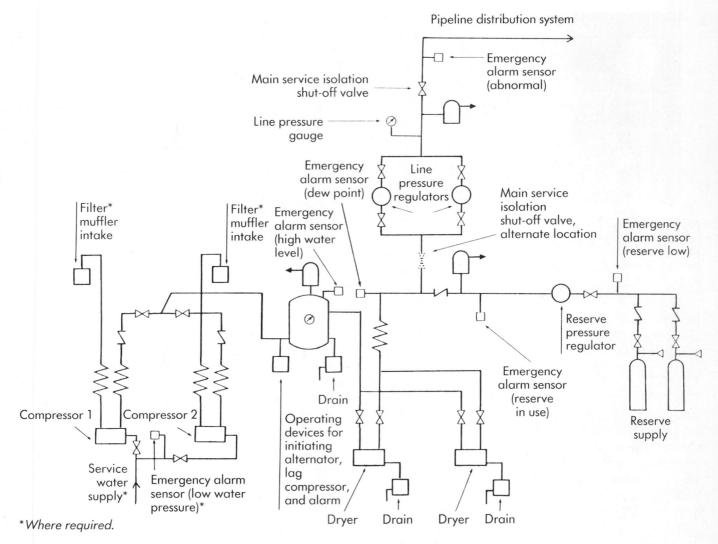

Fig. 1-18. A typical duplex medical air compressor system. Compressors at *lower left* draw in ambient air (it is critical that these air intakes not be located near any source of air pollution, such as a garage or the exhaust from the facility's vacuum system) and send high-pressure air to a holding tank. This air is dried and filtered on its way to pressure regulators, which deliver gas at about 55 psig into the pipeline system. (Reproduced with permission from CSA Standard Z305.1-M1984, Nonflammable medical gas piping systems, Rexdale, Ont, 1984, Canadian Standards Association.)

cated away from any street, or other, exhaust. It is particularly important that the pumps be located away from the hospital's vacuum system exhaust. The air must first be thoroughly dried to remove water vapor and filtered to remove dirt, oil, and other contaminants. The condensed water is then properly disposed of (to eliminate potential breeding grounds for bacteria, such as those causing Legionnaire's disease). The piping should not be exposed to subfreezing temperatures. Valves, pressure regulators, and alarms analogous to those in oxygen supply systems are needed.

Nitrous oxide

Specific standards exist for nitrous oxide systems, and certain portions of the more general standards of the NFPA and CSA are applicable as well.[16] A nitrous oxide central supply system may or may not be warranted, depending on the expected daily use of nitrous oxide. If there is sufficient demand for nitrous oxide, such a system might be cost-effective compared to attaching small cylinders to each anesthesia machine. Even though anesthesiologists are the only people who utilize the nitrous oxide system, they must delegate the responsibility for the operation and maintenance of the central nitrous oxide system to other hospital personnel.

Nitrous oxide central supply systems are usually of the cylinder-manifold type, as shown in Fig. 1-11. Again, it is necessary to have two separate banks of cylinders with an automatic crossover. Large institutions, however, may need a bulk liquid storage system similar to the one used

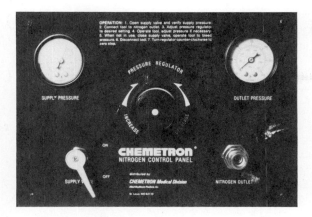

Fig. 1-19. An operating room control panel for nitrogen. The outlet pressure of nitrogen can be controlled by the variable pressure regulator. In this manner, the exact pressure can be set to meet the demands of the piece of equipment that is being powered.

for oxygen and shown in Fig. 1-16. In this case, the storage of liquid nitrous oxide requires an insulated container similar to that used for liquid oxygen.

Nitrogen

Even though a nitrogen central supply system is designed to supply gas only for powering operating room equipment, it is still subject to the same types of standards outlined above. Nitrogen supply systems are frequently smaller than those for nitrous oxide but are of essentially the same design, whereby a series of H cylinders are connected by a manifold (pressure header) system that feeds a pressure regulator. A typical nitrogen control panel is illustrated in Fig. 1-19. Again, since this system will service the operating room, it is important to delegate responsibility for maintenance. Although relatively uncommon, some systems are designed to mix central nitrogen with oxygen to create medical air. It is also possible to store nitrogen as a liquid for a centrally supplied system.

Central vacuum system

Although not a source of medical gas, the central vacuum system is no less important and demands the same attention to detail as a medical gas system. Inadequate or failed suction can be disastrous in the face of a surgical or anesthetic crisis.

Certain standards exist for the central vacuum source and vacuum piping system; the Canadian standards are considered the most complete and current.[13] Major operating rooms must have enough suction to remove 99 L of air per minute. Smaller operating rooms ("minor rooms") and locations outside the OR require only 57 or 28 L/min. Factors such as normal wall suction (-7 psig), total flow of the system, and the length of the longest run of pipe must be considered in order to maintain adequate suction. There must be two independent vacuum pumps, each one capable of handling the peak load alone. An automatic switch-

ing device distributes the load under normal conditions and shifts automatically if one unit fails. Emergency power connections are essential. The pumps must be located away from oxygen and nitrous oxide storage. There must be traps to collect and safely dispose of any solid or liquid contaminants introduced into the system, and the system piping must not be exposed to low temperatures (to prevent condensation). The type and location of the vacuum system exhaust is specified and must not be near the intake for the medical air compressor.

MEDICAL GAS PIPELINES

Medical gas must travel through a pipeline to reach its designated point of use. The potential for serious injury to a patient from a medical gas pipeline mishap has led to the development of detailed standards.[12,13]

Planning

In any new construction the physicians need to provide the architects and engineers with the number and desired locations of the gas outlets. Anesthesiologists need to decide if they want one or two sets of wall outlets for anesthesia gases in each operating room, and/or some sort of ceiling mounted distribution of the gases. Representatives from all of the departments that will be using the system should be involved in planning the location of the outlets. A basic layout for a portion of a piping system is illustrated in Fig. 1-20. Extensive planning is necessary for each separate medical gas pipeline. Anesthesiologists must be aware of all appropriate requirements. For example, each anesthetizing location must have a separate shut-off valve (Fig. 1-21), and other areas such as the Post Anesthesia Care Unit (PACU) require zone shut-off valves.

Detailed standards must be followed with respect to the specific type of pipe used (usually seamless copper tubing), as well as the cleaning, soldering, and supporting of the pipe within walls.[8,12,13] In addition, pipelines must be protected (for example, by enclosure in conduits), especially when they run underground. The various pipes located inside risers and walls must be labeled in a specific way and at given intervals.

Once drafted, the plans must be examined to verify that all standards have been met. Given the fact that the construction of medical gas pipelines is relatively uncommon, it is possible that a given engineering, architectural, or building firm has never before constructed one. Any changes made in the plans should be recorded in the "as built" drawings. This enables hospital personnel to know the exact location of the pipes should problems arise.

Additions to existing systems

Even more difficult than planning a new medical gas pipeline system is adding to an existing system. In addition to all the planning outlined above, the interaction between the old facility and the new one must be considered. The central supply system may need to be expanded to in-

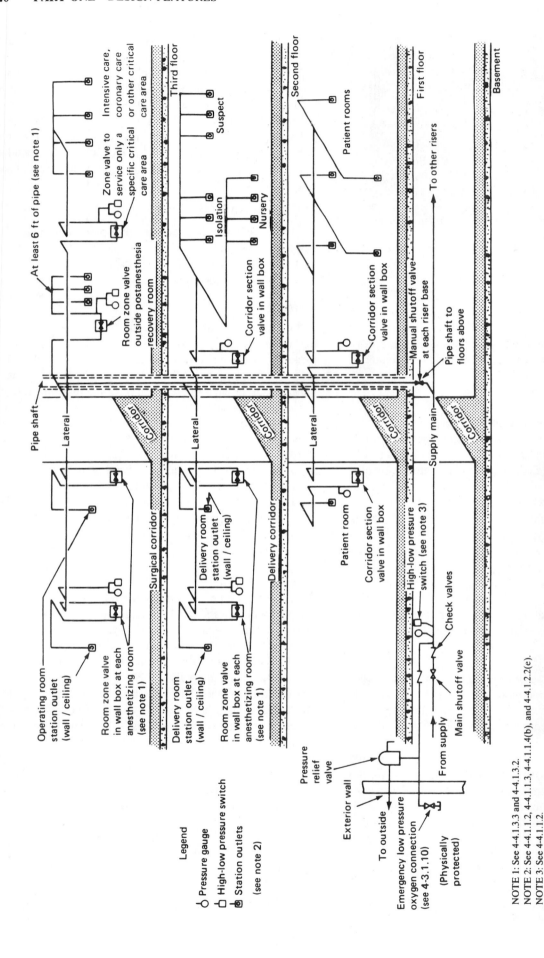

Fig. 1-20. A representative portion of the pipeline system for oxygen in a hospital facility. Note that separate similar designs are needed for the other medical gases. (Reprinted with permission from NFPA 99-1990, Health Care Facilities. Copyright © 1990, National Fire Protection Association. Quincy, MA 02269. This reprinted material is not the complete and official position of the National Fire Protection Association on the referenced subject, which is represented only by the standard in its entirety.)

NOTE 1: See 4-4.1.3.3 and 4-4.1.3.2.
NOTE 2: See 4-4.1.1.2, 4-4.1.1.3, 4-4.1.1.4(b), and 4-4.1.2.2(e).
NOTE 3: See 4-4.1.1.2.

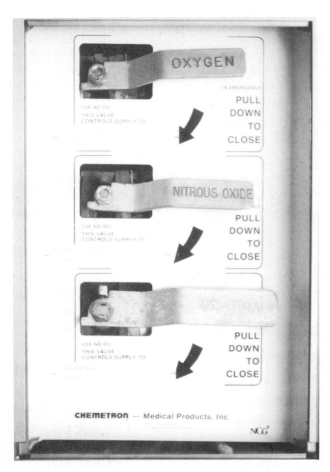

Fig. 1-21. Typical shut-off valves for the gases supplied in operating rooms. Each gas must have its own shut-off valve, and a separate series of valves must be present for each operating room.

clude new pipeline systems, which may necessitate the difficult task of shutting down the existing pipeline system. Extreme precision is required for such an operation. Again, procedural standards exist for either modifying or adding to existing systems.[13]

Installation and testing

Installation of a pipeline should be overseen by a representative from the medical facility, and the testing should actively involve several individuals who will be using the system. Prior to installation, the copper tubing used for the medical gas pipeline must be clean and free of contamination. The lengths of pipe must be stored with both ends sealed with rubber or plastic caps to prevent contamination. After the pipelines have been installed, but before the outlet valves are installed at each gas outlet location, the pipeline must be "blown free" of any particulate matter with high pressure gas.

The system involves pressure regulators that function to maintain normal outlet pressure (e.g., 55 psig for oxygen). Also, there must be pressure relief devices that automatically vent the gas if the pressure increases by 50% above the normal operating pressure. High- and low-pressure alarms and shut-off valves are required at various locations throughout the system. The locations of all of these should be marked on a map of the institution.

The pipeline terminates at various locations within the hospital. At these termination points a connector is installed to allow the interface of various pieces of medical equipment (i.e., anesthesia machine or ventilator). The connectors installed at each outlet of the pipeline are subject to detailed requirements.[12,13] Two basic types of connectors are used. One is the quick-coupler, which is made by several manufacturers and allows for rapid connection and disconnection of fittings and hoses (Figs. 1-22 and 1-23). The other is a noninterchangeable thread system, called the Diameter Index Safety System (DISS)[5] (Fig.

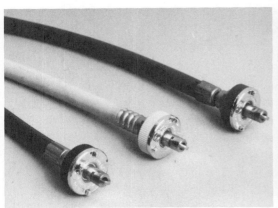
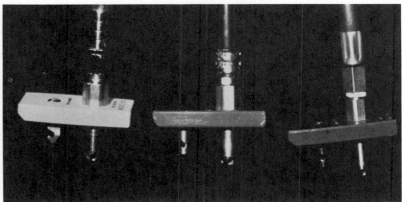

Fig. 1-22. Examples of two common types of quick couplers used in hospitals. Note that each is specific for the individual gas. The quick coupler and the attached hose should be color-coded for the specific gas.

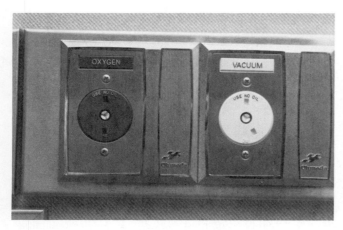

Fig. 1-23. The wall connection for oxygen and vacuum in a safety-keyed quick-connect system. The Ohmeda quick-connect system is illustrated. In this system, each gas is assigned two specific pins, with corresponding inlet holes within the circumference of the circle. In this manner, the connection is made gas-specific.

1-24). Both of these systems have gas-specific fittings to prevent incorrect connections. Improper use of a gas outlet or use of an incorrect fitting essentially defeats the purpose of the built-in safeguards of the system. Accordingly, the station outlets must have back-up automatic shut-off valves in case the quick-coupler is damaged or removed. All outlets, hoses, and quick-couplers should be properly labeled and color coded.

Gas outlets in the operating room may be located in either the wall or the ceiling. If the gas hoses are run along the floor, then they must be made of noncompressible materials to prevent obstruction in case the hose is run over by a piece of heavy equipment. Outlets may be suspended from the ceiling in columns or freestanding hose drops (Fig. 1-25), or they may be integrated into a multiservice gas boom (Fig. 1-26). These gas booms can be configured with all the anesthetic gases, as well as vacuum, electrical outlets, mass spectrometer connections, and even a telephone. They can be rotated to several different positions and raised or lowered electrically as necessary.

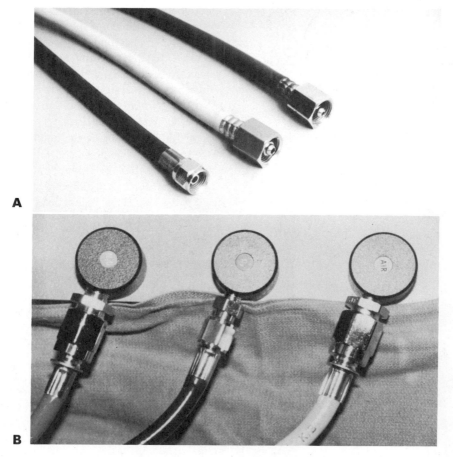

Fig. 1-24. A, Examples of the diameter index safety system (DISS). These are threaded connections in which the diameters of the threads are specific for each of the gases. **B,** Connection made to DISS fittings on the anesthesia machine.

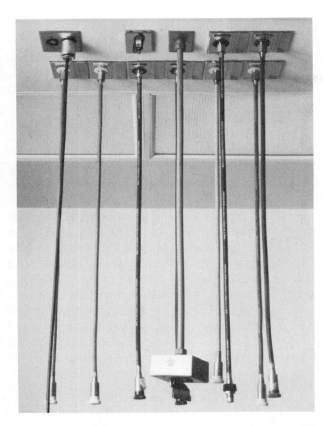

Fig. 1-25. Free-standing hose drops in an operating room. Note the proximal ends of the hoses (nearest to ceiling) have DISS connections, and the distal ends (nearest to the anesthesia machine) have quick-coupler connections.

Testing of the pipeline begins after the couplers have been installed. Before the walls are closed, the pipeline is subjected to 150 psig and each joint examined for leaks. The system then undergoes a 24-hour standing pressure test whereby the system is filled with gas to at least 150 psig, disconnected from the gas source, and closed. If the pressure is the same after 24 hours, there are no leaks. Cross-connection testing involves pressurizing each pipeline system separately with test gas and verifying that only the outlets of that particular system (for example, compressed air) have pressure. This is particularly important when additions or modifications are made to existing pipeline systems. After the correct connections have been verified, each pipeline is connected to its own central supply of gas. The pipelines are then purged with their own gases. The content of gas from each and every station outlet must then be analyzed. An oxygen analyzer can be used for the oxygen (100%) and medical air (21%) outlets. The concentrations of nitrous oxide and nitrogen must be 100% according to chromatography or other appropriate analysis. Once the testing has been completed, the facility can accept responsibility for it from the contractor. Anesthesiologists should certainly be involved in verifying the correctness of the gas supplies. Major problems with new systems have been identified by anesthesiologists after the system was "certified" safe for use.[17] Australia has a rigorous "permit to work system" modeled after a similar system in the United Kingdom, with specific steps that must be followed before gas supplies can be used.[18,19]

Contamination of medical gas pipelines has become a subject of concern.[8] Rigorous standards have been developed to prevent contamination. Gas samples should be taken at the same time from both the source of the system and the most distant station outlet. If analysis by gas chro-

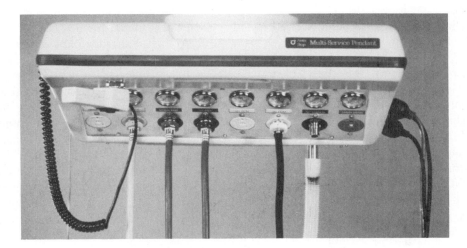

Fig. 1-26. The distribution head for a multiservice gas boom. Compressed gases, vacuum, line pressure monitoring gauges, and electrical connections can all be integrated at one location. The articulated arm can be raised or lowered electrically, and it can be rotated in an arc of nearly 360°. (Reproduced courtesy of Ohmeda, a Division of BOC Health Care, Inc.)

matography demonstrates that contaminants are present above the maximum allowable level, then the system should be purged and retested. If purging the system fails to solve the problem, extensive troubleshooting may be necessary. Detailed records of all testing must be maintained and should be available for inspection by the JCAHO. Once the testing has been satisfactorily completed, the system is ready for use.

HAZARDS OF MEDICAL GAS DELIVERY SYSTEMS

A number of deaths have occurred as a result of incorrect installation or malfunction of medical gas delivery systems. The exact number is not known, however, because the medical literature contains very few publications on medical gas delivery systems. Physicians and administrators may be reluctant to discuss or publish details of accidents occurring at their facility. Often, only personnel within the medical facility are aware of an accident. If the accident is either serious or results in litigation, it may be reported in the lay press. It is probable, however, that many if not most of the accidents involving medical gas delivery systems are not reported at all. This may actually prevent the dissemination of valuable information that could help to prevent future accidents. One attempt was made to learn about problems with bulk gas delivery systems by conducting a survey of hospitals with anesthesia residency training programs.[20] One third of the hospitals responding reported problems, three of which were deaths. In this survey, a total of 76 malfunctions in medical gas delivery systems were reported by a group of 59 institutions. Half of these involved insufficient oxygen pressure, crossed pipelines, depletion of central supply gas, failure of alarms, pipeline leaks, and freezing of gas regulators. Insufficient oxygen pressure most frequently occurred because pipelines were damaged during unrelated hospital construction projects, such as resurfacing a parking lot above a buried pipeline. Another frequent problem was debris or other material in pipelines, which could be eliminated by adhering to the prescribed procedures for testing newly installed gas piping systems.

In the United Kingdom between 1964 and 1973, 29 deaths or permanent complications were reported to the Medical Defence Union (a malpractice insurance company). These resulted from problems in either the gas supply or anesthetic apparatus.[21] Three of the cases were the result of either an error or failure in piped oxygen supplies, and two were caused by contaminated nitrous oxide.

Errors on the part of commercial suppliers when filling liquid oxygen bulk reservoirs have endangered patients, and in at least one instance they have actually harmed a patient. A supplier succeeded in filling a liquid oxygen reservoir with liquid nitrogen, bypassing the indexed non-interchangeable safety valve connection, which is designed to prevent such an occurrence.[22] A hypoxic gas mixture was thus delivered to anesthetized patients. Fortunately, however, the ensuing problems were quickly recognized and a catastrophe averted by a switch to tank oxygen supply. In another more recent episode, two patients received a hypoxic gas mixture that led to the death of one of the patients.[23] In this case a 100-L container of "liquid oxygen" was delivered and connected to the hospital's gas pipeline about 1 hour before the patients were anesthetized. This container of "liquid oxygen" actually contained almost pure nitrogen. It is interesting to note that no inspired oxygen analyzer was in use at the time of the accident.

Several other types of problems with bulk oxygen delivery systems have also been reported. In one case, the delivery of a large volume of liquid oxygen caused a sudden drop in the temperature of the system, which resulted in a regulator freezing in a low-pressure mode.[24] Insufficient oxygen pressure was the result. Attempts to correct this problem quickly revealed that a low-pressure alarm had been disconnected during a recent modification of the system. In an attempt to restore regulator function, several maneuvers were performed that actually worsened the situation by allowing excessive pressure (100 psig) into the hospital pipeline. This caused reducing valves on anesthesia machines to rupture. In this case, injury to patients was avoided by the quick thinking of the anesthesiologists in the operating room. A more tragic incident involved a child who suffered a cardiac arrest and subsequent brain damage when an oxygen pipeline valve was simply turned off.[25] Another case of a hypoxic mixture coming from oxygen outlets involved a problem with the regulator in the oxygen pipeline. The regulator failed, causing a decreased oxygen pressure that then allowed high-pressure compressed air to enter the oxygen system through an air-oxygen blender connected to both outlets in the neonatal intensive care unit.[26]

Accidental cross-connecting of pipelines represents a clear threat to patients that has been recognized for some time.[27,28,29] Exposure of a patient to an incorrect gas proves the inadequacy of the testing of that pipeline. An additional source of error may arise when the pipeline is connected to the anesthesia machine. According to one report, several deaths were caused by the connection of the nitrous oxide pipeline to the oxygen inlet on the anesthesia machine (and the corresponding connection of the oxygen pipeline to the nitrous oxide inlet).[30] In other instances, repair of the hoses that run from the outlet to the machine led to the interchange of the oxygen and nitrous oxide female Schraeder (quick-couple) adapters. As a result, the nitrous oxide pipeline was connected to the oxygen inlet, causing, among other catastrophes, the death of one patient.[31,32]

One published report concerning contamination of gas pipeline systems involves a newly constructed hospital building.[8] During cross-connection testing of the gas pipelines, a distinct "organic chemical" odor was detected. Gas chromatography revealed the presence of a volatile hydrocarbon at a concentration of 10 ppm. Four days of purging reduced this contaminant to 0.1 ppm in the oxygen and 0.4 ppm in the medical air pipelines. The original outlet tests also revealed that a fine, black powder was being expelled from gas outlets. Subsequent investigation revealed that during installation the ends of the pipe segment were color coded with spray paint. Later, when the pipe ends were being prepared for soldering, they were sanded down, and the paint particles settled inside the pipeline. This particulate contamination was eliminated by the purging process.

Contamination of a hospital oxygen pipeline system by other chemicals has also been reported. This has occurred when the solution used to clean the oxygen supply tubing between the supply tank and the hospital pipeline had not been flushed out.[33] In this case, all of the hospital outlets had to be shut down and patients had to be switched to tank supplies while the problem was identified and the pipeline system was flushed out with fresh oxygen.

A commercial firm that conducts tests of new hospital gas pipelines conducted a study of 10 hospitals in which a total of 1668 gas outlets were examined. At 7 hospitals, all outlets failed the gas purity tests. Of the total of 1668 outlets, 331 (20%) failed for a variety of reasons, such as unacceptably high moisture, volatile hydrocarbons, halogenated hydrocarbon solvents, unidentified odors, and particulate matter (such as solder flux). It appears that contamination of new medical gas pipelines is a common problem and one that merits close attention.

Although the potential hazards of using medical gas delivery systems are many, they are largely preventable. Close attention to the applicable standards prevents most problems.

PROCEDURES

When a new medical gas delivery system is constructed, both the medical staff and the plant engineering department must be involved in all stages of the process. This prevents building into the system inadequacies or inconveniences that might otherwise limit its value and may even create a hazard. The medical facility must clearly designate the lines of responsibility for the medical gas delivery system among the hospital staff members. One suggestion is for institutions to have four departments (i.e., plant engineering, maintenance, anesthesia, and respiratory therapy) and to delegate responsibility for the gas delivery systems to one or more members of each department. Each member of the group should possess a thorough understanding of the institution's systems and be able to manage any problem that might occur.

Excellent communication must be established with the firm that supplies the bulk gas. The gas supplier should furnish the hospital with a list of people to contact in an emergency and should also notify the institution whenever a bulk gas delivery is to be made. In this way, the delivery can be overseen by the appropriate committee member. Had this been done in certain situations, several of the problems already cited would have been avoided.

Communication between the supplier and the hospital's representatives is important when the gas delivery system undergoes any work. In addition, representatives from both the institution and the supplier should be aware of any construction that might affect the gas system. In one case, such precautions could have prevented crushing of the underground pipes of an oxygen bulk supply system during resurfacing of a hospital parking lot.[20] The hospital needs to develop protocols and designate a responsible person to respond to medical gas alarms (including a complete failure of the oxygen system). That such plans are necessary is shown by a situation in which a sudden tornado caused the total destruction of one hospital's central bulk oxygen supply.[34]

Interdepartmental communication is also critical. All affected departments must be notified when the gas supply system is to be shut off for repair or periodic maintenance. A near-crisis situation arose when an engineering department shut down piped oxygen supplies during the operating schedule without notifying anyone else in the hospital.[20] Following repair or maintenance, a qualified person should inspect the system before it is put back into service. The patient death due to interchanged Schraeder connectors could have been prevented had this procedure been followed.

Anesthesia providers are often complacent about their gas supply until either a problem or a catastrophe occurs. Almost all injuries to patients and problems related to medical gases are preventable, even those caused by natural disasters. Building and maintaining a safe medical gas system takes a great deal of effort on the part of many individuals but is well worth the cost.

REFERENCES

1. Safe handling of compressed gas in containers, publication P-1, ed 7, Arlington, Va, 1984, Compressed Gas Association.
2. Characteristics and safe handling of medical gases, publication P-2, ed 7, Arlington, Va, 1989, Compressed Gas Association.
3. *Compressed gas containers.* In Dorsch JA and Dorsch SE, *Understanding anesthesia equipment,* ed 2, Baltimore, 1984, Williams & Wilkins, pp 10-14.
4. American National, Canadian, and Compressed Gas Association standard for compressed gas cylinder valve outlet and inlet connections, publication V-1, ed 6, Arlington, Va, 1987, Compressed Gas Association.
5. Diameter index safety system, publication V-5, ed 3, Arlington, Va, 1989, Compressed Gas Association.
6. Pressure relief device standards: part 1, cylinders for compressed gases, publication S-1.1, ed 7, Arlington, Va, 1989, Compresssed Gas Association.
7. Feeley TW, Bancroft ML, Brooks RA et al: Potential hazards of compressed gas cylinders: a review, *Anesthesiology* 48:72-74, 1978.
8. Eichhorn JH, Bancroft ML, Laasberg H et al: Contamination of medical gas and water pipelines in a new hospital building, *Anesthesiology* 46:286-289, 1977.

9. Slack GD: *Medical gas and vacuum systems,* Chicago, 1989, American Hospital Association.

10. Eichhorn JH: Medical gas delivery systems. In Lisbon A, editor: Anesthetic considerations in setting up a new medical facility, *Int Anesthesiol Clin* 19(2):1-26, 1981.

11. Bulk oxygen systems at consumer sites, NFPA 50, Quincy, Mass, 1990, National Fire Protection Association.

12. Health care facilities, NFPA 99, Quincy, Mass, 1990, National Fire Protection Association, pp 41–67.

13. Nonflammable medical gas piping systems, Z305.1-M1984, Rexdale, Ont, 1984, Canadian Standards Association.

14. *Medical gas piping systems.* In Dorsch JA and Dorsch SE, *Understanding anesthesia equipment,* ed 2, Baltimore, 1984, Williams & Wilkins, pp 16-37.

15. Bancroft ML, duMoulin GC, Hedley-Whyte J: Hazards of hospital bulk oxygen delivery systems, *Anesthesiology* 52:504-510, 1980.

16. Standard for nitrous oxide systems at consumer sites, publications G-8.1, Arlington, Va, 1990, Compressed Gas Association.

17. Krenis LJ, Berkowitz DA: Errors in installation of a new gas delivery system found after certification, *Anesthesiology* 62:677-678, 1985.

18. Seed RF: The permit to work system, *Anaesth Intensive Care* 10:353-358, 1982.

19. Howell RSC: Piped medical gas and vacuum systems, *Anaesthesia* 35:679-698, 1980.

20. Feeley TW, Hedley-Whyte J: Bulk oxygen and nitrous oxide delivery systems: design and dangers, *Anesthesiology* 44:301-305, 1976.

21. Wylie WD: "There, but for the grace of God. . . .", *Ann R Coll Surg Engl* 56:171-180, 1975.

22. Sprague DH, Archer GW: Intraoperative hypoxia from an erroneously filled liquid oxygen reservoir, *Anesthesiology* 42:360-362, 1975.

23. Holland R: "Wrong gas" disaster in Hong Kong, *Anesthesia Patient Safety Foundation Newsletter* 4(3):26, 1989.

24. Feeley TW, McClelland KJ, Malhotra IV: The hazards of bulk oxygen delivery systems, *Lancet* 1:1416-1418, 1975.

25. Epstein RM, Rackow H, Lee AA et al: Prevention of accidental breathing of anoxic gas mixtures during anesthesia, *Anesthesiology* 23:1-4, 1962.

26. Carley RH, Houghton IT, Park GR: A near disaster from piped gases, *Anaesthesia* 39:891-893, 1984.

27. N$_2$O asphyxia, *Lancet* 1:848, 1974 (editorial).

28. The Westminster inquiry, *Lancet* 2:175-176, 1977 (editorial).

29. Macintosh R: Wrongly connected gas pipelines, *Lancet* 2:307, 1977.

30. McCormick JM: National fire protection codes—1968, *Anesth Analg* 47:538-545, 1968.

31. Mazze RI: Therapeutic misadventures with oxygen delivery systems: the need for continuous in-line oxygen monitors, *Anesth Analg* 51:787-792, 1972.

32. Robinson JS: A continuing saga of piped medical gas supply, *Anaesthesia* 34:66-70, 1979.

33. Gilmour IJ, McComb C, Palahniuk RJ: Contamination of a hospital oxygen supply, *Anesth Analg* 71:302-304, 1990.

34. Johnson DL: Central oxygen supply versus mother nature, *Respir Care* 20:1043, 1975.

Chapter 2

THE ANESTHESIA MACHINE

James B. Eisenkraft, M.D.

The modern anesthesia machine is the result of a continuous evolutionary process. New features have been added as the result of advances in technology and system design, as well as a growing understanding of patient safety considerations. The current voluntary consensus standard that describes the features of a contemporary machine is published by the American Society for Testing and Materials (ASTM) and designated F1161-88.[1] This document, approved in July 1988 and published in March 1989, is entitled, "Standard Specification for Minimum Performance and Safety Requirements for Components and Systems of Anesthesia Gas Machines." It specifies the minimum performance and safety requirements to be used in the design of anesthesia gas machines for human use in order to enhance the safety of the patient and operator.[1] This standard supersedes the Z79.8-1979 anesthesia machine standard published in 1979 by the American National Standards Institute.[2] The F1161-88 is a consensus standard adopted voluntarily by the machine manufacturers. Certain accrediting and licensing bodies may, however, choose to adopt such standards in whole or in part and make them *requirements* for machines used in a particular locality. A summary of the important new aspects addressed in the F1161-88 standard is provided later in this chapter.

Presently, in the United States, the two largest manufacturers of anesthesia delivery systems (machines, ventilators, vaporizers, scavenging systems) are North American Dräger* and Ohmeda.† This chapter reviews the features of a basic anesthesia delivery system, making reference to the Dräger and Ohmeda products where appropriate (Figs. 2-1 and 2-2). The flow of compressed gases from their points of entry into the machine, through the various components to their exit at the common gas outlet is described. The function of each component is discussed so that the effects of failure of that component, as well as the rationale for the various machine checkout procedures, can be appreciated. This approach provides a framework from which to diagnose problems arising with the machine. It is emphasized at the outset that the individual machine manufacturer's Operator and Service Manuals represent the most comprehensive reference for any specific model of machine, and the reader is strongly encouraged to review the relevant manual(s).

*Telford, Pa.
†A Division of BOC Health Care Inc., Madison, Wis.

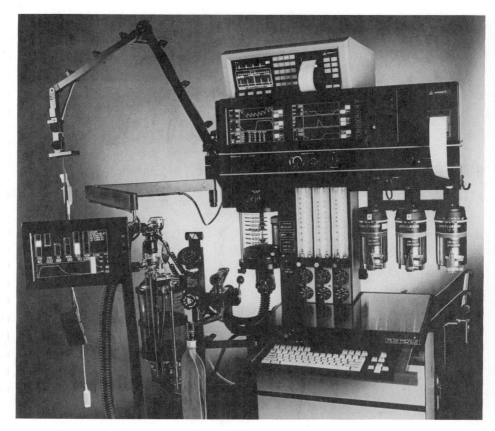

Fig. 2-1. Narkomed 4 anesthesia system. (Courtesy of North American Dräger, Inc, Telford, Pa.)

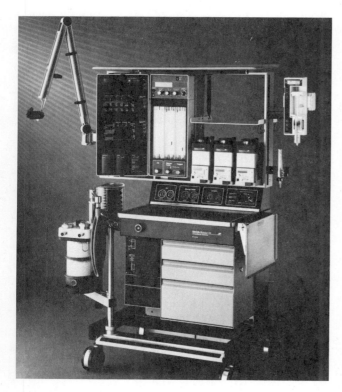

Fig. 2-2. Ohmeda Modulus CD anesthesia system. (Courtesy of Ohmeda, a Division of BOC Health Care, Inc, Madison, Wis.)

THE BASIC ANESTHESIA MACHINE

The flow arrangements of a basic two-gas anesthesia machine are shown in Fig. 2-3. The machine receives each of the two basic gases, oxygen and nitrous oxide, from two supply sources: a tank or cylinder source, and a pipeline source. The storage and supply of these gases to the operating room is described in Chapter 1.

The basic functions of any anesthesia machine are to receive compressed gases from their supplies and to create a gas mixture of known composition and flow rate at the common gas outlet. The relationship between pressure and flow is stated in Ohm's law:

$$\text{Flow} = \frac{\text{Pressure}}{\text{Resistance}}$$

The flow of gases from high-pressure sources through the machine to exit the common gas outlet at pressures approximating atmospheric therefore requires changes in pressure or resistance or both to achieve the stated goal. Modern anesthesia machines also incorporate certain safety features designed to prevent the delivery of a hypoxic mixture to the patient circuit. These features include the oxygen supply pressure failure alarm, fail-safe system, and gas flow proportioning systems.

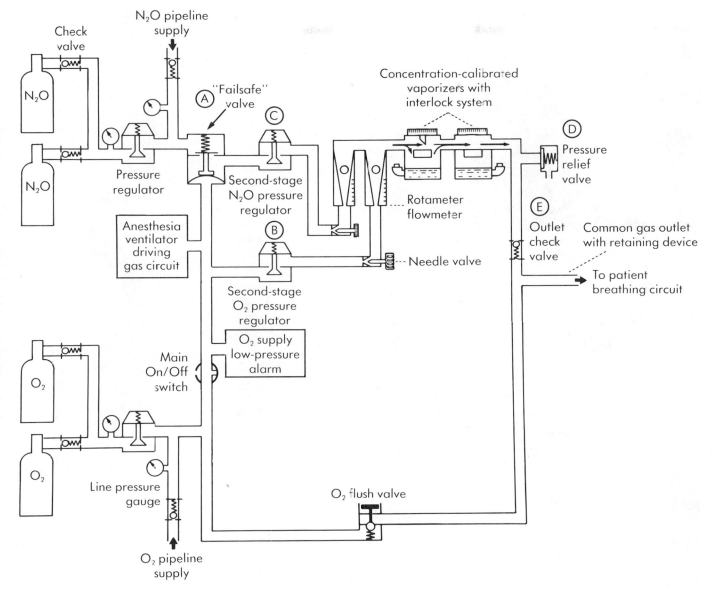

Fig. 2-3. Schematic of flow arrangements of a contemporary anesthesia machine. **A,** The fail-safe valve in Ohmeda machines is termed a pressure sensor shut-off valve; in Dräger machines it is the oxygen failure protection device (OFPD). **B,** Second-stage oxygen pressure regulator is used in Ohmeda (but not Dräger Narkomed) machines. **C,** Second-stage nitrous oxide pressure regulator is used in Ohmeda Modulus machines having the Link 25 Proportion Limiting System; not used in Dräger machines. **D,** Pressure relief valve used in certain Ohmeda machines (see Table 2-1); not used in Dräger machines. **E,** Outlet check valve used in Ohmeda machines except Modulus II Plus and Modulus CD models (see Table 2-1); not used in Dräger machines. The oxygen take-off for the anesthesia ventilator driving gas circuit is *downstream* of the main on/off switch in Dräger machines, as shown here. In Ohmeda machines, the take-off is *upstream* of the main on/off switch. (Adapted from *Check-out: a guide for preoperative inspection of an anesthesia machine,* ASA, 1987. Reproduced by permission of the American Society of Anesthesiologists, 520 N. Northwest Highway, Park Ridge, Ill.)

OXYGEN

Pipeline oxygen is supplied to the wall outlets in the OR at a pressure of 50 to 55 psig.* The wall outlet connectors are gas-specific, according to their manufacturer.

*Psig = pounds per square inch gauge pressure. Psia = pounds per square inch absolute pressure. 0 psig = 14.7 psia.

Thus for any individual manufacturer (e.g., Ohmeda, Chemetron, Schraeder) the medical gas wall outlets and connectors are noninterchangeable among the medical gases or the vacuum (Figs. 2-4 and 2-5). A conductive rubber hose carries the pipeline oxygen from the wall outlet to the anesthesia machine's oxygen inlet. At the ma-

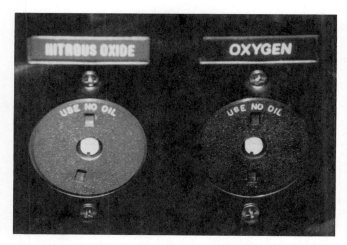

Fig. 2-4. Medical gas–specific wall outlet connectors by Ohmeda, a Division of BOC Health Care, Inc., Madison, Wis.

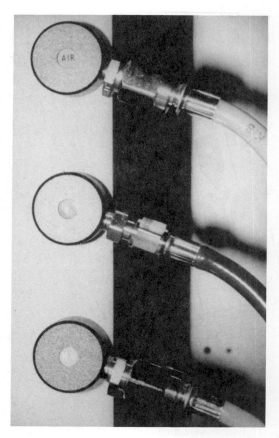

Fig. 2-6. Diameter indexed safety system (DISS). From above are shown the connectors at the machine end of the medical gas hoses for air, oxygen, and nitrous oxide. Note that the connectors are of different diameters, making them gas-specific.

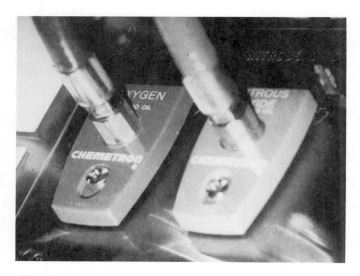

Fig. 2-5. Medical gas–specific pipeline hose connectors by Chemetron, Medical Division, Allied Health Care Products, St. Louis, Mo.

chine end the pipeline connectors are gas-specific by national standard. This is the Diameter Index Safety System (DISS), which assures that the correct gas enters the correct part of the anesthesia machine (Fig. 2-6).[3] The machine's oxygen pipeline inlet incorporates a check valve, which prevents leakage of oxygen from the machine if the pipeline is not connected and the oxygen tanks are in use (Fig. 2-7). Failure of this valve causes leakage of oxygen from the machine. Downstream of the pipeline inlet in the machine is a pressure gauge that records the pipeline gas supply pressure (Fig. 2-3).

Tank oxygen is supplied to the machine from the backup E cylinders, which are attached via the oxygen hanger yokes. The medical gas pin-index system ensures that only an oxygen tank fits correctly into an oxygen hanger yoke (see Chapter 1 and Fig. 2-8).[4] A cylinder

should never be force-fitted to a hanger yoke. Obviously the pin-index system, a safety feature, should never be violated. Such violation is possible, however—one or both pins can be extracted from the yoke, or several plastic washers can be used to separate the tank's gas outlet from the hanger yoke so that the yoke pins do not reach the tank. Such practice is to be condemned.

The pressure in a full oxygen tank is approximately 1900 psig (Chapter 1). Oxygen enters the hanger yoke at this pressure and then passes through a strainer nipple (Fig. 2-9) designed to prevent dirt or other particles from entering the machine. The oxygen then flows past a hanger yoke ("floating") check valve to enter the anesthesia machine at high pressure (Fig. 2-9).

Several considerations apply *before* a tank is hung in a yoke. First, the plastic wrapper that surrounds the tank valve must be removed. Then the valve is opened slowly, "cracked," to allow gas to exit the tank and blow out any particles of dirt that may be lodged in the outlet. The tank is then hung in the yoke. The gas outlet hole is aligned with the strainer nipple, and the two yoke pins are aligned with the corresponding holes in the tank. The tank should never be turned through 180° and then hung in the yoke

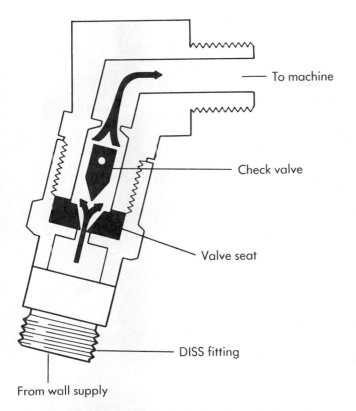

— To machine

— Check valve

— Valve seat

— DISS fitting

From wall supply

Fig. 2-7. Machine pipeline inlet check valve. The flow of oxygen from the wall supply opens the pipeline inlet valve. If the wall supply hose were disconnected and the tank oxygen were in use, pressure of oxygen in the machine would force the check valve to its seated position, preventing loss of oxygen via this connector. (From Bowie E, Huffman LM: *The anesthesia machine: essentials for understanding,* Madison, Wis, 1985, Ohmeda, a Division of BOC Health Care, Inc. Reproduced by permission.)

since the T-handle screw could, if tightened, damage the tank valve stem pressure relief mechanism (see Chapter 1).

Most machines have two hanger yokes for oxygen. Once O_2 has passed through the check valve, the two hanger yokes are interconnected by high-pressure tubing, to which an oxygen pressure gauge is also connected (Fig. 2-10). This gauge measures the pressure of the oxygen cylinder supply connected via the hanger yoke(s). On many machines both yokes may share one pressure gauge. In this case, in order to measure the tank pressure, the pipeline supply is first disconnected from the machine and both tanks turned off. Next the oxygen flush button is depressed to drain all oxygen from the machine. The tank and pipeline gauge readings should both fall to zero. One tank is then turned on, and its pressure is noted on the gauge. The tank is then turned off. The oxygen flush button is again depressed, and the tank gauge pressure falls to zero. The second tank is then opened, and its pressure is noted. The second tank is then closed, and the oxygen flush button is depressed. The pipeline connector is then reattached to the wall oxygen outlet.

As noted previously, there is a check valve in each oxygen hanger yoke, designed to prevent oxygen from flowing out of the machine through the strainer nipple. This valve prevents loss of gas via the hanger yoke if there is no oxygen tank hanging in one yoke but an oxygen tank in the other yoke is being used to supply the machine (Fig. 2-10). These valves also prevent transfilling of one oxygen tank to the other if two tanks are hanging on the machine and both are on. Thus, if one tank were full and the other empty, but both were open, oxygen would tend to flow from the full tank to the empty one, were it not for this

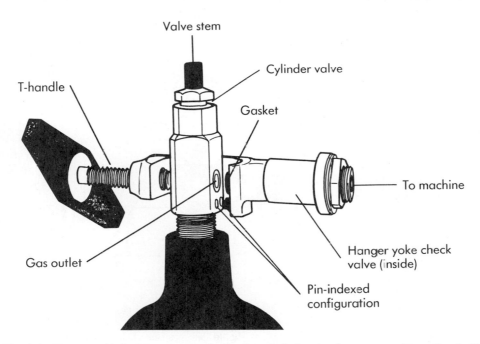

Valve stem

T-handle

— Cylinder valve

Gasket

— To machine

Gas outlet

Hanger yoke check valve (inside)

Pin-indexed configuration

Fig. 2-8. Hanger yoke for an oxygen tank showing pin-indexed safety system. (From Bowie E, Huffman LM: *The anesthesia machine: essentials for understanding,* Madison, Wis, 1985, Ohmeda, a Division of BOC Health Care, Inc. Reproduced by permission.)

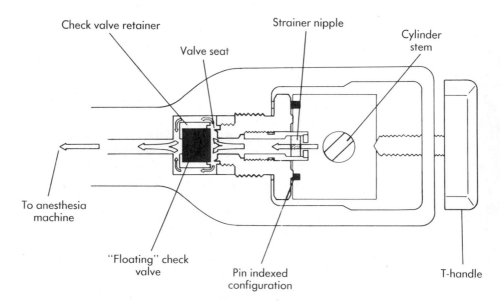

Fig. 2-9. Hanger yoke showing flow of oxygen from the tank through the strainer nipple into the machine. (From Bowie E, Huffman LM: *The anesthesia machine: essentials for understanding,* Madison, Wis, 1985, Ohmeda, a Division of BOC Health Care, Inc. Reproduced by permission.)

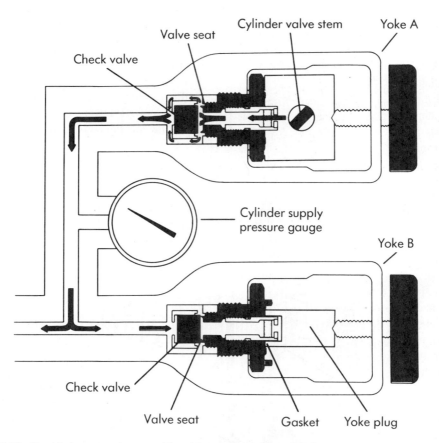

Fig. 2-10. Double hanger yoke assembly with oxygen tank hanging in yoke A. Gas flows into the machine via the floating check valve. Gas cannot escape via yoke *B* because (a) the oxygen pressure closes the check valve and (b) if any gas should leak past the check valve, its flow is prevented by the yoke plug, which has been tightened into yoke B, occluding the yoke nipple. (From Bowie E, Huffman LM: *The anesthesia machine: essentials for understanding,* Madison, Wis, 1985, Ohmeda, a Division of BOC Health Care, Inc. Reproduced by permission.)

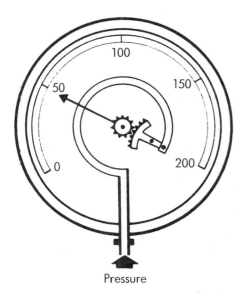

100

150

50

0

200

Pressure

Fig. 2-11. Bourdon tube gauge. Pressure applied to the inside of the curved tube causes it to straighten and thereby move a pointer across a scale. (Adapted with permission from Parbrook GD, Davis PD, Parbrook EO: *Basic physics and measurement in anesthesia,* 1992, Butterworth-Heinemann Limited, Oxford and the author.)

check valve. If the check valve were not present, the transfilling and sudden compression of oxygen into the empty cylinder could cause a rapid rise in the temperatures of the pipes, gauge, and tank, with an associated risk of fire. This is known as an adiabatic change (the state of a gas is altered without the gas being permitted to exchange heat energy with its surroundings).[5] See also Chapter 1.

If there are two hanger yokes for oxygen but only one tank is hanging, a yoke plug should be inserted and tightened in the empty yoke. Thus in the event that the oxygen check valve leaks, loss of oxygen from the empty yoke is prevented by the yoke plug.

The pressure gauges used in the machine to measure pipeline supply pressure or tank supply pressure (Fig. 2-3) are of the Bourdon tube design. In principle, the Bourdon tube is a coiled metal tube, sealed at its inner end and open to the gas pressure at its outer end (Fig. 2-11). As gas pressure rises, the coiled tube tends to straighten out, or uncoil. A pointer attached to the inner-sealed end thereby moves across a scale calibrated in units of pressure. If the Bourdon tube were to burst, the inside of the gauge could be exposed to high pressure. The gauge is therefore constructed with a special heavy glass window and a safety back designed to act as a pressure fuse so that gas is released from the back of the casing if there is a sudden rise in pressure. The cylinder and pipeline pressure gauges for the gases supplied to the machine are generally situated in a panel on the front of the anesthesia machine (Fig. 2-12).

Cylinder pressure regulator

A pressure regulator is a device that converts a variable, high input gas pressure to a constant, lower output pressure. As mentioned above, tank oxygen enters the machine at pressures of up to 1900 psig, depending on how full the tank is. These variable, high input pressures are reduced to a constant, lower output pressure of 45 psig by the oxygen cylinder pressure regulator, sometimes termed the first-stage regulator (see Fig. 2-3). As noted in Fig. 2-10, the tank oxygen from both yokes flows to a common pathway leading to the inlet of the regulator. One regulator serves the two oxygen hanger yokes and is to be found under the machine's work surface.

A diagram that illustrates the principles of action of the regulator is shown in Fig. 2-13. This is described as a direct-acting regulator since the high-pressure gas tends to open the valve. In an indirect-acting regulator the high-pressure gas tends to close the valve. Essentially, the regulator works by balancing the force of a spring against the forces due to the gas pressures acting on a diaphragm. Oxygen at tank pressure enters the high-pressure inlet and is applied over a small area to the valve seat (Fig. 2-13). Valve opening is opposed by a return spring. The valve seat is connected by a thrust pin to a diaphragm in the low-pressure chamber of the regulator. Upward movement of the diaphragm is opposed by a spring whose tension is adjusted at the factory to exert a pressure of 45 psig on the diaphragm. The adjustment of this spring is such that oxygen may flow from the high-pressure inlet, across the valve seat, and into the low-pressure chamber. If pressure in the low-pressure chamber exceeds 45 psig, the diaphragm moves upward and closes down the valve opening, halting the flow of oxygen from high- to low-pressure chambers until the gas pressure exerted on the diaphragm falls below 45 psig. The pressure in the low-pressure chamber and the low-pressure piping of the machine when supplied by the tanks is thereby kept at a constant 45 psig. A cessation of flow from the low-pressure chamber, as would occur if the oxygen flowmeter were closed down, causes pressure to build up here, closing the regulator valve and halting the flow of gas from the cylinder into the regulator.

Failure of the pressure-reduction function of a regulator can transmit excessively high pressure (up to 1900 psig) to the machine low-pressure system (see Fig. 2-13). To protect against such occurrences, the F1161-88 standard requires the regulator to incorporate a pressure-relief valve in the low-pressure chamber, whereby excess pressures are vented to atmosphere.[1] If the diaphragm should rupture or develop a hole, the regulator would fail and gas would escape around the adjustment screw and spring. The high flow of escaping oxygen makes a loud sound, alerting the anesthesiologist to the possibility of a regulator failure. Such a hole represents a significant leak in the low-pressure system through which oxygen would be lost. Reference to Fig. 2-3 shows that even if the tanks were turned off but the pipeline supply were in use, a ruptured diaphragm in the regulator would cause loss of oxygen from the machine's low-pressure system and a possible failure

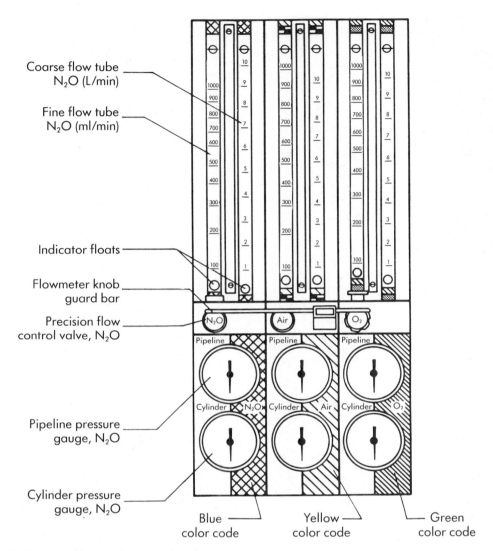

Coarse flow tube
N₂O (L/min)

Fine flow tube
N₂O (ml/min)

Indicator floats

Flowmeter knob
guard bar

Precision flow
control valve, N₂O

Pipeline pressure
gauge, N₂O

Cylinder pressure
gauge, N₂O

Blue
color code

Yellow
color code

Green
color code

Fig. 2-12. Pressure gauges for tank *(lower gauges)* and pipeline *(upper gauges)* gas supplies on Dräger Narkomed machine. (Reproduced by permission of North American Dräger, Inc, Telford, Pa.)

of oxygen supply to the flowmeters. Such a machine should be withdrawn from service until the problem has been corrected by an authorized service technician. Meanwhile, oxygen may be supplied to the patient by a self-inflating (Ambu) bag connected to a portable supply of oxygen (e.g., a transport oxygen cylinder with its own pressure-reducing valve and flowmeter). The F1161-88 standard sets out minimum performance standards for pressure regulators in the anesthesia machine.[1]

Oxygen supply to the machine low-pressure system

Oxygen is normally supplied to the pipeline connector inlet at pressures of 50 to 55 psig, while the tank oxygen supply is regulated to enter at 40 to 45 psig. This difference in supply pressures is deliberate. Thus, if the pipeline is connected and the oxygen tanks are open, oxygen will

be preferentially drawn from the pipeline supply. This is because the higher pressure (50 to 55 psig) from the pipeline supply closes the valve in the first-stage oxygen regulator, thereby preventing the flow of oxygen from the tank. However, there are times, such as during heavy usage of oxygen, when the pipeline pressure may fall below 45 psig, in which case oxygen would be drawn from the tanks if they were left open. Thus, once the tank supply has been checked it should be turned off to prevent loss of the backup oxygen supply. If it is left open, oxygen could also leak around the plastic washer between the tank and the yoke.

An awareness of the differential in supply pressures of oxygen to the machine is essential. Thus, if a pipeline crossover is suspected (e.g., a hypoxic gas is flowing through the oxygen pipeline to the piping in the machine),

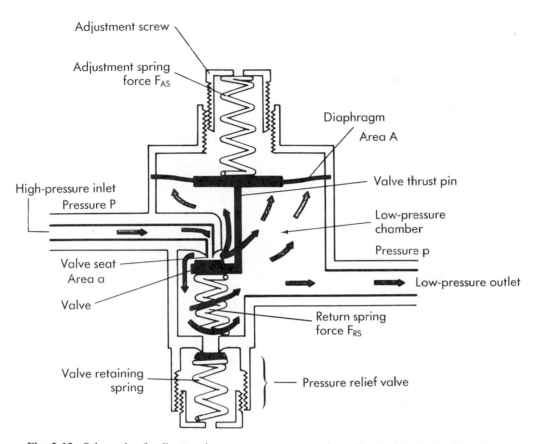

Fig. 2-13. Schematic of a direct-acting oxygen pressure regulator. In principle the regulator functions by balancing forces acting on the diaphragm. Gas under high pressure *(P)* enters the regulator and is applied to the valve over the area of the seat *(a)*. Because force = pressure × area, the force due to high-pressure gas is $P \times a$. Valve opening is initially opposed by the force of the return spring, F_{RS}. Because of the small area of the valve orifice, gas flowing through it enters the next chamber at a lower pressure *(p)*. This lower pressure is applied over the large area of the diaphragm *(A)* as a force of $p \times A$. Upward movement of the diaphragm is opposed by the force of the adjustment spring F_{AS}. The valve and diaphragm are connected by a thrust pin and so move as one unit according to the forces applied in either direction. In equilibrium, the forces acting on the diaphragm are equal; thus $(P \times a) + F_{AS} = (p \times A) + F_{RS}$. The reduced pressure $p = [(F_{AS} - F_{RS}) + (P \times a)]/A$. The regulator is designed such that p is fairly constant despite changes in P. (Adapted from Bowie E, Huffman LM: *The anesthesia machine: essentials for understanding,* Madison, Wis, 1985, Ohmeda, a Division of BOC Health Care, Inc. Reproduced by permission.)

the pipeline supply must be disconnected from the machine if the backup oxygen supply is to be used. For example, if a hypoxic gas (say nitrous oxide) is accidentally used to supply the oxygen pipeline at a supply pressure of greater than 45 psig, this prevents the anesthesiologist from delivering the true oxygen from the backup tanks. This is because the pressure from the wall supply is greater than that from the first-stage oxygen regulator.

Flow pathways for oxygen in the low-pressure system

Oxygen, having entered the machine low-pressure system at 50 to 55 psig (pipeline) or 45 psig (tank regulator), can flow or pressurize in five directions (Figs. 2-3 and 2-14).

Oxygen flush. As soon as any oxygen supply is connected to the machine, depression of the oxygen flush button results in flow of oxygen to the machine common gas outlet at 35 to 75 L/min.[1] Reference to Fig. 2-3 shows that this pathway bypasses the main on/off switch and that the pressure at the common gas outlet could rise, up to the supply pressure to the machine, unless some pressure relief mechanism is present (see the section on the Common Gas Outlet and Outlet Check Valves). Extreme caution is therefore necessary when the oxygen flush is used, so as not to cause barotrauma.

The F1161-88 standard requires that the oxygen flush valve be self-closing and that it be designed to minimize unintended operation by equipment or personnel acciden-

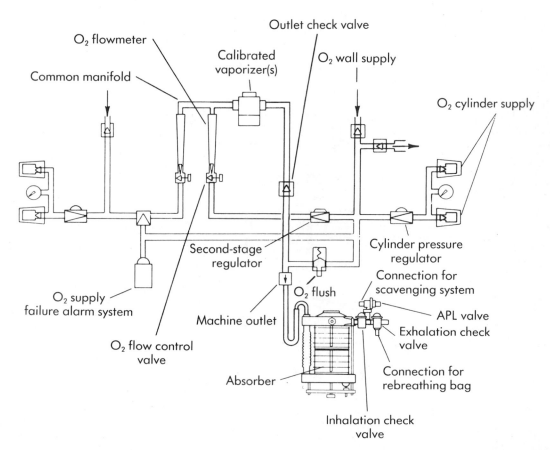

Fig. 2-14. Schematic showing paths for oxygen flow or pressurization in an Ohmeda machine. APL = adjustable pressure limiting ("pop-off") valve. (From Bowie E, Huffman LM: *The anesthesia machine: essentials for understanding,* Madison, Wis, 1985, Ohmeda, a Division of BOC Health Care, Inc. Reproduced by permission.)

tally pressing against it.[1] A modern design of oxygen flush button is shown in Fig. 2-15. Note that the button is recessed in a housing to prevent accidental depression and that the valve is self-closing. Unless otherwise stated, oxygen flows to or pressurizes the following components only when the main on/off switch is in the on position (See Fig. 2-3).

Oxygen supply failure alarm system. Oxygen pressurizes an oxygen supply failure alarm system such that if the supply pressure falls (usually below 30 psig) an alarm is triggered (see Figs. 2-3 and 2-14). The Ohmeda Modulus I, Modulus II, and Excel machines use a canister pressurized with oxygen. This canister emits an audible alarm for at least 7 seconds when the pressure falls below threshold. In Dräger Narkomed and in Ohmeda Modulus II Plus and Modulus CD machines, a pressure-operated electrical switch ensures a continuous audible alarm whenever the oxygen supply pressure falls below the threshold setting.[6,7,8,9]

The F1161-88 standard requires that whenever oxygen supply pressure falls below the manufacturer-specified threshold, a medium-priority alarm shall be activated within 5 seconds. After the alarm has been activated it may be released by the user for a period not to exceed 120 seconds but shall be reset automatically upon restoration of oxygen supply pressure to a level above the alarm threshold.[1]

Pneumatically powered anesthesia ventilator. Oxygen at a pressure of 50 to 55 psig (pipeline) or 45 psig (tanks) is used as the power source for pneumatically driven anesthesia ventilators, such as the Ohmeda 7000, the Ohmeda 7800 series, and the Dräger AV-E. In Ohmeda machines the ventilator connection is such that when the connection is made the valve opens, permitting compressed oxygen to flow to the ventilator (Fig. 2-16). In Dräger Narkomed machines the oxygen take-off to drive the ventilator is *downstream* of the machine main on/off switch so that the Dräger AV-E ventilator cannot be operated if the machine is turned off (see Fig. 2-3, item 6). In Ohmeda machines the oxygen take-off to the ventilator circuit is *upstream* of the main on/off switch. It should be noted that when in use such ventilators consume large quantities of oxygen. If the machine is being supplied by a backup E cylinder, the cylinder's contents are exhausted

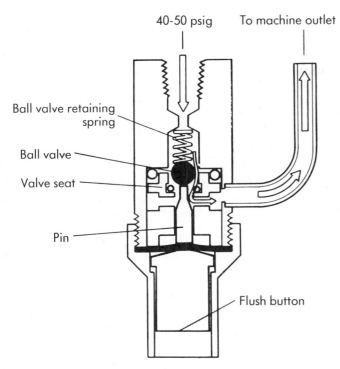

40-50 psig   To machine outlet

Ball valve retaining spring

Ball valve

Valve seat

Pin

Flush button

Fig. 2-15. Schematic of oxygen flush valve in closed position. Note that it is recessed to prevent accidental activation. (From Bowie E, Huffman LM: *The anesthesia machine: essentials for understanding,* Madison, Wis, 1985, Ohmeda, a Division of BOC Health Care, Inc. Reproduced by permission.)

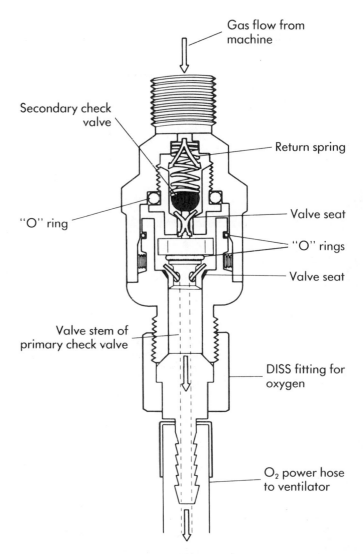

Gas flow from machine

Secondary check valve

Return spring

"O" ring

Valve seat

"O" rings

Valve seat

Valve stem of primary check valve

DISS fitting for oxygen

O_2 power hose to ventilator

Fig. 2-16. Oxygen power outlet to ventilator. While the diameter indexed safety system, DISS, fitting on the ventilator's oxygen supply hose is screwed on to the connector, the valve is lifted from its seat, permitting oxygen to flow to the ventilator's power hose. (From Bowie E, Huffman LM: *The anesthesia machine: essentials for understanding,* Madison, Wis, 1985, Ohmeda, a Division of BOC Health Care, Inc. Reproduced by permission.)

rapidly because, in addition to supplying oxygen to the patient circuit, it is also being depleted by a "thirsty" ventilator. In those ventilators that use 100% oxygen as the driving gas (e.g., Ohmeda 7000, Ohmeda 7800, Air Shields), the ventilator oxygen consumption is in excess of the minute ventilation set on the ventilator (i.e., Rate × Bellows Tidal Volume). The Dräger AV-E is more economical in terms of oxygen because it uses oxygen to drive a venturi that entrains air. The air-oxygen mixture is then used as the ultimate driving gas that enters the ventilator bellows housing (see Chapter 6).[6,10]

Fail-safe valves. When the main on/off switch is in the on position (Fig. 2-3), oxygen pressurizes and holds open a pressure-sensor shut-off valve. These valves reduce or interrupt the supply of nitrous oxide and other gases (e.g., carbon dioxide, helium, air) to their flowmeters if the oxygen supply pressure falls below the threshold setting. This valve, in relation to control of the nitrous oxide supply, is the so-called fail-safe system designed to prevent the unintentional delivery of a hypoxic mixture to the flowmeters. Turning the machine main on/off switch to the off position allows the oxygen pressure in parts of the machine downstream of the switch (normally 45-55 psig) to be vented to the atmosphere. The resulting decrease in oxygen pressure causes the fail safe valves to interrupt the supply of all other gases to their flow control valves. The

design of the fail-safe system differs between the Dräger and Ohmeda machines.

In Ohmeda machines, when the oxygen supply pressure falls below 20 to 25 psig, flow of nitrous oxide and other gases to their flowmeters is interrupted. The pressure sensor shut-off valve used by Ohmeda is an "all-or-nothing" threshold arrangement, open at oxygen pressures greater than 20 to 25 psig and closed at pressures below 20 psig (Fig. 2-17).[7,8,9]

The fail-safe valve in Dräger Narkomed machines is called an oxygen failure protection device (OFPD) and, as in the Ohmeda systems, there is one for each of the other gases supplied to the machine (Fig. 2-18). As the oxygen

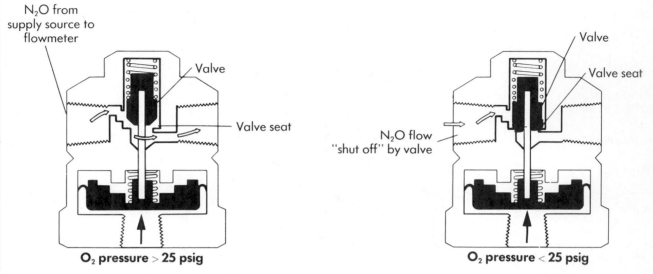

Fig. 2-17. Ohmeda pressure sensor shut-off valve. If oxygen supply pressure on the diaphragm exceeds threshold (in this case 25 psig) the valve is lifted from its seat and nitrous oxide can flow to its flowmeter. If the oxygen supply pressure falls below the threshold setting (the valve return spring pressure) the valve is no longer held off its seat and interrupts the flow of nitrous oxide to its flowmeter. There is a pressure sensor shut-off valve for each gas (other than oxygen) supplied to the machine. (From Bowie E, Huffman LM: *The anesthesia machine: essentials for understanding,* Madison, Wis, 1985, Ohmeda, a Division of BOC Health Care, Inc. Reproduced by permission.)

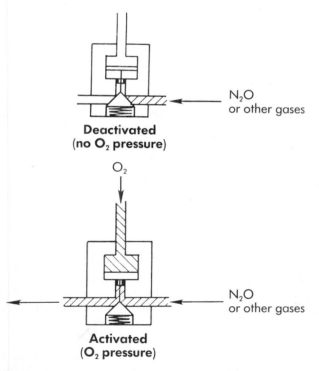

Fig. 2-18. Dräger oxygen failure protection device (OFPD). As the supply pressure of oxygen decreases from the normal value of 55 psig, the OFPD proportionally decreases the nitrous oxide supply pressure to the nitrous oxide flowmeter. The nitrous oxide flow is interrupted completely when oxygen supply pressure is 12 ± 4 psig. There is an OFPD for each gas (other than oxygen) supplied to the machine. Thus, a four-gas machine would have three OFPDs. (Reproduced by permission of North American Dräger, Inc, Telford, Pa.)

supply pressure falls, OFPDs proportionately reduce the supply pressure of other gases to their flowmeters. The supply of nitrous oxide and other gases is completely interrupted when the oxygen supply pressure falls to below 12 ± 4 psig.[6]

It must be recognized that both designs of fail-safe valve ensure that at low or zero oxygen supply pressures only oxygen may be delivered to the machine's common gas outlet. However, as long as there is an adequate oxygen supply *pressure,* other gases may flow to their flowmeters. The fail-safe system does not ensure oxygen *flow* at its flowmeter, only a supply *pressure* to the oxygen flowmeter. Thus a normally functioning fail-safe system permits flow of 100% nitrous oxide provided the machine has an adequate oxygen supply *pressure.* The term fail-safe therefore represents something of a misnomer, since it does not ensure oxygen *flow* (Fig. 2-19).

Flowmeters. Oxygen flows to the oxygen flow control valve and flowmeter(s) (rotameters). Supply pressure to the oxygen flowmeters differs in Ohmeda and Dräger machines.

In contemporary Ohmeda machines the oxygen supply pressure to the flowmeters is regulated to about 14 psig by a second-stage regulator. This regulator (Figs. 2-3 and 2-14) ensures a constant supply pressure to the Ohmeda oxygen flowmeter. Thus, even if the oxygen supply pressure to the machine decreases below 45 to 50 psig, as long as it exceeds 14 psig the flow set on the oxygen flowmeter is maintained. Without this regulator, if the oxygen supply pressure were to fall, the oxygen flow at the flowmeter

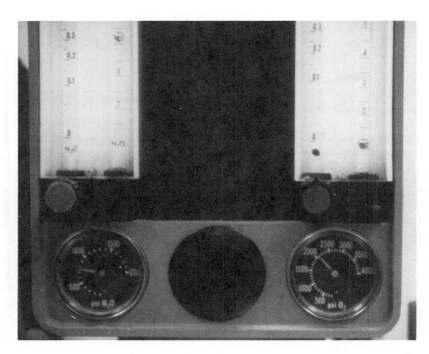

Fig. 2-19. Limitations of the fail-safe system. In this machine, because the supply pressure of oxygen is adequate (2000 psig from the tank and therefore 45 psig in the machine), nitrous oxide may flow to its flowmeter and beyond (4 L/min) even though the oxygen flow control valve is turned off and no oxygen is flowing. The term "fail safe" is therefore somewhat of a misnomer.

would decrease and, if another gas (e.g., nitrous oxide) was also being used, a hypoxic gas mixture could result at the flowmeter manifold.

The second-stage oxygen regulator used in Ohmeda machines is similar in terms of principle of operation to that of the first-stage regulator (Fig. 2-13). However, because it normally handles lower pressures than the first-stage regulator, it does not require or incorporate a pressure-relief valve.[9]

The design of the Dräger Narkomed anesthesia machine does not use a second-stage oxygen pressure-regulator valve (Fig. 2-3). Dräger Narkomed machines have OFPDs that interface the supply pressure of oxygen with those of nitrous oxide and each of the other gases supplied to the machine.[6] The OFPD consists of a seat-nozzle assembly connected to a spring-loaded piston (Fig. 2-18). When deactivated, the spring is expanded, forcing the nozzle against the seat so that no gas can flow through the device to the flowmeter. As oxygen pressure increases, it is applied to the piston, which in turn forces the nozzle away from its seat so that gas can flow through the OFPD. The OFPD responds to oxygen pressure changes such that as pressure falls, the other gas flows will fall in proportion. When the oxygen supply pressure is less than 12 ± 4 psig, the OFPD is closed completely.[6] A decrease in oxygen supply pressure causes a proportionate decrease in the supply pressures of each of the other gases to their flowmeters. As the oxygen supply pressure and flow decrease, all other gas flows are decreased in proportion in order to pre-

vent the creation of a hypoxic gas mixture at the flowmeter level (see the preceding section). The operation of the OFPD can be demonstrated as follows: With the Dräger Narkomed machine supplied from the pipeline oxygen (55 psig), set 6 L/min flows of both nitrous oxide and oxygen. If the pipeline oxygen is now disconnected and the tank oxygen supply opened (45 psig), the flows of both oxygen and nitrous oxide will be observed to have decreased at the rotameters.

The use (Ohmeda) or non-use (Dräger) of a second-stage oxygen regulator affects the total gas flow emerging from the common gas outlet of the machine if the oxygen supply pressure falls. In an Ohmeda machine, as long as the oxygen supply pressure exceeds 14 psig all gas flows are maintained at the original flowmeter settings. In a Dräger Narkomed machine, if the oxygen supply pressure falls from normal (45 to 55 psig) all gas flows decrease in proportion via the OFPDs. A decrease in total gas flow from the machine's common gas outlet might result in rebreathing, depending upon the anesthetic circuit in use. A rebreathing (Mapleson A-F) system is affected more than is a circle system with a carbon dioxide absorber.

NITROUS OXIDE

Like oxygen, nitrous oxide (N_2O) may be supplied to the machine either from the pipeline system at 50 to 55 psig or from the backup E cylinder supply on the machine itself. Nitrous oxide from the tank supply enters the nitrous oxide–specific yokes at pressures of up to 745 psig (at 20° C) and then passes through a first-stage regulator similar to that for oxygen. This regulator reduces this pressure to 40 to 45 psig (see Fig. 2-3). The pin-index safety system is designed to ensure that only a nitrous oxide tank may hang in a nitrous oxide hanger yoke. As with oxygen, a check valve in each yoke prevents the back flow of nitrous oxide if no tank is hung in the yoke. (See Fig. 2-10.)

The nitrous oxide pipeline is supplied from liquid nitrous oxide or from banks of large tanks of nitrous oxide, usually H cylinders (see Chapter 1). The pressure in the pipeline is regulated to 50 to 55 psig to supply the outlets in the operating room. Once it enters the anesthesia machine, nitrous oxide must flow past the fail-safe valve in order to reach its flow control valve and rotameter.

In Ohmeda Modulus anesthesia machines which have the Link-25 Proportion Limiting System, a second-stage nitrous oxide regulator further reduces gas pressure so that nitrous oxide is supplied to its flowmeter at a nominal 26 psig (Fig. 2-3).[7] The actual downstream pressure of this second-stage nitrous oxide regulator is adjusted at the factory or by an Ohmeda field service representative to ensure correct functioning of the proportioning system.

OTHER MEDICAL GASES

If another medical gas, such as air and/or helium or carbon dioxide, is supplied to the machine, the arrangements are similar to those for the nitrous oxide supply. Thus for the pipeline supply there is a DISS gas-specific connector, and for the tank supply there is a pin-indexed gas-specific hanger yoke. Supply pressure gauges are generally provided for the supply source (pipeline, tank), and a fail-safe valve controls the flow of each gas to its flowmeter, according to the oxygen supply pressure to the machine.

ANESTHESIA MACHINE GAS-PIPING SYSTEM

Within the anesthesia machine, piping conducts compressed gases from their points of entry into the machine, between the various components, and to the common gas outlet. The F1161-88 standard requires that this piping be capable of withstanding four times the intended service pressure without rupturing.[1] It further specifies that between the cylinders or the pipeline inlet and the flow control valves the maximum leakage of each gas shall not exceed 10 ml/min at normal working pressure.[1] "The maximum permissible leakage rate on all gas services between the flow control valves and the common gas outlet shall be 30 ml/min at a pressure of 30 cm H_2O with the vaporizers in both the ON and OFF position."[1] The standard requires that gas piping connectors be noninterchangeable or that the content of each pipe be identifiable by a marking at each junction.[1] Such a system is designed to prevent crossover of gases within the machine.

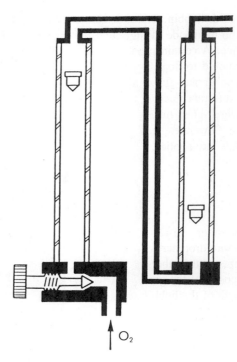

Fig. 2-20. Flowmeters arranged in series. The oxygen flows first through a rotameter where low flows (<1 L/min) are measured and then through a rotameter where high flows are measured. (From Schreiber PJ: *Anesthesia systems,* Telford, Pa, 1985, North American Dräger Inc. Reproduced by permission.)

FLOWMETERS

The proportions of oxygen and nitrous oxide, and other medical gases controlled by the machine, as well as total gas flows delivered to the common gas outlet, are adjusted by means of flow control valves and flowmeters (rotameters). There may be one rotameter, or two rotameters (Fig. 2-20) in series for each gas.[1] If two are present for any gas, the first permits accurate measurement of low flows (usually up to 1 L/min), and the second permits measurement of higher flows (of up to 10 or 12 L/min). The F1161-88 standard requires that each flowmeter be calibrated for discharge through the common gas outlet into a standard atmosphere (760 mmHg) at 20° C.[1] In North America the oxygen flowmeter is positioned on the right side of a rotameter bank downstream of the other flowmeters and closest to the common gas outlet (Figs. 2-3 and 2-14). In the event of a leak in one of the other flowmeter tubes, this position is the least likely to result in a hypoxic mixture.[11] Where oxygen and other gases are delivered by their flowmeters into a common manifold, the oxygen is delivered downstream of all other gases.[1]

Rotameters are examples of constant pressure, variable orifice flowmeters, and their operation is based upon the principle of the Thorpe tube.[5] Each rotameter consists of a tapered glass tube that has a small cross-sectional diameter at the bottom and a wider diameter at the top and that contains a ball or bobbin. The area between the outside of the bobbin and the inside of the glass tube represents the variable orifice. A certain pressure difference across the bobbin is required to float the bobbin. As the orifice widens, greater and greater flows are required to create the same pressure difference across the bobbin, which floats higher in the tapered glass tube.

At low flow rates, gas flow is essentially laminar and Poiseuille's law applies.[5] Thus

$$\text{Flow} = \frac{\pi p r^4}{8vl}$$

where:

$\pi =$ A constant, 3.142
$p =$ Pressure drop across the bobbin
$r =$ Radius of the tube
$v =$ Viscosity of the gas
$l =$ Length of the bobbin or float

When the orifice is larger and flows are greater, turbulence occurs, in which case

$$\text{Flow} \propto p \propto r^2 \propto \text{length}^{-1} \propto \frac{1}{\sqrt{\text{density}}}.$$

Thus flowmeters use a physical property of the gas to measure flow. In the case of low flows, when flow is laminar, the property used is the viscosity of the gas. At high flows, when flow is turbulent or orificial, gas density is used to measure flow.[5]

Rotameters are precision instruments. Flow tubes are manufactured for specific gases, calibrated with a unique float, and are meant to be used within a certain range of temperatures and pressures. Flowmeters are not interchangeable among gases, and if a gas is passed through a rotameter for which it has not been calibrated, the flows shown are likely incorrect. Theoretical exceptions to this are that at *low* flows, flow rates of gases with *similar viscosities* are read identically (e.g., oxygen and helium, 202 and 194 micropoise, respectively); and at *high flows*, gases of *similar density* (e.g., nitrous oxide and carbon dioxide, both of which have molecular weights of 44) are read identically. Again, it is emphasized that flowmeters are *not* interchangeable among medical gases and for the recent Ohmeda machines, they are now manufactured so that they cannot be interchanged.[7,8]

The gas flow to the rotameter tube is controlled by a touch- and color-coded knob, which is linked to a needle valve (Fig. 2-21). In the United States the oxygen control knob is color-coded green (as is everything related to oxygen), is fluted, and is larger in diameter than the other gas flow control knobs.[1] The nitrous oxide control knob is smaller, color-coded blue, and is not fluted (Fig. 2-22).

Manufacturers of anesthesia machines offer as an option an oxygen flow that, when the machine's main on/off switch is turned on (i.e., the machine is capable of delivering an anesthetic), cannot be completely discontinued.

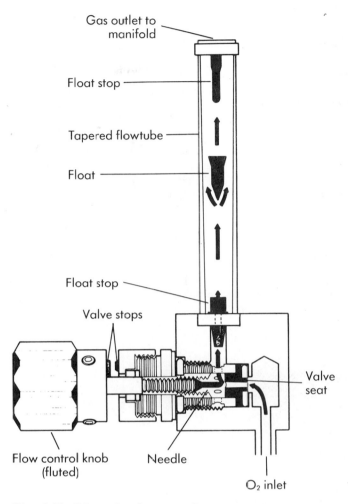

Fig. 2-21. Schematic of oxygen flowmeter and flow control valve. Other designs may use a ball rather than the elongated float shown. Note that the flow control knob for oxygen is fluted (touch coded) to distinguish it from the other knobs, which are knurled. Minimum oxygen flow is achieved by means of valve stops in this Ohmeda flow control system. (From Bowie E, Huffman LM: *The anesthesia machine: essentials for understanding*, Madison, Wis, 1985, Ohmeda, a Division of BOC Health Care, Inc. Reproduced by permission.)

This is because either a valve stop is provided to ensure a minimum oxygen flow of 200 to 300 ml/min past the partially open needle valve (Ohmeda, see Fig. 2-21), or a gas flow resistor is provided, which permits a similar flow of 200 to 300 ml/min to bypass a totally closed oxygen flow-control needle valve (Dräger Narkomed, see Fig. 2-23).[6] In Dräger Narkomed machines, the minimum-oxygen-flow feature functions only in the O_2/N_2O mode but not in the ALL GASES mode.[6]

The F1161-88 standard also requires that each flowmeter assembly be clearly and permanently marked with the appropriate color, the unit of measure used, and the name or chemical symbol of the gas it measures. The manufacturer should ensure that the flowmeters and tubes are not interchangeable among the different gas flowmeter locations or between different locations (i.e., high and low

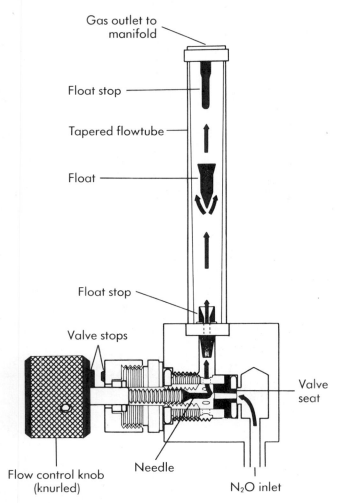

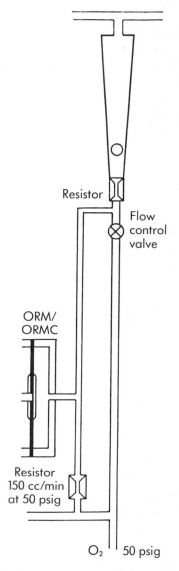

Fig. 2-22. Nitrous oxide flowmeter and control knob. The flowmeter is essentially the same as for oxygen, but the flow control knob is smaller and knurled. (From Bowie E, Huffman LM: *The anesthesia machine: essentials for understanding,* Madison, Wis, 1985, Ohmeda, a Division of BOC Health Care, Inc. Reproduced by permission.)

flows) of the same gas. Flowmeters may also be pin-indexed to eliminate the possibility of installing a flowmeter intended for a different gas.[1] This system is not required by the standard but is used in contemporary Ohmeda anesthesia machines (Fig. 2-24).

Flowmeter tubes are fragile and are therefore protected on the machine by a plastic window. Individual flow control knobs may also be protected from accidental alterations in setting by a bar that extends across the front of them (Fig. 2-25). This design is used in Dräger Narkomed machines.

In order to obtain a true reading of flow, the rotameter tubes must be kept vertical to prevent the ball or bobbin from touching the sides of the glass tube. The flow should be read at the middle of the ball or the top of the bobbin. The ball or bobbin is more likely to stick at low flows and where the tube is narrowest. Electrostatic charges and dirt

Fig. 2-23. Minimum oxygen flow on Dräger Narkomed machine is achieved by a bypass resistor. In the Narkomed machines there are no stops on the flow control knob, so that the oxygen flow control valve can be closed completely. Minimum oxygen flow is achieved when oxygen bypasses the flow control valve through a resistor designed to permit a flow of 150 ml/min when the supply pressure is 50 psig. (Reproduced by permission of North American Dräger, Inc, Telford, Pa.)

may also interfere with the bobbin's free movement. In this respect a ball is superior to a bobbin in that a ball is less likely to stick.

Flowmeters are individually calibrated by the manufacturer against a master flowmeter for each gas. Each master flowmeter was, in turn, calibrated with a bubble meter system.[12] In clinical practice, flowmeter calibration is most easily checked by setting gas flows to produce desired nitrous oxide–oxygen concentrations and checking with a gas analyzer the composition of the gas mixture emerging from the machine's common gas outlet.

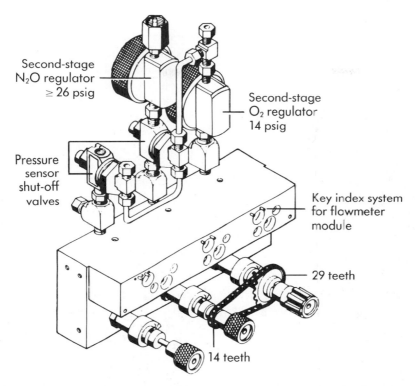

Fig. 2-24. Ohmeda Link 25 Proportion Limiting System. Note the use of a key index system for flowmeter modules in Ohmeda Modulus machines. (Reproduced by permission of Ohmeda, a Division of BOC Health Care, Inc, Madison, Wis.)

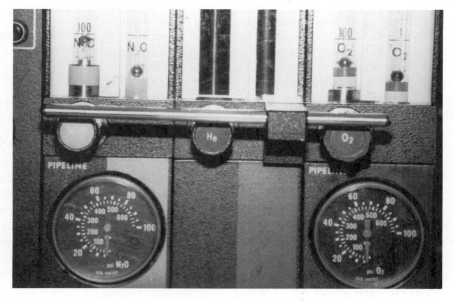

Fig. 2-25. Dräger Narkomed machines are provided with a bar in front of the flow control knobs to protect against accidental alterations in setting.

OXYGEN RATIO MONITORING AND PROPORTIONING SYSTEMS

A major consideration in the design of contemporary anesthesia machines is the prevention of delivery of a hypoxic gas mixture to the patient. The fail-safe system described above only serves to interrupt (Ohmeda) or proportionately reduce and ultimately interrupt (Dräger OFPD) the supplies of nitrous oxide and other gases (e.g., air, carbon dioxide, helium) to their flowmeters if the oxygen supply *pressure* to the machine falls. It does not prevent delivery of a hypoxic mixture to the common gas outlet, and the term "fail safe" is therefore somewhat of a misnomer.

In contemporary machines, oxygen and nitrous oxide flow controls are physically interlinked either mechanically (Ohmeda machines) or mechanically and pneumatically (recent Dräger Narkomed machines), so that a fresh gas mixture containing at least 25% oxygen is created at the level of the rotameters when nitrous oxide and oxygen are being used.[6,7,8] Older anesthesia machines, such as the Boyle 50 and the original Dräger Narkomed, did not have the oxygen and nitrous oxide flow controls interlinked. Therefore, as long as a normal oxygen supply pressure was connected to the machine, a hypoxic gas mixture (i.e., 100% nitrous oxide) could be delivered to the patient merely because the oxygen was not turned on at the flow control valve. In this case, the fail-safe is functioning normally but does not prevent the user from incorrectly setting the flow controls to deliver a hypoxic mixture. It is essential to be aware of this because these machines may still be in use (see Fig. 2-19).

Ohmeda anesthesia machines use the Link-25 Proportion Limiting Control System to ensure an adequate percentage of oxygen in the gas mixture created.[7,8] In this system the openings of the oxygen and nitrous oxide flow control valves are proportioned, while the supply pressures of these gases to their flow control valves are precisely regulated by second-stage (low pressure) regulators. Thus a gear with 14 teeth is integral with the nitrous oxide flow control spindle, while a gear with 29 teeth "floats" on a threaded oxygen flow control valve spindle (Fig. 2-24). The two gears are connected by a precision stainless steel link chain. For every 2.07 revolutions of the nitrous oxide flow control spindle, an oxygen flow control, set to the lowest oxygen flow, rotates once because of the 14:29 ratio of gear teeth. Because the gear on the oxygen flow control spindle is thread-mounted so that it can ride (float) on the control valve spindle (rather than being integral with the spindle), oxygen flow can be increased independently of that of nitrous oxide. However, regardless of the oxygen flow set, if the flow of nitrous oxide is increased sufficiently, the gear on the oxygen spindle will engage with the oxygen flow control knob, causing it to rotate and open the needle valve and thereby causing the oxygen flow to increase.[7,8] If nitrous oxide flow is now decreased, the oxygen flow remains high unless it is deliberately reduced by the user. The proportion 75% nitrous oxide to 25% oxygen is completed because the nitrous oxide flow control valve is supplied from a second-stage gas regulator that reduces nitrous oxide pressure to a nominal 26 psig (adjusted as previously described) before it reaches the flow control valve, whereas the oxygen flow control valve is supplied at a pressure of 14 psig from a second-stage oxygen regulator (Figs. 2-3 and 2-24). The Link 25 System permits the nitrous oxide and oxygen flow control valves to be set independently of one another but, whenever a setting of nitrous oxide concentration more than 75% is attempted, the oxygen flow is automatically increased to maintain at least 25% oxygen in the resulting mixture. This system thus *increases the minimum flow of oxygen according to the nitrous oxide flow setting.*[7,8]

It should be noted that the Link-25 System interconnects only the nitrous oxide and oxygen flow control valves. If the anesthesia machine has flow controls for other gases, such as helium or air (see Fig. 2-24), a gas mixture containing less than 25% oxygen could be set at the level of the flow meters. This potential hazard is addressed on recent Ohmeda machines by supplying helium in tanks containing a mixture of helium and oxygen (75%:25%).

In Dräger Narkomed machines, the Oxygen Ratio Monitor Controller (ORMC) (Fig. 2-26) serves to limit the flow of nitrous oxide according to the oxygen *flow* and creates a mixture of at least 25% oxygen at the flowmeter level when these two gases are being used.[6,13,14] At oxygen flow rates of less than 1 L/min, even higher concentrations of oxygen are delivered. In addition, an alarm is activated when the ORMC is functioning to prevent a hypoxic mixture when the Dräger Narkomed machine is used in the N_2O/O_2 mode but not in the ALL GASES mode (i.e., when air, helium, etc. might be switched into the system).[14]

The ORMC works as follows: As oxygen flows past its flow control valve and up the rotameter tube, it encounters a resistor that creates a back pressure, which is applied to the oxygen diaphragm (Fig. 2-26). As nitrous oxide flows past its flow control valve and up the rotameter tube, it too encounters a resistor that causes a back pressure on the nitrous oxide diaphragm. The two diaphragms are linked by a connecting shaft whose ultimate position depends on the relative back pressures, and therefore flows, of nitrous oxide and oxygen. One end of the connecting shaft controls the orifice of a slave valve, which in turn controls the supply pressure of nitrous oxide to its flow control valve. When the oxygen flow is high, the shaft moves to the left and opens the slave control valve. Conversely, if the flow of nitrous oxide is increased excessively, the shaft moves to the right, closing the slave valve orifice and limiting the supply pressure, and thereby the flow, of nitrous oxide to its flow control valve. When the ORMC is acting to prevent a hypoxic mixture, the leaf spring contacts (Fig.

2-26) are closed, triggering an alarm. This alarm is disabled when the machine is in the ALL GASES mode, but the ORMC will continue to prevent delivery of a hypoxic mixture when nitrous oxide and oxygen are used.[6,13]

The Dräger ORMC differs from the Ohmeda Link-25 Proportioning Limiting System in a number of ways. First, the ORMC does not use second-stage oxygen and nitrous oxide regulators. Second, the ORMC serves to limit the flow of nitrous oxide according to the flow of oxygen, whereas the Link-25 System increases the flow of oxygen as the nitrous oxide flow is increased. Like the Link-25 System, the ORMC functions only between nitrous oxide and oxygen, and there is no interlinking of oxygen with other gases (such as air or helium) that might be delivered by the machine. Thus when a third or fourth gas is in use, the proportioning systems afford no protection against a hypoxic mixture at the common gas outlet. Although of elegant design, both the ORMC and Link-25 systems are subject to mechanical and/or pneumatic failure (see Chapter 16) and should be tested according to the manufacturer's instructions during the pre-use machine checkout.[7,13] Furthermore, if the systems are functioning correctly, they ensure adequacy of only >25% oxygen at the flowmeter

level. An oxygen leak downstream of the flowmeters could result in a hypoxic mixture emerging from the machine common gas outlet. *An oxygen analyzer in the patient circuit is therefore essential if a potentially hypoxic mixture is to be detected and thereby prevented.*

VAPORIZER MANIFOLDS

After individual gas flows have been measured by their respective rotameters, a mixture of the gases is created in a manifold downstream of the flowmeters. From here the gas mixture flows to the vaporizer manifold, where concentration-calibrated vaporizers are mounted on the machine. In the North American Dräger Narkomed machines, the Vapor 19.1 vaporizers are permanently mounted (and not designed to be removed by the user). These Dräger vaporizers are mounted in series; that is, fresh gas flows through each vaporizer (albeit via a bypass channel) on its way to the common gas outlet. An interlock device ensures that only one vaporizer can be turned on at any one time.

Ohmeda machines are equipped with Tec series vaporizers that are designed to be easily removable by the user. The Ohmeda vaporizer manifold is designed such that no

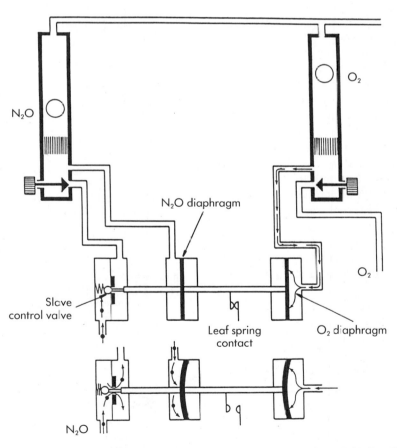

Fig. 2-26. North American Dräger Oxygen Ratio Monitor Controller. (From Schreiber PJ: *Anesthesia systems,* Telford, Pa, 1985, North American Dräger Inc. Reproduced by permission.)

gas from the flowmeters enters any part of a vaporizer that is turned off, not even the vaporizer's bypass channel. The Ohmeda vaporizers are therefore not mounted in series. When a Tec vaporizer is turned on, fresh gas enters only that vaporizer. (For more details, see Chapter 3.)

Machines on which no vaporizers have been mounted are available as "clean machines" for use with patients susceptible to malignant hyperthermia. In a Dräger Narkomed machine, this involves replacing the usual vaporizer mounts with a length of metal tubing connecting the flowmeter manifold to the common gas outlet of the machine. An Ohmeda machine with Selectatec System may be made "clean" simply by removing all the vaporizers and then flushing the machine with oxygen from the oxygen flowmeter. The oxygen flush should not be used for this purpose because this flow would by-pass the vaporizer manifold, which would therefore not be "cleaned." (See Fig. 2-3.)

COMMON GAS OUTLET AND OUTLET CHECK VALVES

The fresh gas mixture produced by the settings of the flowmeters for oxygen, nitrous oxide, and/or other gases, and vapor from one concentration-calibrated vaporizer exit the machine via the common gas outlet. In the Ohmeda Modulus I, Modulus II, and Excel machines there is (1) an outlet check valve (Fig. 2-27) and (2) a pressure relief valve (Fig. 2-3).[8] The outlet check valve is situated between the vaporizers and the common gas outlet. The pressure relief valve, as its name suggests, prevents the build-up of excessive pressures upstream of the outlet check valve. In some Ohmeda machines (Excel, Modulus I with Selectatec Switch) the pressure relief valve is located downstream of the outlet check valve. In all machines, these components are located upstream from where the oxygen flush flow would join to pass to the common gas outlet. The use or nonuse of an outlet check valve varies among the various models of machine. The pressure relief mechanism and its location with respect to an outlet check valve, if present, also varies. The arrangements used in some recent models of machine are summarized in Table 2-1. Readers are encouraged to review the schematic of their own particular machines to understand the configuration of their system.

The purpose of the outlet check valve is to prevent reverse gas flow, a situation that could cause gas to go back into the vaporizer ("pumping effect") if the vaporizer did not have its own outlet check valve or specialized design. This effect, if not prevented, causes increased concentrations of anesthetic agent output (see Chapter 3).

Dräger Narkomed machines are designed so that an outlet check valve is not required. The pumping effect is eliminated by the special design of the Vapor 19.1 vaporizer. The Ohmeda Modulus II Plus and Modulus CD machines are equipped with Ohmeda TEC 4 or TEC 5 vapor-

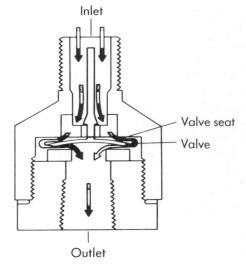

Open position

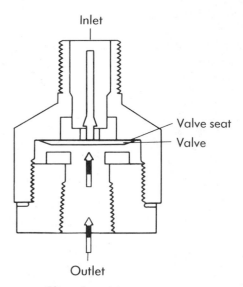

Closed position

Fig. 2-27. Machine outlet check valve located between the vaporizer and the common gas outlet. This valve is present on Ohmeda Modulus I, Modulus II, and Excel machines but not on Ohmeda Modulus II Plus, Modulus CD, or Dräger Narkomed machines. The valve is designed to permit gas flow from the vaporizers to the common gas outlet, and to prevent reverse gas flow, which might cause a pumping effect on the vaporizer. Increased pressure at the common gas outlet causes closure of the valve. (From Bowie E, Huffman LM: *The anesthesia machine: essentials for understanding,* Madison, Wis, 1985, Ohmeda, a Division of BOC Health Care, Inc. Reproduced by permission.)

izers, which incorporate a baffle system and a specially designed manifold to prevent the pumping effect. This makes an outlet check valve unnecessary in these machines. Nevertheless, the Ohmeda Modulus II Plus and Modulus CD machines do have a pressure relief valve upstream of the common gas outlet.[7,15] Dräger Narkomed

Table 2-1. Outlet check valve and pressure relief arrangements in recent model Ohmeda and North American Dräger machines

		Pressure relief valve		
Machine model	Outlet check valve	Present/Absent	Minimum opening ("cracking") pressure*	Location with respect to outlet check valve
Ohmeda Modulus I	Present	Present	2.3-2.9 psig	Upstream
Modulus I with Selectatec Switch	Present	Present	2.3-2.9 psig	Downstream
Modulus II	Present	Present	2.3-2.9 psig	Upstream
Modulus II Plus	Absent	Present	2.3-2.9 psig	Not applicable
Modulus CD	Absent	Present	2.3-2.9 psig	Not applicable
Excel	Present	Present	5 psig	Downstream
North American Dräger	Absent†	Via Vapor ‡9.1 vaporizer‡	Approx. 18 psig	Not applicable

*Minimum opening pressure psig.
†Some *older* model Dräger machines may use a check valve in the vaporizer outlet (see Chapter 3).
‡Pressure relief is via a special mechanism in the Vapor 19.1 vaporizer.

machines do not have a separate pressure relief valve. In these machines pressure relief, if required, takes place when the pressure exceeds 18 psig through the specially designed Vapor 19.1 vaporizers. The presence or absence of an outlet check valve and pressure relief valve is of some significance when it comes to leak-testing the low pressure system of the anesthesia machine, and it also affects the performance of a transtracheal jet ventilating system connected to the common gas outlet (see below).

Transtracheal jet ventilation systems are configured by anesthesiologists for use in an emergency. These systems can be connected to the machine common gas outlet via a 15-mm connector and ventilation is achieved by intermittent depression of the oxygen flush button.[16,17,18] The driving pressure of such systems is limited by the threshold opening pressure of the pressure relief mechanism, if present (see Fig. 2-3 and Table 2-1). In the case of Ohmeda Modulus II Plus or Modulus CD machines, the pressure relief valve opens at 2.2 to 2.9 psig. In the case of Dräger Narkomed machines equipped with Vapor 19.1 vaporizers, it opens at 18 psig. In the case of Ohmeda Modulus I and Ohmeda Modulus II machines (outlet check valve present), and Dräger Narkomed machines without vaporizers (no pressure relief system), the driving pressure is 45 to 55 psig, depending on whether the tank or pipeline oxygen supply to the machine is in use (Fig. 2-3). The "cracking" pressure of the relief mechanisms (i.e., the pressure at which the relief valve first begins to open) provides some guide to the potential driving pressure available for the transtracheal ventilating system. In practice, pressures a little higher than the "cracking" pressure are generated because of both the flow restriction offered by the relief valve and that offered by the ventilating system. It should be noted, however, that anesthesia machine oxygen flush systems were not designed or intended by

the manufacturers to be used for transtracheal jet ventilation and because of this are not labeled for this use. It is preferable to purchase a purpose-built transtracheal jet ventilation system designed to be connected via a pressure-reducing valve and toggle switch, to a separate 50 psig oxygen source.

The F1161-88 standard requires machines to have only one common gas outlet. When that common gas outlet is connected to the breathing system by a fresh gas supply hose (the usual arrangement in most ORs), the common gas outlet must be provided with a manufacturer-specific retaining device.[1] The purpose of the retaining device is to help prevent disconnection or misconnections between the machine's common gas outlet and the patient circuit that could injure the patient. Thus a disconnection here could result in entrainment of room air, which might result in a hypoxic mixture in the circuit as well as failure of delivery of inhaled anesthetic. Dräger Narkomed machines have a bar type of retaining device (Fig. 2-28), and Ohmeda machines use a spring-loaded bayonet-fitting retaining device.[7,15] The F1161-88 standard requires that the common gas outlet have a 15-mm female fitting or a 15/22-mm coaxial fitting. It must not incorporate a 19-mm, 23-mm or 30-mm conical fitting because these are specific for other parts of the delivery system (i.e., the patient circuit and the scavenging system). (See Chapter 16.)

ANESTHESIA MACHINE LOW-PRESSURE SYSTEM CHECKOUT

The anesthesia delivery system should be checked each day before the first case, and whenever any change has been made to the system. Such changes include replacing the ventilator bellows or anesthesia circuit and moving the anesthesia machine within the operating room. Moving the

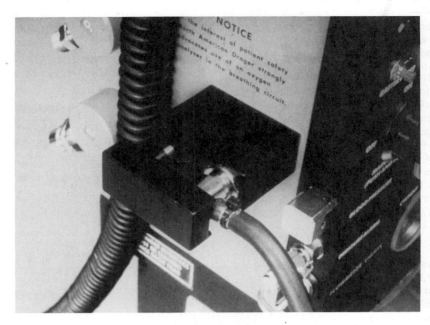

Fig. 2-28. Common gas outlet retaining device on a Dräger Narkomed machine, designed to prevent accidental disconnection of the hose connecting the common gas outlet to the patient circuit.

machine may cause kinking or compression of tubing, which in turn may produce interference with gas delivery, ventilator function, or waste gas scavenging. Thus, in addition to a complete checkout at the start of each day, a shortened checkout of the delivery system should precede each case.

In August 1986, the Food and Drug Administration (FDA) published its "Anesthesia Apparatus Checkout Recommendations," which are shown in Table 2-2.[19] This checklist is currently under review and being revised.* Meanwhile, this checkout applies as a general guideline only and the FDA encourages users to modify this checkout "to accommodate differences in equipment design and variations in local clinical practice. . . . Users should refer to the operators manual for special procedures or precautions." In this respect, the user must understand the basic arrangement and functions of the components of the anesthesia machine so as to apply the correct checkout procedure. This will become apparent in the following sections. The reader should also review Chapters 16 and 22.

Testing for Leaks in the Anesthesia Machine and Breathing System

Item 16 in the FDA 1986 checklist (Table 2-2) describes what should be performed prior to each case. This checkout evaluates the components of the delivery system that are downstream of the flowmeters, and should detect *gross* leaks that may be due to cracked rotameter tubes,

leaking gaskets and vaporizers, and leaks in the anesthesia circuit. In this generic test, the adjustable pressure-limiting (APL or "pop-off") valve is closed and the patient circuit is occluded at the patient end (item 16a). The system is then filled via the oxygen flush until the reservoir bag is just full but there is negligible pressure in the system. Oxygen flow is set to 5 L/min (item 16b). Oxygen flow is then slowly decreased until pressure no longer rises above about 20 cm H_2O (Fig. 2-29). This set flow is said to approximate the total rate of gas leak, which should be no greater than a few hundred ml/min (item 16c). The reservoir bag should then be squeezed to a pressure of about 50 cm H_2O to verify that the system is gas-tight (item 16d). If there is a large enough leak, the circuit pressure may fall to zero (Fig. 2-30).

The advantages of this test routine are that it can be performed quickly and that it checks the patient circuit as well as the low-pressure components of the machine in those models that do not have an outlet check valve. Disadvantages of this routine are that it is relatively insensitive to small leaks and that, in those machines that have an outlet check valve (e.g., Ohmeda Modulus I, Modulus II, Excel models), only the patient circuit downstream of the outlet check valve is tested for leaks.

The generic checkout is insensitive because it is dependent on volume. Thus in this test a large volume of gas (i.e., that contained in the circuit tubing, absorber, and reservoir bag) is compressed. One then observes the circuit pressure gauge for any changes. The term *compliance* expresses the relationship between volume and pressure and is defined as change in volume per unit change in pressure. Because of the large volume of gas compressed and the

*Lees DE: FDA Preanesthesia Checklist Being Evaluated, Revised, Anesthesia Patient Safety Foundation Newsletter 6:25, 1991. A draft of the 1992 FDA checklist is shown in Table 22-3.

Table 2-2. Anesthesia apparatus checkout recommendations (as published by the FDA, August 1986)

This checkout, or a reasonable equivalent, should be conducted before administering anesthesia. This is a guideline which users are encouraged to modify to accommodate differences in equipment design and variations in local clinical practice. Such local modifications should have appropriate peer review. Users should refer to the operators manual for special procedures or precautions.

†1. INSPECT ANESTHESIA MACHINE FOR:
machine identification number
valid inspection sticker
undamaged flowmeters, vaporizers, gauges, supply hoses
complete, undamaged breathing system with adequate CO_2 absorbent
correct mounting of cylinders in yokes
presence of cylinder wrench

†2. INSPECT AND TURN ON:
electrical equipment requiring warm-up. (ECG/pressure monitor, oxygen monitor, etc.)

†3. CONNECT WASTE GAS SCAVENGING SYSTEM:
adjust vacuum as required

†4. CHECK THAT:
flow-control valves are off
vaporizers are off
vaporizers are filled (not overfilled)
filler caps are sealed tightly
CO_2 absorber by-pass (if any) is off

†5. CHECK OXYGEN (O_2) CYLINDER SUPPLIES:
a. Disconnect pipeline supply (if connected) and return cylinder and pipeline pressure gauges to zero with O_2 flush valve.
b. Open O_2 cylinder; check pressure; close cylinder and observe gauge for evidence of high pressure leak.
c. With the O_2 flush valve, flush to empty piping.
d. Repeat as in b. and c. above for second O_2 cylinder, if present.
e. Replace any cylinder less than about 600 psig. At least one should be nearly full.
f. Open less full cylinder.

†6. TURN ON MASTER SWITCH (if present)

†7. CHECK NITROUS OXIDE (N_2O) AND OTHER GAS CYLINDER SUPPLIES:
Use same procedure as described in 5a. & b. above, but open and *CLOSE* flow-control valve to empty piping.
Note: N_2O pressure below 745 psig. indicates that the cylinder is less than 1/4 full.

†8. TEST FLOWMETERS:
a. Check that float is at bottom of tube with flow-control valves closed (or at min. O_2 flow if so equipped).
b. Adjust flow of all gases through their full range and check for erratic movements of floats.

†9. TEST RATIO PROTECTION/WARNING SYSTEM (if present):
Attempt to create hypoxic O_2/N_2O mixture, and verify correct change in gas flows and/or alarm.

†10. TEST O_2 PRESSURE FAILURE SYSTEM:
a. Set O_2 and other gas flows to mid-range.
b. Close O_2 cylinder and flush to release O_2 pressure.
c. Verify that all flows fall to zero. Open O_2 cylinder.
d. Close all other cylinders and bleed piping pressures.
e. Close O_2 cylinder and bleed piping pressure.
f. CLOSE FLOW-CONTROL VALVES.

†11. TEST CENTRAL PIPELINE GAS SUPPLIES:
a. Inspect supply hoses (should not be cracked or worn).
b. Connect supply hoses, verifying correct color coding.
c. Adjust all flows to at least mid-range.
d. Verify that supply pressures hold (45-55 psig.).
e. Shut off flow-control valves.

†12. ADD ANY ACCESSORY EQUIPMENT TO THE BREATHING SYSTEM:
Add PEEP valve, humidifier, etc., if they might be used (if necessary remove after step 18 until needed).

13. CALIBRATE O_2 MONITOR:
†a. Calibrate O_2 monitor to read 21% in room air.
†b. Test low alarm.
c. Occlude breathing system at patient end; fill and empty system several times with 100% O_2.
d. Check that monitor reading is nearly 100%.

14. SNIFF INSPIRATORY GAS:
There should be no odor.

†15. CHECK UNDIRECTIONAL VALVES:
a. Inhale and exhale through a surgical mask into the breathing system (each limb individually, if possible).
b. Verify unidirectional flow in each limb.
c. Reconnect tubing firmly.

‡16. TEST FOR LEAKS IN MACHINE AND BREATHING SYSTEM:
a. Close APL (pop-off) valve and occlude system at patient end.
b. Fill system via O_2 flush until bag just full, but negligible pressure in system. Set O_2 flow to 5 L/min.
c. Slowly decrease O_2 flow until pressure *no longer rises* above about 20 cm H_2O. This approximates total leak rate, which should be no greater than a few hundred ml/min. (less for closed circuit techniques).
CAUTION: Check valves in some machines make it imperative to measure flow in step c. above when pressure *just stops rising*.
d. Squeeze bag to pressure of about 50 cm H_2O and verify that system is tight.

17. EXHAUST VALVE AND SCAVENGER SYSTEM:
a. Open APL valve and observe release of pressure.
b. Occlude breathing system at patient end and verify that negligible positive or negative pressure appears with either zero or 5 L/min. flow and exhaust relief valve (if present) opens with flush flow.

18. TEST VENTILATOR:
a. If switching valve is present, test function in both bag and ventilator mode.
b. Close APL valve if necessary and occlude system at patient end.
c. Test for leaks and pressure relief by appropriate cycling (exact procedure will vary with type of ventilator).
d. Attach reservoir bag at mask fitting, fill system and cycle ventilator. Assure filling/emptying of bag.

19. CHECK FOR APPROPRIATE LEVEL OF PATIENT SUCTION.

20. CHECK, CONNECT, AND CALIBRATE OTHER ELECTRONIC MONITORS.

21. CHECK FINAL POSITION OF ALL CONTROLS.

22. TURN ON AND SET OTHER APPROPRIATE ALARMS FOR EQUIPMENT TO BE USED.
(Perform next two steps as soon as is practical)

23. SET O_2 MONITOR ALARM LIMITS.

24. SET AIRWAY PRESSURE AND/OR VOLUME MONITOR ALARM LIMITS (if adjustable).

---

†If an anesthetist uses the same machine in successive cases, these steps need not be repeated or may be abbreviated after the initial checkout.
‡A vaporizer leak can only be detected if the vaporizer is turned on during this test. Even then, a relatively small but clinically significant leak may still be obscured.

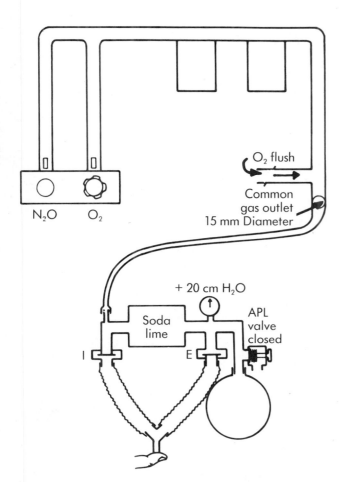

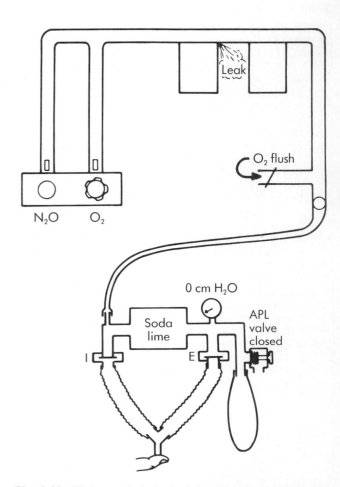

Fig. 2-29. Generic (FDA 1986 checklist item 16) leak test in a machine with no outlet check valve. In this case a pressure of 20 cm of water is sustained, indicating that both the patient circuit and low-pressure parts of the machine are gas-tight. (From Eisenkraft JB: *The anesthesia delivery system, part II.* In *Progress in anesthesiology, vol 3,* Chapter 8, 1989. Reproduced by permission of the Dannemiller Memorial Educational Foundation, San Antonio, Tex.)

Fig. 2-30. FDA generic leak check in a machine with no outlet check valve. A leak at the vaporizer mount results in failure of the system to hold pressure, which in this case has fallen to zero. Such a leak would not be detectable if an outlet check valve were present because pressure applied at the common gas outlet would not be transmitted into the vaporizer manifold. (From Eisenkraft JB: *The anesthesia delivery system, part II.* In *Progress in anesthesiology, vol 3,* Chapter 8, 1989. Reproduced by permission of the Dannemiller Memorial Educational Foundation, San Antonio, Tex.)

high compliance of the distensible reservoir bag, relatively large changes in volume (i.e., leaks) may exist with minimal changes in pressure. The anesthesiologist performing the check is looking for a pressure drop as an indicator of gas leakage; however, relatively large leaks may go undetected by this test.

The second limitation of the FDA 1986 generic checkout is related to the presence or absence of an outlet check valve. Application of the generic leak check in this situation tests only for leaks in components downstream of the outlet check valve (Fig. 2-31). Furthermore, in the past, certain anesthesia delivery systems *configured by the user* placed a free-standing vaporizer in series between the common gas outlet of the machine and the fresh gas inlet of the patient circuit. Some of these free-standing vaporizers incorporated their own outlet check valve (see Chapter 3) to prevent a pumping effect on the vaporizer. If such an

arrangement is being used, the generic leak check will test only up to this check valve in the outlet of the vaporizer. The use of in-series free-standing vaporizers is not described in the F1161-88 standard and should be avoided. Further, because free-standing vaporizers were placed downstream of the machine's common gas outlet, use of the oxygen flush would cause a bolus of potent inhaled agent to be delivered to the patient circuit. Also, the tubing connections can be disrupted by the use of the high pressures associated with use of the oxygen flush. A disconnect between the common gas outlet of the machine and the free-standing vaporizer could also cause a leak and/or a low-concentration oxygen mixture to develop in the patient circuit during controlled ventilation, hence the current requirement for a retaining device.[1] In addition,

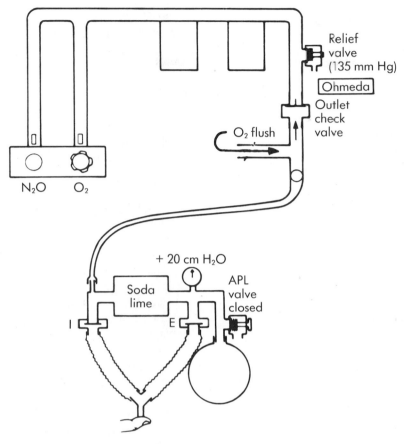

Fig. 2-31. Application of FDA generic leak check to a system with an outlet check valve. In this case application of a positive back pressure of 20 cm of water causes the check valve to close, so that only those components downstream of the valve are being leak-tested. (From Eisenkraft JB: *The anesthesia delivery system, part II.* In *Progress in anesthesiology, vol 3,* Chapter 8, 1989. Reproduced by permission of the Dannemiller Memorial Educational Foundation, San Antonio, Tex.)

any vaporizer exclusion system (interlock) would be compromised with a free-standing arrangement. Again, it is emphasized that *the use of free-standing vaporizers is not recommended and may be hazardous.* (See Chapter 16.)

The limitations of the FDA generic leak check make it obvious that specialized leak checks of the low-pressure system must be utilized; the machine operator's manual should be consulted for details. Those tests described for the Dräger Narkomed and Ohmeda machines are briefly reviewed in the following sections to illustrate the differences in system design, function, and checkout.

Dräger Narkomed Machines: No Outlet Check Valve

North American Dräger recommends the following test procedure for checking the anesthesia breathing system and fresh gas delivery system.[13] In this test, all gas flow control (flowmeter) valves are closed and the machine system main power switch is turned to STANDBY or OFF. In this position no gas should flow to the flowmeters or from the common gas outlet. All vaporizer concentration dials

are set to ZERO concentration. The inspiratory and expiratory valves are short-circuited with 22-mm-diameter circuit hose (Fig. 2-32). The shortest possible length of hose should be used to minimize contained gas volume. The MANUAL/AUTOMATIC selector valve is set to the MANUAL (Bag) position. The APL ("pop-off") valve is closed (turned fully clockwise). The reservoir bag is removed and the test terminal is attached to the bag mount (see Fig. 2-32). A sphygmomanometer squeeze bulb is connected to the hose barb on the test terminal. It is now apparent that the total volume of the circuit components has been drastically reduced by the removal of the circle system tubing [a circle with each limb 152 cm (5 feet) in length has a volume of about 1200 ml] and the reservoir bag (3 L). The sphygmomanometer bulb is squeezed by hand until the pressure shown at the breathing system pressure gauge indicates a pressure higher than 50 cm H_2O. The gauge is then observed for a pressure drop. The manufacturer's specification demands that 30 seconds or longer shall be required for a pressure decrease from 50 to 30 cm

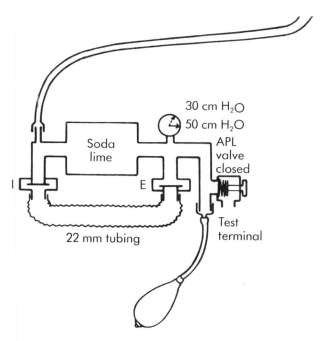

Fig. 2-32. Dräger Narkomed positive pressure leak check. Thirty seconds or longer should be required for a pressure decrease from 50 to 30 cm of water. (From Eisenkraft JB: *The anesthesia delivery system, part II.* In *Progress in anesthesiology, vol 3,* Chapter 8, 1989. Reproduced by permission of the Dannemiller Memorial Educational Foundation, San Antonio, Tex.)

H_2O.[14] Because the volume of gas being compressed in this test is minimal, small gas leaks will result in a decrease in pressure that is observable on the circuit pressure gauge.

The *positive pressure leak check* should be repeated sequentially with each vaporizer turned ON and set at any concentration above 0.4%. This checks for leaks in individual vaporizers (e.g., filler caps, selector switches, vaporizer mounts).[13]

It should be noted that the test specifications given in this section apply to an anesthesia breathing system without accessories (e.g., volumeter, sidestream gas analyzer, and other adapters).[6,13] Test limits will be exceeded when accessory items are included in the test (the supplier of the accessory items should be contacted for leak specifications).

Leaks in the patient circuit components can be distinguished from leaks in the low-pressure part of the Narkomed machine (no outlet check valve) as follows. If a leak has been identified with the combined circuit-machine positive-pressure leak check as described above, the sphygmomanometer bulb can be connected to the machine's common gas outlet with a 15-mm (endotracheal tube) connector and to a pressure gauge with a three-way stopcock. With this arrangement only the machine (as opposed to machine and circuit in the previous test) is pressurized to 50 cm H_2O, and a decrease in pressure indicates a leak within the machine upstream of the common gas outlet.

This test is possible because no outlet check valve is present in Dräger Narkomed machines.

Ohmeda Machines With Outlet Check Valve Present

In certain of the Ohmeda machines, the presence of an outlet check valve complicates positive-pressure testing of the machine's low-pressure system (Fig. 2-31). Application of positive pressure downstream of the valve causes it to close, and only components downstream of this valve (i.e., downstream of the common gas outlet) are checked for leaks. Positive-pressure ventilation and opening of the oxygen flush valve cause the check valve to close (see Figs. 2-3 and 2-27). For this reason, Ohmeda describes a *negative pressure leak test* performed with a special suction bulb device, which is supplied with each machine to which this test applies (Fig. 2-33).[8,15]

First, the adequacy of the leak testing device should be checked by sealing the inlet connector of the bulb and squeezing the bulb until it is collapsed. The bulb is then released and the time taken to reinflate is observed. If reinflation occurs in less than 60 seconds, the device should be replaced.[8,15] The device is checked periodically (at times of machine servicing) to ensure that the vacuum produced by the evacuated bulb is at least negative 65 mmHg (Fig. 2-33).

The device is then used to check the machine as follows.[8,15] First, the anesthesia machine's system master switch and all vaporizers are turned OFF so that no gases are flowing in the low-pressure parts of the machine. Each gas supply is then opened by turning on the back-up cylinder valves or by connecting the pipeline supply. The flow control valves (rotameters) are turned fully OPEN. Thus, with the master switch turned off and the flowmeters open, no gas is flowing, but the entire system is accessible for testing. The negative-pressure leak-testing bulb is attached to the machine's common gas outlet via a 15-mm connector. The hand bulb is repeatedly squeezed and released until it remains collapsed. If the bulb reinflates within 30 seconds (Fig. 2-34), a leak of as little as 30 ml/min is present. The test procedure is repeated with each vaporizer turned to the ON position to look for leaks in the individual vaporizers. If the source is not easily correctable, the machine should be withdrawn from service. When the leak tests are completed, the negative-pressure bulb is removed from the common gas outlet. Because the leak check described is conducted with all of the flow control valves open, components up to and including the machine's main ON/OFF control switch are also tested for leaks.

The negative leak check described for Ohmeda machines results in the outlet check valve being held open by the −65 mmHg vacuum (Figs. 2-33 and 2-34) and air or gas being sucked into the system through any leaks. If such leaks were present while the machine was in service, anesthesia gases would escape from the system. If, following testing, the anesthesia machine is found to have a leak,

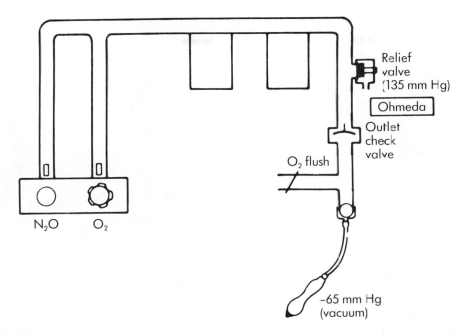

Fig. 2-33. Ohmeda negative pressure leak check. (From Eisenkraft JB: *The anesthesia delivery system, part II*. In *Progress in anesthesiology, vol 3*, Chapter 8, 1989. Reproduced by permission of the Dannemiller Memorial Educational Foundation, San Antonio, Tex.)

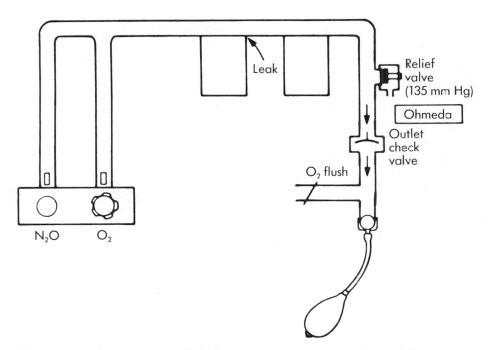

Fig. 2-34. Ohmeda negative pressure leak check. In the presence of a leak into the machine, the evacuated bulb reinflates. (From Eisenkraft JB: *The anesthesia delivery system, part II*. In *Progress in anesthesiology, vol 3*, Chapter 8, 1989. Reproduced by permission of the Dannemiller Memorial Educational Foundation, San Antonio, Tex.)

it should be withdrawn from use until an authorized agent has repaired the leak, rechecked the system, and certified that it is fit to be put back into clinical service.

Ohmeda machines without outlet check valve present

Ohmeda Modulus II Plus and Modulus CD have no outlet check valve. Although the most recently introduced Ohmeda models (Modulus II Plus, Modulus CD) *do not* have an outlet check valve, Ohmeda recommends use of the *negative* leak-test procedure as described above to check for leaks in these models.[7,20] Indeed, the negative-pressure leak-check device could, in principle, be used to check for leaks in a Dräger Narkomed machine, but North American Dräger has not (to date) provided specifications for the application of such a leak-check device on their products (see also Chapter 22 and Table 22-3).

ELECTRICAL SYSTEM

Contemporary anesthesia machines, although basically pneumatic, also incorporate electrical systems. Recent Dräger and Ohmeda machines require connection to an electrical power supply. Turning the main switch on (Fig. 2-35) energizes the electrical systems of the machine and mechanically opens the flow of gases to the flowmeters (provided gas supply pressure is adequate) so that the machine is capable of delivering an anesthetic. The electrical system powers the alarms and monitors on the machine as well as the ventilator control system. If the machine's electrical system were to fail completely, the flow of gases to the flowmeters continues uninterrupted as long as the machine's main on/off switch is turned on. In the event that the AC power supply to the machine fails, a 12-V battery back-up system provides power to the machine's monitors, alarms, and ventilator controls. When fully charged, the battery supply provides power for 30 to 45 minutes in most machines. Full charge of the battery, however, depends on keeping the machine's AC power cord plugged into an energized electrical receptacle. A battery test indicator is provided on the machine to check for the status of the reserve power battery (Fig. 2-35). Contemporary anesthesia machines are frequently equipped with a number of convenience receptacles or outlets to provide AC power to other monitors (e.g., blood pressure, pulse oximeter). These receptacles are energized via the machine's main AC power cord.

The presence of several electrical systems on the machine necessitates that each circuit be protected from overload. This is achieved by using circuit breakers, which vary in number according to the number of circuits present (Fig. 2-36). In principle, however, one circuit breaker protects the machine's main AC power supply, one (or more) protect(s) the convenience receptacles, and one (or more) protect(s) the low-voltage (12-V) DC circuits. It is not uncommon for circuit breakers on the machine to be tripped.

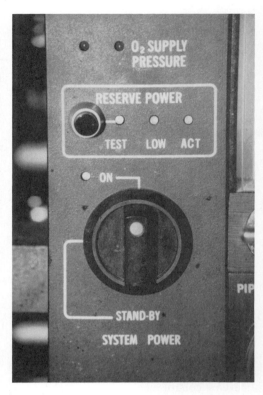

Fig. 2-35. System power switch on Dräger Narkomed machine. Note reserve power (battery) test button and low power indicator warning lights.

Commonly this is due to overloading a convenience receptacle, for example, by connecting an OR table's power cord to it. In this case other convenience receptacles on the same circuit will have their power interrupted. The anesthesiologist should be familiar with the power supply capabilities of the receptacles and the power demands of any equipment connected to them as well as with the location (not always obvious) and function of the circuit breakers on the machine. The manufacturer's operator's manual should be consulted for details on specific models.

ANESTHESIA MACHINE STANDARD (ASTM F1161-88)

The most recent anesthesia machine standard is the ASTM F1161-88.[1] Contemporary North American Dräger and Ohmeda machines far exceed this standard, and both companies offer an evaluation program that advises users on upgrading or replacing older equipment that may no longer be considered acceptable.

Important aspects of the recent F1161-88 standard are listed below. The reader is encouraged to review the original document for further details.

Flow control (section 9.1)

Only one flow adjustment control for each gas delivered to the common gas outlet shall be provided. Thus, banks of flowmeters in parallel with separate high- and low-flow

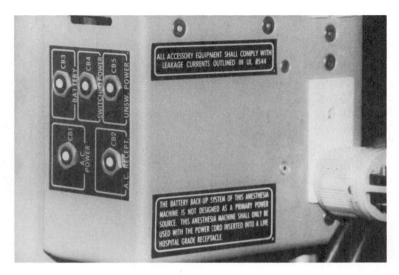

Fig. 2-36. Convenience receptacles (AC power outlets) and circuit breakers on Dräger Narkomed 2A machine. The location of the receptacles and circuit breakers varies among the various models of anesthesia machines.

controls for the same gas are now considered obsolete and may be dangerous. Some new anesthesia machines include a separate flow control and nipple for oxygen (for Monitored Anesthesia Care [MAC] cases). This does not violate the standard since this oxygen is not being delivered to the common gas outlet.

Concentration-calibrated vaporizers (section 12.1)

All vaporizers located within the fresh gas circuit shall be concentration calibrated. Control of the vapor concentration shall be provided by means of calibrated knobs or dials (12.1.1). Measured flow vaporizers (Copper Kettle, Verni-Trol) are not mentioned and therefore are no longer to be considered contemporary.

Common gas outlet (section 13.1.1)

When the common gas outlet is connected to the breathing system by a fresh gas supply hose, the common gas outlet shall be provided with a retaining device. The outlet should have a manufacturer-specific fitting.

Alarms (section 16)

Alarm characteristics of monitors should be categorized as high, medium, or low priority. The alarms should be distinguishable audibly and visually, and the operator response should be immediate (high priority), prompt (medium priority), or an awareness (low priority). Contemporary machines should therefore incorporate an integrated and prioritized alarm system. (See also Chapter 17.)

Oxygen supply precautions (section 17)

The machine shall be designed so that whenever the oxygen supply pressure is reduced from normal (manufacturer-specified) and until flow ceases, the set oxygen *concen-*

tration shall not decrease at the common gas outlet. The anesthesia circuit's oxygen concentration shall be measured and the analyzer will annunciate a high priority alarm when the concentration falls below the preset threshold. The contemporary machine is designed so that the oxygen analyzer is enabled and functioning any time the machine is capable of delivering an anesthetic mixture.

Ventilatory monitoring (section 18)

The anesthesia machine shall have breathing pressure monitoring as well as either exhaled volume or ventilatory carbon dioxide monitoring. The alarms associated with these monitors are to be enabled and functioning automatically whenever the machine is in use.

REFERENCES

1. Standard specification for minimum performance and safety requirements for components and systems of anesthesia gas machines, F1161-88, Philadelphia, Pa, March 1989, American Society for Testing and Materials.
2. Minimum performance and safety requirements for components and systems of continuous flow anesthesia machines for human use, ANSI Z79.8.-1979, New York, 1979, American National Standards Institute.
3. Diameter-index safety system, CGA V-5, New York, 1978, Compressed Gas Association.
4. Compressed gas cylinder valve outlet and inlet connections, pamphlet V-1, New York, 1977, Compressed Gas Association.
5. Parbrook GD, Davis PD, Parbrook EO: *Basic physics and measurement in anesthesia,* ed 2, Norwalk, Conn, 1986, Appleton-Century-Crofts.
6. Narkomed 3 anesthesia system technical service manual, Telford, Pa, 1988, North American Dräger.
7. Modulus II Plus anesthesia machine: preoperative checklists; operation and maintenance manual. Madison, Wis, October 1988, Ohmeda.

8. Modulus II anesthesia system: operation and maintenance manual. Madison, Wis, August 1987, Ohmeda.

9. Bowie E, Huffman LM: *The anesthesia machine: essentials for understanding*, Madison, Wis, 1985, Ohmeda, The BOC Group.

10. Raessler KL, Kretzman WE, Gravenstein N: O_2 consumption by anesthesia ventilators, *Anesthesiology* 69(3A):271, 1988.

11. Eger EI II, Hylton RR, Irwin RH et al: Anesthetic flow meter sequence—a cause for hypoxia, *Anesthesiology* 24:396, 1963.

12. Dorsch JA, Dorsch SE: *Understanding anesthesia equipment,* ed 2, Baltimore, Md, 1984, Williams & Wilkins.

13. Narkomed 3 anesthesia system: operator's instruction manual, Telford, Pa, 1986, North American Dräger.

14. Schreiber P: Safety guidelines for anesthesia systems, Telford, Pa, 1985, North American Dräger.

15. Modulus II system service manual, Madison, Wis, May 1985, Ohmeda.

16. Benumof JL, Scheller MS: The importance of transtracheal jet ventilation in the management of the difficult airway, *Anesthesiology* 71:769-778, 1989.

17. Delaney WA, Kaiser R: Percutaneous transtracheal jet ventilation made easy, *Anesthesiology* 74:952, 1991.

18. Gaughan S, Benumof JL, Ozaki G: Can an anesthesia machine flush valve provide for effective jet ventilation? *Anesthesiology* 75:3A, A130, 1991 (abstract).

19. Anesthesia apparatus checkout recommendations, Rockville, Md, 1986, Food and Drug Administration.

20. Modulus CD anesthesia system: operation and maintenance manual, Madison, Wis, 1991, Ohmeda.

Chapter 3

ANESTHESIA VAPORIZERS

James B. Eisenkraft, M.D.

GENERAL PRINCIPLES

Vapor is the gaseous phase of a substance that is a liquid at room temperature and atmospheric pressure.[1] Anesthesia vaporizers are devices that facilitate the change of a liquid anesthetic into its vapor phase and add a controlled amount of this vapor to the flow of gases passing to the patient circuit.

The anesthesiologist should be familiar with the principles of vaporization of potent inhaled agents as well as their application in both the construction and use of anesthesia vaporizers designed to be placed in the fresh gas circuit. The most recent (1989) voluntary consensus standard for anesthesia machines (ASTM F1161-88) requires that all vaporizers located within the fresh gas circuit be concentration-calibrated and that control of the vapor concentration be provided by means of calibrated knobs or dials.[2] The measured flow systems (Copper Kettle, Verni-Trol), not mentioned in the Standard,[2] are therefore now considered by most to be obsolete, although military field anesthesia machines still use such systems (see Chapter 29 and Fig. 29-1). The principles of measured flow systems are discussed in this chapter, because they form a basis for understanding the contemporary concentration-calibrated variable bypass vaporizers for isoflurane, enflurane, and halothane.

At this time, two new potent inhaled agents are undergoing clinical investigation in the United States. These agents are sevoflurane* and desflurane.† The physical properties of sevoflurane with regard to vaporization are similar to those of enflurane. The principles of operation of the sevoflurane concentration-calibrated vaporizer are therefore identical to those of the enflurane vaporizer. On the other hand, desflurane has certain physical properties that make it much more volatile and preclude its administration by way of conventional concentration-calibrated variable bypass vaporizer technology. The special consid-

---

*Maruishi Pharmaceutical Co Ltd, Osaka, Japan.
†Anaquest, Inc, Liberty Corner, NJ.

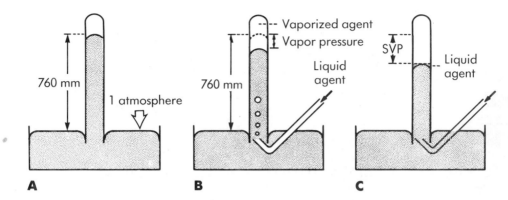

Fig. 3-1. Measurement of vapor pressures using a simple Fortin barometer. (From Eisenkraft JB: *Vaporizers and vaporization of volatile anesthetics.* In *Progress in anesthesiology, vol 2,* San Antonio, Tex, 1989, Dannemiller Memorial Educational Foundation. Reproduced by permission.)

erations for vaporizing desflurane are therefore discussed in a separate section at the end of this chapter.

VAPOR, EVAPORATION, AND VAPOR PRESSURE

When placed in a closed container at atmospheric pressure (760 mmHg) and room temperature (20° C), a potent inhaled anesthetic such as halothane is in liquid form. Some halothane molecules escape from the surface of the liquid to enter the space above as a vapor. At constant temperature, an equilibrium is established between the molecules in the vapor phase and those in the liquid phase. The molecules in the vapor phase are in constant motion, striking the walls of the container to exert a *vapor pressure*. An increase in temperature causes more molecules to enter the vapor phase (evaporate), resulting in an increase in vapor pressure. The gas phase above the liquid is said to be saturated when it contains all the halothane vapor that it can hold at a given temperature. The pressure from this halothane vapor is referred to as its *saturated vapor pressure* (SVP) at that temperature.

Measurement of vapor pressure

The following description is intended to provide an understanding of how, in principle, SVP could be measured in a simple laboratory experiment. Figure 3-1, *A* shows a Fortin barometer, which is essentially a long test tube filled with mercury and inverted into a trough containing mercury. When the barometer tube is vertical, the mercury in the tube falls to a certain level, leaving a vacuum above the mercury meniscus. In this system, the pressure at the surface of the mercury in the trough is atmospheric. Because pressures at a given depth in a communicating system of liquids are equal, the pressure at the surface of the mercury in the trough is equal to the pressure exerted by the column of mercury. In this example, atmospheric pressure is said to be equivalent to 760 mm Hg because this is the height of the column of mercury in the tube.

In Fig. 3-1, *B* halothane liquid is introduced at the bottom of the mercury column from whence it floats to the top and then evaporates in the vacuum. The halothane vapor exerts a pressure, causing a fall in the mercury column by an amount equivalent to the vapor pressure exerted. If liquid halothane is added until a small amount remains unevaporated on the top of the mercury column (Fig. 3-1, *C*), the space above the column must be fully saturated with vapor, and the pressure now exerted by the vapor is the SVP at that temperature. Additional liquid halothane will not affect the vapor pressure. If this experiment is repeated at different temperatures, a graph can be constructed that plots saturated vapor pressure against temperature. Such curves for some of the volatile anesthetic agents are shown in Fig. 3-2. More modern and sophisticated technologies for measuring the partial pressure or SVP of gases and vapors are described in Chapter 8.

Boiling point

The saturated pressure exerted by the vapor phase of a potent volatile agent depends only on the volatile agent and the ambient temperature. The temperature at which vapor pressure becomes equal to ambient (atmospheric) pressure and at which all of the liquid agent changes to the vapor phase is the liquid's *boiling point*. The most volatile agents are those with the highest SVPs. Therefore, at any given temperature these agents also have the lowest boiling points (e.g., desflurane and diethyl ether boil at 23.5° C and 35° C, respectively, at an ambient pressure of 760 mm Hg). Boiling point decreases with falling ambient barometric pressure, such as occurs at high altitude.

Units of vapor concentration

The presence of anesthetic vapor may be quantified either (1) as an absolute pressure, expressed in mm Hg, or (2) in volumes percent (i.e., volumes of vapor per 100 volumes of total gas). From Dalton's law (see the following section), volumes percent can be calculated as the frac-

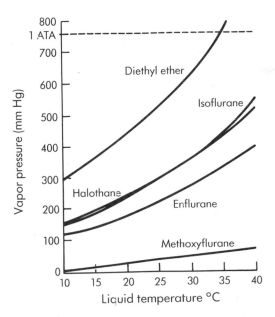

Fig. 3-2. Vapor pressure curves for diethyl ether, isoflurane, halothane, enflurane, and methoxyflurane. (From Eisenkraft JB: *Vaporizers and vaporization of volatile anesthetics.* In *Progress in anesthesiology, vol 2,* San Antonio, Tex, 1989, Dannemiller Memorial Educational Foundation. Reproduced by permission.)

Table 3-1. Expression of MAC (vol %) of agent in oxygen as a partial pressure (mm Hg) (assuming an ambient pressure of 760 mm Hg)

Agent	MAC (vol %)		P_{MAC1} (mm Hg)
Halothane	0.75×760	=	5.7
Enflurane	1.68×760	=	12.8
Isoflurane	1.15×760	=	8.7
Methoxyflurane	0.16×760	=	1.2
Sevoflurane*	1.7×760	=	12.9
Desflurane†	6.0×760	=	45.6
Desflurane†	7.25×760	=	55.1

*From Katoh T, Ikeda K: *Anesthesiology* 66:301, 1987.
†From Rampil IJ, et al: MAC is age-related. Ages: 18-30 yr, 7.25%; 31-65, 6.0%. *Anesthesiology* 74:429, 1991.

tional partial pressure of the agent, that is, (partial pressure due to vapor/total ambient pressure) × 100%.

Dalton's law of partial pressures

Dalton's law states that the pressure exerted by a mixture of gases (or gases and vapors) enclosed in a given space is equal to the sum of the pressures that each gas or vapor would exert if it alone occupied the container.[3] A gas or vapor exerts its pressure independently of the pressure of the other gases present. For example, in a container of dry air at atmospheric pressure (760 mm Hg) with oxygen representing 21% of all gases present, the pressure exerted by the oxygen (its partial pressure) is 21% × 760, or 159.6 mm Hg. Consider now the same air at a pressure of 760 mm Hg and fully saturated with water vapor at 37° C (normal body temperature). Because vapor pressure depends on temperature, the SVP for water at 37° C is 47 mm Hg. The pressure due to oxygen is now 21% of 713 (i.e., 760 − 47) mm Hg. The partial pressure of oxygen is therefore 149.7 mm Hg.

It should be noted that volumes percent expresses the relative ratio or proportion (%) of gas molecules in a mixture, and partial pressure (mm Hg) represents an absolute value. Anesthetic uptake and potency are related directly to partial pressure and only indirectly to volumes percent. This distinction will become more apparent when hyperbaric and hypobaric conditions are considered.

Minimum alveolar concentration

The minimum alveolar concentration (MAC) of a potent inhaled anesthetic agent is the concentration that produces immobility in 50% of patients undergoing a standard surgical incision. Used as a measure of anesthetic potency or depth, MAC is commonly expressed as volumes percent of alveolar (end-tidal) gas at one atmosphere pressure at sea level (i.e., 760 mm Hg). Table 3-1 shows how MAC expressed in familiar volumes percent can be expressed as a partial pressure in mm Hg. Anesthesiologists should learn to think of MAC in terms of partial pressure rather than in terms of volumes percent because it is the partial pressure (tension) of the anesthetic in the brain which is responsible for the depth of anesthesia. This concept has been advocated by Fink,[4] who suggested the term *minimum alveolar pressure (MAP),* and James and White,[5] who suggested *minimum alveolar partial pressure (MAPP).* In this chapter the term P_{MAC1} (Table 3-1) is used to express the partial pressure of a potent inhaled agent at a concentration of 1 MAC. Thus 1 MAC halothane is equivalent to a P_{MAC1} of 5.7 mm Hg (see Table 3-1).

Latent heat of vaporization

Vaporization requires energy to transform molecules from the liquid phase to the vapor phase. This energy, called the latent heat of vaporization, is defined as the amount of heat (calories) required to convert a unit mass (grams) of liquid into vapor.[3] The latent heats of vaporization at 20° C of halothane, enflurane and isoflurane are 35, 42 and 41 cal/g, respectively. The heat of vaporization is inversely related to ambient temperature in such a way that at lower temperatures, more heat is required for vaporization. Heat required to vaporize anesthetic agents is drawn from the remaining liquid and the surroundings. As vapor is generated and heat energy is lost, the temperatures of the vaporizer and the liquid fall. This causes the vapor pressure of the anesthetic to fall and results in decreased

Table 3-2. Physical properties of potent inhaled volatile agents

Agent	Halothane	Enflurane	Isoflurane	Methoxyflurane	Sevoflurane	Desflurane
Structure	$CHBrClCF_3$	$CHFClCF_2OCHF_2$	$CF_2HOCHClCF_3$	$CHCl_2CF_2OCH_3$	$CH_2FOCH(CF_3)_2$	$CF_2HOCFHCF_3$
Molecular wt.	197.4	184.5	184.5	165.0	200	168
Boiling point at 760 mm Hg (° C)	50.2	56.5	48.5	104.7	58.5	23.5
SVP at 20° C (mm Hg)	243	175	238	20.3	160	664
SV Concn. at 20° C and 1 ATA† (vol %)	32	23	31	2.7	21	87
MAC at 1 ATA† (vol %)	0.75	1.68	1.15	0.16	1.7	6-7.25*
P_{MAC1} (mm Hg)	5.7	12.8	8.7	1.22	12.9	46-55*
Specific gravity of liquid at 20° C	1.86	1.52	1.50	1.41	1.51	1.45
ml vapor per g liquid at 20° C	123	130	130	145	120	143
ml vapor per ml liquid at 20° C	226	196	195	204	182	207

*Age-related.

†1 ATA = one atmosphere absolute pressure (760 mm Hg)

vaporizer output if no compensatory mechanism is provided. These compensatory mechanisms are described in a later section.

Specific heat

Specific heat is the quantity of heat (calories) required to raise the temperature of a unit mass (grams) of a substance by one degree of temperature (1° C).[3] Heat must be supplied to the liquid anesthetic in the vaporizer to maintain the liquid's temperature during the evaporation process, when heat is being lost.

Specific heat is also important when it comes to vaporizer construction material. Thus temperature changes are more gradual for materials with a high specific heat than for those with a low specific heat, for the same amount of heat lost through vaporization. Thermal capacity, defined as the product of specific heat and mass, represents the amount of heat stored in the vaporizer body.[3]

Also of importance is the construction material's ability to conduct heat from the environment to the liquid anesthetic. This ability, called thermal conductivity, is defined as the rate at which heat is transmitted through a substance. In order for the liquid anesthetic to remain at a relatively constant temperature, the vaporizer should be constructed from materials with a high specific heat and high thermal conductivity. In this respect, copper comes close to the ideal—hence the Copper Kettle vaporizer. More recently, bronze and stainless steel have been used in vaporizer construction.

REGULATING VAPORIZER OUTPUT: VARIABLE BYPASS VERSUS MEASURED FLOW

The saturated vapor pressures of halothane, enflurane, and isoflurane at room temperature are 243 mm Hg, 175 mm Hg, and 241 mm Hg, respectively. Dividing the SVP by ambient pressure (760 mm Hg) gives the saturated vapor concentration as a percentage of one atmosphere. This is an application of Dalton's law (discussed earlier). The saturated vapor concentrations of halothane, enflurane, and isoflurane are therefore 32%, 23%, and 31%, respectively; these concentrations are far in excess of those required clinically (Fig. 3-2; Table 3-2). Thus first the vaporizer creates a saturated vapor in equilibrium with the liquid agent, and second the vapor is diluted by a bypass gas flow. This results in clinically safe and useful concentrations. If this were not done, the agent could be delivered in a lethal concentration to the anesthesia circuit.

Contemporary anesthesia vaporizers are concentration-calibrated and of the variable bypass design.[2] In a variable bypass vaporizer (e.g., Tec series from Ohmeda, Dräger Vapor 19.1) the total fresh gas flow from the anesthesia machine flowmeters passes to the vaporizer (Fig. 3-3). The vaporizer splits the incoming gas flow between two pathways. The smaller flow enters the vaporizing chamber of the vaporizer and emerges with the anesthetic agent at its saturated vapor concentration. The larger bypass flow is eventually mixed with the vaporizing chamber's output and results in the desired or "dialed-in" concentration (Fig. 3-3).

In the *measured flow* (non–concentration-calibrated) vaporizers (e.g., Copper Kettle* or Verni-Trol†), a measured flow of oxygen is selected on a separate flowmeter to pass to the vaporizer, from which vapor emerges at its SVP (Fig. 3-4). This flow is then diluted by an additional measured flow of gases (i.e., oxygen, nitrous oxide, air, etc.) from other flowmeters on the anesthesia machine (Fig. 3-4). With this type of arrangement, calculations are

*Foregger/Puritan-Bennett.

†Ohio Medical Products (now Ohmeda), Madison, Wis.

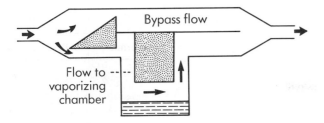

Fig. 3-3. Schematic of concentration-calibrated variable bypass design of vaporizer. (From Eisenkraft JB: *Vaporizers and vaporization of volatile anesthetics.* In *Progress in anesthesiology, vol 2,* San Antonio, Tex, 1989, Dannemiller Memorial Educational Foundation. Reproduced by permission.)

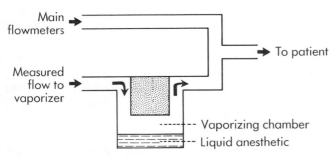

Fig. 3-4. Schematic of measured flow vaporizing arrangement. These are "bubble-through" vaporizers. (From Eisenkraft JB: *Vaporizers and vaporization of volatile anesthetics.* In *Progress in anesthesiology, vol 2,* San Antonio, Tex, 1989, Dannemiller Memorial Educational Foundation. Reproduced by permission.)

necessary to determine the anesthetic vapor concentration in the emerging gas mixture.

With either type of vaporizing system, there must be an efficient method to create a saturated vapor in the vaporizing chamber. This is achieved by having a large surface area for evaporation. Flow-over vaporizers (e.g., Drägerwerk Vapor 19.1 and Ohmeda Tec series vaporizers) increase the surface area using wicks and baffles. In bubble-through vaporizers (e.g., Copper Kettle and Verni-Trol), oxygen is bubbled through the liquid agent. In order to increase the surface area tiny bubbles are created by passing the oxygen through a sintered bronze disc (in the Copper Kettle) that creates large areas of liquid-gas interface over which evaporation of the agent can occur quickly.

Calculation of vaporizer output

At a constant room temperature of 20° C, the saturated vapor pressures of the commonly used potent inhaled agents are (1) halothane, 243 mm Hg; (2) enflurane, 175 mm Hg; and (3) isoflurane, 238 mm Hg, (Table 3-2). If ambient pressure is 760 mm Hg, then these SVPs represent (243/760) = 32% halothane, (175/760) = 23% enflurane, and (239/760) = 31% isoflurane, each in terms of volumes percent of one atmosphere (760 mm Hg).

A concept fundamental to understanding vaporizer function is that under steady state conditions, if a certain volume of *carrier gas* flows from the machine into a va-

porizing chamber over a certain period of time, that same volume of carrier gas exits the chamber over the same period of time. However, due to the addition of vaporized anesthetic agent, the total volume exiting the chamber is greater than that entering. In the vaporizing chamber, anesthetic vapor at its SVP constitutes a mandatory fractional volume of the atmosphere (i.e., 32% in a halothane vaporizer at 20° C and 760 mm Hg ambient pressure). Therefore, the volume of carrier gas constitutes the difference between 100% of the atmosphere in the vaporizing chamber and that due to the anesthetic vapor. In the case of halothane (20° C and 760 mm Hg pressure) the carrier gas represents, at any time, 68% of the atmosphere in the vaporizing chamber. Thus if 100 ml of carrier gas flows per minute through a vaporizing chamber containing halothane, carrier gas represents 68% (100 − 32%) of the atmosphere, and the remaining 32% is halothane vapor. By simple proportions, the volume of halothane vapor can be calculated to be 47 ml ([100/68] × 32). In other words, if 100 ml of carrier gas flows into the vaporizing chamber per minute, the same 100 ml of carrier gas will emerge together with 47 ml of halothane vapor per minute. Another way of expressing this is

$$\frac{\text{SVP agent (mm Hg)}}{\text{Total pressure (mm Hg)}}$$

$$= \frac{\text{Agent vapor (x ml)}}{\text{Carrier gas (y ml) + Agent vapor (x ml)}}$$

$$= \frac{\text{Volume of agent vapor}}{\text{Total volume leaving vaporizer}}$$

For halothane in the above example, $y = 100$ ml/min; therefore,

$$\frac{243}{760} = \frac{x}{100 + x}$$

from which x can be calculated to be 47 ml.

Conversely, if x is known, the carrier gas flow y can be calculated. Thus at steady state the total volume of gas leaving the vaporizing chamber is larger than the total volume that entered, the additional volume being anesthetic vapor at its saturated vapor concentration.

Measured flow vaporizers (Copper Kettle, Verni-Trol)

Although measured flow vaporizers are not mentioned in the latest anesthesia machine standard, it is helpful to first review the function of, for example, the Copper Kettle. Suppose the anesthesiologist wishes to deliver 1% (vol/vol) halothane to the patient circuit with a total fresh-gas flow rate of 5 L/min (Fig. 3-5). This requires the vaporizer to evolve 50 ml of halothane vapor per minute (1% × 5000 ml).

In the vaporizing chamber, halothane represents 32% of the atmosphere, assuming a constant temperature of 20° C and a constant saturated vapor pressure of 243 mm Hg.

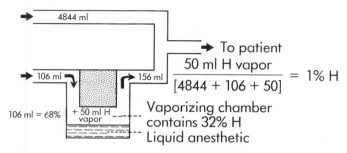

4844 ml

To patient

$$\frac{50 \text{ ml H vapor}}{[4844 + 106 + 50]} = 1\% \text{ H}$$

106 ml → ↙ 156 ml

106 ml = 68%   + 50 ml H vapor

Vaporizing chamber contains 32% H Liquid anesthetic

In practice mainflow is set to 5 L/min, vaporizer flow is set to 100 ml/min and H output is 0.913%, i.e., 47 ml H vapor diluted in [5000 + 100 + 47] ml

Fig. 3-5. Preparation of 1% halothane by volume using a measured flow vaporizing system. (From Eisenkraft JB: *Vaporizers and vaporization of volatile anesthetics.* In *Progress in anesthesiology, vol 2,* San Antonio, Tex, 1989, Dannemiller Memorial Educational Foundation. Reproduced by permission.)

Now if 50 ml of halothane vapor represents 32%, the carrier gas (oxygen) must represent the other 68% (100 − 32%). Thus

$$\frac{50}{32} = \frac{x}{68}$$

$$x = \frac{50}{32} \times 68$$

$$x = 106 \text{ ml}$$

Alternatively,

$$\frac{243}{760} = \frac{50}{y + 50} = 106 \text{ ml}$$

where y = carrier gas (oxygen) flow.

Thus if 106 ml/min of oxygen flows into a Copper Kettle vaporizer, 156 ml/min of gas emerges, of which 50 ml is halothane vapor and 106 ml is the oxygen that flowed into the vaporizer. This vaporizer output of 156 ml/min must be diluted by an additional fresh gas flow of 4844 (5000−156) ml/min to create a halothane mixture of *exactly* 1% (because 50 ml of halothane diluted in a total volume of 5000 ml gives 1% halothane by volume).

In clinical practice, however, the anesthesia provider would likely set flows of 100 ml/min to the Copper Kettle vaporizer and 5 L/min of fresh gas on the main flowmeters, which results in a little less than 1% halothane (actually 47/5147 = 0.91%). Multiples of either of these flows are used to create other concentrations of halothane from a Copper Kettle. Thus a 100-ml/min oxygen flow to the vaporizer and 2500 ml/min on the main flow meters gives approximately 2% halothane (actually 1.78%). It is important to realize that if there is oxygen flow only to the Copper Kettle vaporizer and no bypass gas flow is set on the main flowmeters, lethal concentrations (approaching 32%) of halothane are delivered to the anesthesia circuit, albeit at low flow rates.

Because halothane and isoflurane have similar vapor pressures at 20° C (Table 3-2), the flows described for halothane are essentially the same as those to set for isoflurane when a 1% concentration of isoflurane is to be produced from a Copper Kettle. A Copper Kettle arrangement is shown in Fig. 3-6.

In the case of enflurane (Fig. 3-7), the measured flow vaporizer contains 23% enflurane vapor (175/760 = 23%). The oxygen flow therefore represents the remaining 77% of the vaporizer's atmosphere. If 1% enflurane is required at a 3-L/min rate of flow, 30 ml/min of enflurane vapor

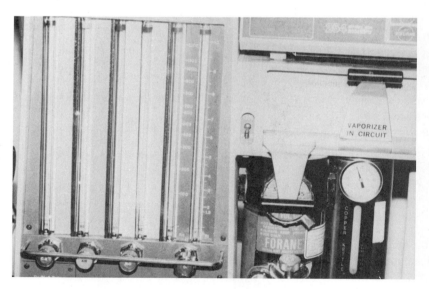

Fig. 3-6. Copper Kettle vaporizing system. Note thermometer and agent level gauge. The oxygen flowmeter knob on the extreme left is marked "C-K" to indicate that it controls oxygen flow to the Copper Kettle. Note also the use of a Puritan Bennett 254 anesthetic agent analyzer to confirm that desired concentrations of agent are being delivered.

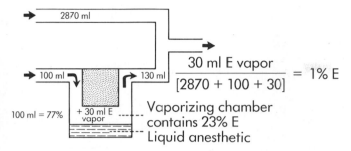

$$\frac{30 \text{ ml E vapor}}{[2870 + 100 + 30]} = 1\% \text{ E}$$

Vaporizing chamber
contains 23% E
Liquid anesthetic

In practice mainflow is set to 3 L/min,
vaporizer flow is set to 100 ml/min,
and E output is 0.96%, i.e., 30 ml E vapor
diluted in [3000 + 100 + 30] ml

Fig. 3-7. Preparation of 1% (vol/vol) enflurane with a measured flow system. (From Eisenkraft JB: *Vaporizers and vaporization of volatile anesthetics.* In *Progress in anesthesiology, vol 2,* San Antonio, Tex, 1989, Dannemiller Memorial Educational Foundation. Reproduced by permission.)

needs to be generated. If 30 ml represents 23% of the atmosphere in the vaporizer, the carrier gas must represent 100 ml/min ([30/23] × 77).

Alternatively, using the formula given previously, we obtain

$$\frac{175}{760} = \frac{30}{30 + y} = 100 \text{ ml/min}$$

where y = oxygen flow to the vaporizer.

Thus if 100 ml/min of oxygen are bubbled through liquid enflurane contained in a measured flow vaporizer, 130 ml/min of gas will emerge, 30 ml/min of which is enflurane vapor. This must be diluted by a fresh gas flow of (3000 − 130) = 2870 ml/min to achieve exactly 1% enflurane. In practice—for example in the Verni-Trol system shown in Fig. 3-8—a bypass gas flow of 3000 ml is set on the main flowmeters to give a resulting enflurane concentration slightly less than 1% (actually 30/3130 = 0.96%).

In the preceding examples, it was necessary to calculate both the oxygen flow to the measured flow vaporizer and the total bypass gas flow needed to produce the desired output concentrations of vapor. This is inconvenient and may give rise to errors. However, it is important to understand the *principles* underlying the calculations because

these vaporizing systems may still be in use in some institutions and are used on military field machines (see Fig. 29-1). Because of the obvious potential for error with a measured flow vaporizing system, the concurrent continuous use of an anesthetic agent monitor with high- and low-concentration alarms is encouraged.[6] Reference to Fig. 3-6 shows a Puritan Bennett 254 infrared agent analyzer in use to measure agent concentration.

Variable bypass

In the concentration-calibrated variable bypass vaporizer, the total flow of gas arriving from the anesthesia machine flowmeters is split between a variable bypass and the vaporizer chamber containing the anesthetic agent (Fig. 3-3). The ratio of these two flows, the *splitting ratio,* depends on the anesthetic agent, temperature, and chosen vapor concentration set to be delivered to the patient circuit.

In the previous section it was calculated that in order to deliver 1% halothane accurately, an incoming total gas flow of 4950 ml/min must be split so that 106 ml enters the vaporizing chamber and 4844 ml enters the bypass (Fig. 3-5). This results in a *splitting ratio* of 46:1 (4844/106) at a temperature of 20° C. A variable bypass vaporizer (e.g., Dräger Vapor 19.1), set to deliver 1% halothane is therefore effectively set to a splitting ratio of 46:1 (Fig. 3-9).

Consider a concentration-calibrated variable bypass enflurane-specific vaporizer set to deliver 2% enflurane. What splitting ratio for incoming gases does this vaporizer achieve? If carrier gas enters the vaporizing chamber at 100 ml/min, enflurane vapor emerges at 30 ml/min and must be diluted in 1500 ml/min of total gas flow to produce a 2% concentration. Thus if carrier gas enters the vaporizer at 1470 ml/min from the flowmeters and splits such that 1370 ml/min enters the bypass while 100 ml/min enters the vaporizing chamber, when the gas flows merge, 2% enflurane is the result. The splitting ratio is 13.7:1 (1370/100) (Fig. 3-10).

Table 3-3 shows the splitting ratios for variable bypass vaporizers used at 20° C. The reader is encouraged to calculate these ratios and to apply them to different total fresh gas flows arriving from the main flowmeters to the inlet of a concentration-calibrated variable bypass vaporizer.

The concentration-calibrated vaporizer is agent-specific and should be used only with the agent for which the unit

Table 3-3. Gas flow splitting ratios at 20° C

	Halothane	Enflurane	Isoflurane	Methoxyflurane	Sevoflurane
1%	46:1	29:1	44:1	1.7:1	25:1
2%	22:1	14:1	21:1	0.36:1	12:1
3%	14:1	9:1	14:1	*	7:1

*Maximum possible is 2.7% at 20° C (see Table 3-2).

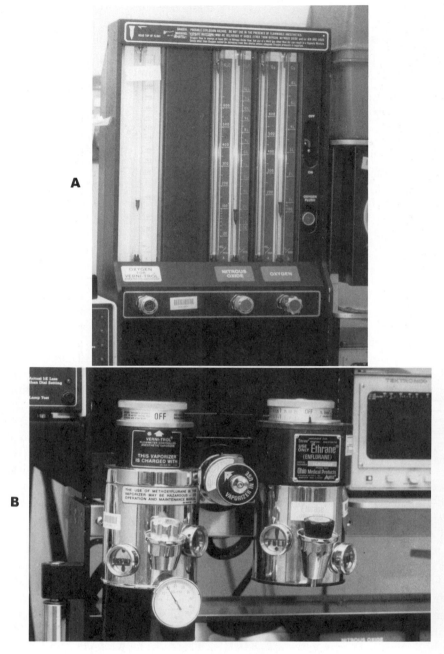

Fig. 3-8. A, Verni-Trol system on Ohio Modulus anesthesia machine set to produce approximately 1% enflurane. Note main flowmeters are set to deliver nitrous oxide at 2 L/min and oxygen at 1 L/min while the oxygen flow to the Verni-Trol vaporizer is 100 ml/min. **B,** Verni-Trol (measured flow) vaporizer is shown on the *left*. A concentration-calibrated enflurane vaporizer is shown on the *right*.

is designed and calibrated. In order to produce a 1% vapor concentration, a halothane vaporizer makes a flow split of 46:1, whereas an enflurane vaporizer makes a flow split of 29:1 (Table 3-3). If an empty enflurane vaporizer set to deliver 1% were filled with halothane, the halothane vapor emerging would be in excess of 1%. Understanding splitting ratios enables prediction of the concentration output of an empty agent-specific variable bypass vaporizer that has been erroneously filled with an agent for which it was not designed.

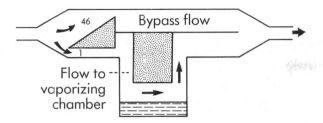

Splitting ratio: Ratio of bypass flow to vaporizing chamber flow

Fig. 3-9. Preparation of 1% (vol/vol) halothane by a variable bypass vaporizer. Although not shown in the diagram, wicks are used to increase the surface area for evaporation. (From Eisenkraft JB: *Vaporizers and vaporization of volatile anesthetics.* In *Progress in anesthesiology, vol 2,* San Antonio, Tex, 1989, Dannemiller Memorial Educational Foundation. Reproduced by permission.)

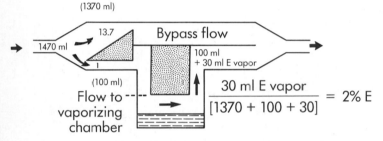

Splitting ratio of 13.7:1 gives 2% E

Fig. 3-10. Preparation of 2% (vol/vol) enflurane by a variable bypass vaporizer. (From Eisenkraft JB: *Vaporizers and vaporization of volatile anesthetics.* In *Progress in anesthesiology, vol 2,* San Antonio, Tex, 1989, Dannemiller Memorial Educational Foundation. Reproduced by permission.)

Efficiency and temperature compensation

Agent-specific concentration-calibrated vaporizers should be located in the fresh gas path between the flowmeter manifold outlet and the common gas outlet on the anesthesia machine.[2] The vaporizers must be capable of accepting a total gas flow of 15 L/min from the machine flowmeters and of delivering a predictable concentration of vapor.[2] However, as the agent is vaporized and the temperature falls, SVP also falls. In the case of a measured flow vaporizer (e.g., Copper Kettle) or an uncompensated variable bypass vaporizer, this results in delivery of less anesthetic vapor to the patient circuit. For this reason, all vaporizing systems must be temperature-compensated, either manually or automatically.

The measured flow vaporizer (e.g., Copper Kettle, Verni-Trol) incorporates a thermometer that measures the temperature of the liquid agent in the vaporizing chamber. A

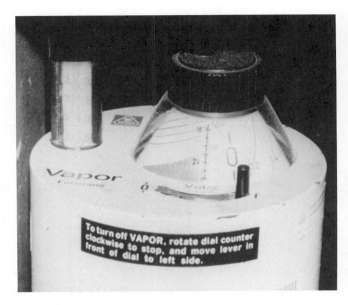

Fig. 3-11. Dräger Vapor vaporizer. Temperature compensation is achieved by reading the temperature from the thermometer and then using the control dial to align the desired output concentration (slanting) line with the marking for ambient temperature.

higher temperature translates to a higher SVP in this chamber. Reference to the vapor pressure curves (Fig. 3-2) enables a re-setting of either oxygen to the vaporizer, or the bypass gas flow, or both, to ensure correct output at the prevailing temperature. Such an arrangement can be tedious, but it does ensure the most accurate and rapid temperature compensation. The Dräger Vapor vaporizer (Fig. 3-11) (as distinguished from the most recent Vapor 19.1 models fitted to contemporary Dräger Narkomed machines) is a variable bypass vaporizer that incorporates a thermometer and a grid of lines on the vaporizer control dial for temperature compensation, whereby the desired output concentration is matched to the temperature of the liquid agent. Turning the control dial changes the size of an orifice in the bypass flow.

Most of the contemporary variable bypass vaporizers (e.g., Ohmeda Tec series, Dräger Vapor 19.1) achieve automatic temperature compensation via a temperature-sensitive valve in the bypass gas flow. When temperature rises, the valve in the bypass opens wider to create a higher splitting ratio. More gas flows through the bypass, and less gas enters the vaporizing chamber. A smaller volume of a higher concentration of vapor emerges from the vaporizing chamber. This vapor, when mixed with an increased bypass gas flow, maintains the vaporizer's output at reasonable constancy when temperature changes are not extreme.

Temperature-sensitive valves vary in design among the different types of vaporizers. Some vaporizers (e.g., Ohio Calibrated Vaporizer) have, in the vaporizing chamber, a

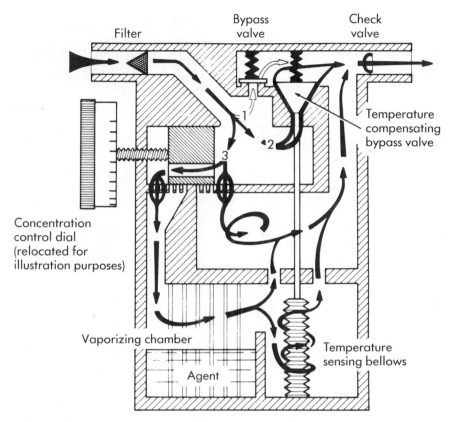

Fig. 3-12. Schematic of Ohio Calibrated Vaporizer. Temperature compensation is achieved by a gas-filled temperature sensing bellows that controls the size of a temperature compensating bypass valve. Note also the check valve in the vaporizer outlet, designed to protect against the pumping effect. (Reproduced by permission of Ohmeda, a Division of BOC Health Care, Inc, Madison, Wis.)

gas-filled bellows linked to a valve in the bypass gas flow (Fig. 3-12).[7] As the temperature increases the bellows expands, causing the valve to open wider. Other vaporizers (e.g., Ohio Tec series) use a bimetallic strip for temperature compensation.[8] This strip is incorporated into a flap valve in the bypass gas flow. The valve is composed of two metals each having a different coefficient of expansion (change in length per unit length per unit change in temperature). Nickel and brass have been used in bimetallic strip valves, brass having a greater coefficient of expansion than nickel. As the temperature rises, one surface of the flap expands more than the other, causing the flap to bend in a manner that opens the valve orifice wider, increasing the bypass flow. The principle of differential expansion of metals is applied similarly in the Dräger Vapor 19.1 vaporizers, where an expansion element increases bypass flow and reduces gas flow in the vaporizing chamber as temperature increases.[9]

The vapor pressures of the volatile anesthetics vary as a function of temperature in a nonlinear manner (see Fig. 3-2). The result is that the vapor output concentration at any given vaporizer dial setting remains constant only within a certain range of temperatures. For example, the Dräger Vapor 19.1 vaporizers are specified as accurate to ±15% of the concentration set when they are used within the temperature range of +15° C to +35° C at one atmosphere of pressure.[10] The boiling point of the volatile anesthetic agent must never be reached in the current variable bypass vaporizers designed for halothane, enflurane, isoflurane, methoxyflurane, and sevoflurane; otherwise, the vapor output concentration would be impossible to control and could be lethal.

In some older vaporizers (e.g., Fluotec Mark II), the temperature compensation valve was contained in the vaporizing chamber itself. The thymol preservatives added to halothane could cause this valve to stick. In later versions of the Fluotec vaporizers, and in other modern vaporizers, these problems have been solved by placement of the temperature compensating valve in the bypass gas flow.

Incorrect filling of vaporizers

Contemporary concentration-calibrated variable bypass anesthesia vaporizers are agent-specific. If an empty vaporizer designed for one agent is filled with an agent for

Table 3-4. Output in volumes percent and MAC (in oxygen) of erroneously filled vaporizers at 22° C

Vaporizers	Liquid	Setting %	Output %	Output MAC
Halothane	Halothane	1.0	1.00	1.25
	Enflurane	1.0	0.62	0.37
	Isoflurane	1.0	0.96	0.84
Enflurane	Enflurane	2.0	2.00	1.19
	Isoflurane	2.0	3.09	2.69
	Halothane	2.0	3.21	4.01
Isoflurane	Isoflurane	1.5	1.50	1.30
	Halothane	1.5	1.56	1.95
	Enflurane	1.5	0.97	0.57

Bruce DL, Linde HW: Vaporization of mixed anesthetic liquids, *Anesthesiology* 60:342-346, 1984 (reproduced by permission).

which it was not intended, the vaporizer's output may be erroneous. Because at room temperature the vaporizing characteristics of halothane and isoflurane are almost identical, this problem at present mainly applies when halothane or isoflurane are interchanged with enflurane.

An even more dangerous situation will occur if a vaporizer designed for methoxyflurane (an agent with an SVP of 20.3 mm Hg at 20° C) is filled with halothane, enflurane, or isoflurane (see Table 3-2). It can be calculated that a methoxyflurane vaporizer filled with halothane and set to deliver 1% methoxyflurane (albeit 6 MAC, see Table 3-2) would deliver 14.8% (20 MAC) halothane. Set to 1 MAC (0.16%) methoxyflurane, the vaporizer makes a flow split of 16:1, similar to that of a halothane or isoflurane variable bypass vaporizer set to deliver just less than 3% (Table 3-3). The use of methoxyflurane recently has become sporadic and greatly diminished, but the anesthesiologist must be aware of this potentially lethal complication where ever methoxyflurane is still administered.

Bruce and Linde[11] reported on the outputs of erroneously filled vaporizers (Table 3-4).* Erroneous filling affects the output concentration and consequently the *potency* output of the vaporizer. In their study, an enflurane vaporizer set to 2% (1.19 MAC) but filled with halothane delivered 3.21% (4.01 MAC) halothane. This is 3.3 times the anticipated anesthetic potency output.

Erroneous filling of vaporizers may be prevented if careful attention is paid to the specific agent and the vaporizer during filling. *Agent-specific keyed* filling mechanisms, analogous to the pin-index safety system for medical gases, are available as options on modern vaporizers. Liquid anesthetic agents are available packaged in bottles that have agent-specific and color-coded collars (Fig. 3-13). One end of an agent-specific filling device fits the collar on the agent bottle, and the other end fits only the vaporizer designed for that liquid agent. Although well-intentioned, these filling devices have not yet gained much

popularity. Such devices are not required by the F1161-88 standard, which states only that the filling mechanism *should* be fitted with a permanently attached, standard, agent-specific, keyed filling device to prevent accidental filling with the wrong agent.[2] Agent-specific filling devices will assume much greater importance when desflurane is introduced into clinical use (see section on desflurane).

Vaporization of mixed anesthetic liquids

Perhaps a more likely scenario is that an agent-specific vaporizer, partially filled with the correct agent, is topped

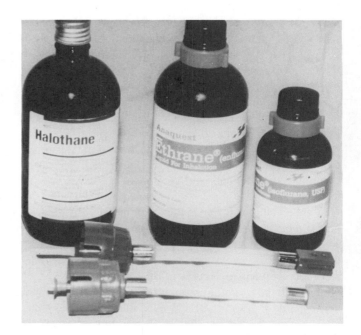

Fig. 3-13. Agent-specific filling devices for enflurane *(lower)* and halothane *(upper)*. The left-hand end of the filling device is designed to fit into an agent-specific collar on the bottle, and the right-hand end is specific for the keyed filling inlet on the vaporizer. Agent-specific collars are shown on the bottles of enflurane and isoflurane. Note the absence of an agent-specific collar on the halothane bottle.

*Note that in this study the MACs of halothane, enflurane and isoflurane were taken to be 0.8%, 1.68%, and 1.14%, respectively.

Table 3-5. Vaporizer output after incorrectly refilling from 25% full to 100% full

Vaporizer	Setting %	Refill liquid	Halothane %	Halothane MAC	Enflurane %	Enflurane MAC	Isoflurane %	Isoflurane MAC	Total MAC
Halothane	1.0	Enflurane	0.33	0.41	0.64	0.38	—	—	0.79
	1.0	Isoflurane	0.41	0.51	—	—	0.90	0.78	1.29
Enflurane	2.0	Halothane	2.43	3.03	0.96	0.57	—	—	3.60
Isoflurane	1.5	Halothane	1.28	1.60	—	—	0.57	0.50	2.10

Bruce DL, Linde HW: Vaporization of mixed anesthetic liquids, *Anesthesiology* 60:342-346, 1984 (reproduced by permission).

up with an incorrect agent.[11] This situation is more complex. It is more difficult to predict vaporizer output, and large errors in concentration of delivered vapor can occur. When mixed, halothane, enflurane, and isoflurane do not react chemically but do influence the extent of each other's ease of vaporization. Halothane facilitates the vaporization of both enflurane and isoflurane and is itself more likely to vaporize in the process.[12] The clinical consequences depend on the potencies of each of the mixed agents as well as on the delivered vapor concentrations.

If a halothane vaporizer 25% full is filled to 100% with isoflurane and set to deliver 1%, the halothane output is 0.41% (0.51 MAC) and the isoflurane output is 0.9% (0.78 MAC) (Table 3-5).[11] In this case, the output potency of 1.29 MAC is not far from the anticipated 1.25 MAC (1% halothane). On the other hand, an enflurane vaporizer that is 25% full and set to deliver 2% (1.19 MAC) enflurane and is filled to 100% with halothane has an output of 2.43% (3.03 MAC) halothane and 0.96% (0.57 MAC) enflurane. This represents a total MAC of 3.60, or more than three times that intended.

It is important to avoid erroneous filling of vaporizers; if an error suspected, the vaporizer should be emptied, flushed using 5 L/min of oxygen (in the case of the Ohmeda Tec 4), with the concentration dial set to the maximum output until no trace of the contaminant is detected in the outflow.[13,14] The vaporizer's temperature should then be allowed to stabilize for 2 hours before it is used clinically with great caution. If the contaminant is not volatile (e.g., water) the vaporizer should be serviced by authorized personnel. Dräger and Ohmeda provide contemporary anesthetic vaporizers with agent-specific filling devices designed to prevent erroneous filling as well as to reduce pollution in the operating room while the vaporizing chamber is filled.

Filling of vaporizers

Vaporizers should be filled only in accordance with their accompanying manufacturer's instructions. Overfilling or tilting (either by tilting a freestanding unit or by tilting the whole anesthesia machine) a vaporizer may result in liquid agent entering parts of the anesthesia delivery system (e.g., vaporizer bypass) designed for gases and va-

por only. This can lead to the delivery of lethal concentrations of the agent to the patient circuit. If a vaporizer has been tilted, liquid agent may have leaked into the gas delivery system. The proper procedure is to flush the vaporizer with a high flow rate of oxygen from the flowmeter (not the oxygen flush, which bypasses the vaporizer), with the vaporizer concentration dial set to the maximum concentration.[10,14] Of course, no patient should be connected to the system during the flushing process. The ASTM F1161-88 standard requires that the anesthetic vapor concentration shall be less than 0.1% after the vaporizer is shut off.[2] Clearly, an anesthetic agent analyzer is essential to check the efficacy of the flush procedure before the vaporizer is used clinically.

Reference to Table 3-2 shows that 1 ml of liquid volatile agent produces approximately 200 ml of vapor at 20° C. The theoretical derivation of this volume is presented later in this chapter. Thus it is easy to see how even small volumes of liquid agent entering the gas delivery system can produce lethal concentrations. For example, if 1 ml of liquid halothane entered the common gas tubing, 20 L of fresh gas would be required to dilute the resulting volume of vapor down to a 1% concentration!

Effect of carrier gas on vaporizer output

The carrier gas used to vaporize the volatile agent in the vaporizing chamber can also affect vaporizer output. Figure 3-14 shows the output concentration from an Ohio enflurane variable bypass vaporizer set to deliver 1% enflurane. For the first 10 minutes (*arrow A*) the carrier gas is 70% nitrous oxide and 30% oxygen, and the vaporizer delivers 1% enflurane. After 10 minutes, (*arrow B*) the carrier gas is changed to nitrogen and oxygen, and the vaporizer output is seen to increase to a peak of about 2.6% at 20 minutes, and then to decrease to 1% by 30 minutes, at which point it stabilizes. At 40 minutes (*arrow C*) the carrier gas is changed back to nitrous oxide and oxygen, and the vaporizer output concentration transiently decreases to 0.75%, and gradually returns to 1% by 55 minutes. At 60 minutes (*arrow D*) the carrier gas is changed back to nitrogen and oxygen, and again the vaporizer output increases as occurred previously (at *arrow B*).

The effect of carrier gas on vaporizer output can be ex-

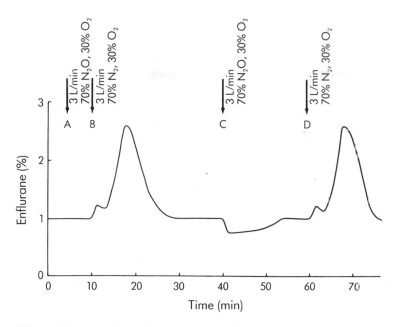

Fig. 3-14. Effect of changing the carrier gas composition (nitrous oxide versus nitrogen) on vaporizer output in an Ohio enflurane vaporizer. (From Scheller MS, Drummond JC: Solubility of N_2O in volatile anesthetics contributes to vaporizer aberrancy when changing carrier gases, *Anesth Analg* 65:88-90, 1986. Reproduced by permission of the International Anesthesia Research Society.)

plained by the solubility of nitrous oxide in a liquid volatile agent. Thus when nitrous oxide and oxygen begin to enter the vaporizing chamber, some nitrous oxide dissolves in the liquid agent and the vaporizing chamber's output *decreases* until the liquid agent has become saturated with nitrous oxide. Conversely, when nitrous oxide is withdrawn as the carrier gas, the nitrous oxide dissolved in the liquid anesthetic comes out of solution and represents, in effect, additional nitrous oxide gas flow to the vaporizing chamber.

The solubility of nitrous oxide in liquid anesthetics is approximately 4.5 ml per ml of liquid anesthetic.[15] Thus 100 ml of halothane liquid, when fully saturated, can dissolve approximately 450 ml of nitrous oxide. When nitrous oxide is discontinued, the volume of nitrous oxide, because it is added (by coming out of solution) to the vaporizing chamber flow over a brief time period, causes the observed *increase* in vaporizer output concentration. This effect is not seen with measured flow vaporizers (e.g., Copper Kettle, Verni-Trol) because in them the carrier gas is always oxygen.[15]

Effects of changes in barometric pressure

Vaporizers are usually used at ambient pressure of 760 mm Hg (one atmosphere at sea level). They may, however, be used under hypobaric conditions—such as at increased altitude—or under hyperbaric conditions—such as in a hyperbaric chamber.[5]

Hypobaric conditions. Few reports are available concerning the use of vaporizers under hypobaric conditions.[5]

The theoretical considerations applying to such use are therefore discussed here. Consider a variable bypass vaporizer set to deliver 1% halothane (1.33 MAC at 760 mm Hg atmospheric pressure), which is being used at an ambient pressure of 500 mm Hg (equivalent to an altitude of approximately 10,000 feet above sea level) and at a temperature of 20° C (see Fig. 3-15). In the vaporizing chamber, halothane has an SVP of 243 mm Hg at a temperature of 20° C; however, this now represents 48.6 volumes percent (243/500). The vaporizer, set to deliver 1% under normal conditions, creates a splitting ratio of 46:1 (see Table 3-3 and Fig. 3-9) between bypass and vaporizing chamber flows.

If the total gas flow to the vaporizer is 4700 ml/min (Fig. 3-15), then 100 ml/min of carrier gas passes through the vaporizing chamber. This now represents 51.4% of the volume there because halothane represents the other 48.6 volumes percent (100 − 51.4). Emerging from the vaporizing chamber is 100 ml/min of carrier gas plus 95 ml/min of halothane vapor ([100/51.4] × 48.6). When the vaporizing chamber and bypass flows merge, the 95 ml/min of halothane vapor are diluted in a total volume of 4795 ml/min (4600 + 100 + 95 ml), giving a halothane concentration of 1.98 volumes percent, or approximately 2% of the (hypobaric) atmosphere by volume. This appears to be double the dialed-in concentration in terms of volumes percent.

However, partial pressures must be considered because it is the *tension* of the anesthetic agent that is important. If halothane represents 1.98% of the gas mixture by volume,

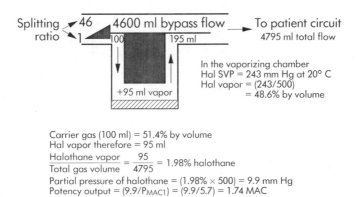

Variable bypass vaporizer set to deliver halothane 1% (1.3 MAC)
at 760 mm Hg (1 ATA).
Consider use at 500 mm Hg ambient pressure (2/3 ATA).

Splitting ratio 46 / 1

4600 ml bypass flow → To patient circuit
4795 ml total flow

100   195 ml

+95 ml vapor

In the vaporizing chamber
Hal SVP = 243 mm Hg at 20° C
Hal vapor = (243/500)
          = 48.6% by volume

Carrier gas (100 ml) = 51.4% by volume
Hal vapor therefore = 95 ml

$\dfrac{\text{Halothane vapor}}{\text{Total gas volume}} = \dfrac{95}{4795} = 1.98\%$ halothane

Partial pressure of halothane = (1.98% × 500) = 9.9 mm Hg
Potency output = $(9.9/P_{MAC1}) = (9.9/5.7) = 1.74$ MAC

Fig. 3-15. Use of a concentration-calibrated vaporizer under hypobaric conditions. (From Eisenkraft JB: *Vaporizers and vaporization of volatile anesthetics.* In *Progress in anesthesiology, vol 2,* San Antonio, Tex, 1989, Dannemiller Memorial Educational Foundation. Reproduced by permission.)

Variable bypass vaporizer set to deliver isoflurane 2% (1.74 MAC)
at 760 mm Hg (1 ATA).
Consider use at 2280 mm Hg ambient pressure (3 ATA).

Splitting ratio 21 / 1

2100 ml bypass flow → To patient circuit
2211.6 ml total flow

100   111.6 ml

+11.6 ml vapor

In the vaporizing chamber
Iso SVP = 238 mm Hg at 20° C
Iso vapor = (238/2280)
          = 10.4% by volume

Carrier gas (100 ml) = 89.6% by volume
Iso vapor therefore = 11.6 ml

$\dfrac{\text{Isoflurane vapor}}{\text{Total gas volume}} = \dfrac{11.6}{2211.6} = 0.52\%$ isoflurane

Partial pressure of isoflurane = (0.52% × 2280) = 11.9 mm Hg
Potency output = $(11.9/P_{MAC1}) = (11.9/8.7) = 1.36$ MAC

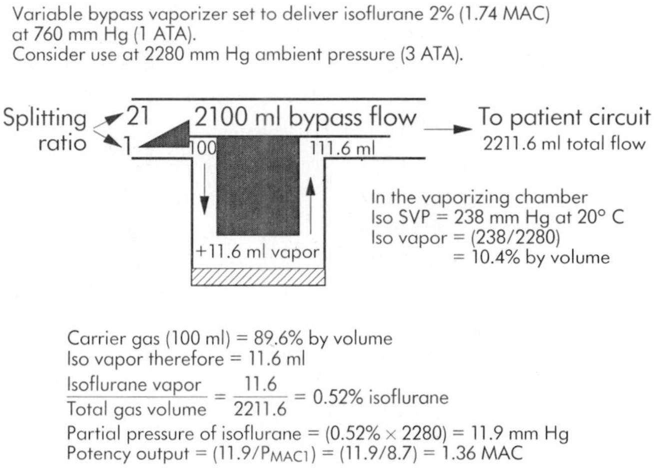

Fig. 3-16. Use of a concentration-calibrated vaporizer under hyperbaric conditions. (From Eisenkraft JB: *Vaporizers and vaporization of volatile anesthetics.* In *Progress in anesthesiology, vol 2,* San Antonio, Tex, 1989, Dannemiller Memorial Educational Foundation. Reproduced by permission.)

its partial pressure in the emerging mixture is 1.98% × 500, or 9.90 mm Hg. In terms of anesthetic potency, this represents 1.74 MAC (9.90/5.7), because the P_{MAC1} of halothane is 5.7 mm Hg (Table 3-1). Thus, in theory, a halothane vaporizer used at a pressure of 500 mm Hg (10,000 feet) set to 1% (vol/vol) delivers twice the set concentration in terms of volumes percent but only 1.3 times the anesthetic potency in MAC (1.74/1.33).

Hyperbaric conditions. Anesthesia vaporizers are occasionally used under hyperbaric conditions. This can occur in a hyperbaric operating chamber or at altitudes below sea level. Consider a variable bypass isoflurane vaporizer set to deliver 2% (1.74 MAC at 760 mm Hg atmospheric pressure) isoflurane vapor: The vaporizer is used at 20° C

under conditions of 3 atmospheres pressure (3 × 760 = 2280 mm Hg), such as may exist in a hyperbaric chamber (Fig. 3-16).

In the vaporizing chamber, the SVP of isoflurane is 238 mm Hg (Table 3-2) and the isoflurane concentration is 10.4 volumes percent (238/2280). A variable bypass isoflurane vaporizer set to deliver 2% creates a splitting ratio of 21:1 for the fresh gas flow (Table 3-3). If the total gas flow to the vaporizer is 2200 ml/min, then 100 ml of carrier gas enters the vaporizing chamber per minute (Fig. 3-16). This 100 ml represents 89.6% of the total gas there (100 − 10.4); the remainder is isoflurane vapor. The amount of isoflurane vapor evolved is ([100/89.6] × 10.4) = 11.6 ml/min. This volume, diluted in (2100 + 100 + 11.6) gives 0.52% (11.6/2211.6) isoflurane vapor by volume. This is 0.26 (0.53/2.0) times the dial setting in terms of volumes percent.

What about potency? The partial pressure of isoflurane in the emerging gas mixture is 11.9 mm Hg (0.52% × 2280). Dividing by the P_{MAC1} for isoflurane of 8.7 mm Hg (Table 3-1) gives a potency output of 1.36 MAC (11.9/8.7). Thus the isoflurane vaporizer, set to deliver 1.74 MAC under conditions of one atmosphere (760 mm Hg) pressure, delivers 1.36 MAC at 3 atmospheres, or approximately 0.8 times the anesthetic potency expected (Fig. 3-16).

These examples show that although changing ambient pressure affects vaporizer output to a significant degree in terms of volumes percent, the effect on anesthetic potency (MAC) is less dramatic. In the examples discussed it was assumed that the set splitting ratios (Table 3-3) remained constant as ambient pressure changed. In reality, however, changes in gas density occur with changes in ambient pressure and can affect the splitting ratios slightly. From a clinical point of view, however, the anesthetic potency output expected for any given vaporizer setting changes little, even though vapor concentration (vol/vol) may be altered considerably.[5,13] Again, it is emphasized that vaporizer output concentration expressed in volumes percent is of limited value unless converted to MAC units according to the concept of partial pressures, as previously described.

Arrangement of vaporizers

Some older anesthesia machines had up to three variable bypass vaporizers arranged in series, making it possible for carrier gas to pass through each vaporizer (albeit all through a bypass chamber) to reach the common gas outlet of the anesthesia machine. Without an interlock system, which permits only one vaporizer to be in use at any time, it was possible to have all three vaporizers turned on simultaneously (Fig. 3-17). Apart from potentially overdosing the patient, the agent from the upstream vaporizer could contaminate the agent(s) in those downstream.[16] During subsequent use, the output of the downstream vaporizer(s) would be contaminated. The resulting concentrations in the emerging gas and vapor mixture would be indeterminate and might even be lethal.

If such an in-series arrangement of vaporizers is present, a vaporizer designed for a less volatile agent (e.g., methoxyflurane) must not be placed downstream relative to more volatile anesthetics (e.g., halothane). In such a case halothane would dissolve in methoxyflurane downstream. If, during subsequent use, the methoxyflurane vaporizer is set to deliver 1% (albeit 6 MAC), in excess of 6% halothane (8 MAC) may also be delivered from the methoxyflurane vaporizer.[16] The most desirable in-series sequence of vaporizers from flowmeter manifold to common gas outlet is therefore methoxyflurane, enflurane, isoflurane, then halothane.

These principles also apply when a free-standing va-

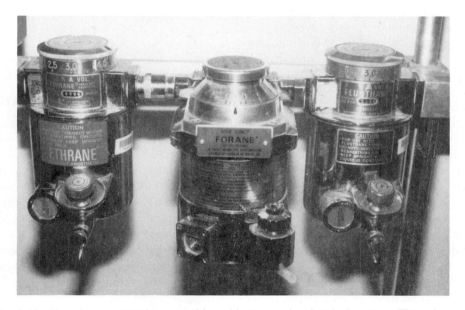

Fig. 3-17. Vaporizers mounted on a machine with no vaporizer interlock system. These three vaporizers are all on, set to deliver 3% agent, and in series. Note also that on the middle vaporizer, concentration is increased by counterclockwise rotation of the dial, which is the modern convention. On the two outer vaporizers, concentration is increased by clockwise rotation of the dial. (From Eisenkraft JB, Sommer RM: *Equipment failure. Anesthesia delivery systems.* In Benumof JL, Saidman LJ editors: *Anesthesia and perioperative complications,* St Louis, Mo, 1991, Mosby–Year Book.)

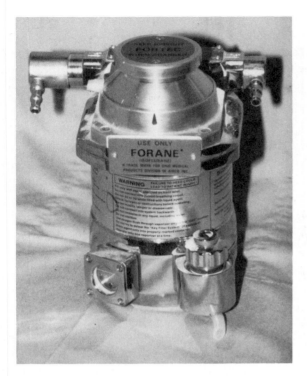

Fig. 3-18. Free-standing concentration-calibrated isoflurane vaporizer. This vaporizer was used in-line between the common gas outlet and the anesthesia circuit. Such potentially dangerous arrangements should not be used.

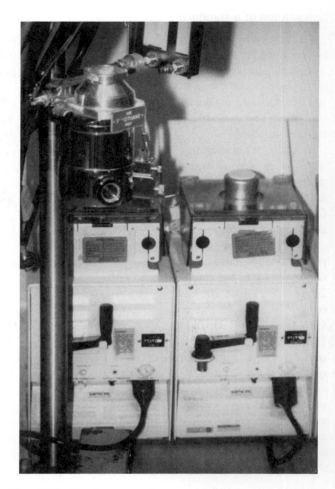

Fig. 3-19. Halothane vaporizer mounted on a cardiopulmonary bypass machine.

porizer is placed in series between the machine common gas outlet and the patient circuit (Fig. 3-18). Such arrangements, configured by the user (and never by the machine manufacturer), are potentially dangerous and should not be used.[17] In addition to the contamination problem by agents upstream, such vaporizers are more easily tipped over. Use of the machine oxygen flush with the free-standing vaporizer on can pump a bolus of agent into the patient circuit, and disconnection of the vaporizer tubing can result in hypoxia in the patient circuit (see Chapter 16). Freestanding vaporizers are, however, routinely used in conjunction with pump oxygenators for cardiopulmonary bypass. In such situations the vaporizer should be securely mounted to the pump (Fig. 3-19) and correct directional flow of gas through the vaporizer confirmed. Such vaporizers are subject to the same routine maintenance and calibration procedures as are all other anesthesia vaporizers.

With contemporary anesthesia machines, only one vaporizer can be on at any given time. To prevent cross-contamination of the contents of one vaporizer with those of another, the F1161-88 standard requires that a system be provided to isolate the vaporizers from one another and to prevent gas from passing through more than one vaporizing chamber.[2] This specification is met by use of an interlock system. Contemporary Dräger and Ohmeda anesthesia machines incorporate manufacturer-specific interlock

systems; these are described in subsequent sections concerning specific vaporizer models.

CALIBRATION AND CHECKING OF VAPORIZER OUTPUTS

Vaporizers should be serviced regularly and their outputs checked to ensure that no malfunction exists. The vaporizer dial is set to deliver a certain concentration of agent, and the actual output concentration is measured by an anesthetic agent analyzer, which samples gas through a connector placed at the common gas outlet of the anesthesia machine.

Currently available methods for practical vapor analysis include mass spectrometry, multiwavelength infrared spectroscopy, laser-Raman scattering, infrared acoustic spectroscopy, lipophilic-coated piezoelectric vibrating crystal, and refractometry. The first three methods allow for identification and quantification of multiple agents in the presence of one another. The last three methods are reliable only in the presence of a single agent that has (already) been *qualitatively* identified to the analyzer. The reader is referred to Chapter 8 for a more detailed discussion of these technologies.

Preparation of a standard vapor concentration

Although the physical methods for measurement mentioned in the previous section may be used to check vaporizer output, the agent analyzers themselves require calibration. For this purpose standard vapor concentrations must be prepared and available for use as the calibration gas standards. The standard mixtures are available from commercial suppliers.

Consider the preparation of a standard mixture of halothane in oxygen. Avogadro's law states that one gram molecule of a gas or vapor will occupy 22.4 L at standard temperature and pressure (STP) (760 mm Hg pressure, 0° C or 273 K).[3] Thus 197.4 g of halothane occupies 22.4 L at STP, and 1 g occupies 22.4/197.4 L.

By Charles' law (the volume of a fixed mass of gas is proportional to absolute temperature if pressure remains constant), 1 g of halothane occupies $[(22.4/197.4) \times (293/273)] = 0.12$ L at 20° C (293 K). One ml of liquid halothane weighs 1.86 g (the specific gravity of halothane is 1.86; see Table 3-2); therefore, 1 ml of liquid halothane generates $[(22.4/197.4) \times (293/273) \times 1.86] = 0.226$ L of vapor. Thus 1 ml of liquid halothane produces 226 ml of vapor at 20° C (see Table 3-2).

By way of this type of calculation, a predetermined volume of liquid agent can be measured accurately with a micropipette, then that volume can be transferred to and vaporized in a chamber of known volume to produce a calibration standard gas mixture.

As discussed earlier, if a vaporizer is tipped on its side and liquid agent enters the bypass chamber or fresh gas piping, small volumes of liquid agent can give rise to very large volumes of vapor.

EFFECT OF USE VARIABLES ON VAPORIZER FUNCTION
Fresh gas flow rate

The output of a concentration-calibrated vaporizer is normally a function of fresh gas inflow rate. Since 1 ml of liquid agent produces about 200 ml of vapor, the consumption of liquid agent per hour can be approximated by the following formula:

$3 \times$ Vaporizer setting (vol %) $\times$ Fresh gas flow rate per minute.

Thus an isoflurane vaporizer set to deliver 1.5% at a flow rate of 4 L/min consumes $3 \times 1.5 \times 4 = 18$ ml of liquid agent per hour.

The output concentrations of modern concentration-calibrated vaporizers (Tec 4, Tec 5, Dräger Vapor 19.1) are virtually independent of the fresh gas flow rate with flows and vaporizer settings in the normal clinical range. At high concentration settings and with high fresh gas flows, output is slightly less than that set on the dial. This is because under these conditions, evaporation of the agent may be incomplete and temperature in the vaporizing chamber will fall. Thus saturation of gas flowing through the vaporizing chamber is incomplete and output falls. The effects of flow rate on vaporizer output are shown for the Ohmeda Tec 5 (Fig. 3-20) and the Dräger Vapor 19.1

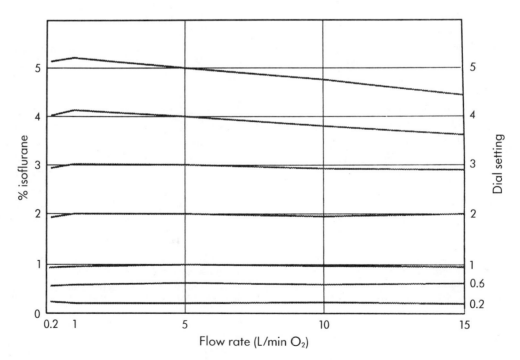

Fig. 3-20. Effect of oxygen flow rate on output concentration of a Tec 5 isoflurane vaporizer at 22° C. (From *Tec 5 operation and maintenance manual,* Madison, Wis, 1989, Ohmeda, a Division of BOC Health Care, Inc. Reproduced by permission.)

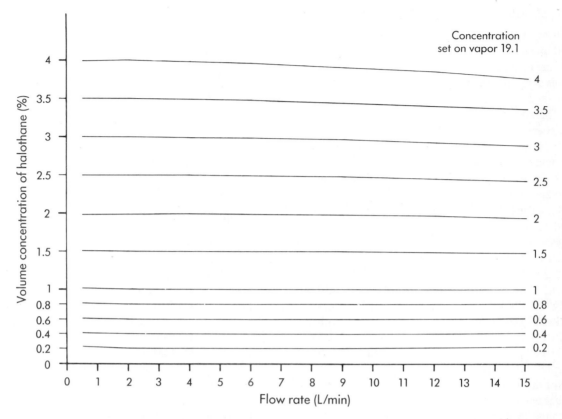

Fig. 3-21. Effect of flow rate of air on output concentration of a Dräger Vapor 19.1 vaporizer. (Reproduced by permission of Drägerwerk AG, Lubeck, Germany.)

(Fig. 3-21). Again, note that this effect is of little clinical significance in most situations.

With some older models of vaporizers (e.g., Ohio Calibrated Vaporizer), the output tended to be less linear with extremes of flow rate. For example, the Ohio Calibrated Vaporizer at low flows (<1 L/min) had an output less than expected (Fig. 3-22), and at flow rates >3 L/min output exceeded expectations. For comparison with more recent models of vaporizers (Figs. 3-20 and 3-21), Fig. 3-22 shows the nonlinearity of the output of the older (and no longer produced) Ohio Calibrated Vaporizers.[7]

Fresh gas composition

It was previously noted that changing the composition of the carrier gas, especially by adding or removing nitrous oxide, temporarily alters vaporizer output.[15] In the case of nitrous oxide, this effect is mainly due to solubility of nitrous oxide, although changes in gas density and viscosity also contribute to changes in output by affecting the flow split between vaporizing chamber and bypass gas flows.

Ohmeda Tec 4 and 5 vaporizers are calibrated using 100% oxygen.[13,14] If the carrier gas is changed to air (or nitrous oxide) the vapor output decreases at low flow rates. At high flow rates and low concentration dial settings, the output may increase slightly.[13,14]

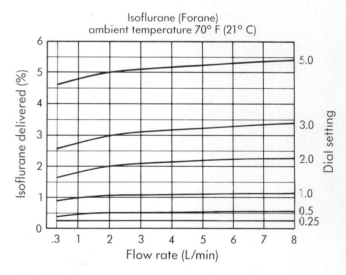

Fig. 3-22. Ohio Calibrated Vaporizer. Performance showing effect of oxygen flow on output concentration. Note nonlinearity of output. (Reproduced by permission of Ohmeda, a Division of BOC Health Care, Inc, Madison, Wis.)

Dräger Vapor 19.1 vaporizers are calibrated using air.[10] If 100% oxygen is then used, the delivered output concentration is approximately 5% to 10% greater than the dial setting (air calibration value). When a mixture of nitrous oxide and oxygen (70:30) is used, the output is 5% to

10% lower than dial setting. In this model of vaporizer, deviations from dial setting increase with lower fresh gas flows, small amounts of agent in the vaporizing chamber, higher concentration dial settings, and extreme changes in the composition of the carrier gas.[10]

Effects of temperature

As previously described, concentration-calibrated vaporizers are temperature-compensated. The effects of changes in temperature are negligible under usual conditions of use. However, if the ambient temperature should exceed the vaporizer's specified range of performance, the vaporizer's output may become high. Indeed, the output may become unpredictable and uncontrolled if the boiling point of the agent is reached. Conversely, if the temperature falls below the specified range for use, the output may be unpredictably low.

Fluctuating back pressure

Fluctuating or intermittent back pressure, or the *pumping effect,* may be applied to the vaporizer by changes in pressure downstream. Such pressure changes may be caused by intermittent positive pressure ventilation (IPPV) in the patient circuit or operation of the oxygen flush control. They may cause changes in gas flow distribution within the vaporizer; these changes lead to increased output if no compensation mechanism exists. The effects of intermittent pressurization are greatest at low flow rates, low concentration settings, when small amounts of liquid agent are present in the vaporizer, and with large and rapid changes in pressure.[10,13] Higher flow rates, higher dial settings, larger volumes of liquid agent in the vaporizer, and smaller, less frequent changes in pressure minimize the pumping effect.

Of the several explanations offered for the pumping effect, the most probable is that during pressurization, gas is compressed in the vaporizer (in both the vaporizing chamber and the bypass). When the pressure decreases, anesthetic vapor leaves the vaporizing chamber through both the normal exit and the vaporizing chamber inlet, to enter the bypass flow. The intermittent addition of vapor to the bypass flow results in the observed intermittent increase in vaporizer output.

Modern vaporizers (Ohmeda Tec 5, Dräger Vapor 19.1) have incorporated certain design features that minimize the significance of the pumping effect (see the next section).[10,13] The Ohio Calibrated Vaporizer has a check valve (Fig. 3-12) in the vaporizer outlet to prevent transmission of rises in downstream pressure.[7] Certain older models of Ohmeda anesthesia machines employ a check valve just upstream of the common gas outlet to prevent retrograde transmission of downstream pressures (see Chapter 2, and Table 2-1). It should be noted, however, that while the check valve is closed, the pressure upstream of it (and hence in the vaporizers) increases because of continuous fresh gas flow from the machine flowmeters.

Thus the use of check valves can limit, but does not totally eliminate, the pumping effect. For this reason, the newest models of anesthesia machine (Ohmeda Modulus II Plus, Ohmeda Modulus CD, all Dräger Narkomed) do not use check valves in their design (see Chapter 2).

CONTEMPORARY VAPORIZERS

Dräger Vapor 19.1. The Dräger Vapor 19.1 vaporizer is used on contemporary Dräger Narkomed anesthesia machines (Fig. 3-23). Up to three such vaporizers may be mounted on the back bar of the Narkomed machine and connected to an interlock system designed to ensure that only one vaporizer or agent is in use at any time (Fig. 3-24). When one vaporizer is turned on, the dials on the others cannot be turned from zero. If one vaporizer should be removed, it must be replaced on the back bar by a special block to ensure continued function of the interlock system. Because failures have been reported,[18] the interlock system's function must be checked periodically (see also Chapter 16).

A schematic of the Dräger Vapor 19.1 vaporizer is shown in Fig. 3-25.[10] With the concentration knob *(3)* in the zero position, the on/off switch *(2)* is closed. Fresh gas enters the vaporizer at the fresh gas inlet *(1)* and leaves via the fresh gas outlet *(10)* without entering the vaporizing parts of the unit. In this off state the inlet and outlet ports of the vaporizing chamber are connected and vented to atmosphere via a hole. The venting prevents pressure

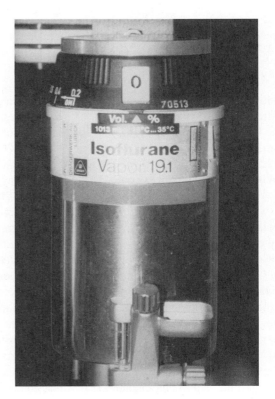

Fig. 3-23. Dräger Vapor 19.1 vaporizer. Note the funnel-fill arrangement. An agent-specific fill mechanism is also available.

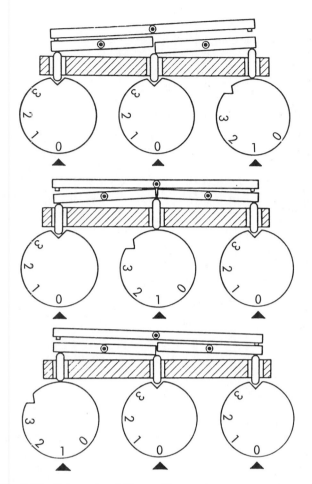

Fig. 3-24. Schematic of Dräger Vapor 19.1 vaporizer interlock system that ensures that only one vaporizer can be in use at any one time. (Reproduced by permission of North American Dräger, Inc, Telford, Pa.)

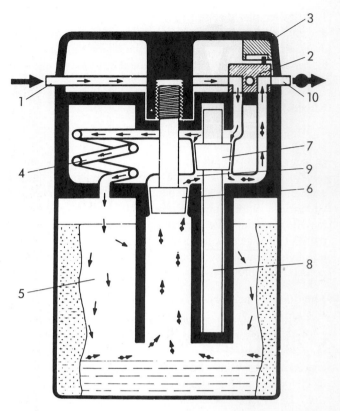

Fig. 3-25. Schematic of Dräger Vapor 19.1 vaporizer. *1* = fresh gas inlet; *2* = on/off switch; *3* = concentration knob; *4* = pressure compensator; *5* = vaporizing chamber; *6* = control cone; *7* = bypass cone; *8* = expansion element; *9* = mixing chamber; *10* = fresh gas outlet. For details of operation, see text. (Reproduced by permission of Drägerwerk AG, Lubeck, Germany.)

buildup in the vaporizing chamber, thereby preventing vapor from being driven (under pressure) into the fresh gas flow. Dräger specifies that venting results in a loss of only 0.5 ml/day of anesthetic at a temperature of 22° C. The vaporizer can be filled only in the off state.[10]

When the concentration knob *(3)* is turned to any volume (%) concentration above 0.2 volume percent, the on/off switch *(2)* opens automatically, allowing the fresh gas to enter the interior of the vaporizer. The gas is immediately divided and follows two different routes. Part of the fresh gas moves through a thermostatically controlled bypass *(7)*, which compensates for temperature changes and maintains the correct volume percent output as selected by the concentration knob *(3)*. The remaining fresh gas moves through a pressure compensator *(4)*, which prevents pressure changes that arise either upstream or downstream from being transmitted into the vaporizer and affecting the vapor output. From the pressure compensator the gas continues into the vaporizing chamber *(5)*, which contains the liquid anesthetic agent that is absorbed and evaporated by

a special wick assembly. As the fresh gas moves through the vaporizing chamber, it becomes fully saturated with anesthetic vapor. The saturated gas leaves the chamber through a control cone *(6)*. The cone is adjustable with the concentration knob *(3)*. The saturated vapor and the fresh gas that did not pass through the vaporizing chamber are combined and leave through the fresh gas outlet *(10)*. The combination of the bypass opening *(7)* and the control cone opening *(6)* determines the volume percent of the vapor output.

In this vaporizer, the pumping effect is prevented by the design of the long spiral inlet tube *(4)* (pressure compensator). When the vaporizing chamber *(5)* becomes decompressed, some anesthetic vapor does enter this spiral, but because of the spiral's length the vapor does not reach the bypass gas flow.

Temperature compensation is achieved by the bypass cone *(7)* and the expansion element *(8)*. When temperature rises, bypass flow increases. Sudden changes in temperature require a compensation time of 6 min/° C in order for concentration output to be maintained within specifications.[10]

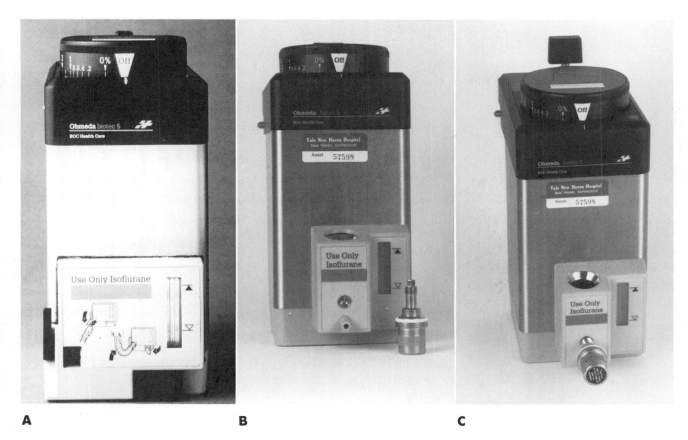

A   **B**   **C**

Fig. 3-26. A, Ohmeda Tec 5 vaporizer with keyed filling system. **B,** Ohmeda Tec 5 vaporizer with funnel-fill system. The filler cap has been removed to show the hexagonal inner end, which is used to drain the vaporizer. **C,** Ohmeda Tec 5 vaporizer with drain key inserted into drain cock. (Courtesy of Ohmeda, a Division of BOC Health Care, Inc, Madison, Wis.)

The Dräger Vapor 19.1 is produced with either a funnel-type (Fig. 3-23) or an agent-specific filling device, and overfilling is not possible because the liquid level is limited by the position of the filling mechanism. The capacity of the vaporizing chamber is approximately 200 ml with dry wicks and 140 ml with wet wicks.[10] This vaporizer does not include an antispill mechanism and should not be tilted more than 45°. If tilted more than this, it should be flushed with a gas flow of 10 L/min with the concentration dial set to maximum prior to clinical use.[10] Drägerwerk states that a flushing time of 5 minutes is usually adequate if the vaporizer has been tilted only briefly and then immediately righted. If it has been tilted for longer, a minimum flush period of 20 minutes is required, during which it is advisable to drain liquid anesthetic from the vaporizing chamber.[10] The manufacturer (Drägerwerk AG, Germany) stipulates in their instruction manual that the vaporizer be inspected and serviced every 6 months by qualified personnel and that an official maintenance record shall be kept.[10] North American Dräger's policy is that vaporizer output be checked bimonthly with a refractometer and that if within specifications, the vaporizer requires no service. The halothane vaporizing chamber is inspected at these times and the vaporizer is returned for service if deemed necessary

by the field service engineer (personal communication, North American Dräger).

Whether in the off or on position, the Dräger 19.1 vaporizer is designed to limit the pressure of the fresh gas supply to a maximum of approximately 18 psig. Thus if the anesthesia common gas outlet should become occluded and the oxygen flush operated, a pressure of 45 to 55 psig could be transmitted retrograde from the common gas outlet back to the flow meters, if not relieved through the Vapor 19.1 vaporizer. Where more than one vaporizer is present (up to three are possible), pressure relief usually occurs through the one closest to the common gas outlet. Thus, even when the vaporizer is turned off, fresh gas continues to flow through the vaporizer unit, albeit not to the vaporizing sections, and therefore has access to the pressure limiting system described above.

Ohmeda Tec 5. The Ohmeda Tec 5 vaporizer,[13] is used on the most recent Ohmeda anesthesia machines (Fig.3-26). Up to three vaporizers may be mounted and locked on a special patented Selectatec manifold. This differs considerably from the Dräger mounting system used in North America in that the Tec vaporizers can be removed easily from the machine.

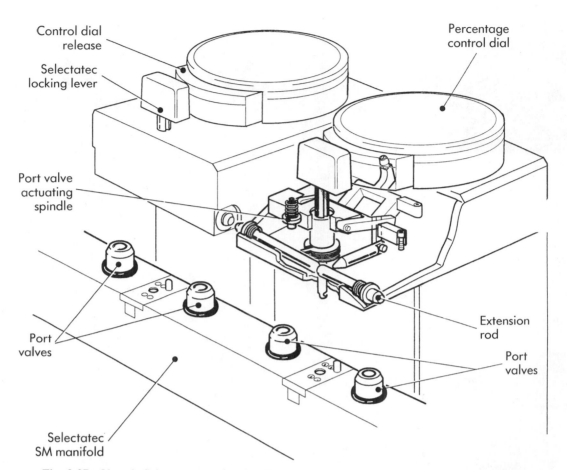

Fig. 3-27. Ohmeda Selectatec vaporizer interlock system. See text for details. The Selectatec SM Manifold is described in Fig. 3-28. (Reproduced by permission of Ohmeda, a Division of BOC Health Care, Inc, Madison, Wis.)

Each Tec 5 vaporizer is locked to the manifold by a Selectatec locking lever. Unless this lever is in the locked position, the concentration control dial release cannot be activated (Fig. 3-27). Once the lever is in the locked position, the dial release can be depressed. This operates the vaporizer interlock mechanism that causes the interlock extension rods to extend laterally to adjacent vaporizers, minimizing the possibility of their being turned on. Simultaneously, the two Selectatec port valve actuating spindles are activated to allow fresh gas to enter the vaporizer. Depressing the control dial release button also enables the control dial to be turned to the desired vapor output concentration. When the control dial is turned to off and the dial release is no longer depressed, the manifold port valves close and the extension rods are retracted, allowing selection of another vaporizer. Thus in the Selectatec system fresh gas enters a vaporizer only when the vaporizer is turned on; otherwise, fresh gas bypasses the vaporizer(s) via a separate channel in the manifold (Fig. 3-28).

Figure 3-29, *A* shows a Tec 5 vaporizer flow diagram, and Fig. 3-29, *B* shows a schematic of the Tec 5. When the concentration dial is set in the zero position, all gas passages are closed except for a channel linking the vaporizer inlet and outlet. When the dial is turned past 0%, the carrier gas stream is split between bypass and vaporizing chamber flows. Bypass gas flows vertically downward from *(a)*, across the base of the sump *(6)*, through the thermostat to *(c)*, and back up the gas transfer manifold via *(d)* to *(e)*. The thermostat or temperature compensating device is located in the base of the vaporizer. It is of the bimetallic strip design, which increases bypass flow as temperature rises and decreases bypass flow as temperature falls.

The fresh gas flowing to the vaporizing chamber flows through an IPPV assembly, designed to minimize the pumping effect, before reaching the vaporizing chamber and wick assembly system. Here it becomes saturated with anesthetic vapor and flows on to combine with the bypass gas flow and exit the vaporizer.

Like the Dräger Vapor 19.1, the Tec 5 incorporates an IPPV chamber to minimize the pumping effect. In the Tec 5 vaporizer, temperature compensation is achieved by a bimetallic strip valve rather than a bypass cone and expansion element. A keyed or a funnel-fill system is available. Although the Tec 5 incorporates an antispill mechanism, if

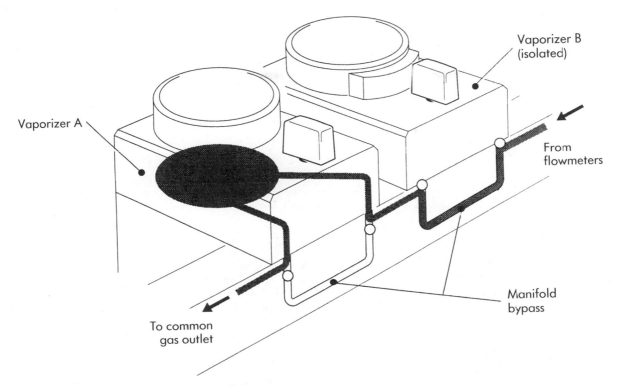

Fig. 3-28. Ohmeda Series-Mounted Manifold (SM) gas circuit. Fresh gas from the machine flowmeters enters the Series-Mounted Manifolds, which incorporate pairs of series-connected, two-way port valves. When a Tec 5 vaporizer is locked onto the manifold and turned on (vaporizer *A*), both associated port valves are opened. Fresh gas from the manifold then flows into the vaporizer through the inlet port valves, and the gas-agent mixture exits via the outlet port valve. When the vaporizer is turned off (vaporizer *B*) or if no vaporizer is fitted to the manifold, each port valve is closed, allowing gas to bypass the vaporizer via the manifold bypass circuit. (Reproduced by permission of Ohmeda, a Division of BOC Health Care, Inc, Madison, Wis.)

the vaporizer is inverted it is recommended that it be purged with carrier gas at 5 L/min for 30 minutes with the dial set to 5%.[13]

The Tec 5 vaporizer has a liquid agent capacity of 300 ml with dry wicks and 225 ml with wet wicks. The vaporizer is calibrated at 22° C with oxygen at 5 L/min.[13] As previously discussed, changes in carrier gas composition may affect agent output concentration.

Ohmeda recommends that the vaporizer be serviced every three years at an authorized service center.[13] Service should include complete disassembly; thorough cleaning; inspection for wear and damage; renewal of wicks, seals, and any worn components; replacement of discontinued parts with more current parts; checking of output, and recalibration if necessary.

Differences between Ohmeda Tec 5 and Tec 4. The Ohmeda Tec 5 vaporizer supersedes the Tec 4 models. Although the principle of operation has not changed, the following changes have been made. The Tec 5 has a larger capacity chamber for agent (Tec 4: 135 ml dry wick, 100 ml wet). The output concentration of the Tec 5 is more linear over wider ranges of flow. The thermostat, which is in

the center of the vaporizer in the Tec 4, is in the base in the Tec 5. There are also improvements in the design and operation of the concentration control dial and the release button in the Tec 5 compared with the Tec 4. Thus, in the Tec 4, pressing the dial release button permits the dial to be turned; rotating the dial past zero activates the interlock mechanism and opens the valve, permitting gas to flow into the vaporizer. In the Tec 5, pressing the dial release button engages the manifold pins and interlock; rotating the dial permits gas to enter the vaporizer. Rotation of the dial in the Tec 5 is therefore easier than in the Tec 4 because it is associated with fewer functions in the Tec 5. Finally, Ohmeda recommends annual service of the Tec 4 vaporizer but triannual for the Tec 5.

Limitations of earlier Selectatec system. As discussed previously, the Selectatec vaporizer extension system relies on vaporizers being adjacent to one another so that extrusion of the extension rods of one vaporizer prevents the other from being turned on. In earlier designs the Selectatec system could be defeated. Thus if the middle one of three vaporizers was removed, the remaining two, not now being adjacent, could both be turned on (Fig.

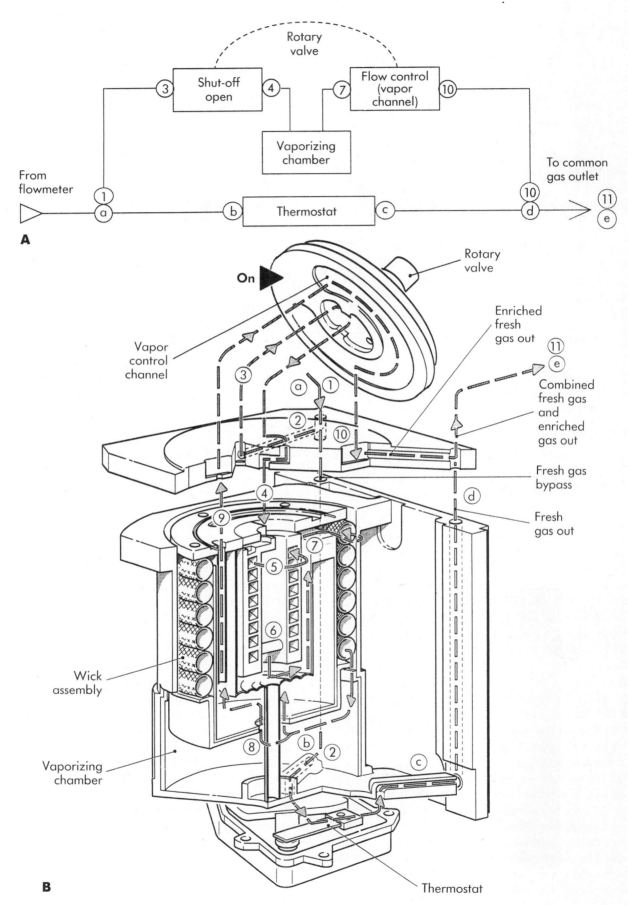

Fig. 3-29. For legend see opposite page.

Fig. 3-29. A, Tec 5 vaporizer flow diagram. **B,** Schematic of Tec 5 vaporizer. Gas flow enters the vaporizer at *(1)*, where it is split into two streams, the bypass circuit and the vaporizing chamber. Gas flows through the bypass circuit vertically downward from *(a)* across the sump base *(b)*, through the thermostat to *(c)*, and back up the gas transfer manifold via *(d)* to *(e)*. Gas flowing to the vaporizing chamber flows from *(1)* across the sump cover *(2)* where it is diverted via *(3)* through the central cavity of the rotary valve and back through the IPPV assembly via *(4)*, *(5)*, and *(6)*. Gas then flows from the IPPV assembly via *(7)* down the tubular wick assembly, where vapor is added, and then flows across the base of the vaporizing chamber above the liquid agent to *(8)*. From here the gas-vapor mixture flows via *(9)* through the sump cover to the proportional radial drug control groove of the rotary valve and back into the sump cover *(10)*, where it merges with gas from the bypass circuit. The total flow then exits the vaporizer into the outlet port of the Selectatec manifold. (Reproduced by permission of Ohmeda, a Division of BOC Health Care, Inc, Madison, Wis.)

3-30). In such a situation one of the two outer vaporizers should be moved to the center position so that the vaporizers can be adjacent.

Selectatec systems manufactured since 1987 and fitted to the Ohmeda Modulus II Plus and subsequent models of Ohmeda anesthesia machines are designed such that if the middle vaporizer is removed (Fig. 3-31), extrusion of the lateral rod of one vaporizer is transmitted to the other via vertical plates joined by a communicating bar. Thus with this contemporary Selectatec system the vaporizer interlock is effective even if the center vaporizer is removed.

DESFLURANE

Desflurane* is a new potent inhaled volatile anesthetic currently undergoing clinical investigation in the United

*Suprane™, Anaquest, Liberty Corner, N.J.

States. The physical properties are shown in Table 3-2. This agent is extremely volatile, having an SVP of 664 mm Hg at 20° C and a boiling point of 23.5° C at an ambient pressure of 760 mm Hg (Fig. 3-32). This presents certain problems related to vaporization and production of a controlled concentration of vapor. There are at least four possible methods for controlling the vapor output concentration of desflurane.

Heated, pressurized measured-flow vaporizing system. This technique is employed in the now discontinued Ohio DM (Direct Metering) 5000 machine.[19] This machine was, however, used for many of the clinical trials of desflurane.

The DM 5000 machine has two important design features that make it suitable for producing controlled concentrations of desflurane. First, it incorporates a heated, measured-flow vaporizer (analogous to a heated Copper

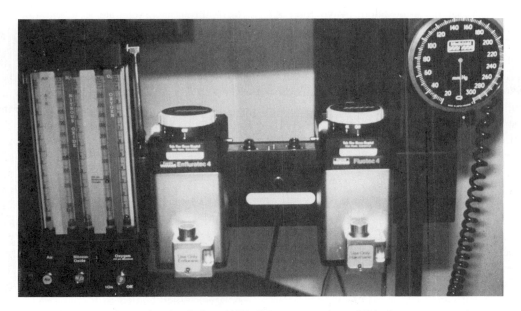

Fig. 3-30. Limitations of early (before 1987) Selectatec systems. With the center vaporizer removed, lateral extension of rods caused by turning on one vaporizer is not transmitted to the other. Thus both vaporizers could be on simultaneously.

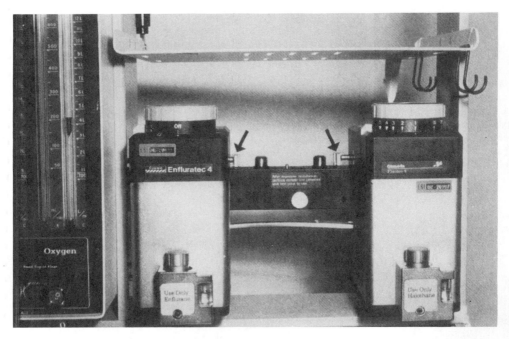

Fig. 3-31. Contemporary Selectatec system. In this design (first fitted to Ohmeda Modulus II machines in 1987) the outward movement of the extension rod of one vaporizer is transmitted via the communicating bars *(arrows)* to prevent the other vaporizer being turned on.

Kettle). Second, the low-pressure parts of the machine between the gas flow-control needle valves and the common gas outlet are maintained at a pressure of 1550 mm Hg. This pressurization is achieved with an altitude compensator valve (also called a back-pressure regulator), located at the common gas outlet. In the DM 5000's vaporizer, desflurane is heated to a temperature of 23 to 25° C, at which its SVP is approximately 770 mm Hg. In the vaporizing chamber desflurane vapor therefore represents 770/1550, or approximately 50%, of the atmosphere by volume. A separate flowmeter is used to control the flow of oxygen to the vaporizer. For each milliliter of oxygen entering the vaporizer, 2 ml of gas emerges, of which 1 ml is desflurane vapor and 1 ml is oxygen. This flowmeter, although actually controlling flow of oxygen to the vaporizer, is calibrated in milliliters desflurane vapor output. A measured-flow arrangement (i.e., main flowmeters for nitrous oxide air, and total flow of oxygen) is used to dilute the desflurane vapor emerging from the vaporizer down to clinically useful concentrations. Upstream of the common gas outlet, the gas mixture (nitrous oxide/air/oxygen/desflurane) is at an absolute pressure of 1550 mm Hg. As it emerges from the machine's common gas outlet to an atmospheric pressure of 760 mm Hg, the volume of the gas mixture doubles (Boyle's law) but the proportions of the components in the original mixture are maintained. Indeed, the DM 5000 flowmeters are calibrated in volumes of gas delivered at atmospheric pressure. As with any measured-flow arrangement, errors in calculation are always a potential hazard.

When such a heated pressurized system is in operation,

an anesthetic agent analyzer should be used continuously to monitor the concentration of the delivered anesthetic, and high-concentration-limit alarms should be enabled to protect against possible overdosing. It is again emphasized that the DM 5000 machine is not available for general clinical use but only for desflurane clinical trials.

Heat liquid to form vapor under pressure. Desflurane can be heated in a sump to >24° C to form a vapor under pressure. This vapor is then metered into the main gas flow through a separate concentration-calibrated vapor flow-control system. A potential limitation of this method is that desflurane vapor might condense to liquid in parts of the delivery system intended only for gas or vapor. A universally heated concentration-calibrated vaporizing system (as distinct from the measured-flow system just described) would address these considerations (see the description of the Tec 6 vaporizer).

Liquid injection. Desflurane liquid in small metered doses can be vaporized into known fresh-gas flows to produce clinically useful concentrations. Thus, 1 ml of liquid desflurane produces 207 ml of desflurane vapor at 20° C (see Table 3-2). This system is analogous to fuel injection systems used in automobile engines and has been used to deliver halothane, enflurane, and isoflurane in certain anesthesia delivery systems, such as the Engstrom ELSA and the Boston Anesthesia Machine (see Chapter 33).

Cooled, variable-bypass concentration-calibrated vaporizer. When cooled to 5° C, desflurane has an SVP of approximately 250 mm Hg (Fig. 3-32), and could thus be administered using a conventional variable-bypass concen-

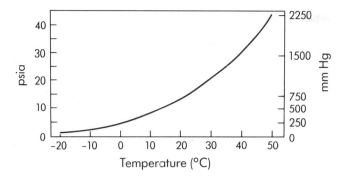

Fig. 3-32. Desflurane (Suprane) saturated vapor pressure in relation to temperature. Compare with Fig. 3-2. (Drawn from data provided by Anaquest, Liberty Corner, NJ.)

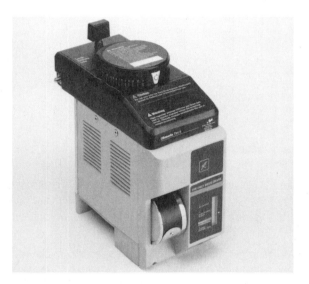

Fig. 3-33. Ohmeda Tec 6 vaporizer for desflurane. (Reproduced by permission of Ohmeda, a Division of BOC Health Care, Inc., Madison, Wis.)

tration-calibrated (Tec type) vaporizer. However, cooling a vaporizer to maintain a constant low temperature presents many technical problems and is energy inefficient.

When desflurane becomes available for general clinical use, it is clear that it will require a vaporizing system that differs from those used for the presently available potent inhaled agents. A desflurane vaporizer will likely use one of the methodologies described above, all of which require a source of energy (electricity). General requirements of the desflurane vaporizer will be that it deliver accurate concentrations over a wide range of gas flows and that it be easily retrofitted to contemporary anesthesia machines by replacement of one of the existing machine-mounted and interlocked vaporizers. Agent-specific filling devices will be essential on bottles of desflurane to ensure that the agent is not accidentally poured into a conventional vaporizer designed for another agent (see Chapter 16). The desflurane vaporizer will also require an agent-specific filling device to ensure that it is never filled with an agent other than desflurane.

Ohmeda Tec 6 vaporizer

At the time of writing (April 1992), desflurane has not been approved for general clinical use by the Food and Drug Administration (FDA). In anticipation of its approval and general clinical use, the Tec 6 vaporizer* has been developed for the controlled administration of desflurane.[20] Prototypes of this vaporizer are currently being used in place of the DM 5000 machine at centers where clinical trials of desflurane are being conducted. The Ohmeda Tec 6 is a concentration-calibrated vaporizer designed to make the clinical administration of desflurane no different from that of any of the other commonly used potent agents in Tec-type vaporizers. The Tec 6 (Fig. 3-33) is very similar in appearance to the Tec 5 vaporizers used for halothane, enflurane, and isoflurane but has a power cord. It is designed to be mounted on an anesthesia machine equipped with a Selectatec manifold. As with other Tec Series vaporizers designed for use with the Selectatec vaporizer mounting system, mechanical interlocks prevent the vaporizer from being turned on if not locked onto the manifold and an interlock device prevents simultaneous use of more than one vaporizer. A manually operated concentration dial is used to set the desired output concentration of desflurane. As with the Tec 4 and 5 vaporizers, a dial release button must first be depressed in order to turn on the vaporizer.

Principles of operation. The principle of operation of the Tec 6 (Fig. 3-34) is that liquid desflurane is heated in a chamber to 39° C to produce desflurane vapor under pressure (approximately 1500 mm Hg; see Fig. 3-32). The variable pressure-regulating valve is continuously adjusted by an output from the pressure sensor to ensure that the pressure of the desflurane vapor entering the rotary valve is the same as the pressure generated by the fresh-gas inflow to a fixed restrictor. The concentration dial and rotary valve control the quantity of desflurane vapor added to the fresh-gas flow so that the dialed-in concentration of desflurane is what emerges from the vaporizer. Thus, unlike other concentration-calibrated vaporizers, such as the Tec 5 and Dräger Vapor 19.1, which are of the variable bypass design (i.e., some fresh gas enters the vaporizing chamber, see Fig. 3-3), in the Tec 6 vaporizer no fresh gas enters the vaporizing chamber.

Design and operational features. The following sections describe in more detail the design and operational features of the Ohmeda Tec 6 vaporizer. A schematic of the Tec 6 is shown in Fig. 3-35. The numbers in parentheses refer to the numbered items in Fig. 3-35.

The vaporizer sump *(1)* is filled with liquid desflurane and when full contains 450 ml of agent *(2)*. The level of the agent is sensed electronically *(3)* and shown on a liquid

*Ohmeda, BOC Health Care, Steeton, West Yorkshire, U.K.

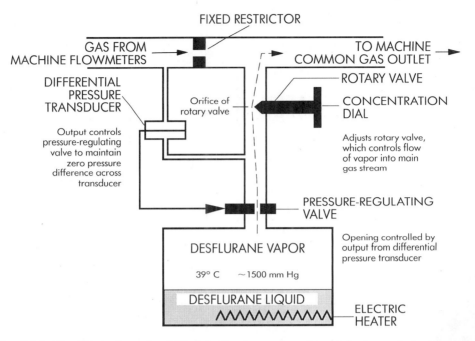

Fig. 3-34. Simplified schematic of Ohmeda Tec 6 vaporizer. Liquid desflurane is heated in the sump to 39° C to produce vapor under pressure (approximately 1500 mmHg). The pressure-regulating valve is continuously adjusted by an output from the differential pressure transducer to ensure that the pressure of the desflurane vapor upstream of the rotary valve is the same as the pressure of the fresh gas inflow to the fixed restrictor. The concentration dial and rotary valve control the quantity of desflurane vapor added to the fresh-gas flow so that emerging from the vaporizer outlet is the dialed-in concentration of desflurane. Thus in the Tec 6 vaporizer no fresh gas enters the desflurane vaporizing chamber. This is in contrast to the other Ohmeda Tec vaporizers, which are of the variable bypass design.

crystal display (LCD)*(23)*. When the vaporizer is energized by connecting the power cord *(26)* to an AC electrical outlet, the 200-watt heater elements *(4)* in the sump heat the liquid agent to 39° C. This creates desflurane vapor under pressure (SVP at 39° C = 1550 mm Hg, see Fig. 3-32). Agent temperature in the sump is monitored by a resistive device and other electronics, which function as a thermostat *(15)* to maintain the temperature at 39° C. During warm-up, a light-emitting diode (LED) display *(19)* on the front panel of the vaporizer indicates that the agent is being heated. While the agent is being heated the shut-off valve *(5)* is held closed, thus containing the vapor in the sump. During this time the pressure transducers *(11,12)* perform a zero check.

Once the desflurane in the sump reaches a temperature of 39° C, the LED *(19)* changes color to indicate that warm-up is completed and the vaporizer is now at operational status. Until this status has been reached, the solenoid dial lock *(8)* keeps the vaporizer dial locked, preventing the dial from being turned from the standby position. Operational status having been attained, the control electronics *(16)* release the dial lock *(8)* and, when the dial is turned from standby, the shut-off valve is opened *(5)*. This permits desflurane vapor under pressure to flow to the pressure-regulating valve *(6)*.

As fresh gas flows through the vaporizer, it encounters a flow restrictor *(10)*, creating a back pressure that is applied to one side of the differential pressure transducer *(11)*. The pressure due to desflurane vapor is applied to the other side of the pressure transducer, which senses any difference between these two pressures and transmits this information to the control electronics *(16)*. The control electronics then adjust the pressure due to the desflurane vapor by opening or closing the pressure-regulating valve *(6)* until there is zero pressure difference across the pressure transducer *(11)*.

The vaporizer concentration control dial and rotary valve *(7)* regulate the actual quantity of desflurane vapor available for addition to the fresh-gas inflow. With a zero pressure differential present across the pressure transducer, the concentration of agent added to the fresh-gas stream is determined almost wholly by the ratio of flow restrictions that the fixed restrictor *(10)* and the rotary valve impose on their respective flows. Rotating the dial *(7)* counterclockwise opens the rotary valve more, permitting more desflurane vapor to mix with the fresh-gas flow, thereby increasing the concentration of vapor output.

In order to prevent condensation of desflurane vapor, in addition to the heating elements in the sump *(4)* there is a 200-watt heating element in the rotary valve plate *(24)* to

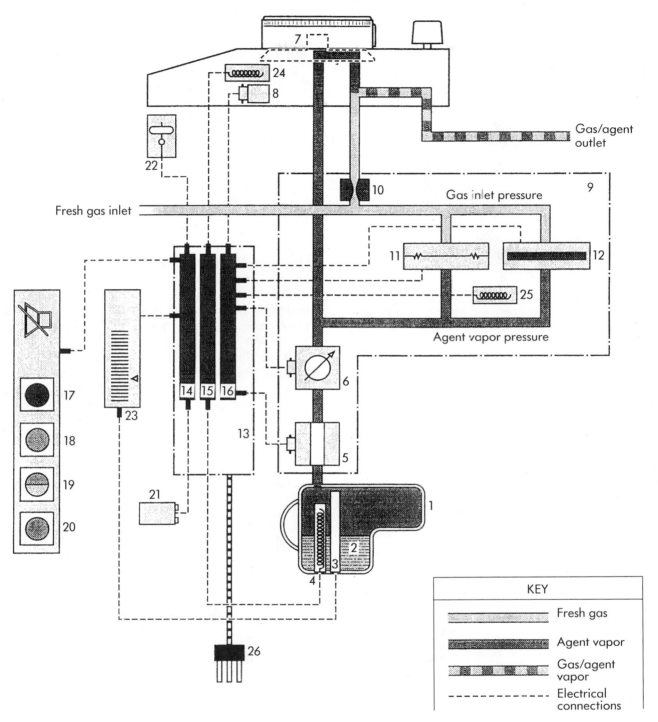

Fig. 3-35. Schematic of Ohmeda Tec 6 desflurane vaporizer. For details of operation, see text. *1,* sump assembly; *2,* liquid desflurane; *3,* level sensor; *4,* sump heaters to heat agent to 39° C; *5,* shut-off valve; *6,* pressure-regulating valve; *7,* concentration dial and rotary valve; *8,* solenoid dial-lock; *9,* vapor control manifold assembly; *10,* fixed restrictor; *11,* pressure transducer; *12,* pressure monitor; *13,* power supply; *14,* alarm electronics printed circuit board (PCB); *15,* heater electronics PCB; *16,* control electronics PCB; *17,* "No output" warning light emitting diode (LED); *18,* "Low agent" warning LED; *19,* "Warm up/operational" LED; *20,* "Alarm battery low" LED; *21,* Back-up battery to power alarms; *22,* tilt switch that shuts down vaporizer if it is tilted excessively; *23,* liquid crystal sump agent level display; *24,* heater to prevent condensation of desflurane in valve plate; *25,* heater to prevent condensation of desflurane in vapor-control manifold; *26,* electrical power cord. (Reproduced from *Provisional Ohmeda Tec 6 vaporizer operation and maintenance manual [April 1992].* By permission of Ohmeda, a Division of BOC Health Care Inc., Madison, Wis.)

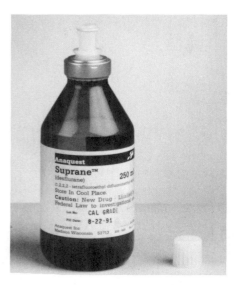

Fig. 3-36. Desflurane (Suprane) bottle. Note the permanently attached agent-specific filling device that normally seals the bottle and whereby the Tec 6 vaporizer can be filled. (Courtesy of Ohmeda, a Division of BOC Health Care Inc., Madison, Wis.)

in the Tec 6 no fresh-gas flow enters the vaporizing chamber. The Tec 6 requires electrical power and incorporates sophisticated electronics to ensure normal operation and a display panel to inform the user about operational status. The Tec 6 vaporizer also incorporates auditory and visual alarms that alert the user to any malfunction. In the event of an AC mains power failure, the vaporizer shuts down automatically and the alarm power supply is then derived from the 9-volt back-up battery. Alarms that may be annunciated include power failure (AC supply), high temperature (>45° C), dry sump, tilt, low temperature (<39° C = warm-up), low drug level (<50 ml), low battery power and vaporizer control system failure.

Filling system. It is essential that desflurane be used only in a vaporizer specifically designed for this agent. Desflurane (Suprane) will be supplied in plastic-coated glass bottles to which a special agent-specific filling device is firmly crimped (Fig. 3-36). The filling device is thus effectively a permanent part of the bottle and incorporates a valve which seals the bottle. The bottle is plastic-coated to prevent loss of agent in the event that the glass becomes cracked. When the vaporizer is at operational status and the agent temperature in the sump is 39° C, the pressure in the sump is approximately 1500 mm Hg (Fig. 3-32). The vaporizer incorporates an agent-specific filling system (Fig. 3-37) that permits filling of the sump at any time. This includes when the vaporizer is first powered up, during warm-up, and while in use, without loss of pressure or agent vapor. If, however, the vaporizer is filled while desflurane is being administered, the fresh-gas flow should be

heat the concentration dial and rotary valve *(7)*, and in the vapor control manifold assembly *(9)* to heat the pressure transducer *(11)* and pressure sensor *(12)*.

Internally, the Ohmeda Tec 6 vaporizer thus differs considerably from the conventional concentration-calibrated vaporizers used for halothane, enflurane, and isoflurane. The latter are of the variable bypass design, whereas

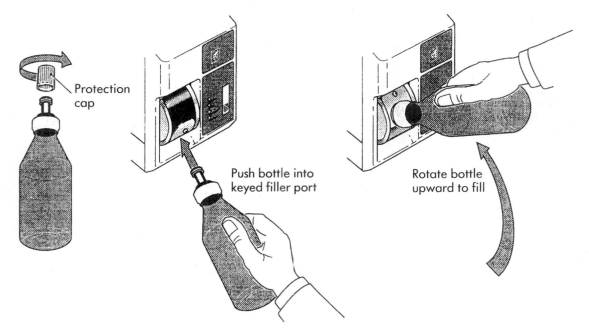

Protection cap

Push bottle into keyed filler port

Rotate bottle upward to fill

Fig. 3-37. Ohmeda Tec 6 vaporizer. Agent-specific filling system for desflurane. (Reproduced from *Provisional Ohmeda Tec 6 vaporizer operation and maintenance manual* [April 1992]. By permission of Ohmeda, a Division of BOC Health Care Inc., Madison, Wis.)

not more than 6 L/min; otherwise, delivered vapor output concentration may decrease.

In order to fill the vaporizer, the protective cap is first removed from the filling device on the agent-specific bottle (Fig. 3-37). The device is then fitted into the filling port on the vaporizer in the lower position and pushed against the spring pressure, into the filler port (Fig. 3-37). The bottle is then rotated upward, thereby locking the bottle to the filler port. When, as a result of upward rotation, the bottle reaches the upper stop, desflurane flows from the bottle, through the filler port, and into the vaporizer sump. The bottle must be held in this position throughout vaporizer filling. During filling, the high pressure (approximately 1500 mm Hg) of vapor at 39° C in the sump is transmitted to the interior of the bottle, which helps drive desflurane liquid into the vaporizer sump. It is because of the high pressure in the sump that the Tec 6 does not incorporate a sight-glass (as used in the other Tec series and Dräger Va-

por 19.1 vaporizers) whereby the agent level can be viewed directly; instead, an agent level sensor is used in the sump and the agent level is displayed on an LCD (Fig. 3-35, *23*) on the vaporizer's front panel. When the LCD level gauge shows the sump to be full, desflurane ceases to flow from the bottle, which is then rotated downward from the upper to the lower (stop) position. This action closes the vaporizer filling valve and prevents loss of pressure from the sump. Once the bottle reaches the lower (stop) position, the bottle is unlocked and released under spring pressure. The valve on the bottle closes automatically to avoid loss or spillage of desflurane. At this time the bottle contains vapor at 39° C and at a pressure of approximately 1500 mm Hg. However, as the bottle and its contents cool down to room temperature (usually 20° C), the pressure in the bottle decreases to approximately atmospheric (see Fig. 3-32 for saturated vapor pressure of desflurane at various temperatures).

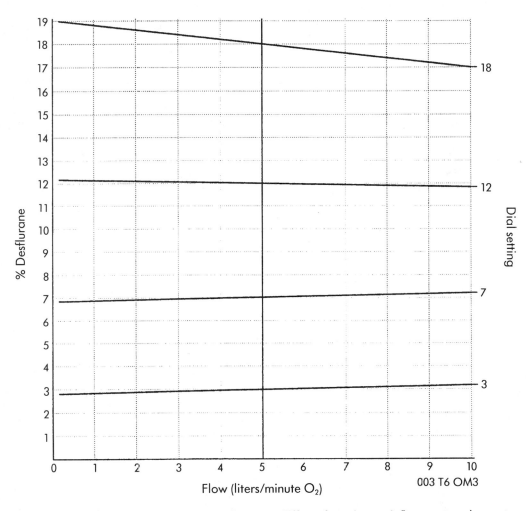

Fig. 3-38. Ohmeda Tec 6 vaporizer performance. Effect of gas (oxygen) flow on vaporizer output. (Reproduced from *Ohmeda Tec 6 vaporizer provisional operation and maintenance manual* [April 1992]. By permission of Ohmeda, a Division BOC Health Care Inc., Madison, Wis.)

Calibration and performance. The concentration dial of the Ohmeda Tec 6 is calibrated for desflurane outputs from 0% to 18% (1% graduations from 0% to 10%; 2% from 10% to 18%) using oxygen as the gas flowing at 5 L/min. The effect of the oxygen flow rate on desflurane output concentration is shown in Fig. 3-38. At oxygen flows of up to 10 L/min and concentration dial settings of up to 12% (approximately 2 MAC) the vaporizer output is extremely accurate. Administration of desflurane should therefore be as easy and convenient as that for the other currently approved potent volatile anesthetics.

FDA approval. The foregoing description applies to the prototype Ohmeda Tec 6 vaporizer. At the time of writing (August 1992) this device was not commercially available and had not yet received FDA approval. It is possible that further modifications may be made before such units are made generally available. The 510(k) application to the FDA for this product is currently under review.

ACKNOWLEDGMENT

The author is most grateful to Ohmeda, a Division of BOC Health Care Inc., Madison, Wis., for providing and permitting the reproduction of technical information concerning the Tec 6 vaporizer.

REFERENCES

1. Hill DW: *Physics applied to anaesthesia,* ed 4, Boston, 1980, Butterworths, p 220.
2. American Society for Testing and Materials: Minimum performance and safety requirements for components and systems of anesthesia gas machines, F1161-88, Philadelphia, Pa, March 1989.
3. Parbrook GD, Davis PD, Parbrook EO: *Basic physics and measurement in anesthesia,* ed 2, Norwalk, Conn, 1986, Appleton-Century-Crofts.
4. Fink BR: How much anesthetic? *Anesthesiology* 34:403-404, 1971.
5. James MFM, White JF: Anesthesia considerations at moderate altitude, *Anesth Analg* 63:1097-1105, 1984.
6. Keenan RL: Volatile agent overdose is potential cause of catastrophe, *Anesthesia Patient Safety Foundation (ASPF) Newsletter* 3(2):13, June 1988.
7. Ohio Medical Products. Operations and maintenance manual, Ohio calibrated vaporizers for ethrane, halothane and forane. Ohmeda (formerly Ohio), Madison, Wis.
8. *Understanding the Tec 4 vaporizer,* Steeton, UK, July 1985, Ohmeda.
9. *Narkomed 3 anesthesia system. Operator's instruction manual,* Telford, Pa, 1986, North America Dräger.
10. *Dräger Vapor 19.1 operating instructions,* Lubeck, Germany, Drägerwerk AG.
11. Bruce DL, Linde HW: Vaporization of mixed anesthesia liquids, *Anesthesiology* 60:342-346, 1984.
12. Korman B, Ritchie IM: Chemistry of halothane-enflurane mixtures applied to anesthesia, *Anesthesiology* 63:152-156, 1985.
13. *Ohmeda Tec 5 continuous flow vaporizer. Operations and maintenance manual,* Madison, Wis, 1989, Ohmeda.
14. *Tec 4 Continuous flow vaporizer. Operations and maintenance manual,* Madison, Wis, 1989, Ohmeda.
15. Scheller MS, Drummond JC: Solubility of N_2O in volatile anesthetics contributes to vaporizer aberrancy when changing carrier gases *Anesth Analg* 65:88-90, 1986.
16. Murray WJ, Zsigmond EK, Fleming P: Contamination of in-series vaporizers with halothane-methoxyflurane, *Anesthesiology* 38:487-489, 1973.
17. Marks WE, Bullard JR: Another hazard of free-standing vaporizers Increased anesthetic concentration with reversed flow of vaporizing gas, *Anesthesiology* 45:445, 1976.
18. Silvasi DL, Haynes A, Brown ACD: Potentially lethal failure of the vapor exclusion system, *Anesthesiology* 71:289-291, 1990.
19. *Ohmeda heated vaporizer anesthesia machine (DM 5000) operation and maintenance manual,* Madison, Wis, 1989, Ohmeda, a Division of BOC Health Care, Inc.
20. *Tec 6 Vaporizer. Operation and maintenance manual,* Ohmeda, A BOC Health Care Company, July 1991, Steeton, UK.

Chapter 4

ANESTHESIA BREATHING SYSTEMS

Theodore Craig Smith, M.D.

The anesthesia machine serves to compound anesthetic gases, vapors, oxygen, air, and (infrequently) other gases, such as helium and carbon dioxide. The patient is the object of delivery of these gas mixtures. The breathing circuit is the interface between the two. It serves to *deliver* the gas mixture from the machine to the patient, to *remove* carbon dioxide, to *exclude* air, and to *condition* temperature and humidity. It converts continuous gas flow from the anesthesia machine to an intermittent flow of breathing, facilitates controlled or assisted respiration, and provides for such other functions as gas sampling, pressure measurements, and spirometric measurements.

The desirable characteristics of a breathing circuit include low resistance to gas flow, minimal rebreathing of the preceding alveolar expirate, removal of carbon dioxide at the rate at which it is produced, rapid changes in delivered gas composition when required, warmed humidification of the inspirate, and safe disposal of waste gases. The components of breathing circuits include the breathing tubing, respiratory valves, reservoir bags, carbon dioxide absorption canisters, a fresh gas inflow site, a pop-off valve leading to a scavenger for excess gas, a Y piece and mask or tube mount, and a mask or tracheal tube. Other devices that may be included are the detecting mechanisms for airway pressure, spirometry, and gas analysis; valves for positive end-expiratory pressure (PEEP); humidifiers; and filters. Vaporizers for potent inhaled agents are no longer placed inside a breathing circuit for reasons of practical safety. These circuit components can be assembled in many ways for specific reasons. Understanding the function of each and the reasons for its use makes rational choices possible.

HISTORICAL DEVELOPMENT OF DEVICES

Breathing circuits have been an important concern from the start. Morton was late to his first public exhibition of "Somniferon" due to a delay in the production of his inhaler. The earliest circuits were mechanically simple; their differences depended on the characteristics of the primary anesthetic agent. Because nitrous oxide and ether anesthetic mixtures were weak or slow to produce anesthesia, it was necessary to exclude air and helpful to include oxygen enrichment. The rapid onset of action and potency of chloroform, on the other hand, demanded accurate control. Certain features became apparent: The ability to assist respiration was advantageous, as was conservation of costly agents and avoidance of large leaks of flammable ones. In the twentieth century, a large number of relatively small but more highly engineered improvements were made as other demands on the breathing circuit were recognized. Dennis Jackson devised the first carbon dioxide absorber to save on the cost of nitrous oxide for animal studies.[1] Ralph Waters brought the idea into the operating room, designing a to-and-fro absorption canister that used soda lime.[2,3] Bryan Sword introduced the first circle breathing circuit in 1930.[4] Thus low-flow absorption systems were already familiar when cyclopropane made them essential. A return to high flows in the United States was brought about by the poor performances of vaporizers for halothane in the 1950s, with the demonstration that such flows could eliminate carbon dioxide without the use of soda lime.[5,6] Today, in addition to factors of convenience and economy, circuits are used to control heat and humidity; to monitor the patient through measurement of tidal volume, respiratory frequency, airway pressure, and inspired and expired gas concentrations; and finally, to control the pollution of the operating room environment by the agents themselves.

Stimulated by Magill's use of a number of pieces of apparatus put together in differing order for differing purposes, Mapleson described a variety of Magill's circuits.[7] The original Ayre's T-piece was modified by innumerable practitioners: the Jackson-Rees circuit represents one such outgrowth.[8] A variety of proprietary nonrebreathing valves were introduced, and the circuits named for them included the Stephen-Slater,[9] the Fink,[6] the Frumin,[11] and the Ruben.[10]

Partial rebreathing and functionally nonrebreathing circuits such as the Bain,[12] Humphrey ADE,[13] and the Lack[14] systems found various proponents. Ingenious switching valves permit transfiguration from one circuit to another.[13] This led to difficulty in remembering which circuit was optimal for what purpose.

The 150-year history of development of the breathing circuit offers to the practitioner a number of choices of breathing circuits. All practical circuits in common use accomplish their goals more or less equivalently, but the simple act of increasing fresh gas flow, for example, may markedly increase the work of breathing.[15] To meet needs conveniently, dependably, and inexpensively, the anesthesiologist needs to understand the functional characteristics of each circuit.

CLASSIFICATIONS OF BREATHING CIRCUITS

A widely used nomenclature developed that classified circuits as open, semiopen, semiclosed, or closed, according to whether a reservoir was used and whether rebreathing occurred. An open system has no reservoir and no rebreathing; a semiopen system has a reservoir but no rebreathing; a semiclosed system has a reservoir and partial rebreathing; and a closed system has a reservoir and complete rebreathing (Box 4-1). Variations on this classification included the type of carbon dioxide absorber and

---

Box 4-1. Classification of breathing circuits

Classification	Examples*
Open	Open-drop ether or Ayre's T piece
Semiopen	Frumin valve system; most self-inflating resuscitator systems
Semiclosed	Magill attachment or Bain system
Closed	Circle system or Waters to-and-fro circuit

*Circuits may function differently at different fresh-gas flows.

---

unidirectional valves used. Because of confusion with this traditional nomenclature, Hamilton recommended its abandonment in favor of a description of the hardware (e.g., circle filter system, coaxial circuit, T-piece) and the gas flow rates being used.[16] Identifying the circuits by eponym (e.g., Adelaid, Bain, Hafnia, Humphrey, Jackson-Rees, Lack, Magill, Waters) did not help in understanding the function or application of the circuit. Almost all anesthesia machines are equipped with some form of a circle breathing circuit (described below) with the facility for carbon dioxide absorption during low-flow anesthesia and carbon dioxide elimination through the pop-off valve during high-flow anesthesia. Because an understanding of *how* circuits work is essential, in this chapter breathing circuits are organized by method of carbon dioxide elimination.

Three methods for removal of carbon dioxide are available:

1. *By chemical absorption of carbon dioxide.* Closed systems (circle or to-and-fro) rely on this technique. Exhaled carbon dioxide is absorbed, and all other exhaled gases are rebreathed. The quantities of fresh oxygen and anesthetics that need to be added are those that replace uptake, metabolic losses, and circuit leaks.[3,17,18]
2. *By dilution with fresh gas.* Because of the intermittent nature of carbon dioxide excretion (during exhalation only) and the continuous inflow of fresh gas, the locations of the inflow site, reservoir bag, and pop-off valves and the choice of inflow rate may all contribute to the efficiency of carbon dioxide removal. When fresh-gas flows are 1 to 1½ times the minute volume (approximately 10 L/min in an adult), dilution alone is sufficient to remove carbon dioxide.[17,19-23] Such systems then behave as if they were nonrebreathing.
3. *By use of valves to separate exhaled gases from inhaled gases.* Systems using nonrebreathing valves are examples of this method of carbon dioxide removal.[6,9,11,24,25] A circuit that by virtue of high flows *behaves as if it were nonrebreathing* is not considered a nonrebreathing circuit in this analysis.

Techniques such as use of open-drop ether or use of a T-piece without a reservoir release exhaled carbon dioxide into the atmosphere. Although similar to the second method above, they are not really "breathing circuits." The

T-pieces with an expiratory reservoir rely on dilution of carbon dioxide by both fresh gas and room air for its removal and have been included in semiclosed circuits below.[26]

COMPONENTS OF A BREATHING CIRCUIT

The circuits described below have many features in common. They connect to the patient's airway through a mask or tracheal tube adapted to the breathing circuit through a Y piece or elbow. They may include tubing through which the patient inspires, exhales, or both. The system may include valves to permit directional gas flow. There is almost always a reservoir bag (a counterlung that moves reciprocally with the patient's lungs). Fresh gas must be supplied to and excessive gas must be removed from the circuit. In some, carbon dioxide is absorbed in a chemical filter. There may be a variety of ancillary devices, such as humidifiers, spirometers, pressure gauges, filters, gas analyzers, positive end-expiratory pressure devices, waste gas scavengers, and mixing and circulating devices.

Connection of the patient to the breathing circuit

Either an anesthesia mask or a tracheal tube connects the circuit to the patient. Masks are made of rubber or clear plastic (to make visible secretions or vomitus). Most have an inflatable or inflated cuff, a pneumatic cushion that seals to the face. Masks come in a variety of sizes and styles to accommodate the wide variety of facial contours. For example, a prominent nasal bridge may prevent a tight fit if the mask's cuff is flat at that point. A prominent chin (mentum) with sunken alveolar ridge causes a leak at the corner of the mouth. The volume of the mask contributes to apparatus dead space. The mask should fit between the interpupillary line over the nose and the groove between the mental process and the alveolar ridge (Fig. 4-1, *A*). The average length of this area is 85 to 90 mm in adults. The newest disposable plastic masks in medium and large sizes are 110 to 140 mm in length. A medium-size mask is too large for most patients unless the fit is made with the cushion over the mental ridge and above the eyebrows, but its very large cushion permits a fairly good seal. Positioning a mask in this way poses the possibility of damage to the ocular and supraorbital nerves from pressure. Choosing from a selection of sizes and styles of mask is more rational than "one size fits all." Masks often have a ring of prongs for attachment to a rubber mask holder; but this mask holder, if pulled too tight, may obstruct the airway. Masks connect to the Y piece or elbow via a 22-mm (⅞ inch) female connection.

Tracheal tubes, standardized by the former Z79 committee of the American National Standards Institute, bear the letters IT (for Implant Tested) or Z79. They are commonly disposable and usually supplied in sterile packages, although no data exist to show this reduces infection.[27]

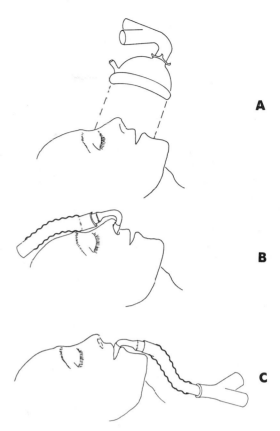

Fig. 4-1. A, A mask's cushion fits over the nose at the interpupillary line and above the mental process. **B,** The tracheal tube is connected to the breathing circuit by a metal or plastic connector that usually fits the tube tightly at one end. Outside diameters of up to 12 mm are commercially available, and all end in a 15-mm slip joint for connection to the circuit. Straight connectors are usual, but 90° curved connectors for oral use and 135° curved connectors for nasal use provide convenient "low-profile" modifications. **C,** This optional malleable 4-inch extension between the connector and the Y piece appears in **B** and **C.**

Important features include a clear plastic material to make visible secretions in the interior, imprinted measures of the distance from the tip to the connector to determine how deeply the tracheal tube is inserted, an inside diameter related to the resistance to breathing, and a relatively large volume nonelastic cuff to distribute a low-pressure seal over a large area of tracheal mucosa.[28] The cuff should be inflated to a volume that just seals the airway at the peak inflation pressure (the just-seal volume) or that just permits a few milliliters of gas to leak past it at peak inflation (the minimal-leak volume). The cuff should inflate symmetrically and should not push the aperture against the tracheal wall. A second opening, the Murphy eye, on the side of the tube near the end is further insurance against obstructions. A tube ending with a diagonal slant or bevel (longer on the right side) and a natural curve of radius 10 to 15 cm facilitates intubation. The tube must then bend in the opposite direction to follow the course of the trachea. This puts pressure on the anterior tracheal wall, the arytenoids, and interarytenoid membrane (which becomes the fulcrum for this change in angulation). Thus the tube must be stiff enough to hold its curve during transglottic insertion yet flexible enough to conform when pushed deeper. The tracheal tube is commonly fitted with a connector which has a 15-mm 1° taper. Although the tube is usually straight, 90° and 135° bends are available: They minimize protrusion of the tube and connector above the face into a surgical field (Fig. 4-1, *B* and *C*). The tube can be cut to the proper length, but the passage of a suction catheter will be difficult and the use of a stylet virtually impossible. Tubes with a second curve 90° over the chin or a reverse curve 135° past the nose (oral and nasal RAE tubes) are of fixed length. The anesthesiologist has no control over the depth to which these tubes are inserted into the trachea (see also Chapter 26).

A variety of special tubes are available, and many more have been introduced at one time or another. The three most commonly used are reinforced tubes, double-lumen tubes, and laser-resistant tubes. Reinforced tubes have a plastic or wire spiral embedded in the wall to resist kinking. Originally designed for suboccipital neurosurgical procedures with the neck flexed acutely forward, they are often used in intraoral surgery when manipulation might compress a soft tube. They are used unnecessarily in a large number of other cases, in which they are problem-prone. The walls of reinforced tubes are thicker than those of other tubes: Thus for a given outside diameter, the smaller inside diameter offers greater resistance to flow. The walls may delaminate, creating valvelike flaps. A small air bubble created by delamination and not visible on initial inspection may expand while nitrous oxide is used. Inflation of a cuff may constrict the lumen below the reinforcement. Reinforced tubes require a stylet for insertion because they are very flexible, but as a result they put less pressure than the other tubes on the posterior laryngeal wall. If the connector is pushed in too far, past the beginning of the spiral reinforcement, it may obstruct the pilot tube to the cuff. If not pushed in far enough, the tube may kink between the spiral and the connector. The older latex tubes collapsed if the molar teeth bore down on them but sprang back to patency when the dental pressure was released. The newer metal tubes can be bitten into near-complete, permanent occlusion.

Double-lumen tubes are useful in thoracic surgery and certain other procedures where separation of the lungs is desired. Originally designed for differential spirometry, they had a left bronchial lumen with a distal cuff, an opening above the cuff to a lumen serving the right lung, and a tracheal cuff just above that. Subsequently, tubes with a right-sided bronchial cuff were designed to permit operation on the left main bronchus. The proximity of the eparterial (right upper lobe) bronchus to the carina requires either an asymmetric cuff or two very small cuffs. Consequently, accurate placement is more difficult. The lumen of these tubes consists of two D-shaped passages over most of their length; consequently double-lumen tubes offer more resistance to breathing than do single-lumen tubes of equivalent diameter. Thus the largest size possible is usually chosen from the available 35, 37, 39, and 41 French size* tubes. A 37-French tube has an outside diameter greater than most 9-mm internal diameter (ID) tubes, and a 41-French tube has an outside diameter greater than that of a 10-mm tube. Double-lumen tubes require special attention for accurate placement.

Tubes with laser-resistant coatings are often used for airway laser surgery. Anesthesiologists craft some by wrapping copper or aluminum foil around the tube: usually ¼-inch adhesive-backed foil is wrapped in a spiral from the cuff to the connector to serve this purpose. Commercially produced tubes use either a metal cover rather like electrical BX cable or a coating of laser-resistant material that usually contains metal. Because these tubes are expensive they may be reused by some anesthesiologists without the manufacturers' approval. No single design of commercially available laser-resistant tube is clearly superior to the hand-wrapped foil covering. Filling the cuff with water instead of air is recommended (see also Chapter 21, Part I).

Breathing tubing

The tubing used in breathing circuits is usually about one meter in length, has a large bore (22-mm diameter) to minimize resistance to gas flow, and has corrugations or spiral reinforcement to permit flexibility without kinking. The internal volume is 400 to 500 ml per meter of length. Although these tubes were formerly made of conductive rubber, disposable plastic tubing has almost completely replaced rubber. Electrical conductivity is no longer necessary when breathing tubing is used with nonflammable agents. The advantage of plastic is that it is light in weight; but it is not biodegradable, and thus it is disposable by design but not by use. Plastic breathing tubes are supplied sterile despite the lack of convincing epidemiologic data.[27,30] By convention, the ends of the tubing are 22 mm internal diameter (ID) and identical in design. Tubing should be inspected before use because manufacturing errors can result in obstruction of the lumen.[31,32] Distensibility of the tubing varies from nearly 0 ml to over 5 ml per meter length per mm Hg of applied pressure; plastic tubing has lower values than rubber (Table 4-1). Apparent distensibility is even greater because of the compression of gas under pressure. This is of the order of 3% of the volume for typical inflation pressures. Inflation of a patient's lungs to 20 mm Hg peak inspiratory pressure compresses

---

*French size is the tube's external circumference in millimeters. Dividing French size by 3 provides an approximation of the *external* diameter in mm. For single-lumen tubes, dividing the French size by 4 gives an approximation of the *internal* diameter.

Table 4-1. Compliance of Ohio anesthesia breathing circuits

Circuit pressure (cm H$_2$O)	Volume (ml)	
	Conductive rubber	Plastic disposable
10	80	30
15	130	100
20	210	190
25	290	320

From Fluidically Controlled Anesthesia Ventilator Operation and Maintenance Manual. Ohio Medical Products (now BOC Health Care, Madison, Wisconsin) 1974.

30 to 150 ml of gas in the tubing.[33] This volume is not delivered to the patient's lungs, but some fraction of it may be measured by a ventilation meter within the circuit, adding a form of apparatus dead space to the system. The exact fraction depends on where the spirometer is placed in the circuit with respect to the valves.

Resistance to gas flow in standard corrugated breathing tubes is exceedingly small (less than 1 mm of water per liter per minute of flow).[34] When it is desirable to have the anesthesia machine at some distance from the patient's head, several tubes may be connected in series with connectors of 7/8-inch (22-mm) outside diameter. Alternatively, extra long tubing is available, including one that can be compressed to 200 ml of volume in about 50 cm of length or can be stretched to nearly 2 meters of length with an 800 ml volume. These "concertina" extensions do not increase the resistance of the system by any appreciable amount and affect the apparatus dead space only by their compliant volume.

The pattern of gas flow through the circuit is almost always turbulent because of the corrugations in the tubing. This promotes both radial mixing and longitudinal mixing. In documenting performance of one circuit, Spoerel[35] has demonstrated complete mixing of dead space and alveolar gas after gas has passed through one meter of such tubing. A change in gas composition at one end (as when the delivered gas is altered at the anesthesia machine) completes a change in the inspired concentration at the patient connection within two to three breaths. The change in inspired concentration is nearly exactly the change in delivered concentration when high fresh-gas flows are used (10 L/min or more). The change decreases to a nearly imperceptible one as inflow is decreased toward that of closed systems.

Lengths of breathing tubing are sometimes used to connect ventilators to the bag mount and to connect to scavenging devices. Optimally, 19-mm connecting ends on the scavenger mounts prevent inappropriate hookups. Tubing of smaller diameter is made for use in circle systems designed specifically for infants and children. Their resis-

tance to gas flow is insignificantly increased. With less compression volume, measured ventilation is more accurate (see also Chapter 26).

Reusable rubber tubing is connected to the mask or tube by a separate Y piece. Disposable sets often incorporate a Y that may or may not be detachable. Such a Y may be rigid, and it may incorporate an angle elbow or a pair of swivel joints. Although the swivel joints are convenient, they offer a greater chance of leaking. Most connectors have negligible leakage, but those with swivels are twice as likely to leak.[36] Any circuit should be tested before use by determining the oxygen inflow required to maintain 20 cm H$_2$O of pressure in the circuit (see also Chapter 22).

Respiratory valves

Unidirectional respiratory valves are incorporated into a breathing circuit in order to direct gas flow. They are commonly discs on knife edges, or rubber flaps or sleeves. The essential characteristics of respiratory valves in breathing circuits are low resistance and high competence.[37,38] The valves must open widely with little pressure and close rapidly and completely with essentially no backflow. Circle and nonrebreathing systems use two nearly identical valves. The inspiratory valve opens on inspiration and closes on expiration, preventing backflow of exhaled gas in the inspiratory limb. The expiratory valve works in a reciprocal fashion to prevent rebreathing. These valves can be mounted anywhere within the expiratory and inspiratory limbs of the circuit. The only critical feature of their location is that one must be placed between the patient and the reservoir bag in each limb. So located and properly functioning, they prevent any part of the circle system from contributing to apparatus dead space.[39] Thus the only apparatus dead space in such a circuit is the distal limb of the Y connector and any tube or mask between it and the patient's airway. The respiratory valves on most modern anesthesia machines are located near or incorporated into the soda lime canister casting along with a fresh-gas inflow site and excess gas (pop-off) valve. In the past, unidirectional valves have been incorporated into the housing of the Y piece to reduce the apparatus dead space effect of compliant volume, but they have fallen into disfavor because of the weight they add to the mask and (more important) because they will cause an obstruction to respiration if they are accidentally incorporated backward to the conventional valves in the circle.[40] When valved Y pieces were used, it was recommended that circle system valves be removed. Failure to reinsert the circle system valves when a normal nonvalved Y piece was used caused needless complications.

The common valves in anesthetic circuits are dome valves consisting of a circular knife edge occluded by a very light disc of slightly larger diameter (Fig. 4-2). When flow is initiated by the patient's inspiratory effort, when

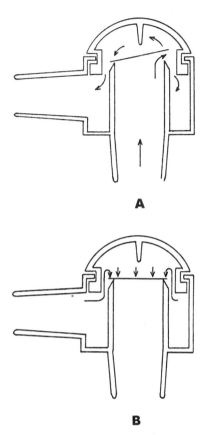

Fig. 4-2. A typical dome valve incorporated into a circle absorber housing. **A,** The valve is in the open position with gas flowing. **B,** Due to back pressure, the plastic disc seats on the knife edge and the valve is closed.

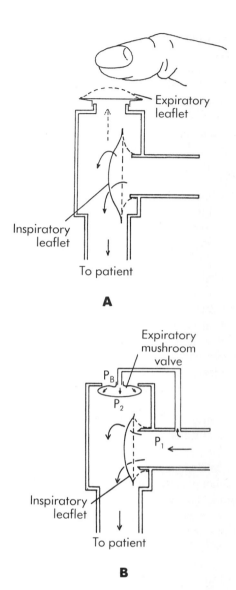

Fig. 4-3. These nonrebreathing valves incorporate two leaflets that open alternately on inspiration or expiration. **A,** In the simplest form the valve functions well during spontaneous ventilation *(solid arrows),* but an attempt to inflate the patient's lungs manually blows open both inspiratory and expiratory leaflets *(dotted arrow)* unless the anesthesiologist simultaneously occludes the expiratory valve with a finger. Several nonrebreathing valves have been designed to overcome the necessity for manual assistance of valve function. **B,** Whenever gas flow opens the inspiratory leaflet, the pressure at point P_1 is greater than at point P_2 or P_B. This pressure difference inflates the mushroom-shaped expiratory balloon, sealing the expiratory limb. If no gas is supplied to the inspiratory limb, spontaneous effort on the part of the patient lowers both P_1 and P_2 well below atmospheric pressure P_B, so that the mushroom valve collapses and the patient inspires room air.

positive pressure is applied to the reservoir bag, or when the ventilator bellows empties, the disc lifts off the knife edge. The disc is contained by a small cage or by the dome itself. It must be hydrophobic so that water condensate does cause it to stick to the knife edge and increase the resistance to opening. Most modern discs are made of hydrophobic plastic and are very light and thin. They require vertical mounting so that the disc will fall properly into the closed position and seal the circuit from backflow. Failure to seal converts a large volume of the circuit into apparatus dead space, resulting in rebreathing. The top of the valve is covered by a removable clear plastic dome so that the disc can be easily seen and periodically cleaned or replaced.

Two respiratory valves create a nonrebreathing system (Fig. 4-3). Nonrebreathing valves permit the patient to inspire from a fresh gas reservoir and exhale into the room or a scavenger. They usually consist of a pair of leaflets, one opening during inspiration and the other during expiration, in the same housing. The early designs (e.g., Digby-Leigh or Steven-Slater) required the anesthesiologist to occlude the expiratory valve with a finger if assisted or controlled ventilation was needed (Fig. 4-3, *A*).[9,24] Inge-

nious designs employing springs, magnets, or flaps automatically close the expiratory valve when respiration is controlled.[41-46] Other designs used the pressure drop across the inspiratory valve to inflate a mushroom-shaped balloon valve (Frumin valve)[11] (Fig. 4-3, *B*) or to depress a dome-shaped cover on the expiratory valve (Fink valve).[6] Resistance is negligible in both of these designs, but the Frumin valve has the marked advantage of collapsing if the inspiratory supply is inadequate, permitting inspiration of room air. The Frumin valve is also lighter in weight and more compact than the others. Some nonrebreathing valves are position-sensitive and must be upright to function properly, and others are not always reliable.[47] Those that use flexible rubber leaflets or collapsible rubber tubing to provide the sealing function are nonpositional. Most nonrebreathing valves connect to masks and/or tracheal tubes, but one can be built into a mask.[46]

Self-inflating resuscitators for air or air/oxygen mixtures use similar valve pairs to control gas flow.[10,48,49] The Ruben valve has an expiratory bobbin-shaped structure that, when open, occludes the inspiratory limb. Anesthetic vapors and secretions tend to expand this bobbin slightly, causing it to jam.[49] Such resuscitator valves should not be used in anesthesia; nor should they be used for transporting patients who are still eliminating anesthetic vapors.

Breathing bags

Breathing bags (reservoir bags or counterlungs) have three principal functions: They serve as a reservoir for anesthetic gases or oxygen from which the patient can inspire; they provide the means for a visual assessment of the existence and rough estimate of the volume of ventilation; and they serve as a means for manual ventilation. A reservoir function is necessary because the anesthesia machines cannot provide the peak inspiratory gas flow needed during normal respiration. While the respiratory minute volume of an anesthetized adult is rarely more than 12 L/min, the peak inspiratory flow rate may reach 50 L/min, and 20 L/min is not uncommon. For example, assume a patient is breathing at a rate of 20 breaths/min with a tidal volume of 500 ml (a minute volume of 10 L/min). If the inspiratory to expiratory (*I:E*) ratio is 1:2, each breath takes one second for inspiration and two seconds for expiration. The tidal volume of 500 ml inspired in one second is an average inspiratory flow (volume per unit time) of 500 ml/sec or 30 L/min. This is many times the commonly used fresh gas flows. The peak flow in mid-inspiration may be 30% to 40% higher.

Assessment of presence and volume of spontaneous ventilation is affected by the fresh gas flow. In low-flow techniques, virtually all the gas inhaled by the patient comes from the reservoir bag: Its excursion thus reflects tidal volume. If the inflow rate from the machine is in excess of 10 L/min, most of the gas inhaled by the patient comes from the fresh gas supply and the reservoir bag shows little excursion. In a spontaneously breathing patient with a circuit gas inflow rate of 6 L/min, nearly half of the tidal volume comes from the inflow, halving the apparent tidal volume as indicated by movement of the bag.

Reservoir bags for anesthesia machines are usually ellipsoidal in shape so that they can be grasped easily with one hand. They are made of nonslippery plastic or latex

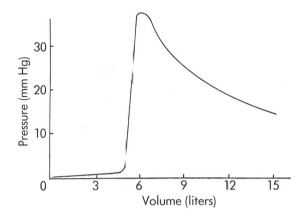

Fig. 4-4. As an anesthesia reservoir bag is filled from its evacuated volume to its nominal volume the pressure increases little, but as the rubber is slightly stretched, a small increase in volume raises the pressure rapidly to some maximum, depending upon the shape and wall thickness of the bag. Further increase in the bag's volume causes a *decrease* in pressure. The falling pressure with rising volume follows Laplace's law, $P = 2T/r$, where P is pressure, the constant T is a function of the bag's thickness and material, and r is the radius.

rubber, in sizes from 0.5 to 6 L. Conductivity is unnecessary. The optimal size is one that holds a volume exceeding the patient's inspiratory capacity; that is, a spontaneous deep breath should not empty the bag. A 3-L bag meets these requirements for most adults and is easy to grasp. Bags with a nipple at the bottom for use as an alternate pop-off site are available but are rarely used.

In circle systems the breathing bag is usually mounted at or near the soda lime canister via a T-shaped fitting, usually near the pop-off valve. The bag may be placed at the end of a third length of corrugated tubing leading from the T-connector, providing some freedom of movement for the anesthesiologist. The pressure-volume characteristics of overinflated bags (Fig. 4-4) become important if the pop-off valve is accidentally left in the closed position and gas inflow continues. Rubber bags become pressure limiting with maximum pressures of 40 to 50 cm H_2O. Prestretching may favorably lower the maximum pressure.[50,51,52] Disposable bags may reach twice the pressure of rubber bags and then rupture abruptly.

Gas inflow and pop-off valves

Gases are delivered from the anesthesia machine to the circuit via thick-walled tubing connected to a nipple incorporated into the circuit. In circle systems this gas inflow nipple is incorporated with the inspiratory unidirectional valve or the soda lime canister housing. Fresh gas inflow may be placed in any portion of the circuit. For circles the preferred inflow site is between the carbon dioxide absorber and the inspiratory valve. The location for other circuits depends on whether breathing is spontaneous, assisted, or controlled because the type of breathing influences the efficiency of carbon dioxide elimination (see below).

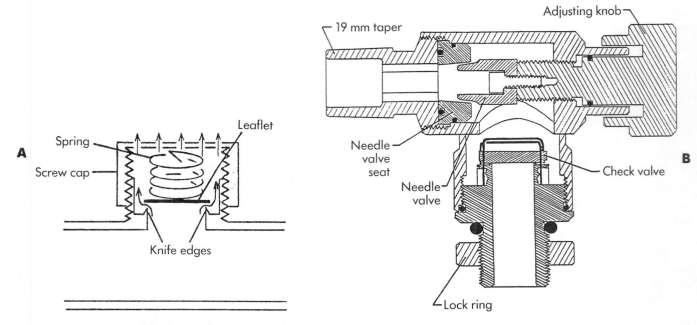

Fig. 4-5. Adjustable pressure limiting (APL or pop-off) valves. **A,** Spring loaded design. When the cap is fully tightened down, the spring is compressed enough to prevent the valve leaflet from lifting at any airway pressure. When the top is loosened and the spring is not compressed at all, the valve opens at a pressure equal to the weight of the leaflet divided by its area, usually less than 1 cm H_2O. **B,** North American Dräger's APL valve design is an adjustable needle valve, the opening of which determines gas flow into the scavenger system. The check valve prevents reverse flow of gas from the scavenger into the patient circuit. (Courtesy of North American Dräger, Inc., Telford, Pa.)

Pop-off valves (overflow, outflow, relief, spill, and adjustable pressure limiting [APL] are synonyms) permit gas to leave the circuit, matching the excess to the inflow of fresh gas. They too may be placed in any portion of a circuit; their efficiency is related in part to the placement of the inflow. There are many different designs, but most are constructed like a dome valve loaded by a spring and screw cap (Fig. 4-5). The valve should open at a pressure of less than 1 cm of water. As the screw cap is tightened down, more and more gas pressure in the circuit is required to open it, permitting PEEP during spontaneous ventilation or pressure-limited controlled respiration. The number of clockwise turns from fully open to fully closed should be one or two. Fewer turns make it difficult to set a desired pressure accurately, and more make it is tedious to use. The exhaust from any of the commonly used pop-off valves can be collected by a scavenging system connected at this point.[53]

The Ohmeda GMS absorber uses an APL valve similar in design to that shown in Fig. 4-5, A, basically a spring-loaded disc. When the spring is fully extended, it exerts a pressure of approximately 1 cm H_2O on the disc to hold the valve closed. This is necessary because connected downstream of the APL valve is the waste-gas scavenging interface. If an *active* scavenging system is used—for example, if suction is applied to the interface—the negative

pressure could potentially be applied to the patient circuit (see Chapter 5). To prevent this the Ohmeda scavenger interface uses a negative pressure relief ("pop-in") valve, which opens at a pressure of -0.25 cm H_2O to allow room air to enter the interface. Thus the greatest negative pressure tending to open the APL valve (-0.25 cm) is less than the least spring tension tending to keep the valve closed (approximately 1.0 cm H_2O). This arrangement protects against application of excess negative pressure (in an active scavenging system) to the breathing circuit. In the fully closed position, the maximum spring pressure applied to the Ohmeda APL valve disc is 75 cm H_2O. Thus, in the manual/bag mode, the circuit pressure in an Ohmeda breathing system is limited to 75 cm H_2O. Note that in the ventilator mode, the circuit pressure is limited by high-pressure-limit settings on the Ohmeda ventilator (up to 120 cm H_2O with the Ohmeda 7800 ventilator; see Chapter 6).

In Dräger anesthesia delivery systems, the design of the APL valve differs from those described above (Fig. 4-5, *B*). This design uses a needle valve instead of a spring-loaded disc. Adjusting the knob of the Dräger APL valve varies the size of the opening between the needle valve and its seat, which in turn adjusts the amount of gas permitted to flow to the scavenger system. A check valve prevents gas from the scavenging system from entering the

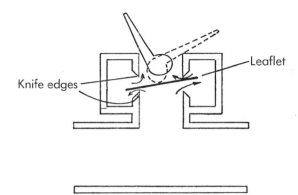

Fig. 4-6. The Steen valve permits gas to exit from a circuit under the slight pressure that occurs during exhalation. A sudden rise in pressure, such as occurs during an assisted or controlled inhalation, however, seals the leaflet against the upper circular knife edge. A lever-operated eccentric cam defeats this effect if desired, and turns the valve into an ordinary pop-off valve that is not spring-loaded.

breathing system. With this design, the needle valve can be totally closed, and therefore it does not function as a true pressure limiter.

Special types of pop-off valves permit spontaneous or assisted respiration without tedious adjustment.[42,54-56] The simplest is the Steen valve (Fig. 4-6), which is essentially two knife-edge valves of the dome type, one inverted over the other, sharing a common disc.[24] A relatively slow flow of gas during the latter part of exhalation (up to 10 L/min) lifts the valve disc at one side only, so that the exhaled gas escapes around the disc. An abrupt increase in pressure lifts the valve vertically, seals it against the upper knife edge, and closes the circuit so that no gas is lost. The Georgia valve adds to the same design a light spring-loading, which increases the range of gas flows that it can exhaust so that it can be used with mechanical ventilators.[57] Most current anesthesia ventilators have such an automatic pop-off valve built in so that gas is exhausted only at end-exhalation (see also Chapter 6).

Carbon dioxide absorption

In partial rebreathing and nonrebreathing systems, carbon dioxide is vented to room air. When a closed system is used, however, the exhaled carbon dioxide must be otherwise removed. Carbon dioxide in the presence of water hydrates to form carbonic acid. When carbonic acid reacts with a metal hydroxide, the reaction is one of neutralization that results in the formation of water, a metal bicarbonate or carbonate, and the generation of heat. This reaction is utilized in anesthesia for carbon dioxide absorption.[58] In the reactions shown below only the molecular forms of the reactants are written. The reactions actually proceed by initial ionization in the thin film of water at the surfaces of the absorbent. In soda lime

$$CO_2 + H_2O \rightarrow H_2CO_3 \quad \text{(1)}$$
$$H_2CO_3 + 2NaOH \rightarrow Na_2CO_3 + 2H_2O \quad \text{(2)}$$
$$H_2CO_3 + 2KOH \rightarrow K_2CO_3 + 2H_2O \quad \text{(3)}$$
$$Na_2CO_3 + Ca(OH)_2 \rightarrow 2NaOH + CaCO_3 \quad \text{(4)}$$
$$\text{(or } K_2CO_3) \qquad \text{(or 2KOH)}$$

In barium hydroxide lime, $Ba(OH)_2$ replaces the NaOH and KOH in equations (2), (3), and (4), and $BaCO_3$ is the product.

"Wet" soda lime is composed of calcium hydroxide (about 80%), sodium hydroxide and potassium hydroxide (about 5%), water (about 15%), and small amounts of inert substances such as silica and clay for hardness. The potassium hydroxide and sodium hydroxide function somewhat like a catalyst to speed the initial reaction, forming sodium and potassium carbonate. The sodium and potassium carbonates react over the course of minutes with the calcium hydroxide to form calcium carbonate and water, regenerating sodium and potassium hydroxides. Soda lime is exhausted when all the hydroxides have become carbonates. Soda lime can absorb 19% of its weight in carbon dioxide.[5] Thus 100 g of soda lime can absorb approximately 26 L of carbon dioxide.

The freshness of soda lime can be determined by feel, taste, and appearance. Fresh granules of soda lime crumble easily between the fingers and have a bitter taste because of their alkaline nature (pH 9–10). In contrast, expended granules are chalky, hard, and have a slightly salty taste. Commonly, organic dyes are added to soda lime to provide a visual indication of its function. As carbonate is formed from the hydroxide, the pH becomes less alkaline and the granules change color: ethyl violet changes from white to blue/violet with exhaustion, ethyl orange from orange to yellow, and cresyl yellow from red to yellow. Ethyl violet is most commonly employed because the color change is vivid and of high contrast at a pH intermediate between NaOH and $CaCO_3$. It can be bleached by intense light, but in the usual OR setting this is not a problem (see also Chapter 16). One can observe a slight fading of color in the zone of active absorption when usage stops. This so-called *regeneration* occurs where the lime is nearly exhausted of calcium hydroxide but has all alkaline hydroxides neutralized.

The color changes only because of the regeneration of a small amount of sodium and potassium hydroxides. Upon the next usage, the expended nature of the soda lime rapidly becomes evident. There is no true regeneration of activity. The color change of indicator lime is not to be relied upon. The anesthesiologist must know what color change is expected of the current absorbent, allow for the effects of regeneration, be cognizant of the effects of preferential gas flow at the surface between the smooth plastic canister and the irregular granules (channeling), and understand the effects of the fresh-gas flows chosen on the time a given charge of soda line can be expected to last. No indicator or rules offer absolute predictions. The use of

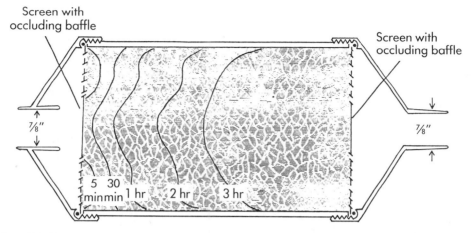

Fig. 4-7. Waters to-and-fro canister. A screen with a central occluding baffle in the to-and-fro canister improves the pattern of soda lime exhaustion. A slip joint at either end permits end-to-end reversal in the breathing circuit. With these two features, 6 to 8 hours of closed circuit anesthesia is possible before inspired carbon dioxide concentration increases above 1%. Typical patterns of soda lime exhaustion are shown by the light lines.

capnometry to detect rising inspired carbon dioxide is a valuable adjunctive technique.

Soda lime is precisely manufactured to maximize its absorptive qualities and to minimize resistance to gas flow.[5] The granules are sized 4 to 8 mesh (they will pass through a strainer having 4 to 8 wires per inch) and have a rough, irregular surface that maximizes the surface-to-volume ratio and that facilitates the rapid diffusion of carbon dioxide through the pores to the voids within the granules.[58-62] About half of the volume of a packed canister is gas. The gas volume of the voids is inversely proportional to the water content of the granules and is 1 to 2 times that of the volume between granules. Soda lime is supplied in quart cartons that will just fill a canister, in disposable canisters, and in bulk containers ranging from 5 pounds to 5 gallons. The volume between granules can be reduced by overzealous packing at the risk of creating "fines" and dust that are irritating. Channeling, preferential flow along the sides of the canister and within the absorbent itself, was a problem with to-and-fro canisters that were often horizontal and improperly packed. The use of baffles, placement so that gas flow is vertical, permanent mounting so the canister is not moved frequently, and avoidance of overly tight packing with unit-sized charges or prepacked cylinders minimize these problems.

Soda lime reacts with trichlorethylene at near room temperature to produce three toxic gases: phosgene, dichloracetylene, and carbon monoxide. Even anesthesia with another agent used in a closed circuit soon after receiving trichlorethylene analgesia was dangerous. The next patient anesthetized with the circuit was also at risk. Fortunately this agent has now been abandoned. Now all new agents are examined for soda lime reactivity. Enflurane re-

acts with soda lime to produce carbon monoxide, but only at (nonclinical) elevated temperatures (see also Chapter 16).

Alternatives to soda lime are available. Lithium hydroxide offers a little more carbon dioxide absorption capacity per unit of volume but over 3 times per unit of weight and is used in submarines. Barium lime hydroxide (Baralyme) contains 20% $Ba(OH)_2$ and little alkali. Its dust is slightly less alkaline when dissolved in water. It is a suitable alternative to soda lime.[63] The end product is barium carbonate as well as calcium carbonate. It is initially pink and turns blue-gray with exhaustion because of two indicator dyes, Mimosa Z and ethyl violet. It is as efficient as soda lime per unit of volume, but because of its density it is half as efficient per unit of mass.

The initial clinical use of soda lime absorption by Ralph Waters was the result of careful and detailed experiments to delineate the optimum size and shape of a to-and-fro canister (Fig. 4-7).[2-4] Three reasons were advanced for preferring the to-and-fro canister: The inspired gas was warmed and humidified by the soda lime; the small volume of the canister permitted rapid change of anesthetic concentration; and the absence of valves and tubes decreased resistance to breathing. These advantages were believed to be worth the awkwardness introduced by the necessity to balance several pounds of warm canister near the patient's face. As advances were made in equipment design these advantages became less important. In time the disadvantage of the to-and-fro canister, including the possibility of gas channeling in poorly packed and maintained canisters (and hence uncertain carbon dioxide absorption,[61] the possibility of dust inhalation,[17] increasing dead space during exhaustion, the propensity for leaks and dis-

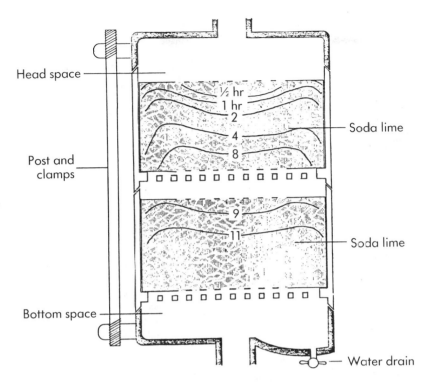

Fig. 4-8. Modern "jumbo" canister. Originated by Elam and Brown, these transparent twin-chambered canisters are now supplied by all producers. Permanently mounted with a vertical gas-flow axis, they eliminate dusting, channeling, and packing problems. Used as intended, changing the exhausted canister only when the second half is exhausted, they utilize the absorptive capacity of soda lime fully, as shown by the lines illustrating patterns of exhaustion. Drop-in, prepacked containers add convenience. The nearly standard shape is 8 cm high and 15 cm in diameter. Because water of condensation may collect at the bottom, forming a caustic lye solution with the dust, a drain valve is an important component. Convenience of opening, closing, and sealing varies with design; but most now have a single-action clamp mechanism. The casting for the top and bottom should be resistant to alkaline corrosion and may incorporate other components of the breathing circuit (e.g., bag mount, inflow site, and valve housings).

connects, and the required frequency of repacking) first limited this system's use to patients with pulmonary infections (for ease of sterilization) and later relegated it largely to museums. However, versions of the Waters canister are still employed as part of pediatric breathing systems, along with valves to change it from to-and-fro to one-way flow. Thus the heating and humidifying contribution are largely retained but the increasing dead space is avoided. Modern "jumbo" canisters (Fig. 4-8) follow the design of the Roswell Park absorber with double chambers to promote efficient use, circular baffles to minimize channeling, clear plastic walls to visualize color change, and mixing space at the top and bottom.[19,58]

Mixing devices

Resistance to gas flow in a modern circle system is less than 1 cm of water per liter per minute of gas flow, one half of a person's normal airway resistance to gas flow.[37,38] Patients, including infants and children, may safely breathe spontaneously from a circle system for prolonged periods. However, before circuit designs permitted

such low resistances, attempts were made to decrease resistance to breathing by providing a continuous flow of gas around the circle, thereby causing the inspiratory and expiratory valves to float open rather than open and close with each breath. Both pumps and Venturi devices (driven by fresh-gas flow) were designed, the most prominent of which was the Revell Circulator.[64,65] Although these devices can decrease dead space and resistance in the apparatus, the potential benefit is small; and in some circumstances these devices may backfire, actually increasing the work of breathing. If the low resistance of modern equipment is still of concern, it can be eliminated by controlled ventilation. Ways to reduce the mean airway pressure during controlled ventilation have been suggested but are not commonly used.[66]

Mixing of the expirate is required to measure carbon dioxide production and physiologic dead space. Standard physiologic testing usually collects all of the expired gas for several minutes in order to mix and measure the mixed expired gas concentrations needed in these calculations (see also Chapter 8). Simply averaging a continuous capnogram will not do: That yields a *time-weighted* average, whereas a *volume-weighted* average is required. To understand the difference, consider what happens toward the end of a respiratory cycle. While the carbon dioxide is increasing slightly, the flow is decreasing rapidly and may become zero at the end-expiratory pause. Carbon dioxide excretion should be the integral of concentration with respect to flow: When flow falls to zero, so does carbon dioxide excretion, but the elevated end-tidal value continues to increase the time-weighted integral of the capnogram. Special volume mixing devices can be used, but the breathing bag or ventilator bellows usually represent suitable sites for such measurements.

Bacterial filters

Many proprietary circuits incorporate one or two filters of pleated paper, foam, or fiber mat designed to trap particles of 1 μm or so (typical of bacterial size but not of viruses). Properly designed, these filters add only slightly to the resistance to gas flow. There is no agreement as to where to place them: when they are located on the inspiratory limb the patient is protected from infective sources in the breathing circuit, and when they are on the expiratory limb the circuit is protected from the patient.[67] However, no data exist to show that either location reduces nosocomial infection.[68] A filter placed at the Y, if it works, permits "disposable" circuits to be reused and can accomplish both tasks. This seems too distasteful to some, and others question the duration of effective filtering action[69] (see also Chapter 23).

The breathing circuit may incorporate a spirometer to measure ventilation, a humidifier to provide warmth and moisture, filters to reduce nosocomial infections, sampling sites for gas analysis, and scavenging devices to control atmospheric contamination by waste gases in the OR. These subjects are discussed in other chapters (see also Chapters 5, 7, 8, 9, and 23).

ANALYSIS OF SPECIFIC CIRCUITS
Circle breathing systems

The basic components of a circle breathing system are an inspiratory and expiratory limb, each with a unidirectional valve, and a reservoir bag or counterlung moving reciprocally with the patient's lungs. The system may be divided into quadrants (Fig. 4-9). The patient and counterlung (but not the absorber!) separate the inspiratory and expiratory limbs of the system; the valves separate the patient from the bag side of the system. The position of the valves within the limbs is not necessarily fixed. They may be anywhere between the patient and the bag with little practical difference in function. They are usually incorporated with the bag mount, pop-off valve, and absorber for manufacturing ease and durability. Even if the valves are moved to other locations, it is convenient to think of four quadrants when analyzing circle systems.

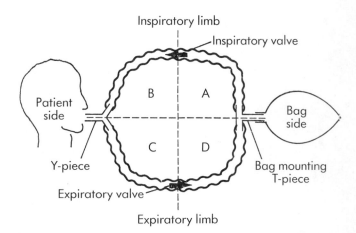

Fig. 4-9. The four quadrants of a basic circle system. Two corrugated breathing tubes connect the patient and the counterlung (a bag or a ventilator bellows). One-way valves are located in the inspiratory limb and in the expiratory limb. The circle is therefore bisected twice, dividing it into four quadrants, *A, B, C,* and *D.* To make a practical circuit for anesthesia, three more essential components must be added: a fresh-gas inflow site, a pop-off valve, and a carbon dioxide absorber.

For practical anesthesia it is necessary to add three other components: a carbon dioxide absorber, a fresh-gas inflow site, and a pop-off valve for venting excess gas. Each of the three may be placed in any of the four quadrants. In theory there are 100 different ways to place three components in four quadrants, but only a few are used.[70] Different manufacturers have used different arrangements, and older designs allowed the user to change the configuration with slight change in function. The optimal configurations for spontaneous and controlled respiration are different.[18] Most current designs are optimal for controlled respiration.

This analysis emphasizes a frequently overlooked or misunderstood point: The absorber is not on the opposite side of the circle from the patient, *the bag is.* Most schematics and diagrams of breathing circuits perpetuate this misconception by showing symmetrical circuit limbs on either side of the absorber. The position of the bag is at neither the inspiratory limb nor the expiratory limb: It separates the two.[39]

Placement of the carbon dioxide absorber, fresh-gas inflow, and pop-off valve. The carbon dioxide absorber may be placed in any of the four quadrants but is almost invariably placed in the inspiratory limb on the bag side so that apparatus resistance to inspiration may be overcome with assisted or controlled ventilation (Fig. 4-10). Placement on the expiratory side (Foregger circles) adds a mild degree of expiratory retard that, like PEEP, may be beneficial for oxygen exchange but increases the risk of barotrauma. A bypass valve to permit carbon dioxide to build up was thought desirable by a majority of anesthesiologists but not by those who build the apparatus.[71] The

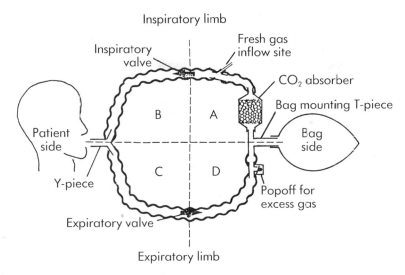

Fig. 4-10. Placement of the carbon dioxide absorber, fresh gas inflow, and pop-off valve. The usual site for the absorber is in the inspiratory limb on the bag side, that is, in quadrant A. The inspiratory valve is usually mechanically attached to the canister but is shown here as it was in Fig. 4-9 for ease of analysis. Fresh-gas inflow is usually on the bag side in the inspiratory limb (quadrant A) downstream from the carbon dioxide absorber. The pop-off valve is usually downstream from the expiratory valve near the bag. It is shown here in quadrant D but could be in A before the carbon dioxide absorber.

carbon dioxide absorber is absolutely necessary in a low fresh gas flow technique because no other method is available to remove carbon dioxide, that is, neither dilution nor exclusion from reinspiration. As fresh-gas flow is increased above gas uptake rates, the other methods become increasingly effective. This is noted by the anesthesiologist as longer intervals before the indicator in soda lime suggests replacing the absorbent. At a 5 L/min fresh-gas flow the absorbent lasts more than twice as long as at 500 ml/minute. This is not an economy because the extra anesthetic gases and vapors cost more than the soda lime saved. In addition to savings on agents, the soda lime has two other beneficial effects. Both expired humidity and heat are partially conserved, and both are optimized as flow decreases.[72,73] The risks of soda lime include airway reaction to inspired alkaline dust (minimized by good design and technique), alkaline "burns" from condensed water and dust spilled from the canister housing, and a breathing circuit with more connections and pieces to go wrong.

Although the inflow site for fresh gas may be placed physically in any of the four quadrants, efficiency and manufacturing convenience are also involved.[13,74] The inflow site is usually incorporated with the other components, that is, the absorber, bag mount, and valves. If the inflow site is located on the patient side of the inspiratory valve (quadrant B, older Foregger circles, Fig. 4-10), gas flows continuously around the circle throughout the respiratory cycle. Thus spirometry in the expiratory limb is inaccurate unless total gas flow is shut off.[75] If inflow is located on the patient side of the expiratory valve (Fig. 4-10,

quadrant C), any carbon dioxide–containing alveolar gas between the Y and the patient is washed into the patient's lungs during inspiration, at the rate of the fresh gas flow. This may be negligible during closed system anesthesia, but it can produce rebreathing of up to half of the previously expired alveolar gas at total flows of 10 L/min. Placement in quadrant D is simply inefficient because some fresh gas will be lost to the pop-off valve in most circles.

Recommended placement is on the bag side of the inspiratory limb between inspiratory valve and absorber (quadrant A, Fig. 4-10). If the absorber housing has appreciable head space, as is common, this inflow site serves to store the continuously delivered fresh gas during exhalation. Gas flows down the inspiratory limb only during inspiration. During expiration fresh gas flows backward toward the absorber, bag, and pop-off valve. Thus fresh gas provides most or all of the respired gas with high-flow techniques, or enriches the oxygen and anesthetic-depleted expiratory gas with low-flow techniques.

The pop-off valve may be placed anywhere in the circle, but some locations are more rational that others. Locating it in the inspiratory limb (Fig. 4-10, quadrants A and B) tends to vent fresh anesthetic and carbon dioxide–free gas. Furthermore, locations in the inspiratory limb on the patient side (quadrant B) permit some carbon dioxide–containing expirate to enter the inspiratory limb during the end of a spontaneous breath. This rebreathing is clearly undesirable. It is mechanically convenient to place the pop-off valve between the expiratory valve and the bag mount, or opposite the bag mount, before the absorber (i.e., in quadrants *D* or *A* but close to the bag mount). Incorporating the pop-off valve into a one-piece absorber/bag mount/expiratory valve/pop-off valve assembly gives convenience and durability.

There is at least theoretic value to sometimes locating the pop-off valve on the patient side at the Y or next to it (quadrant *C,* Fig. 4-10). During spontaneous inspiration, the pressure at this site is below atmospheric and the pop-off valve is closed. During exhalation, the pressure is just slightly above atmospheric and gas flows to the reservoir bag until it is distended to its nominal volume. Then the pressure in the entire circuit increases as fresh-gas inflow and exhalation from the patient continue, opening the pop-off valve. The gas vented is primarily carbon dioxide-rich, oxygen-depleted and anesthetic-depleted end-tidal gas. However, the situation is reversed during assisted or controlled ventilation. During inspiration, the pressure in the circuit at the Y piece is positive with respect to atmospheric. A pop-off valve located at the Y piece would dump fresh gas, and one near the bag would dump a mixture of dead-space and end-tidal gas. Two pop-off valves on the same circuit double the risk of hypoventilation when ventilation is changed to mechanical because the anesthesiologist may fail to close both. For this reason pop-off valves at the Y piece are no longer used.

Flow and concentration. The gas mixture inspired by a patient breathing from a circle system is determined by the fresh-gas inflow, the configuration of the circle, the respiratory pattern, and the uptake by the patient of oxygen and anesthetics. At fresh-gas inflow rates exceeding minute ventilation, the circle behaves like a nonrebreathing system. The concentration of inspired gas closely approaches that being delivered from the gas flowmeters on the machine. As flow is progressively decreased, a disparity between fresh-gas inflow and actual inspired concentration of anesthetics increases.

In a closed system, in which inflow just matches loss from the system, the composition of reinspired gas is not predictable from the inflow concentration of gases.[76] Inspired and expired gases differ because of uptake of oxygen and anesthetic and excretion of carbon dioxide. Oxygen concentration in mixed-expired gas is usually about 4% or 5% lower than that in inspired gas. Although oxygen uptake remains relatively constant during anesthesia (about 200 ml/min STPD* in the average adult, provided that body temperature does not change appreciably), anesthetic uptake varies: It is greatest at the start of anesthesia and decreases with time. If oxygen concentration is maintained constant during closed system anesthesia, the flowmeter values reflect oxygen *consumption* and anesthetic uptake by the patient, rather than inspired *concentrations.* When nitrous oxide is used in closed system anesthesia,

the oxygen tension or concentration in the circle must be monitored continuously, because nitrous oxide uptake declines while oxygen uptake does not. The inspired gas mixture may become hypoxic if the nitrous oxide inflow is not gradually decreased. Whether it is necessary to measure the concentration of potent volatile anesthetics during closed system anesthesia remains controversial: Some believe that it is necessary, and others prefer to monitor anesthetic depth and patient responses clinically (see also Chapter 30).

Semiclosed systems: Mapleson classifications

Mapleson configurations of Magill circuits are characterized by a reservoir that can be filled by fresh gas, expired gas, or both. They may or may not have a pop-off valve, but it does not prevent rebreathing. Carbon dioxide is eliminated by both dilution and efficient arrangement of the circuit components (see below) and is critically affected by total fresh-gas flow and the pattern of respiration. The pattern of respiration includes the respiratory rate, tidal volume, dead space, I:E time ratios, and the inspiratory and expiratory flow patterns. The earliest semiclosed systems consisted of a bag attached to a mask by an elbow or by a length of breathing tubing if it was desirable to move the large bag away from the face. The inlet for fresh gas was a nipple on the elbow or through the tail of the bag. A pop-off valve was placed either at the bag's tail or at the elbow. The bag ideally contained a volume approximating the patient's inspiratory capacity (about 3 L in an adult) to permit spontaneous deep breaths without the feeling of suffocation. Gas flows totaling 1 to 2 times the minute volume were used.[8,74] Mapleson organized the various configurations into five typical ones, and he added a sixth later, as shown in Fig. 4-11.[7,26] Each of these breathing systems may be thought of as lying somewhere along the continuum shown in Table 4-2.

In Table 4-2, the far right situation represents complete rebreathing and is of use only in the study of respiratory control and for treating hiccoughs. The original Mapleson B and C configurations lie midway on the continuum and are judged to have no particular merit, except perhaps for[2] brief procedures or to transport patients while supplemental oxygen is administered and breathing is augmented.

None of the Mapleson systems meets the requirements on the far left, but with optimal configuration and high fresh-gas flow they may approach it. Efficiency of the systems in this context can be translated as the lowest fresh-gas flow that will assure normal removal of carbon dioxide, thereby minimizing rebreathing. There is normally a partial pressure difference for carbon dioxide such that

$$\text{Alveolar} > \text{Mixed expired} > \text{Inspired}$$
$$\text{P}_{A}\text{CO}_2 > \text{P}_{\overline{E}}\text{CO}_2 > \text{P}_{I}\text{CO}_2$$

---

*STPD = standard temperature and pressure, dry.

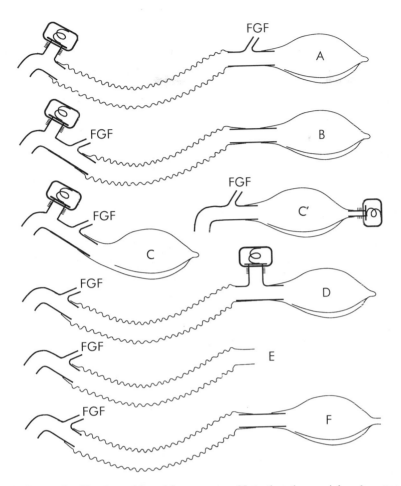

Fig. 4-11. Mapleson classification of breathing systems. Note that the semiclosed systems *(top four)* contain most of the components of a circle system—tubing, connectors, bag, fresh-gas inflow, and pop-off site. They lack carbon dioxide absorbers because carbon dioxide is lowered by addition of fresh gas and elimination of carbon dioxide–rich gas preferentially through the pop-off valve. They also lack separate inspiratory and expiratory limbs: One tubing serves both purposes.

The Mapleson A system (Magill attachment) is optimal for spontaneous respiration. The Mapleson C system is a simple bag and mask. Moving the pop-off to the bag tail is a major improvement (*C'*) because this permits more mixing of fresh and exhaled gas than the Mapleson C (this modification, not one of Mapleson's, has been added by the author). The *B* circuit is wasteful of fresh gas in both spontaneous and controlled respiration. The *D* is similar to the *A* except that it exchanges the inflow and pop-off sites. *A* is optimal for spontaneous breathing and *D* for controlled breathing.

The Mapleson E system is essentially an Ayre's T piece to which has been added a reservoir. If the reservoir is short, it is an open, not a semiclosed, system. It is simple but lacks the convenience of a bag for ventilatory assistance or control. A bag can be added to it (Mapleson F, or Jackson-Rees modification), but because the system still lacks an adjustable pop-off valve, assistance or control of respiration is not convenient.

All of these circuits share a common advantage. Vigorous hyperventilation cannot reduce the patient's carbon dioxide tension much below normal if the fresh-gas flows are kept between one and two times the patient's normal respiratory minute volume.

Table 4-2. The spectrum of carbon dioxide elimination

Maximum carbon dioxide elimination	To	Maximum carbon dioxide retention
No mixing of fresh and alveolar gas	Complete mixing of fresh and alveolar gas	No mixing of fresh and alveolar gas
Fresh gas goes to the patient	The mixture is inhaled	Alveolar gas is rebreathed
Alveolar gas goes to the pop-off valve	Fresh gas and mixed gas are "popped off" simultaneously	Fresh gas goes to the pop-off valve
DESIRABLE	ACCEPTABLE	UNDESIRABLE

The most efficient configurations place the pop-off valve where the highest concentration of carbon dioxide is to be found during the phase of breathing when the circuit pressure is above atmospheric. This occurs at end-expiration during spontaneous breathing and during inspiration with manually assisted or controlled breathing.

A great deal of attention has been devoted to determining the lowest gas flow that can be safely used in clinical anesthesia. There have been a variety of claims for the various circuits and for proprietary modifications of the circuits (e.g., Bain, Humphrey, Lack, Mara F). Unfortunately much of the published work suffers from one or more of the following flaws:

1. Theoretical analyses that embody unrealistic assumptions about mixing and breathing pattern, especially the I:E ratio and expiratory flow.
2. Model studies that embody nonphysiologic states, particularly lack of responsiveness to carbon dioxide and simplified flow patterns.
3. Studies in awake volunteers whose metabolic rates and physiologic responses differ from those of anesthetized patients.
4. Imprecise end points, such as "rebreathing of carbon dioxide" identified by capnography, rather than an increase in alveolar or arterial carbon dioxide concentration.

There is, however, this area of agreement: Systems classified as Mapleson A (Magill attachment, Lack, and Humphrey A) are most efficient for spontaneous unassisted ventilation, and those classified as Mapleson D, E, or F (Jackson-Rees, Bain, Humphrey DE) are most efficient for assisted or controlled ventilation.

A general criticism of the published analyses of breathing circuits is a failure to distinguish between the quantity of reinspired carbon dioxide and minimum inspired carbon dioxide tension. The most common instrumentation, a capnograph, displays a signal of airway concentration as a function of time. Thus if airway carbon dioxide falls slowly with inspiration, just reaching zero near end-inspiration, it is interpreted as no rebreathing, even though a significant amount of carbon dioxide has been reinspired. Conversely, if airway carbon dioxide falls to a low but nonzero concentration for all of inspiration, there may be quite adequate carbon dioxide excretion despite "rebreathing" if total ventilation is increased. Inspired carbon dioxide is properly calculated as the integral of instantaneous flow times instantaneous carbon dioxide concentration, which is difficult or impossible to measure with simple instrumentation. A better analysis is based on the equation of defining alveolar ventilation ($\dot{V}_A$):

$$\dot{V}_A = \frac{\dot{V}_{CO_2}}{F_ACO_2} \qquad (5)$$

$$\dot{V}_A = \dot{V}_E - (V_{DS} \times f) \qquad (6)$$

Equation 5 states that alveolar ventilation is the quotient of carbon dioxide production and alveolar fractional concentration of carbon dioxide. Because F_ACO_2 is proportional to P_ACO_2, a specific PCO_2 defines one and only one $\dot{V}_A$ in a given patient. Equation 6 demonstrates that any increase in dead space ventilation ($V_{DS} \times f$) can be accommodated by an equivalent increase in minute volume ($\dot{V}_E$), keeping alveolar ventilation, and hence carbon dioxide elimination, constant. Any amount of carbon dioxide may be rebreathed, at a concentration equal to or below alveolar carbon dioxide, if an increase in minute volume maintains alveolar ventilation.

Even if instantaneous PCO_2 reaches zero near end-inspiration, a significant volume of carbon dioxide may be rebreathed, requiring an appropriate increase in minute volume. A numerical example may help clarify this. Consider a patient needing 4 L/min of $\dot{V}_A$ with F_ACO_2 of 0.05 (5%) and a current $\dot{V}_E$ of 6 L/min with a respiratory rate (f) of 20/min. The patient could rebreathe 2.5% carbon dioxide and keep F_ACO_2 at 0.05 (5%) if the apparent alveolar ventilation doubled to 8 L/min. If the dead space ventilation did not change (it probably would, but not much depending on whether tidal volume or f was increased), a total minute volume of 10 L would suffice. Clearly an inspired carbon dioxide load can be compensated for. Note that at the ventilatory response to carbon dioxide sensitivity of an awake person (slope of 2 L/min/mm Hg) this would require a rise of less than 2 mm Hg in P_ACO_2. However, at a sensitivity to carbon dioxide frequently seen in an anesthetized person (e.g., 0.5 L/min/mm Hg), the carbon dioxide tension would have to rise nearly 8 mm Hg. Thus there is a real difference between spontaneous breathing, where ventilation is set by the patient's P_ACO_2 and responsiveness, and controlled ventilation, where minute volume is set by the anesthesiologist.

Any gas mixture containing carbon dioxide can be considered to consist of a fraction of carbon dioxide-free gas and a fraction of alveolar gas. Any rebreathing of alveolar gas is simply added dead space and can be compensated for by increasing overall ventilation. For example, given 4 L/min of alveolar ventilation and 2 L/min of dead space ventilation, what will happen if one suddenly inspires 1% carbon dioxide? Each unit of alveolar ventilation now "holds" only 4/5 of the lung-produced carbon dioxide that it used to, so that increasing alveolar ventilation by 5/4 will result in the same carbon dioxide elimination as before.

Mapleson A configurations and carbon dioxide removal. Consider first the Mapleson A circuit shown in Fig. 4-12. The assumptions for this model include spontaneous breathing with a rate of 20/min, tidal volume of 400 ml, I:E ratio of 1:2, a sinusoidal inspiratory flow averaging 24 L/min, a near exponential expiratory flow with a

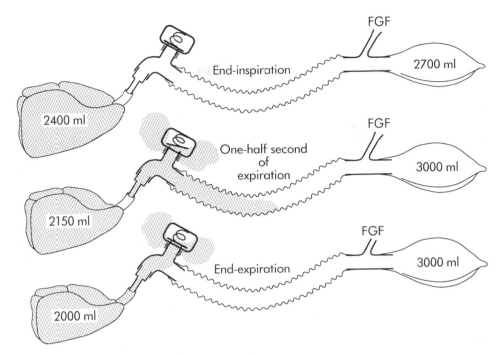

Fig. 4-12. Mapleson A circuit, spontaneous breathing. In this Mapleson A circuit, the stippled areas indicate carbon dioxide–containing gas: (*top*) The end of a normal spontaneous inspiration for a normal adult patient. As the patient begins to exhale, first carbon dioxide–free gas flows from the upper dead space, and then increasingly carbon dioxide–rich gas flows into the corrugated tube and, together with continuing fresh-gas flow, fills the bag one half second later (*middle*). The rest of the expirate goes out through the pop-off valve, along with carbon dioxide–containing gas in the tubing, which is pushed toward the pop-off valve by the fresh-gas flow. Optimally, at end-expiration (*bottom*) the circuit has largely been flushed of carbon dioxide.

half time of less than 0.5 second, a functional residual capacity (FRC) of 2400 ml, a fresh-gas flow of 6 L/min, a bag of 3 L nominal volume at the pop-off valve opening pressure, and a corrugated tube of 500 ml volume. The top diagram shows the condition at end-inspiration, after the lung has inspired 400 ml over one second, consisting of 100 ml of fresh gas flow and 300 ml from the circuit. All of the circuit has been flushed with fresh gas, and carbon dioxide is found only in alveolar gas (stippled area). In the first 0.5 second of exhalation, 250 ml of gas are expired, and together with 50 ml of fresh gas have distended the reservoir bag to 3 L and just opened the pop-off valve (middle diagram Fig. 4-12). Carbon dioxide–containing alveolar gas has penetrated part way down the breathing tube. The exact distance depends on the dead space, the shape and volume of zones I and II of the capnogram (see Chapter 10 and Fig. 10-1 for capnogram zones), and the longitudinal mixing (cone-like flow pattern) in the tube. In the next one and one half seconds of expiration, the rest of the expired alveolar gas (150 ml) has gone out through the pop-off valve and 150 ml of fresh gas has flushed the carbon dioxide–containing expirate in the breathing tube back and out through the pop-off valve. If the sum of the

fresh-gas flow (150 ml) and the carbon dioxide–free dead space gas from zone I exceeds the penetration of zone II and alveolar gas, one has the end-expiratory situation shown in the lowest diagram of Fig. 4-12. This is generally true when fresh-gas flow exceeds 55% of the respiratory minute volume.[77,78] In this particular model, about 100 ml of fresh gas exits the pop-off valve with each breath, as well as the carbon dioxide–containing alveolar expirate. In studies of anesthetized people, the fresh-gas flow that maintains carbon dioxide homeostasis in Mapleson A circuits used with spontaneous breathing has been found to be 70% to 100% of the minute volume, depending on the many covariables.[78-80]

During assisted or controlled ventilation, two different things happen to decrease efficiency. First the bag must be squeezed during inspiration to deliver the entire tidal volume (400 ml) and to vent the fresh-gas flow that comes in over an entire respiratory cycle (in this case 1/20 of 6 L/min, or 300 ml). Now all of the expired tidal volume flows into the breathing tubing accompanied and then followed by the continued fresh-gas flow during the end-expiratory pause. During the next compression, some alveolar gas may reenter the airway until the circuit pressure

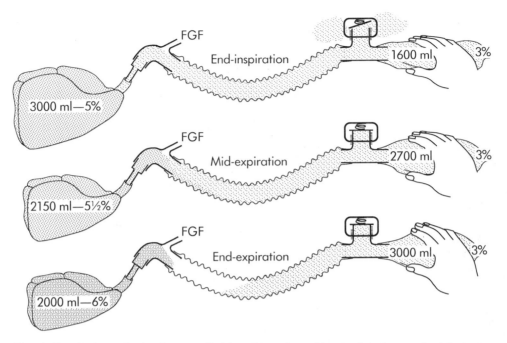

Fig. 4-13. Mapleson D circuit, controlled breathing. At end-inspiration the anesthesiologist has squeezed the bag from its nominal volume of 3 L down to 1600 ml. Of this amount, 800 ml went into the patient's lungs along with 200 ml of fresh gas, and 600 ml of the bag's contents (with about 3% carbon dioxide) left the circuit through the pop-off valve *(top)*. During the next 2 seconds the patient exhales nearly all of the tidal volume (900 ml), and this with the continuing fresh-gas flow fills the bag *(middle)*. Because of the fresh-gas flow, the bag's carbon dioxide concentration content is diluted below alveolar gas. Further, the patient's expiratory flow diminishes toward the end-expiratory pause, and the fresh gas flows into the patient end of the circuit. This is the gas that will enter the patient's lungs first on the next inspiration *(bottom)*.

rises to the threshold of the pop-off valve. Thereafter, some carbon dioxide and some fresh gas go both to the lung and to the pop-off valve. Intuitively, one can appreciate that the effect would depend on the rate of compression of the bag, that is, the inspiratory flow, the lung and chest wall compliance, airway resistance, the volume of dead space, the I:E timing, and the fresh-gas flow. Thus during assisted ventilation the Mapleson A circuit is far less efficient than during spontaneous ventilation in terms of preventing rebreathing.

Mapleson D configurations and carbon dioxide removal. A typical circuit for controlled ventilation is shown in Fig. 4-13. The assumptions for this model are a fresh-gas flow of 6 L/min, a minute volume of 10 L using V_T of 1000 ml and rate of 10, an FRC of 2000 ml, an expiratory flow nearly exponential with 0.5 second half-time, an I:E ratio of 1:2, and a peak inspiratory gas flow rate of 30 L/min. At inspiration the bag is squeezed to deliver 1000 ml to the patient in 2 seconds and to blow 600 ml out the pop-off valve. Because in these 2 seconds 200 ml of fresh gas entered, one has the state shown in the top panel of Fig. 4-13.

Now the patient exhales. At 2 seconds the patient has exhaled 900 ml, which is diluted with 200 ml of fresh gas

as it enters the circuit. This has refilled the bag to 2700 ml. In the next 2 seconds of expiration, the rest of the tidal volume, 100 ml, and 200 ml more of fresh gas have filled the breathing tubing and the bag has regained its initial volume of 3 L. The lungs now contain 6% carbon dioxide (it has been slowly increasing due to continued carbon dioxide delivery to a progressively smaller alveolar volume). The bag contains 3% carbon dioxide, but in the breathing tubing the concentration falls toward zero, the fresh gas F_ICO_2. In fact, if ⅔ of the fresh-gas flow is washed into the lungs, it will provide 4 L/min of carbon dioxide–free alveolar ventilation and the $PaCO_2$ will be normal, *despite obvious rebreathing of some carbon dioxide.* Studies of anesthetized people in fact show normal carbon dioxide homeostasis with a fresh-gas flow of 70% of total minute ventilation in Mapleson D circuits during controlled breathing if minute volume is 150 ml/kg or greater.[12,81]

Proprietary semiclosed systems. Although a variety of pieces of anesthesia hardware can be used to assemble the Mapleson circuits A through F, several specific circuits with eponymic identities have been introduced that offer specific advantages. These include the Jackson-Rees, the Bain, the Lack, the Mera F, and the Humphrey ADE. The

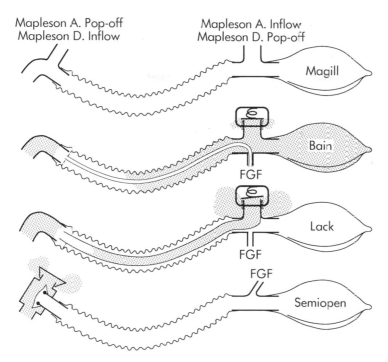

Fig. 4-14. Comparison of the Mapleson A and D circuits with the Bain, Lack and semiopen circuits. *(top)* A schematic of the Mapleson A and D circuits with an indication for placement of the inflow and pop-off valves that distinguish A from D. The Bain circuit *(next panel)* shown at end-expiration, utilizes a small-bore fresh-gas delivery tube to deliver fresh gas to the patient end of the circuit. The Lack circuit *(third panel)* looks similar externally, but the inner tube is now an expiratory limb delivering expired gas to the pop-off valve at the bag end. In a semiopen circuit *(bottom)* the breathing tube is *inspiratory,* and all expired gas exits at the valve. Only fresh gas is found in the tubing.

last four are conveniently coaxial: They have a tube-within-a-tube arrangement that moves the physical location of the fresh-gas inflow and/or the expiratory valve away from the patient-connection elbow, while variously preserving the advantages of the A, D, or F circuits. The Bain and Lack circuits are shown in Fig. 4-14.

The Bain circuit is basically a coaxial Mapleson D. Instead of a separate small-bore tube for delivery of fresh gas to the patient elbow, the delivery tube enters the corrugated expiratory tube near the bag mount and pop-off valve and runs coaxially to the patient end, where the end is secured by a plastic "spider" in the center of the tube. Thus fresh gas is delivered at the patient end and the pop-off valve exhausts gas at the bag end of the corrugated tube, a Mapleson D arrangement. Various recommendations for fresh-gas flow (FGF) have been published. One commercial brand has a package insert recommending an FGF of 100 ml/kg/min. Such recommendations often were based on instantaneous inspired carbon dioxide concentration being zero for some portion of the cycle. However, with suitably augmented ventilation (150 ml/kg or more instead of the 90 ml/kg for a normal person at rest), adequate carbon dioxide elimination results from an FGF of 70 ml/kg/min during assisted or controlled ventila-

tion.[12,35,81] Spontaneous ventilation, although not recommended for prolonged periods, requires a greater flow, up to 150 ml/kg/min.[25,82,83]

The Bain circuit may malfunction if the central tube (fresh gas delivery) becomes disconnected, either where it enters the corrugated outer tube or from its retaining spider at the patient end. Either disconnection effectively increases the apparatus dead space and, for any given minute volume, reduces alveolar ventilation accordingly.[84] Disconnection at the bag end is by far the more serious problem. Inspection may disclose this, but either case may not be identified by inspection alone. Two tests have been proposed. One test utilizes a very low oxygen flow (50 ml/min) and occlusion of the inner tube with a finger or plunger from a small disposable syringe.[85] The flowmeter bobbin should fall with occlusion of the inner tube. Alternatively, filling the reservoir bag with gas and operating the oxygen flush will normally create a Venturi effect that partially empties the bag.[86] (For further discussion of Bain circuits and testing their integrity, see Chapter 26.)

The Lack circuit (coaxial Mapleson A) appears similar to the Bain circuit externally: Near the bag are both a pop-off valve and a fresh-gas inflow nipple. However, the central tube is larger in diameter and serves as an *expiratory* limb, leading from a "spider" that centers it coaxially to the pop-off valve.[14] The circuit is long enough that this central tube has a volume of 500 ml. Fresh gas flows between the external corrugated tube and the central tube to the patient connection end. This is essentially a Mapleson A circuit and is optimal for spontaneous breathing. Figure 4-14 shows the Lack system at end-expiration. The first part of exhalation has passed retrograde between the corrugated hose and inner tube toward the bag, which is simultaneously filling with fresh gas. Because this first part contains little or no carbon dioxide, little carbon dioxide is found in the outer channel. When the bag reaches its nominal volume, the pressure rises enough to open the pop-off valve, and for the rest of exhalation carbon dioxide–rich gas passes into the inner channel. If expiratory flow falls to nearly zero (at end-expiratory pause), fresh gas flows toward the patient through the outer channel and even into the inner tube, pushing alveolar gas out through the pop-off valve. Any carbon dioxide remaining in the inner tube is not rebreathed during the subsequent inspiration because the expiratory valve closes and little gas flows backward in the inner (expiratory) tubing. Reports that the Lack system is more efficient, equally efficient, or less efficient than a Magill attachment may be found in the literature, but the differences are always small.[79,87,88] Fresh-gas flow of 70% of minute volume results in negligible carbon dioxide rebreathing. Note that with spontaneous breathing, increasing fresh-gas flow is of little value in lowering arterial PCO_2, which is set by the patient's respiratory control state.

The Humphrey ADE circuit is now available as a coaxial circuit 1.6 m long with a 15-mm inner tube of 300 ml volume and a 28-mm outer tube of 700 ml volume.[89] A fixed, machine-mounted valving assembly with one control lever permits selection of either a Mapleson A or D configuration. With modern anesthesia ventilators that exhaust excess gas at end-expiration, the system becomes a Mapleson E, hence the suffix ADE.[89] The disadvantage of forgetting to switch the lever, and the ubiquitous circle systems in hospitals in the United States, have led to greater interest outside than inside the United States. A notable exception is the work of Artru and Katz,[90] who studied patients and used a rise in end-tidal rather than inspired carbon dioxide concentration as the criterion for rebreathing. They found that with an appropriate lever setting, an FGF of 66 ml/kg/min prevented a rise in end-tidal carbon dioxide during both spontaneous and controlled breathing.

The Mera F system, introduced in Japan in 1978, uses a modern circle canister-valve assembly as the mounting for a coaxial Bain-like circuit. Byrick, et al.[83] found at 100 ml/kg/min FGF it functioned as well as the standard Bain circuit. During controlled respiration, this FGF kept $PACO_2$ at 45 mm Hg (± 9) during light anesthesia despite a lower minute volume, because of a slightly improved capture of

dead space gas for reinspiration. The Mera F tubing is quite suitable for the Humphrey ADE single-lever hardware.

The Jackson-Rees breathing circuit is a modification of Ayre's T piece, which is used in pediatric anesthesia worldwide. It adds a corrugated tube, a bag, and sometimes a variable-spring-loaded valve to the expiratory limb of the T. Mapleson added it to his classification system as F in 1975.[26] Nightingale, et al.[23] have pointed out that if the volume of the expiratory limb exceeds the tidal volume, then Mapleson D, E, and F systems function identically during spontaneous breathing and should be supplied with an FGF of 100 ml/kg or more per minute. Further, if the Jackson-Rees system is assembled with a spring-loaded valve in the tail of the bag, it becomes a Mapleson D and can be used with controlled ventilation with an FGF of 70 ml/kg/min (and augmented minute volume, of course).

Semiopen systems

Semiopen systems, also known as nonrebreathing systems, eliminate carbon dioxide by use of two valves that exclude rebreathing. The reservoir bag contains pure fresh gas, which must of course be supplied at rates at or above the current respiratory minute volume. Apparatus dead space is minimized if the pair of valves, one opening on inspiration and one on expiration, are incorporated into one small-volume assembly near the mask or tracheal tube (Fig. 4-3, *B*). The valves must be designed to open with little pressure and close quickly with the change in gas flow between inspiration and expiration. Clever design permits the pressure drop across the inspiratory valve to positively close the expiratory valve, making transition from spontaneous to controlled breathing automatic: All the anesthesiologist has to do is squeeze the bag. The Frumin and Fink valves were once commonly used in anesthesia. Ruben valves and others still find application in self-inflating resuscitator bag-valve assemblies. Most mechanical ventilators used postoperatively and in intensive care units also employ such circuits, actively closing the expiratory valve by the machine pressure generated to start inspiration. Gas masks and SCUBA (self-contained underwater breathing apparatus) gear are other examples of nonrebreathing circuits, as were the intermittent-flow anesthesia machines of earlier times. The major advantages of semiopen circuits were the relative accuracy of flowmeters at high gas flow (assuring inspired gas concentrations) and the ability to measure respiratory minute volume by setting fresh-gas flow to keep the breathing bag just partly distended at each end-expiration. With currently available instrumentation neither advantage is of much value. Semiopen systems could be heated, humidified, and scavenged as readily as could semiclosed systems[53,91-94] but often required a higher FGF, typically 80 to 100 ml/kg/min.

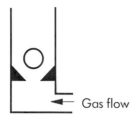

Fig. 4-15. Weighted-ball design free-standing PEEP valve. This is designed to be mounted vertically in the expiratory limb of a circle just upstream of the exhalation unidirectional valve.

POSITIVE END-EXPIRATORY PRESSURE

In order to improve oxygenation, the application of positive end-expiratory pressure (PEEP) to a breathing system may be required. PEEP may be achieved by adding a free-standing PEEP valve (e.g., Boehringer valve, Boehringer Laboratories, Wynnewood, Pa.) between the expiratory limb of a circle system and the expiratory unidirectional valve. A schematic of such a valve is shown in Fig. 4-15. Thus a weighted ball must be lifted off its seat by the gas flow. The weight of the ball determines the amount of PEEP, and valves are available for application of various levels of PEEP including 2.5, 5, 10, 15, and 20 cm H_2O. Such valves can be used in series to create any desired level of PEEP. It is essential that they be placed correctly (vertically) in the expiratory limb. If placed in the inspiratory limb, they would totally obstruct the circuit (see Chapter 16). Also, if not mounted vertically they can malfunction.

Both North American Dräger and Ohmeda offer PEEP valves as options in their anesthesia breathing systems. These valves are purpose-designed and built into the system so as to prevent erroneous placement. The Ohmeda PEEP valve is essentially a spring-loaded expiratory unidirectional valve that is adjustable between 2 and 20 cm H_2O. It is essential that the PEEP valve be installed only on the exhalation unidirectional valve, and *never* on the inhalation unidirectional valve. Thus, in Fig. 4-2, if an adjustable spring were placed between the valve disc and the dome, it would tend to prevent the opening of the disc, thereby requiring a higher pressure upstream for gas to flow across the valve. Adjusting spring tension with the calibrated knob thereby adjusts the level of PEEP applied to the circuit between the inspiratory valve and the expiratory unidirectional PEEP valve (Fig. 4-16). In the Ohmeda GMS Absorber system the pressure in the circuit is sensed just downstream of the inspiratory unidirectional valve so that the circuit pressure gauge and any alarms will detect the presence of PEEP in the circuit (see also Chapters 9 and 16).

With an Ohmeda GMS absorber in the APL or bag mode, and with the patient breathing spontaneously, the setting on the APL valve must be higher than the PEEP

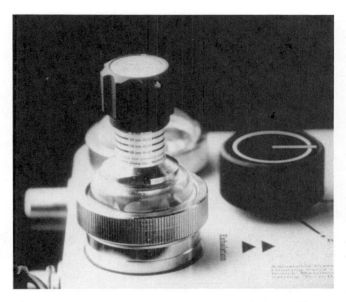

Fig. 4-16. Ohmeda PEEP valve. This is essentially a calibrated spring-loaded exhalation unidirectional valve. (Courtesy of Ohmeda, BOC Health Care, Inc., Madison, Wis.)

setting. If this is not done, inadequate tidal volumes may be delivered to the patient during inspiration. Ohmeda also warns that the PEEP valve should be installed into the GMS absorber only when the use of PEEP is anticipated for that case. It should be removed when not in use; otherwise, deposits from the breathing circuit can collect in the valve mechanism, causing it to malfunction (see also Chapter 16).[95] The use of PEEP in the patient circuit may result in a significant decrease in delivered tidal volume. Factors that influence the tidal volume delivered to the patient include patient circuit pressure (affected by PEEP), compliance, and resistance. The ventilation must be appropriately adjusted to compensate for any decrease in tidal volume that is caused by the addition of PEEP.[98]

North American Dräger delivery systems use a PEEP valve based upon magnetic principles. Thus, instead of using the force of a weighted ball or of a spring, the force of attraction between two magnets is used to adjust the pressure needed to open the valve (Fig. 4-17). Because this valve is located between the patient circuit and the selector block that houses the switch for manual (bag) or automatic (ventilator) mode, it must permit bidirectional flow so that during a positive pressure inspiration, gas flows from the reservoir bag or ventilator bellows, through the valve, and to the patient circuit via a spring-loaded one-way valve (Fig. 4-18). Upon exhalation, the one-way valve closes and gas pressure must now overcome the force of attraction between the two magnets to open the valve and flow to the bag or ventilator bellows (Fig. 4-19). The Dräger PEEP valve is not calibrated, but the knob is marked to show direction of rotation for increasing or decreasing PEEP. A slide-switch is incorporated into the latest ver-

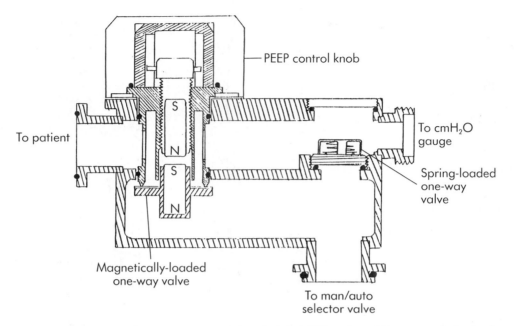

Fig. 4-17. North American Dräger magnetic principle PEEP valve. Adjustment of the knob moves a magnet closer to or further away from a magnetic one-way valve through which exhalation occurs. N and S refer to the north and south poles of the magnets. (Courtesy of North American Dräger, Inc., Telford, Pa.)

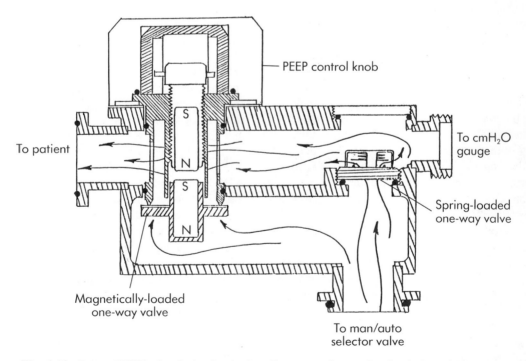

Fig. 4-18. Dräger PEEP valve during inspiration. Gas cannot flow to the circuit through the magnetic one-way valve; instead, it flows through the spring-loaded one-way valve. (Courtesy of North American Dräger, Inc., Telford, Pa.)

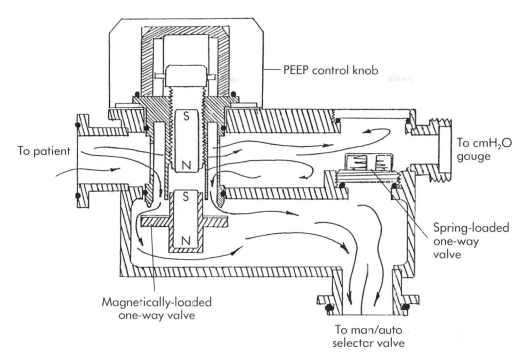

Fig. 4-19. Dräger PEEP valve during exhalation. As the patient exhales, gas enters the PEEP valve. It cannot flow through the spring-loaded one-way valve, and the magnetic one-way valve is closed. As the patient continues to exhale, pressure rises above the force of attraction between the magnets, causing the magnetic one-way valve to open and allow gas to flow to the manual/automatic selector switch. (Courtesy of North American Dräger, Inc., Telford, Pa.)

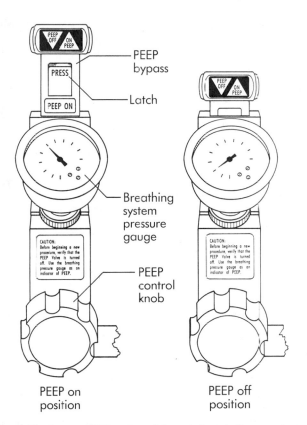

Fig. 4-20. Dräger PEEP valve slide-switch to indicate and control the on/off function of the PEEP valve. (Courtesy of North American Dräger, Inc., Telford, Pa.)

sion of this valve to control and clearly indicate whether the PEEP valve is on or off (Fig. 4-20).

The location of the PEEP valve in relation to the expiratory unidirectional valve (free-standing valve or Ohmeda PEEP valve) or in the manual/automatic switch block (North American Dräger) permits application of PEEP to the patient circuit during all modes of ventilation, that is, spontaneous, assisted, controlled, and automatic. In this location the circuit pressure gauge and alarms sensing pressure at the absorber will detect the presence and level of PEEP applied (see also Chapter 16).

CIRCUIT MALFUNCTION AND SAFETY

Despite continued improvement in the design and function of anesthesia machines and related equipment, accidents resulting from their misuse or malfunction continue to occur.[96-98] Preventable anesthesia mishaps are largely due to equipment failures or to human errors. Some of the problems are not serious, but many have such a potential. Two are common: breathing circuit disconnections and unintentional changes in gas flow. Either can cause serious or even lethal effects. From these and similar analyses come important recommendations that anesthesiologists and manufacturers of anesthesia equipment should heed. First, it is essential that anesthesiologists be thoroughly familiar with and understand the function of the equipment that they use. Second, a routine for checking equipment before using it each time is essential. Third, the design of a piece of equipment should be as simple as possible. Needless elaboration may serve only to confuse the user and detract from the basic utility of the device. Finally, not all potential equipment malfunctions or errors in their use can be anticipated: Anesthesiologists must be constantly vigilant for their possible occurrence and be prepared to manage their consequences (see also Chapter 16).

REFERENCES

1. Jackson DE: A new method for the production of general analgesia and anesthesia with a description of the apparatus used, *J Lab Clin Med* 1:1-12, 1915.
2. Waters RM: Clinical scope and utility of carbon dioxide filtration in inhalation anesthesia, *Anesth Analg* 3:20-26, 1924.
3. Waters RM: Carbon dioxide absorption technique in anesthesia, *Ann Surg* 103:38-45, 1936.
4. Sword BC: The closed circle method of administration of gas anesthesia, *Anesth Analg* 9:198-202, 1930.
5. WR Grace & Co, Dewey and Almy Chemical Division: *The Sodasorb manual of carbon dioxide absorption*, New York, 1962.
6. Fink BR: A non-rebreathing valve of new design, *Anesthesiology* 15:471-474, 1954.
7. Mapleson WW: The elimination of rebreathing in various semiclosed anaesthetic systems. *Br J Anaesth* 26:323-332, 1954.
8. Sykes MK: Rebreathing circuits: a review, *Br J Anaesth* 40:666-674, 1968.
9. Stephen CR, Slater HM: A nonresisting nonrebreathing valve, *Anesthesiology* 9:550-552, 1948.
10. Ruben H: Anaesthesia system with eliminated spill valve adjustment and without lung rupture risk, *Acta Anaesthesiol Scand* 28:310-314, 1984.
11. Frumin MJ, Lee ASJ, Papper EM: New valve for non-rebreathing systems, *Anesthesiology* 20:383-385, 1959.
12. Bain JA, Spoerel WE: A streamlined anaesthetic system, *Can Anaesth Soc J* 19:426-435, 1972.
13. Dixon J, Chakrabarti MK, Morgan M: An assessment of the Humphrey ADE anaesthesia system in the Mapleson A mode during spontaneous ventilation, *Anaesthesia* 39:593-596, 1984.
14. Lack JA: Theatre pollution control, *Anaesthesia* 31:259-262, 1976.
15. Kay B, Beaty PCW, Healy TEJ, et al: Change in the work of breathing imposed by five anaesthetic breathing systems, *Br J Anaesth* 55:1239-1246, 1983.
16. Hamilton WK: Nomenclature of inhalation anesthetic systems, *Anesthesiology* 25:3-5, 1964.
17. Tenpas RH, Brown ES, Elam JO: Carbon dioxide absorption. The circle versus the to-and-fro, *Anesthesiology* 19:231-239, 1958.
18. Eger EI, Ethans CT: The effects of inflow, overflow and valve placement on economy of the circle system, *Anesthesiology* 29:93-100, 1968.
19. Brown ES, Seniff AM, Elam JO: Carbon dioxide elimination in semiclosed systems, *Anesthesiology* 25:31-36, 1964.
20. de Silva AJC: Normocapnic ventilation using the circle system, *Can Anaesth Soc J* 23:657-666, 1976.
21. Keenan RL, Boyan CP: How rebreathing anaesthetic systems control Paco$_2$: studies with a mechanical and a mathematical model, *Can Anaesth Soc J* 25:117-121, 1978.
22. Ladegaard-Petersen HJ: A circle system without carbon dioxide absorption, *Acta Anaesthesiol Scand* 22:281-286, 1978.
23. Nightingale DA, Richards CC, Gress A: An evaluation of rebreathing in a modified T-piece system during controlled ventilation of anaesthetized children, *Br J Anaesth* 37:762-771, 1965.
24. Steen SN, Chen JL: Automatic non-rebreathing valve circuits: some principles and modifications, *Br J Anaesth* 35:379-382, 1963.
25. Spoerel WE: Rebreathing and end-tidal CO$_2$ during spontaneous breathing with the Bain Circuit, *Can Anaesth Soc J* 30:148-154, 1983.
26. Willis BA, Pender JW, Mapleson WW: Rebreathing in a T-piece volunteer and theoretical studies of the Jackson-Rees modification of Ayre's T-piece during spontaneous respiration, *Br J Anaesth* 47:1239-1246, 1975.
27. Feeley TW, Hamilton WK, Xavier B, et al: Sterile anesthesia breathing circuits do not prevent postoperative pulmonary infection, *Anesthesiology* 54:369-372, 1981.
28. Chandler M: Pressure changes in tracheal tube cuffs, *Anaesthesia* 41:287-293, 1986.
29. Rampil IJ. Anesthetic considerations for laser surgery, *Anesth Analg* 74:424-435, 1992.
30. Parmley JB, Tahir AH, Dascomb HE, et al: Disposable versus reusable rebreathing circuits: advantages, disadvantages, hazards and bacteriologic studies, *Anesth Analg* 51:888-894, 1972.
31. Berry FA, Eastwood DW: Serious defects in "simple" equipment, *Anesthesiology* 28:471, 1967.
32. Cozantis OA, Tahkuman O: Aneurysm of ventilator tubing, *Anaesthesia* 26:235-236, 1971.
33. Bushman JA, Collins JM: The estimation of gas losses in ventilator tubing, *Anaesthesia* 22:664-667, 1967.
34. Proctor DF: Studies of respiratory air flow: resistance to air flow through anesthetic apparatus, *Bull Johns Hopkins Hosp* 96:49-58, 1955.
35. Spoerel WE: Rebreathing and carbon dioxide elimination with the Bain circuit, *Can Anaesth Soc J* 27:357-361, 1980.
36. Wang J-S, Hung W-T, Lin C-Y: Leakage of disposable breathing circuits, *J Clin Anesth* 4:111-115, 1992.
37. Foregger R: The classification and performance of respiratory valves, *Anesthesiology* 20:296-308, 1959.
38. Hunt KH: Resistance in respiratory valves and canisters, *Anesthesiology* 16:190-205, 1955.
39. Eger EI, II: *Anesthetic systems: construction and function*. In Eger EI, II, editor: *Anesthetic uptake and action*, Baltimore, 1974, Williams and Wilkins.
40. Dogu TS, Davis HS: Hazards of inadvertently opposed valves, *Anesthesiology* 33:122-123, 1970.
41. Hirano T, Saito T: A new automatic nonrebreathing valve, *Anesthesiology* 31:84-85, 1969.
42. Horn B: Valve for assisted or controlled ventilation, *Anesthesiology* 21:83, 1960.
43. Lewis G: Nonrebreathing valve, *Anesthesiology* 17:618-619, 1956.
44. Newton GW, Howill WK, Stephen CR: A piston-type nonrebreathing valve, *Anesthesiology* 16:1037-1038, 1955.
45. Ruben H: A new nonrebreathing valve, *Anesthesiology* 16:643-645, 1955.
46. Stephen CR, Slater HM: A nonrebreathing mask, *Anesthesiology* 13:226-229, 1952.
47. Loehning RW, Davis G, Safar P: Rebreathing with "nonrebreathing valves," *Anesthesiology* 25:854-856, 1964.
48. Redick LF, Dunbar RW, MacDougal DC, et al: An evaluation of hand operated self-inflating resuscitation equipment, *Anesth Analg* 49:28-32, 1970.
49. Wisborg K, Jacobsen E: Functional disorders of Ruben and Ambu-E valves after dismantling and cleaning, *Anesthesiology* 42:633-634, 1975.
50. Johnston RE, Smith TC: Rebreathing bags as pressure limiting devices, *Anesthesiology* 38:192-194, 1973.
51. Waters DJ: Use and misuse of a pressure-limiting bag, *Anaesthesia* 22:322-325, 1967.
52. Woolmer R, Lind B: Rebreathing with a semiclosed system, *Br J Anaesth* 26:316-322, 1954.
53. Lecky JH: The mechanical aspects of anesthetic pollution control, *Anesth Analg* 56:769-774, 1977.

54. Lee S: A new popoff valve, *Anesthesiology* 25:240-242, 1964.
55. Linker GS, Holaday DA, Waltuck B: A simply constructed automatic pressure relief valve, *Anesthesiology* 32:563-564, 1970.
56. Mitchell JV, Epstein HG: A pressure-operated inflating valve, *Anaesthesia* 21:277-281, 1966.
57. Smith RH, Volpitto PP: Volume ventilator valve, *Anesthesiology* 20:885-886, 1959.
58. Brown, ES, Elam JO: Practical aspects of carbon dioxide absorption, *NY State J Med* 55:3436-3442, 1955.
59. Adriani J, Rovenstine EA: Experimental studies in carbon dioxide absorbers for anesthesia, *Anesthesiology* 2:1-19, 1941.
60. Brown ES: The activity and surface area of fresh soda lime, *Anesthesiology* 19:208-212, 1958.
61. Brown ES: Voids, pores and total air space of carbon dioxide absorbents, *Anesthesiology* 19:1-6, 1958.
62. Brown ES, Bakamjian V, Seniff AM: Performance of absorbents: effects of moisture, *Anesthesiology* 20:613-617, 1959.
63. Kitborn MG: Preliminary clinical report on a new carbon dioxide absorbent—baralyme, *Anesthesiology* 2:621-637, 1941.
64. Revell DG: An improved circulator for closed circle anaesthesia, *Can Anaesth Soc J* 6:104-107, 1959.
65. Neff WB, Burke SF, Thompson R: A venturi circulator for anesthetic systems, *Anesthesiology* 29:838-841, 1968.
66. Eger EI, Hamilton WK: Positive-negative pressure ventilation with a modified Ayre's T-piece, *Anesthesiology* 19:611-618, 1958.
67. Mazze RI: Bacterial air filters, *Anesthesiology* 54:359-360, 1981.
68. Garibaldi RA, Britt MR, Webster C, et al: Failure of bacterial filters to reduce the incidence of pneumonia after inhalation anesthesia, *Anesthesiology* 54:364-368, 1981.
69. Dryden GE, Dryden SR, Brown DG, et al: Performance of bacterial filters, *Respir Care* 25:1127-1135, 1980.
70. Harper M, Eger EI II: A comparison of the efficiency of three anesthesia circle systems, *Anesth Analg* 55:724-729, 1976.
71. Neufeld PD, Johnson DL: Results of the Canadian Anaesthetists' Society opinion survey on anaesthetic equipment, *Can Anaesth Soc J:* 30:469-473, 1983.
72. Chalon J, Kao ZL, Dolorico VN, et al: Humidity output of the circle absorber system, *Anesthesiology* 38:458-465, 1973.
73. Dery R, Pelletier J, Jacques A, et al: Humidity in anesthesiology. II. Evolution of heat and moisture in the large CO_2 absorbers, *Can Anaesth Soc J* 14:205-219, 1967.
74. Molyneux L, Pask EA: The flow of gases in a semiclosed anaesthetic system, *Br J Anaesth* 23:81-91, 1951.
75. Briere C, Patoine JG, Audet R: Inaccurate ventimetry by fresh gas inlet position, *Can Anaesth Soc J* 21:117-119, 1974.
76. Smith TC: Nitrous oxide and low inflow circle system, *Anesthesiology* 27:266-271, 1966.
77. Norman J, Adams AP, Sykes MK: Rebreathing with the Magill attachment, *Anaesthesia* 23:75-81, 1968.
78. Kain ML, Nunn JF: Fresh gas economics of the Magill circuit, *Anesthesiology* 29:964-974, 1968.

79. Humphrey D: The Lack, Magill and Bain anaesthetic breathing systems: a direct comparison in spontaneously breathing anaesthetized adults, *J R Soc Med* 75:513-524, 1982.
80. Ungerer MJ: A comparison between the Bain and Magill anaesthetic systems during spontaneous breathing, *Can Anaesth Soc J* 25:122-124, 1978.
81. Bain JA, Spoerel WE: Prediction of arterial carbon dioxide tension during controlled ventilation with a modified Mapleson D system, *Can Anaesth Soc J* 22:34-38, 1975.
82. Byrick RJ: Respiratory compensation during spontaneous ventilation with the Bain circuit, *Can Anaesth Soc J* 27:96-104, 1980.
83. Byrick JJ, Janssen E, Yamashita, M: Rebreathing and co-axial circuits, *Anaesthesia* 32:294, 1977.
84. Paterson JG, Vanhooydonk V: A hazard associated with improper connection of the Bain breathing circuit, *Can Anaesth Soc J* 22:373-377, 1975.
85. Foex P, Crampton Smith A: A test for co-axial circuits. *Anaesthesia* 32:294, 1977.
86. Pethick SL: *Can Anaesth Soc J* 22:115, 1975 (correspondence).
87. Barnes PK, Conway CM, Purcell GRG: The Lack anaesthetic system, *Anaesthesia* 35:393-394, 1980.
88. Noh M, Walters F, Norman J: A comparison of the Lack and Bain semi-closed circuits in spontaneous respiration, *Br J Anaesth* 49:512, 1977.
89. Humphrey D, Brock-Utne JG, Downing JW: Single lever Humphrey A.D.E. low flow universal anaesthetic breathing system. Part I, *Can Anaesth Soc J* 33:698-709, 1986. Part II, *Can Anaesth Soc J* 33:710-718, 1986.
90. Artru A, Katz RA: Evaluation of the Humphrey A.D.E. breathing system, *Can J Anaesth* 34:484-488, 1987.
91. Bruce, DL: A simple way to vent anesthetic gases, *Anesth Analg* 52:595-598, 1973.
92. Dery R, Pelletier J, Jacques A, et al: Humidity in anesthesiology. III. Heat and moisture patterns in the respiratory tract during anesthesia with the semi-closed system, *Can Anaesth Soc J* 14:287-298, 1967.
93. Gedeon A, Mebius C: The hygroscopic condenser humidifier, *Anaesthesia* 34:1043-1047, 1979.
94. MacKanying N, Chalon J: Humidification of anesthetic gases for children, *Anesth Analg* 53:387-391, 1974.
95. GMS PEEP Valve. Operation and Maintanance Manual. Madison, Wis, 1991, Ohmeda, a Division of BOC Health Care, Inc.
96. Cooper JB, Newbower RS, Kitz RJ: An analysis of major errors and equipment failures in anesthesia management, *Anesthesiology* 60:34-42, 1984.
97. Eger EI, Epstein RM: Hazards of anesthetic equipment, *Anesthesiology* 25:490-504, 1964.
98. Wyant GM: *Mechanical misadventures in anaesthesia*, Toronto, 1978, University of Toronto Press.

Chapter 5

WASTE ANESTHETIC GAS SPILLAGE AND SCAVENGING SYSTEMS

Isaac Azar, M.D.
James B. Eisenkraft, M.D.

TRACE CONCENTRATIONS OF ANESTHETICS AS POLLUTANTS

Concern over trace concentrations of anesthetic gases dates to 1967, when Vaisman[1] reported a survey of 354 anesthesiologists in Russia. All worked in poorly ventilated operating rooms and used nitrous oxide, halothane, and ether. Of the total, 303 responded to the survey; and of these, 110 were female. Among female responders there were 31 pregnancies, 18 of which ended in spontaneous abortion. One pregnancy resulted in a congenitally abnormal child. Vaisman concluded that these problems in pregnancy—as well as other reported effects, such as nau-

*Parts of this chapter are adapted with permission from Azar I: *Waste anesthetic gas spillage and scavenging systems.* In Cottrell JE editor: *Occupational hazards to OR and recovery room personnel,* Boston, 1981, Little, Brown; and from Eisenkraft JB: *Operating room pollution.* In Eisenkraft JB editor: *Progress in anesthesiology, vol 1,* 1987, Dannemiller Memorial Educational Foundation, San Antonio, Tex.

sea, irritability, and fatigue—were due to a combination of chronic inhalation of anesthetic vapors, emotional strain, and excessive workload.[1] Although uncontrolled and largely anecdotal, this study drew attention to the possibility that trace concentrations of anesthetics may be harmful. The matter was taken up by investigators in the United Kingdom[2,3] and in Scandinavia,[4] and their results appeared to confirm Vaisman's findings.

In 1970 the United States Congress passed the Occupational Safety and Health Act,[5] the purpose of which was to ensure "safe and healthful working conditions, for all men and women in the nation." The Act established the National Institute for Occupational Safety and Health (NIOSH), which has the responsibility of conducting and funding research in exposure hazards and recommending safety standards. The Act also established the Occupational Safety and Health Administration (OSHA), which, after due procedure, would enact into law and then enforce NIOSH recommended standards.[6] NIOSH funded a number of studies, one of which was the national survey of occupational disease among operating room (OR) workers, conducted in conjunction with the American Society of Anesthesiologists' (ASA) Ad Hoc Committee on Waste Anesthetic Gases. This study surveyed 49,000 potentially exposed [members of the ASA, American Association of Nurse Anesthetists (AANA), Association of Operating Room Nurses (AORN), Association of Operating Room Technicians (AORT)] and 26,000 unexposed (members of the American Academy of Pediatrics, American Nurses Association) personnel.[7] The results, published in 1974, showed an increased reported incidence among females of spontaneous abortion, liver and kidney disease, and cancer, and a higher reported incidence of congenital abnormalities in the offspring of exposed women. Among the exposed males, the incidence of cancer did not increase, but that of hepatic disease did. NIOSH sponsored further related studies, including investigations of the effects of trace anesthetic vapors on perceptual skills[8,9] and of methods for reducing exposure to waste gases.[10]

In March 1977, NIOSH published *Criteria for a recommended standard; exposure to waste anesthetic gases and vapors.*[11] This report estimated that 214,000 workers were potentially exposed on a day-to-day basis to trace concentrations of anesthetic gases. The document reviewed all the data then available and found that, although not completely definitive, the evidence strongly suggested a relationship between health hazards and trace concentrations of anesthetic gases. No relationship of cause and effect was established, and no safe exposure levels could be identified. However, the document recommended that risks should be minimized as much as possible by maintaining "exposures as low as is technically feasible." The document also recommended measures to reduce exposure and to monitor exposure levels, and extensive record-keeping regarding the health of OR personnel.

NIOSH recommended environmental limits for the upper boundary of exposure as follows: "Occupational exposure to halogenated anesthetic agents shall be controlled so that no worker is exposed at concentrations greater than 2 ppm (parts per million) of any halogenated anesthetic agent. . . . When such agents are used in combination with nitrous oxide, levels of the halogenated agent well below 2 ppm are achievable. In most situations, control of nitrous oxide to a time-weighted average (TWA) concentration of 25 ppm during the anesthetic administration period will result in levels of approximately 0.5 ppm of the halogenated agent. . . . Occupational exposure to nitrous oxide when used as the sole anesthetic agent, shall be controlled so that no worker is exposed at TWA concentrations greater than 25 ppm during anesthetic administration. Available data indicate that with current control technology, exposure levels of 50 ppm, and less for nitrous oxide are attainable in dental offices."[11]

These recommended exposure limits were based on two pieces of work. First, Whitcher, et al[10] showed that these levels were readily attainable in the operating room when certain precautionary measures were taken. Second, Bruce and Bach[12] found no decrement in the psychomotor capacities of volunteers exposed for 4 hours at these levels.

To provide a perspective on what ppm means, consider that the presence of 25 ppm of nitrous oxide in the atmosphere represents a concentration of one four-hundredth of 1%:

$$100\% \ N_2O \text{ is one million parts per million (by volume)}$$
$$100\% \ N_2O = 10^6 \text{ ppm}$$
$$1\% \ N_2O = 10,000 \text{ ppm}$$
$$(1/100) \times 1\% \ N_2O = 100 \text{ ppm}$$
$$(1/400) \times 1\% \ N_2O = 25 \text{ ppm}$$

Two ppm of halothane represents a concentration of one five-thousandth of 1% halothane.

$$100 \text{ ppm} = (1/100) \times 1\% \text{ halothane}$$
$$2 \text{ ppm} = (1/100 \times 1/50) \times 1\%$$
$$= (1/5000) \times 1\% = 0.0002\%$$
$$0.5 \text{ ppm} = (1/20,000) \times 1\% = 0.00005\%$$

To express in terms of anesthetic potency, divide by the MAC of halothane (0.76%).

$$2 \text{ ppm} = 0.0002\% = \frac{(2 \times 10^{-4})}{0.76} \text{ MAC}$$

or 0.00026 MAC halothane

What levels of trace anesthetics may be found in the operating room? When no attempt has been made to reduce leakage of or to scavenge waste gases, trace gas levels of 400 to 600 ppm of nitrous oxide and from 5 to 10 ppm of halogenated agents may be detected.[11] Effective scavenging alone can reduce these levels more than tenfold.

The volume of nitrous oxide that must be released into an OR in order to reach the NIOSH maximum recommended limit of 25 ppm is easily calculated. Assume an

OR has the dimensions 5 meters (wide) $\times$ 5 meters (long) $\times$ 4 meters (high). Volume of OR is therefore given by:

$$500 \text{ cm} \times 500 \text{ cm} \times 400 \text{ cm}$$
$$\text{or } (5 \times 10^2) \times (5 \times 10^2) \times (4 \times 10^2)$$
$$\text{or } (5 \times 5 \times 4) \times 10^6 \text{ ml}$$
$$\text{or } 100 \times 10^6 \text{ ml}$$

NIOSH limit is $25/10^6$. If the OR volume is 100×10^6, this limit is reached by release of

$$(25 \times 100) = 2500 \text{ ml of N}_2\text{O}.$$

This calculation assumes uniform mixing of all gases and no ventilation or air conditioning of the OR. If it is assumed that the OR ventilation system produces 12 air changes per hour, it is apparent that a nitrous oxide leakage rate of 500 ml/min will serve to maintain the atmospheric nitrous oxide level at 25 ppm. In the OR described previously, 2.5 L of N_2O would be necessary to produce 25 ppm. If an OR has 12 air changes per hour, each air change takes 5 minutes. A leakage rate of 2.5 L N_2O per 5 minutes $(2.5/5) = 0.5$ L N_2O/min.

Anesthetic pollution is not limited only to the OR. Significant contamination may occur in the corridors of an OR suite, in the anesthesia workroom, and in the nitrous oxide storage area. Poorly ventilated postanesthesia care units may also be contaminated with exhaled anesthetic agents.[13]

SOURCES OF ANESTHETIC GAS SPILLAGE

Potential sources of anesthetic gas spillage are the adjustable pressure limiting valve, the high- and low-pressure systems of the anesthesia machine, the anesthesia ventilator, cryosurgery, and other miscellaneous sources.

The adjustable pressure limiting valve

The adjustable pressure limiting (APL) or "pop-off" valve of the anesthesia breathing circuit is the outlet for waste anesthetic gases during spontaneous or assisted ventilation. Depending on the inflow rate of fresh gas, more than 5 L of gas can exit the circuit through this valve every minute. The effect of such spillage on the level of anesthetic pollution in the OR is given by the equation

$$C = (L \times 60 \times 10^6)/(NV)$$

where:

C = OR pollutant level in parts per million
L = Pollutant spillage in liters per minute
V = OR total air volume in liters
N = Number of air exchanges per hour

For example, if $L = 3$ L/min, $V = 126,000$ L, and $N = 10$ exchanges per hour, then

$$C = (3 \times 60 \times 10^6)/(10 \times 126,000) = 142 \text{ ppm}$$

Particularly large volumes of anesthetic gases are discharged through the relief valve of nonrebreathing systems, such as the Jackson-Rees circuit (Mapleson D). Without scavenging and proper room ventilation, nitrous oxide levels as high as 2000 ppm have been found in the breathing zone of anesthesiologists.[14]

The high-pressure system of the anesthesia machine

The high-pressure system of the anesthesia machine includes the nitrous oxide central supply pipeline, the reserve tanks, and the internal piping of the machine that leads to the nitrous oxide flowmeter (Fig. 5-1). The pressure in this system is 50 to 70 psig. Leaks therefore are likely to contribute significantly to the pollution of the OR. Common sources of high-pressure leaks are defective connectors in the nitrous oxide central supply line (Fig. 5-1) and defective yokes for the nitrous oxide reserve tanks (Fig. 5-1). In one OR suite, major high-pressure leaks were detected in 50% of the anesthesia machines.[15] When the OR is not being used, background nitrous oxide pollution is caused primarily by high-pressure leaks.

The low-pressure system of the anesthesia machine

The low-pressure system of the anesthesia machine includes the nitrous oxide flowmeter, the vaporizers, the fresh gas delivery tubing (from the anesthesia machine to the breathing circuit) (Fig. 5-2, F), the carbon dioxide absorber (Fig. 5-2, E), the breathing hoses (Fig. 5-2, D), the unidirectional valves, the ventilator, and the various components of the scavenging system. Leaks occur most commonly in the carbon dioxide absorber because of loose screws, worn gaskets, granules of soda lime on the gaskets, and an open petcock. Other leaks may occur as a result of breaks in the rubber and plastic components of the breathing circuit, loose domes on the unidirectional valves (Fig. 5-2, A and B), or a poorly fitting oxygen sensor (Fig. 5-2, C) in the breathing circuit. Particularly prone to leakage are disposable breathing circuits, especially those of the swivel type, due to imperfections in the manufacturing process.[16] Although vaporizers are usually gas-tight, they too occasionally leak as a result of loose mounts or defective seals and gaskets.

A direct linear relationship exists between the peak pressure in the breathing circuit and the amount of gas that escapes through a leak in the low-pressure system: the higher the pressure, the greater the leak. Despite effective scavenging, as much as 2 L/min may leak from the breathing circuit, raising the nitrous oxide level in the air because of 100 to 200 ppm.

The scavenging system itself may be a source of pollution. The rubber parts and safety valves may leak anesthetic gases, or improperly sized hoses (i.e., 22-mm diameter) may have been "adapted" to fit the 19-mm scavenger connections. The system may also be overloaded because of inadequate vacuum or ventilation systems, and consequently the waste gases are spilled into the air.

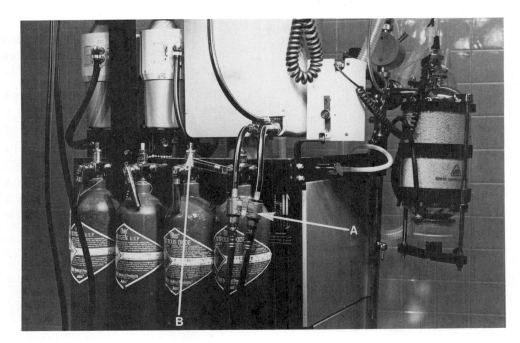

Fig. 5-1. Sources of leaks in the high-pressure system: **A,** quick connector; **B,** yoke of nitrous oxide reserve tank.

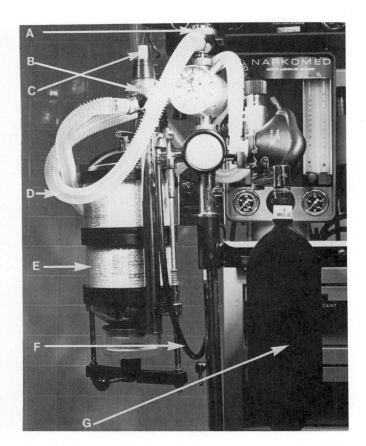

Fig. 5-2. Sources of leaks in the low-pressure system: **A** and **B,** domes of the unidirectional valves; **C,** oxygen sensor; **D,** breathing hoses; **E,** Carbon dioxide absorber; **F,** delivery tube, and **G,** breathing bag.

The anesthesia ventilator

The anesthesia ventilator may be a major source of leakage. Some ventilators leak internally, causing anesthetic gases to mix with the nonscavenged driving gas of the ventilator. In one case, the OR nitrous oxide level rose from 5 ppm to 80 ppm each time the ventilator was used.

Errors in anesthesia technique

With a leak-proofed anesthesia machine and an effective scavenging system, 94% to 99% of all OR anesthetic pollution is caused by errors in anesthesia technique.[17] The following errors contribute significantly to anesthetic pollution:

1. Insufflation and old-fashioned techniques such as open-drop anesthesia cause extensive OR pollution.
2. Turning the nitrous oxide flowmeter and/or a vaporizer on while the breathing circuit is not attached to the patient causes direct spillage of anesthetic gases into room air. This often occurs at the beginning and end of anesthesia administration, and during intubation. The anesthesiologist should turn off both the vaporizer and the oxygen and nitrous oxide flowmeters; otherwise, anesthetic-laden gas in the circuit will flow into the room.
3. A poorly fitting face mask permits leakage of anesthetic gases around the rim.
4. An uncuffed tracheal tube that is too small in relation to the tracheal diameter, or a poorly seated cuffed tracheal tube, may allow anesthetic gases to leak and spill into the room air.

5. Upon conclusion of surgery, if a deeply anesthetized patient is disconnected from the breathing circuit, relatively high concentrations of anesthetic gases can be exhaled into the room air.
6. Inadvertent spillage of liquid volatile anesthetic agent while a vaporizer is refilled adds vapor to room air (each ml of spilled liquid adds about 200 ml of vapor).
7. Emptying the breathing circuit of anesthetic gases while the circuit is disconnected from the patient spills anesthetic gases directly into the room air.

Cryosurgery

Cryosurgery, used by gynecologists, ophthalmologists, otolaryngologists, and dermatologists, is a major source of OR pollution.[18] A jet of 20 to 90 L/min of liquid nitrous oxide is used as a surgical tool. The liquid rapidly evaporates, raising the level of nitrous oxide in the air. Air contamination with nitrous oxide is particularly high when cryosurgery is used in a small, poorly ventilated office.[19]

Miscellaneous sources of anesthetic pollution

During cardiopulmonary bypass the pump oxygenator may not be scavenged. When a potent volatile anesthetic agent is used during bypass, the waste anesthetic gas is often discharged into the OR air. Diffusion of anesthetic vapors from rubber and plastic goods in the anesthesia workroom may represent another cause of anesthetic pollution. As much as 300 ml of anesthetic vapor may be released from a used breathing circuit.[17]

A minor cause of anesthetic pollution is diffusion of anesthetic gases from the surgical wound and the patient's skin. The concentration of halothane in the air immediately over the operating field was found to be 3 to 6 times higher than in the OR air. Higher levels were also found under the surgical drapes, possibly due to diffusion of halothane from the patient's skin.[20]

An infrequent cause of OR pollution is the inadvertent crossing of the fresh-air and exhaust ducts of the OR ventilation system. In addition, installing the system exhaust port in a position upwind from the fresh-air intake may result in contamination of all ORs supplied by that ventilation system.

OPERATING ROOM VENTILATION SYSTEMS

The OR ventilation system is the single most important factor in reducing anesthetic air pollution. Unventilated ORs are four times as contaminated as those with proper ventilation.

The components of a typical OR ventilation system include:

1. Fresh-air intake from outside
2. Central pump
3. Series of filters
4. Air conditioning units
5. Manifold that distributes fresh air to the ORs
6. Manifold that collects air from the ORs
7. Fresh-air inflow port in each OR

The OR fresh-air inflow port is located in the ceiling, and the outflow port is located on an adjacent wall 6 inches above the floor. Generally, OR ventilation systems are one of two types: nonrecirculating or recirculating. The following sections describe the various features of each system.

The nonrecirculating ventilation system

Most ORs are equipped with nonrecirculating ventilation systems (Fig. 5-3). This type of system pumps fresh air into the OR from the outside and removes stale air. The number of air exchanges per hour varies significantly between ORs. A survey of one OR suite showed the number of air exchanges to vary between less than 5 and more than 30 per hour among the various rooms.

The number of air exchanges per hour is an important determinant of the level of anesthetic pollution in the OR. A rate of 10 or more exchanges per hour is recommended. Lower rates might permit creation of *hot spots* (air pockets highly contaminated by anesthetics), and higher rates may create air turbulence and cause discomfort to OR personnel.

The air flow pattern in the OR, as well as the location of the anesthesia machine in relation to the air flow, also influences the level of anesthesia pollution (Fig. 5-4). When air flow generates floor-to-ceiling eddies causing extensive air mixing, hot spots are reduced in size and number. On the other hand, hot spots are more likely to form with laminar air flow, which reduces air mixing.

The recirculating ventilation system

A recirculating ventilation system partially recirculates stale air. Each air exchange consists of part filtered and conditioned stale air and part fresh outdoor air. This is more economical than the nonrecirculating system because it requires less air conditioning. The recirculating system is particularly popular in locations with extremely hot or cold climates. Because filtering does not cleanse air of anesthetic gases, a recirculating system may contaminate clean ORs by recirculating polluted air from contaminated ORs to clean ORs.

WASTE GAS SCAVENGING SYSTEMS

Modern anesthesia machines are factory-equipped with scavenging systems. However, some machines not equipped with such systems may still be in use. The Joint Commission on Accreditation of Healthcare Organizations (JCAHO)* requires availability and use of scavenging sys-

*JCAHO Accreditation manual for hospitals, vol 1, standards, SA.1.4.3.3.1, Oakbrook Terrace, Il, 1991, JCAHO.

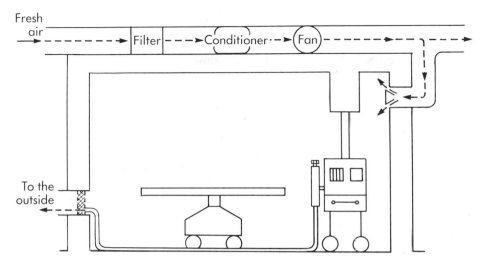

Fig. 5-3. A nonrecirculating ventilation system serving as passive disposal route for anesthetic waste gases. (From Whitcher CE, Piziali R, Sher R, et al: *Development and evaluation of methods for elimination of waste anesthetic gases and vapors in hospitals*. HEW (NIOSH) Publication No. 75-137. Washington, DC, 1975, US Government Printing Office.)

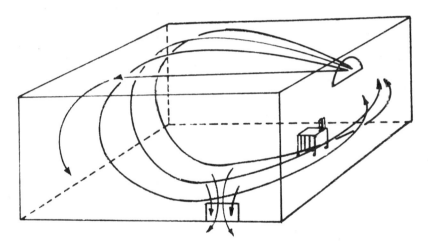

Fig. 5-4. Operating room air flow pattern with ceiling-to-floor eddy. (From Berner O: Concentration and elimination of anaesthetic gases in operating theatres, *Acta Anaesthesiol Scand* 22:46, 1978.)

tems. Some anesthesia personnel discharge the waste anesthesia gases toward the floor, believing that the heavier-than-air anesthetic gases form a layer on the floor and flow out via the OR ventilation system. In reality, waste anesthetic gases are effectively mixed with room air by air eddies created by OR traffic. When the anesthesia machine is equipped with a properly functioning scavenging system, the air pollution by waste gases in the OR is reduced by 90%.

General properties of scavenging systems

An anesthesia scavenging system collects the waste anesthetic gases from the breathing circuit and discards them. A properly designed and assembled system will not affect the dynamics of the breathing circuit; nor will it af-

fect ventilation and oxygenation of the patient. The American National Standards Institute (ANSI) document ANSI Z.79.11-1982 provides minimal performance and safety criteria to serve as guidelines for the manufacturer of equipment that removes excess anesthetic gases from the working environment.[21] This standard, published in 1982, will soon be superseded by a document from the American Society for Testing and Materials (ASTM).

A typical scavenging system consists of (1) a relief valve whereby gas leaves the circuit, (2) tubing to conduct the gas to a scavenging interface, (3) the interface, and (4) a disposal line. Scavenging systems are classified as either active or passive. In an active scavenging system, a substantial negative pressure (hospital vacuum) is applied to the disposal line connected to the interface. The waste gas

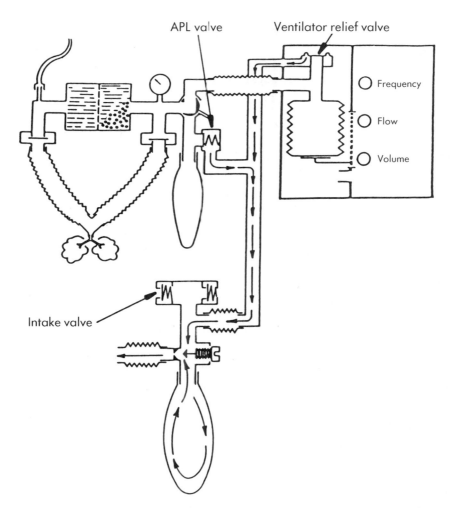

Fig. 5-5. Points of exit for waste gas from a typical circle system. APL = Adjustable pressure limiting. (Reproduced by permission of North American Dräger, Inc, Telford, Pa.)

is literally sucked away from the interface. In a passive scavenging system, the waste gases flow under their own pressure, via a wide-bore tube, to the OR ventilation outlet grille.

Adjustable pressure limiting and ventilator pressure relief valves

When a circle system is in use with spontaneous or controlled ventilation, waste gases leave the circuit via the adjustable pressure limiting (APL), or "pop-off," valve (Fig. 5-5). This valve is usually of the spring-loaded design such that a minimum amount of positive pressure is needed for gas to exit the circuit (see also Chapter 4). The APL valve has a single exhaust port (Figs. 5-6 and 5-7). In order to avoid accidental connection to the breathing circuit, this port should be a 19-mm male fitting with a 1:40 conical shape.

When an anesthesia ventilator is in use, the APL valve is out of circuit and gas exits the circle at end-exhalation via the ventilator pressure relief (PR) valve (Fig. 5-5). During inspiration, this valve is normally held closed by

positive pressure transmitted from the ventilator driving gas circuit. The exhaust port of the PR valve is also 19 mm in diameter to connect to the 19-mm tubing that conducts waste gas from both the PR and APL valves to the scavenger interface.

Conducting tube

Conducting tubing conducts the waste gases from the APL or PR valve to the scavenging interface. It is specified to be of 19 mm or 30 mm diameter and rigid enough to prevent kinking.[21]

The scavenging interface

The scavenging system interfaces the gas flowing out of the patient circuit with the hospital's suction or evacuation system. Scavenging systems may be open or closed.

Closed reservoir systems

Closed systems use spring-loaded valves to ensure that excessively high or low pressures are not applied to the patient circuit (Figs. 5-8 and 5-9). Thus, if the system were

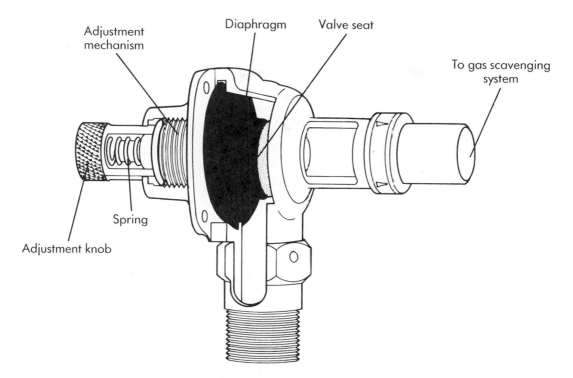

Fig. 5-6. The Ohmeda APL valve. (From Bowie E, Huffman LM: *The anesthesia machine: essentials for understanding, 1985.* Reproduced by permission of Ohmeda, a Division of BOC Healthcare, Inc, Madison, Wis.)

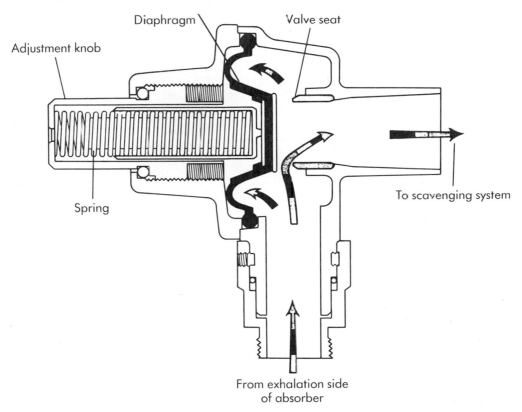

Fig. 5-7. Schematic of Ohmeda APL valve. Note that it is a spring-loaded valve in contrast with the needle valve design used by North American Dräger (see Fig. 4-5B). (From Bowie E, Huffman LM: *The anesthesia machine: essentials for understanding,* 1985. Reproduced by permission of Ohmeda, a Division of BOC Healthcare, Inc, Madison, Wis.)

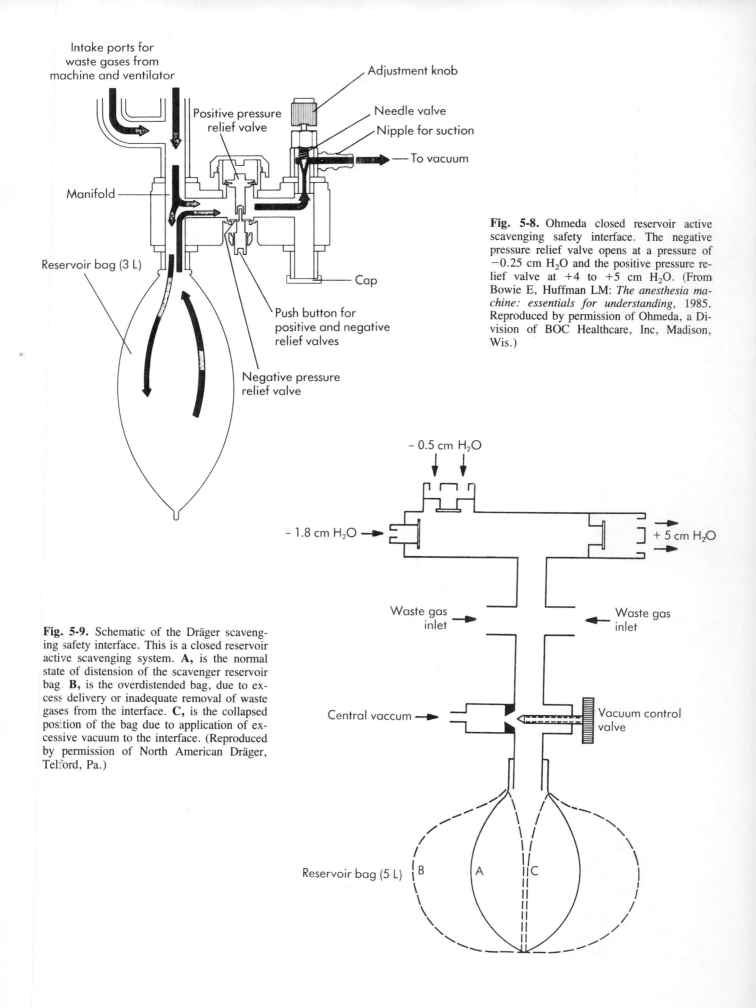

Intake ports for
waste gases from
machine and ventilator

Adjustment knob

Positive pressure
relief valve

Needle valve

Nipple for suction

To vacuum

Manifold

Reservoir bag (3 L)

Cap

Push button for
positive and negative
relief valves

Negative pressure
relief valve

Fig. 5-8. Ohmeda closed reservoir active scavenging safety interface. The negative pressure relief valve opens at a pressure of -0.25 cm H_2O and the positive pressure relief valve at $+4$ to $+5$ cm H_2O. (From Bowie E, Huffman LM: *The anesthesia machine: essentials for understanding,* 1985. Reproduced by permission of Ohmeda, a Division of BOC Healthcare, Inc, Madison, Wis.)

Fig. 5-9. Schematic of the Dräger scavenging safety interface. This is a closed reservoir active scavenging system. **A,** is the normal state of distension of the scavenger reservoir bag. **B,** is the overdistended bag, due to excess delivery or inadequate removal of waste gases from the interface. **C,** is the collapsed position of the bag due to application of excessive vacuum to the interface. (Reproduced by permission of North American Dräger, Telford, Pa.)

-0.5 cm H_2O

-1.8 cm H_2O

$+5$ cm H_2O

Waste gas
inlet

Waste gas
inlet

Central vaccum

Vacuum control
valve

Reservoir bag (5 L)

B   A   C

not connected to suction, excess pressure in the interface due to gas entering it from the circuit would be vented to the OR via the positive pressure relief valve (the "pop-off" opens at about +5 cm H_2O). In the event that excessive suction were to be applied to the circuit, one (Ohmeda interface, Fig. 5-8) or two (Dräger closed interface, Fig. 5-9) negative pressure relief ("pop-in") valves (−0.5 to −1.8 cm H_2O), depending on the system, would open to preferentially suck in room air and to minimize the potential application of negative pressure to the patient circuit. Figure 5-10 shows an Ohmeda closed reservoir interface connected to an OR ventilation duct. No vacuum is connected to the interface, and the needle valve is closed. This is an example of a passive scavenging system.

A reservoir bag is incorporated into the closed reservoir interface assemblies for the following purposes:

1. To contain the flow of waste anesthetic gases during exhalation and thus avoid overwhelming the disposal route with gas.
2. To serve as a visual indicator of a properly functioning disposal route (active or passive). An overdistended bag indicates an occluded disposal route or a weak vacuum; a collapsed bag indicates an excessive vacuum. With normal operation the bag should fill during exhalation, and empty during inhalation. This is because gas is normally added to the interface from the circuit only during exhalation.

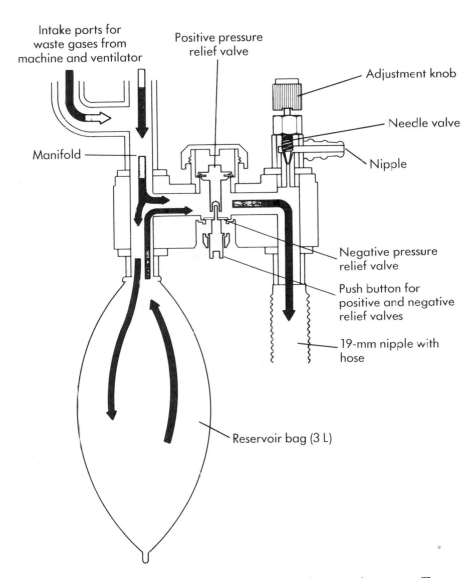

Fig. 5-10. Ohmeda closed reservoir scavenging interface used as a passive system. The vacuum is not connected (compare with Figure 5-8), and gas flows passively to the OR exhaust ventilation duct. (From Bowie E, Huffman LM: *The anesthesia machine: essentials for understanding,* 1985. Reproduced by permission of Ohmeda, a Division of BOC Healthcare, Inc, Madison, Wis.)

Open reservoir systems

Open reservoir scavenging interfaces are valveless (Figs. 5-11 through 5-13) and use continually open relief ports to provide positive and negative pressure relief.[22] In the Dräger open reservoir interface (Fig. 5-11), the reservoir canister contains the excess waste gas and thereby accommodates a range of waste gas flow rates from the patient circuit. Because this type of interface depends on relief ports for pressure relief, care must be taken to ensure that these ports remain unoccluded at all times. Another design of open reservoir system uses a tube-within-a-tube assembly (Fig. 5-12), which is essentially similar in principle of operation to the Dräger open reservoir interface described above.

A reservoir bag is sometimes incorporated in the open reservoir design of interface assembly for the same reasons given for its inclusion in the closed reservoir design.

Disposal routes

Waste anesthetic gases may be disposed of by active disposal routes (wall suction or a dedicated evacuation system) or passive disposal routes (the OR ventilation system or a through-the-wall conduit) (Fig. 5-14).

Active disposal routes. When waste anesthetic gases are disposed of by way of wall suction, the following requirements should be met:

1. The wall suction should be capable of drawing at least 30 L/min^{-1} of air.
2. The scavenging interface should be equipped with at least one negative pressure relief valve (closed reservoir) or ports open to the atmosphere (open reservoir).
3. The exhaust port of the wall suction should be at a safe distance from the breathing zone of personnel.
4. Explosive anesthetic gases should not be used (National Fire Protection Association regulations).

It is preferable to have a separate, dedicated vacuum system for waste anesthetic gases because, when the wall suction system is used, it has the following disadvantages:

1. The strength of the wall suction may not be sufficient to meet the needs of both the anesthesiologist and the surgeon in addition to the needs of the scavenging system. Diverting 20 L/min of air to the scavenging system reduces the intensity of the remaining vacuum by 25%, which may not be adequate to meet the needs of the anesthesiologist.[17]
2. Waste anesthetic gases may damage the vacuum system's machinery.

Passive disposal routes

The OR ventilation system. When used for disposal of waste anesthetic gases, the OR ventilation system should meet the following requirements:

1. It must be of the nonrecirculating type.
2. It must supply at least 10 room air exchanges per hour.

The hose leading from the scavenging interface to the ventilation outflow port should be kept off the floor to avoid accidental occlusion. If placed on the floor, the hose should be rigid enough to remain patent under a pressure of 10 kg/cm (Fig. 5-15).

Through-the-wall disposal. With a passive through-the-wall disposal system, waste anesthetic gases flow through a duct in the wall, window, ceiling, or floor toward the outside. Because OR ventilation results in a slight positive pressure in the OR with respect the outside, gases flow naturally into disposal ducts connected to the outside. A potential danger of such a disposal route is occlusion of the exhaust port by ice, nesting birds, or insects. Gusty winds may generate positive pressure at the exhaust port and interfere with the disposal of the waste anesthetic gases. These problems can be avoided by directing the exhaust port downward and shielding it with a wired screen. Also, an air flow indicator should be installed in the tubing between the anesthesia machine and the wall to confirm the proper direction of gas flow.

Scavenging the anesthesia ventilator

Modern anesthesia ventilators are factory-equipped with a disposal system that directs waste anesthetic gases to the anesthesia machine's scavenging system (Fig. 5-5). Older designs of anesthesia ventilator, however, often discharge waste anesthetic gases directly into the ORs ambient air or do not have a standard 19-mm scavenging connection. Also, older ventilators are often fraught with internal leaks, which mix the anesthetic gases with the ventilator's driving gas. This significantly increases the volume of gas that must be disposed of with each breath and might therefore overwhelm the capacity of the scavenging system, resulting in spillage of anesthetic gases. Some manufacturers offer special kits to leak-proof old ventilators and refit them with a proper scavenging system. For example, the original Air Shields Ventimeter* can be retrofitted so that the driving gas is separated from the waste anesthetic gases, thus enabling the waste gases to be scavenged from a 19-mm connector. Their use is highly recommended.

Scavenging nonrebreathing (pediatric) anesthesia systems

Scavenging a nonrebreathing anesthesia system is best accomplished by connecting its exhalation port to the scavenging system of the anesthesia machine. The pediatric Jackson-Rees system can be scavenged by connecting either the open tail of its breathing bag or the relief valve (if one is used) directly to the scavenging interface of the anesthesia machine. The breathing bag can be scavenged by a series of improvised tubings and adaptors (Fig. 5-16) or by a commercial valve, such as the Dupaco or the Ohio bag tail valve. Vital Signs manufactures a scavenging re-

*Hatboro, Pa.

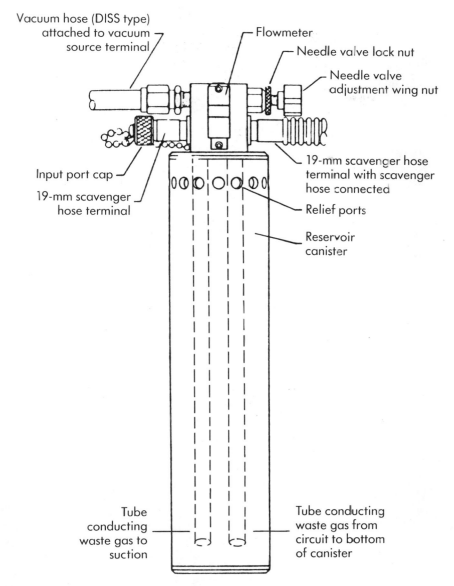

Vacuum hose (DISS type) attached to vacuum source terminal

Flowmeter

Needle valve lock nut

Needle valve adjustment wing nut

Input port cap

19-mm scavenger hose terminal

19-mm scavenger hose terminal with scavenger hose connected

Relief ports

Reservoir canister

Tube conducting waste gas to suction

Tube conducting waste gas from circuit to bottom of canister

Fig. 5-11. Dräger open reservoir scavenging system. (Reproduced by permission of North American Dräger, Inc, Telford, Pa.)

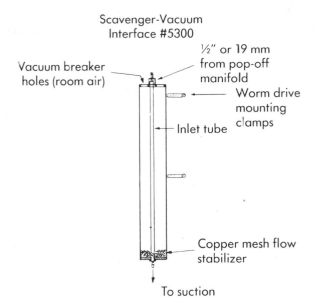

Scavenger-Vacuum Interface #5300

½" or 19 mm from pop-off manifold

Vacuum breaker holes (room air)

Worm drive mounting clamps

Inlet tube

Copper mesh flow stabilizer

To suction

Fig. 5-12. Tube-within-a-tube assembly type of open reservoir scavenging system. (Reproduced by permission of Boehringer Laboratories, Wynnewood, Pa.)

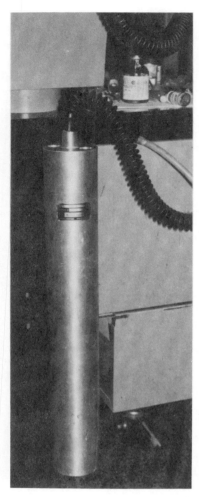

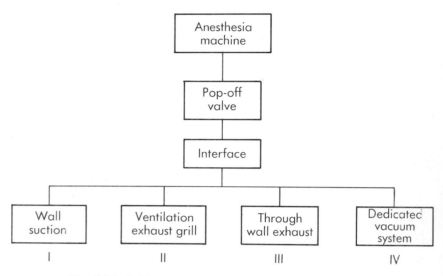

Fig. 5-14. Guide to selection of waste anesthetic gas cleanup.

Fig. 5-13. Boehringer open reservoir scavenger-vacuum safety interface. (Reproduced by permission of Boehringer Laboratories, Wynnewood, Pa.)

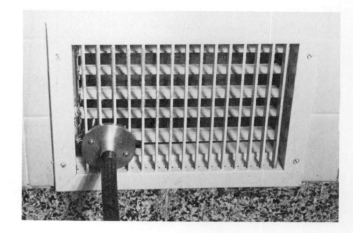

Fig. 5-15. Exhaust grille adaptor for passive disposal of waste anesthetic gases via the OR ventilation system.

lief valve that can be used with all Mapleson systems, including the Jackson-Rees pediatric modification (Fig. 5-17). This relief valve can be easily connected to the scavenging interface of the anesthesia machine.

Scavenging cryosurgical units

Newer models of nitrous oxide cryosurgical units are equipped with built-in scavenging systems. Older models, however, are not scavenged and spill large amounts of nitrous oxide gas into the OR ambient air. Fitting older units with scavenging systems is strongly recommended.

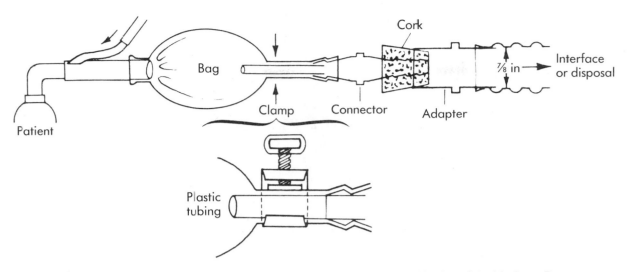

Fig. 5-16. Connection of scavenging interface to a Jackson-Rees modification of the Mapleson D system. (From Whitcher CE, Piziali R, Sher R, et al: *Development and evaluation of methods for elimination of waste anesthetic gases and vapors in hospitals.* HEW (NIOSH) Publication No. 75-137. Washington, DC, 1975, U.S. Government Printing Office.)

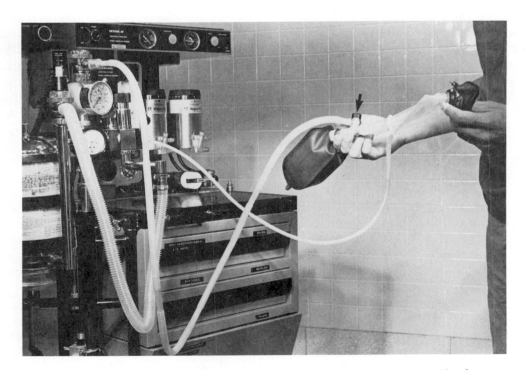

Fig. 5-17. The Vital Signs pediatric Gasovac *(arrow)* connected to the expiration side of a scavenged breathing circuit of an anesthesia machine. Note that the breathing bag was removed and its port is connected to the inspiratory side of the breathing circuit. This forces the waste anesthetic gases to flow one way, toward the scavenging system.

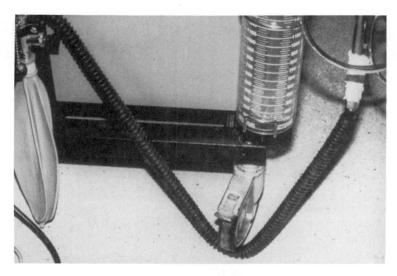

Fig. 5-18. Occlusion of 19-mm scavenger hose conducting gas from the outlets of the APL and PR valves to the closed reservoir active scavenging system. Note that the reservoir bag is collapsed. This situation can lead to high pressure in the breathing circuit and barotrauma.

HAZARDS OF SCAVENGING

Scavenging of the anesthesia breathing circuit increases the complexity, and consequently the hazards, of administering anesthesia. If the scavenging interface were mistakenly bypassed, or if it malfunctioned, excessive positive or negative pressure in the scavenging system could be transmitted directly to the breathing circuit. This might cause circulatory embarrassment and pulmonary barotrauma to the patient. Excessive negative pressure may be caused by unopposed vacuum, and excessive positive pressure may be caused by occlusion of the connecting tubing (Fig. 5-18) (see also Chapter 16).

Scavenging mishaps are usually caused by human error, negligence, or both. In one case, a one-way metallic connector was assembled in reverse, obstructing the disposal line and causing excessive positive pressure in the breathing circuit.[23] No pressure-relief valve had been incorporated into the system. In another case, the perforated connector of a tube-within-a-tube assembly was accidentally replaced with one that had no perforations.[24] The unopposed negative pressure in the scavenging system shut off the ventilator's exhalation valve and caused excessive positive pressure in the breathing circuit. The patient sustained a bilateral pneumothorax and subcutaneous emphysema.

In yet another case, the expiratory breathing hose was mistakenly attached to the scavenging port of the relief valve, causing an abrupt rise in the pressure of the breathing circuit.[25] Accidental occlusion of the disposal line by the wheels of the anesthesia machine has also been reported.[25]

The inherent vulnerability of scavenging systems has been the cause of some mishaps. In one case, the negative pressure relief valve failed to open despite excessive negative pressure in the system, causing the patient circuit reservoir bag to collapse.[26] In another case, ice buildup in the exhaust port of a passive through-the-wall disposal route was apparently the cause of pneumothorax and death in a laboratory animal.[27] In yet another case, a plastic bag was sucked in by the perforated connector of an active disposal route.[28] This occluded the perforations and led to unopposed negative pressure in the breathing circuit.

Whenever abnormal pressure exists in the breathing circuit, the scavenging system should be checked immediately for possible malfunction. If a malfunction is suspected, the system should immediately be disconnected from the breathing circuit.

ANESTHETIC LEAK-DETECTION AND LEAK-PROOFING PROGRAM

The scavenging system removes only waste anesthetic gases that are captured from the relief valve. Spillage from other sources is not evacuated by the scavenging system and depends solely on the OR's ventilation system for disposal. In spite of a properly functioning scavenging system, the pollution level in the OR may be above the maximal levels recommended by NIOSH.

In order to reduce the level of anesthetic pollution in the OR, the anesthesia machine should be tested regularly for leaks. If found, leaks should be corrected as soon as possible. Errors in anesthetic technique leading to spillage of anesthetic gases should be corrected as well.

To detect and prevent anesthetic leaks, a leak-detecting and leak-proofing program should be adopted in every OR suite. The results should be documented, and the records should be maintained indefinitely (Fig. 5-19). These records are useful for equipment maintenance follow-up and for compliance with recommendations of government agencies and accrediting organizations. The records can potentially also be used for legal defense.

Testing the high-pressure system for leaks

Testing of the high-pressure system of the anesthesia machine for leaks begins with the quick connector in the nitrous oxide central supply line. The connector is submerged under water or rinsed with liquid soap (Fig. 5-20). The appearance of gas bubbles indicates a leak. Liquid soap can also be used to detect leaks in the yokes of the reserve nitrous oxide tanks. Faulty quick connectors should be repaired or replaced immediately. The yokes of the reserve tanks should be tightened, and defective washers should be replaced (Fig. 5-21).

Next, the nitrous oxide high-pressure system inside the anesthesia machine is tested. The nitrous oxide central supply hose is disconnected from the machine. A reserve nitrous oxide tank is used to pressurize the nitrous oxide system, and the tank is then turned off. The nitrous oxide system pressure, as indicated by the nitrous oxide pressure gauge, is then recorded and rechecked 1 hour later. A significant drop in pressure suggests a leak inside the machine, between the nitrous oxide reserve tank and the nitrous oxide flowmeter.

In one study, significant high-pressure nitrous oxide leaks were detected in 50% of the anesthesia machines.[17] After the leaks were corrected, the background nitrous oxide level in the OR suite decreased from 19 ppm to 0.2 ppm.

Internal nitrous oxide leaks are difficult to correct and should be left to the manufacturer's maintenance service. It is recommended that the high-pressure nitrous oxide system be tested by departmental anesthesia technicians once a month and serviced by the manufacturer once every 4 months.

Testing the low-pressure system for leaks (See also Chapter 22)

The following procedure is recommended for testing the low-pressure system for leaks:

1. Remove the breathing hoses and bag from the anesthesia breathing circuit.
2. Interconnect the two unidirectional valves using a short piece of corrugated hose.
3. Close the APL valve tight; remove the reservoir bag and occlude the bag mount opening. This minimizes the compliance of the low-pressure system.
4. Slowly turn on the oxygen flowmeter until the breathing circuit pressure gauge indicates 40 cm H_2O.
5. Record the rate of oxygen flow necessary to maintain this pressure for 30 seconds. This rate of flow is equal to the low-pressure system's leak rate. The

low-pressure leak rate generally should not exceed 200 ml/min, which would contribute no more than 4 ppm of nitrous oxide air pollution to an average sized OR.

The low-pressure system generally should be tested and serviced by departmental technical personnel at least once a week, as well as whenever the carbon dioxide absorber, unidirectional valves, or other component of the breathing circuit is replaced.

Correcting errors in the anesthetic technique

The following precautions in anesthetic technique will significantly reduce the spillage of anesthetic gases:

1. All gases and vaporizers should be turned off when the patient is not connected to the breathing circuit (i.e., during intubation).
2. The face mask should be carefully selected and firmly held against the patient's face.
3. The tracheal tube should be carefully selected. Except for pediatric patients, no leak should be allowed around the cuff.
4. Upon conclusion of anesthesia, when the breathing bag is emptied of anesthetic gases, the breathing circuit should be attached to the patient with the relief valve held wide open. This should direct the contents of the bag into the scavenging system.
5. After completion of surgery, and while still deeply anesthetized, the patient should remain connected to the breathing circuit, breathing 100% oxygen for a few minutes. This will direct the exhaled anesthetic gases to the scavenging system of the anesthesia machine.
6. Vaporizers should be refilled in the evening when the OR is not being used. This reduces the risk of exposing OR personnel to anesthetic vapors from accidental spillage of volatile anesthetic liquid while the vaporizers are refilled. Also, the use of agent-specific filling devices reduces the amount of volatile anesthetic agent that is spilled (see Chapter 3).

Miscellaneous preventive measures

The OR ventilation system should be serviced regularly to ensure optimal function. Hospital engineers should check the filters for cleanliness and the dampers for proper position and balance. If the system is allowed to deteriorate, the number of air exchanges per hour decreases gradually and the level of anesthetic pollution increases. Also, the function of the hospital vacuum should be checked at regular intervals to ensure adequate negative pressure and flow capacity.

In the postanesthesia care unit, the level of nitrous oxide in the air is directly related to room ventilation and number of patients in the unit. If ventilation is maintained at the rate of 500 m³ of fresh air per patient per hour, the mean nitrous oxide level in the room is about 10 ppm.[20]

BETH ISRAEL MEDICAL CENTER
Department of Anesthesiology

High-pressure test

Date	Room No.	Machine No.	N$_2$O connectors		Machine pressure		Comments
			Distal	Proximal	Initial	After 1 hr	

A

1. Perform test during first week of each month.
2. Record N$_2$O connector leaks on a 0-to-3 scale.
3. Record machine pressures in psi.   Technician _____

BETH ISRAEL MEDICAL CENTER
Department of Anesthesiology

Low-pressure test

Date	Room No.	Machine No.	Initial leak rate	Corrected rate	Leak sites

B

Report leak rate in cc O$_2$/min at a circuit pressure of 40 cm H$_2$O.

Technician _____

Fig. 5-19. Examples of forms for documenting **A,** high-pressure leak testing, **B,** low-pressure leak testing.

BETH ISRAEL MEDICAL CENTER
Department of Anesthesiology

**Operating room ventilation and trace N₂O levels
(quarterly report)**

Room No.	Machine No.	Air exchanges per hr	N₂O (ppm) Background*	Active room	Comments

C

*Operating room inactive at least 2 hours

Date _____

Technician _____

Fig. 5-19, cont'd. C, Quarterly OR ventilation and testing for nitrous oxide pollution.

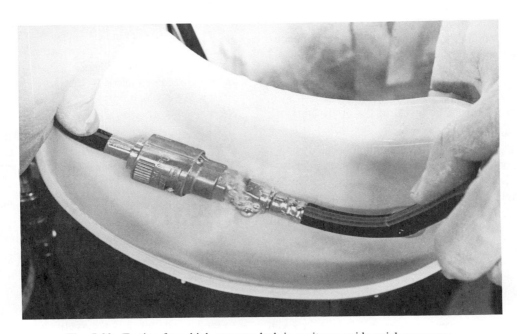

Fig. 5-20. Testing for a high-pressure leak in a nitrous oxide quick connector.

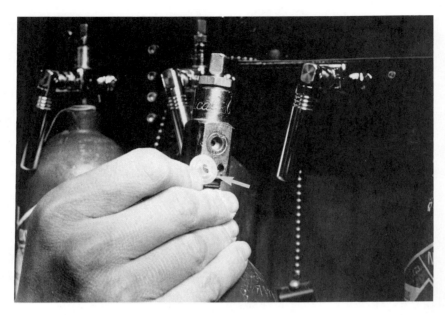

Fig. 5-21. High-pressure leak caused by a defective washer *(arrow)* on the yoke of a nitrous oxide reserve tank.

MONITORING OF ANESTHETIC POLLUTION AND PERSONNEL EXPOSURE

Regular analysis of the level of anesthetic pollution is necessary in order to meet the following objectives:

1. To determine whether or not the leak-detecting and leak-proofing program is effective.
2. To uncover occult leaks from unexpected sites.
3. To document compliance with NIOSH recommendations for maximum levels of anesthetic pollution.
4. To document the existence of safe working conditions in the OR suite.

Monitoring trace anesthetic levels in the operating room

The levels of both nitrous oxide and halogenated agents in the OR can be determined individually. Infrared analyzers can detect trace levels of anesthetic agents. These devices are capable of measuring not only nitrous oxide but all of the volatile anesthetics. A basic model, such as the MIRAN 203,* can be purchased for approximately $6500 and measures any single anesthetic agent. It can be upgraded to measure any of the other anesthetic gases for $600 to $900 per gas. The MIRAN 1B2, a top-of-the-line analyzer, is capable of analyzing 116 different gases. Not only can all of the anesthetic agents be tested for, but various other toxic substances, such as ethylene oxide, can also be measured. Although this device costs approximately $17,000, it may be well worth the investment be-

*The Foxboro Co., E. Bridgewater, Mass.

cause it can be used in many different areas of the hospital.

Because the level of halogenated agents in OR air is closely related to that of nitrous oxide, the level of the halogenated agent can be extrapolated from that of nitrous oxide, as follows:

$$\frac{\% \text{ H in FGI}}{\% \text{ N}_2\text{O in FGI}} = \frac{\text{ppm H in RA}}{\text{ppm N}_2\text{O in RA}}$$

where:

H = Halogenated agent
FGI = Fresh gas inflow
RA = Room air

Measurements of anesthetic pollution are reliable only if the anesthetic gases are evenly distributed in the ambient air. The uniformity of distribution depends on the following factors:

1. Number of room air exchanges per hour.
2. Flow pattern of room ventilation.
3. Placement of the anesthesia machine in relation to the ventilation flow.
4. Traffic patterns of personnel in the OR.

When the number of room air exchanges is greater than 10/hr, the anesthetic gases are fairly evenly distributed in room air. The air near the ventilation outflow grille represents the mean level of the trace anesthetic gases in the room.[20]

Optimum reduction of air contamination is achieved by certain control measures supported by an air-monitoring program. The monitoring is essential and ensures the efficacy of control measures, the identification of leaks or defects in technique, and documentation of compliance with the recommended standard. NIOSH recommends that monitoring be done either by a knowledgeable person familiar with techniques of sampling or by an industrial hygienist.[11] Monitoring requires both sampling and analysis. Analysis may be performed by infrared methods or gas chromatography, either inside or outside the hospital.

Sampling methods

Two decisions must be made with regard to sampling: where to do it and when to do it.

Where to sample. Monitoring personal exposure by sampling the atmosphere in the face mask area of exposed personnel is not required by the NIOSH recommended standard,[11] although perhaps this method offers the most pertinent information on individual exposure. Sampling in the immediate work area of the most highly exposed person, the anesthesiologist, is recommended. A recent study has shown that measuring nitrous oxide at the level of the anesthesia machine's shelf correlates well with personal sampling when levels of nitrous oxide are below 35 ppm.[29] Shelf-level measurement is certainly more practical than personal sampling.

General area sampling is valid if complete air mixing has been demonstrated previously in the operating room. In a room where all leakage is under effective control, gas concentrations may be uniform, making this kind of sampling appropriate. This type of sampling may be most appropriate in the empty OR to detect background leakage.

When to sample. The timing of sampling is also critical to obtaining representative exposure concentrations. There are essentially three types of temporal sampling: grab sampling, time-weighted average (TWA) sampling, and continuous sampling.

Grab sampling. Grab sampling is useful for monitoring steady-state conditions—for example, high-pressure leakage from nitrous oxide lines, which produces baseline nitrous oxide levels. With this technique, an air sample from the empty operating room is taken for subsequent analysis. Inert containers are available for this purpose from Boehringer Laboratories.* The container is sealed and mailed to the company for analysis of the contents. Delay in obtaining the results is one disadvantage. Another is that, because anesthetic leakage tends to be intermittent, the value of such sampling is obviously limited (Fig. 5-22).

Time-weighted average sampling. The TWA sample is obtained by pumping ambient air continuously into an inert bag at a constant, low rate of flow, usually around 4 L/hr. The bag has a capacity of 20 to 30 L. The result-

*Wynnewood, Pa.

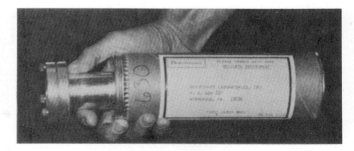

Fig. 5-22. Grab sample container for off-site analysis. (Reproduced by permission of Boehringer Laboratories, Wynnewood, Pa.)

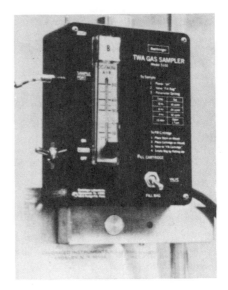

Fig. 5-23. Time-weighted averaging pump. (Reproduced by permission of Boehringer Laboratories, Wynnewood, Pa.)

ing concentration in the bag therefore represents an average exposure over the collection period. Commercially available TWA gas sampling systems provide TWA concentrations over periods of 1 to 8 hours. The sampling pump can be mounted on a pole in the OR (Fig. 5-23). Aliquots of a collected TWA sample can be analyzed in-house or mailed in the inert containers used in grab sampling (Fig. 5-22) to a central testing laboratory. The TWA for personal exposure can also be obtained from a battery-powered sampling pump and collection bag worn by the anesthesiologist. Clearly, however, wearing a bag and pump is inconvenient. Knowledge of the TWA concentrations is useful for documentation purposes, because the recommended standard refers to a TWA concentration of 25 ppm, although the time period for collection is not specified.[11]

Continuous sampling. Use of the portable infrared analyzer, which is capable of continuous sampling, is the best method for monitoring the OR atmosphere (Figs. 5-24

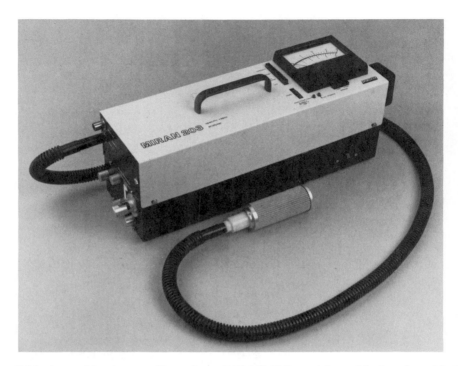

Fig. 5-24. A portable nitrous oxide analyzer (MIRAN 203) used for quick detection of leaks. (Courtesy of The Foxboro Co, East Bridgewater, Mass.)

and 5-25). Because this device offers a continuous readout, it can be used for detection of leaks, demonstration of errors in anesthetic technique, and determination of trace gas levels. Analyzers operate on the principle that most gases present unique infrared absorption spectra. For example, the infrared absorption spectrum for nitrous oxide peaks at around 4.5 μm (See Fig. 8-2).

These infrared analyzers work in the following manner: A pump perfuses a cell with OR air. To measure nitrous oxide, the infrared source generates a light beam that is filtered to pass the infrared component at around 4.5 μm. The beam is transmitted through the sample cell and sensed by a detector. The higher the concentration of nitrous oxide, the more infrared radiation is absorbed and the less is the energy sensed at the detector. The signal is processed and displayed in ppm nitrous oxide. Infrared analysis can detect concentrations in parts per 100 million. The sensitivity of the instrument is a function of the path length of the infrared beam through the sample of gas. Path lengths of 20 m or more produce very high sensitivity. Infrared analyzers can also be used to measure trace concentrations of halogenated agents (see Table 5-1), although they are less reliable for this purpose because these agents have overlapping absorption spectra.

It is clear from the foregoing that the trace concentrations of anesthetics in question are well below the concentrations used for clinical anesthesia. For this reason, the analyzers used to monitor clinically useful concentrations of anesthetic gases (e.g., mass spectrometry, infrared gas

Table 5-1. Infrared analyzer detection limits

Agent	Minimum detectable concentration
Nitrous oxide	0.07 ppm
Halothane	0.08 ppm
Enflurane	0.01 ppm
Isoflurane	0.02 ppm
Methoxyflurane	0.07 ppm

From Syrjala RJ, et al: *The analysis of anesthetic gases with MIRAN infrared analyzers*, South Norwalk, Conn, 1977, Foxboro Analytical.

analysis, Raman spectroscopy) are not sensitive enough for monitoring the OR atmosphere.

By using a chart recorder connected to the output of an infrared trace concentration gas analyzer, a continuous plot of the nitrous oxide concentration in room air can be obtained during anesthesia. The value of this type of monitoring is quite obvious. Instantaneous peaks on the chart reflect a high level of leakage of the gas, such as may be due to adjustment of a face mask. Alternatively the chart may reflect a leak in some other part of the system. Also, because levels of waste gases do fluctuate, this approach is more reliable than a grab sample for measuring concentrations that may be inhaled by personnel in the OR.

TWA concentrations may be obtained from the infrared trace concentration gas analyzer by integrating the output, i.e.: determining the area under the time-concentration curve and dividing by the time. This can be done by counting the

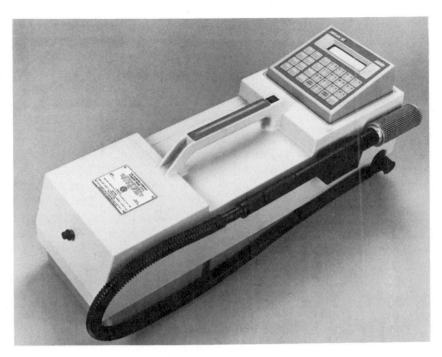

Fig. 5-25. MIRAN 1B2 Portable Ambient Air Analyzer. (Courtesy of the Foxboro Co, East Bridgewater, Mass.)

squares (in a chart record) or with a planimeter. The integration for nitrous oxide can also be derived electronically using a microcomputer. This provides a continuously updated TWA concentration and is relatively inexpensive. If a peak concentration suggestive of a leak in the system is sensed, the analyzer, acting as a leak detector, can "sniff out" the source of the leak.

The ideal air-monitoring program should measure all anesthetic gases employed in the OR. The recommended standard, however, requires monitoring only of the most frequently used agent, because following recommended work practices and control procedures will reduce all agents proportionately.[11] Thus nitrous oxide can be monitored and acts as a tracer for the potent agents that may be administered along with it in some fixed proportion. However, in rooms where nitrous oxide is rarely used (i.e., cardiac ORs), this technique is not satisfactory. In these rooms the halogenated agents must be monitored specifically.

The passive diffusion monitor. A relatively new approach to monitoring OR pollution is the passive diffusion monitor. The Nitrox Dosimeter* is an example. Although this device is designed for monitoring personal exposure, it can also be used for area sampling. In concept, the device is similar to the radiation badges worn by personnel in x-ray departments to monitor their exposure to radiation (Fig. 5-26). The dosimeter is a tube in which a molecular

*R.S. Landauer Co., Glenwood, Ill.

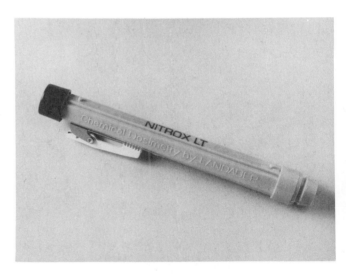

Fig. 5-26. A passive diffusion monitor, the Nitrox Dosimeter. (Courtesy of RS Landauer Co, Glenwood, Ill.)

sieve traps nitrous oxide. The tube, worn by the person whose exposure is being checked, must be uncapped at the beginning of the period of exposure to nitrous oxide and capped at the end. It is designed to sample over a period of 40 hours, and the wearer must keep a record of the exposure time. The effective air sampling rate is about 5 ml/hr. The dosimeter, labeled with the individual's name and period of exposure, is returned to the company for analysis. Analysis involves heating the dosimeter to drive off the nitrous oxide trapped in the molecular sieve, followed by infrared analysis. Results are expressed in TWA form, ppm-hr. These dosimeters are remarkably accurate: When tested against continuous TWA sampling with an infrared analyzer, they show a correlation coefficient close to 1.0.

Biological exposure

Sonander, et al [30] working in Sweden have attempted to correlate biological exposure as measured by analysis of urine samples from exposed OR personnel with technical exposure as measured by gas sampling. They studied 4 anesthesiologists and 25 nurse anesthetists. Urine samples were obtained early in the day, before OR work began, and then some 8 hours later in the work day. These personnel also wore personal sampling pumps so that TWA exposure concentrations could be obtained. The nitrous oxide concentrations in the gas above the urine in the collection containers, measured by gas chromatography, showed a good correlation ($r = 0.97$) with technical exposure measurements. The authors suggested that this method of analyzing urine gas provides a useful means of assessing biological exposure during routine anesthetic work. [30]

Ideal monitoring and current practice

How frequently should the OR be monitored? The recommended standard[11] requires repetitive sampling quarterly in locations in which mixed-inhalation anesthetic agents are used and whenever ventilation, anesthetic equipment, or scavenging techniques are modified. Ideally, monitoring should be performed quite frequently, even continuously; but continuous monitoring is impractical and very expensive.

Empty ORs, out of use for at least 2 hours, should be surveyed to detect background leakage from equipment high-pressure systems. The rooms should be resurveyed later in the day and while in use to detect actual working exposure levels. If high levels are detected, some explanation should be sought; and remedial action should be taken and documented as soon as possible. High levels intraoperatively may, however, represent an unavoidable sequela of the anesthetic technique in use at the time of monitoring.

Multipoint infrared analyzer

One solution to the problem of monitoring the OR atmosphere is the use of a multipoint infrared analyzer, for example, the MIRAN 981 or 983 Multipoint Ambient Air Monitoring System (Fig. 5-27).[31] Sampling ports are located in each OR, and plastic tubing conveys air from the OR to the intake manifold of the gas analyzer. A microcomputer and solenoid valve system select the test location so that a sample of that room's air is analyzed. This system, analogous to the now-familiar multiplexed mass spectrometry systems in common use for monitoring gases in

the anesthesia circuit, has long been used in industry to monitor for hazardous gases (e.g., ethylene oxide). With such a system, data can be transmitted back to the OR whose atmosphere is being sampled to indicate whether excessive concentrations of nitrous oxide are present. The system also lends itself to the production of permanent records. Unfortunately, because of their cost, these systems have not gained much popularity for use in ORs.

Olfaction

Although the anesthesiologist is the ultimate monitor of the patient in the operating room, the senses are not very effective at detecting trace concentrations of anesthetics. The olfactory thresholds for nitrous oxide and halothane are 10% to 30% (100,000 to 300,000 ppm) and 0.005% to 0.01% (50 to 100 ppm), respectively.[32] The nose is very sensitive to the smell of methoxyflurane and can detect 0.1 to 2 ppm of this agent.

ARE TRACE CONCENTRATIONS OF ANESTHETICS HAZARDOUS?

Although there are at present no formal requirements for monitoring the OR atmosphere for waste anesthetic gases, there are recommendations.[33] The NIOSH-recommended limits have not yet been enacted into law by OSHA, and it is quite likely that they never will be. Such a law has been opposed by both hospitals and anesthesiologists because the recommendations are considered by many to be unreasonable. There are several reasons for this.

First, the limits are recommended on the basis of the work of Whitcher, et al,[10] who had shown that these levels were readily achievable; but this was subsequently shown not to be true.[34] In 1979, they reported data to the effect that even when all reduction measures were taken, exposure levels depended very much on the anesthetic technique used. Thus, when a mask was used, mean levels of 180 ppm nitrous oxide were found. When the patients underwent tracheal intubation, mean levels of 16 ppm were achieved. Should all anesthetized patients therefore undergo tracheal intubation so that this arbitrary level can be maintained? Obviously not. Clearly each technique has its associated degree of atmospheric contamination. An inhalational induction of a pediatric patient would certainly violate the recommended standard; yet it has obvious advantages for the patient. Second, the results of tests of psychomotor activity conducted by Bruce and Bach,[12] which also formed a basis for the recommended standard, have not been substantiated by other workers, all of whom found no effects at much higher trace concentrations of anesthetics.[35,36] Third, no "safe" trace level has ever been demonstrated for any of the anesthetics in use.

An even more fundamental issue still remains unresolved: Are trace levels of anesthetics really hazardous?

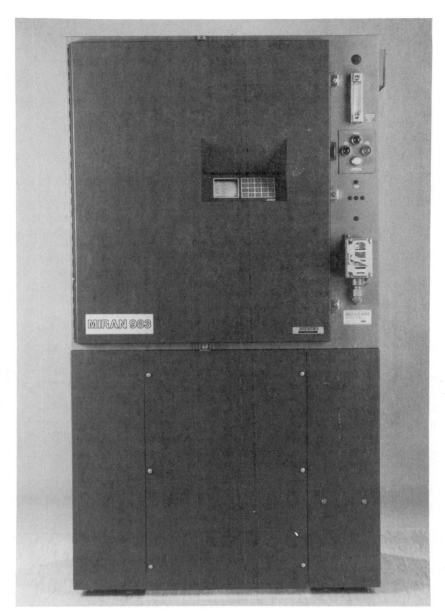

Fig. 5-27. MIRAN 983 single-component multipoint ambient air monitoring system. (Reproduced by permission of The Foxboro Co, East Bridgewater, Mass.)

Certainly no cause-effect relationship has ever been demonstrated.[11,37,38] The studies to date that have incriminated anesthetics have all been based on questionnaire surveys sent to people who were assumed either to have been exposed to trace anesthetics in the operating room (e.g., members of the ASA, AANA) or not to have been so exposed (e.g., pediatricians). Such studies are notoriously unreliable. They are wide open to responder bias, and such bias may explain all of the observed differences to date between "exposed" and "unexposed" personnel.[38]

That such bias exists in these studies was very clearly demonstrated by Axelsson and Rylander,[39] who studied a total of 655 pregnancies among workers in one Swedish hospital. Following a postal questionnaire survey, they checked the accuracy of the responses they received against the respondents' medical records. They found that all women who suffered miscarriages and who worked at sites with exposure to anesthetic gases correctly reported their work sites and miscarriages, whereas one third of all miscarriages by women who were not so exposed during pregnancy went unreported in the questionnaire. The authors concluded that their study draws attention to the methodologic difficulties in using questionnaires to study pregnancy outcome and pinpoints the importance of responder bias.

The Epistat report

The ASA Ad Hoc Committee on Effects of Trace Anesthetic Agents on Health of Operating Room Personnel retained a group of epidemiologists and statisticians, the Epistat Group, to review all the available data pertaining to health hazards among OR workers. They reviewed 17 published reports.[40] Four were excluded from further consideration because they did not present data on the specific outcomes under evaluation; five more were excluded because they did not used comparable control groups. Data from two studies among dentists and dental assistants were also excluded because the exposure of these personnel to anesthetic gases differs substantially from that of OR personnel. Thus data from only six studies were considered worthy of scrutiny. The group's report found that the only health hazard consistently reported among female OR workers was an increased relative risk of spontaneous abortion.

The authors observed that, on the basis of the available data, the relative risk for spontaneous abortion among exposed women is approximately 1.3, or 33% greater than for nonexposed women. The authors further stated that the magnitude of this increase is well within the range that might be due to bias or uncontrolled confounding variables (such as responder bias), and that epidemiologic data currently available are insufficient for developing standards or setting exposure limits. Furthermore, even if this increased relative risk were true, it should be viewed in perspective. For example, maternal smoking of one pack of cigarettes per day increases the spontaneous abortion rate by 80% and maternal consumption of alcohol may increase the rate by 200%.[41]

The report urged that future studies be "prospective cohort studies, with careful documentation of type, amount and duration of exposure, meticulous and uniform follow-up and thorough ascertainment and confirmation following pre-defined criteria, of out-come events."[40] This is to avoid previous methodological errors.

To date, trace concentrations of anesthetics have been neither fully incriminated nor fully exonerated as causes of the reported health problems of OR workers. However, absence of evidence does not constitute evidence of absence; and although the possibility of a hazard does exist, measures should be continued both to reduce exposure and to monitor the effects of these measures. This is certainly recommended by all concerned agencies, including NIOSH, the American Hospital Association (AHA), the Joint Commission on Accreditation of Healthcare Organizations (JCAHO), and the American Society of Anesthesiologists (ASA). The ASA Ad Hoc Committee on Effects of Trace Anesthetic Agents on Health of Operating Room Personnel emphasizes that the administration of anesthesia and the safety of the patient are their primary goals, and that pollution control must be of secondary concern.[42] Further studies are necessary to resolve fully the question of whether anesthetics are pollutants, and the answer may well never be known. In determining adequacy and appropriateness of waste gas scavenging systems, current recommended standards should be reviewed and adopted.[21]

REFERENCES

1. Vaisman AI: Working conditions in surgery and their effect on the health of anesthesiologists (in Russian), *Eskp, Khir Anesthezio!* 3:44-49, 1967.
2. Knill-Jones RP, Rodrigues LV, Moir DD, et al: Anaesthetic practice and pregnancy: controlled survey of women anaesthetists in the United Kingdom, *Lancet* ii:1326, 1972.
3. Knill-Jones RP, Newman BJ, Spence AA: Anaesthetic practice and pregnancy: controlled survey of male anaesthetists in the United Kingdom, *Lancet* ii:807, 1975.
4. Askrog V, Harvald B: Teratogen effekt of inhalations anaestitika, *Nord Med* 83:498, 1970.
5. Occupational Safety and Health Act of 1970, Public Law 91-596, 91st Congress, S. 2193, Dec. 29, 1970.
6. *All about OSHA.* (revised) US Department of Labor. OSHA Publication 2056, 1982.
7. Cohen EN, Brown BW, Bruce DL: Occupational disease among operating room personnel: a national study, *Anesthesiology* 41:321-340, 1974.
8. Bruce DL, Bach MJ, Arbit J: Trace anesthetic effects on perceptual, cognitive and motor skills, *Anesthesiology* 40:453-458, 1974.
9. Bruce DL, Bach MJ: *Trace effects of anesthetic gases on behavioral performance of operating room personnel.* Cincinnati, US Department of HEW, Public Health Service, Center for Disease Control, National Institute for Occupational Safety and Health, HEW Publication No (NIOSH)76-169, 1976.
10. Whitcher CE, Piziali R, Sher R, et al: *Development and evaluation of methods for the elimination of waste anesthetic gases and vapors in hospitals.* Cincinnati, US Department of HEW, Public Health Service, Center for Disease Control, National Institute for Occupational Safety and Health, HEW Publication No (NIOSH)75-137, 1975.
11. *Criteria for a recommended standard: occupational exposure to waste anesthetic gases and vapors.* Cincinnati, US Department of HEW, Public Health Service, Center for Disease Control, National Institute for Occupational Safety and Health, Publication No 77-140, 1977.
12. Bruce DL, Bach MJ: Effects of trace anaesthetic gases on behavioral performance of volunteers, *Br J Anaesth* 48:871-875, 1976.
13. Pfaffli P, Nikki P, Ahlman K: Concentration of anaesthetic gases in recovery rooms, *Br J Anaesth* 44:230, 1972.
14. Mehta S, Burton P, Simms JS: Monitoring of occupational exposure to nitrous oxide, *Can Anaesth Soc J* 25:419, 1978.
15. Lecky JH: The mechanical aspects of anesthetic pollution control, *Anesth Analg* 56:769, 1977.
16. Cottrell JE, Chalon J, Turndorf H: Faulty anesthesia circuits: a source of environmental pollution in the operating room, *Anesth Analg* 56:359, 1977.
17. Whitcher CE, Piziali R, Sher R, et al: *Development and evaluation of methods for elimination of waste anesthetic gases and vapors in hospitals.* Washington, DC, US Government Printing Office, HEW (NIOSH) Publication No 75-137, 1975.
18. Wray RP: A source of non-anesthetic nitrous oxide in operating room air, *Anesthesiology* 52:88, 1980.
19. ECRI Health Devices Program: *Nitrous oxide exhausted from cryosurgical units,* Plymouth Meeting, Pa, Oct 17, 1979, ECRI.
20. Berner O: Concentration and elimination of anesthetic gases in operating theaters, *Acta Anaesthesiol Scand* 22:46, 1978.
21. American National Standards Institute: American national standard for anesthetic equipment: scavenging systems for excess anesthetic gases, ANSI Z.79.11-1982, New York, 1982.

22. *Open reservoir scavenger. operation and maintenance manual,* Telford, Pa, 1986, North American Dräger.

23. Hamilton RC, Byrne J: Another cause of gas scavenging line obstruction, *Anesthesiology* 51:365, 1979 (correspondence).

24. Abramowitz M, McGill WA: Hazard of an anesthetic scavenging device, *Anesthesiology* 51:276, 1979 (correspondence).

25. Tavakol M, Habeeb A: Two hazards of gas scavenging, *Anesth Analg* 57:286, 1978.

26. Mor ZF, Stein FF, Orkin LR: A possible hazard in the use of a scavenging system, *Anesthesiology* 47:302, 1977.

27. Hagerdal M, Lecky JH: Anesthetic death of an experimental animal related to scavenging system malfunction, *Anesthesiology* 47:522, 1977.

28. Patel KD, Fazleali YD: A potential hazard of the Dräger scavenging interface system for wall suction, *Anesth Analg* 58:327, 1979.

29. Kaarakka P, Malischke PR, Kreul JF: Alternative sites for measuring breathing zone nitrous oxide levels, *Anesthesiology* 55S:A139, 1981.

30. Sonander H, Stenquist O, Nilsson K: Nitrous oxide exposure during routine anaesthetic work: measurement of biologic exposure from urine samples and technical exposure by bag sampling, *Acta Anaesthesiol Scand* 29:203-208, 1985.

31. Russell MW, Hummel RS, Meeks C: Real time monitoring of trace nitrous oxide levels with microcomputer controlled system, *Anesthesiology* 61:A168, 1984 (abstract).

32. Halsey MJ, Chand S, Dluzewski AR, et al: Olfactory thresholds: detection of operating room contamination, *Br J Anaesth* 49:510-511, 1977.

33. Mazze RI: Waste anesthetic gases and the regulatory agencies, *Anesthesiology* 52:248-256, 1980.

34. Whitcher CE, Siukola LVM: Occupational exposure, education and sampling methods, *Anesthesiology* (suppl S336);p51, 1979.

35. Gambill AF, McCallum RN, Henrichs TF: Psychomotor performance following exposure to trace concentrations of inhalation anesthetics, *Anesth Analg* 58:475-482, 1979.

36. Frankhuizen JL, Vlek CAJ, Burm AGL, et al: Failure to replicate negative effects of trace anaesthetics on mental performance, *Br J Anaesth* 50:229-234, 1978.

37. Ferstandig LR: Trace concentrations of anesthetic gases: a critical review of their disease potential, *Anesth Analg* 57:328-345, 1978.

38. Ferstandig LR: Trace concentrations of anaesthetic gases, *Acta Anaesthesiol Scand Suppl* 75:33-42, 1982.

39. Axelsson G, Rylander R: Exposure to anaesthetic gases and spontaneous abortion: response bias in a postal questionnaire study, *Int J Epidemiol* 11:250-256, 1982.

40. Hennekens CH, Colton T, Rosner B, et al: *Evaluation of the epidemiologic evidence for occupational hazards of anesthetic gases,* Park Ridge, Ill, 1982, American Society of Anesthesiologists.

41. Buring JE, Hennekens CH, Mayrent SL, et al: Health experiences of operating room personnel, *Anesthesiology* 62:325-330, 1985.

42. *Waste anesthetic gases in operating room air: a suggested program to reduce personnel exposure,* Park Ridge, Ill, 1980, American Society of Anesthesiologists.

Chapter 6

ANESTHESIA VENTILATORS

Alan W. Grogono, M.D.
Joe T. Travis, M.D.

An anesthesia ventilator has to function in conjunction with the other components of the anesthesia delivery system. Its performance may, therefore, be affected by the machine, the patient circuit, the patient, and the effects of the anesthetic. The factors that will be considered here will be limited to those that can be understood and examined from a viewpoint that is proximal to the terminal bronchiole. Therefore, although ventilation is markedly affected by various pathophysiological changes (e.g., ventilation/perfusion mismatch, shock, or pneumothorax) these changes are best reviewed as an aspect of physiology rather than of equipment.

Since the 1960s the use of intermittent positive-pressure ventilation (IPPV) in anesthesia practice has become widespread. Today's observer might wrongly conclude that the development and research had occurred recently. However, much of the necessary experimentation and design took place much earlier. The brief historical review that follows illustrates how long ago the principles were established.

HISTORY

The early recorded attempts to ventilate a person artificially date to the 1400s. Baker[1] has found records referring to the resuscitation of a newborn with expired air (i.e. mouth-to-mouth resuscitation) as early as 1472. He also refers to a report of the successful resuscitation of an asphyxiated miner in 1744. Paracelsus suggested the use of the fireplace bellows to inflate the lungs artificially and is credited with the first such use in 1530.[2] The use of the bellows became accepted practice in attempts to revive victims of drowning, especially in Denmark, during the mid to late 1700s. Detailed procedures were developed, including a monetary reward system, for those who reported the drowning and initiated the prescribed techniques.

In 1891, George Fell, a professor of physiology at the University of Niagara in Buffalo, devised a hand-operated bellows for artificial ventilation and resuscitation.[3] The

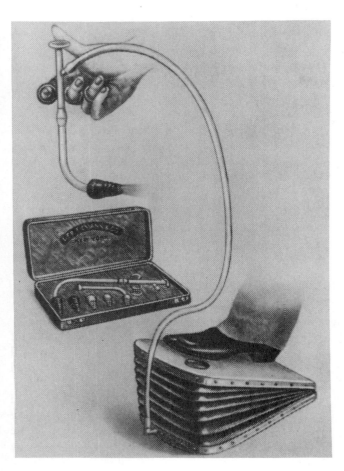

Fig. 6-1. Fell-O'Dwyer apparatus. (Reproduced with permission from Mushin WW, Rendell-Baker L, Thompson PW, et al: *Automatic ventilation of the lungs,* ed 3, Oxford, 1980, Blackwell Scientific.)

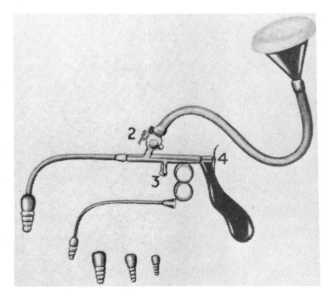

Fig. 6-2. Matas modification of Fell-O'Dwyer apparatus. (Reproduced with permission from Mushin WW, Rendell-Baker L, Thompson PW, et al: *Automatic ventilation of the lungs,* ed 3, Oxford, 1980, Blackwell Scientific.)

bellows, connected via rubber tubing to a valve device and a mask, was utilized to ventilate the patient. The operator simultaneously manipulated the bellows and the valve. The valve closed the circuit allowing forced inspiration with bellows compression in one position and opened the circuit to air in the other position allowing passive exhalation to the room. He successfully treated several cases of opium overdosage using this apparatus. Earlier, in 1887, O'Dwyer[4] had reported the successful use of endoral tubes in treating cases of diphtheria. His metal tubes were fashioned with conical ends that were wedged into the glottis producing a seal. In 1896, O'Dwyer combined his endoral tubes with the Fell apparatus creating the Fell-O'Dwyer device[5] (Fig. 6-1). He simplified the valve device by replacing the valve mechanism with a simple opening that the operator would cover with a thumb during the inspiratory phase and release during expiration. The patient could also breathe spontaneously through the hole. The hand-operated bellows was later replaced with a foot-operated version.

Early attempts at thoracic surgery were foiled by the development of a pneumothorax in the spontaneously breathing patient, resulting in a high mortality rate. Physiology experiments, however, had demonstrated that the lungs could be successfully ventilated with positive pressure while the chest was open. Andreas Vesalius (1515–1564) published *de Humani Corporis Fabrica,* in 1555, in which he described the placing of a reed into the opened trachea of an animal and then maintaining the animal's life by blowing into the reed while the animal's chest was opened.[6] Robert Hooke repeated these experiments in 1667 utilizing a bellows placed into the trachea to successfully ventilate the lungs of a dog.[7] Aware of these experiments, it was natural for the surgeons of the late 1890s to attempt this technique of ventilation for chest surgery. In France in 1896, Tuffier and Hallion[8] were able to partially resect the lung of a patient whose trachea they intubated blindly with a cuffed tracheal tube and ventilated during the surgery. Rudolph Matas[9] of New Orleans utilized the Fell-O'Dwyer device to resect an area of the chest wall in a patient in 1898. He subsequently modified the device to allow the administration of anesthetic vapor (Fig. 6-2). Compared to the dog, intubation of the trachea in the human proved to be a much more difficult task, hence these methods were not widely utilized at the time.

Attempting to circumvent the difficulties of tracheal intubation, Sauerbruch, in 1904, developed the negative pressure operating chamber (Fig. 6-3). The patient's head protruded from the chamber and was exposed to atmospheric pressure; when the patient's body was exposed to subatmospheric pressure inside the chamber, inspiration would occur. This system required that the surgeon be in the chamber with the patient, which created a whole new set of problems. Further development of negative pressure

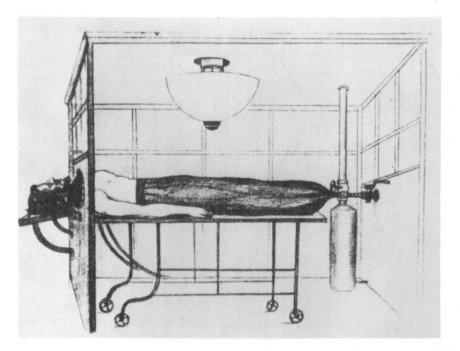

Fig. 6-3. Sauerbruch's negative pressure operating chamber. (Reproduced with permission from Mushin WW, Rendell-Baker L, Thompson PW, et al: *Automatic ventilation of the lungs,* ed 3, Oxford, 1980, Blackwell Scientific.)

ventilation devices resulted in the "iron lung" by Drinker and Shaw,[10] which was widely used to treat patients suffering from respiratory failure during the polio epidemics. Brauer's solution to the problem of providing ventilation without intubation was to introduce, in 1905, a positive-pressure chamber that enclosed the patient's head, producing an air-tight seal at the neck[11] (Fig. 6-4).

The techniques of tracheal ventilation remained largely unused until after World War I. At that time Magill began utilizing these techniques for head and neck surgery.[12] Eventually Guedel and Treweek[13] would report success in creating a quiet surgical field by the apnea resulting from the combination of deep ether anesthesia with hypocapnia produced by hyperventilation. This technique was responsible for creating a greater acceptance of tracheal intubation and controlled ventilation. The introduction of curare into clinical practice in 1942 created an even greater ease in providing a quiet surgical field, but at the same time demanded complete control of the airway and ventilation of the patient.

UNDERSTANDING INTERMITTENT POSITIVE-PRESSURE VENTILATION (IPPV)

Gas exchange

It is an advantage to make a clear distinction between the elimination of carbon dioxide and the intake of oxygen even though these two processes are interrelated at the metabolic level, in transport by hemoglobin, and in the control of ventilation. Carbon dioxide elimination depends on ventilation and, therefore, the ventilation achieved determines the $PaCO_2$. By contrast, oxygenation can be facilitated by enriching the inspired air and, accordingly, may be largely independent of ventilation.

Carbon dioxide equilibrium. The quantity of carbon dioxide produced normally dictates the minute ventilation. With the exception of using cardiopulmonary bypass or an extracorporeal membrane oxygenator (ECMO), there is no satisfactory alternative method for eliminating carbon dioxide. Breathing is essential. Normally, in the absence of disease, high altitude, and pharmacological intervention, spontaneous ventilation results in a $PaCO_2$ close to 40 mm Hg. The quantitative relationship between carbon dioxide production and minute ventilation is, however, often poorly understood.

Carbon dioxide production. A resting adult weighing 70 kg produces about 0.008 gram molecules (moles) of carbon dioxide per minute. At standard temperature (0° C) and pressure (760 mm Hg), one mole of any gas occupies 22.4 liters. Therefore 0.008 moles occupies about 180 ml. At body temperature (37° C) this is about 200 ml.

> CO_2 production per minute is 0.008 moles.
> At 760 mm Hg, and at 37° C, this is 200 ml.

Carbon dioxide elimination. Expressing carbon dioxide production either in moles or in milliliters at atmospheric pressure provides no insight into the quantity of

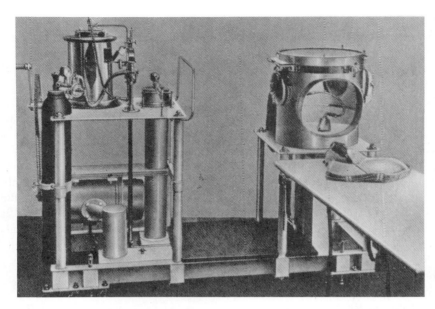

Fig. 6-4. Brauer's positive pressure apparatus. (Reproduced with permission from Mushin WW, Rendell-Baker L, Thompson PW, et al: *Automatic ventilation of the lungs,* ed 3, Oxford, 1980, Blackwell Scientific.)

ventilation required to maintain homeostasis. More helpful information is provided when the same quantity of carbon dioxide is expressed at different partial pressures using Boyle's law (see Table 6-1).

The volume of carbon dioxide shown at each partial pressure in Table 6-1 is the volume occupied by the metabolic production for 1 minute (0.008 moles). At each pressure the volume shown is the volume of carbon dioxide produced and is, therefore, the least alveolar ventilation per minute that is capable of eliminating the carbon dioxide produced. Any smaller alveolar ventilation is insufficient to allow the carbon dioxide to escape at that partial pressure.

The patient's minute volume is made up of both the alveolar ventilation and the dead space. Normally, the physiological dead space is one third of the minute volume. For an alveolar minute ventilation of 4000 ml, the required total minute ventilation is, therefore, 6000 ml. The mixed expired carbon dioxide has a partial pressure of about 25 mm Hg.

It should be noted that during IPPV under anesthesia, the physiological dead space typically increases to approximately 45% of the tidal volume. The same alveolar ventilation of 4000 ml/min thus requires a total minute ventilation of about 7250 ml, which will eliminate a mixed expired partial pressure for carbon dioxide of about 21 mm Hg.

Oxygen uptake. At rest the adult human (70 kg) has an oxygen consumption of about 250 ml/min. Strictly speaking, ventilation is not essential for oxygenation. When the patient is breathing oxygen, the pulmonary reservoir represents about 10 minutes worth of metabolic consumption. More than this, if an oxygenated, apneic patient

Table 6-1. The same metabolic production of carbon dioxide expressed at different partial pressures. Each volume represents the minimum alveolar ventilation capable of achieving that partial pressure of carbon dioxide

	Partial pressure (mm Hg)	Volume occupied (ml)
Normal atmospheric pressure	760	200
One tenth atmospheric or double alveolar partial pressure	76	2000
Normal alveolar partial pressure	38	4000
Half alveolar partial pressure	19	8000

is connected to an oxygen supply (apneic oxygenation) then oxygenation is unlimited; survival is now limited by carbon dioxide accumulation, not by hypoxia.

The clear distinction between carbon dioxide elimination and oxygenation emphasizes the relationship between carbon dioxide elimination and ventilation, and also rationalizes the therapy of hypoxia. When the patient's oxygenation is inadequate, there is an understandable temptation to adjust either the ventilator or the inspired oxygen tension. The appropriate response is to first examine, and then treat, the patient. Varying the ventilation is not the therapy for hypoxia, nor is an increased inspired oxygen concentration the therapy for deteriorating lung function. An increase in inspired partial pressure of oxygen may become necessary but should be employed only if other attempts to improve lung function fail.

Net effect of respiratory quotient (RQ). Respiratory quotient is the ratio between carbon dioxide production and oxygen consumption. The production of carbon dioxide, e.g., 200 ml each minute, is normally slightly less than the oxygen consumption, e.g., 250 ml (RQ, 200/250 = 0.8). This discrepancy has interesting implications. Because the minute volume inspired is slightly greater than that exhaled, there is a continuing, small, net inward movement of gas into the lung. As a result the partial pressure of nitrogen, or nitrous oxide, is slightly greater in the lung than in the inspired gas and, of necessity, there is an equal reduction in the space that would have been available for the respiratory gases, carbon dioxide and oxygen. With an RQ of 0.8, the sum of the alveolar, or arterial, partial pressures for carbon dioxide and oxygen will, therefore, always be slightly less than the humidified inspired oxygen tension (P_IO_2 = 0.21 × [760 − 47] = 149 mm Hg) instead of being exactly equal to it: P_AO_2 (100) + P_ACO_2 (40) = 140 mm Hg and is not equal to P_IO_2 (149 mm Hg).

Lung function during anesthesia and mechanical ventilation

Disadvantages. During intermittent positive-pressure ventilation (IPPV) under anesthesia, lung function is commonly adversely affected. This may be caused by many factors including atelectasis due to immobilization and absence of sighing; retention of secretions due to cough suppression, ciliary damage, and inspissation of secretions by dry gases; creation of additional physiological dead space by positive end-expiratory pressure (PEEP); and increased ventilation-perfusion mismatching due to anesthetic-induced inhibition of hypoxic pulmonary vasoconstriction. Tracheal suction provides an additional cause for hypoxia; the benefits of removing secretions from the airway tend to be offset by the removal of some of the oxygen and the entry of nitrogen, the negative pressure that may promote atelectasis, and the initiation of coughing and straining, both of which tend to increase metabolic rate and lower cardiac output.

Advantages. Tracheal intubation protects the airway from secretions; mechanical ventilation with muscular relaxation diminishes the work of breathing; and ventilation with inhalational anesthetics may relieve bronchospasm. In addition, poor function of an abnormal lung can be improved during anesthesia by using the appropriate pattern of ventilation. Examples of this are given in the section *Intermittent positive-pressure ventilation waveforms.*

Types of ventilation

More variations of IPPV are utilized in critical care than in the operating room. Occasionally a patient in a critical care unit requiring anesthesia is dependent on a specific pattern of ventilation. When this occurs it is often preferable to bring the ventilator with the patient and use it dur-

ing the procedure, because an anesthesia ventilator may be unable to provide the same pattern of IPPV. The principal varieties of ventilation are reviewed below.

Spontaneous ventilation. Spontaneous ventilation causes minimal variation in intrathoracic pressure (Fig. 6-5). During periods of spontaneous ventilation under anesthesia, it is desirable to maintain low pressure in the breathing circuit; this maximizes the minute ventilation and provides the least obstruction to venous return to the thorax. Patients with compromised lung function and a tendency to atelectasis may benefit from continuous positive airway pressure (CPAP). With a mask that fits well over the face and using very high gas flows, this positive pressure may be maintained throughout the ventilatory cycle. More commonly the pressure falls toward atmospheric pressure during inspiration.

Controlled ventilation. Controlled ventilation is employed where paralysis, sedation, or weakness from any cause impairs the patient's ability to initiate breaths. During general anesthesia this is the mode of intermittent positive-pressure ventilation most commonly employed.

Assisted ventilation. In assisted ventilation, each breath is triggered by the patient. The patient, therefore, determines the minute volume delivered. Assisted ventilation may be useful when weaning patients from IPPV. The penalty is that a subatmospheric phase is usually required to initiate each breath. This may be deleterious in a patient who requires significant positive end-expiratory pressure (PEEP).

Intermittent mandatory ventilation. Intermittent mandatory ventilation (IMV) provides a few mandatory breaths per minute and, thus, a minute volume below that required by the patient's metabolic rate. This technique provides an alternative to assisted ventilation and allows the patient to exercise the muscles of ventilation when being weaned from ventilatory support.

Synchronized intermittent mandatory ventilation. Synchronized intermittent mandatory ventilation (SIMV) differs from IMV in that the mechanically supported breaths are initiated (triggered) by the patient's effort. If the patient becomes apneic, IMV will be provided, but the synchronization diminishes the likelihood that the patient's spontaneous effort will oppose the mechanical breath.

Airway pressure release ventilation. Airway pressure release ventilation (APRV) implies that positive pressure is maintained continuously (like uninterrupted CPAP) and that each breath is achieved by briefly interrupting the pressure supply and, thus, allowing the patient to exhale before reapplying the pressure.

Pressure support ventilation. Pressure support ventilation (PSV) provides triggered ventilation with a maintained positive pressure and no subatmospheric phase. When the patient initiates inspiratory flow, the ventilator promptly responds with an increase in pressure and an adequate breath.

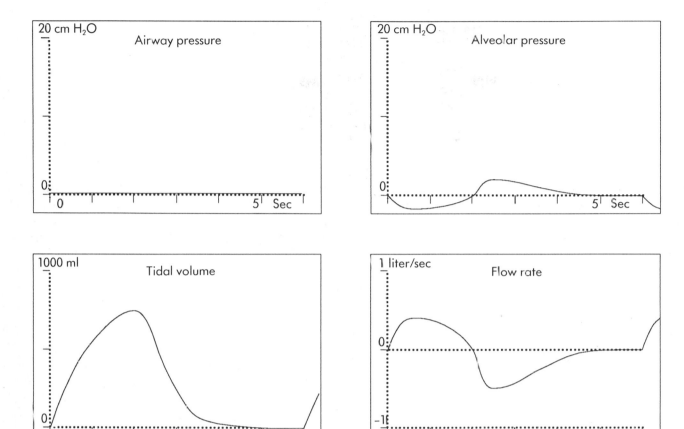

Fig. 6-5. Pressure, volume, and flow in normal spontaneous breathing.

Jet ventilation. High pressure air, oxygen, or anesthetic gas from a blender may be intermittently blown into the airway to achieve ventilation. This can be accomplished with no tracheal tube or via a Carden[14] tube that is a specially constructed short tube inserted beyond the vocal cords to direct the jet. In either case the surgeon is able to operate on the upper airway with minimal interference to visualization. If a metal cannula is employed, the size to deliver the gas is approximately 16 gauge. The pressure required may be as high as 2 or 3 atm. The effect of the jet is critically influenced by the alignment of the cannula. If aimed carelessly at the pharyngeal wall instead of axially toward the larynx, inadequate inspiratory pressure may be achieved. Conversely, excessive inspiratory pressure can also be achieved. Therefore, auscultation with a precordial stethoscope and close observation of the patient's chest wall are required.

Other types of IPPV. High frequency jet ventilation is occasionally of use; for example, it may achieve adequate ventilation in a patient with a significant bronchopleural fistula. Intermittent negative pressure ventilation has been utilized in anesthesia machines (RPR Pesty, Paris, France) but is accompanied by disadvantages and has not been utilized in other equipment.

Other methods of augmenting ventilation. Extrathoracic negative pressure has been employed in cuirass ventilators[15] and in tank ventilators such as the iron lung.[16] Gravity has been used in rocking beds, which utilize the weight of the abdominal contents to augment ventilation.

Machine compliance

There may be a large discrepancy between the tidal volume that is actually delivered to the patient and the tidal volume that has been preset, or is judged by, the movement of a bellows. This discrepancy occurs in all ventilators and anesthesia machines (except PhysioFlex, see below and also Chapter 33) because some of each breath is retained in the machine due to compression of the gas itself and the elasticity of the hoses of the circuit. It is essential to understand the origin and the magnitude of machine compliance because it ranges from being inconsequential to being of overriding importance. Machine compliance is greatest and most variable in machines in which an external ventilator is connected to a circuit that includes a soda lime absorber and a humidifier. This is because the compressible volume is large, there is a greater total length of compliant breathing hose, and the change in pressure during each breath affects the gas in the entire circuit, including the bellows. It is the magnitude of this volume that is responsible for much of the machine compliance.

The total volume of the gas that may be compressed in the circuit often exceeds 6 liters. Knowing this volume makes it possible to estimate the volume of each breath lost due to compression. For every 10 cm H_2O pressure, approximately 1% of the compressible volume is retained in the circuit instead of going to the patient. This is because 1 atm (760 mm Hg) is a pressure of approximately 1000 cm H_2O. A rise in the pressure in the circuit of 1000 cm H_2O would be caused by the addition of 100% more gas to the circuit; an increase of only 10 cm H_2O would, therefore, be caused by a 1% addition of gas.

In adults the potential loss due to compression and stretching is commonly balanced by the magnitude of the fresh gas flow from the anesthesia machine. For example a fresh gas flow of 6 L/min (100 ml/sec) will add, during an inspiratory period of 2 seconds, about 200 ml of fresh gas to the circuit. This is usually sufficient to offset the loss due to machine compliance, a loss that is relatively small compared to normal adult tidal volumes.

In children such losses can dominate the small tidal volumes required, partly because fresh gas flows may be reduced and partly because inspiratory times may be very brief allowing little time for fresh gas to be added to the circuit (see also Chapter 26). The clinical implications of this problem are discussed below.

VENTILATOR CLASSIFICATION

Many schemes have been employed for classifying ventilators. The most useful provide information about the ventilator's behavior. Two principal classifications are discussed here: the first describes the circuit and its characteristics; the second describes the ventilator's response to changes in the patient.

Machine and ventilator circuits

The relationship between the anesthesia ventilator and the breathing circuit is critical. The design determines the requirement for the fresh gas flow and for the settings of the ventilator. The principal features that require consideration are the presence or absence of carbon dioxide absorption, and the relationship between the ventilator and the breathing circuit.

No absorption of carbon dioxide, external ventilator. When a Mapleson D[17] circuit (i.e., a Bain[18] circuit) is employed, the reservoir bag can be replaced by attaching a ventilator. There is no absorption of carbon dioxide and, therefore, a high fresh gas flow rate is required. The Mapleson D circuit is moderately wasteful in that fresh gas escapes via the ventilator during exhalation. However, during the pause between breaths, as fresh gas flows into the exhalation hose, it displaces the previous breath further away from the patient and is stored. The next ventilator breath then uses some of this stored gas and some fresh gas (see also Chapter 4).

When using this circuit it is common to recommend that the ventilator be set to provide a relatively generous minute volume, e.g., 10 L/min; this ensures appreciable mixing of alveolar gas with circuit gas. The fresh gas flow rate governs the amount of this mixture containing carbon dioxide, which has to escape from the circuit between breaths. The effective ventilation is, therefore, regulated by the fresh gas flow. When utilizing this system it is important to differentiate between the *minute volume* as set on the ventilator; the *minute volume* set on the fresh gas flowmeters, which may be used to regulate carbon dioxide elimination; and the effective *minute volume* as judged by the patient's $PaCO_2$. Analysis of this effective minute volume is complicated by the fact that the inspired gas may well contain some carbon dioxide.

No absorption of carbon dioxide, integral ventilator
Stored fresh gas. Several ventilators store the fresh gas flow and intermittently release this gas to the patient. In these ventilators, the flow of anesthetic gases (the minute volume) is stored in a reservoir, usually a bellows that is pressurized by means of a weight or springs. When the bellows has filled, the expiratory valve closes and the inspiratory valve opens to allow the stored fresh gas to flow to the patient. When the bellows has emptied the valve positions are reversed to allow the patient to exhale. These designs are known as minute volume dividers; for example, Manley (B.O.C. Medishield, London, U.K.),[19] Minivent (Minivent, London, U.K.),[20] R.P.R. (Pesty-Technomed S.A., Montreuil, France),[21] and Barnet (no longer in production).[22] They utilize no soda lime absorber, and they operate as nonrebreathing systems. The fresh gas flow is equal to the minute volume and, accordingly, the patient's ventilation is regulated by adjustment of the fresh gas flow. Some of these designs (Manley, Minivent) also derive all their power from this fresh gas flow and require no electrical power.

No stored fresh gas. One anesthesia ventilator (Takaoka[23]) also utilizes the power of the fresh gas flow but stores no fresh gas between breaths. During inspiration the flow of anesthetic gases is directed to the patient with the expiratory valve closed. When the expiratory valve opens, the fresh gas and the patient's exhalation both exit from the ventilator. The fresh gas flow is thus wasted between breaths and necessitates high fresh gas flow rates to achieve adequate ventilation (e.g., 15 L/min). This design functions as though a thumb were used to intermittently cover the exhalation limb of a T-piece adapter.

Absorption of carbon dioxide, external ventilator. The closed circuit with soda lime absorption is connected to an external ventilator. This is the most common arrangement in the United States. It permits low fresh gas flows to be utilized and provides an intact closed circuit available for manual ventilation if the mechanical ventilator fails. However, there is a large compressible volume composed of the bellows, the ventilator hose, the soda lime canister, and the patient circuit hoses. Consequently,

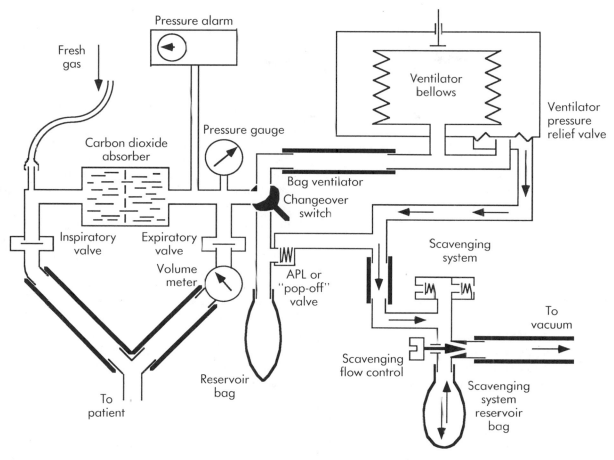

Fig. 6-6. Circuit showing changeover (or selector) switch to exclude the APL or "pop-off" valve during controlled ventilation. (Reproduced with permission from Schreiber P, *Safety guidelines for anesthesia systems,* 1985. North American Dräger, Inc. Telford, Pa.)

the circuit compliance may be as high as 10 ml/cm H_2O.

Proper arrangement of the components of the circuit and ventilator contributes to satisfactory performance. In sequence, between the expiratory valve and the inspiratory valve, there should be the pressure limiting valve (APL or "pop-off") and connection for the ventilator or bag; next the absorber; and finally the fresh gas inflow connection. In newer designs (see Fig. 6-6) the pressure relief valve is automatically excluded from the circuit when the ventilator is selected. Older ventilators still in widespread use, however, may unintentionally be used with the APL valve partially or completely open.

Absorption of carbon dioxide, integral ventilator. The recent introduction of new anesthesia machines in Holland (see A New Anesthesia Machine: The PhysioFlex, below, and Chapter 33) suggests that there may be advantages to be gained by making the ventilator an integral component of the anesthesia circuit. In this design there is a valveless circuit in which a fan continually circulates the gases through the soda lime, the ventilator chamber(s), and the patient hoses. This arrangement permits the volume of the circuit to be reduced. The design also automat-

ically measures the circuit compliance and incorporates this information so that it is the patient's actual minute volume and tidal volume that are calculated and displayed.

Stable versus unstable classification

The following classification of intermittent positive-pressure ventilators[24] focuses on the concerns of the clinician: what should the clinician expect to observe when there is a change in compliance or airway resistance, or when a leak develops; that is, "What happens to the ventilation when the patient changes?" The three critically important features of IPPV are the minute volume, the tidal volume, and the inspiratory flow rate. Each of these three lends itself to being analyzed in this way: do they remain stable in the face of changing conditions?

For each feature the same approach is used: will that feature be *stable* or *unstable* in response to a change in the patient, that is, if the patient's compliance decreases, will the ventilator be able to maintain the same performance? This approach to classification emphasizes the importance of understanding the interaction between the machine and the patient.

The distinction between stable and unstable also provides a rational basis for understanding existing classifications, for approaching an unfamiliar ventilator, and for analyzing and understanding the behavior that may be anticipated. The approach also explains the difference between two readily confused terms: pressure preset (unstable tidal volume) and pressure generator (unstable inspiratory flow rate).

The classification is most useful and reliable for adult ventilators where losses due to the circuit compliance are not usually significant. Although such losses may be between 7 and 10 ml/cm H_2O, or around 100 to 200 ml per breath, in adults these losses are considerably less than the tidal volume and are commonly offset by a comparably high fresh gas flow, which replaces volume during the inspiratory phase (see Machine compliance above). With smaller patients fresh gas flows may be less and the loss of gas in the circuit due to gas compression and stretching of the hoses becomes more significant; in neonates such losses may be critical (see also Chapter 26).

In adults, logic would appear to favor "stable" settings of volume and flow, which will change little as the patient changes. Reliance can be placed on monitoring the pressure to indicate such changes. In neonates, by contrast, airway obstruction could cause a critical change in delivered tidal volume with little observable change in pressure. In neonates a pressure preset machine may be preferable because there are advantages in knowing that an appropriate pressure is achieved with each breath. Monitoring then focuses on knowing that adequate exchange is actually occurring. Safe monitoring, especially for the smallest patients, requires capnometry, tidal volume determined from flow measurements made at the tracheal tube connector, or frequent blood gas analysis.

Minute volume: stable versus unstable. A stable, or reliable, minute volume is in general a desirable property in a ventilator. The minute volume is the most significant feature of IPPV. Some ventilators permit the minute volume to be directly set. When this is so it is reasonable to expect the minute volume to remain stable. In such machines the minute volume changes little in response to changes in the patient's compliance or airway resistance.

Setting the minute volume may be achieved where there is a single control for this purpose or where the minute volume of fresh anesthetic gas first drives the ventilator and is then divided into breaths by the machine (e.g., Manley ventilator[19]). The same stable minute volume is usually preset in other ways, typically as a result of setting the respiratory rate in combination with a stable tidal volume.

By contrast there are ventilators in which the minute volume is inherently unstable; changes in the patient's compliance and airway resistance are associated with proportional change in the ventilation. Most pressure preset ventilators behave like this. In addition many volume preset machines can be made to behave similarly by reducing the setting of the maximum pressure control. Then, instead of behaving like a tidal volume stable machine (volume preset) they will behave like a tidal volume unstable machine (pressure preset).

Tidal volume: stable versus unstable. A ventilator that delivers a stable tidal volume is volume preset (Fig. 6-7). The implication is that changes in the patient's compliance or airway resistance have a negligible effect on the tidal volume. By contrast, any leak of gas from the circuit results in a decrease in the delivered tidal volume, and this decrease is comparable to the size of the leak. Various mechanisms have been employed to achieve a stable tidal volume. They include a bellows that is mechanically driven over a preset range, a bellows whose movement trips a switch, and a constant inspiratory flow for a timed inspiratory period. In a tidal volume preset machine, it is appropriate to monitor the pressure. Variations in the patient will be reflected by comparable changes in pressure. Ideally, both the peak and the plateau pressures should be measured if they are provided. The plateau represents the effect of compliance and the difference between the two pressures represents the effect of airway resistance.

An unstable tidal volume occurs when the pressure is preset or where the pressure safety limit is markedly reduced (Fig. 6-7). In these ventilators, changes in the patient's compliance or airway resistance cause significant alterations in the patient's tidal volume. Again the effect of a leak is different; in pressure preset ventilators, provided the preset pressure is achieved, moderate leaks have

	Behavior	Best monitor	Effect on tidal volume of increased		
			Compliance	Resistance	Leak
Volume preset	Stable tidal volume	Pressure	Ø	Ø	↓
Pressure preset	Unstable tidal volume	Volume	↑	↓	Ø

Fig. 6-7. Ventilator classification by tidal volume.

	Behavior	Best monitor	Effect on inspiratory flow of increased		
			Compliance	Resistance	Leak
Flow generator	Stable inspiratory flow	Pressure	∅	∅	↓
Pressure generator	Unstable inspiratory flow	Inspiratory flow	↑	↓	∅

Fig. 6-8. Ventilator classification by inspiratory flow.

little effect on the tidal volume. Pressure preset behavior occurs, for example, in ventilators with a relatively light weight driving the bellows down or where the pressure during inspiration is measured and is used to determine the end of the inspiratory phase. In a pressure preset machine it is appropriate to monitor the tidal volume because alterations will reflect changes in the patient.

Inspiratory flow: stable versus unstable. A ventilator that provides a stable inspiratory flow is termed a flow generator (Fig. 6-8). The inspiratory flow rate is controlled by the ventilator and resists changes in the patient's compliance or airway resistance, although some machines vary the actual flow rate during the inspiratory phase. As in the case of the tidal volume, however, the effect of a leak is different. The leak represents a loss of the preset flow and, therefore, causes a decrease in inspiratory flow. Mechanisms that result in stable inspiratory flows include mechanically driven pistons or bellows, high pressure gas released through a valve, or pipeline pressure delivered via a flowmeter.

An unstable inspiratory flow occurs in pressure generator ventilators (Fig. 6-8). The relatively low pressure available during the inspiratory phase is insufficient to resist changes in the patient's compliance or airway resistance. Modest leaks, however, have little effect provided that the intended pressure is maintained. Examples of mechanisms that act as pressure generators include a weight acting on a bellows to generate a low pressure, for example, 15 to 40 cm H_2O, or a Venturi that entrains room air to produce similar pressures.

This classification provides a basis to help explain the difference between two commonly confused terms: pressure preset and pressure generator. Pressure preset (unstable tidal volume) is contrasted with volume preset and both refer to control of the tidal volume (Fig. 6-7), whereas pressure generator (unstable inspiratory flow rate) is contrasted with flow generator, and both of these terms refer to control of the inspiratory flow rate (Fig. 6-8). It is possible for a ventilator to be constructed that has any one of the four possible combinations of these variables (i.e., pressure preset flow generator, pressure preset pressure generator, volume preset flow generator, or volume preset pressure generator).

Other classifications

Cycling. Ventilators have also been classified according to their cycling mechanism (e.g., volume, time, pressure, or flow), the intention being to afford insight into function. It is, however, less satisfactory for this purpose than the volume preset versus pressure preset (stable versus unstable above) because similar behavior is provided by mechanisms that sound very different. For example, a stable tidal volume can be provided either by a volume-cycled ventilator or by a time-cycled ventilator which is also a constant flow generator. Conversely an unstable tidal volume could be provided by a pressure-cycled ventilator or by a time-cycled ventilator which is also a pressure generator. Because of such ambiguities the classification is mentioned here for completeness but is not advocated for clinical description.

Bellows ascending or descending. The ventilator bellows may be classified according to its direction of travel during exhalation. When disconnected from a patient, an ascending bellows tends to collapse to an empty position, whereas a descending (hanging) bellows tends to descend to a fully expanded position because its own weight tends to draw in room air. Should a leak or a partial disconnect occur, a descending bellows may continue to move almost normally, whereas an ascending bellows tends to collapse and remain stationary in the presence of a leak (see also Chapter 16). Adequate leak detection equipment minimizes the importance of this distinction, and future designs could obviate the value of this distinction by eliminating the presence of a bellows altogether (see description of PhysioFlex anesthesia machine below and in Chapter 33).

Power. Ventilators are often classified according to their source of power (e.g., electric or pneumatic). Unless the location of intended use predicates in favor of one or the other, this classification is of little importance to the user and usually offers no insight into the clinical behavior of the equipment.

Single or double circuit. Some ventilators provide a single circuit and either pass the driving gas on to the patient to ventilate the lungs (e.g., the Takaoka,[23] or minute volume dividers such as the Manley[19]), or they are mechanically powered and drive the gas to the patient without the need for a separate pneumatic circuit (e.g., the Emerson[11]). Other ventilators employ two separate circuits: in the first is the driving gas, usually compressed oxygen or air, which provides the power; the second circuit contains the anesthetic gas mixture used to ventilate the patient's lungs. The single circuit machine offers simplicity. The double circuit machine allows the use of a closed circuit but necessitates the use of a bellows, diaphragm, or membrane to separate the two circuits.

Other features. An anesthesia ventilator may or may not be capable of providing a number of other features such as positive end-expiratory pressure (PEEP), expiratory retard, inspiratory plateau or hold, and triggering in response to a patient's efforts. With the possible exception of triggering, which is rarely of use in modern anesthesia practice, these features are useful in specific circumstances but probably do not warrant use for classification.

CONTROLLED VENTILATION: THE VARIABLES

Interrelationship of variables

Many of the respiratory variables depend on each other. Minute volume ($\dot{V}_E$), tidal volume (V_T), and respiratory rate (f) are interrelated:

$$\dot{V}_E = V_T \times F$$

The time that is devoted to the inspiratory phase (T_I) consists of two parts: inspiration and plateau (T_{plat}). The inspiratory phase (T_I) and the respiratory rate (f) determine the inspiratory: expiratory ratio (R):

$$R = \frac{1}{\dfrac{60}{f \times T_I} - 1}$$

$$T_I = \frac{60 \times R}{(R + 1) \times f}$$

$$f = \frac{60 \times R}{(R + 1) \times T_I}$$

The inspiratory flow rate ($\dot{V}_I$) in liters/minute depends on V_T and the time available for inspiration before the plateau ($T_I - T_{plat}$):

$$\dot{V}_I = \frac{V_T \times 60}{T_I - T_{plat}}$$

These interrelationships invite analysis of the different variables. Which one is most important? Which should be preset? If the manufacturer provides different controls, is there still an advantage in considering these principal variables? In descending order of importance the principal four are $\dot{V}_E$, V_T, $\dot{V}_I$, and T_{plat}. Each of these four variables is important in its own right. They represent the ventilation, the size of each breath, the rate of inspiratory gas flow, and the time available for gas redistribution in the lung. As a byproduct they also determine the less important variables: f, R, T_I, and the expiratory period (T_E). Except for

the possible addition of PEEP, or expiratory retard, they have defined the ventilatory cycle. Three of these main variables are either volumes or flows, which is appropriate considering that ventilation is the process under consideration; the only time is the duration of the inspiratory plateau. Unfortunately ventilator manufacturers show little uniformity in their approach to providing controls. Nevertheless, to have these four parameters in mind when setting a ventilator provides a logical framework. It also diminishes the emphasis on parameters that are not in themselves critical.

Principal ventilator variables

Minute volume. The object of ventilation is to maintain an appropriate minute ventilation. In resting healthy human beings, minute volumes range from about 1 L/min at birth to about 12 L/min in larger adults. Anesthesiologists should be familiar with the range of minute volumes normally encountered in anesthesia practice. The range in adults is usually between about 5 and 10 L/min (Table 6-2). The values in this table provide a range within which to work and which facilitate the initial settings of a ventilator. Values can be inferred for other individuals (e.g., a young adult who is only of medium size, would require about 1 L/min less). It should be noted, however, that this Table 6-2 slightly truncates the extremes. There are a few very large young athletic adults who have ventilatory requirements that exceed the values shown by 1 to 2 L/min. There are a few emaciated elderly patients who require 1 to 2 L/min less. Nevertheless, this simple table can be used to predict initial ventilatory requirements.

Another method commonly used is to provide 10 ml/kg at a rate of 10 breaths per minute. This makes no allowance for the influence of gender, age, or metabolic requirements. It should be remembered that during surgery the combined effects of muscle relaxants, anesthesia, and hypothermia may significantly lower the metabolic rate and, hence, the carbon dioxide production and the ventilation required. By contrast, healing wounds, sepsis, thyrotoxicosis, and recovery from major trauma are examples of conditions that may significantly increase the metabolic rate.

The minute volume can be set directly on some anesthesia ventilators. Even when such a control is not provided, it is prudent to calculate the minute volume being administered to the patient. This reduces the chance of administering grossly inappropriate ventilation. It also facilitates the adjustment of a ventilator to correct an abnormal $PaCO_2$ using the following relationship: when a ventilator is adjusted, the minute volume multiplied by the $PaCO_2$ remains approximately constant:

$$\dot{V}_E \times PaCO_2 = K$$

Tidal volume. In resting healthy human beings, the tidal volume ranges from about 20 ml at birth to a little over 1 L in large athletes. Although the majority of ventilators allow direct setting of the tidal volume, it is less im-

Table 6-2. Average minute volume (liters) in anesthetized adults

	Male	Female
Large young adult	10	9
Middle age and size	8	7
Small and aged	6	5

portant than the minute volume and is rarely critical. For a given minute volume, a wide range of tidal volumes and respiratory rates are usually well tolerated. When the tidal volume is being preset, the airway pressure should be monitored to reflect changes in the patient.

In anesthesia it is customary to employ larger volumes and, therefore, slower rates, for example, 6 to 10 breaths per minute. This expands alveoli and leaves longer gaps between breaths for the surgeon to work peacefully in the thorax or upper abdomen. By contrast, extracorporeal shock wave lithotripsy is more effective if the renal stone undergoes minimal movement and it is common to employ reduced tidal volumes at a high respiratory rate, for example, 20 to 25 breaths per minute. (See also Chapter 27.)

Inspiratory flow. The inspiratory flow rate at rest ranges from about 2.5 L/min to about 50 L/min. In adults the range is about 10 to 50 L/min (about 200 to 1000 ml/sec). The actual value for the inspiratory flow is often not calibrated and is rarely measured.

Inspiratory plateau. An inspiratory plateau allows time for redistribution of gas between alveoli with different compliances and airway resistances. It also allows for the compliance (C) to be estimated or calculated

$$C = \frac{V_T}{P_{plat}}$$

In healthy lungs the plateau is not usually required. If unnecessarily protracted it may even be hazardous; prolonged raised intrathoracic pressure may diminish venous return to the thorax and compromise cardiac output.

Inspiratory pressure (preset, pop-off, or dependent). In ventilators that are inherently pressure preset, the pressure does not vary in response to changes in the patient and the tidal volume is *unstable* (see classification above). The tidal volume is monitored to detect changes in the patient's compliance or airway resistance.

In volume preset machines the inspiratory pressure is a dependent variable. It is used as a monitor of the patient's compliance and the airway resistance. In volume preset machines there is also an inspiratory pressure limit valve (pop-off or safety valve), that may be adjusted. If this pressure limit is set too low it will alter the behavior of the machine; instead of retaining the fundamental tidal-volume stable (volume preset) behavior, it will now function as a tidal-volume unstable (pressure preset) machine. It is this ability to use an adult ventilator in this pressure preset mode that can make an adult ventilator safer for use in small children (see also Chapter 26).

Intermittent positive-pressure ventilation waveforms

Volume, pressure, and flow. The normal waveforms obtained during spontaneous breathing are shown in Fig. 6-5. The *volume* waveform represents the expansion of the lung with respect to time. The pressure at the mouth is atmospheric throughout; there is a little change in the alveolar pressure and the flow rate shows a sinusoidal pattern.

During IPPV (Figs. 6-9 and 6-10) the volume waveform is positive (above zero) throughout the cycle, rising during inhalation and falling back toward zero during exhalation. The waveform is almost indistinguishable from the *pressure* waveform in the alveoli. This is because the compliance of the lung is essentially linear in the range of pulmonary expansion used clinically. At the mouth, however, the *pressure* waveform is somewhat different. The pressure during inspiration is slightly higher representing the additional pressure required to overcome airway resistance, and during the expiratory phase the mouth pressure is normally zero because the patient is usually permitted unobstructed exhalation.

The *flow* waveform is conventionally biphasic with a positive (upward) waveform during inspiration and a negative (downward) waveform to represent the reversal of flow during exhalation. In a constant flow generator (stable inspiratory flow) the inspiratory flow rate is approximately a rectangular wave (Fig. 6-9). In a constant pressure generator (unstable flow) the inspiratory flow rate declines exponentially as the pressure differential diminishes during the inspiratory phase (Fig. 6-10).

Several variations in waveform are employed in anesthesia. In the next section they are illustrated by means of alveolar pressure graphs which, as stated above, are usually very similar to volume waveforms. The waveforms are representative of a constant flow generator. Figure 6-11 shows the normal waveform for comparison with the others which follow it.

Positive end-expiratory pressure

Benefit. When the closing volume of the lung (i.e., lung volume at which small airways begin to close) is greater than the functional residual capacity, alveoli collapse during each respiratory cycle. This collapse can be prevented by maintaining the volume of the lung above the closing volume. PEEP has this effect (Fig. 6-12). It acts as "pneumatic scaffolding" to support the volume of the lung between each breath and, thus, minimize the risk of alveolar closure.

Risk. Cardiac output depends on the adequacy of the venous return to the thorax. A raised pressure during the expiratory period can have a critical effect on the mean intrathoracic pressure. In a normal patient with zero PEEP, intermittent positive-pressure ventilation (IPPV) elevates the mean intrathoracic pressure by 2 to 3 cm H_2O. Application of even modest PEEP, for example, 5 cm H_2O, more than doubles this increase in the mean intrathoracic pressure. In a patient with a reduced blood volume, such a change can compromise venous return.

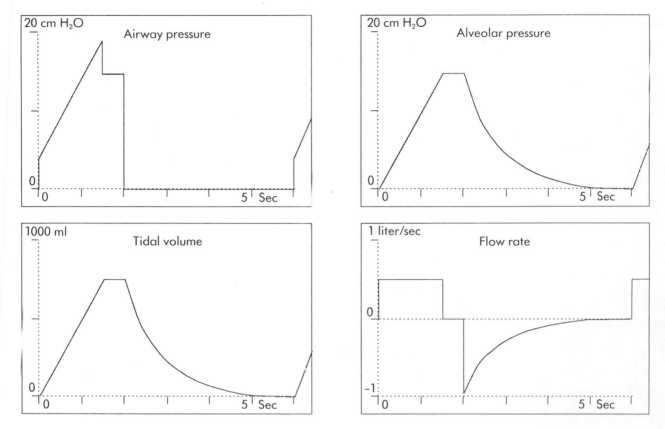

Fig. 6-9. Pressure, volume, and flow during IPPV with a constant flow generator.

Expiratory retard

Benefit. Airway closure during exhalation occurs in asthma and in chronic obstructive pulmonary disease. The loss of elasticity in the lung tissue allows intrapleural pressure to collapse small airways. Forceful voluntary effort to exhale may actually exacerbate such expiratory obstruction (air trapping). Paradoxically, an obstruction at the mouth (the pursed lips, or "whistle" of a patient with chronic obstructive pulmonary disease) assists exhalation by preventing airway collapse. Some ventilators offer an expiratory retard but it is rarely of critical value in anesthetized patients (Fig. 6-13).

Risk. Ventilators that incorporate an expiratory retard feature may also permit the operator to mechanically or manually initiate rapid breathing. In such circumstances there may be insufficient time for exhalation to occur. A "staircase" rise in intrathoracic volume and pressure may occur with impairment of venous return and, possibly, some risk of pulmonary damage.

Prolonged inspiratory phase

Benefit. A prolonged inspiratory phase creates a calmer motion for the surgeon operating in the thorax or upper abdomen (Fig. 6-14). This ventilatory pattern also allows more time for gas redistribution in the lung. This can be useful in chronic obstructive pulmonary disease with ventilatory maldistribution although a more rapid inflation fol-

lowed by an inspiratory plateau may be even more useful for this purpose (see below).

Risk. The disadvantages of prolonging the inspiratory period are usually negligible. It does allow less time for exhalation and may cause small increases in the mean intrathoracic pressure.

Shortened inspiratory phase

Benefit. The shorter the inspiratory period, the less is the impact on the mean intrathoracic pressure (Fig. 6-15). In a hypovolemic, hypotensive patient it is appropriate to try shortening the inspiratory period, although greater benefit may result from a reduction in the overall ventilation.

Risk. In the patient with chronic obstructive pulmonary disease, the reduction may provide too little time for adequate gas redistribution; too rapid an inspiratory flow may also cause regional hyperinflation with the risk of barotrauma; and the jerky pattern of ventilation may also be more disturbing to the surgeon working in the thorax or upper abdomen.

Inspiratory plateau

Benefit. A plateau, or pause, provides the best conditions for gas redistribution in the lung and is, for a small number of compromised patients, of critical value (Fig. 6-16). In addition, the plateau provides an opportunity to observe the airway pressure without gas flow. This plateau

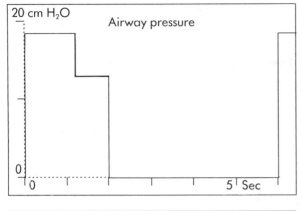

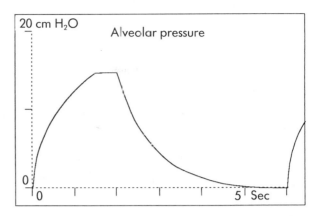

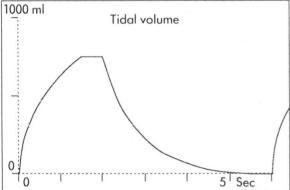

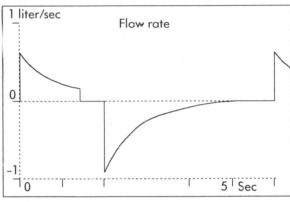

Fig. 6-10. Pressure, volume, and flow during IPPV with a constant pressure generator.

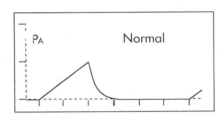

Fig. 6-11. Normal alveolar pressure (P_A) waveform.

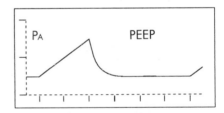

Fig. 6-12. Effect of positive end-expiratory pressure (PEEP) on alveolar pressure (P_A).

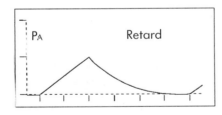

Fig. 6-13. Expiratory retard. Effect on alveolar pressure (P_A).

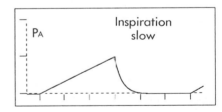

Fig. 6-14. Prolonged inspiratory phase. Effect on alveolar pressure (P_A).

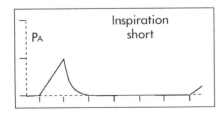

Fig. 6-15. Shortened inspiratory phase. Effect on alveolar pressure (P_A).

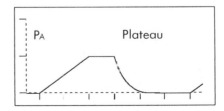

Fig. 6-16. Inspiratory plateau or hold. Effect on alveolar pressure (P_A).

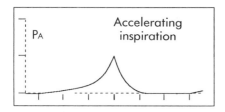

Fig. 6-17. Accelerating inspiration. Effect on alveolar pressure (P_A).

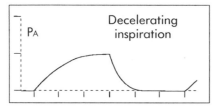

Fig. 6-18. Decelerating inspiration. Effect on alveolar pressure (P_A).

pressure is a measure of the total thoracic compliance (volume of gas per cm H_2O).

Risk. An inspiratory plateau provides a prolonged period of raised intrathoracic pressure and, therefore, raises the mean intrathoracic pressure. Prolonged high intrathoracic pressures may compromise venous return to the thorax and, therefore, diminish cardiac output.

Variations of inspiratory flow pattern. Various attempts have been made to improve pulmonary function during IPPV by modifying the flow rate during the inspiratory phase. For example, accelerating inspiration (Fig. 6-17) which provides an inspiratory flow rate that starts slowly and accelerates, has been advocated as minimizing the effect of IPPV on the mean intrathoracic pressure. It is probably of little benefit, as a greater reduction in the mean intrathoracic pressure can be achieved by maintaining a rapid flow rate throughout the inspiratory period. There is also an obvious similarity between the accompanying diagram and the diagram for shortened inspiratory phase (see Fig. 6-15). Decelerating inspiration (Fig. 6-18) provides an inspiratory flow that starts rapidly and diminishes, allowing rapid filling of the lungs followed by time for redistribution. Although this waveform might benefit the patient with chronic obstructive pulmonary disease, the benefit is probably better provided by an inspiratory plateau. There is an obvious similarity between the accompanying diagram and that for the inspiratory plateau (Fig. 6-15).

CHARACTERISTICS OF AN IDEAL VENTILATOR

The nature of clinical practice ensures that ventilator design is subject to continuous modification. The problems that occur during anesthesia will naturally initiate improvements. Unfortunately, this process often tends to eliminate the minor problems without even raising questions about

more fundamental flaws in the design. Indeed, the process of making these minor corrections may actually sanction basic faults; their reappearance in successive versions actually reaffirms the inevitability of their presence. The paragraphs that follow describe the characteristics of an ideal ventilator. An attempt has been made to categorize them into four groups: *general features* that would be desirable in any mechanical device; *ventilation features* that define its performance; *current requirements* necessitated by inherent flaws in design; and *future features* realizable in anticipated designs.

General features

Like any other mechanical device, a ventilator should be reliable, and convenient to operate, and its controls should be accurate. Many current designs are somewhat inconvenient to operate, for example, two controls must be operated to turn the anesthesia ventilator on and control knobs may be inaccurate. Ventilators should also be economical. If the ventilator is driven by compressed gas, then a mechanism should be incorporated to conserve the gas. For example, in recent North American Dräger ventilators, a venturi is utilized to decrease the consumption of oxygen used to drive the ventilator bellows. This has the additional benefit of reducing the fluctuation in the fresh oxygen flow, which is frequently observed as a ventilator cycles.

Ventilation features

The anesthesia ventilator should be capable of ventilating patients of all ages and who may have normal or abnormal pulmonary function. For all age groups the ventilator should be capable of providing satisfactory IPPV and should be capable of achieving the minute volumes, tidal volumes, and inspiratory flow rates given previously. There should be sufficient power, and the pressure limit should be adjustable to permit peak inflation pressures of 60 to 80 cm H_2O. The inspiratory phase should be capable of providing an adjustable plateau or pause after the inspiratory flow has ceased. The expiratory phase should offer PEEP and, perhaps, an expiratory retard. Ideally, humidification and heating should be integral in the machine. Unfortunately, this is technically difficult and therefore, with existing machines, humidification requires an extrinsic device.

Current requirements

Some design details exist only to solve problems that are inherent to existing equipment. For example, it is generally accepted that an ascending bellows design is preferable. This is because it enables leaks to be detected more readily. If, however, ventilators never leaked, or if they employed reliable leak detection alarms, the direction of bellows movement would be of little consequence. The valves in existing closed circuits are essential to the satisfactory function of an external, closed-circuit ventilator. Each valve must be light in weight; must rest on a delicate, thin, annular valve mount; must be contained by a metal frame/guide; and must be enclosed in a transparent housing. Scavenging systems are required because of concern about pollution in the operating room, and they have been refined to minimize the risk of excessive positive or negative pressure being applied to the patient circuit. A change-over switch converts the breathing circuit from manual to automatic ventilation but, until recently, did not exclude the circuit adjustable pressure limiting (APL) valve from the automatic mode. In addition, the switch still does not simultaneously turn the ventilator power on or off (see Fig. 6-6).

These features are of interest because their presence would be obviated by appropriate changes in design. Such changes include: incorporating adequate leak detection; eliminating the necessity for the bellows, the scavenging system and the valves in the closed circuit; and providing a ventilator on/off switch that also converts the circuit to and from the manual/bag mode of use. The incorporation of these changes may characterize future designs.

Ideally, the volume of the breathing circuit should be minimal to reduce the system compliance; however, this is difficult to achieve in existing designs because of the size, layout, and distensibility of the various circuit components. An alternative strategy is to compensate for system compliance as discussed below.

Future features

Future anesthesia ventilators should be designed to function as a closed circuit for reasons of economy and to reduce pollution. The ventilator and the humidifier should be integral parts of the anesthesia circuit itself to minimize the number of components and connections and to reduce the compressible volume.

The ventilator should incorporate sufficient artificial intelligence to assist the user. For example, the equipment's compliance factor should be known, or measured by the equipment, so that minute volume, tidal volume, and inspiratory flow rate can all be set accurately. When first turned on, and between cases, the equipment should automatically reset itself so that it provides frequently used, safe settings (e.g., normal adult settings for IPPV, no PEEP, no retard, short inspiratory plateau, no trigger). There should be numerical, graphical, and trend displays with alarms for various parameters including ventilatory parameters (pressure, volume, flow, and capnogram); metabolic information (oxygen consumption, carbon dioxide production, and respiratory quotient); and pulmonary mechanics (compliance, airways resistance, and leaks).

As ventilator design changes, familiar features such as the bellows and the sound that most ventilators currently make may disappear. The bellows and the noise made by each ventilator breath afford useful monitoring informa-

tion. However, with modern methods of monitoring, such as capnometry and pulse oximetry, the value of these time-honored methods may be questioned: it may be necessary to introduce artificially created sound to reassure the operator; it may even prove possible to enjoy silence and trust that alarms and warnings will alert the operator if performance departs from preset values.

CURRENT DESIGNS OF ANESTHESIA VENTILATORS

The anesthesia ventilators selected for detailed description are those that are currently in common use in the United States (North American Dräger, Ohmeda). Understandably, most anesthesia delivery systems in current use have many similarities; the requirement for safety indicates a need for familiarity, and the small total size of the market makes major change prohibitively expensive. Several attempts have been made to use new technology to introduce radically new designs and features into anesthesia machines; until recently no very radical change has successfully come to market. One recent experimental design[25] incorporated modern computing technology and attempted to maintain a familiar feel by simulating accepted features such as flowmeters. Another new microprocessor-controlled anesthesia machine[26] was designed so that the user could switch between most of the known types of breathing circuits. Such developments reveal a marriage to existing concepts that in itself tends to limit innovation. Nevertheless the steady improvement in computers and our growing confidence in their abilities suggest that radically new designs will eventually appear (see also Chapter 33).

North American Dräger AV-E

Classification. The North American Dräger anesthesia ventilator (North American Dräger, Telford, PA)[27] currently marketed in the United States is the AV-E (anesthesia ventilator electronic). It is the standard ventilator supplied with the North American Dräger Narkomed 2A, Narkomed 2B, Narkomed 3, and Narkomed 4 anesthesia machines (Fig. 6-19) and is not available as a free-standing unit. The control mechanism of the ventilator is housed in the anesthesia machine above the flowmeters with the control switches located on a panel in the front of this area. The AV-E utilizes compressed oxygen to drive the ventilatory process and electrical power for the timing circuits and control of the solenoid valves. Driving gas and ventilatory gas remain separated at all points in the system. Tidal volume is preset by the user and internal electronic circuits control the timing of breaths. The machine therefore provides a stable minute volume, stable tidal volume, and stable inspiratory flow rate. The duration of the inspiratory plateau is also adjustable by varying the inspiratory/expiratory ratio.

Operation. The operator has access to five controls governing the operation of the ventilator. The dial power

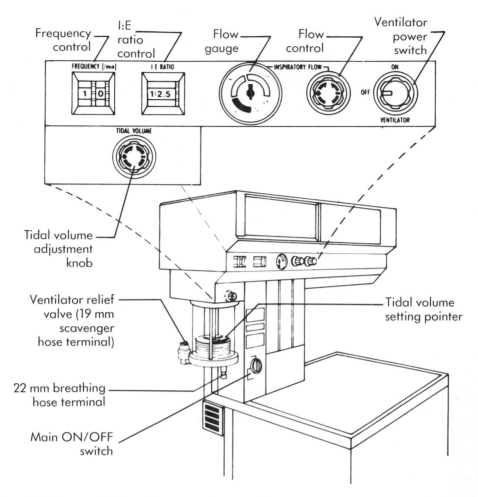

Fig. 6-19. Dräger AV-E ventilator on a Dräger Narkomed anesthesia machine. (Courtesy of North American Dräger, Inc., Telford, Pa.)

switch has an "off" position and two "on" positions. The upper "on" position is intended for normal ventilator use. The lower position changes the circuit low pressure alarm from the normal 15 second delay to a 60 second delay. This lower position is selected when extremely low frequency ventilation is used along with a high I:E ratio resulting in an expiratory time greater than 15 seconds, thus preventing false alarms under those conditions. A thumb wheel is provided that allows the operator to select the I:E ratio from 1:1 to 1:4.5 in eight increments. The frequency of ventilation is also controlled in the range of 1 to 99 breaths per minute using a thumb wheel. The tidal volume is controlled at the bellows, located to the left of the anesthesia machine (Fig. 6-19). A locking device prevents accidental changes in the tidal volume. The locking bar is depressed and the desired tidal volume is selected by rotating the control knob. A plate inside the bellows housing roughly indicates the selected tidal volume on a scale printed on the chamber. The flow rate adjustment knob al-

lows continuous adjustment of the inspiratory flow with the delivered flow rate displayed on an adjacent gauge. The flow rate adjustment controls the flow rate of driving gas into the bellows housing and hence the rate at which the bellows is compressed. It is possible for the flow rate to be set such that the full tidal volume is not delivered to the patient. An excessively high peak inspiratory pressure may result from setting the inspiratory flow rate too high. Decreases in lung compliance may create a situation in which ventilation is reduced when a previously adequate flow rate setting becomes inadequate as the compliance of the lungs decreases. The user should periodically inspect for full compression of the bellows.

Recommended operation procedure. North American Dräger recommends the following sequence for adjusting the controls of the AV-E:[28]

1. Adjust the tidal volume to the desired setting.
2. Adjust the breaths per minute to the desired frequency.

3. Set the I:E ratio.
4. Turn on the power switch.
5. Set the manual-automatic valve to the Auto position (this simultaneously switches the manual bag and pop-off valve out of the circuit and the ventilator into the circuit, Fig. 6-6). The flow control setting must then be adjusted so that the bellows empties completely by the end of the inspiratory phase (Fig. 6-19).

Ventilator function. Figure 6-20 is a schematic of the Dräger AV-E in the inspiratory phase. Oxygen from a pipeline or tank is provided to the ventilator at a pressure of approximately 50 psig. The inspiratory cycle begins with the opening of the solenoid control valve by the electronic control portion of the machine. The electronics determine the timing of the valve opening and closing based on the setting that the operator has selected. The solenoid valve is the electromechanical link between the control and pneumatic portions of the ventilator. The opening of the solenoid valve releases pressure, which opens the control valve to allow oxygen to flow through the flow regulator at a rate determined by the user (see above discussion). The power relief valve is held closed by the pressure of the oxygen. The oxygen flows through the venturi, entraining room air to aid in the driving of the bellows. This ingenious mechanism allows almost 80% of the driving gas to come from room air, reducing the oxygen required and the oxygen supply pressure decrease. The final gas mixture entering the bellows housing and compressing the bellows has an oxygen concentration of about 35%.[27] As the chamber containing the bellows is pressurized, the ventilator relief valve is closed by the increasing pressure, closing the connection of the patient circuit to the scavenging circuit. The bellows is forced downward driving the contained gas into the breathing circuit. As the bellows reaches its full compression, excess pressure in the driving system is relieved through the venturi port and air is no longer entrained into the system. After complete bellows compression there is an inspiratory pause until the end of the inspiratory phase.

The changeover from inspiratory phase to expiratory phase occurs when the solenoid valve closes (Fig. 6-21). The control valve then closes and oxygen ceases to flow to the venturi. The power relief valve opens allowing the pressure in the bellows chamber to fall. The bellows then rises passively as the patient exhales. The fall in pressure in the chamber around the bellows allows the ventilator relief valve to open. When the pressure in the bellows exceeds the 2 cm H_2O back pressure exerted by the relief ball-valve (Fig. 6-21), the excess gas is released from the breathing circuit to the scavenging system. Although contemporary Dräger AV-E ventilators all have ascending bellows, there are still a few older models in use with hanging bellows (Fig. 6-22).

There are a few potential problems that are peculiar to the Dräger AV-E design. If a leak develops in the ventilator bellows, there is a risk that driving gas will enter the breathing circuit. In many designs such a leak introduces oxygen and diminishes the anesthetic concentration. In the Dräger design, because air is entrained into the driving gas circuit, a leak introduces nitrogen into the gas being breathed from the patient circuit. A rising nitrogen concentration in the end-tidal gas could be open to misinterpretation as evidence of an air embolism. Another potential source of problems is the ventilator relief valve pilot line (Figs. 6-20, 6-21, and 6-22). This tube has to be patent to permit exhalation. If this tube becomes kinked, exhalation is obstructed and pulmonary barotrauma is possible.[29]

Basic Dräger AV-E ventilators are not pressure limited, but a pressure limit control is available from North American Dräger, Inc., and it may be retrofitted to certain ascending bellows design AV-E units. The pressure limit control device works by sensing the pressure in the patient circuit at the bellows and, whenever the threshold high pressure set limit is exceeded, a valve in the driving gas circuit opens to vent driving gas to the atmosphere. In this way the driving gas pressure is limited, and thereby the pressure of gas in the patient circuit, for the remainder of the inspiratory time.

It is important to note the significance of the muffler in the function of the Dräger AV-E ventilator (Figs. 6-20 and 6-21). The entrained room air must pass unimpeded through this device during the inspiratory cycle; likewise all of the driving gas must exit through the muffler during the expiratory cycle. Any debris or impediment to flow will hinder the proper functioning of the ventilator and result in residual pressure developing in the system, which may prevent the relief valve from opening and creating an increase in the patient's airway pressure.[30] (See also Chapter 16.)

Alarm system. The alarm system of the AV-E is integrated into the central alarm system of the Dräger Narkomed anesthesia machine. The location and alarm method varies with the particular model of machine on which the ventilator is installed. A high pressure alarm sounds whenever circuit pressure exceeds +65 cm H_2O. The subatmospheric pressure alarm is triggered when the pressure in the circuit decreases to 10 cm H_2O below atmospheric pressure. This condition may exist if the scavenging system is malfunctioning, if the fresh gas flow is inadequate, or if the patient is inhaling against an obstruction. The continuing pressure alarm is designed to alert the user should the airway pressure remain above 18 cm H_2O pressure for more than 10 seconds. A blocked or closed pop-off valve, malfunctioning ventilator pressure relief valve, or an obstruction in the scavenging system may create a continuing pressure situation. The minimum ventilation pressure functions as a "disconnect" alarm, indicating that the amplitude of the pressure wave during inspiration did not achieve the selected minimum. The

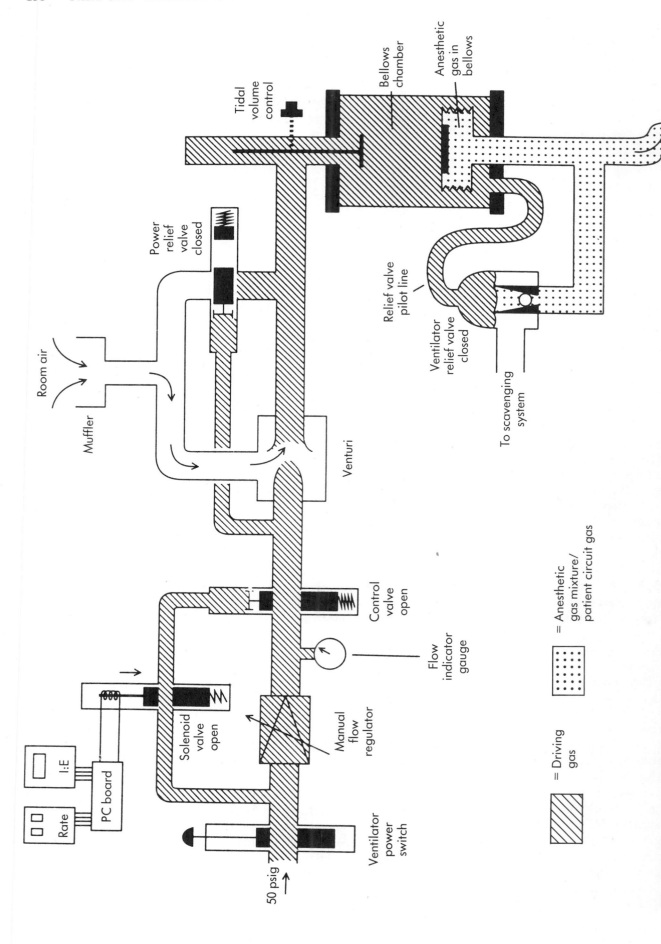

Fig. 6-20. The Dräger AV-E in the inspiratory phase. (Reproduced with permission from Andrews JJ: *Anesthesia systems*. In Barash PG, Cullen BP, Stoelting RK, editors: Clinical anesthesia, J.B. Lippincott, 1989, Philadelphia, pp 505-542.)

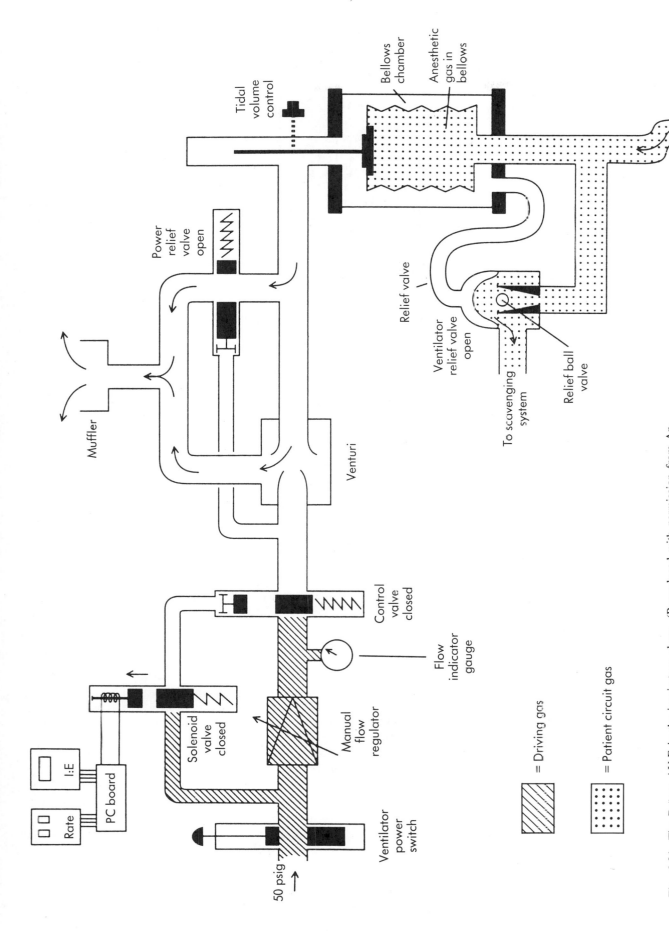

Fig. 6-21. The Dräger AV-E in the inspiratory phase. (Reproduced with permission from Andrews JJ: *Anesthesia systems.* In Barash PG, Cullen BP, Stoelting RK, editors: Clinical anesthesia, J.B. Lippincott, 1989, Philadelphia, pp 505-542.)

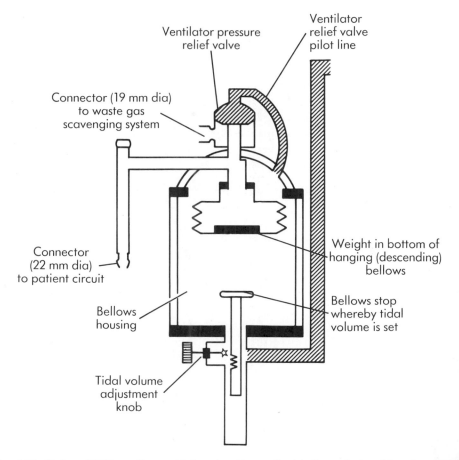

Fig. 6-22. Dräger AV-E ventilator with hanging (descending) bellows design. Note that the bellows *descends* during exhalation and that there is no PEEP ball-valve in the ventilator relief valve. (Diagram courtesy of J.B. Eisenkraft, M.D.)

user is able to select 8, 12, or 26 cm H_2O and should select the highest value that is below the peak inspiratory pressure. In the most recent version, any minimum pressure setting can be selected by the user with a continuously adjustable control.

Ohmeda 7000

Classification. The Ohmeda 7000 ventilator is incorporated into Ohmeda anesthesia machines and is also available as a free-standing unit (see Fig. 6-23).[31] This ventilator consists of two distinct modules: the control assembly and the bellows assembly. The control assembly is typically either mounted directly under and attached to the bellows assembly in a free-standing application (Fig. 6-23) or mounted separately on the anesthesia machine. The Ohmeda 7000 utilizes compressed oxygen to drive the ventilatory process and electrical power for the timing circuits and control of the solenoid valves. Driving gas and ventilatory gas remain separated at all points in the system. Minute ventilation is preset by the user and internal circuits control the timing of breaths based on the user-defined parameters of respiratory rate and I:E ratio.

Operation. Control of the Ohmeda 7000 is through two toggle switches and three dial knobs (Fig. 6-23). One toggle switch is provided to turn the ventilator on or off; the second controls a sigh option for the machine. The sigh function produces a "sigh" breath of approximately 150% of the preset tidal volume on every 65th breath. Unlike the AV-E, the tidal volume is not directly controlled in the Ohmeda 7000; rather the minute ventilation and respiratory rate are set using continuously adjustable dial knobs. The machine then calculates the appropriate tidal volume to deliver. A dial is also provided to adjust the I:E ratio of the ventilator. The internal circuitry uses this input to calculate the appropriate flow rate of compressed oxygen into the bellows chamber. A "manual cycle" push button allows the user to cycle the ventilator, and a "lamp test" button illuminates the alarm lights to verify that the bulbs are functioning.

Recommended operation procedure. The Ohmeda operation manual recommends the following sequence for operation of the 7000:[31]

1. Set the desired values for minute volume, rate, and I:E ratio on the control dials.

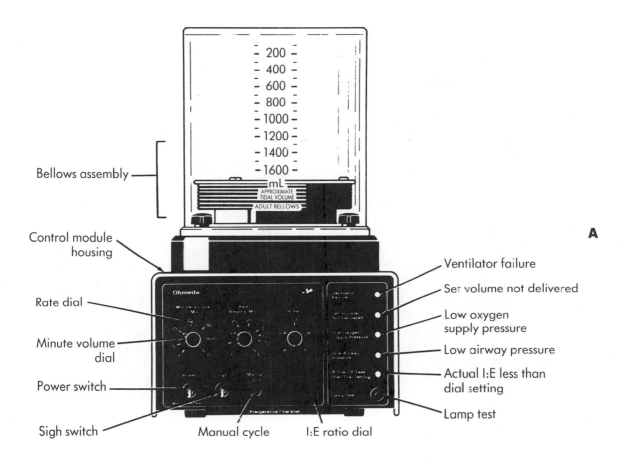

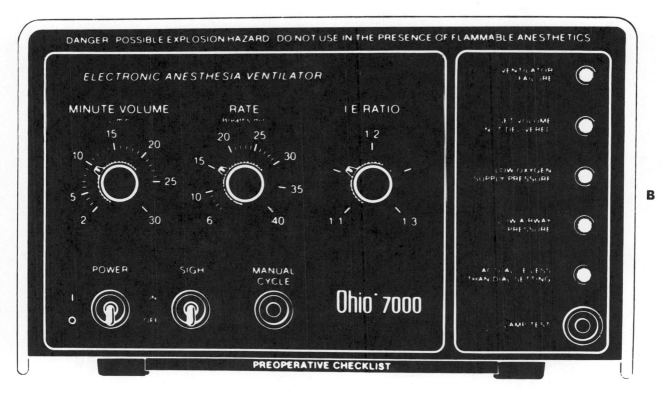

Fig. 6-23. A, The Ohmeda 7000 Ventilator. **B,** Close-up of the control panel of the Ohmeda 7000 Ventilator. (Permission granted by Ohmeda, A Division of BOC Health Care, Inc., Madison, Wis.)

2. With the power switch off, use the anesthesia system's oxygen flush valve to fill the bellows. Maintain an oxygen flow that is sufficient to keep the bellows fully extended.
3. Switch the power on.
4. Compare the ventilator minute volume setting to the volume monitor reading.

Ventilator function. Internally the Ohmeda 7000 differs in many ways from the Dräger AV-E (see description above). Like the AV-E the driving gas is compressed oxygen from either a wall source or a tank source regulated to approximately 50 psig. A very accurate, internal gas regulator further reduces this driving gas pressure to 38 psig. After being regulated down to this reduced pressure the gas is then passed to a set of five solenoid valves in parallel. Each solenoid valve controls the flow of oxygen to a "tuned" orifice. The solenoid valves control the amount of gas per minute flowing through the corresponding orifices. By precisely opening and closing selected solenoid valves the volume of oxygen corresponding to the calculated tidal volume and at the correct overall flow rate is delivered. From the five orifices the oxygen flows to a collection chamber and then to the bellows chamber. The collection chamber is fitted with a pressure relief valve, venting to the atmosphere at approximately 65 cm H_2O (Fig. 6-24).

The driving gas (compressed oxygen) enters the bellows chamber driving the bellows down, and thereby delivering the gas contained in the bellows to the patient circuit (Fig. 6-25). Unlike the Dräger AV-E, the volume of driving gas reaching the chamber is in a one-to-one ratio with the tidal volume set and is 100% oxygen. As the tidal volume delivered is determined by the driving gas volume entering the bellows chamber, the bellows does not fully descend except when delivering the maximal tidal volume of 1600 ml (see Fig. 6-23). This is in contrast to the Dräger AV-E in which each properly delivered tidal volume results in a complete emptying of the bellows. This design difference explains why the AV-E's tidal volume scale begins at the bottom of the bellows chamber and increases upward. The 7000 is calibrated from the top of the bellows chamber down and does not require a limiting mechanism to determine the tidal volume. Like the Dräger AV-E, the Ohmeda 7000 has a pop-off valve mechanism in the bellows assembly (Fig. 6-25) to vent the excess gas in the circuit to the scavenging system at end-expiration after the bellows

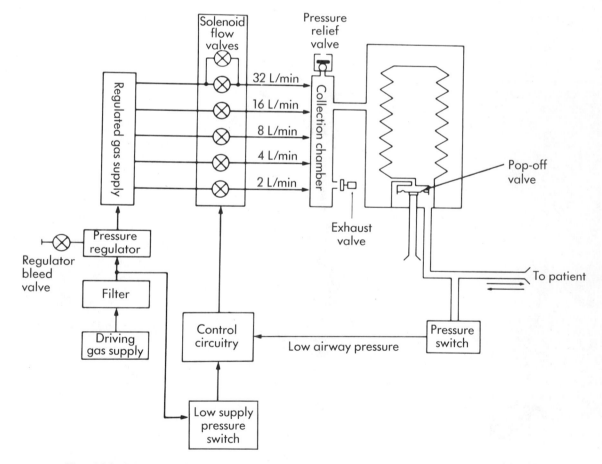

Fig. 6-24. Schematic of operation of the Ohmeda 7000 Ventilator. (Permission granted by Ohmeda, A Division of BOC Health Care, Inc., Madison, Wis.)

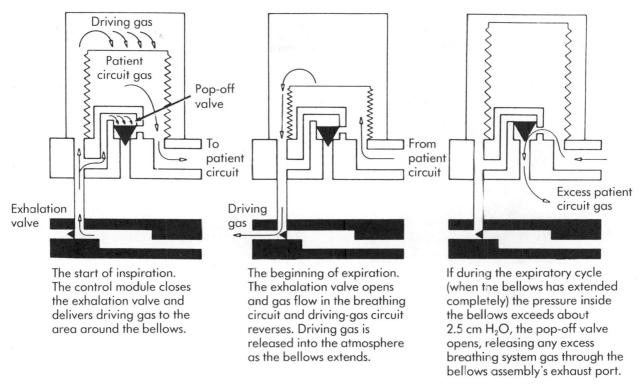

The start of inspiration. The control module closes the exhalation valve and delivers driving gas to the area around the bellows.

The beginning of expiration. The exhalation valve opens and gas flow in the breathing circuit and driving-gas circuit reverses. Driving gas is released into the atmosphere as the bellows extends.

If during the expiratory cycle (when the bellows has extended completely) the pressure inside the bellows exceeds about 2.5 cm H_2O, the pop-off valve opens, releasing any excess breathing system gas through the bellows assembly's exhaust port.

Fig. 6-25. The inspiratory and expiratory phases of the Ohmeda 7000 Ventilator. (Permission granted by Ohmeda, A Division of BOC Health Care, Inc., Madison, Wis.)

has refilled. This pop-off valve requires a pressure of 2.5 cm H_2O to open. The valve is closed during inspiration by the pressure of the driving gas in the bellows chamber. At the end of the inspiratory phase, the control circuitry opens a pressure relief valve venting the driving gas and allowing passive exhalation into the bellows (Fig. 6-25). The Ohmeda pressure relief valve is flush-mounted inside the bottom of the bellows. Unlike the Dräger AV-E, this design does not require a relief valve pilot line (Figs. 6-20, 6-21, and 6-22).

Alarm system. The alarm display of the Ohmeda 7000 ventilator consists of a column of five red lights located on the far right side of the control panel (Fig. 6-23). An audible tone sounds when an alarm condition occurs. The alarms are labeled and function as follows:

"Ventilator Failure" alarms when the unit detects a critical internal failure.

"Set Volume Not Delivered" alarms when the user has selected a minute ventilation and respiratory rate combination that requires a tidal volume greater than can be delivered by the ventilator.

"Low Oxygen Supply Pressure" alarms when the pressure in the driving gas line falls below 40 psig. Continued operation with a low gas supply results in a minute volume of less than that set on the control panel.

"Low Airway Pressure" alarms if the airway pressure does not reach 6 cm H_2O after two or three ventilator cycles. It functions as a circuit low pressure alarm.

"Actual I:E Less Than Dial Setting" alarms when the settings are adjusted in such a way that the required output exceeds the capability of the machine.

Ohmeda 7800 series ventilators

Classification. The Ohmeda 7800 (Fig. 6-26)[32] is the most recent and advanced ventilator from Ohmeda. It is available in several configurations. The 7800 is available as a stand-alone unit, as an accessory to the Excel anesthesia machine, or as a retrofit to update an existing Modulus II anesthesia machine. The 7810 is provided as an integral part of the Modulus II Plus anesthesia machine, and the 7850 is the ventilator incorporated in the Ohmeda Modulus CD system. The ventilator is an electronically controlled, pneumatically driven, tidal volume preset ventilator. As a result of the accuracy of microprocessor control this ventilator is able to deliver tidal volumes from 50 ml to 1500 ml without changing the bellows assembly. Ventilatory monitoring in the form of both tidal volume, minute volume, and inspired oxygen concentration have been incorporated into the ventilator, so that if the ventilator should fail so also might these monitors (see also Chapter 16).

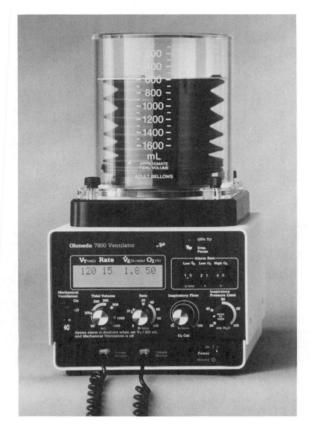

Fig. 6-26. The Ohmeda 7800 ventilator. (Permission granted by Ohmeda, A Division of BOC Health Care, Inc., Madison, Wis.)

Operation. The user controls the 7800 through an on/off toggle switch, two buttons, and four dial knobs (Fig. 6-26). A liquid-crystal display screen provides information to the user concerning several aspects of ventilator function. On the top line of the display, exhaled tidal volume, respiratory rate, expired minute ventilation, and inspired oxygen concentration are shown. A second line of the display is used for control messages and alarm conditions. Adjusting, or merely even touching one of the control knobs, results in that control's setting being displayed on the second line of the display screen. (If wearing gloves, it is necessary to turn the knob slightly to view the display).

Unlike the Ohmeda 7000, the user directly selects the tidal volume, not the minute ventilation. Respiratory rate is also controlled by a dial-type knob. The inspiratory flow rate is continuously adjustable from 10 to 100 liters per minute; however the liquid crystal screen displays the I:E ratio as the inspiratory flow rate is changed. A control knob is provided to limit the maximum inspiratory pressure generated by the ventilator. Should the pressure in the circuit exceed this limit, the control circuitry terminates the inspiration, immediately switches to exhalation, and produces an alarm condition. Adjustments to the inspiratory pressure limit also change the sustained pressure

alarm limit; the limit is set to one half of the selected maximum inspiratory pressure up to a maximum of 30 cm H_2O. The sustained pressure alarm is annunciated when the limit is exceeded for 15 seconds.

An inspiratory pause button is present and pressing it adds an inspiratory pause to the end of the inspiratory cycle equal to 25 percent of the inspiratory time. As the inspiratory time is lengthened and the expiratory time reduced by adding this pause, the I:E ratio naturally falls. Push wheels are used to set the alarm limits for high and low inspired oxygen concentration, and low minute ventilation.

Recommended operation procedure. Initiation of operation of the Ohmeda 7800 series ventilators is very similar to that of the Ohmeda 7000. Of notable difference is the determination of tidal volume rather than minute volume as already mentioned, and the selection of alarm limits for the built-in volume and oxygen monitors of the 7800.

Ventilator function. Like other ventilators, the driving gas to the Ohmeda 7800 series ventilators is usually from a pipeline oxygen source delivered between 35 and 75 psig. The driving gas pressure is regulated down to 26 psig and delivered to a pneumatic manifold. Inside the pneumatic manifold a flow control valve controls the driving gas volume that flows to the bellows chamber. The flow control valve has a variable orifice allowing the microprocessor to vary precisely the flow rate and volume delivered to the bellows assembly. The determination of the correct flow rate and volume are made by the microprocessor based on the settings the user has selected. A secondary regulator provides pneumatic power to the exhalation valve, which closes during inhalation and opens during exhalation to vent the driving gas as the bellows reexpands (Fig. 6-27).

Like the Ohmeda 7000 ventilator, a pop-off valve is present inside the bellows to release excess gas from the patient circuit at end-exhalation once the bellows is full. During inspiration this valve is held closed by the pressure of the driving gas. Various internal sensors allow the ventilator to monitor its own function to ensure correct operation and alert the user to failures or alarm conditions. The circuitry for the oxygen sensor is inside the ventilator control housing, but a remote sensor in the patient circuit is required. This sensor is to be located at the inspiratory limb of the circle breathing system. A flow sensor is also located in the patient circle breathing system on the expiratory limb. The output from this sensor is processed by the ventilator and the exhaled tidal volume and minute ventilation are displayed on the liquid-crystal display screen. This information can also be used to alert the user to circuit disconnects.

Alarm system. The design of the Ohmeda 7800 series ventilators represents a departure from previous designs in that the feedback to the user is through messages displayed on the liquid crystal display screen as opposed to dedicated

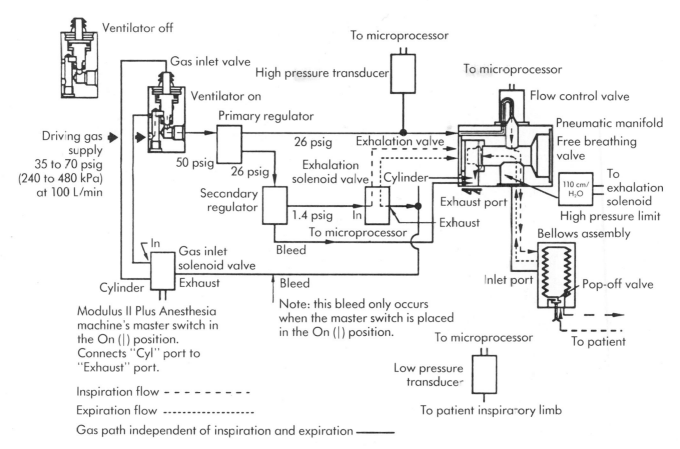

Fig. 6-27. The Ohmeda 7800 ventilator schematic of operation. (Permission granted by Ohmeda, A Division of BOC Health Care, Inc., Madison, Wis.)

lights each indicating a specific condition. Future changes in the software of the ventilator may produce changes in the conditions detected and the messages displayed. Software version 1 provides the ventilator with at least 25 alarm or alert warnings for the user. The user should consult the specific manual for the details of the particular version being used.[32]

Older designs of anesthesia ventilators

The Ohio Anesthesia Ventilator, introduced in 1973; the Ohio V5 (1979); the Ohio V5A (1983); and the Dräger AV share several design characteristics.[11] The use of these ventilators is decreasing as they are gradually retired; however, as they are occasionally encountered, a brief discussion is justified. These machines are purely pneumatically driven and controlled, requiring no electrical power supply for operation. Internal control of cycling is achieved through a fluidic control mechanism, the discussion of which is beyond the scope of this text but is described elsewhere.[33] They all possess descending (hanging) bellows with a stop mechanism to set the tidal volume. A disconnect alarm was built into some of these ventilators; however, the threshold was such that if a resistance exists

in the circuit, the unit may be unable to detect a disconnect. The Dräger AV is controlled through two dial knobs: one sets the respiratory rate, the other the flow rate into the bellows chamber. The tidal volume is determined at the bellows chamber.

A very different control system is utilized in the Ohio Anesthesia Ventilator.[11] The respiratory rate is determined indirectly by a combination of the "expiratory time" and the "inspiratory flow rate" controls. Expiratory time controls the duration of the expiratory phase of the respiratory cycle, that is, the time between the end of one inspiration and the beginning of the next. The inspiratory flow rate alters both the time of the inspiratory phase and the peak airway pressure achieved. The combined setting of the inspiratory time and the expiratory time determines the I:E ratio as well as the duration of a single respiratory cycle, which is the reciprocal of the respiratory rate. A control is provided for the expiratory flow rate; however, unlike the inspiratory flow rate this does not alter the time of the expiratory phase. The expiratory flow rate must be set with caution as breath "stacking" with greater and greater airway pressure may occur if the expiratory flow rate is low enough to prevent complete exhalation before the initiation

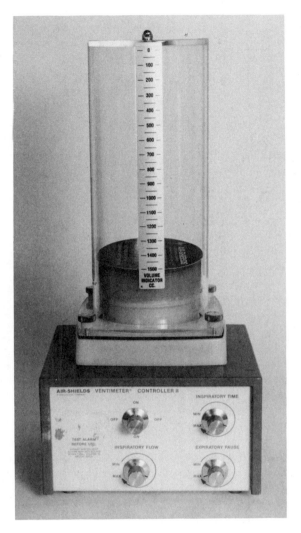

Fig. 6-28. The Air-Shields Ventimeter Controller II.

of the next inspiratory cycle. Maximum inspiratory pressure is controlled through an appropriately labeled knob. The ventilator exhausts any remaining gas when the selected pressure is reached regardless of whether the full tidal volume is delivered or not. A manual cycling button is present. Provision is made for the ventilator to act in an assist mode; it will sense the initiation of a spontaneous respiratory effort by the patient and at an adjustable level, trigger a breath.

The Ohio V5 in many ways represents a simplification of the Ohio Anesthesia Ventilator. The controls are reduced to an "On-Off" switch, an "Inspiratory Flow" knob, an "Expiratory Time" knob, and a "Manual Cycle" button. Tidal volume is controlled at the bellows. The hazard of breath stacking is eliminated by not allowing the expiratory rate to be reduced. The V5A is very similar to the V5. It has an optional pediatric bellows assembly available.

The Air-Shields Ventimeter Controller II (Air-Shields Inc., Hatboro, Pa) is a pneumatically powered ventilator for use in conjunction with an anesthesia machine (Fig. 6-28). The machine functions as an external ventilator for use with a closed circuit with carbon dioxide absorption. Controls are provided for inspiratory flow rate, inspiratory time, and expiratory time. By means of these controls, because the inspiratory flow rate is stable, this ventilator effectively provides a stable minute volume and a stable tidal volume although neither of these is directly preset. The driving gas is compressed air or oxygen obtained from the hospital pipeline. The flow of this gas to drive the bellows is controlled by an inspiratory flow control knob. The cycling of the ventilator is controlled by varying the time for inspiration and the time for expiration. These two controls adjust the time taken for pressure to build up and then diminish in a chamber in the pneumatic timing unit. These are the only controls on the Ventimeter II. Previous models of this ventilator had a manual inflating bag, a switch to permit patient triggering of ventilation, and a switch to add negative pressure to exhalation. These extra features have been eliminated from the current model because they were of little practical value and could confuse the operator.

A new anesthesia machine: the PhysioFlex

The PhysioFlex (Physio BV, Amsterdam, The Netherlands)[34] anesthesia machine bears little resemblance to existing equipment (Figs. 6-29 and 6-30; see also Chapter 33). It is designed to function as a closed-circuit machine. This almost eliminates pollution, it makes for economical operation, and it facilitates accurate measurement of the gases used by measuring the amount required to replenish that used each minute. Thus oxygen and nitrous oxide consumptions are displayed continuously.

The circuit (Fig. 6-29) is significantly different from existing closed circuits. There are no valves because a modern version of the Revell Circulator[35] circulates gas around the circuit at a flow rate of 70 L/min. The concentration of gases and volatile agents are measured and are replenished as needed. Gases are admitted via computer-controlled valves; potent inhaled volatile agents are introduced by automatic injection to maintain the selected end-tidal concentration. Soda lime absorbs carbon dioxide, and when required, the concentration of volatile agents may be reduced by switching some of the gas stream through an activated charcoal filter.

The ventilator consists of four membrane chambers, only one of which is represented in Fig. 6-29. The actual number of membrane chambers in use is selected automatically by the computer depending on the size of the breath required. All the closed circuit gas flows continuously through the membrane chamber(s) of the ventilator. These features of the design reduce the internal volume and the machine compliance. On start-up the machine automatically measures its own compliance; this allows the computer to maintain accurately the values that the operator set

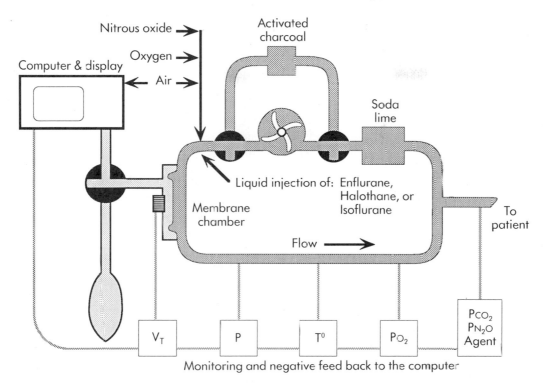

Fig. 6-29. Schematic diagram of the PhysioFlex Anesthesia Machine. (Physio BV Amsterdam, The Netherlands.)

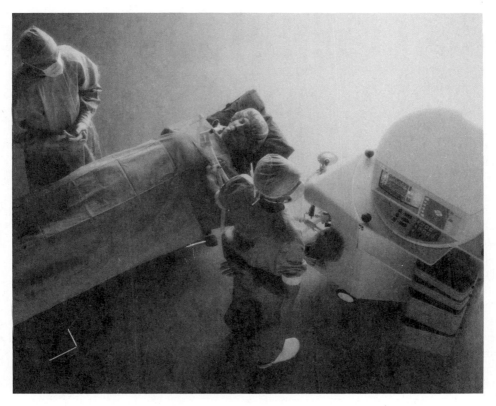

Fig. 6-30. PhysioFlex Anesthesia Machine. (Physio BV Amsterdam, The Netherlands.)

for the patient's minute volume, tidal volume, and inspiratory flowrate.

The PhysioFlex anesthesia machine incorporates radical changes in layout, design, and function; many familiar features have been eliminated. This machine indicates possible trends in the design of anesthesia machines and stimulates a reappraisal of existing anesthesia equipment, much of which is currently tolerated because of general familiarity with it, reluctance to incur major expense, and current fear of liability litigation. It is probably no accident that the PhysioFlex machine has been developed and marketed in a country, The Netherlands, with a lower incidence of such litigation.

MATCHING THE VENTILATOR TO THE PATIENT

Certain pathological or physiological conditions may determine the ventilator, the mode, or the pattern of ventilation employed. The age of the patient may influence the choice of ventilator. The size of the bellows and hoses should preferably be matched to the patient. For example, it is desirable to employ equipment with the very smallest volume when neonates are being ventilated. Nevertheless, even with this precaution, there may be an enormous discrepancy between the tidal volume preset and the tidal volume delivered. Machine compliance should be assumed to exceed 5 ml/cm H_2O. Thus if a neonate were ventilated with a low fresh gas flow it may be necessary to set the bellows to at least 100 ml to achieve a tidal volume of 20 ml. In such circumstances the ventilator should be regarded as a device that reliably produces the correct pressure with each breath (pressure preset, see above) rather than as a volume preset machine (see also Chapter 26).

Various types of lung pathology may dictate particular methods or patterns of ventilation. Some patients with chronic obstructive pulmonary disease or asthma may benefit from prolongation of the expiratory pause to allow time for complete lung emptying. On the other hand patients with restrictive lung disease may not be able to tolerate large tidal volumes, with the associated high inflation pressures, and will benefit from more frequent smaller breaths. A patient with emphysematous bullae should not be exposed to either large tidal volumes with their attendant risks of stretching and rupture, or to excessively rapid inspiratory flow rates with the risks of uneven filling and rupture of a bulla. A patient with a leak due to a bronchopleural fistula can present significant problems during IPPV and may require high frequency jet ventilation, with or without conventional IPPV.

There are occasions when a ventilator or a specific pattern of ventilation may suit a patient particularly well or may even be critical to survival. When surgery is indicated in such circumstances, it may be easiest to transfer the ventilator to the operating room together with the patient. Administering anesthetic gases in such a situation may be impractical. Any necessary sedation or anesthesia will then be administered intravenously and a useful approximation to a given pattern of ventilation can be provided manually or by appropriately setting an anesthesia ventilator. However, some anesthesia ventilators still in use have appreciable limitations and may, for example, be unable to provide an inspiratory plateau, an expiratory retard, high peak inflation pressure, or a high level of positive end-expiratory pressure.

HAZARDS AND THEIR PREVENTION

The major unavoidable risk associated with the use of an anesthesia ventilator is unexpected cessation of ventilation. Interruption in IPPV should always be detected by appropriate monitoring and constant vigilance (see Chapter 16). If the defect is obvious, an attempt at immediate correction is appropriate (e.g., reattach hose, insert electric plug, reconnect monitor). However, unless the malfunction is immediately corrected, the nonfunctioning equipment should be removed for repair and immediately replaced with a functioning unit. An operating room is not the place to effect repairs, and an anesthetized patient deserves undivided attention. A simple trustworthy technique should be used to ventilate the patient, such as a self-inflating bag and mask, or mouth-to-tube ventilation. Although some malfunctions may be puzzling or confusing, most can be anticipated or prevented by appropriate precautions. Some of the more common hazards, adverse effects of IPPV, and their prevention, are considered below.

Sequelae of intermittent positive-pressure ventilation

Some adverse effects are associated more or less routinely with the use of anesthesia ventilators and may occur in susceptible individuals even though the ventilator is functioning correctly. These hazards are important because, as they can occur with a normally functioning ventilator, they should be anticipated with vigilance and prevented if possible.

1. Hypothermia and drying of the secretions both occur because dry gas is commonly inspired during general anesthesia. Drying occurs in the trachea and bronchi, heat is lost due to vaporization of water, and the temperature of the patient may fall. In lengthy cases humidification is strongly recommended (see Chapter 7).
2. Hypercarbia or hypocarbia may occur due to incorrect setting of the ventilator.
3. Hypotension may be caused by excessive ventilation associated with hypocarbia and raised intrathoracic pressure; this is especially likely to occur soon after induction.
4. Barotrauma from excessive transpulmonary pressure is always a possibility during IPPV. This is especially likely in the presence of chronic obstructive

pulmonary disease with either large tidal volumes or excessively rapid inspiratory flow rates.

Operator errors

Errors due to inappropriate setting of the controls are usually readily corrected if recognized. There are various examples of which the first three are the most important, probably the most common, and all too often not promptly detected:

1. There may be failure to turn the ventilator *on* or return the manual/automatic changeover switch to *ventilate* after a period of manual ventilation.
2. There may be failure to close the adjustable pressure-limiting (pop-off) valve when initiating or resuming IPPV.
3. There may be failure to attach the ventilator hose to the absorber assembly.
4. Rate or volume may be inappropriate, e.g., when an adult patient follows a pediatric case.
5. The pressure may be set too low to deliver the preset tidal volume.
6. If a trigger is installed it may be set at so sensitive a level that rapid breathing is initiated with insufficient expiratory pause. This may cause hyperventilation, raise intrathoracic pressure, and decrease cardiac output.
7. If an expiratory retard is installed it may be too tightly closed; rapid IPPV or frequent use of a manual trigger button may then cause breath-stacking or barotrauma.
8. The PEEP valve may be left turned up. If unrecognized this can raise the mean intrathoracic pressure and cause hypotension or barotrauma.
9. Excessive fresh gas flow may contribute to an increase in the inspired tidal volume and contribute to hyperventilation.
10. The tidal volume may be set too low to overcome the machine compliance so that the ventilator merely compresses the gas in the circuit; a total obstruction may pass unnoticed.
11. Alarm systems are too commonly inactivated.
12. Finally, when a problem arises, undue reliance on manual ventilation can jeopardize the patient. A common response to a suspected ventilator failure is to initiate manual ventilation. This permits a rapid evaluation of breath sounds, circuit integrity, patient compliance, and airway resistance, all of which should be completed within a few breaths. There is a temptation, however, to continue with this manual ventilation introducing a real risk of producing significant hyperventilation. Caution should therefore be exercised to ensure that manual ventilation is not unnecessarily protracted. In addition to being excessive, it occupies the operator's attention and hands thus preventing attention to other possible causes or courses of action.

Equipment malfunction

1. Some ventilators can stall in inspiration causing sustained high intrapulmonary pressure, e.g., the Ohio Anesthesia Ventilator.
2. The ventilator bellows can deteriorate and develop a leak. Oxygen from the driving circuit may then enter the breathing circuit via the ventilator, elevate the concentration of oxygen in the circuit, and dilute the anesthetic concentration. Conversely, with the Dräger AV-E, air can enter the circuit and decrease the delivered FIO_2.
3. An external PEEP valve can be unintentionally inserted in the inspiratory limb. This totally obstructs inspiration and, unless recognized, can cause negative intrapulmonary pressures, pulmonary edema, and death.
4. The valves in the breathing circuit may stick in the closed position and cause obstruction to inspiration or to expiration. In addition, a valve could stick open and cause rebreathing.
5. The pipeline oxygen supply may fail, necessitating the use of the tanks. An "E" size cylinder normally lasts for some hours. However, when supplying a ventilator as well as the breathing circuit it may last only 30 to 40 minutes.
6. Problems can occur with the scavenging system including inappropriate connection, valve malfunction, and occlusion of the scavenging hose. These may interfere with the escape of gas from the circuit and allow the development of excess pressure, or may apply negative pressure to the circuit.
7. A wrong connection can occur in which confusion occurs between the hoses for circuit, the ventilator, or the scavenger.
8. The timing mechanism can fail with the ventilator in the expiratory phase. In this case the bellows is fully distended and the low pressure alarm will not sound. Only an apnea alarm will be activated in this circumstance.

Cross infection

Several authors have studied the risk of cross infection arising from the use of ventilators and anesthesia circuits. Cross infection has occurred; cases have been reported in which the repeated use of the same piece of airway equipment has transferred infection between patients.[36] Soda lime absorbers cannot be regarded as a barrier to the transmission of bacteria. Indeed, bacteria (e.g., pseudomonas) has been cultured from soda lime absorbers.[37] Nevertheless, with the older type of nondisposable circuits, adequate infection control was achieved by washing with suitable decontamination fluids.[38] The subsequent widespread introduction of disposable circuits has obviated the need for such decontamination: bacteria are not disseminated during quiet breathing[39] nor do the machine and circuit disseminate organisms.[40] (See also Chapter 23.)

The concern caused recently by AIDS, and the greater risk posed by hepatitis B, warrants a vigilance about controlling cross contamination in all aspects of anesthesia care. A new organism might appear with the morbidity of these diseases and the ease of transmission that characterizes some of the childhood viral diseases. An example of the potential for risk in a hospital setting was provided by the epidemic of Ebola Fever in Zaire in 1981.[41] Admittedly these cases of African hemorrhagic fever were spread principally by the reuse of intravenous equipment, but the overwhelming mortality that accompanied this disease, even among the staff of the hospital, provides appropriate emphasis on the requirement for routine precautions. Precautions that prevent cross contamination appear to offer appropriate safety for airway equipment and anesthesia delivery systems. The use of disposable circuits appears to afford patients adequate safety; actual sterility is hard to achieve.

Preoperative precautions

An anesthesia ventilator should be inspected and tested prior to use. For the purposes of this section it is assumed that the remaining parts of the anesthesia machine are tested and working. These notes, therefore, focus on the ventilator and its circuit. The equipment should respond appropriately to the following tests before use:

1. The circuit holds a sustained pressure in the manual mode (tests for circuit leak).
2. The ventilator inflates a reservoir bag attached to the Y-adapter (tests mechanical function and connections).
3. Inspiratory and expiratory valves lift and seat correctly during controlled ventilation of this rebreathing bag.
4. Against occlusion, the ventilator's inspiratory phase reaches an appropriate high pressure and does not exceed it (tests pressure is adequate and safety relief valve is working).
5. With the ventilator off and the circuit occluded, the previously filled bellows does not collapse (tests integrity of bellows in ascending bellows).
6. The bellows moves when the patient breathes spontaneously into the circuit with the ventilator connected (circuit integrity and no valves stuck).

Intraoperative evaluation

When anesthesiologists are monitoring IPPV, they routinely hear and observe several functions to confirm that the ventilator is working normally. Confirmation depends upon some, or all, of the following:

1. The breath sounds via an esophageal or precordial stethoscope are normal.

2. The oxygenation of the patient is satisfactory as judged by pulse oximetry.
3. The clinical condition and the vital signs of the patient are satisfactory.
4. The function of the ventilator itself sounds normal.
5. The bellows moves evenly over the preset range and reaches both ends of its travel.
6. The hoses of the circuit and ventilator expand and contract with the pressure of each inspiration and expiration.
7. The pressure gauge shows the expected peak and plateau pressures.
8. Condensation forms and clears in the tracheal tube (unless external humidification is employed).
9. Capnography shows a normal level of end-tidal carbon dioxide with a normal waveform.
10. All alarms are enabled, operational, and silent.

REFERENCES

1. Baker AB: *Early attempts at expired air respiration, intubation and manual ventilation.* In Atkinson RS, Boulton TB, editors: *The history of anaesthesia,* London, 1987, Royal Society of Medicine. pp 372-374.
2. Gordon AS: *History and evolution of modern resuscitation techniques.* In Gordon AS, editor: *Cardiopulmonary resuscitation conference proceedings,* Washington, DC, 1966, National Academy of Sciences, pp 7-32.
3. Fell GE: Forced respiration, *JAMA* 16:325-330, 1891.
4. O'Dwyer J: Fifty cases of croup in private practice treated by intubation of the larynx, with a description of the method and of the dangers incident thereto, *Med Rec* 32:557-561, 1887.
5. Hochberrg LA: *Thoracic surgery before the 20th century,* New York, 1960, Vantage Press, pp 684-697.
6. Vesalius A: *De humani corporis fabrica libri septem,* Basileae. Ex Off. Ioannis Oporini, 1543.
7. Mushin WW, Rendell-Baker L: *The principles of thoracic anaesthesia,* Oxford, 1953, Blackwell, pp 28-30.
8. Tuffier T, Hallion L: Intrathoracic operations with artificial respiration by insufflation, *C R Soc Biol (Paris)* 48:951, 1896.
9. Matas R: Artificial respiration by direct intralaryngeal intubation with a new graduated air-pump, in its applications to medical and surgical practice, *Am Med* 3:97, 1902.
10. Drinker P, Shaw L: An apparatus for the prolonged administration of artificial respiration, *J Clin Invest* 7:229, 1929.
11. Mushin WW, Rendell-Baker L, Thompson PW, et al: *Automatic ventilation of the lungs,* Oxford, 1980, Blackwell Scientific.
12. Magill IW: Development of endotracheal anaesthesia, *Proc R Soc Med* 22:83-88, 1928.
13. Guedel AE, Treweek DN: Ether apnoeas, *Anesth Analg* 13:253-264, 1934.
14. Carden E, Vest HR: Further advances in anesthetic techniques for microlaryngeal surgery. *Anesth Analg* 53:584-587, 1974.
15. Collier CR, Affeldt JE: Ventilatory efficiency of the cuirass respirator in totally paralyzed chronic poliomyelitis patients, *J Appl Physiol* 6:531, 1954.
16. Drinker P, McKhann L: The use of a new apparatus for prolonged administration of artificial respiration, *JAMA* 92:1658, 1929.
17. Mapleson WW: The elimination of rebreathing in various semiclosed anaesthetic systems. *Br J Anaesth* 26:323, 1954.
18. Bain JA, Spoerel WE: A streamlined anaesthetic system, *Can Anaesth Soc J* 20:426, 1972.
19. Manley RW: A new mechanical ventilator, *Anaesthesic* 16:317, 1961.

20. Cohen AD: The Minivent respirator, *Anaesthesia* 21:563, 1966.

21. Mollaret P, Pocidalo JJ: Présentation d'un respirateur artificiel à pressions positive et négative avec pause réglable (R.P.R.), *C R Soc Biol (Paris)* 150:1898, 1956.

22. Mushin WW, Rendell-Baker L, Thompson PW, et al: *The 'Barnet' Mark III Ventilator.* In *Automatic ventilation of the lungs,* Oxford, 1980, Blackwell, pp 312-330.

23. Takaoka K: Respirador automatico de Takaoka. *Rev Bras Anestesiologia* 14:390, 1964.

24. Grogono AW: The classification of intermittent positive pressure ventilators, *Br J Anaesth* 44:405-407, 1972.

25. Cooper JB, Newbower RS, Moore JW, et al: A new anesthesia delivery system, *Anesthesiology* 49:310-318, 1978.

26. Sykes MK, Sugg BR, Hahn CEW, et al: A new microprocessor controlled anaesthetic machine, *Br J Anaesth* 62:445-455, 1989.

27. Dräger AV-E. Anesthesia ventilator specifications and equipment manual. Telford, Pa, 1986, North American Dräger Inc.

28. Dräger AV-E. Anesthesia ventilator instruction manual. Telford, Pa, 1984, North American Dräger, Inc.

29. Eisenkraft JB. Potential for barotrauma or hypoventilation with the Dräger AV-E ventilator, *J Clin Anesth* 1:452-456, 1989.

30. Roth S, Tweedie E, Sommer RM: Excessive airway pressure due to a malfunctioning anesthesia ventilator, *Anesthesiology* 65:532, 1986.

31. Ohmeda: 7000 electronic anesthesia ventilator. Operation and maintenance manual. Madison, Wis, 1988, Ohmeda, A Division of BOC Health Care, Inc.

32. Ohmeda: 7800 Ventilator. Service manual. Madison, Wis, 1990, Ohmeda, A Division of BOC Health Care, Inc.

33. Hill DW. *Physics applied to anaesthesia,* ed 4, Boston, 1980, Butterworths, pp 155-162.

34. Verkaik APK, Erdmann MD: Respiratory diagnostic possibilities during closed circuit anaesthesia, *Acta Anaesthesiol Belg* 41:177-188, 1990.

35. Revell DG: An improved circulator for closed circle anaesthesia, *Can Anaesth Soc J* 6:104-107, 1959.

36. Walter CW: Cross-infection and the anesthesiologist, twelfth annual Baxter-Travenol lecture, *Anesth Analg* 53:631-644, 1974.

37. Dryden GE: Uncleaned anesthesia equipment, JAMA 233:1297-1298, 1975.

38. Nielsen H, Jacobsen JB, Stokke DB, et al: Cross-infection from contaminated anaesthetic equipment. *Anaesthesia* 35:703-708, 1980.

39. du Moulin GC, Hedley-Whyte J: Bacterial interactions between anesthesiologists, their patients, and equipment, *Anesthesiology* 57:37-41, 1982.

40. du Moulin GC, Saubermann, AJ: The anesthesia machine and circle system are not likely to be sources of bacterial contamination, *Anesthesiology* 47:353-358, 1977.

41. Knipe DM: *Molecular genetics of animal viruses.* In Fields BN, editor: *Virology,* New York, 1985, Raven Press, pp 129-144.

Chapter 7

HUMIDIFICATION AND HUMIDIFIERS

Sivam Ramanathan, M.D.

Moisture and humidity are vital components of our environment. The air that we breathe contains moisture. Proper control of environmental humidity in health care facilities is essential to assure the comfort of patients and staff. Similarly, the inspired humidity must be regulated to minimize the harmful effects of inspiring dry gas during anesthesia. This chapter outlines the hazards of improper levels of environmental and inspired humidity together with methods and equipment by which humidification can be optimized for these purposes.

PHYSICAL PRINCIPLES OF WATER VAPORIZATION

The amount of evaporation of liquid water is directly proportional to its temperature. If the ambient temperature is less than the water temperature, the water vapor recondenses into liquid water, leading to a *rainout*. The amount of water that can be held as vapor in any atmosphere depends on the ambient temperature. A warmer atmosphere can hold more water vapor than a cooler one. Saturated humidity, the maximum amount of water vapor that can be held in the gaseous phase by a given atmosphere, is dependent on temperature.[1,2,3]

The relationship between the temperature of a liquid and its vapor pressure is described by the vapor-pressure–temperature diagram[1,2,3] (Fig. 7-1). Any liquid at its boiling point exerts a saturated vapor pressure (SVP) equal to atmospheric pressure, assuming that the temperature of the liquid is equal to the temperature of the atmosphere.[3] Thus at 100° C (boiling point) water exerts an SVP of 760 mm Hg at sea level. The SVP-temperature curve for water can be described mathematically by the exponential equation $P_{H_2O} = 6.03 \times e^{0.0053t}$, where t equals the temperature of water vapor between 28 and 45° C.[4] Many computer programs use this equation to calculate SVP to determine the intrapulmonary shunt fraction and other pulmonary physiology indices, such as oxygen consumption and alveolar gas uptake.[4] The Antoine equation is used to describe the

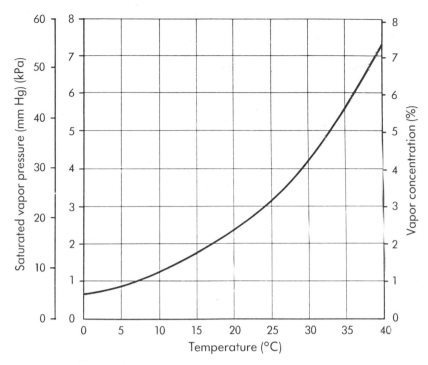

Fig. 7-1. Saturated water vapor-pressure–temperature diagram. (Reproduced from Mushin W, Jones P: *Physics for the anaesthetist,* ed 4, Boston, 1987, Blackwell Scientific.)

relationship between SVP and the temperature of many volatile anesthetics and water over a wider range of temperature, from −20 to 100° C. The Antoine equation is

$$\log_{10} (SVP) = A - \frac{B}{t + C}$$

where *A, B,* and *C* are constants for each liquid.[3]

Saturated humidity is related to the maximum vapor capacity, whereas absolute humidity is the actual amount of water contained in a given volume of gas at a given temperature and pressure.[1,2,3] Relative humidity (RH) is the ratio of the absolute humidity to the saturated humidity at a given temperature. Absolute humidity is expressed in grams of water vapor per cubic meter of gas (g/m³) or, more conveniently, as milligrams of water vapor per liter of gas (mg/L).[1,2,3,5] Note that grams of water per cubic meter of gas is the same as milligrams of water per liter of gas.[1]

RH is expressed as a percentage. In practice, RH may be readily measured with a simple hygrometer. If RH, ambient temperature, and atmospheric pressure are known, the absolute humidity can be calculated from the laws of Charles and Avogadro.[1,2,3] The following example describes the conversion of RH to absolute humidity. For instance, the RH of a given volume of air is 60% at 23° C and at an atmospheric pressure of 760 mm Hg.

1. The actual water vapor pressure = (RH × SVP at 23° C)/100 = 60 × 21.1/100 = 12.66 mm Hg.

2. The volume percent of water vapor = 12.66/760 = 1.66% (from Dalton's law of partial pressures). (Substitute the actual atmospheric pressure if different.)
3. Each liter of gas thus contains 16.6 ml of water vapor.
4. According to Avogadro's law, 18 g of water (1 g molecular weight) occupies 22.4 L of volume as vapor at 0° C and 760 mm Hg.
5. At 23° C, the same amount of water occupies 24.3 L (22.4 × [296/273]), assuming an atmospheric pressure of 760 mm Hg (by Charles' law: volume is proportional to absolute temperature if pressure is constant).
6. The weight of 1 L of water vapor is 0.741 g at 23° C (i.e., 18/24.3).
7. The weight of 16.66 ml of water vapor is 12.3 mg (i.e., 0.741 × 16.66), an absolute humidity of 12.3 mg of water vapor per liter of gas. In other words each liter of gas at an RH of 60% contains 12.3 mg of water, and at full saturation it contains 20.5 mg.

The pulmonary alveolar water-vapor pressure, which is fully saturated at 37° C, exerts an SVP of 47 mm Hg. This represents 6.18 ml (47/760) of water vapor per 100 ml of gas volume, 61.8 ml of water vapor per liter of gas volume, or 44 mg of water per liter of gas at 760 mm Hg atmospheric pressure. The 44 mg of water per liter of gas is derived as follows: At 37° C and a P_{H_2O} of 47 mm Hg,

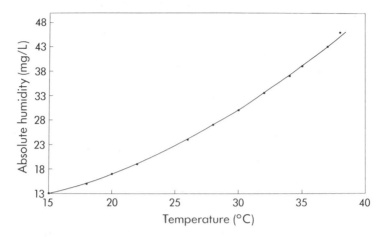

Fig. 7-2. The relationship between absolute humidity and temperature. Note that the curve resembles the vapor pressure–temperature diagram for water shown in Fig. 7-1.

there are 61.8 ml of water vapor per liter of gas (see above). By Charles' law, at standard temperature and pressure (STP) this volume is $(61.8 \times [273/310]) = 54.4$ ml (or 0.0544 L), where 310 is the absolute temperature scale equivalent of $37°$ C. By Avogadro's law, 18 g of water vapor at STP occupies 22.4 L. Therefore 0.0544 L of water vapor weighs $(18 \times [0.0544/22.4]) = 0.044$ g, or 44 mg. Throughout this chapter, the absolute humidity content will be expressed as mg/L of gas. The saturated-humidity–temperature diagram is shown in Fig. 7-2.

Correction of partial pressure of respiratory gases

Dalton's law of partial pressures states that in a mixture of gases, each gas exerts a partial pressure as if it alone occupies the container. The total pressure of the mixture equals the sum of the individual partial pressures. In that gas mixture, the ratio of the partial pressure of any component gas to the total pressure is the same as the ratio of its partial volume to the total volume.[2,3] The partial pressure of water vapor is determined by temperature and not by atmospheric pressure.

Because the body's temperature normally remains constant, the SVP of water in the lower respiratory tract is also constant; the SVP is 47 mm Hg at $37°$ C. By convention, the tracheal composition of a respiratory gas mixture is calculated assuming dilution with water vapor.[3,6] The volume or partial pressure fraction of a component gas in the trachea is less than in the original mixture before it entered the upper respiratory tract. For instance $P_{\text{Trach } O_2} = ([P_{\text{ambient}} - 47] \times 0.209)$ mm Hg, where 47 mm Hg is the SVP of water in the alveoli and 0.209 is the fractional concentration of oxygen in the atmospheric air. The values for partial pressure of oxygen before and after entry into the trachea are, therefore, 159 (760×0.209) and 149 (713×0.209) mm Hg, respectively. Thus there is a 5% decrease in the partial pressure of inspired oxygen as a result of the addition of water vapor. The same considerations apply to

the calculation of the tracheal composition of inhaled anesthetic vapors and other respiratory gases. The dilution of oxygen with water vapor assumes paramount importance at high altitudes because the partial pressure of oxygen diminishes with decreasing ambient pressure, whereas the SVP of water depends only on temperature and therefore does not change.[3]

HUMIDITY AND TEMPERATURE IN THE AIRWAY

The function of the upper air passages is to heat and humidify the incoming gases (Table 7-1).[7] During spontaneous nose breathing, the inhaled gases enter the airway at a temperature of $23°$ C and a RH of 60%. They are rapidly warmed and humidified before they reach the carina.[7] The temperature and humidity of exhaled gases measured at the level of the incisor teeth are less than those of alveolar gases. The difference in the humidity and temperature between the alveolar and exhaled gases accounts for 50% of the normal insensible water loss in adults and 15% of the daily water loss (Table 7-2).[8] When a tracheal tube is present, the inspired gas bypasses the air passages. Inhaling dry gases during anesthesia contributes to significant heat loss (Table 7-1).[7]

HEAT LOSS DURING ANESTHESIA

Breathing dry gases during anesthesia leads to heat loss in two ways: (1) thermal energy is required to raise the temperature of gases inhaled at room temperature to that of the body, and (2) energy is expended by the body to increase the water content of the unhumidified dry gases. Because the specific heat of gas mixtures is negligible (0.0003 cal/cm^3 of oxygen), heat loss by the first process is usually less than that by the second.[2,3] However, when the tracheobronchial/pulmonary apparatus adds water to the dry gases, significant energy is expended in the form of latent heat of vaporization of water (580 cal/g of water).

Table 7-1. Airway relative humidity and temperature

	Upper airway*				Alveolus			
	Temperature °C		Relative Humidity %		Temperature °C		Relative Humidity %	
	Insp.	Exp.	Insp.	Exp.	Insp.	Exp.	Insp.	Exp.
Nose breathing	23	32	60	75	37	37	100	100
Tracheal tube	25	32	0	87	37	37	100	100

From Dick W: Aspects of humidification: requirements and techniques, *Int Anesthesiol Clin* 12:217, 1991.
*Note that the differences in alveolar and upper airway temperatures account for the normally occurring respiratory heat loss, which amounts to 30% to 50% of the insensible water loss. When the inspired gases are not humidified during anesthesia, the heat loss can be substantial. Also note the ability of the air passages to raise the humidity and temperature of the inspired gases before they reach the alveoli.

Table 7-2. Daily water loss(ml)

	Normal temperature	Hot weather	Heavy exercise
Insensible loss			
Skin	350	350	350
Respiratory tract	350	250	650
Urine	1400	1200	500
Sweat	100	1400	5000
Feces	100	100	100
TOTALS	2300	3300	6600

From Guyton AC: Partition of the body fluids: osmotic equilibria between extracellular and intracellular fluids. In Guyton AC, editor: *Textbook of medical physiology*, Philadelphia, 1986, WB Saunders, pp 382-392.

The following example calculates heat loss during anesthesia in a patient who receives unhumidified gases via a circle system at a ventilatory volume of 7 L/min.[2,3] After 1 hour of anesthesia, the inspired relative humidity reaches 60% at 20° C, whereas the patient exhales into the circuit gases saturated with water vapor at 32° C (the temperature of the gases inside the tracheal tube in situ at the level of the incisor teeth):

Absolute inspired humidity	10.2 mg/L (from Fig. 7-2)
Absolute expired humidity	33.5 mg/L (from Fig. 7-2)
Water added to gases by the patient	23.3 mg/L (33.5 − 10.2)
Amount of water lost per minute	163.1 mg (23.3 mg/L × 7L)
Amount of water lost per hour	9.8 g (163.1 × 60)
Latent heat of vaporization per hour	5684 calories (9.8 × 580)

Heat lost in warming the inspired gases is 1512 calories, calculated by (0.0003 × 12 × 7000 × 60), where 0.0003 represents the specific heat of oxygen, 12 represents the number of degrees through which the temperature of the inspired gas must be raised (32 − 20), and 7000 is the volume per minute. Total calorie cost per hour is therefore 7196 calories, or 7.196 kcal = 30 kJ (kilojoules) [i.e., 7.196 kcal × 4.18 kJ/kcal.]

PULMONARY DEFENSE MECHANISMS AND HUMIDITY

Lack of humidity interferes with the function of the pulmonary defense mechanisms against inhaled pathogens. The mucous blanket that covers the upper and lower airways constitutes a major nonspecific aerodynamic pulmonary defense mechanism.[9] Particles that are deposited in the airway become trapped by the upper airway's mucus. In addition, highly soluble irritant gases, such as sulphur dioxide, ozone, ammonia, and chlorine, may dissolve in the upper airway's mucous blanket. The gases dissolve to produce their respective acids, which are neutralized by the polyionic organic molecules found in the secretions. The mucous blanket that covers the lower airway constitutes a 7-μm-thick "conveyer belt" (Fig. 7-3).[10] The blanket, which consists of an outer layer and an inner layer, functions as a sol-gel. The inner, sol, portion, which consists of thin periciliary fluid, remains in contact with the shafts of the cilia. The outer tier of thick mucus remains in contact with the claws of the cilia. The cilia beat sequentially at a rate of 100 to 1500 cycles/min, giving rise to metachronal waves (Fig. 7-3).[11] Each metachronal wave consists of an effector stroke, during which the cilia come into contact with the undersurface of the gel phase, followed by a recovery phase. The mucous blanket moves at an ever-increasing rate over the cilia toward the proximal airways. The velocity of the mucus ranges from 1 mm/min in the small airways to 5 to 20 mm/min in the larger ones.[9,12] In the subglottic area, the tracheal stream diverges to pass the posterior laryngeal commissure. Once at the glottis, the mucus is expectorated or swallowed.

The mucous secretions of the airway consist of 95% water and 1% each of protein, carbohydrate, lipid (including surfactant), and other organic materials.[13] The principal proteins are enzymes including lysozyme, α_1-antitrypsin, proteinases, collagenases, and elastases. Thrombin and lactoferrin are also present. α_1-Antitrypsin inhibits bacterial enzymes, and lactoferrin is a potent bacteriostatic agent.

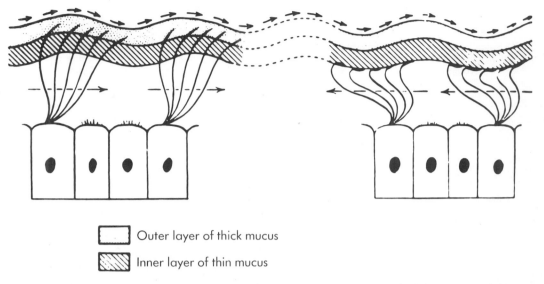

☐ Outer layer of thick mucus

▨ Inner layer of thin mucus

Fig. 7-3. The two-tier mucous conveyer belt. The outer layer consists of thick mucus, and the inner layer consists of thin mucous. (From Churchill-Davidson HC: *A Practice of Anaesthesia,* Chicago, 1984, Year Book Medical Publishers Inc., p. 5. Used by permission.)

Several disease states, hypoxia, hypercarbia, and pharmacologic agents affect mucociliary transport. Temperature and humidity also affect mucociliary transport. The conveyer belt functions efficiently at an RH of 80 to 90% at 32 to 33° C, values normally found in the upper airway (Table 7-1).[7,9]

ENVIRONMENTAL HUMIDITY

Maintaining proper levels of environmental humidity is essential not only to prevent buildup of static electricity in the operating room but also to provide optimum working conditions for health care personnel.

Prevention of static electrification

Static electricity is a potential source of ignition in the operating room. Static electricity forms as a result of accumulation of opposite charges on two insulated objects that are separated from each other. Static electrical sparks discharge when the accumulated charges are conducted away to the earth.[2,3] The slower the separation of the two insulated objects from one other (e.g., a blanket being pulled off an operating table mattress), the slower is the rate of accumulation of static charge, thus minimizing the chances for the buildup of a high potential capable of discharging to earth.[2,3,14] When RH is optimal, a thin film of moisture forms over several contiguous surfaces. The impurities (carbonic acid ions) contained in water impart electrical conductivity to these surfaces.[2] The entire insulated surface coated with this water film remains at the same potential, thus preventing buildup of static potential. In addition, optimum RH level helps maintain the conductivity of the terrazzo type of operating room flooring.[2,3,14] Explo-

sions occur more frequently when the RH is below 60%. An RH of 60% does not result in an uncomfortable temperature-humidity index as long as the ambient temperature does not rise above 22° C. Low air humidity explains the increased static sparks ("carpet shock") noted in the winter. Many operating rooms are equipped with a hygrometer that records RH on a circular chart.

Indirect health effects of environmental humidity

Indoor environmental RH in the range of 40% to 70% minimizes the survival and/or the infectivity of bacteria and viruses.[15] High or low RH outside this range is associated with an increased incidence of respiratory infections and absenteeism in the workplace. The population of allergenic mites and fungi increases when the environmental RH humidity exceeds 80%. The RH also affects the formation of several irritants from building materials and poorly vented cooking gas. These irritants include off-gassing of formaldehyde from indoor building materials, and the formation of sulfuric acid, sulfates, nitrous acid, nitric acid, and ozone.[15] These chemicals are suspected of playing an etiologic role in respiratory illness. Itching, dermatoses, and eczema are associated with low indoor RH. Figure 7-4 summarizes the optimum RH ranges that minimize adverse health effects.[15]

Minienvironment under the drapes. For conscious patients, local humidity and temperature increase under the drapes during ophthalmic surgery because of the impermeability of the disposable drapes.[16] Under the drapes, the temperature of the air can rise 5° C and the humidity can rise 30% above ambient levels, thus producing an uncomfortable temperature-humidity index around the patient's

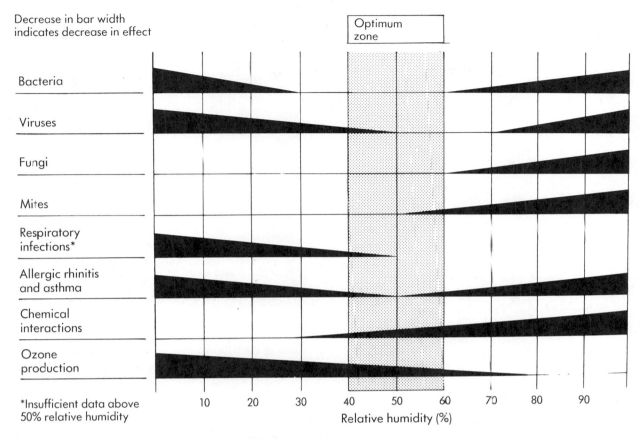

Fig. 7-4. Optimum relative humidity range for minimizing adverse health effects. (From Arundel AV, Sterling EM, Biggin JH, et al: Indirect health effects of relative humidity in indoor environments, *Environ Health Perspect* 65:351, 1986. Reproduced by permission.)

head and neck. The increase in humidity also increases the minienvironmental carbon dioxide concentration to 3.5% and decreases the available oxygen concentration to 17.5%.[16] Flushing the minienvironment with air or oxygen via a specially constructed drape support (attached to a suction-evacuation system) has been shown to improve the atmospheric conditions under the drapes.[16]

MEASUREMENT OF HUMIDITY

The instruments used to measure relative humidity are called hygrometers. Several different types of hygrometer exist.

Wet and dry bulb thermometers

Two thermometers placed next to each other form one type of hygrometer. One end of a wick wraps around the bulb of one thermometer, and the other end of the wick dips in water. The evaporation of water from the wick decreases the wrapped thermometer's temperature reading. The rate of cooling depends on the moisture content of the surrounding air. The difference in readings between the wet and dry thermometers is noted. This difference is then used to read RH values from a table. Sling psychrometers

are based on the same principle, but in this case cooling is done by whirling the entire unit.[2,3]

Dew-point hygrometer

The dew point is the temperature at which the ambient air is fully saturated with water vapor. The dew-point hygrometer consists of a silver tube containing ether and a thermometer to measure the temperature of the ether. Air is pumped through the ether with a squeeze bulb to cool the ether. When the dew point is reached, water begins to condense on the outside of the tube. The higher the moisture content of the ambient air, the higher is the dew point. Suppose the temperature at dew point is 10° C: The SVP of water at this temperature is approximately 10 mm Hg, and the SVP at the ambient temperature of 20° C is 18 mm Hg (Fig. 7-1). The RH of the air is therefore 56% (i.e., 10/18).

Electric dew-point hygrometer

In the electric dew-point hygrometer, a beam of light is reflected into a photoelectric cell by a mirror cooled by an air conditioning coil. The temperatures of the ambient air and the mirror are measured. When the mirror starts to

Humidity sensor

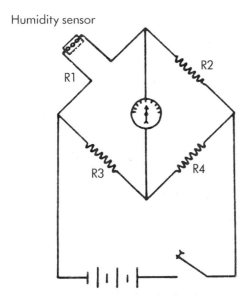

Fig. 7-5. Electric hygrometer with lithium carbonate sensor. Humidity sensor placed in Wheatstone bridge. When the resistances $R_1/R_3 = R_2/R_4$, no current passes through the bridge and the galvanometer reads zero. If dry gases reach the sensor, the hygroscopic sensor loses water and its resistance rises; if moist gases reach the sensor, its resistance falls. (From Chalon J, Ali M, Turndorf H, et al: *Humidification of anesthetic gases*, Springfield, Ill, 1981, Charles C Thomas. Reproduced by permission.)

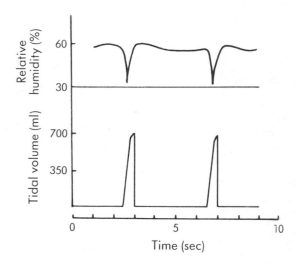

Fig. 7-6. Simultaneous pneumotachogram and hygrotachogram of the Bain circuit at a fresh gas flow of 4.9 L/min and a minute volume of 8.4 L/min. During a positive pressure inspiration dry fresh gas flows past the humidity sensor into the tracheal tube, causing the observed decrease in RH during inspiration. (From Ramanathan S, Chalon J, Capan L, et al: Rebreathing characteristics of the Bain anesthesia circuit, *Anesth Analg* 56:822, 1977. Reproduced by permission.)

fog, the water globules condensing on the mirror deflect the reflected incident light onto a photoelectric cell connected to a light meter. Very compact fiberoptic systems are available.[1]

Hair hygrometer

The hair hygrometer, which is useful to measure RH between 15% and 85%, is commonly used to measure humidity in operating rooms and neonatal incubators. Human hair lengthens as ambient humidity increases. The increase in length, magnified by a system of levers, is used to move a pen across a circular chart bearing calibrations in RH.[2,3,14]

Electric hygrometer with Dunsmore sensor

The electric hygrometer uses a Dunsmore sensor which consists of a bifilar palladium wire wound on an insulated core. The wire is coated with hygroscopic film.[1] The sensor is mounted on a Wheatstone bridge (Fig. 7-5). The galvanometer reads zero current when the bridge is balanced. The resistance of the sensor rises when dry gases flow through the sensor housing and decreases when moist gases flow. The changes in the galvanometer reading are converted into RH readings by way of nomograms provided by the manufacturer.[1] Electric hygrometers use different sensors for different ranges of RH. The narrow-range sensors are free from hysteresis. The major

advantage of the instrument is its fast response, which makes possible the recording of instantaneous exhaled or inhaled RH hygrotachograms (Fig. 7-6).[17] If the sensor becomes wet with liquid water, the hygrometer reading freezes at full scale until the sensor is dry. The instrument is available as a desk-top model in the form of the Hygro-Temperature Controller.*

The above-mentioned methods are used to measure water vapor concentration. However, they are not useful for measuring the content of liquid water present as aerosols. This can be done by (1) noting the weight gain of a dry sponge following exposure to the atmosphere containing droplets or (2) noting the total loss per minute of water volume from a nebulizer and dividing it by the minute ventilation.[18]

IMPORTANCE OF HUMIDITY

Both insufficient humidity and excessive humidity are associated with significant hazards.

Insufficient humidity

When the upper airway is bypassed with a tracheal tube or a tracheostomy, the entire task of humidifying and warming the inspired air falls on the lower airways. The inhalation of cold, dry gases leads to ciliary immobility, twisting, and tangling; inspissation of secretions; and tracheal encrustation.[9] The encrusted secretions interfere with

---

*Hygrodynamics Division of Newport Scientific Inc., 8246 East Sandy Court, Jessup City, Md. 20794.

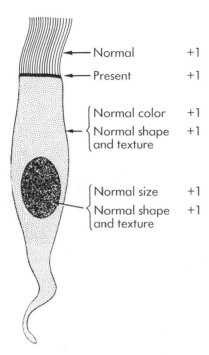

Normal   +1

Present   +1

Normal color   +1

Normal shape
and texture   +1

Normal size   +1

Normal shape
and texture   +1

Fig. 7-7. Scoring system for the assessment of cellular damage. (From Chalon J, Loew D, Malebranche J: Effects of dry anesthetic gases on tracheobronchial ciliated epithelium, Anesthesiology 37:338, 1972. Used by permission of JB Lippincott.)

the ability of the trachea to add heat and moisture, and the dry inhaled gas starts to affect the more distal airways. As this phenomenon slowly extends into the distal airways, it causes an increase in local resistance to air flow, which ultimately results in a ventilation/perfusion abnormality.[9,19,20] Mucosal inflammation, microatelectasis, decreased pulmonary compliance, and decreased functional residual capacity soon follow.

In 1961, Burton[21] was the first to show that breathing dry gas caused tracheal mucous membrane damage in dogs. In the same year, using cinemicroscopic techniques, Toremalm[22] demonstrated altered mucus flow when dry gas was inhaled by rats. The use of heat and moisture exchangers maintained mucous flow in his experiments. Marfatia, et al.[23] showed that breathing dry gas caused a reduction in body weight and histopathologic damage to the tracheal mucosa in rabbits.

Chalon, et al.[24] introduced a simple method for quantitating tracheal damage produced by unhumidified gases. They used a point-scoring system to assess cellular integrity. The procedure is performed as follows: Tracheal aspirates are obtained by suctioning the tracheal tube with a suction catheter. The aspirate is stained with Papanicolaou stain. The stained smears are examined under a microscope, and the cellular integrity is assessed via a point-scoring system. One point is given for the presence of each of the following features: normal cilia, normal end plate, normal cytoplasmic color (blue by Papanicolaou

stain), normal cytomorphology, normal nuclear size, and normal nuclear morphology (Fig. 7-7).[24] Thus each cell can score a maximum of six points. Two hundred cells are counted from each study. When dry gases are breathed, the mean score decreases, signifying damage to the tracheal epithelium. No such changes occur when the inhaled gases contain saturated humidity at 32° C, even after 4 hours of anesthesia (Fig. 7-8).[1,24-27]

Breathing unhumidified gases decreases body temperature, especially during abdominal surgery, when the peritoneum acts as a heat and moisture exchanger. Because patients are generally poikilothermic under general anesthesia, their body temperature tends to drift towards the ambient. The decrease in body temperature is more dramatic when infants breathe unhumidified gases.[5] Compared to adults, the rate of decrease in body temperature is approximately three times faster in infants breathing dry air.[5,28] Thus, delivering saturated humidity in the inspired air tends to minimize decreases in body temperature in infants and children. Chalon, et al.[26] showed that the use of fully saturated gases at 32° C virtually eliminated the heat loss that commonly occurs during anesthesia and surgery when dry gases are inhaled. Postoperative shivering was not seen in patients who breathed fully saturated gases. In the same study, Chalon, et al. reported a reduced rate of postoperative complications. The rate of postoperative complications was quantified in their study via a point-scoring system based on the presence of postoperative fever >38.3° C; chest signs such as rales, diminished air entry, and cough; and roentgenographic evidence of atelectasis (Fig. 7-8). Other authors have confirmed the beneficial effects of humidification on body temperature.[29] The possible harmful effects produced by the lack of humidification are summarized in Box 7-1.

Box 7-1. Hazards of underhumidification

1. Changes in tracheal cytology
2. Increase in sputum viscosity
3. Loss of mucous belt function
4. Loss of ciliary function
5. Desiccation of respiratory mucosa
6. Inspissation, encrustation, and retention of secretions
7. Mucous plugs in the airways
8. Decreased pulmonary compliance
9. Atelectasis (radiologically demonstrated)
10. Increased airway resistance
11. Decreased functional residual capacity
12. Increased pulmonary shunting
13. Loss of surfactant function
14. Increased desquamation of cells into the tracheal lumen
15. Squamous cell metaplasia
16. Hypothermia

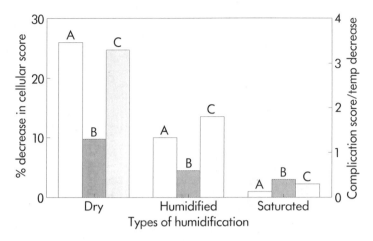

Fig. 7-8. A, Percent decrease in the tracheal cellular score *(left y-axis);* B, postoperative complication score and C, intraoperative temperature *(temp)* decrease *(right y-axis).* (Based on Chalon J, Patel C, Ali M, et al: Humidity and the anesthetized patient, *Anesthesiology* 50:195, 1979.)

Excessive humidity

Excessive levels of humidity in the anesthetic circuit are also associated with problems. Condensed water in the circuit forms a nidus for bacterial growth, thus necessitating repeated sterilization of all pieces of anesthesia equipment.[30] Aerosols are more likely than water vapor to transmit pathogens. Vaporized water can carry 4000 times the heat capacity of dry gases. Moritz, et al.[31] showed that the presence of water vapor (steam) increased the likelihood of thermal injury to the air passages of dogs inhaling hot gases. Klein and Graves[32] reported "hot pot tracheitis" from a malfunctioning heated humidifier. Heated humidifiers pose another hazard in that if the thermostat fails, both steam and boiling water droplets may enter the airway.[1] (See also Chapter 16.) Thus it is necessary to monitor the temperature of the gases close to the tracheal tube when heated humidifiers are used.[1]

Excessive levels of humidity may also cause heat and water gain, which is particularly hazardous in infants and small children.[33,34] Ultrasonic nebulizers are especially dangerous in this regard.[31] Other pulmonary hazards of overhumidification resemble those produced by underhumidification. They include degeneration of the cilia,[35] increased secretions,[36] atelectasis,[37] a decrease in functional residual capacity and static compliance,[38] and diminished surfactant activity.[37]

The use of aerosols for humidification reportedly increases airway resistance to gas flow due to the formation of standing waves in the liquid layer.[39] Heat retention has been reported with the use of the Water's to-and-fro soda lime canister because of its proximity to the patient.[40] The hazards of excessive humidification are summarized in Box 7-2.

Box 7-2. Hazards of overhumidification

1. Increased airway resistance (aerosol humidifiers)
2. Hyperthermia
3. Airway thermal burns
4. Positive water balance
5. Infection or growth of organisms
6. Altered ciliary epithelium
7. Altered pulmonary function
8. Altered surfactant function
9. Atelectasis

Excessive humidity and capnometry

Excessive humidity can damage a capnometer. Several methods are used to prevent entry of water into the capnometer. For example, water-separating tampons containing silica gel can trap water. Simple mechanical water traps in which the gases are required to make a 180° turn are used in some models. The less dense gases make the turn more readily and are aspirated into the measuring circuit. The water-laden heavier gases decelerate upon negotiating the curve and consequently lose the water droplets into the trap chamber.[41] A sampling tube, constructed of an ion exchange resin called Nafion is used in some models. This resin allows water vapor to diffuse out to the atmosphere and minimizes the chances of water entry into the capnometer.[42] (See also Chapter 8.)

IDEAL HUMIDITY LEVELS

An inspired absolute humidity of 28 to 32 mg/L is associated with minimum heat loss and minimal damage to tracheal epithelium when anesthesia lasts longer than 1 hour.[1,25] For shorter lengths of time, a humidity level of at least 12 mg/L is required to prevent cellular damage. Assuming that a patient who has undergone tracheal intubation loses moisture at full saturation at 32° C (34 mg/L of water), it is only logical to replace the moisture that is lost. Ideal environmental relative humidity is 40% to 60% at 22 to 23° C.

HUMIDITY IN ANESTHESIA CIRCUITS

This section describes the humidity output of several anesthesia circuits. It also briefly discusses how these circuits may be humidified.

Sources of humidity in anesthesia circuits

Water is removed intentionally from commercial medical gases to prevent clogging of pressure regulators.[1] However, the anesthetic circuit is never completely dry, even in the absence of exogenously added humidity. Some moisture always finds its way into the circuit. Previous use of the ventilator or the circuit, the mechanical dead space of the circuit, and the use of soda lime, which incorporates moisture (approximately 15% by weight), are the initial sources of humidity in the circle system.[1] In rebreathing systems, such as the Bain circuit, the patient's exhaled moisture is used to rehumidify the inspired gases. In the circle system, the patient's exhaled moisture is wasted because the inspiratory and expiratory streams are separate. However, over the course of time, the humidity of the inspired gases rises as a result of water being added from the neutralization reaction of soda lime by the patient's exhaled carbon dioxide[1,43] (Fig. 7-9, see also Chapter 4). In an average-sized adult, the RH reaches about 60% at room temperature in 100 minutes. An RH of 60% is associated with decreased cellular damage to the trachea when compared with dry gases.[24,26] However, an RH of 100% at 32° C is required to prevent heat loss and tracheal cellular damage. Thus the reaction of neutralization is an inadequate supplier of humidity. Drastic design changes are necessary to conserve heat and moisture in the circle system. Smaller patients with a lower carbon dioxide output generate less humidity from the soda lime. This is particularly true of pediatric circle systems (see Chapter 26). The design changes in the existing systems capable of conserving heat and moisture are described in the next section.

Contrary to the circle systems, circuits that involve rebreathing, such as the Mapleson D, start with a higher humidity so long as the fresh-gas flow is 70 ml/kg. The conventional flow rates recommended by Mapleson for preventing carbon dioxide rebreathing (i.e., 2.5 to 3 times the minute ventilation) dry out the system. Circuits that employ nonrebreathing valves contain only minimal levels of humidity because the exhaled moisture is lost to the surroundings.[1]

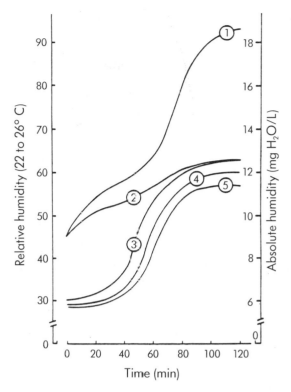

Fig. 7-9. Rise in the inspiratory humidity of a circle absorber. The study was done on a model of a patient. Exhaled carbon dioxide and moisture were added to the model. *Curve 1*, Fresh-gas ventilation = 6 L/min, $\dot{V}CO_2$ = 200 ml (simulates closed-circuit anesthesia). The $\dot{V}CO_2$ represents the carbon dioxide output of an average-sized patient. *Curve 2*, Previously used semiclosed system at a fresh-gas flow of = 5 L/min. *Curve 3*, Previously unused dry semiclosed system. Note the higher starting humidity with the previously used system. *Curve 4*, The cascade humidifier is omitted from the model to assess the contribution made by the exhaled moisture to the inspired humidity. Lack of exhaled moisture leads to lower initial and final inspired humidity levels in the circuit. *Curve 5*, $\dot{V}CO_2$ = 100 ml/min to simulate a small patient. The initial moisture in an unused system is derived from the soda lime, which contains moisture. (From Chalon J, Ali M, Turndorf H, et al: *Humidification of anesthetic gases,* Springfield, Ill, 1981, Charles C Thomas. Used by permission.)

Humidification of the circle system

There are many ways of increasing the humidity of the circle system when used with an adult patient. These include (1) decreasing the fresh-gas inflow, (2) improving the design of the circuit so that it will preserve moisture and heat, and (3) adding exogenous humidity. Each of these methods has advantages and disadvantages.

Decreasing the fresh-gas inflow. The lower the fresh-gas flow (FGF) the higher is the inspired humidity. When the FGF is decreased to 500 ml/min (for example, in closed-circuit anesthesia), 60% RH is reached in 40 minutes, and at stabilization almost 90% RH is achieved at 22 to 24° C—approximately 33% higher than the corresponding values for a 5-L FGF (Fig. 7-9).[1,43] Bengston, et al.[44,45] showed that the temperature of the inspired gases is 6.8° C warmer with an absolute humidity of 28 mg/L at steady state when the closed system is in use. The moisture liberated from the neutralization reaction of the soda lime is not diluted to the same extent with the reduced FGF as it is with a conventional 5-L flow. Because of the separation of inhaled and exhaled gas streams, the minute ventilation does not affect the humidity significantly so long as the FGF remains the same.[1] However, because the use of reduced FGF requires careful monitoring of FIO_2, the technique of closed-circuit anesthesia is not recommended for the novice. The reduction in FGF with a view to increasing inspired humidity in Mapleson D systems will have disastrous consequences. Any system that uses biologic heat and moisture for rehumidification is perhaps best suited for use in the operating room because it avoids electrical hazards associated with the use of exogenous humidifiers.

Improving the design of the system. The commercially available circle systems are poorly designed to con-

serve heat and moisture. Several improvements have been advocated, but the commercial manufacturers have not been interested in incorporating the improvements suggested in various publications. It is beyond the scope of this discussion to describe all of the design changes recommended in the literature; however, a few are mentioned in the following subsections.

Diverting the fresh-gas flow through the soda lime. Diverting the FGF through the soda lime can increase the inspired humidity because the dry fresh gases will absorb the moisture stored in the soda lime before it reaches the inspiratory limb. In conventional circle systems the FGF enters the circuit close to the inspiratory limb, which bypasses the soda lime (Fig. 7-10, *A*). The modification described will raise the inspired humidity by 250% (Fig. 7-10, *B*).[1] This is particularly true of pediatric circle systems.

Coaxial circuit. In this modification of the circle system, the inspiratory limb is placed within the expiratory limb. The exhaled gases keep the inhaled gases warm.[46] This system delivers an inspired humidity 20% higher than

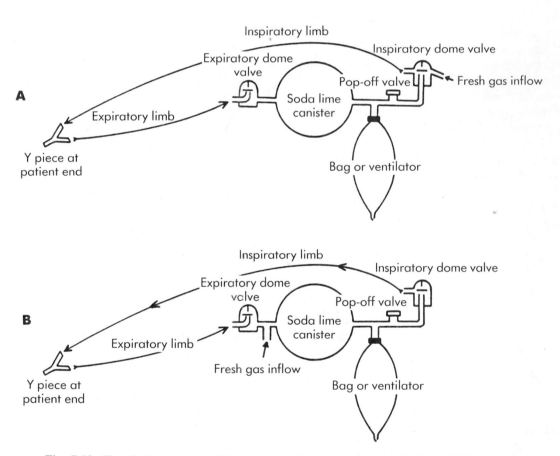

Fig. 7-10. The circle system. **A,** The conventional configuration, in which the FGF enters the circuit through the inspiratory dome valve; **B,** principle of increasing inspired humidity by channeling the fresh gas inflow through the soda lime canister. (Modified from Chalon J, Ali M, Turndorf H, et al: *Humidification of anesthetic gases,* Springfield, Ill, 1981, Charles C Thomas. Used by permission.)

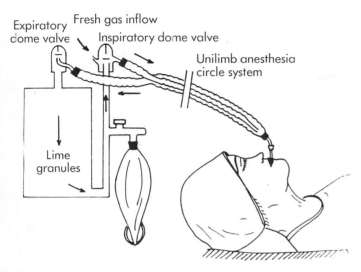

Fig. 7-11. Unilimb (coaxial) anesthesia circuit in which the exhaled gases warm the inhaled gases. (From Ramanathan S, Chalon J, Turndorf H: A compact, well-humidified breathing circuit for the circle system, *Anesthesiology* 44:238, 1976. Used by permission of JB Lippincott.)

the conventional circle. In the coaxial circuit, the temperature of the inhaled gases will be approximately 3.5° C warmer than room temperature (Fig. 7-11).

Relocating the conduit tube. The metal tube along which the gases travel from the soda lime canister to the patient circuit usually lies outside the soda lime, leading to the cooling of gases. If the conduit tube is placed within the center of the soda lime, the gases can be kept warm, thus preventing rainout and cooling.[47] Other modifications include using a coaxial circuit with this system together with redirected FGF to achieve maximum humidity (Fig. 7-12).[1,46] This modified circle system develops excellent humidity levels (Fig. 7-13).

Water vaporizer in the soda lime absorber. Another simple way of improving humidity in the circle absorber is to place a water vaporizer inside the soda lime (Fig. 7-14). The water warmed by the hot soda lime provides reasonable levels of humidity (Fig. 7-15).[48] Using an unwarmed humidifier leads to rapid cooling of water and thence to loss of humidifying efficiency. The humidity levels attained in various circuits in use are given in Table 7-3.

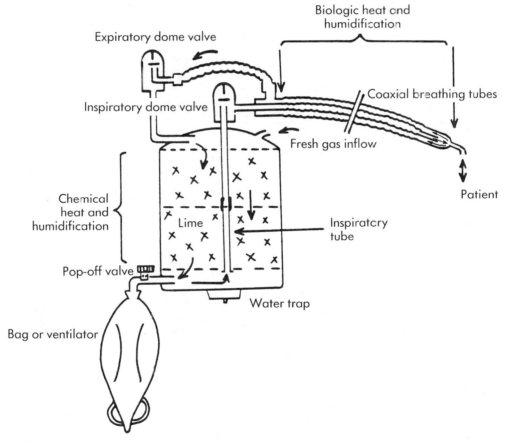

Fig. 7-12. Circle absorber system modified to utilize biologic heat and humidification. The inspiratory tube that delivers the gases to the inspiratory dome valve is situated within the soda lime. In addition, a unilimb circuit is used to increase efficiency. This arrangement prevents the heat loss and water rainout that may happen in a conventional absorber system, in which the inspiratory tube is placed outside the soda lime. Note that the FGF is passed through the lime granules. (From Chalon J, Patel C, Ramanathan S: Humidification of the circle absorber system, *Anesthesiology* 48:142, 1978. Used by permission of JB Lippincott.)

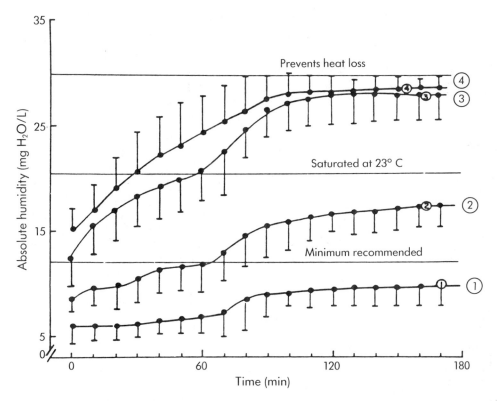

Fig. 7-13. Humidity output of the conventional circle compared to that of the circle system shown in Figure 7-12. *Curve 1,* Conventional system at an FGF of 5 L/min with a ventilation of 6 L/min. *Curve 2,* Modified system (Fig. 7-12) with the FGF flowing through the inspiratory dome valve. *Curve 3,* FGF being passed through the lime granules. *Curve 4,* Same as in *curve 3* with FGF reduced to 1.5 L/min. (From Chalon J, Patel C, Ramanathan S: Humidification of the circle absorber system, *Anesthesiology* 48:142, 1978. Used by permission of JB Lippincott.)

Insulating the circuit. In the Raincoat circuit,* the expiratory and inspiratory limbs of the anesthesia circuit are insulated by a plastic sleeve with a view to preventing rainout. The humidity level may reach the same value as in the unilimb circuit described above.

Heat and moisture exchangers. The "artificial noses," or heat and moisture exchangers, can be used to humidify inspired gases.[5,49-56] In addition, the Pall Ultipore† breathing filter reportedly functions as a bacterial filter, protecting the circuit from bacterial and viral contamination.[5] (See also Chapters 4 and 23.) Because water does not condense inside the filter, reaerosolization of bacterial aerosols occurs only occasionally. Water condensation is a major problem with hot water humidifiers.[53] However, the antibacterial properties of these filters cannot be fully relied on, and the anesthesiologist must fully implement other infection-control procedures to protect the patient.[5,57] The pore size in the Pall filter is approximately

0.2 μm, which allows water vapor, but not liquid water, to pass through.[49] These filters condense the moisture from the exhaled humidity and return it to the patient during inhalation. However, the humidifying efficiency decreases when large tidal volumes are used.[51] In the Pall Ultipore filter, the filtering medium is made up entirely of ceramic fiber and the filtering surface has a much larger hygrophobic medium (Fig. 7-16).[56] The medium has to be completely hygrophobic so that the small pores do not become blocked with water droplets.[3] Several different types of hygroscopic media are used in different commercial brands: corrugated aluminum or paper, felt, cellulose sponge, stainless-steel fibers, or porous plastic foam. The artificial noses are inexpensive and disposable and do not require external electric power to operate. Used during tracheal anesthesia, they deliver between 28 and 30 mg/L of water at about 28 to 30° C (Fig. 7-17),[49,55] which is quite adequate to prevent damage to tracheal cells and heat loss.[49]

In canine studies, the artificial nose has been shown to minimize damage to the tracheal epithelium following 10 days of spontaneous breathing via tracheostomy.[58] How-

*Raincoat Corporation, Louisville, Ky.
†Pall Conserve Heat and Moisture Exchanger, Pall Biomedical Inc., Fajardo, Puerto Rico.

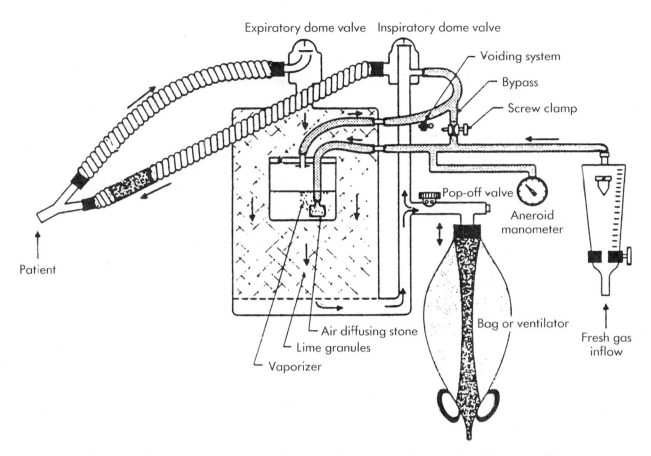

Fig. 7-14. Water vaporizer placed inside a soda lime canister. Note that by adjustment of the screw clamp on the bypass, the flow through the humidifier and thus the humidity output of the system can be controlled. (From Chalon J, Ramanathan S: Water vaporizer heated by the reaction of neutralization by carbon dioxide, *Anesthesiology* 41:401, 1974. Used by permission of JB Lippincott.)

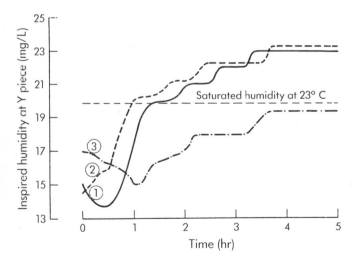

Fig. 7-15. *Curve 1,* Humidity output of the system described in Fig. 7-14 for average-sized patient at an FGF of 5 L/min. *Curve 2,* The humidity output in a large patient. *Curve 3,* The humidity output in a small patient with a carbon dioxide output of 100 ml/min. (From Chalon J, Ramanathan S: Water vaporizer heated by the reaction of neutralization by carbon dioxide, *Anesthesiology* 41:401, 1974. Used by permission of JB Lippincott.)

ever, the artificial nose may not deliver adequate humidity to patients mechanically ventilated via a tracheostomy in the intensive care unit. Martin, et al.[59] found that with long-term use during mechanical ventilation of tracheotomized patients, the Pall filter did not deliver adequate humidity, leading to clogging of the tracheostomy tube and the formation of tenacious secretions. Other problems with these units include addition of dead space[55] and possible airway obstruction when they become soiled with vomitus, secretions, or pulmonary edema fluid. Occasionally the heat and moisture exchange units can leak gas under high pressure.

Hot water systems. When gases are bubbled through water the efficiency of humidification rapidly decreases as the water cools. The water's temperature must be maintained by way of either biologic heat or electrical energy. Very high temperature settings of the humidifier will cause rainout of water droplets in those portions of the circuit remote from, and therefore cooler than, the humidifier. Heated wires placed in the anesthesia circuit are used to circumvent this problem. Two examples are described in the following subsections.

Table 7-3. Humidity levels in different anesthesia circuits

Systems	mg/L of water
Existing systems	
Adult circle	
Semiclosed	5-18
Closed	18
Bloomquist circle (pediatric)	0.5-11
Bloomquist (redirected FGF)	3-26
Columbia pediatric circle	3-19
Bain circuit	13-20
Jackson-Rees circuit	
Spontaneous ventilation	2.5
Controlled ventilation	8
Modifications	
Coaxial circuit on absorber	7-20
Raincoat circuit	?7-20
Vaporizer in soda lime	19-23
New absorber*	
FGF in inspiratory limb	17
FGF through the soda lime	28
Add-ons	
Heat and moisture exchangers ("artificial noses")	28
Hot water humidifiers	34
Hot water humidifiers with hose heaters	44

*New absorber is constructed with the conduit pipe through the soda lime and bears the coaxial circuit.

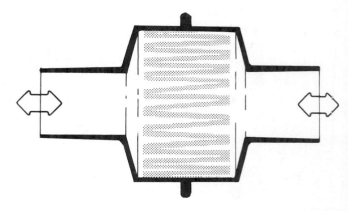

Fig. 7-16. Pall Ultipore heat and moisture exchanger. (From Mushin W, Jones P: *Physics for the anaesthetist*, ed 4, Boston, 1980, Blackwell Scientific Publications. Used by permission.)

Cascade humidifier. The cascade humidifier* is a thermostatically controlled humidifier in which the inspired gas is passed through the hot water as small bubbles, which have a greater surface area than larger bubbles. The bubbles are generated by a special process known as the *cascade process* (Fig. 7-18). There are two ways of inserting the humidifier into the system: (1) The FGF can be passed through the humidifier before it enters the circle or

*Manufactured, for example, by the Puritan-Bennett Corp., Los Angeles, Calif.

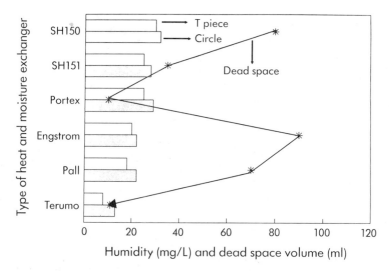

Fig. 7-17. Humidity output and dead space volume in different commercial brands of heat and moisture exchangers when used with T-piece breathing circuit or circle system. *SH 150*, Siemens SH 150; *SH 151*, Siemens SH 151; *Portex*, Portex Humid-Vent; *Pall*, Pall Ultipore; *Engstrom*, Engstrom Edith; *Terumo*, Terumo Breathaid. (Based on Turtle MJ, Ilsley AH, Rutten AJ, et al: Equipment: an evaluation of six disposable heat and moisture exchangers, *Anaesth Intensive Care* 15:317, 1987.)

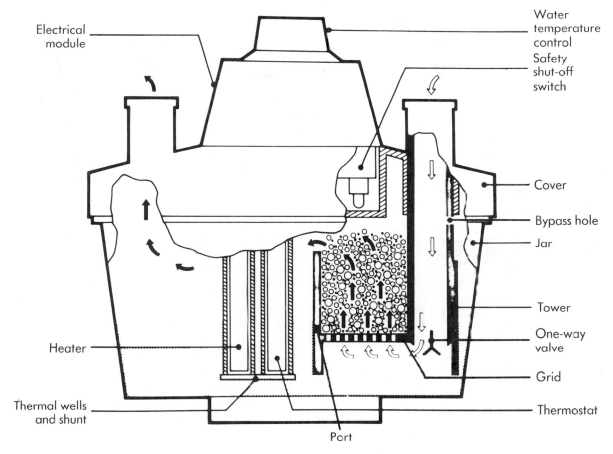

Fig. 7-18. Cascade humidifier system. Gas enters the inlet through a one-way valve and bubbles upward through the grid. When the patient makes a respiratory effort, the negative pressure is transmitted through the sensing port to start an assisted breath. Without the sensing port, the negative pressure must be equal to the depth of the water in the humidifier. (From Op't Holt T: Aerosol generators and humidifiers. In Barnes TA, Lisbon A, editors: *Respiratory Care Practice*, Chicago, 1988, Mosby–Year Book. Used with permission.)

other system. The temperature of the gases exiting the humidifier is set by adjusting the thermostat of the humidifier so that the temperature near the Y-piece reads 32° C, at which temperature the fully saturated gases will carry approximately 33 mg/L of water. Temperatures >32° C are usually associated with a significant rainout. (2) When the cascade humidifier is used in an adult circle absorber system, it can be placed in the inspiratory limb or it can be used to humidify the fresh gas, as is the case with the Jackson-Rees system. The outlet temperature of the gases, whether they be inspired or fresh, must be monitored carefully to prevent overheating and rainout.

Units with heated wire to prevent rainout. Increasing the water temperature to raise humidity causes rainout in those portions of the circuit remote from the heater. Some units incorporate an electrically heated wire that maintains the temperature of the gases downstream, thus preventing rainout. The gases pass over or bubble through heated wa-

ter. A thermistor probe is used to measure temperature at the patient end and at the outlet of the humidifier. If one of the temperatures exceeds a set limit, the unit is automatically deactivated (Fig. 7-19). The units are always provided with high-humidity, low-humidity, and temperature alarms. These units can generate humidity levels in excess of 40 mg/L (saturated vapor at 37° C). Several makes and models are available, and some units have the thermistor probe located outside the inspiratory tube. The MR630 dual-mode heated respiratory humidifier,* in which the thermistor probe is situated outside the breathing tube, is an example of a dual servo unit. Alarms are provided for overheating, low temperature, and disconnects (low pressure). The units can be used to humidify, for example, an adult circle system (Fig. 7-20, *A*), an intensive care unit ventilator circuit (Fig. 7-20, *B*), or pediatric Mapleson

*Fisher and Paykel, 25 Carbine Road, PO Box 14348, Panmure, Auckland, New Zealand.

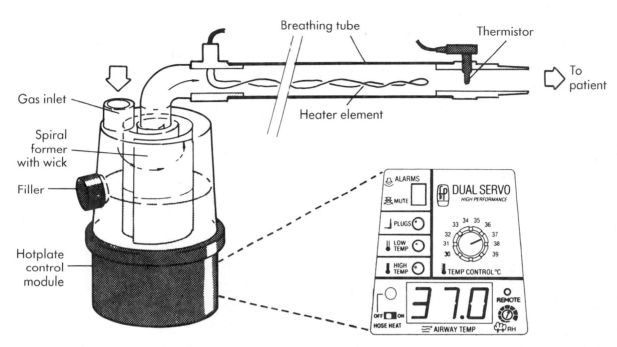

Fig. 7-19. Fisher and Paykel humidifier system with heater element in the breathing tube. The unit shown has a spiral aluminum scroll and paper wick to increase evaporation during high flows. Also shown are the alarms and the relative humidity control. Other vaporizing assemblies without the wick are available. Resistance across the unit is 0.1 to 0.2 cm H_2O/30 L/min. (From Mushin W, Jones P: *Physics for the Anaesthetist*, ed 4, Boston, 1987, Blackwell Scientific Publications. Used by permission.)

Table 7-4. Temperature and humidity settings and delivered humidity of the Fisher and Paykel heated wire humidifiers

Set temp.*	RH setting	Outlet temp.	Proximal temp.	Outlet AH† mg/L	Proximal AH mg/L
37	−2	35	37	39.6	35.8
37	−1	36	37	41.7	37.7
37	0	37	37	43.9	39.8
37	+1	38	37	46.2	41.9
37	+2	39	37	48.6	44.1

*Set temperature is the temperature set for the patient end of the tube.
†AH is absolute humidity. The RH setting is used to adjust the temperature difference between the outlet and the Y-piece. When the temperature of the Y-piece is greater than the outlet temperature, the AH reaching the patient decreases. When the Y-piece temperature is less, the AH increases.

Systems (Fig. 7-20, *C, D*). The circle system is humidified by inclusion of the humidifier and the heated hose as a part of the inspiratory limb. T-piece systems, such as the Mapleson D, E, and F, may be humidified by passage of the FGF through the humidifier.[60]

The units are very efficient at delivering saturated humidity at body temperature. In the Fisher and Paykel unit, the amount of humidity received by the patient can be roughly regulated by means of an RH control (Fig. 7-19), which is really a temperature regulator. This regulator permits a temperature differential of −2 to +2° C to be maintained between the humidifier and the Y-piece at the patient end (Fig. 7-20). Setting the RH control at −2 will maintain the Y-piece temperature 2° C warmer than the

humidifier outlet temperature. Assuming that the Y-piece temperature is set at 37° C, a setting of −2 on the RH control will maintain a humidifier temperature of 35° C, a difference of 2° C (Table 7-4). The increase in temperature at the Y-piece will reduce the RH from 100% to 82% (because the water content remains the same). At a setting of 0, the humidifier and the Y-piece will be at the same temperature, and at a setting of +2, the humidifier will be warmer than the Y-piece. These devices have been shown to increase the central body temperature in children by 0.25° C.[60]

Different types of disposable and reusable water chambers are available for this humidifier. They include a chamber with wick, a general purpose pass-over type of

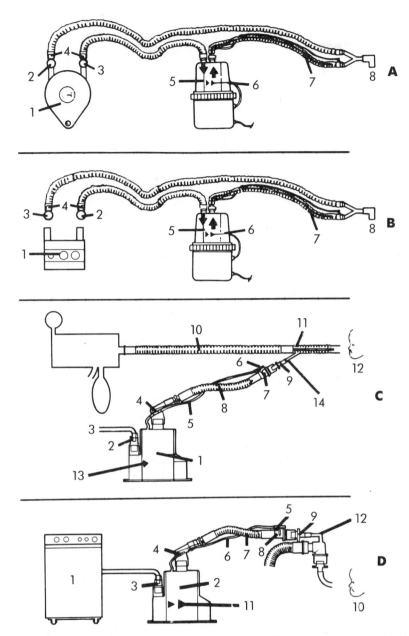

Fig. 7-20. Placement of the Fisher and Paykel humidifier in different situations: **A,** Adult circle. *1,* Absorber; *2* and *3,* expiratory and inspiratory valves; *4,* breathing circuit; *5,* humidifier; *6,* water fill mark; *7,* breathing circuit with heater wire. **B,** Ventilators. *1,* Ventilator. **C,** Bain circuit. *1,* Humidifier; *3,* FGF entering the humidifier; *4* through *6,* proximal and distal temperature sensors; *7,* temperature sensor housing; *8,* pediatric delivery hose with heater wire; *9* and *14,* Bain circuit FGF; *11,* Bain circuit. **D,** Jackson-Rees circuit. *1,* Anesthesia machine. The rest of the attachments are similar to the Bain circuit attachments. (From package insert, Dual Servo Humidifier Fisher and Paykel, Auckland, New Zealand.)

chamber, a low-compressible-volume chamber for neonatal and pediatric use, and a chamber with a hydrophobic auto water-feed mechanism. These humidifiers are more efficient at maintaining body temperature in children than are the artificial noses.[60-62] However, the presence of an electrically heated wire in the inspiratory hose can lead to

mishaps, including (1) electrical hazard due to the close proximity of the electrically heated element to the patient's heart, and (2) thermostat failure and/or inadequate gas flow, leading to overheating. It must be remembered that steam has an enormous thermal capacity and that any accidental overheating will soon result in thermal injury to the

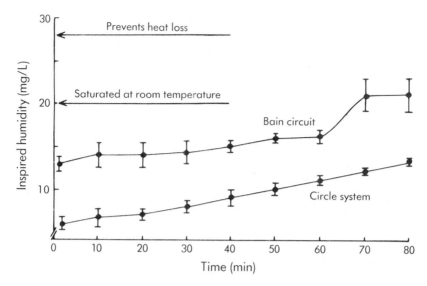

Fig. 7-21. Humidity output of the Bain circuit at FGF 4.9 L/min and a minute volume of 8.4 L. The humidity output of the circle system is shown for comparison. (Used with permission from Ramnathan S, et al: Rebreathing characteristics of the Bain anesthesia circuit, *Anesth Analg* 56:822, 1977.)

trachea. Accidental circuit disconnects and bacterial colonization in the humidifier chamber are additional hazards.

The Bain circuit. The Bain circuit (Fig. 7-20, *C*) is a coaxial version of the Mapleson D system in which the FGF is delivered close to the patient via a gas delivery tube placed inside the exhalation breathing tube. The coaxial breathing circuit, simple and lightweight, is particularly useful in head and neck operations. Although Mapleson recommended an FGF of 2.5 to 3 times the normal minute ventilation with this type of circuit, the inventors of the circuit recommended that an FGF of 70 to 80 ml/kg (at a minute volume of 140 ml/kg) may be sufficient to maintain normocarbia.[63,64] The circuit delivers higher levels of humidification than a conventional absorber because the entire breathing tube acts as a heat and moisture exchanger (Fig. 7-21). The humidity ranges from 12 mg/L at the start of anesthesia to 20 mg/L at stabilization.[17] However, rebreathing of moisture is also associated with rebreathing of exhaled carbon dioxide. Increasing the minute volume without altering the FGF will lead to an increase in inspired humidity and increased inspired carbon dioxide tension.[17,65]

AEROSOL GENERATORS

Vaporizer humidifiers deliver water vapor, whereas nebulizers deliver small particles of water. Nebulizers may be used for humidifying inspired gases and for delivering aerosolized bronchodilators, corticosteroids, and cromolyn sodium. The aerodynamic diameter (particle size) is important in determining in which part of the airway the water particles will be deposited. Particles <1 μm in diameter can reach the alveoli with ease. Particles between 1 and 3 μm reach the bronchioles;[5] particles between 3 and 5 μm are arrested in the main trachea and the bronchi; and

particles between 5 and 10 μm are deposited in the pharynx. Thus particles <5 μm are said to be in the respirable range.[1,66] Particles <0.5 μm are exhaled without being deposited. A light scatterer (Bausch and Lomb) is used to measure particle size.[1] Many aerosols contain particles of heterodisperse aerodynamic diameters, and the index mass median aerodynamic diameter is used to describe their collective performance characteristics.[66] For humidification, larger particles of up to 3 to 5 μm are acceptable. Particle size may not remain constant as the aerosol moves through the airway. The other important factor that influences the life of the microdroplet is the RH of the medium. When the RH is >80% the evaporation rate of the particle slows considerably.[67] Volatile aerosol particles, such as those delivered by metered-dose inhalers, shrink in size because of evaporation in the airway.[68] Hygroscopic particles containing sodium chloride enlarge as they travel through the airway. The aerosol generators are mainly of two types: compressed-gas nebulizers and ultrasonic nebulizers.

Compressed-gas nebulizers

In the compressed-gas nebulizer, a gas jet stream emerges from a constricted orifice and is directed across a capillary tube (Fig. 7-22, *top, middle*). The subatmospheric pressure (Bernoulli effect) generated by the jet draws water from the capillary and nebulizes it. Additional humidity can be provided if the nebulizer is also heated. Large nebulizers with large reservoirs are used to humidify supplemental oxygen. A graded orifice at the top of the humidifier allows air entrainment, whereas units with small reservoirs are used to deliver drug aerosols (Fig. 7-22). Hydrosphere nebulizers make use of the Baffington principle to nebulize the water (Fig. 7-22, *bottom*). A thin film of water coats the surface of a glass sphere. A gas jet

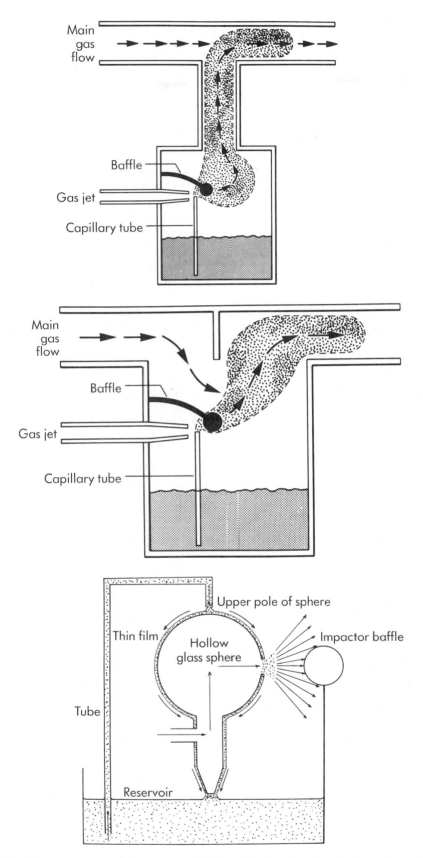

Fig. 7-22. Side stream *(top)*, main stream *(middle)*, and hydrosphere jet nebulizers *(bottom)*. The hydrosphere nebulizer uses the Baffington principle. (From Op't Holt T: *Aerosol generators and humidifiers.* In Barnes TA, Lisbon A, editors: *Respiratory care practice,* Chicago, 1988, Mosby–Year Book. Used by permission.)

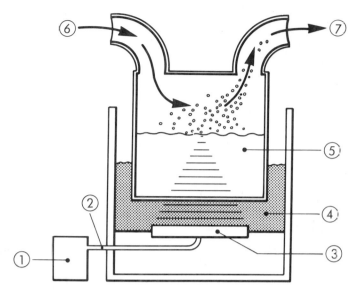

Fig. 7-23. Ultrasonic nebulizer. *1*, Electric generator; *2*, cable; *3*, piezoelectric crystal; *4*, couplant chamber; *5*, solution cup (water cup); *6*, carrier gas inlet; *7*, aerosol outlet. (From Op't Holt T: *Aerosol generators and humidifiers.* In Barnes TA, Lisbon A, editors: *Respiratory care practice,* Chicago, 1988, Mosby–Year Book. Used by permission.)

exiting from within the sphere propels the water onto a baffle and breaks it into small particles, 3 to 5 μm in size (Fig. 7-22, *bottom*). The Bird 500 unit* is an example of a compressed-gas nebulizer. It delivers a particle size of 0.5 to 3 μm at a water content of 12 to 32 mg/L.

Ultrasonic nebulizers

The rapid oscillations of a piezoelectric crystal (1.5 MHz) can be used to break water into small particles (Figure 7-23). The water can be either placed on top of the piezoelectric transducer or slowly dripped onto the transducer. A blower may be used to propel the water particles into the patient circuit. The ultrasonic nebulizer produces a humidity level of 25 to 48 mg/L with a water particle size of 2.8 to 4.0 μm.[1] The De Vilbiss Series 800† is an example of an ultrasonic nebulizer.

When correctly set, nebulizers can deliver large quantities of water. To what extent the water droplets reach the lower airway is debatable. The use of nebulizers for humidifying inspired gases during anesthesia is not very practical because of the complexity in channeling the nebulizer flow through the humidifier.[69] The use of ultrasonic nebulizers, although employed in the 1960s for this purpose, has been superseded by hot pot humidifiers. Because of their ability to deliver liquid water, these nebulizers have been implicated in producing positive water balance,[70] increased alveolar-arterial oxygen partial pressure gradient (A-a DO$_2$),[71] increased airway resistance,[72] and

*Bird Products Corp., Palm Springs, CA 92262
†DeVilbiss Co., Somerset, PA 15501

fungal contamination.[73] Another hazard associated with the use of this device has been reported recently. When tap water is used for humidification, indoor contamination with heavy metal particles increases significantly.[74]

Metered-dose inhalers

Metered-dose inhalers (MDI) are self contained and are powered by chlorofluorocarbon propellants (Freons), which are easily liquefied under pressure. They are nontoxic and nonflammable and have ideal suitable thermodynamic properties.[66] Medical aerosol consumption is only 0.5% of the total chlorofluorocarbon use and therefore contributes only insignificantly to atmospheric ozone depletion.[75] However, the search is under way for ozone-friendly propellants. Dry powder inhalers may provide the answer.[66]

The MDIs are extensively used in the treatment of asthma to deliver cromolyn sodium, β$_2$-mimetic drugs, and corticosteroids. Even under the best possible conditions, only 10% of the drug delivered by the MDI reaches the lungs.[76] Provision of an aerosol holding chamber generally improves the availability of the drug.[66,76] The chamber, which is 5 cm long and 10 cm wide, is placed approximately 20 cm away from the tracheal tube (Fig. 7-24, *C*) and forms a reservoir for the aerosol from which the drug is eventually inhaled. At least four MDI puffs are delivered into the chamber when bronchodilator therapy is required for treating bronchial spasm in anesthetized patients or in patients requiring mechanical ventilation in the intensive care unit. The actual number of puffs is determined by the total dose of the drug to be delivered. The MDI is 3 to 4 times more efficient in delivering drug to the lung than are jet nebulizers.[76] A jet nebulizer may be inserted into the inspiratory side of the circuit to deliver bronchodilator (Fig. 7-24, *D*). The ideal distance between the tracheal tube and the location of the nebulizer is approximately 70 cm (Fig. 7-24, *D*). Moving the jet nebulizer closer to the patient may not necessarily improve deposition in the lung and, indeed, may decrease it.[76,77] There are two reason for this: (1) Placing the nebulizer close to the patient allows the aerosol to drift into the expiratory tube, only to be blown away by the exhaled gases; and (2) the segment of inspiratory tube between the nebulizer and the Y-piece can function as an aerosol holding chamber.[77]

HUMIDIFICATION DURING JET VENTILATION

High- or low-frequency jet ventilation (HFJV or LFJV) delivers gases at high flow rates, and the unhumidified jet will cause rather rapid damage to tracheal cells, heat loss, and viscid secretions.[78] At a driving pressure of 35 psig and a frequency of 100 cycles/min, the HFJV mode delivers approximately 15 L of dry gas. In addition, an entrainment flow that needs to be humidified is provided during jet ventilation. Because a pressure of 20 to 50 psig is required to drive the jet, a tremendous back-pressure will be generated in conventional humidifiers. In addition, passing

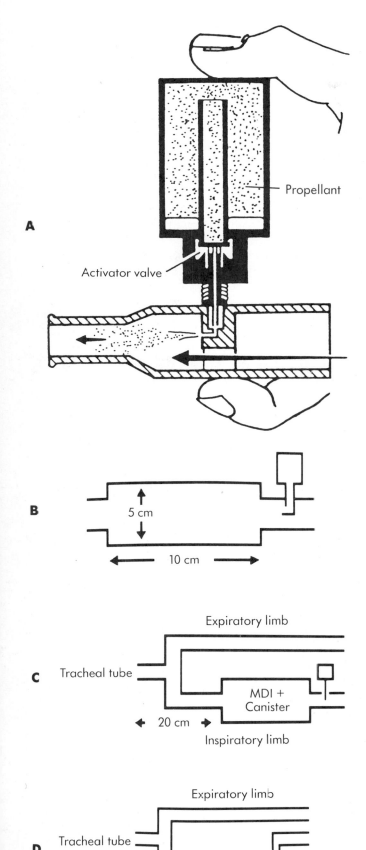

A

Propellant

Activator valve

B

5 cm

10 cm

C

Expiratory limb

Tracheal tube

MDI +
Canister

20 cm

Inspiratory limb

D

Expiratory limb

Tracheal tube

70 cm

Inspiratory limb

Nebulizer

Fig. 7-24. A, Metered dose inhaler. (From Ward JJ, Helmholz HF: Applied humidity and aerosol therapy. In Burton GG, Hodgkin JE, Ward JJ, editors: *Respiratory care,* Philadelphia, 1991, JB Lippincott) Placement of MDI or gas nebulizer in the patient circuit. **B,** Aerosol holding chamber (AHC) with the MDI installed; **C,** the MDI-AHC assembly placed in the patient circuit; **D,** the placement of a jet nebulizer in the patient circuit. (From Fuller HD, Dolovich MB, Posmituck G, et al: Pressurized aerosol versus jet aerosol delivery, *Am Rev Respir Dis* 141:440, 1990. Used by permission.)

the jet through a conventional humidifier will attenuate the jet effect.

The task of humidifying the entrainment flow can be accomplished easily with a heated humidifier. Humidifying the entrainment flow alone is not sufficient because the main jet will dry out the entrained stream.[79] The main jet is humidified by infusing 0.9% saline at a known rate into one limb of a Y-piece, and the jet nozzle is connected through the other limb. A constant infusion pump, which can function at increased outlet pressure (IVAC type of pump*), can be used to deliver the liquid into the jet nozzle (Fig. 7-25).

When catheter jet ventilation is used, the force of the jet may be used to entrain water.[18] An epidural catheter with a single terminal hole is inserted into the jet catheter until its tip reaches a point 0.5 cm from the jet catheter opening (Fig. 7-26). The remaining, free end of the epidural catheter is brought out of the jet catheter via a Y-piece. The jet ventilator is connected to the free opening in the Y-piece. When the jet is activated, the Venturi effect makes the epidural catheter function as an injector. By adjusting the distance between the patient end of the epidural catheter and the jet catheter, the quantity of water entrained can be regulated between 8 and 44 mg/L (Fig. 7-27).

HUMIDIFICATION IN PEDIATRIC SYSTEMS

Lack of inspired humidity causes serious problems in children. The respiratory water loss is significantly greater in children than in adults. In addition, because of the smaller size of the airways, children develop airway clogging more readily than adults when breathing dry gas. Pediatric circle systems were introduced into anesthesia with the mistaken belief that the reaction of neutralization of soda lime would provide moisture. The circle systems for pediatric use are discussed in Chapter 26. Because children excrete only small amounts of carbon dioxide, the humidity output of these circle systems is inadequate.[80,81] To prevent heat loss, extra humidity must be provided either by way of heated water baths (Fig. 7-20) or heat and moisture exchangers.[60,61,82] The Jackson-Rees circuit is essentially a dry system because of the excessive FGF required to eliminate rebreathing. For prolonged cases, ei-

*IVAC Corp., San Diego, CA 92121

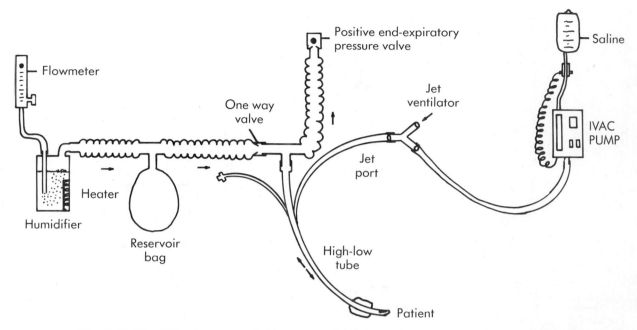

Fig. 7-25. Humidification system for high-frequency jet ventilation. Note that both the main jet and the entrainment flows are humidified. (From Sladen A, Guntapalli K, Marquez J, et al: High-frequency jet ventilation in the postoperative period: a review of 100 patients, *Crit Care Med* 12:782, 1984.)

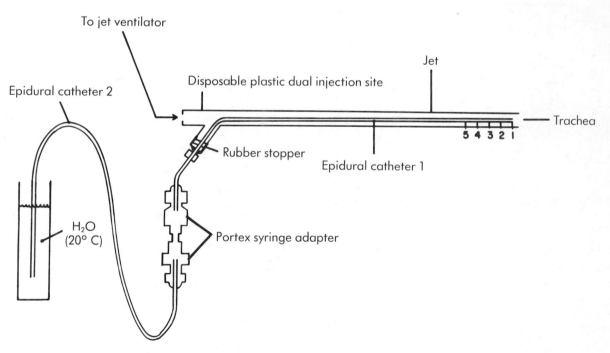

Fig. 7-26. Humidification system for catheter jet ventilation. *1, 2, 3, 4,* and *5,* are indelible marks on the catheter; the humidity level can be controlled by positioning the injector catheter opposite one of these markings. (From Ramanathan S, Arismendy JR, Gandhi S, et al: Coaxial catheter for humidification during jet ventilation, *Anesth Analg* 61:689, 1982. Used by permission.)

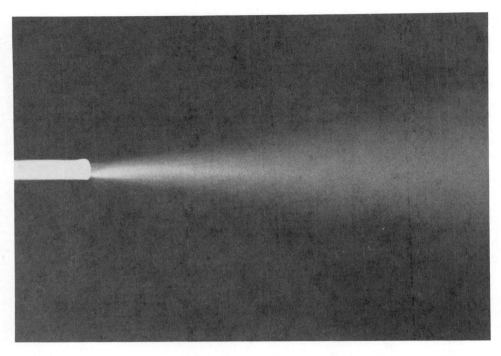

Fig. 7-27. Nebulization produced by the system in Fig. 7-26. (From Ramanathan S, Arismendy JR, Gandhi S, et al: Coaxial catheter for humidification during jet ventilation, *Anesth Analg* 61:689, 1982. Used by permission.)

ther heated humidification or heat and moisture exchangers must be provided. Humidification of the circle system and the Jackson-Rees system is shown in Fig. 7-20, *A* and *D*.

Medical gases are completely dry. Prolonged breathing of dry gases can lead to morbidity and heat loss. Excessive humidification may lead to water intoxication, positive heat balance, and bacterial colonization. Several humidity systems are commercially available. Systems that efficiently utilize the patient's exhaled humidity and warmth are preferable to those that employ electrical energy. For practical purposes, an inspired humidity of 32 mg/dL is adequate in preventing heat loss and tracheal cytologic damage. Humidity in excess of these levels is unphysiologic. For short-term clinical use, the heat and moisture exchangers are suitable; and for prolonged use, one of the hot water humidifiers may be used.

REFERENCES

1. Chalon J, Ali M, Turndorf H, et al: *Humidification of anesthetic gases,* Springfield, Ill, 1981, Charles C Thomas.
2. Hill DW: *Physics applied to anaesthesia,* ed 4, Boston, 1980, Butterworths.
3. Mushin W, Jones P: *Physics for the anaesthetist,* ed 4, Boston, 1987, Blackwell Scientific Publications.
4. Siegel D, Ramanathan S, Chalon J, et al: An improved program to calculate intrapulmonary shunting, *Crit Care Med* 7:282, 1979.
5. Shelly MP, Lloyd GM, Park GR: A review of the mechanisms and methods of humidification of inspired gases, *Intensive Care Med* 14:1-9, 1988.
6. Nunn JF: *Oxygen.* In *Applied respiratory physiology.* Boston, 1977, Butterworths, pp 375-444.
7. Dick W: Aspects of humidification: requirements and techniques, *Int Anesthesiol Clin* 12:217-239, 1991.
8. Guyton AC: *Partition of the body fluids: osmotic equilibria between extracellular and intracellular fluids.* In Guyton AC, editor: *Textbook of medical physiology,* Philadelphia, 1986, WB Saunders.
9. Grande CM, Ramanathan S, Turndorf H: The structural correlates of airway function. *Problems in Anesthesia* 2:175, 1988.
10. Linton RAF: *Structure and function of the respiratory tract in relation to anaesthesia.* In Churchill-Davidson HC, editor: *A practice of anaesthesia,* Chicago, 1984, Year Book Medical Publishers, pp 3-30.
11. Sleigh MA: Some aspects of the comparative physiology of cilia, *Am Rev Respir Dis* 93:16, 1966.
12. Newhouse M, Sanchis J, Bienstock J, et al: Lung defense mechanisms. I, *N Engl J Med* 295:990-998, 1976.
13. Breeze R, Turk M: Cellular structure, function, and organization in the lower respiratory tract, *Environ Health Perspect* 55:3, 1984.
14. Sykes MK, Vickers MD, Hull CJ, et al: *Principles of clinical measurement,* ed 2, Oxford, 1981, Blackwell.
15. Arundel AV, Sterling EM, Biggin JH, et al: Indirect health effects of relative humidity in indoor environments, *Environ Health Perspect* 65:351, 1986.
16. Ramanathan S, Capan L, Chalon J, et al: Minienvironmental changes under the drapes of patients undergoing awake eye surgery, *Anesthesiology* 48:286, 1978.
17. Ramanathan S, Chalon J, Capan L, et al: Rebreathing characteristics of the Bain anesthesia circuit, *Anesth Analg* 56:822, 1977.
18. Ramanathan S, Arismendy JR, Gandhi S, et al: Coaxial catheter for humidification during jet ventilation, *Anesth Analg* 61:689, 1982.
19. Klainer AS, Turndorf H: Surface alterations due to endotracheal intubation, *Am J Med* 58:674, 1975.

20. Proctor D: State of the art—The upper airways—The larynx and trachea, *Am Rev Respir Dis* 115:315, 1977.
21. Burton J: Effects of dry anaesthetic gases on the respiratory mucous membrane, *Lancet* 1:235, 1962.
22. Toremalm N: Airflow patterns and ciliary activity in trachea after tracheotomy, *Acta Otolaryngol* 53:442, 1961.
23. Marfatia S, Donahoe P, Hendrin W: Effect of dry and humidified gases on the respiratory epithelium in rabbits, *J Pediatr Surg* 10:583, 1975.
24. Chalon J, Loew D, Malebranche J: Effects of dry anesthetic gases on tracheobronchial ciliated epithelium, *Anesthesiology* 37:338, 1972.
25. Chalon J, Ali M, Ramanathan S, et al: The humidification of anaesthetic gases: its importance and control, *Can Anaesth Soc J* 26:361, 1979.
26. Chalon J, Patel C, Ali M, et al: Humidity and the anesthetized patient, *Anesthesiology* 50:195, 1979.
27. Chalon J, Tayyab M, Ramanathan S: Cytology of respiratory epithelium as a predictor of respiratory complications after operations, *Chest* 67:32, 1975.
28. Fonkalsrud EW, Calmes S, Barcliff LT, et al: Reduction of operative heat loss and pulmonary secretions in neonates by use of heated and humidified anesthetic gases, *J Cardiovasc Surg* 80:718, 1980.
29. Stone DR, Downs J, Paul W, et al: Adult body temperature and heated humidification of anesthetic gases during general anesthesia, *Anesth Analg* 60:736, 1981.
30. Lumley J: Decontamination of anaesthetic equipment and ventilators, *Br J Anaesth* 48:3, 1976.
31. Moritz AR, Henriques FC, McLean R: The effects of inhaled heat on air passages and lungs: an experimental investigation, *Am J Pathol* 21:311, 1945.
32. Klein EF, Graves SA: Hot pot tracheitis, *Chest* 65:225, 1974.
33. Walker JEC, Wells RE, Merril EW: Heat and water exchange in the respiratory tract, *Am J Med* 30:259, 1961.
34. Tamer MA, Modell JH, Reiffell CN: Hyponatremia secondary to aerosol therapy on newborn infant, *J Pediatr* 77:1051, 1970.
35. Dery R: Humidity in anesthesiology. IV. Determination of alveolar humidity and temperature in the dog, *Can Anaesth Soc J* 30:259, 1971.
36. Knudsen J, Lombholdt N, Wisborg K: Postoperative complications using dry and humidified anaesthetic gases, *Br J Anaesth* 45:363, 1973.
37. Tsueda T, Noguchi H, Takima Y, et al: Optimum humidification of air administered to a tracheostomy in dogs, *Br J Anaesth* 49:965, 1977.
38. Noguchi H, Takumi Y, Aochi O: A study of humidification in tracheostomized dogs, *Anesthesiology* 45:844, 1973.
39. Jones JG, Clarke SW, Oliver RW: Two phase gas-liquid flow in the airways, *Br J Anaesth* 41:192, 1969.
40. Clarke RE, Orkin LR, Rovenstine EA: Body temperature in anesthetized man: effect of environmental temperature, humidity and anesthesia system, *JAMA* 154:311, 1954.
41. Mogue LR, Rantala B: Capnometers, *J Clin Monit* 4:115, 1988.
42. Deluty SH: Capnography: how does it work and what can we learn from it? *Progress in Anesthesiology,* 4:273, 1990.
43. Chalon J, Kao ZL, Dolorico VN, et al: Humidity output of the circle absorber system. *Anesthesiology* 38:458, 1973.
44. Bengtson JP, Bengtson A, Stenquist O: The circle system as a humidifier, *Br J Anaesth* 63:453, 1989.
45. Bengtson JP, Sonander H, Stenquist O: Preservation of humidity and heat of respiratory gases during anaesthesia: a laboratory investigation, *Acta Anaesthesiol Scand* 31:127, 1987.
46. Ramanathan S, Chalon J, Turndorf H: A compact, well-humidified breathing circuit for the circle system, *Anesthesiology* 44:238, 1976.
47. Chalon J, Patel C, Ramanathan S: Humidification of the circle absorber system, *Anesthesiology* 48:142, 1978.

48. Chalon J, Ramanathan S: Water vaporizer heated by the reaction of neutralization by carbon dioxide, *Anesthesiology* 41:401, 1974.
49. Chalon J, Markham JP, Ali MM, et al: The Pall Ultipore Breathing Circuit Filter: an efficient heat and moisture exchanger, *Anesth Analg* 63:566, 1984.
50. Court MH, Dodman NH, Seeler DC: Inhalation therapy oxygen administration, humidification, and aerosol therapy, *Vet Clin North Am: Small Anim Pract* 15:1043, 1985.
51. Eckerbom B, Lindholm CE: Performance evaluation of six heat and moisture exchangers according to the Draft International Standard (ISO/DIS 9360), *Acta Anaesthesiol Scand* 34:404, 1990.
52. Op't Holt T: *Aerosol generators and humidifiers.* In Barnes TA, Lisbon A, editors: *Respiratory care practice,* Chicago, 1988, Mosby–Year Book, pp 356-405.
53. Saravolatz LD, Pohlod DJ, Conway W, et al: Lack of bacterial aerosols associated with heat and moisture exchangers. *Am Rev Respir Dis* 134:214, 1986.
54. Scanlan C: *Humidity and aerosol therapy.* In Scanlan CL, Spearman CB, Sheldon RL, et al, editors: *Egan's fundamentals of respiratory care,* St Louis, 1990, Mosby–Year Book, pp 557-583.
55. Turtle MJ, Ilsley AH, Rutten AJ, et al: Equipment: an evaluation of six disposable heat and moisture exchangers, *Anaesth Intensive Care* 15:317, 1987.
56. Ward JJ, Helmholz HF: *Applied humidity and aerosol therapy.* In Burton GG, Hodgkin JE, Ward JJ, editors: *Respiratory care,* Philadelphia, 1991, JB Lippincott, pp 355-396.
57. Bygdeman S, von Euler C, Nystrom B: Moisture exchangers do not prevent patient contamination of ventilators: a microbiological study, *Acta Anaesthesiol Scand* 28:591, 1984.
58. Myer CM, Hubbell RN, McDonald JS, et al: Study of humidification potential of a heat and moisture exchanger in tracheostomized dogs, *Ann Otol Rhinol Laryngol* 97:322, 1988.
59. Martin CM, Perrin G, Gevaudan MJ, et al: Heat and moisture exchangers and vaporizing humidifiers in the intensive care unit, *Chest* 97:144-149, 1990.
60. Bissonnette B, Sessler DI, Laflamme P: Passive and active inspired gas humidification in infants and children, *Anesthesiology* 71:350, 1989.
61. Bissonnette B, Sessler DI: Passive or active inspired gas humidification increases thermal steady-state temperatures in anesthetized infants, *Anesth Analg* 69:783, 1989.
62. Youngberg J, Graybar G, Subaiya L, et al: Maintaining body temperature during anesthesia with a servo-controlled heated humidifier, *South Med J* 78:814, 1985.
63. Bain JA, Spoerel WE: A streamlined anesthetic system, *Can Anaesth Soc J* 196:426, 1972.
64. Bain JA, Spoerel WE: Flow requirements for a modified Mapleson D system during controlled ventilation, *Can Anaesth Soc J* 20:629, 1973.
65. Ramanathan S, Chalon J, Rothblatt A, et al: Effects of minute volume increases on the rebreathing characteristics of the Bain anaesthesia circuit during controlled ventilation, *Acta Anaesthesiol Scand* 24:93, 1980.
66. Newman SP: Aerosol inhaler, *Br Med J* 300:1286, 1990.
67. Robinson JS: *Humidification.* In Scurr C, Feldman S, editors: *Scientific foundations of anaesthesia,* Chicago, 1974, William Heinemann, pp 488-496.
68. Johnson CE: Principles of nebulizer-delivered drug therapy for asthma, *Am J Hosp Pharm* 46:1845, 1989.
69. Tayyab MA, Ambiavagar M, Chalon J: Water nebulization in a nonrebreathing system during anesthesia, *Can Anaesth Soc J* 20:728, 1973.
70. Swenson O, Grana L, Hausam T: Use of ultrasonic nebulizer during anesthesia, *J Pediatr Surg* 6:554, 1971.

71. Modell J, Moya F, Ruiz B: Blood gas and electrolyte determinations during exposure to ultrasonic nebulized aerosols, *Br J Anaesth* 40:20, 1968.

72. Waltrmath CL, Erbguth PH, Sunderland WA: Increased respiratory resistance after ultrasonic nebulization of anesthesia gas, *Anesthesiology* 39:547, 1973.

73. Gemma H, Sato A, Chida K, et al: Two cases of hypersensitivity pneumonitis due to contamination of an ultrasonic humidifier, *Nippon Kyobu Shikkan Gakkai Zasshi* 29:710, 1991.

74. Fidler AH: Air humidifiers: beneficial or a hazard? *Off Gesundheitwes* 51:764, 1989.

75. Newman SP: Metered dose pressurized aerosols and the ozone layer, *Eur J Respir Dis* 3:495, 1990.

76. Fuller HD, Dolovich MB, Posmituck G, et al: Pressurized aerosol versus jet aerosol delivery, *Am Rev Respir Dis* 141:440, 1990.

77. Hughes JM, Sacz J: Effects of nebulizer mode and position in a mechanical ventilator circuit on dose and efficiency, *Respir Care* 32:1131, 1987.

78. Doyle HJ, Napolitano AE, Lippman R, et al: Different humidification systems for high-frequency jet ventilation, *Crit Care Med* 12:815, 1984.

79. Sladen A, Guntupalli K, Marquez J, et al: High-frequency jet ventilation in the postoperative period: a review of 100 patients, *Crit Care Med* 12:782, 1984.

80. Ramanathan S, Chalon J, Turndorf H: Humidity output of the Bloomquist infant circle, *Anesthesiology* 43:679, 1975.

81. Ramanathan S, Chalon J, Rand P: Humidity output of the Columbia pediatric circle, *Anesth Analg* 55:887, 1976.

82. Bissonnette B, Sessler DI, LaFlamme P: Intraoperative temperature monitoring sites in infants and children and the effect of inspired gas warming on esophageal temperature, *Anesth Analg* 69:192, 1989.

Part II

SYSTEM MONITORS

Chapter 8

MONITORING GASES IN THE ANESTHESIA DELIVERY SYSTEM

James B. Eisenkraft, M.D.
Daniel B. Raemer, Ph.D.

Although the technology whereby gases can be analyzed has long been available, only relatively recently has intraoperative monitoring of respired gases become widespread. Modern systems are accurate and reliable, have rapid response times, and are becoming less expensive as competition among their manufacturers increases. Anesthesiologists who are aiming to make their practices state-of-the-art are often now required to make significant (financial) decisions as to which monitor they should purchase, and they may be overwhelmed by technical and other commercial information. This chapter provides a framework for the understanding of the methods whereby gases are analyzed and the important basic differences among the various systems. Some important applications of respiratory gas monitoring are also discussed.

The respiratory gases of most interest to the anesthesiologist include oxygen, carbon dioxide, nitrous oxide, and the potent inhaled anesthetic agents. Other gases that may be of relevance in certain situations are nitrogen and helium. Numerous gas monitors offer various options to the user. Ultimately, these monitors use one or more of a limited number of technologies to make the analysis and present the data. A basic understanding of the principles involved in gas monitoring naturally leads to an understanding of the applications and limitations of each technology and, therefore, each device.

SAMPLING SYSTEMS

In order for a monitor to analyze gas, either the gas must be brought to the analyzer or the analyzer must be brought to the gas. All anesthesia circuits include at least one oxygen analyzer. This is usually located in the vicinity of the inspiratory unidirectional valve in the circle system or in the fresh-gas supply of a rebreathing system. These analyzers are of either the fuel cell or the polarographic type, and gas passes over the sensor that measures the oxygen concentration.

To monitor the gases actually respired by the patient, gas sampling from the airway is required. The gas to be analyzed can be continuously sampled from the patient's airway and conducted via fine-bore tubing to the analyzer unit. Such a design is termed a side-stream, or diverting, system because the gas is diverted from the airway for analysis elsewhere.

Diverting or side-stream systems

Advantages of the diverting type of analyzers are that they are remote from the patient, that they can be of any size, and that therefore they offer more versatility in terms of monitoring capabilities. Disadvantages include problems of the catheter sampling system (such as clogging with secretions or water), kinking, failure of the aspirator pump, long response time, and artifacts when the gas sampling rate is poorly matched to respired gas flow rates. Thus if a diverting system is used with a very small patient (neonate) and the gas sampling rate exceeds the patient's expiratory gas-flow rate, then artifacts may be produced. If an uncuffed tracheal tube is used and there is a leak between the tube and the trachea, the sampling pump may suck air into the tracheal tube. In addition, fresh gas from the circuit may dilute the patient's exhaled gas if the sampling rate far exceeds expiratory flow rate. Ideally, the gas sampling rate should be appropriate for the patient and for the circuit used. Some diverting systems can aspirate up to 500 ml of gas per minute. This may limit the ability to use low-flow or closed circuit anesthesia techniques. Indeed, if the gas sampling rate exceeds the fresh gas inflow rate, negative pressures can be created in the patient circuit. Some diverting systems offer the possibility of returning gas to the patient circuit once it has been analyzed; alternatively, the gas can be conducted to a waste-gas scavenging system for appropriate disposal. In certain diverting analyzers (e.g., Datex Capnomac*) that incorporate a paramagnetic oxygen sensor, room air is required to make the oxygen analysis. This air is added (at a rate of 10 ml/min) to the gas exiting the monitor and potentially returned to the patient circuit. This could create a problem during closed circuit anesthesia, because nitrogen (at a rate of 8 ml/min) is added to the circuit. (See also Chapters 16 and 26.)

*Datex, Tewksbury, Mass.

Nondiverting or main-stream systems

The alternative to a diverting system for airway gas monitoring is a main-stream, or nondiverting, arrangement. This is presently available only for monitoring carbon dioxide via infrared technology. Although these analyzers overcome the gas sampling problem, they require a special airway adapter and analysis module to be placed in the circuit near to the patient. These modules are vulnerable to damage and are not inexpensive to replace. New designs, however, are light in weight, have low deadspace, and use solid-state technology to improve performance. In addition, modules placed in the airway are subject to interference by water vapor, secretions, and blood. Because condensed water blocks all infrared wavelengths, leaving too little source intensity to make a measurement, the main-stream cuvette's window is heated (usually to 41° C) to prevent such condensation and interference. All presently available multigas analyzers are of the diverting or side-stream variety.

ANALYSIS SYSTEMS

The respiratory tract and the anesthesia delivery system both contain respired gases in the form of molecules. Gas molecules are in constant motion, and when they strike the walls of the container they give rise to pressure (defined as force per unit area); the more gas molecules present, the greater is the pressure exerted. Dalton's law of partial pressures states that the total pressure exerted by a mixture of gases is equal to the arithmetic sum of the partial pressures exerted by each gas in the mixture. The total pressure of all gases in the anesthesia system at sea level is 760 mm Hg. Respiratory gas analyzers may display data in mm Hg or as volumes percent, but it is important to understand in principle how the measurement was made. The reader should understand the difference between partial pressure (mm Hg), which is an absolute term, and volumes percent, which is an expression of a proportion, or ratio.

How many molecules? (partial pressure)

An analysis system that is based on quantifying a specific property of a gas molecule in effect determines in absolute terms the number of molecules of that gas that are present, that is, mm Hg. Gas molecules that are composed of two or more dissimilar atoms have bonds between their component atoms. Certain wavelengths of infrared radiation excite the molecules, stretching or distorting these bonds, which also absorb the radiation. Monatomic gases, such as helium and argon, or gases whose molecules are composed of two similar atoms, such as oxygen and nitrogen, do not absorb infrared radiation. Carbon dioxide molecules absorb infrared radiation at a wavelength of 4.3 μm. The more molecules of carbon dioxide that are present, the more radiation at 4.3 μm is absorbed. This property of the carbon dioxide molecule is applied in the infrared carbon dioxide analyzer. Because the amount of radiation absorbed is a function of the *number of molecules* present, it is, therefore, also a function of partial pressure. Thus, infrared analyzers measure partial pressure.

In the analysis of gases by Raman spectroscopy (Ohmeda Rascal II), a helium-neon laser emits monochromatic light at a wavelength of 633 nm. When this light interacts with the intramolecular bonds of specific gas molecules, it is scattered and re-emitted at wavelengths different from that of the incident light. Each re-emission wavelength is characteristic of specific gas molecules present in the gas mixture and therefore is a function of their partial pressure. Thus, Raman spectroscopy measures partial pressure.

When the partial pressure of each component of a gas mixture is known, a reading in volumes percent can be computed as

$$\frac{\text{Partial pressure of the component gas (mm Hg)}}{\text{Total pressure of all gases (mm Hg)}} \times 100\%$$

An adequate number of molecules of the gas(es) to be measured (i.e., adequate partial pressure) must be present to facilitate gas analysis by Raman and infrared methods. These systems must also be pressure compensated if analyses are being made at ambient pressures other than those used for the original calibration of the system.

What proportion? (volumes percent)

Another approach to gas analysis is to separate the molecular components of a gas mixture and determine what proportion each gas contributes to the total. This approach is applied in mass spectrometry. Thus, if in a sample of gas containing 100 molecules there were 30 molecules of oxygen, oxygen would represent 30% of the gas sample and therefore might reasonably be assumed to represent 30% of the original gas mixture being analyzed. The result is expressed as 30 volumes percent, or as a fractional concentration (0.30). This system does not measure *partial pressures;* it measures only *proportions.* If the system is provided with an actual pressure reading to be made equivalent to 100%, the basic measured proportions can be converted to readings in mm Hg. In the above example, if 100% were made equivalent to 760 mm Hg, oxygen would have a calculated partial pressure of (760 × 30%) = 228 mm Hg.

These fundamental differences in the approach to analysis should be borne in mind when the sections that follow are read and, more important, when the data presented by these monitors are interpreted in a clinical setting.

MASS SPECTROMETRY

The mass spectrometer is an instrument that allows the identification and quantification, on a breath-by-breath basis, of all of the gases commonly encountered during the administration of an inhalational anesthetic. These gases include oxygen, nitrogen, nitrous oxide, halothane, enflurane, and isoflurane; other agents, such as helium, sevoflurane, argon, and desflurane, may be added or substituted if desired. Although the technology of mass spectrometry has been available for many years, analyzer units for dedication to a single patient are too expensive for routine use in each OR. In 1981, the concept of a shared, or multiplexed, system was introduced.[1] Such an arrangement permits one central analyzer to function as part of a computerized multiplexed system that can serve up to 31 patient sampling locations (ORs and recovery room or intensive care unit beds) on a time-shared basis. This section presents the principles of operation, applications, and limitations of the two shared mass spectrometry systems currently available for use in the OR and intensive care areas. These are the System for Anesthetic and Respiratory Analysis (SARA)* and the Marquette Advantage (MA) System.† At the center of each system is the analyzer unit itself. Although the SARA and MA systems are basically similar in principle, they do differ in certain details.

Principles of operation

The mass spectrometer analyzer unit separates the components of a stream of charged particles (ions) into a spectrum according to their mass/charge ratios. The relative abundance of ions at certain specific mass/charge ratios is determined and is related to the fractional composition of the original gas mixture. The creation and manipulation of ions is carried out in a high vacuum (10^{-5} mm Hg) to avoid interference by outside air and to minimize random collisions among the ions and residual gases.

The most common design of mass spectrometer is the magnetic sector analyzer,[2] so called because it uses a permanent magnet to separate the ion beam into its component ion spectra (Fig. 8-1). A stream of gas to be analyzed is continuously drawn by a sampling pump from a patient airway connector via a long nylon catheter. During transit through the sampling catheter, the pressure drops from atmospheric (usually 760 mm Hg) in the patient circuit to approximately 40 mm Hg by the inlet of the analyzer unit. A very small amount of the gas actually sampled from the circuit (approximately 10^{-6} ml/sec) enters the analyzer unit's high-vacuum system through the molecular inlet leak. The gas molecules are then bombarded by an electron beam which causes some of the molecules to lose one or more electrons and become positively charged ions. Thus an oxygen molecule (O_2) might lose one electron and become an oxygen ion ($O_2{}^+$) with one positive charge. The mass/charge ratio would therefore be 32/1, or 32. If the oxygen molecule lost two electrons, it would gain two

*PPG Biomedical Systems, Lenexa, Kan.

†Marquette Electronics, Inc., Anesthesia and Respiratory Care Division, Milwaukee, Wis.

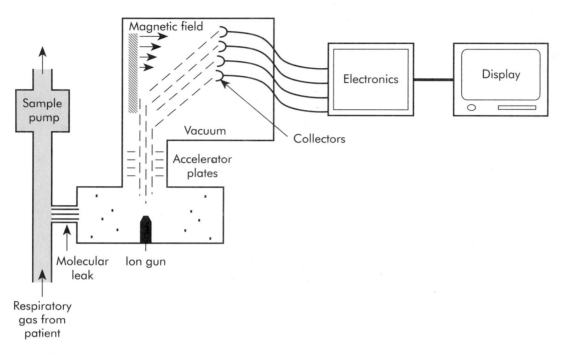

Fig. 8-1. Diagram of a magnetic sector respiratory mass spectrometer. The respiratory gas is sampled and drawn over a molecular leak. Gas molecules enter a vacuum chamber (through the molecular inlet leak), where they are ionized and electrically accelerated. A magnetic field deflects the ions. The mass and charge of the ions determine their trajectory, and metal dish collectors are placed to detect them. The electrical currents produced by the ions impacting the collectors are processed; the composition is computed; and the results are displayed. (From Raemer DB: *Monitoring respiratory function.* In Rogers MC, Tinker JH, Covino BJ, Longnecker DE, editors: *Principles and practice of anesthesiology,* St. Louis, 1992, Mosby–Year Book.)

positive charges and the resulting ion (O_2^{++}) would have a mass/charge ratio of 32/2, or 16.

This process of electron bombardment also causes large molecules (e.g., halothane, enflurane, isoflurane) to become fragmented, or "cracked," into smaller, positively charged ions. The positive ions created in the analyzer are then focused into a beam by the electrostatic fields in the ion source, directed through a slit to define an exact shape for the beam, and accelerated and directed into the field of the permanent magnet. The magnetic field influences the direction of the ions, causing each ion species to curve in a trajectory whose arc is related to its mass/charge ratio. The effect is to create several separate ion beams exiting the magnetic field. The separated beams are directed to individual collectors, which detect the ion current and transmit it to amplifiers that create output voltages in relation to the abundance of the ion species detected. The collector plates are positioned so that ions with specific mass/charge ratios strike specific collectors. The heaviest ions are deflected the least and travel the furthest before striking a collector (Fig. 8-1). Collectors for these heavy ions are therefore located furthest from the ion source. Summing and other computer circuitry measures the total voltage from all of the collector circuits as well as the individual voltages from each collector. Total voltage is considered equivalent

to 100% of the analyzed gas mixture. Individual gas collector circuit voltages are expressed as percentages of the total voltage, and displayed as percentages of the sampled gas mixture. Thus if the voltage from the oxygen collector circuit (mass/charge ratio 32) represented 30% of the total voltage from all of the collector circuits, oxygen would be read as constituting 30% of the total gas mixture analyzed.

The MA and SARA systems use magnetic sector analyzers that have up to eight collectors and therefore can detect and analyze up to eight different gases or ion species. Most of the mass spectrometers in common clinical use, however, use only seven collectors, i.e., for oxygen, carbon dioxide, nitrogen, nitrous oxide, enflurane, halothane and isoflurane. A collector for argon or one other gas is available at extra cost. The position of the collector is determined by the mass/charge ratio of the ion species to be detected. Nitrogen ions with one positive charge have a mass/charge ratio of 28, and singly-charged oxygen ions have a mass/charge ratio of 32. Nitrogen and oxygen are therefore detected by collectors in these positions (28 and 32, respectively).

The situation becomes a little more complicated when it comes to distinguishing among compounds that, when ionized and singly-charged, have the same mass/charge ratio. Thus carbon dioxide and nitrous oxide both have molecular weights of 44 and, when ionized, are both detected and indistinguishable from each other by a collector in the 44 position. Similarly, enflurane and isoflurane are isomers; both have molecular weights of 184.5 and are indistinguishable by a collector in the 184.5 position. The mass spectrometer, however, is able to overcome this problem. When compounds enter the analyzer, the parent molecule fragments or "cracks," and breakdown products are formed in fixed proportion to the quantitative presence of the parent compound. These fragments are also ionized and can be detected by the collector system; thus the parent molecule is identified and quantified. Thus carbon dioxide is broken down, in part, to carbon, and C^+ ions are formed; whereas nitrous oxide is broken down, in part, to nitric oxide, and NO^+ ions are formed. This provides the means to separate, both qualitatively and quantitatively, nitrous oxide from carbon dioxide. The SARA system measures carbon dioxide by detecting C^+ ions by a collector for a mass/charge ratio of 12, and it measures nitrous oxide by detecting NO^+ ions with a mass/charge ratio of 30. The SARA system analyzes and quantifies halothane, enflurane and isoflurane by detecting ionized fragments of the parent halothane, enflurane, and isoflurane molecules, which have mass/charge ratios of 118, 68, and 51, respectively.

In the MA system the sum total of N_2O^+ and CO_2^+ ions is measured by a collector for mass/charge ratio 44, and the contribution due to CO_2^+ is subtracted using information from a collector for mass/charge ratio at the 12 position, which detects C^+ ions and thereby infers the proportion of carbon dioxide. Collectors for mass/charge ratios 117, 69, and 87 are used to detect fragments of halothane, enflurane, and isoflurane, respectively (Table 8-1). The rapid handling of information from the several collectors to calculate the relative abundances of agents with similar mass/charge ratios requires a sophisticated computer program.[3]

The mass spectrometer functions as a proportioning system for the components of a gas mixture and assumes that all of the gases present have been detected when it displays each of the components of the mixture as a *percentage* of the total. If ambient (atmospheric) pressure information is entered into the software, the measured percentages or proportions can be converted to readings in mm Hg (i.e., partial pressures). It must be remembered that the mass spectrometer does not measure partial pressures; it calculates them from the measured proportions and the atmospheric pressure information that must be supplied to it.

Usually, because the mass spectrometer is sampling respired gases from the patient circuit, the total pressure entered is ambient minus 47 mm Hg, the latter representing the saturated vapor pressure of water at body temperature (37° C). Thus, at sea level (760 mm Hg), a pressure of 713 mm Hg would be entered into the mass spectrometer software to be apportioned among the gases present. The

Table 8-1. Fixed collector mass spectrometer monitoring of anesthetic and respiratory gases

	Mass-to-charge ratio monitored	
Compound	Marquette Advantage MGA-1100	SARA/Medspect II
Halothane	117	118
Enflurane	69	67-69
Isoflurane	87	51
Oxygen	32	32
Nitrous oxide	44	30
Nitrogen	28	28
Carbon dioxide	12,44	12

Information obtained from the manufacturers.

mass spectrometer readings, when displayed in mm Hg, represent somewhat of a compromise because inspired gas is usually not fully saturated with water vapor, whereas expired gas usually is. If an incorrect value for total ambient pressure is entered into the mass spectrometer software, all readings in mm Hg will be incorrect, but the readings in volumes percent will be correct. Thus suppose that the end-tidal carbon dioxide is measured as 5% by the mass spectrometer and that ambient pressure is 760 mm Hg. The reading in mm Hg will be 35.65 [i.e., $(760 - 47) \times 5\%$]. If a value of 500 mm Hg is entered instead of 713, the reading in mm Hg will be 25 (i.e., $500 \times 5\%$). In any case of doubt, the clinician should use the reading in percent. In some systems, any user at any patient's station can change the ambient pressure entry for the whole network.

The mass spectrometer will display erroneous readings when a gas that is not detected by the collector plate system is present in the mixture being analyzed. Thus in the presence of helium, which has a mass/charge ratio of 4, the usual seven agents will be summed to 100% as if helium were not present. In the presence of 50% helium, all readings given would, therefore, be approximately twice their real values in the original gas mixture, and this error would apply to readings in both the volumes percent and mm Hg display modes.[4] If a gas not detected by the mass spectrometer is present in sufficient amount, the total ion current from all of the collectors will be less than if all of the ions were detected. If it is substantially less, an alarm message may be generated. If measurement of helium is desired (e.g., for determination of functional residual capacity by helium dilution or if helium is used during anesthesia for laser surgery) the capability to detect and quantify this gas may be added to the MA system. Use of helium in the mass spectrometer does, however, saturate the ion pump in the high-vacuum chamber more quickly, necessitating more frequent replacement of this pump.

As each ion makes contact with a collector, it recovers its lost electron and becomes a neutral gas molecule once again. These molecules, together with nonionized components of the original sample, are removed by the ion pump. The design of the pump varies from unit to unit; the MA system uses a tantalum plate and a titanium plate to absorb the ions. As the pump becomes saturated the ability to create a vacuum is gradually lost. In the MA system, this requires a cartridge change about once a year.

The mass spectrometer analyzer unit has a very rapid response time and can display data for all seven gases continuously and in real time. Computer algorithms have been created to detect maximum and minimum carbon dioxide levels and, thereby, to identify inspiration and end-expiration. Other gases measured simultaneously at these points in time can be displayed as inspired and end-expired values. The computer system also permits the entry of concentration limits and activation of alarms when these limits are exceeded. Mass spectrometer analyzer units should be moved as little as possible and should be left on to maintain the high vacuum. In the standby mode, the vacuum pump continues to maintain a low pressure but the ion gun is turned off.

Shared mass spectrometry systems

Multiplexing permits the sharing of one (expensive) gas analyzer among up to 31 sampling locations or stations. For the SARA and MA systems, the sampling locations must be within about 200 feet of the central analyzer unit. Gas is continually sampled from the patient circuit through a T connector or elbow adapter, via a capillary tube to a headwall plate located in the wall or ceiling. This plate has two connections; one accepts the capillary sampling tube and the other an electrical cable that transmits information to and from a monitor display unit by the sampling station or bedside. From the headwall plate, a long sampling catheter leads to the inlet selector unit (ISU) (the MA system uses a rotary valve; the SARA system uses individual three-way solenoid valves) at the location of the central analyzer. At any moment, these electronically controlled valves direct the gas from one sampling site into the mass spectrometer unit for analysis and the gas from the other sites to a waste-gas scavenging system. The valve system may also be connected to one or more tanks of calibration gas mixtures for periodic calibration and balancing of the system.

In the basic SARA system, all patient catheters are continuously sampled at a rate of 120 ml/min by a sampling pump. When the lumen of one of these catheters is opened via the sampling valve system to the mass spectrometer for gas analysis, the gas sample in this catheter is drawn into the analyzer unit (past the molecular leak) and analyzed at a rate of 240 ml/min, that is, double that of the basic gas sampling rate. This permits analysis of stored line data in less time.[1] This is analogous to tape-recording a lecture at normal speed and then playing back the tape at double speed. Playback time is half that of the original lecture.

In the MA system, all catheters are continuously sampled at 240 ml/min, and when the patient whose sample is to be analyzed is connected (via the motorized rotary valve) to the analyzer, the gas is drawn into the analyzer (past the molecular inlet leak) also at 240 ml/min. In the MA system, because the sampling and the analysis rates are equal, the capnogram and respiratory rate can be displayed in real time. In the basic SARA system, however, because the sampling and analysis rates differ, respiratory rate the is not displayed and a real-time capnogram is not available.

In a shared system, the gas from each sampling location is directed in sequence by the valve system to the mass spectrometer for analysis. The time between analyses at any particular location therefore depends on (1) the number of breaths analyzed from each sampling location (i.e., dwell time); (2) the number of sampling locations in use; (3) the priority settings; and (4) in the case of "stat" samples, the distance between sampling locations and the analyzer.

Dwell time

The dwell time is the time that the analyzer spends analyzing the gas from a specific sampling location. It therefore depends on the algorithm for breath detection and on the patient's respiratory rate. The SARA system determines breaths by measuring maximum and minimum carbon dioxide levels. Inspiration is defined at the minimum carbon dioxide level, and the values of all other gases are then determined. Increases in carbon dioxide levels are followed until a plateau is reached, at which point end-expired values are recognized and determined. The MA system detects breaths when certain dynamic carbon dioxide thresholds are crossed by the carbon dioxide level in the sampled gas. Both the SARA and MA mass spectrometry systems are usually configured to detect two breaths before they automatically switch to the next sampling location. Thus for the MA system, if the respiratory rate were 12 per minute, the dwell time for two breaths would be about 10 seconds. If the rate were slower, dwell time would be longer because analysis occurs in real time. With 20 locations on line, it may take 5 or more minutes (30 × 10 seconds) before data are updated at any one sampling location. For the SARA system, because analysis is performed at twice the usual gas sampling rate, two breaths are detected and analyzed in half the time the MA system would take, and so data on individual patients are more frequently updated. Thus the dwell time of the MA system is longer than that of the SARA system. The MA system, however, allows the user to vary the dwell time for each sampling location according to the number of breaths to be detected or by setting a dwell time limit. Both the MA and SARA systems use a central computer or microprocessor to transmit data to the screen display units at each patient's bedside. A keypad system on or by the screen permits entry of commands, patient data, and alarm limits. A central printer is usually provided for the creation of a permanent record of the data stored during the time the patient was being monitored.

Priority settings enable the anesthesiologist to obtain a "stat" gas analysis for a patient. In the stat mode, the electronic multiplexing valve system is commanded to sample from the stat location, usually for a period of 30 seconds, although this period may be varied by the user. Frequent use of this mode will obviously delay updating of information at the other sampling locations. The systems can also be programmed to sample certain locations more frequently than others. Thus a Neuroscan package (available with the SARA system) permits the sampling frequency of selected rooms (maximum of two) to be increased by 50%. This may facilitate the detection of air emboli during neurosurgery, albeit at the cost of less frequent gas analysis at other sampling locations. This is partially offset by the shorter dwell time and more frequent scanning of all locations by the SARA as compared with the MA system. In the case of a stat analysis command, there is a time delay between the command and the display of data pertaining to the gas composition sampled from the circuit at that moment. This delay is, to some extent, a function of the distance between the sampling location and the central analyzer unit.

Applications of gas analysis in the operating room

The mass spectrometer represents a fairly comprehensive gas analysis system for the OR. Before other types of monitors are discussed, some of the potential applications and limitations of the available mass spectrometry systems are briefly reviewed. The two multiplexed mass spectrometry systems described (MA and SARA) display the inspired and end-tidal concentrations of the gases analyzed either in volumes percent or in mm Hg. They also display a carbon dioxide waveform (capnogram) in real time (MA system) or simulated (basic SARA system). Trends of inspired and end-expired concentrations and their differences (inspired minus expired) are available for all gases. In addition, the MA system displays the respiratory rate.

Carbon dioxide. Capnometry and capnography are discussed in detail in Chapter 10, but some important and some additional considerations are discussed in this section. The continuous measurement of carbon dioxide (capnometry) permits the identification of inspiration and expiration as well as display of the carbon dioxide waveform (capnogram). When carbon dioxide is at a minimum, inspiration is identified and the composition of the inspired gas mixture is determined. When carbon dioxide is at a maximum, end-expiration is identified and the composition of end-tidal (alveolar) gas is determined. An increase in inspired carbon dioxide may be due to addition of carbon dioxide to the circuit from a carbon dioxide flowmeter on the machine; it may be due to rebreathing, such as caused

by exhausted soda lime or a malfunctioning unidirectional valve; or it may be artifactual.

End-expired or end-tidal carbon dioxide ($PE'CO_2$) is a valuable monitor of delivery to, and removal of, carbon dioxide in the lungs. If ventilation and perfusion are well matched ($V/Q = 1.0$), end-expired carbon dioxide approximates arterial carbon dioxide ($PaCO_2$). In the presence of constant ventilation, $PE'CO_2$ decreases when perfusion to the lungs is decreased, as may occur in shock, low-cardiac output states, pulmonary embolism, air embolism, and cardiac arrest. In such cases, $PaCO_2$ increases in association with a sudden decrease in $PE'CO_2$. Changes in gas exchange result in a more gradual decrease in $PE'CO_2$. Such changes may be due to atelectasis, pneumothorax, and endobronchial intubation. An increase in alveolar ventilation associated with normal V/Q ratios will result in a decreased $PE'CO_2$ in association with decreased $PaCO_2$. Low $PaCO_2$ is also associated with hypothermia and decreased carbon dioxide production.

Increases in $PE'CO_2$ together with increases in $PaCO_2$ are associated with decreases in alveolar ventilation, increased carbon dioxide production (e.g., malignant hyperthermia or convulsions), increased transport of carbon dioxide to the lungs (such as after cardiopulmonary resuscitation), following the administration of bicarbonate, following tourniquet release, or after insufflation of carbon dioxide (laparoscopy). Obstruction to ventilation (e.g., a kinked tracheal tube or bronchospasm) may cause carbon dioxide retention and an increase in $PE'CO_2$. Such causes should be diagnosable from the capnogram. Perhaps the most common use of $PE'CO_2$ is in evaluating the adequacy of ventilation, although the value of this is limited in situations of abnormal V/Q. Monitoring of $PE'CO_2$ and visualization of the capnogram over a 30-second (stat) period can allow immediate identification of esophageal intubation,[5,6] circuit disconnects, tracheal tube obstructions, and ventilator failure. Failure to detect a carbon dioxide waveform within a certain time period during a room scan leads to annunciation of an audible alarm, alerting that no breath has been detected.

End-tidal carbon dioxide ($PE'CO_2$) should not be confused with mixed-expired carbon dioxide ($P\bar{E}CO_2$).[7] The latter represents the *average* concentration of carbon dioxide in the total of the expired gas volume collected over a period of time. Mixed expired gas is composed of both dead space and alveolar gas. End-tidal carbon dioxide usually represents alveolar carbon dioxide ($PACO_2$). Calculation of the ratio of physiologic dead space to tidal volume using the Bohr equation requires a knowledge of mixed expired carbon dioxide. Thus $V_D/V_T = [(PaCO_2 - P\bar{E}CO_2)/PaCO_2]$. Use of $PE'CO_2$ in place of $P\bar{E}CO_2$ results in an estimation of the alveolar dead space, which is but one component of the physiologic dead space.[7]

The inspired carbon dioxide ($PICO_2$) in the anesthesia circuit is normally zero. Detection of carbon dioxide in the inspired gas raises the possibility of accidental administration of carbon dioxide rebreathing due to exhausted soda lime, a unidirectional valve stuck in the open position, miscalibration of the capnograph, or some other problem that requires identification.

An increased $PICO_2$ value may also occur artifactually at rapid respiratory rates and represents a limitation of the frequency response of the sampling system. When respiratory rates exceed about 30/min, there is a tendency for the breaths, which are stored in the catheter between the patient sampling port and the central mass spectrometer unit, to "smear" into one another. As a result, the inspired carbon dioxide appears greater than actual (should be zero) and the end-expired carbon dioxide is less than actual. The size of the error is directly related to respiratory frequency and to the length of the sampling catheter.[8] It has been suggested that for critical situations in which respiratory rates exceed 40/min, a shared mass spectrometer may not be adequate for the measurement of carbon dioxide because of the errors introduced by long sampling catheters. In cases of doubt, arterial blood should be analyzed for $PaCO_2$.[8]

Oxygen. The monitoring of inspired oxygen helps ensure that the oxygen delivery system is adequate. All anesthesia delivery systems should, however, have a separate and continuous monitor of oxygen in addition to the intermittent monitoring that may be provided by a multiplexed mass spectrometer. These analyzers are discussed in a subsequent section.

The mass spectrometer measures and displays inspired and end-tidal oxygen concentrations. It has been suggested that monitoring of FIO_2 and $FE'O_2$ permits estimation of metabolic rate or oxygen consumption ($\dot{V}O_2$) of the patient, and that $\dot{V}O_2 = \dot{V}_{exp} \times (FIO_2 - FE'O_2)$, where $\dot{V}_{exp}$ is the expired minute volume read from the spirometer in the expiratory limb of the anesthesia circle, and FIO_2 (inspired oxygen) and $FE'O_2$ (end-tidal oxygen) (or %) are obtained from the mass spectrometer. Such an approach does not provide an accurate estimate of $\dot{V}O_2$ for the following reason. Minute oxygen uptake by the lungs is given by

$$\dot{V}O_2 = (\dot{V}_{insp} \times FIO_2) - (\dot{V}_{exp} \times FEO_2),$$

where $\dot{V}_{insp}$ is the inspired minute volume and FIO_2 is the inspired oxygen fraction; therefore, $\dot{V}_{insp} \times FIO_2$) is the total amount of oxygen entering the lungs per minute. $\dot{V}_{exp}$ is the expired minute volume and FEO_2 is the *mixed expired* oxygen fraction; therefore $\dot{V}_{exp} \times FEO_2$) is the total amount of oxygen leaving the lungs per minute. The volumes $\dot{V}_{insp}$ and $\dot{V}_{exp}$ are not identical, and FEO_2 is not the same as $FE'O_2$. For similar reasons, $\dot{V}CO_2$ cannot be accurately estimated from $FICO_2$ and $FE'CO_2$ as displayed by the mass spectrometer. Nevertheless, calculations of $\dot{V}_{exp} \times (FIO_2 - FE'O_2)$ and $\dot{V}_{exp} \times (FE'CO_2 - FICO_2)$ are an interesting exercise and may be of some value in terms of following trends.[9]

Nitrogen. The mass spectrometer measures and displays inspired and end-tidal nitrogen. Monitoring of end-tidal nitrogen is useful in ensuring denitrogenation prior to a rapid sequence induction of anesthesia. In a patient who has been denitrogenated, detection of nitrogen in end-tidal ($E'N_2$) gas is a sensitive means for detecting air entering the cardiorespiratory system. Sources of air embolism include open veins during pelvic, thoracic, and intracranial surgery, the latter particularly in the sitting position. The monitoring of $E'N_2$ is as sensitive as the precordial Doppler in detecting air embolism (0.1 ml/kg).[10] Detection of $E'N_2$ is a useful way of confirming air embolism that has otherwise been suspected because of a decrease in $E'CO_2$. By way of $E'N_2$, estimations have been made of the size of the air embolus.[11] Detection of any inspired nitrogen in the circuit of a denitrogenated patient usually indicates an equipment fault causing an air leak either into the anesthesia system or into the mass spectrometry sampling system itself.

Potent inhaled agents. Mass spectrometry permits the monitoring of the three potent agents halothane, enflurane, and isoflurane simultaneously and in the presence of one another. New agents, such as sevoflurane and desflurane, can be added if desired. Monitoring inspired and end-tidal halothane, enflurane, or isoflurane is useful in determining uptake of anesthetic agent, establishment of a steady state ($FI = FE'$), and washout of the agent. Knowledge of end-tidal agent concentration may permit more rapid awakening of the patient and aid in the diagnosis of postoperative apneas.

Vaporizer function and content can be checked. Thus, accuracy of vaporizer calibrations and outputs can be determined by sampling from the common gas outlet of the anesthesia machine (closest convenient sampling point to the vaporizer output). Obviously, when gas is sampled from this site no capnogram will be detected, so that selection of a special analysis or real-time mode on the mass spectrometer may be required in order to perform this function. If a vaporizer contains more than one agent (halothane, enflurane, or isoflurane, all agents will be detected and quantified.

Erroneous readings for the potent inhaled agents have been reported in association with aerosol propellants used to nebulize beta-adrenergic agonist drugs (e.g., albuterol) being introduced into the airway for the treatment of bronchospasm. The aerosol propellants contain fluorocarbons, which are "cracked" and ionized by the electron beam in the mass spectrometer. These ions are detected by the isoflurane collector in the MA system, giving rise to erroneously high reported levels of isoflurane. The SARA system displays an erroneously high enflurane level. Although the clinician should have an awareness of these potential artifacts, they are generally of very short duration, usually affecting only one breath.[12,13,14]

As has been described for carbon dioxide, at high respiratory frequencies and use of long sampling catheters, the inspired and expired concentrations of the potent inhaled agents reported by the mass spectrometer may also be erroneous. This phenomenon has been described for halothane at respiratory rates greater than 32/min.[15]

Limitations

When shared mass spectrometry systems were first introduced, it was suggested that the costs would be justified if (1) patient safety were enhanced; (2) closed circuit anesthesia systems could be used routinely, decreasing the cost of anesthetic gases; (3) resident education would be improved; and (4) clinical research on anesthetized patients would be facilitated.[1]

Safety. All of the functions of a multiplexed mass spectrometry system can now be provided by other dedicated monitors, as described in subsequent sections of this chapter. Certainly the mass spectrometer cannot replace a continuous oxygen monitor or a circuit low-pressure or volume alarm. In October, 1986, the American Society of Anesthesiologists (ASA) approved Standards for Basic Intraoperative Monitoring (last updated in October, 1991). The Standards are not fulfilled by a shared mass spectrometry system; nor is such a system required by the Standards. Although there are reports of life-threatening situations having been detected by mass spectrometers, to date no large study has demonstrated an actual increase in safety by use of this monitoring modality. One small study[16] has attempted to define the clinical utility of mass spectrometry. In this study, 339 patients were monitored by a Perkin Elmer Advantage 1100 System.* In half of the cases the anesthesiologists were blinded to the gas analysis data, but in the other half the anesthesiologists were given access to the data. In all cases, the mass spectrometry patient data were collected in a computer. Certain error and gross error limits for the inspired and end-expired gas values were entered into the computer, and the numbers and types of errors and gross errors in each group were determined. The results showed no significant differences between the two groups in the number of errors or gross errors for carbon dioxide, nitrogen, or inhaled anesthetics, and the anesthesiologists who were blinded to the data missed no major clinical events.

Cooper, et al.[17] have analyzed a total of 1089 descriptions of preventable critical incidents occurring during anesthesia, of which 70 resulted in a substantive negative outcome (SNO), ranging from extended hospital stays and permanent patient damage to death. The 70 incidents with SNO were subdivided into technical (28), judgmental (23), monitoring/vigilance (13), and other (6 equipment failure, monitoring error). Jameson[18] has further analyzed the subgroups and suggested that 36/70 (or 51.5%) of incidents with SNO would have been detectable by frequent mass spectrometry monitoring.

*Perkin-Elmer, Pomona, Calif. This division of Perkin-Elmer is now owned by the Marquette Gas Analysis Corp., and the new Advantage systems carry the brand name of Marquette.

Clearly, a major limitation of the multiplexed systems is that they are shared. Although this may help to reduce the cost, it also limits the frequency of respiratory gas analyses for each patient. In response to this, and considering that continuous monitoring of carbon dioxide is of greatest interest and importance and in many locales is now mandated, the manufacturers of the shared systems made available as relatively inexpensive add-on options, infrared continuous detection systems for carbon dioxide, which are placed in series between the patient capillary sampling tube and the headwall adapter at each sampling location. As gas is continuously being sampled from all the patients (at 120 or 240 ml/min) the in-line carbon dioxide detector provides a continuous qualitative indication of the presence of carbon dioxide. These detectors (Lifewatch in the MA system and Precheck in the SARA system) relay their information back to the bedside patient monitor. In the Lifewatch system, the central mass spectrometer provides carbon dioxide calibration points to the infrared analyzer, which can then give a quantitative estimation of carbon dioxide and respiratory rate as well as a real-time calibrated capnogram. The most recent version of Lifewatch for the MA system is Lifewatch Plus. This version incorporates new software that enables capnometry (i.e., measurement of PCO_2) as well as capnography independent of the main mass spectrometry unit. Other modifications include clips to stabilize the measurement cuvette within the unit and mounting of the Lifewatch Plus unit on the rear of the main display unit. These modifications are designed to improve the reliability of these infrared units.

The latest version of the MA system is the MGApc, which incorporates a disc drive for data storage and a paramagnetic rapid-response oxygen analyzer. The system also features an autostart function, which automatically turns on the monitor in the sampling location upon the detection of a few breaths. If no breaths are detected for a full 5-minute period, implying that no patient is connected to the system, that sampling location automatically shuts down. This MA system samples circuit gas at a rate of approximately 340 ml/min. Of this, 240 ml/min are directed via Lifewatch Plus to the mass spectrometer analyzer unit and 100 ml/min are directed to a paramagnetic oxygen analyzer in the display unit.

The SARA CAP PLUS system is a combination of a free-standing continuous carbon dioxide and nitrous oxide infrared gas analyzer together with a galvanic cell oxygen analyzer, which interfaces with the SARA mass spectrometry system for subsequent analysis of carbon dioxide, nitrous oxide, oxygen, nitrogen, halothane, enflurane, and isoflurane. Thus the problems of the basic shared system have been addressed, in part, by the addition of dedicated infrared and oxygen analyzers to the display units at the patient bedside.

In the SARA CAP PLUS system gas in the patient circuit is sampled normally at a rate of 200 ml/min, of which

100 ml/min passes to the mass spectrometer sampling system and 100 ml/min to the infrared system for continuous capnography. When the sampling location is connected via the multiplexing valve system to the mass spectrometer analyzer for gas analysis, the sampling rate increases by 100 ml/min to 300 ml/min. This permits a flow of 200 ml/min to the mass spectrometer analyzer unit while maintaining the flow of 100 ml/min to the infrared system.

Some large facilities have two mass spectrometry systems installed, each one serving half of the total number of ORs. In the event that one system fails, the deprived ORs can be connected to the remaining functioning mass spectrometry system. This facilitates continued monitoring during failure of one unit.[19]

Cost. In theory the cost of a shared mass spectrometry system would be offset to some extent by the use of low-flow anesthesia systems. Because the mass spectrometer samples circuit gas at 120 to 240 ml/min (even more in the more recent, modified systems), its use may be limited in closed circuit anesthesia. In low-flow situations, fresh gas flow should be increased to satisfy the additional sampling requirements of the mass spectrometer. Gas sampled by a multiplexed mass spectrometer system obviously cannot be returned to the patient circuit. The multiplexed mass spectrometer may also be of limited value in pediatric situations, where very small tidal volumes are being used.[20] In such situations, artifactual capnograms may be obtained, depending on the type of circuit and the gas sampling location used. The most accurate capnogram is obtained with a sampling point as close to the patient as possible. (See also Chapter 26.)

Education. Although it has not been documented as producing changes in resident education, the gas analysis information provided by the mass spectrometer certainly lends itself to educational applications and an appreciation of the scientific basis of anesthesia practice.

Research. Mass spectrometry systems, and now other technologies for gas analysis, facilitate clinical research, as evidenced by the frequency of their use in many recently reported studies. In this respect, as in its patient care role, regular calibration and servicing are essential to avoid failures and erroneous data.

Dedicated (stand-alone) mass spectrometry systems

Stand-alone mass spectrometers have been developed (Ohmeda 6000, Masstron Specmate, Paradygm Solo) for dedicated use for one patient, rather than sharing a multiplexed system. The Ohmeda 6000 Multigas Analyzer* is a quadrupole filter type of mass spectrometer. It works on the principle that a controlled electrostatic field can prevent all but a narrow range with regard to mass/charge ratio of charged particles (ions) from reaching a target. An

*Ohmeda, Madison, Wis.

electrostatic field is created by four electrically conducting parallel rods. Opposite pairs of surfaces are connected. To the two pairs of rods are applied equal but opposite potentials, each of which has direct current (DC) and radiofrequency voltage components. Gas enters the unit and is ionized, and the ions are injected down the longitudinal axis between the four rods. In their course the ions are exposed to oscillating electrostatic fields so that when the voltages applied across the rods are varied, only ions of selected mass/charge ratio reach the target at the end of the quadrupole chamber. The number of hits on the collector is detected for each ion mass/charge ratio or species sought and apportioned to indicate the composition of the gas sample analyzed. This cycle of filtering out all but one mass/charge ratio of ion and then measuring its abundance is repeated until each component of the mixture of gases has been analyzed. The process occurs so rapidly as to appear almost instantaneous, and the response times of this type of analyzer are almost identical to those of the magnetic sector units. In the Ohmeda 6000 unit, the gas sampling rate is fixed at 30 ml/min. One potential advantage of a quadrupole system is that it can be adapted to measure new or additional agents by changes in software only.

The lower gas sampling rate of the Ohmeda 6000 (30 ml/min) may better facilitate its use for pediatric patients and with low-flow anesthesia. The Ohmeda unit is a dedicated analyzer made to be used continuously with one patient, and thus it provides information that would be only intermittently available from the shared systems. Although many of these units are in service, this analyzer is no longer in production. The two other stand-alone mass spectrometers (Masstron Specmate and Paradygm Solo) were displayed at national meetings but have never been marketed.

INFRARED ANALYZERS

Measuring energy absorbed from a narrow band of wavelengths of infrared light passing through a gas sample is called infrared spectroscopy. Carbon dioxide, nitrous oxide, water, and potent volatile anesthetic agents absorb infrared energy when their atoms rotate or vibrate asymmetrically, resulting in a change in dipole moment (i.e., the charge disribution within the molecule). The nonpolar molecules argon, nitrogen, helium, xenon, and oxygen do not absorb infrared energy. Because the number of molecules in the path of the infrared energy determines the total absorption, infrared analyzers measure the partial pressure of a gas.

The respiratory and anesthetic gases exhibit absorption of infrared radiation at unique bands in the spectrum (Fig. 8-2). Carbon dioxide absorbs strongly between 4.2 and 4.4 μm. Nitrous oxide absorbs strongly between 4.4 and 4.6 μm and less strongly at 3.9 μm. Anesthetic agents have strong absorption bands at 3.3 μm and throughout the

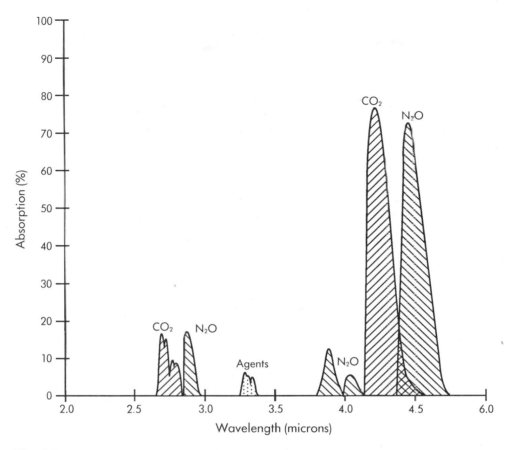

Fig. 8-2. Absorption bands of respiratory gases in the infrared spectrum. (From Raemer DB: *Monitoring respiratory function.* In Rogers MC, Tinker JH, Covino BG, Longnecker DE, editors: *Principles and practice of anesthesiology,* St. Louis, 1992, Mosby–Year Book.)

range 9 to 12 μm. Because of the proximity of the nitrous oxide and carbon dioxide absorption bands, some carbon dioxide analyzers are affected by high concentrations of nitrous oxide.[21]

A separate phenomenon, called collision broadening, may affect infrared analyzer measurements. Molecular collisions result in a change in the dipole moment of the gas being analyzed. Thus the infrared absorption band is broadened and the apparent absorption at the measurement wavelength is altered.[22] In a typical infrared carbon dioxide analyzer, 95% oxygen causes a 0.5% decline in the measured carbon dioxide. Nitrous oxide causes a more substantial increase of about 0.1% carbon dioxide per 10% nitrous oxide due to collision broadening. Some analyzers automatically compensate for the effect of collision broadening by measuring or estimating concentrations of interfering gases.

Figure 8-3 shows a block diagram of an infrared analyzer that consists of five systems: infrared light source, optical path, signal detector, signal processor, and gas sampler. Light sources made of tungsten wires or ceramic resistive materials heated to 1500 to 4000K emit energy over a broad wavelength range that includes the absorption spectrum of the respiratory gases. Because energy output of infrared light sources tends to drift, optical systems have been designed to stabilize the analyzers. Three common designs are distinguished by their use of single or dual infrared beams and by their use of positive or negative filtering.[23]

Single-beam positive filter

In one single-beam positive filter design, precision optical bandpass filters mounted on a wheel spinning at 40 to 250 revolutions per minute sequentially interrupt a single infrared beam. The beam retains energy at a narrow band of wavelengths during each interruption. For each gas of interest, a pair of bandpass filters are selected at an absorption peak and at a reference wavelength where relatively little absorption occurs. The chopped infrared beam then passes through a cuvette containing the sample gas. The ratio of intensity of the infrared beam for each pair of filters is proportional to the partial pressure of the gas and is

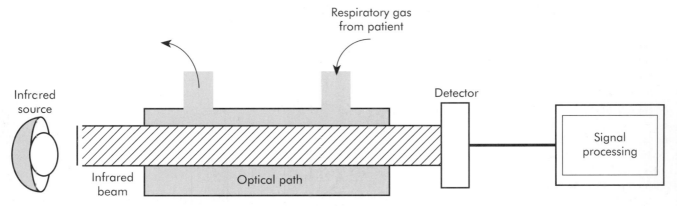

Fig. 8-3. Block diagram of an infrared respiratory gas analyzer. An infrared source emits a beam that passes through an optical path. The respiratory gas from the patient is sampled and passes through the optical path. An infrared detector filters the beam and measures the infrared wavelength absorbed by the gas sample. The electrical signal from the detector is processed to report the gas composition in mm Hg. This value can be converted (automatically) to a reading in volumes percent if the ambient pressure is known. (From Raemer DB: *Monitoring respiratory function.* In Rogers MC, Tinker JH, Covino BG, Longnecker DE, editors: *Principles and practice of anesthesiology,* St. Louis, 1992, Mosby–Year Book.)

insensitive to changes in the intensity of the infrared source.

Another single-beam positive filter design uses stationary optical filters instead of a spinning filter wheel. The pairs of filters are mounted close together within the circumference of the infrared beam. A separate infrared detector for each filter is used to measure the infrared intensity. As before, the ratio of intensity at the absorption peak and reference wavelength is used to calculate the partial pressure of each gas in the sample.

Single-beam negative filter

In the single-beam negative filter design, the filters are usually gas-filled cells mounted in a spinning wheel. During each interruption, the infrared beam retains energy at all wavelengths except those absorbed by the gas. The chopped infrared beam then passes through a cuvette containing the sample gas. Analogous to the positive filter design described previously, the ratio of infrared beam intensity for each pair of filter cells is proportional to the partial pressure of the gas and is insensitive to changes in intensity of the infrared source.

Dual-beam positive filter

In the dual-beam positive filter design, the infrared energy from the source is split into two parallel beams. One beam passes through the sample gas, and the other passes through a reference gas. A spinning blade passes through the beams and sequentially interrupts one, the other, then both. The two beams are optically focused to a single point, where a bandpass optical filter selected at the absorption peak of the gas of interest is mounted over a single detector. As before, the ratios of the intensities of the sample and reference beams are proportional to the partial pressure of the gas.

Detection of infrared radiation

For measuring carbon dioxide, nitrous oxide, and sometimes anesthetic agents, a radiation-sensitive solid state material, lead selenide, is commonly used as a detector. Lead selenide is quite sensitive to changes in temperature. Thus it is usually thermostatically cooled or temperature-compensated.[24]

Anesthetic agents, and occasionally carbon dioxide and nitrous oxide, are sometimes measured with another detector type, the Luft cell. This detector uses a chamber filled with gas that expands as infrared radiation enters the chamber and is absorbed. A flexible wall of the chamber acts as a diaphragm that moves as the gas expands, and a microphone converts the motion to an electrical signal.[25]

The signal processor converts the measured electrical currents to display gas partial pressure. First, the ratios of detector currents at various points in the spinning wheel's progress (or from multiple detectors) are computed. Next, electronic scaling and filtering are applied. Finally, linearization according to a look-up table containing the point-by-point conversion from electrical voltage to gas partial pressure is accomplished by a microprocessor. Compensation for cross-sensitivity or interference between gases can be accomplished by the microprocessor following linearization.

Infrared wavelength and agent specificity

In general, infrared analyzers must use a specific wavelength of radiation for each gas to be measured. Thus carbon dioxide is measured using a wavelength of 4.3 μm and nitrous oxide using 3.9 μm. Some agent analyzers (e.g., the Datex PB 254)[26] use a wavelength of 3.3 μm to measure the three potent inhaled anesthetics (halothane, enflurane, and isoflurane), but use of a single wavelength does not permit differentiation among these agents. When such a system is used the analyzer must be programmed by the user for the particular agent being administered. This action sets the appropriate gain in the software program, and the displayed reading will be accurate for the one agent in use. Obviously, programming such an analyzer for the wrong agent, or use of mixed agents, will lead to erroneous readings of agent concentration.

Infrared analyzers can be made to be agent-specific (i.e., have the facility to both identify and quantify mixed agents in the presence of one another) by measurement of each agent at a separate specific wavelength. The Nellcor 2500 Monitor* incorporates individual wavelength filters in the range of 9 to 11 μm for halothane, enflurane, and isoflurane to provide agent specificity. The Datex Capnomac Ultima† with agent identification uses a proprietary technology called sweeping spectrum analysis, whereby infrared absorbance in the range of 3.3 μm is continuously scanned. Although all potent agents absorb infrared radiation of wavelength 3.3 μm, continuously scanning through wavelengths from slightly above to slightly below 3.3 μm reveals that the patterns of absorbance over this narrow range differ among the agents. Sweeping spectrum analysis involves scanning 30 distinct data points on the wave pattern at a rate of 25 Hz. The information is compared with a known reference to identify the agents in use, each of which has a characteristic fingerprint, or scan. The agent is thus identified by its absorbance fingerprint and then quantified according to the amount of absorbance.

Sampling systems and infrared analysis

The principles of gas sampling systems are described at the beginning of this chapter. Main-stream capnometers locate a cuvette directly in the patient's respiratory gas stream. An infrared optical measurement device is fitted over the cuvette, which is heated to about 41° C to prevent condensation on its windows. Advantages of the main-stream monitors include convenience, no need for waste gas disposal, and no compensation needed for water vapor. Bulkiness, vibration, and fragility of the sensor are limitations of these monitors. At present, main-stream analyzers are available only for carbon dioxide. This technology is used in the Novametrix Model 1260 capnograph.‡

Side-stream instruments continuously withdraw between 50 and 500 ml/min from the breathing circuit through narrow-gauge sample tubing to the optical system, where the measurement is made. Side-stream monitors are sometimes considered more versatile than the main-stream

monitors because they can be used to measure more gas species, their tubing is less cumbersome in the breathing circuit, and fragile optical components are less exposed and vulnerable to damage. The disadvantages of side-stream monitors are a slower response time and the need to deal with liquid water and water vapor. Water vapor from the breathing circuit condenses on its way to the sample cuvette and can interfere with optical transmission. Nafion tubing, a semipermeable polymer that selectively allows water vapor to pass from its interior to the relatively dry exterior, is sometimes used to eliminate water vapor.[27] A water trap is usually interposed between the patient sampling catheter and the analyzer to protect the optical system from liquid water and body fluids.[28]

Infrared photoacoustic spectrometer

Figure 8-4 shows the photoacoustic spectrometer, which is similar to the basic infrared spectrometer. Infrared energy is passed through optical filters that select narrow-wavelength bands corresponding to the absorption characteristics of the respiratory gases. Carbon dioxide is measured at a wavelength of 4.3 μm, nitrous oxide at 3.9 μm, and the potent inhaled agents at a wavelength between 10.3 and 13.0 μm.[29] Evenly spaced windows are located along the circumference of a rotating wheel. The optical components are located astride the wheel along one of its radii. Thus a series of infrared beams pulse on and off at particular frequencies according to the rotation rate of the wheel and the spacing of the windows. The gas flowing through the measurement cuvette is exposed to the pulsed infrared beams. As each gas absorbs the pulsating infrared energy in its absorption band, it expands and contracts at that frequency. The resulting sound waves are detected with a microphone. The partial pressure of each gas in the sample is then proportional to the amplitude (or "volume") of the measured sound.

The photoacoustic technique has the distinct advantage over other infrared methods in that a simple microphone detector can be used to measure all of the infrared-absorbing gases. However, this device is sensitive to interference from loud noises and vibration. Also, because only one wavelength is used to measure the potent inhaled anesthetics (halothane, enflurane, and isoflurane), the monitor cannot distinguish among the agents and must be programmed for the one that is in use. Erroneous readings might arise in the presence of mixed anesthetic agents. This technology is used in the Brüel and Kjaer Anesthetic Gas Monitor 1304.*[30]

RAMAN SPECTROMETER

When light strikes gas molecules, most of the energy scattered is absorbed and re-emitted in the same direction and at the same wavelength as the incoming beam

*Nellcor, Inc., Hayward, Calif.
†Datex, Tewksbury, Mass.
‡Novametrix Medical Systems, Inc., Wallingford, Conn.

*Brüel and Kjaer Instruments, Marlboro, Mass.

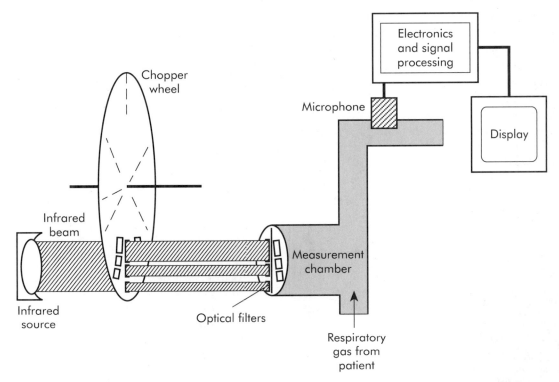

Fig. 8-4. Schematic diagram of a photoacoustic spectrometer. An infrared source emits a beam that passes through a spinning chopper wheel that has several rows of circumferential slots. The interrupted infrared beams then pass through optical filters that select specific wavelengths of light chosen to be at the absorption peaks of the gases to be measured. Each interrupted infrared light beam impinges on its respective gas in the measurement chamber, causing vibration of the gas as energy is absorbed and released from the molecules. The vibration frequency of each gas is dependent on the spacing of its slots on the chopper wheel. A microphone converts the gas vibration frequencies and amplitudes into electrical signals that are converted to the gas concentrations for display. (From Raemer DB: *Monitoring respiratory function*. In Rogers MC, Tinker JH, Covino BG, Longnecker DE, editors: *Principles and practice of anesthesiology*, St. Louis, 1992, Mosby–Year Book.)

(Rayleigh scattering).[31] At room temperature, about 1/1,000,000 of the energy is scattered at a longer wavelength, producing a so called red-shifted spectrum. This Raman scattering can be used to measure the constituents of a gas mixture. Unlike infrared spectroscopy, Raman scattering is not limited to gas species that are polar. The gases carbon dioxide, oxygen, nitrogen, water vapor, nitrous oxide, and the anesthetic agents all exhibit Raman activity. Monatomic gases such as helium, xenon, and argon, which lack intramolecular bonds, do not exhibit Raman activity.

As shown in Fig. 8-5, the medical Raman spectrometer uses a helium-neon laser (wavelength 633 nm) to produce the incoming light beam. The measurement cuvette is located in the cavity of the laser so that the gas molecules are struck repeatedly by the beam. This results in enough Raman scattering to be collected and processed by the optical detection system. Photomultiplier tubes count the scattered photons at the characteristic Raman-shifted wavelength for each gas. Thus the Raman spectrometer measures the partial pressures of the gases in its measure-

ment cuvette. Measurements are converted electronically to the desired units of measure and displayed on a screen. Raman spectroscopy is the principle of operation of the RASCAL II.*

COLORIMETRIC CARBON DIOXIDE DETECTORS

Because carbon dioxide in solution is acidic, pH-sensitive dyes can be used to detect and measure its presence. A colorimetric carbon dioxide detector (FEF END-TIDAL CO_2 DETECTOR†) is designed to be interposed between the tracheal tube and breathing circuit. Respiratory gas passes through a hydrophobic filter and a piece of filter paper that is visible through a plastic window. The detector itself consists of a piece of filter paper permeated with an aqueous solution containing metacresol purple, a pH-sensitive dye. Carbon dioxide from the expired breath dissolves

*Ohmeda, Boulder, Colo.
†Fenem, Inc., New York.

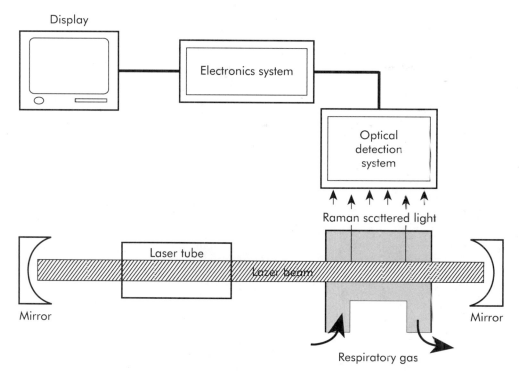

Fig. 8-5. Block diagram of a Raman scattering respiratory gas analyzer. A laser tube generates a monochromatic light beam that is contained within a cavity by mirrors. The respiratory gas from the patient is sampled and passes through the laser beam. The gas molecules scatter a small amount of light at wavelengths different from that of the incoming beam. The wavelength shift is characteristic of the gas species. The scattered light is detected, and the gas composition is computed and displayed to the user in the appropriate units of measure. (From Raemer DB: *Monitoring respiratory function.* In Rogers MC, Tinker JH, Covino BG, Longnecker DE, editors: *Principles and practice of anesthesiology,* St. Louis, 1992, Mosby–Year Book.)

in the aqueous solution, changing the color of the dye from purple to yellow. The degree of color change is dependent on the concentration of carbon dioxide. Upon inspiration of carbon dioxide–free gas, carbon dioxide leaves the solution and the color of the indicator returns to its resting (purple) state. The system is calibrated to provide an approximate indication of expired carbon dioxide concentration that can be discerned by comparison of the indicator color with a graduated color scale printed on the device's housing. This type of detector is intended to be used to confirm tracheal intubation, and one study has verified its efficacy in this regard.[32] Another study has questioned the sensitivity and rapidity of the device as a means to assess the correct placement of a tracheal tube.[33] A study in children found that this detector effectively confirms clinical signs of tracheal intubation when capnography is unavailable.[34]

WATER VAPOR AND ACCURACY OF CAPNOMETERS

Water vapor may be an important factor in the accuracy of a carbon dioxide analyzer. Most side-stream carbon di-

oxide analyzers report ambient temperature and pressure, dry (ATPD) values for PCO_2 by using Nafion* tubing to remove water vapor from the sample. Severinghaus[35] has recommended that carbon dioxide analyzers report their results at body temperature and pressure, saturated (BTPS), so that end-tidal values are close to conventionally reported alveolar gas partial pressure. The error in reporting PCO_2 at ATPD when it should be reported at BTPS is about 2.5 mm Hg.

Carbon dioxide values reported in ATPD can be converted to BTPS by decreasing the dry gas reading by the fraction $(P_{ATM} - 47)/P_{ATM}$, where P_{ATM} is the atmospheric pressure in mm Hg and 47 mm Hg is the vapor pressure of water at 37° C. A few carbon dioxide analyzers perform this conversion automatically for the user.

Main-stream analyzers naturally report readings near BTPS.[36] Depending on breathing circuit conditions, a small decrease from body temperature may result in the analyzer reading slightly less (<0.5 mm Hg) than BTPS values.

*Perma Pure, Inc., Toms River, NJ.

PIEZOELECTRIC ANALYSIS OF ANESTHETIC AGENTS

The concentration of potent inhaled anesthetics can be measured via piezoelectric crystal technology. A lipophilic coated piezoelectric quartz crystal undergoes changes in natural resonant frequency when exposed to such lipid-soluble agents as the potent inhaled anesthetics. This change in frequency is directly proportional to the partial pressure of the agent. This technology is used in the Vital Signs* analyzer and in the Biochem 8100 Anesthetic Agent Monitor.† These are side-stream or diverting analyzers. Advantages of this technology include a short warm-up time (2 minutes), better signal-to-noise ratio, and small offset drift. Disadvantages include lack of agent specificity and sensitivity to water vapor.[37]

*ICOR Ab, Bromma, Sweden.
†Biochem International, Inc., Waukesha, Wis.

OXYGEN ANALYZERS

The fraction of inspired oxygen (FIO_2) or fraction of expired oxygen (FEO_2) from an anesthesia breathing circuit is monitored with an oxygen analyzer. Three types of oxygen analyzers are in common use for monitoring: those based on (1) a polarographic sensor, (2) a fuel or galvanic cell, and (3) a paramagnetic sensor. In addition to these methods, multigas analyzers using mass spectroscopy or Raman spectroscopy measure oxygen and are sometimes used as oxygen monitors.

Polarographic sensor

The polarographic oxygen sensor (Fig. 8-6) consists of a noble-metal electrode (usually platinum) and a reference electrode in an electrolyte bath. An electrical potential difference of −0.6 to −0.8 volts is applied across the electrodes, thus polarizing them. The sensor is exposed to the breathing circuit via an oxygen-permeable membrane (usu-

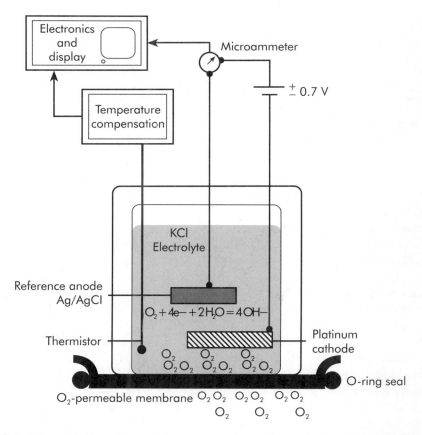

Fig. 8-6. Schematic of a polarographic oxygen analyzer. Oxygen in the gas sample permeates a teflon or polyethylene membrane and enters a potassium chloride electrolyte solution. When a potential of 0.7 volts from a battery is impressed across a platinum cathode and reference anode, current flows through the circuit in proportion to the availability of oxygen. The measured current is thus linearly related to the oxygen tension of the gas sample. Temperature compensation is required for accurate measurement. (From Raemer DB: *Monitoring respiratory function.* In Rogers MC, Tinker JH, Covino BG, Longnecker DE, editors: *Principles and practice of anesthesiology,* St. Louis, 1992, Mosby–Year Book.)

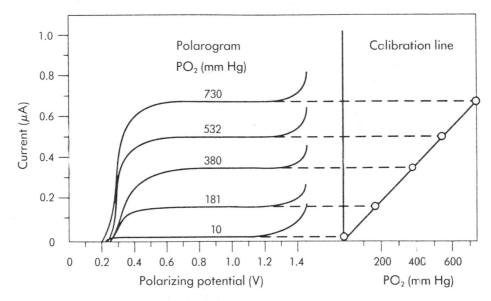

Fig. 8-7. The relationship between polarizing potential and current for different oxygen partial pressures. Within the operational range of polarization potential, the current resulting from oxygen reduction is almost linear with the supply of oxygen molecules at the electrode surface. (From Raemer DB, Philip JH: *Monitoring anesthetic and respiratory gases.* In Blitt CD, editor: *Monitoring in anesthesia and critical care medicine,* New York, 1990, Churchill-Livingstone.)

ally teflon). Oxygen molecules traverse the membrane at a rate proportional to their partial pressure in the breathing circuit. The sensor consumes the oxygen molecules according to the following two-step redox (reduction-oxidation) reaction:

$$O_2 + 2\ H_2O + 2\ e^- \rightarrow H_2O_2 + 2\ OH^-$$
$$H_2O_2 + 2\ e^- \rightarrow 2\ OH^-$$

For every molecule of oxygen reduced, four electrons are supplied by the electrical circuit. Thus, the current, having been determined by the availability of oxygen molecules, is directly proportional to the partial pressure of oxygen in the breathing circuit (Fig. 8-7). Measurement of the current and conversion to units of oxygen pressure (mm Hg) or equivalent concentration (percent) can easily be accomplished electronically and the results displayed on a digital (numeric) or analog (needle) meter.

Fuel cell

The fuel cell or galvanic cell is basically an oxygen battery consisting of a noble metal cathode and a lead anode in a potassium hydroxide electrolyte bath (Fig. 8-8). As in the polarographic electrode, an oxygen-permeable membrane is exposed to the breathing circuit. Oxygen is reduced at the cathode according to the following reaction:

$$O_2 + 2\ H_2O + 4\ e^- \rightarrow 4\ OH^-$$

The following reaction occurs at the anode:

$$2\ Pb + 6\ OH^- \rightarrow 2\ PbO_2H^- + 2\ H_2O + 4\ e^-$$

Thus, a voltage develops which is proportional to the oxy-

gen partial pressure. No polarization potential is required. The galvanic sensor voltage can be measured and electronically scaled to units of partial pressure or equivalent concentration (percent) and displayed.

Paramagnetic analyzer

The paramagnetic oxygen sensor utilizes the strong, positive magnetic susceptibility of the gaseous oxygen molecule to measure oxygen concentration. Because it has two electrons in unpaired orbits, the oxygen molecule is attracted by a magnetic field. Modern paramagnetic oxygen sensors utilize this property by measuring a pressure differential between a stream of reference gas (air) and one of the measured gas as the streams are exposed to a changing magnetic field (Fig. 8-9). An electromagnet is rapidly switched off and on, creating a changing magnetic field between its poles. The electromagnet is designed to have its poles in close proximity, forming a narrow gap. The streams of sample and reference gas have different oxygen partial pressures, and the pressure between the entrance and exit of the respective gas streams differs slightly because of the magnetic force on the oxygen molecules. A sensitive pressure transducer is used to convert this force to an electrical signal. The electrical signal can then be filtered appropriately and used to display the oxygen pressure or equivalent concentration (i.e., in percent). Paramagnetic oxygen analysis is used in the Datex Capnomac and Puritan Bennett 250 series multigas analyzers.[26]

The paramagnetic property of oxygen is also utilized in the magnetoacoustic measurement of oxygen. This technology is applied in the Brüel and Kjaer Anesthetic Gas

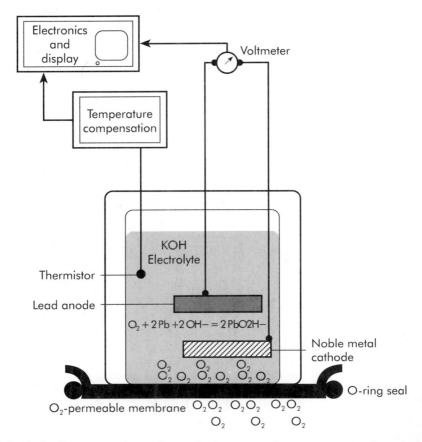

Fig. 8-8. Fuel cell oxygen analyzer. Oxygen in the gas sample permeates a membrane and enters a potassium hydroxide electrolyte solution. A potential is established between a lead anode and noble metal cathode as oxygen is supplied to the anode. The measured voltage between the electrodes is proportional to the oxygen tension of the gas sample. Temperature compensation is required for accurate measurement. (From Raemer DB: *Monitoring respiratory function.* In Rogers MC, Tinker JH, Covino BG, Longnecker DE, editors: *Principles and practice of anesthesiology,* St. Louis, 1992, Mosby–Year Book.)

Monitor Type 1304* (Fig. 8-10).[30] The gas sample containing oxygen is exposed to an alternating magnetic field. This causes the gas to expand and contract, generating a pressure wave that is proportional to the oxygen concentration. The pressure wave is detected as a sound wave by a sensitive microphone. Because the frequency of oscillation of the magnetic field differs from the three frequencies used to pulsate the infrared radiation (used by infrared-photoacoustic spectroscopy to make the measurements of carbon dioxide, nitrous oxide, and anesthetic agent), the oxygen sound signal is detected by the same microphone that is used to measure the other respired gases. The amplitude of the oxygen pressure wave gives an absolute measurement of oxygen concentration in mm Hg. In order to ensure accuracy, the measurement oxygen signal from the gas sample is compared with a reference oxygen signal. The reference oxygen signal is generated by having the sampling pump draw both patient and reference gas (room air at 10 ml/min) to unite in the same switched magnetic field (Fig. 8-10). The pressure wave due to the reference gas is detected by a separate microphone. Because the concentration of room air in the reference flow is known (21% of ambient atmospheric pressure in mm Hg), the oxygen concentration in the gas sample can be measured by comparison of the measurement signal with the reference signal.[30]

Calibration of oxygen analyzers

All oxygen analyzers require periodic calibration. Because all analyzers produce an electrical signal proportional to oxygen pressure, the constant of proportionality (gain) must be determined. Generally, the electrical signal in the presence of 0% oxygen is known to be near zero. Thus no offset correction is required. In the case of the polarographic or fuel cell analyzer, the gain changes with time because of changes in electrolyte, electrode, and membrane. The gain of the paramagnetic sensor changes with temperature, humidity, and pneumatic factors. Calibration with a known gas, either room air (21% oxygen) or 100% oxygen, before each use is practical. In some cases,

*Brüel & Kjaer, Naerum, Denmark and Marlborough, Mass.

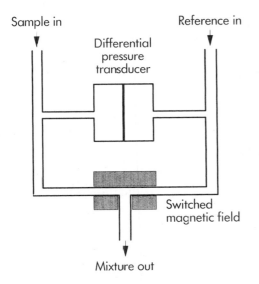

Fig. 8-9. Paramagnetic oxygen analyzer. The sample and reference gas streams converge in a rapidly changing magnetic field. Because the two streams have different oxygen tensions (i.e., different numbers of oxygen molecules) a pressure differential is created across a sensitive pressure transducer. The transducer converts this force to an electrical signal that is displayed as oxygen partial pressure or converted to a reading in volumes percent.

the oxygen analyzer performs its own periodic computer-controlled automatic calibration process.

Response time of oxygen analyzers

The response time differs among oxygen analyzers. Polarographic and fuel cell analyzers respond quite slowly to changes in oxygen pressure in the breathing circuit because of their dependence on membrane diffusion. Response times are generally on the order of 20 to 30 seconds, prohibiting breath-by-breath measurements. The TED R-15 Oxygen Sensor* is a galvanic fuel cell specified to have a 90% response time of less than 15 seconds. Some analyzers use a single fuel cell to measure inspired and expired concentration by directing the gas to the sensor with a valve. The valve is timed according to a carbon dioxide waveform to direct only inspired gas to the sensor for several sequential breaths. Then the valve is limited to direct only expired gas to the sensor for several breaths. Thus, both inspired and expired concentrations are displayed, albeit averaged over several breaths. The paramagnetic analyzer, having no membrane, can respond on a

*Teledyne Electronic Devices, City of Industry, Calif.

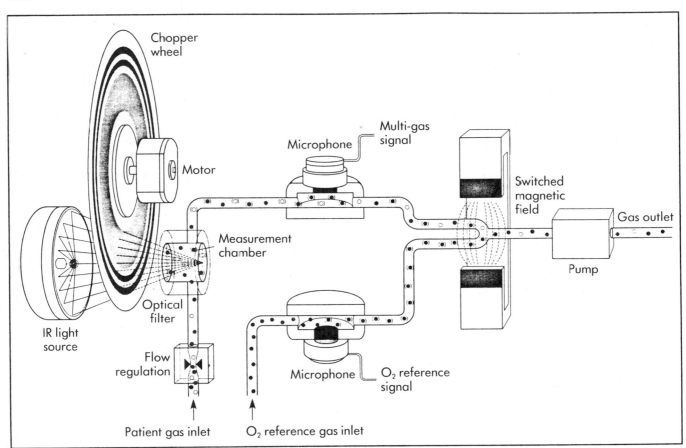

Fig. 8-10. Magnetoacoustic measurement of oxygen and photoacoustic measurement of carbon dioxide, nitrous oxide, and anesthetic agents as used in the Brüel & Kjaer Anesthetic Gas Monitor Type 1304. (Reproduced by permission of Brüel & Kjaer Instruments, Inc.. Marlborough, Mass.)

Table 8-2. Common respiratory gases and the technologies whereby they are commonly measured

Gas/Technology	O_2	CO_2	N_2O	AA	N_2	He	Ar
Mass spectroscopy	X	X	X	X	X	X	X
Raman spectroscopy	X	X	X	X	X		
IR-light spectroscopy		X	X	x*			
IR-photoacoustic		X	X	x*			
Piezoelectric resonance				X			
Polarography	X						
Fuel cell	X						
Paramagnetic	X						
Magnetoacoustic	X						

*Agent specific if at least one wavelength per anesthetic agent (AA) is used.

breath-by-breath basis. Sampling from the breathing circuit Y piece, the paramagnetic oxygen analyzer can measure both inspired and expired oxygen concentrations and display the real-time waveforms (oxygram). The magnetoacoustic oxygen analyzer has a 10% to 90% rise time of <250 msec, permitting real-time monitoring of oxygen concentration at high respiratory rates.

Respiratory gases in the anesthesia delivery system can be analyzed via a number of modern technologies, each of which is based on application of some specific physical property of the gas molecule. The analysis methods and their applications are summarized in Table 8-2. In interpreting gas analysis data, the anesthesiologist should understand the principles of how the data were obtained so that erroneous data can be identified and, if necessary, rejected.

REFERENCES

1. Ozanne GM, Young WG, Mazzei WJ, et al: Multipatient anesthetic mass spectrometry, *Anesthesiology* 55:62-70, 1981.
2. Watson JT: *Introduction to mass spectrometry,* New York, 1985, Raven Press
3. Davis WOM, Spence AA: Modification of the MGA200 mass spectrometer to enable measurement of anaesthesia gas mixtures, *Br J Anaesth* 51:987-988, 1979.
4. Siegel M, Gravenstein N: Evaluation of helium interference with mass spectrometry, *Anesth Analg* 67:887-889, 1988.
5. Sum Ping ST: Esophageal intubation, *Anesth Analg* 66:483, 1987.
6. Salzarulo HH, Leiman BC, Katz J, et al: Carbon dioxide detection and esophageal intubation, *Anesth Analg* 67:195, 1988.
7. Nunn JF: *Applied respiratory physiology,* ed 3, Boston, 1987, Butterworths.
8. Scamman FL, Fishbaugh JK: Frequency response of long mass-spectrometer sampling catheters, *Anesthesiology* 65:422-425, 1986.
9. Eisenkraft JB, Neustein SM, et al: Estimation of $\dot{V}o_2$ during aortic cross clamping: Mass spectrometry versus Fick. Paper presented at the Society of Cardiovascular Anesthesiologists annual meeting, San Antonio, Texas, May 1991 (abstract).
10. Matjasko MJ, Petrozza P, Mackenzie CF: Sensitivity of end-tidal nitrogen in venous air embolism detection in dogs, *Anesthesiology* 63:418-423, 1985.
11. Severinghaus JW: Air embolism detected by mass spectrometry. Paper presented at McGill University Annual Review Course in Anesthesiology, June 1982.

12. Gravenstein N, Theisen GJ, Knudsen AK: Misleading mass spectrometer reading caused by an aerosol propellant, *Anesthesiology* 62:70-72, 1985.
13. Elliot WR, Raemer DB, Goldman DB, et al: The effects of bronchodilator-inhaler aerosol propellants on respiratory gas monitors, *J Clin Monit* 7:175-180, 1991.
14. Kharasch ED, Silvarajan M: Aerosol propellant interference with clinical mass spectrometers, *J Clin Monit* 7:172-174, 1991.
15. Scamman FL: High frequency response of a central mass spectrometer system to halothane, *Anesthesiology* 67:A174, 1987 (abstract).
16. Guffin AV, Shamsi A, Marlar K, et al: Clinical utility of respiratory gas, monitoring by mass spectrometry, *Anesthesiology* 67:A174, 1987 (abstract).
17. Cooper JB, Newbower RS, Kitz RJ: An analysis of major errors and equipment failures in anesthesia management, *Anesthesiology* 60:34-42, 1984.
18. Jameson LC: *Applications of mass spectrometry: ASA refresher course No 226,* Park Ridge, Ill, 1986, American Society of Anesthesiologists.
19. Steinbrook RA, Elliott WR, Goldman DB, et al: Linking mass spectrometers to provide continuing monitoring during system failure, *J Clin Monit* 7:271-273, 1991.
20. Sasse FJ: Can we trust end-tidal carbon dioxide measurement in infants? *J Clin Monit* 1:147-148, 1985 (editorial).
21. Severinghaus JW, Larson CP, Eger EI: Correction factors for infrared carbon dioxide pressure broadening by nitrogen, nitrous oxide, and cyclopropane, *Anesthesiology* 22:429-432, 1961.
22. Nielsen JR, Thornton V, Dale EB: The absorption laws for gases in the infrared, *Reviews of Modern Physics* 16:307-324, 1944.
23. Raemer DB, Philip JH: *Monitoring anesthetic and respiratory gases.* In Blitt CD: *Monitoring in anesthesia and critical care medicine,* New York, 1990, Churchill-Livingstone, pp 373-386.
24. Hudson RD Jr: *Infrared system engineering,* New York, 1969, Wiley, pp 264-303.
25. Luft K: Uber eine neue methode der registrierenden gasanalyse mit hilfe der absorbtion ultratoter strahlen ohne spektrale zerlegnung, *Z Techn Phys* 24:97, 1943.
26. *PB 254 Owners Manual,* Wilmington, Mass, 1985, Puritan-Bennett Corp.
27. Kertzman J: Paper 73425, Instrument Society of America, Analytical Instrumentation Division, 121, 1973.
28. Evaluation: carbon dioxide monitors, *ECRI Health Dev* 15:255-271, 1986.
29. Møllgaard K: Acoustic gas measurement, *Biomedical Instrumentation and Technology* 23:495-497, 1989.
30. *Anesthetic Gas Monitor 1304: product data.* Marlborough, Mass, 1989 Brüel & Kjaer Instruments.
31. Westenskow DR, Smith KW, Coleman DL, et al: Clinical evaluation of a Raman scattering multiple gas analyzer for the operating room, *Anesthesiology* 70:350-355, 1989.
32. Goldberg JS, Rawle RP, Zehnder JL, et al: Colorimetric end-tidal carbon dioxide monitoring for tracheal intubation, *Anesth Analg* 70:191-194, 1990.
33. Sum Ping ST, Mehta MP, Symreng T: Accuracy of the FEF CO_2 detector in the assessment of endotracheal tube placement, *Anesth Analg* 74:415-419, 1992.
34. Kelly JS, Wilhoit RD, Brown RE, et al: Efficacy of the FEF colorimetric end-tidal carbon dioxide detector in children, *Anesth Analg* 75:45-50, 1992.
35. Severinghaus JW: Water vapor calibration errors in some capnometers: respiratory conventions misunderstood by manufacturers? *Anesthesiology* 70:996-998, 1989.
36. Raemer DB, Calalang I: Accuracy of end-tidal carbon dioxide tension analyzers, *J Clin Monit* 7:195-208, 1991.
37. Westenskow DR, Silva FH: Laboratory evaluation of the vital signs (ICOR) piezoelectric anesthetic agent analyzer, *J Clin Monit* 7:189-194, 1991.

Chapter 9

MONITORING VENTILATION

Daniel B. Raemer, Ph.D.

Safe and effective management of the respiratory system during anesthesia requires substantial monitoring. The modalities for monitoring ventilation include arterial blood gas analysis; respiratory gas analysis; oximetry; and pressure, flow, and volume measurement. This chapter deals with pressure, flow, and volume measurement in relation to respired gases only; the other modalities are discussed elsewhere (see Chapters 8, 11 and 16).

In this chapter, first, the clinical implications of pressure, flow, and volume measurement during anesthesia are discussed. Second, the physics of gases are reviewed in order to explain the principles of operation and the limitations of instruments used to measure pressure and flow. Third, the specific devices used for these measurements are described.

CLINICAL IMPLICATIONS

Monitoring pressure and volume of the respiratory system during anesthesia is an important component of the efficacious management of ventilation. The utility of this monitoring is threefold. First, the safety of ventilation is enhanced. Second, setting and verifying appropriate ventilatory parameters to achieve effective gas exchange is as-

sisted. Finally, the mechanics of the respiratory system may be appreciated.

Safety of ventilation

Measurement of airway pressure and gas flow can detect many mishaps in the breathing circuit, including leaks, disconnections, and obstructions. A pressure manometer, either mechanical or electromechanical, is generally used to measure breathing circuit pressure and is often capable of detecting ventilatory mishaps. During positive-pressure ventilation, peak inspiratory pressure (PIP) usually exceeds 15 cm H_2O and sometimes reaches 60 cm H_2O depending on several factors, including the breathing circuit compliance, airway resistance (mostly in the tracheal tube adapter), the patient's total thoracic compliance, the ventilator's driving pressure, and the location of the sensing site in the circuit.[1] Nonetheless, a complete disconnection in the breathing circuit usually causes a loss of the positive-pressure swings, and the pressure gauge will show greatly diminished or absent peak pressures. Similarly, the breathing circuit can be obstructed by foreign bodies,[2] as well as by mucous plugs, blood, or other substances produced by the patient. Obstructions can also be caused by kinking of the expiratory tubing,[3] faults in the anesthesia machine,[4,5] or manufacturing defects in the breathing circuit system.[6,7] Misplacement of free-standing one-way valves—for example, positive end-expiratory pressure (PEEP) valves not specifically designed for and built into the breathing circuit—can also obstruct the breathing circuit, and they should be used with caution.[8] Observed changes in breathing circuit pressure depend on the location of the pressure monitor tap, the location of the obstruction, and the mode of ventilation. When the pressure monitor tap is located on the ventilator side of an inspiratory obstruction, the manometer will display high peak pressure in the breathing circuit, up to the capability of the ventilator. The manometer pressure returns to baseline during the expiratory phase. Note that the maximum pressure deliverable by anesthesia ventilators is limited to between 55 cm H_2O and 120 cm H_2O.[9] If the obstruction is located on the expiratory limb of the breathing circuit, the result is a stepwise increase in pressure with each inspiration, up to the pressure capability of the ventilator. The manometer's gauge pressure will not return to baseline during the expiratory phase (see also Chapter 16).

A respiratory gas-flow or volume meter in an anesthesia breathing circuit can also be an excellent detector of ventilation mishaps. Generally, flow or volume diminishes in the face of a circuit leak, disconnection, or obstruction. The readings of the flowmeter depend on its location relative to the problem, the degree of obstruction or disconnection, the mode of ventilation, and the presence or absence of patient respiratory efforts.

Effective gas exchange

The delivery of gas to and from the patient should be monitored to ensure adequate lung expansion, oxygen delivery, and carbon dioxide elimination. Inspired gas volume expands the lung and prevents closure of airways (atelectasis) and shunting;[10] fills the mechanical, anatomic, and alveolar dead spaces; compensates for gas compression and distension of the breathing circuit; delivers oxygen to the alveolar space to meet the metabolic demands of the patient; and, during expiration, must be adequate to eliminate the carbon dioxide produced by metabolism.

During anesthesia, anatomic and alveolar dead spaces, which increase with age, may represent one third to one half of tidal volume.[11] In an adult, the anatomic dead space is normally about 170 ml and includes the pharynx, trachea, and major conducting airways. When a patient has undergone tracheal intubation, all of the pharyngeal volume and most of the tracheal volume are bypassed, thereby reducing the anatomic dead space to about 130 ml.[12] Alternatively, a face mask adds approximately 100 ml to the dead space.[13] Typically, the loss of volume due to compression and circuit distension is about 150 ml.[1] In the extreme, a rubber circle breathing circuit for an adult, including a heated humidifier with a PIP of 50 cm H_2O, can have a compression and compliance volume of ap-

proximately 700 ml.[14] The average resting metabolic oxygen consumption of an adult male is about 3.3 ml/kg/min.[15] During general anesthesia with muscle relaxation and surgery, this value is reduced to an estimated 85% of basal oxygen consumption (2.8 ml/kg/min). Because the inspired gas volume essentially determines expired gas volume, either may be used to assess the adequacy of ventilation for gas exchange.

Breathing circuit pressures may be monitored to evaluate the inspired gas volume being delivered. Peak inspiratory pressure is dependent on both the resistance to flow of the breathing system and the compliance of the breathing system and thorax. Peak inspiratory pressure is generally in a range from about 5 to 40 cm H_2O. Very low PIP indicates either a very compliant breathing circuit, extremely compliant lungs, a significant leak in the system, low inspired tidal volume (V_T), or a low flow rate of fresh-gas delivery. Abnormally high PIP indicates that either the respiratory system is extremely noncompliant, the resistance in the breathing circuit or airway is increased, or inspiratory gas flow is high. In addition to PIP, an airway plateau pressure can be determined during an end-inspiratory pause. Measuring plateau pressure requires the presence of a period of zero flow during the inspiratory phase, which depends on ventilator settings (i.e., V_T, ratio of inspiratory time to expiratory time, respiratory rate). In the absence of flow, only compliance of the breathing system and the lungs, and not flow resistance, contribute to the plateau pressure. An abnormally low plateau pressure indicates that the V_T is not filling the system or that the respiratory system is very compliant. A high plateau pressure indicates that the lung or respiratory system is overfilled or unusually stiff.

Monitoring volume usually provides a reasonable estimate of alveolar ventilation; expired volume is often used to guide adjustment of the mechanical ventilator or of manual ventilation. Nominally, minute ventilation must be increased to 1.5 to 3 times the required alveolar ventilation to compensate for dead space. When a pressure-preset mechanical ventilator is used, the volume of inspired or expired respiratory gas should be measured to estimate alveolar ventilation (see also Chapter 6).

Respiratory volumes and flows are always, by convention, reported at body temperature (37° C) and barometric pressure (P_B), saturated (BTPS). When the absolute quantity of gas is of importance, such as during measurement of oxygen consumption or carbon dioxide production, measurements are reported at standard temperature and pressure, dry (STPD). In an anesthesia breathing circuit, expiratory gas is often measured at ambient temperature and pressure and is fully saturated with water vapor (ATPS). Inspired gas is usually at ambient temperature and pressure, dry (ATPD). It may be warmer and somewhat humidified, however, due to rebreathing and the heat and moisture generated from carbon dioxide absorption; if this is so, the conditions are essentially unknown during measurement. Active heated humidification of an anesthesia breathing circuit brings the gas close to BTPS conditions. If the volume or flow analyzer does not make the appropriate conversions to BTPS automatically, then the user should apply the appropriate formulas to the measured data (see the discussion of physics of gases in this chapter).

The mechanics of the respiratory system

The resistance and compliance of the respiratory system during anesthesia can be evaluated by monitoring the appropriate pressures and volumes. Three forces must be overcome to ventilate the lung[16]: First, elastic forces are developed in tissues of the lung and chest wall when a volume change occurs. Elastic forces are independent of gas flow and are thus static forces. Second, flow resistance forces occur due to fluid friction (viscosity) that develops when gas flows within airways. Flow resistive forces require gas movement and are therefore dynamic forces. Third, inertial forces depend on the mass of the tissue and gases and result when gases or tissues are accelerated. Inertial forces are generally of minor importance and are usually ignored. During spontaneous ventilation, work is performed by the respiratory muscles to overcome these static and dynamic forces. During positive-pressure ventilation, the mechanical ventilator performs the work needed to overcome these forces.

The transmural pressure across the lung, the difference between the pressure at the airway opening (P_{ao}) and the pleural pressure (P_{pl}), is known as the transpulmonary pressure (P_L). Unfortunately, direct measurement of P_{pl} is not easy. However, the esophageal pressure (P_{es}) has been shown to approximate the pleural pressure under many circumstances and can be measured with a balloon catheter.[17] The difference between P_{ao} and the ambient pressure is defined as the transrespiratory pressure (P_{trs}).

Compliance is the change in volume relative to the change in pressure. The compliance of the lung (C_L), chest wall (C_W), and respiratory system (C_{rs}) as a whole can be measured. Compliance is determined by measuring the appropriate pressure and the volume at two points when the flow is zero. Nominally, zero flow exists at end-expiration and end-inspiration. The ratio of the change in transpulmonary pressure to the change in volume between these two points in the respiratory cycle is C_L. By substituting P_{trs} for P_L in the measurement, C_{rs} can be measured. Now C_W can be determined algebraically: Because

$$\frac{1}{C_{rs}} = \frac{1}{C_L} + \frac{1}{C_W}$$

rearranging gives

$$C_W = \frac{C_L \times C_{rs}}{C_L - C_{rs}}$$

Note that in measuring compliance, it is assumed that there is no active muscular activity at the time of zero gas flow.

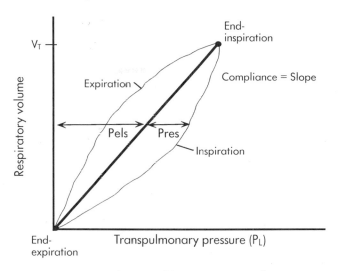

Fig. 9-1. Plot of respiratory volume versus transpulmonary pressure, P_L, during a single spontaneous breath. The inspiratory phase follows the curve on the right upward and terminates at end-inspiration, where the volume is V_T. The expiratory phase follows the left curve downward to end-expiration. The slope of the line connecting the points of zero flow, nominally end-expiration and end-inspiration, is the compliance, C_L. The pressure along this line separates the pressure due to elastic losses (P_{els}) from the pressure due to resistive losses (P_{res}).

The compliance can be used to separate the pressure responsible for elastic work (W_{el}) from that responsible for flow resistive work (W_{fr}). Figure 9-1 is a plot of volume versus P_L during a single spontaneous breath. The pressure used to overcome elastic forces is shown as P_{els}, and the pressure used to overcome flow resistive forces is shown as P_{res}. The line connecting end-inspiration and end-expiration separates these pressures and has a slope of C_L.

During anesthesia, C_{rs} is generally less than in the awake state by about 20% and is approximately 0.1 L/cm H_2O.[18] Most of this reduction is attributed to about a 50% decrease in C_L to about 0.15 L/cm H_2O.

The resistance of the respiratory system (R_L) can be determined from the measured flow and pressure. The resistance is computed as

$$R_L = \frac{P_L}{\dot{V}}$$

and the transrespiratory resistance can be determined by substituting P_{trs} for P_L in the measurement.

Generally, after induction of anesthesia and placement of a tracheal tube, R_L increases by about 50% to a value of approximately 5 cm H_2O/L/s.

The work done by the respiratory system (W_{rs}) is the sum of W_{el} and W_{fr}. Work is the product of pressure and volume; thus W_{el} can be calculated as

$$W_{el} = \frac{V_T^2}{2 \times C_L}$$

Table 9-1. Physical properties of respiratory and anesthetic gases at standard temperature and pressure (STP)

Gas or vapor	Density (kg/m³)	Viscosity (kg/m/s)
Air	1.3	171.7
Argon	1.8	213.3
Carbon dioxide	2.0	141.6
Helium	0.2	187.7
Nitrogen	1.3	168.0
Nitrous oxide	2.0	137.9
Oxygen	1.4	190.9
Water	0.8	96.8
Desflurane	7.5	
Enflurane	8.2	
Halothane	8.8	
Isoflurane	8.2	
Sevoflurane	8.9	

To determine W_{fr}, the inspiratory volume is integrated with respect to pressure and the integral is subtracted from W_{el} as follows:

$$W_{fr} = W_{el} - \int V_I \, dp$$

Work is defined as force times distance. The Système International (SI) unit of work is the joule (J), and 1 J = 1 newton (N) × 1 meter (m).

PHYSICS OF GASES

Physical properties of gases and vapors respired during anesthesia are important factors in the measurement of their pressure, volume, and flow. Under standard conditions of pressure and temperature (0° C, 1 atm pressure), the respiratory gases, oxygen, nitrogen, nitrous oxide, water vapor, air, and anesthetic vapors behave as ideal gases; they occupy 22.4 L/mole. The densities of the gases and vapors respired during anesthesia are shown in Table 9-1.

Pressure is the force resulting from the kinetic energy of a gas. The thermodynamic state of a gas can be described at any given time by the variables volume, pressure, temperature, and quantity (moles). Generally, the *Ideal Gas Law* defines this relationship:

$$P = \frac{n \times R \times T}{V}$$

where

P = Pressure in pascals (Pa). 1 kilopascal (kPa) is approximately 7.5 mm Hg)
n = Number of moles of the gas
R = Universal gas constant ($R = 8.314$ J/mole/K)
T = Temperature in Kelvin (K)
V = Volume occupied in m³.

(NOTE: The units of measure used are according to the Système International [SI]. In clinical medicine, especially in the United States, other systems of measurement are often used.) The Ideal Gas Law is a nineteenth century generalization of three earlier, well-known relationships:

1. At a constant temperature, the pressure and volume are inversely proportional to each other (*Boyle's law*).
2. At a constant pressure, the volume of a gas is directly proportional to absolute temperature (*Charles' law*).
3. At a constant volume, the pressure of a gas is directly proportional to absolute temperature (*Gay-Lussac's law*).

When two or more gases occupy the same volume, the partial pressure of a gas is the pressure exerted by a gas as if it occupied the volume by itself. Furthermore, Dalton's law states that the sum of the partial pressures of the gases in a mixture occupying the same volume equals the total pressure.

Vapor is a term that describes the gaseous state of substances that are liquids at room temperature and pressure. Vapor pressure, the pressure of the gas in equilibrium with the liquid phase of the substance, is a function only of absolute temperature. Water vapor pressure is 47 mm Hg (6.3 kPa) at 37° C and is approximately 17.5 mm Hg (2.3 kPa) at 20° C. (See also Chapters 3 and 7).

The implications for making clinical measurements of pressure and volume of respired gases follow from the Ideal Gas Law, Dalton's law, and the principle of vapor pressure. The conditions of the system (temperature and either pressure or volume) must be stated to make the measured variable useful. The following formulas are used to convert gas volume *(V)* from common conditions during measurement at ATPS to BTPS and STPD. ATPS to BTPS:

$$V_{BTPS} = V_{ATPS} \times \frac{310}{273 + T_{am}} \times \frac{P_B - P_{H_2O}}{P_B - 47}$$

BTPS to STPD:

$$V_{STPD} = V_{BTPS} \times \frac{273}{310} \times \frac{P_B - 47}{760}$$

ATPS to STPD:

$$V_{STPD} = V_{ATPS} \times \frac{273}{273 + T_{am}} \times \frac{P_B - P_{H_2O}}{760}$$

where

T_{am} = Ambient temperature in ° C
P_B = Barometric pressure in mm Hg
P_{H_2O} = Vapor pressure of water at T_{am} in mm Hg.

When nonstandard measurement conditions exist, the appropriate application of the Ideal Gas Law, Dalton's law, and a table of vapor pressure of water[19] should suffice.

When a pressure difference exists between one region and another, gas flows along that gradient. The volume of gas that flows is dependent on the viscosity of the gas. As the gas flows, intermolecular forces act tangentially to the direction of flow. In a cylindrical pipe, the intermolecular force between the pipe and the gas ensures that the velocity of the gas at the wall is zero. Away from the wall, the gas at the next molecular layer experiences friction with the layer of stationary gas. Each subsequent molecular layer away from the wall exhibits friction with adjacent layers. This friction, called the viscosity, is characterized by a parameter called the coefficient of viscosity. Viscosity of a gas increases with temperature and (slightly) with pressure. The viscosity of air increases by about 4% as the temperature increases from ambient to body temperature.[20] Table 9-1 contains nominal values for the coefficients of viscosity for the common anesthetic and respiratory gases.

The flow of a gas in a cylindrical pipe can often be considered laminar flow. The principal characteristic of laminar flow is that the velocity of gas molecules increases toward the center of the pipe. In fact, the profile of velocity is essentially parabolic (Fig. 9-2). Laminar flow in an ideal pipe is described by the Hagen-Poiseuille equation:

$$F = \frac{\pi \times r^4 \times \Delta P}{8 \times \eta \times l}$$

where

F = Flow
r = Radius of the pipe
ΔP = Pressure difference between the entry and exit of the pipe
η = Viscosity of the gas
l = Length of the pipe.

Note that the flow is directly proportional to the pressure difference.

When the flow of a gas in a pipe is disturbed so that it is no longer laminar, turbulent flow is the result. One major characteristic of fully developed turbulent flow is that the flow profile is almost flat (Fig. 9-2). That is, the velocity of the gas molecules along a slice through the pipe is about the same (except very near the walls). The effect of viscosity on the flow profile is minimal. In addition, the relationship between gas flow and the pressure difference (inlet − outlet) is a polynomial:

$$F = \frac{\Delta P^{0.5}}{A}$$

where A is a constant; A is a function of the density of the gas but must be determined empirically because it is also dependent on geometric factors. The polynomial relationship implies that under turbulent conditions, the pressure difference must be increased by a substantially greater degree to achieve an increase in flow than under laminar conditions.

The distinction of flow conditions between laminar and turbulent is complex. In general, the flow makes a transition between laminar and turbulent at a critical velocity.

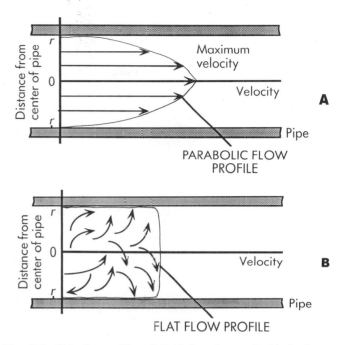

Fig. 9-2. Velocity profiles of fluid flow in a cylindrical pipe. The velocity is plotted against distance from the center of the pipe. **A,** depicts laminar flow, showing the parabolic velocity profile. **B,** depicts turbulent flow, showing the essentially flat flow profile produced.

For an ideal pipe, this critical velocity, v_c, is described by

$$v_c = \frac{k \times \eta}{d \times \rho}$$

where

k = Reynolds number, a dimensionless quantity
d = Diameter of the ideal pipe
ρ = Density of the gas

The value of k is approximately 2000 for water but is considerably less for gases. Laminar and turbulent flows can coexist, and they often do in the respiratory system.[21] Another place where flow will be turbulent is at an orifice where the length of the flow region is less than its radius.

MONITORS OF PRESSURE, FLOW, AND VOLUME
Pressure manometers

Manometers that measure respiratory gas pressure include calibrated liquid columns, analog gauges, strain gauges, electromechanical transducers, solid state transducers, and spring-loaded pressure switches. Calibrated liquid columns, such as those shown in Fig. 9-3, measure pressure relative to the force due to gravity on the liquid. From basic principles of physics, the height, h, of a liquid column opposed by a pressure P is independent of the area

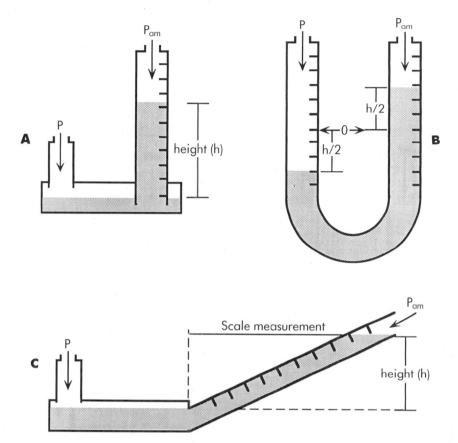

Fig. 9-3. Three types of liquid column gauge manometers. **A,** A single-tube manometer. The height of the column, *h,* reflects the pressure difference between *P* and P_{am}. A small decline in the level of the fluid in the vessel as fluid rises in the measurement tube is minimized when the surface area of the liquid vessel is much larger than the cross-sectional area of the tube. Alternatively, the scale graduations can be adjusted to compensate for the declining level of fluid in the vessel. **B,** A U-tube manometer. The change in the height of each of the fluid columns from zero must be summed to give the total difference in height between the columns. **C,** Slant-tube manometer for measuring small pressures. The small change in the height of the column is magnified on the scale in the horizontal direction. The pressure can be determined with more resolution than in the vertical column manometer. *P,* Applied pressure; P_{am}, ambient pressure.

of the column and is given by

$$h = \frac{P}{g \times \rho}$$

where

P = Pressure
g = Acceleration due to gravity (9.81 m/s²)
ρ = Density of the liquid.

Given the density of the liquid in the column, the scale can be calibrated in units of pressure accordingly. For measuring the small pressures sometimes seen in the respiratory system, the sensitivity of fluid-filled columns can be enhanced by use of liquid with low density or by slanting the tube as shown in Fig. 9-3, *C*. Due to the mass and viscosity of the liquid, the response of fluid-filled columns is inadequate to measure dynamic respiratory pressures.

Analog gauges are commonly used to measure and display the pressure in the respiratory system. The gauge itself is based on a Bourdon tube (Fig. 9-4), diaphragm, or bellows. In the Bourdon tube design, an indicator needle mechanism is attached to the closed, free end of a curved piece of flattened, soft, metal tubing. The open end of the tubing is in communication with the breathing circuit. Pressure in the circuit causes the flattened tubing to become more circular, thus uncoiling the tubing and moving the indicator needle mechanism. A small adjustment screw is often used to align the indicator needle to the zero-pressure mark when ambient pressure is applied. A high-quality Bourdon tube is accurate and reliable and requires no mechanical stop at zero. Excessive pressures can bend the malleable tubing or indicator needle mechanism, thus rendering the tube inoperable.

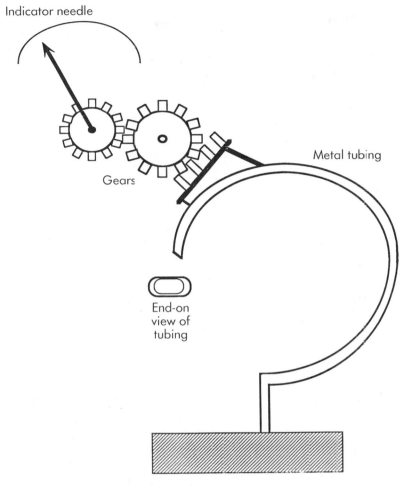

Fig. 9-4. Schematic representation of a Bourdon tube pressure gauge.

Electromechanical transducers are often used for measurements in the respiratory system, especially in conjunction with such flowmeters as pneumotachometers and Pitot tubes. The most common electromechanical transducer is the metal or semiconductor strain gauge. When a metal wire or thin segment of semiconductor material is stretched within its elastic limit, its resistance is altered due to dimensional changes and a change in the material's resistivity. The change in resistivity is called the piezoresistive effect. Fine wires made from such alloys as constantan, nichrome, and karma are particularly appropriate for metal strain gauges. In one common design, the bonded-wire strain gauge, the wires are cemented to a backing (Fig. 9-5). A flexible diaphragm attached to the bonded-wire strain gauge is exposed to the pressure to be measured on one side and the ambient pressure on the other. As the diaphragm bends, the wires are stretched and the change in resistance corresponding to the change in pressure can be measured. In another design (Fig. 9-6), two pairs of wires are attached to posts of two structural members that can move with respect to each other. One of the structural members is mechanically attached to a pressure-sensing diaphragm. When the diaphragm moves due to im-

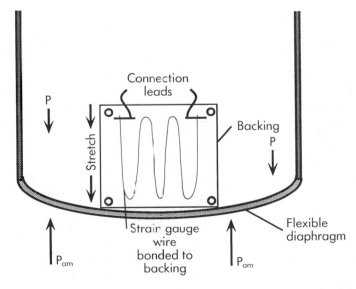

Fig. 9-5. Top view of a bonded-wire strain gauge. A length of metal strain gauge wire is cemented to a backing that is fixed at one end. When pressure is applied to the flexible diaphragm, the backing and strain gauge wire are stretched. The resulting change in resistance of the wire is measured and displayed as a change in pressure. P, Applied pressure; P_{am}, ambient pressure.

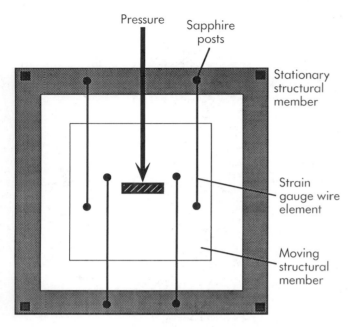

Fig. 9-6. Top view of an unbonded-wire strain gauge. Lengths of strain gauge wire are stretched between posts on two supporting structural members. The outer structural member is stationary. When pressure is applied in the direction shown, the center structural member moves incrementally. One pair of strain gauge wires stretches further while the other relaxes. The resulting change in resistance of the four elements is measured in a Wheatstone bridge circuit and displayed as pressure.

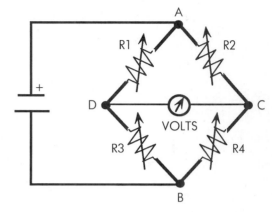

Fig. 9-7. Wheatstone bridge electrical circuit for strain gauge transducers. Voltage from a battery or other source is applied between points A and B. One or more of the variable resistors shown in the circuit (R_1 to R_4) are resistance elements of the transducer. The remaining resistor values are chosen so that the voltage difference measured between points C and D is very small, or "balanced", when zero pressure is applied to the transducer. As the pressure applied to the transducer changes, the bridge becomes "unbalanced" and a voltage difference appears between points C and D. Appropriate assignment of resistance elements and temperature-sensitive elements as the resistors in the bridge can result in highly sensitive, temperature-compensated measurement.

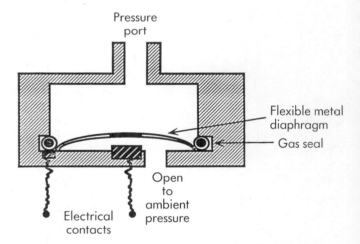

Fig. 9-8. Schematic cross section of a pressure switch. The pressure of the gas at the pressure port forces a metal diaphragm to make an electrical contact when the pressure exceeds a certain value. Some pressure switches have a spring and adjustment screw to allow calibration of the switching pressure threshold.

pinging pressure, two of the wires are stretched and the other pair are relaxed. The changes in the resistances of the four wires are then measured. In the semiconductor strain gauge, the materials used are usually crystals of silicon or germanium. A flexible diaphragm is etched into the crystal by way of integrated circuit techniques. A system of four silicon elements is produced in the diaphragm in such a way that the elements change predictably in resistance value as the diaphragm is deformed. During manufacture, the resistance elements are dimensionally trimmed with a laser so that no further calibration is required. The advantage of semiconductor materials is that they exhibit 50 to 100 times the change in resistance per unit of strain compared to metals.[22] However, the temperature sensitivity is substantially greater in semiconductor gauges and accurate compensation is a major factor in their design.

In both the metal and semiconductor strain gauges, the change in resistance of the elements is measured via an electrical circuit called a Wheatstone bridge (Fig. 9-7). This arrangement is particularly useful for three reasons. First, the Wheatstone bridge allows the simultaneous measurement of resistance changes in multiple elements when they are used as legs of the bridge. Second, temperature compensation can be incorporated directly into the bridge by way of metal or semiconductor elements that are sensitive to temperature but not exposed to the strain. Third, a

small change in resistance can be measured as a relative change in voltage near zero between the two balance points of the bridge.

Pressure switches, often used to monitor breathing circuit pressures, are used in systems that detect excessive pressure, circuit integrity, and circuit obstruction. The pressure switch is designed in such a way that the breathing circuit pressure is opposed by a linear spring or spring-metal diaphragm (Fig. 9-8). In the diaphragm switch, when the pressure exceeds a threshold, the diaphragm is bent to a point where an electrical contact is made. The electrical contact is then used by an electrical circuit to detect breathing circuit pressure in excess of the specified value. An adjustment screw is sometimes provided to change the spring force and hence the threshold pressure value.

Flowmeters

Several types of respiratory flowmeters are used in anesthesia systems to monitor respiratory flow and volume. Typically, flowmeters are used to monitor tidal volume and minute volume. Occasionally, flowmeters capable of measuring instantaneous flow are used.

The vane anemometer, originally introduced into respiratory measurement by Wright,[23] is commonly used to measure tidal volume and minute ventilation. This device uses a low-mass rotating vane in the gas stream. Gas molecules colliding with the blades of the vane transfer their momentum in the direction of flow and cause the vane to rotate. In the mechanical version, the rotation of the vane is connected to the dial via a gear mechanism, much like

that in a watch. In an electronic implementation (Fig. 9-9), two pairs of light emitting diodes (LED) and silicon photodetectors are used to measure the rate and direction of the vane's rotation. The rotation rate is integrated electronically to determine the volume of gas passing the transducer over time.

Several physical factors limit the accuracy of the vane anemometer.[24] Because the principle of operation is momentum, the density of the gas affects the measurement. The gas flow is directed to the blades of the vane by tangential slots; hence the viscosity of the gas also influences the measurement. Furthermore, inertia and momentum of the vane are problematic. Accuracy is poor at low flows because of inertia and at high flows because of momentum. The accuracy of the Wright respirometer has been shown to be within ±10% during anesthesia, but the modern electronic vane anemometer has not been evaluated in this setting. Electronic vane anemometers have been evaluated for pulmonary function testing and have demonstrated moderate accuracy during most maneuvers.[25]

A sealed volumeter (Fig. 9-10) is used in some systems to measure tidal volume and minute ventilation. This de-

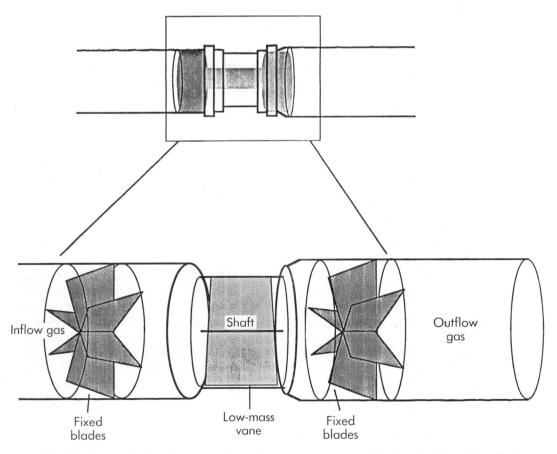

Fig. 9-9. Schematic drawing of an electronic vane anemometer. Gas flow is directed by fixed vanes at the inlet. Swirling gas causes a low-mass vane to spin. Light emitting diodes are positioned to detect the revolutions of the vane, which are converted into a flow measurement. This is the principle of operation of spirometers used in contemporary Ohmeda anesthesia systems.

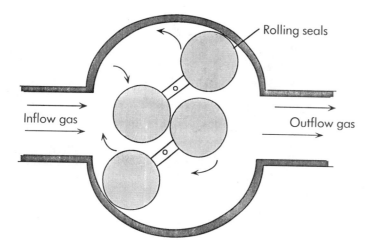

Fig. 9-10. Schematic drawing of a sealed volumeter. Polystyrene rotating elements form a seal against the interior of the volumeter. Gas flow rotates the elements, transferring fixed volumes of gas from the inlet to the outlet. Measured volume is displayed on a gauge mechanically connected to the rotating element shaft (mechanical spirometer). If the number of fixed volumes of gas transferred is measured electronically, measured volume may be read on a remote display. This is the principle of operation of the Drägerwerk AG volumeter (Spiromed).

vice consists of a pair of rotating elements in the gas-flow path, configured much like a circular door at the entrance of an office building. A fixed volume of gas is passed across the transducer with each quarter rotation of the elements. A seal is formed between the polystyrene rotating elements and the interior wall of the tube.

The sealed volumeter provides substantially more resistance to flow than does the vane anemometer. The accuracy of the volumeter is affected by gas density and by the inertia of the rotating elements. However, it is not influenced substantially by the flow pattern of the gas. The number of fixed volumes of gas transferred from inlet to outlet is measured mechanically or electronically and displayed on an integral scale (mechanical spirometer) or on a remote display (electronic spirometer). The accuracy of the volumeter has not been independently evaluated in an anesthesia setting.

The principle of operation of the pneumotachometer is to measure the loss of energy of the flowing gas as it passes through a resistive element. The resistive element is designed to ensure that the flow of the gas is laminar so that the energy loss is completely due to viscosity and the flow is directly proportional to pressure. The energy loss is measured as a pressure difference from the inlet to the outlet of the resistive element. The most common type of resistive element, designed by Fleish,[26] consists of narrow, parallel metal tubes aligned in the direction of the flow (Fig. 9-11). Nominally, for laminar flow, the pneumotachometer obeys the Hagen-Poiseuille law:

$$F = \frac{\pi \times r^4 \times (P_1 - P_2)}{8 \times l \times \eta}$$

where

F = Gas flow
r and l = Radius and length of the element, respectively
P_1 and P_2 = Inlet and outlet pressures, respectively
η = Viscosity of the gas.

Thus the measurement of flow is independent of gas density and total pressure (except for a slight effect of pressure on viscosity).

Fleish pneumotachometers are available in various sizes (resistances) to accommodate the appropriate flow range. The resistance of the element must be chosen so that the pressure difference produced in the flow range of interest is large enough to be measured accurately by the available pressure transducer. Too resistive an element will impede ventilation. The Fleish pneumotachometer usually uses a heating element to raise the temperature of the device to about 40° C, thus preventing condensation of the moist expired gas.

The pressure across the resistive element is measured using a differential pressure transducer with sufficient sensitivity and frequency response. The transducer must be nulled ("zeroed") electronically by reserving a measurement made with zero flow. The pressure difference is typically in the range of 2 cm H_2O. Pressure transducer output readings tend to drift and the measured signal is small; therefore, they must be renulled periodically. For vigorous ventilatory flows, the rate of change in gas flow is great and the frequency response of the transducer must be adequate to follow these changes. A pressure transducer used for pneumotachometry usually has a frequency response that is flat up to 40 Hz.[27]

The respiratory volume is computed by integrating the flow with respect to time (because Flow = Volume/Time). Traditionally, the integration was performed by way of an analog circuit. Computerized systems now perform the integration by digital summation. In either case, the pneumotachometer is calibrated by setting a gain coefficient according to a volume produced by manually discharging a calibrated (usually 1-L) syringe through the device. Often the calibration syringe is emptied several times at different rates to simulate the range of flows expected.

In practice, the characteristics of the Fleish pneumotachometer are dependent on the geometry of the tubing on the upstream side of the resistive element.[28] This results in a distinctly nonlinear deviation from Poiseuille's law.

The viscosity of gases in the respiratory mixture must be taken into consideration for the measurement of flow to be accurate. Consider that the viscosity of a gas mixture of 88.81% oxygen, 1.61% nitrogen, and 9.58% carbon dioxide is 9.1% greater than that of air.[29] Thus substantial errors can result if this factor is not considered. Although viscosity of gas mixtures is not strictly the weighted sum of the individual viscosities of the pure gases, many researchers have used this approach. The error resulting from this assumption is generally less than 1%. Temperature is considered to have a linear effect on the viscosity of

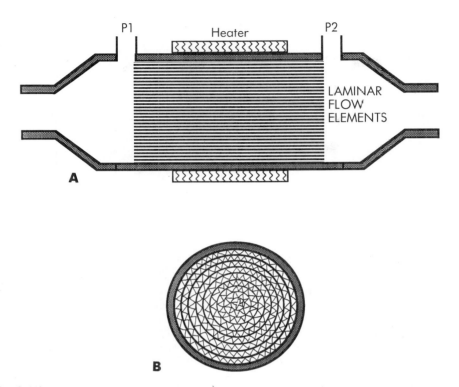

Fig. 9-11. Two cross-sectional views of a Fleish pneumotachometer. **A,** is a longitudinal cross section showing the parallel paths that constitute the laminar flow resistance element. Pressure ports P1 and P2 are used to measure the differential pressure across the resistance element. The Fleish pneumotachometer is generally bidirectional. A heating element surrounds the device and is used to prevent condensation forming within the elements. **B,** is a cross section of the laminar flow elements. The commercial pneumotachometer is constructed from aluminum, and the resistance elements have a roughly triangular appearance.

respiratory gases in the range of 20 to 40° C, although the linear coefficient is different for each gas.[30]

The other disadvantage of the pneumotachometer in an anesthesia circuit is its propensity to accumulate mucus and water in its narrow tubes. It must be repeatedly calibrated because its effective resistance changes with fouling. In addition, the pneumotachometer must be cleaned and sterilized between uses.

Another device for measuring gas flow that has been used in anesthesia is the Pitot tube (Fig. 9-12). This device measures the difference in kinetic energy of the gas impinging on a pressure port facing the direction of the flow and on a pressure port perpendicular to the flow.[31] The pressure difference, nominally proportional to the square of the flow rate, is sensitive to the density of the gas. Viscous losses around the pressure ports and small pressure differences at low flows are limitations of the Pitot tube flowmeter.

Recently, devices using both the pneumotachometer principle and the Pitot tube have been introduced for use in clinical anesthesia. An increased sensitivity and range are provided by this combined technique. However, the effects of density and viscosity on the measurement must be carefully considered. Combining respiratory gas composi-

tion monitoring with Pitot tube flow monitoring technology has the promise of accomplishing the appropriate compensations (see Fig. 9-13). A commercially available device that combines all of these technologies to display respired gas composition as well as pressures, flows, volumes, compliance, and pressure-volume and volume-flow relationships (Fig. 9-14) at the patient connector is now available.

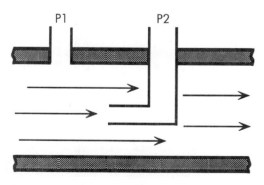

Fig. 9-12. Longitudinal cross section of a Pitot tube flowmeter. The pressure (P_2) measured at port P2 facing the flow direction is greater than the pressure (P_1) measured at port P1 due to the kinetic energy of the gas impinging on the port. The pressure difference ($P_2 - P_1$) is proportional to the square of the flow rate.

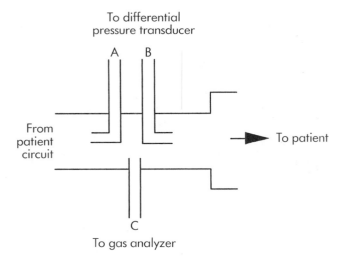

Fig. 9-13. Longitudinal cross section of a side-stream gas analyzer and spirometry adapter. This uses two Pitot tubes (*A* and *B*) facing in opposite directions in the airway adapter. The pressure differential is used to measure flow and flow direction (i.e., inspiration and expiration). Respiratory gas is continuously sampled via port *C* and analyzed for composition. The results of the analysis are used to correct the flow readings for density and viscosity. Absolute airway pressure is also continuously measured via ports *A* and *B*. This technology is used in the Datex Capnomac Ultima Monitor (Datex Medical Instrumentation, Tewksbury, Mass.).

Monitoring respiratory system pressure and gas flow is important for effective anesthesia management. Pressure and flow monitoring can enhance safety by detecting or confirming potential ventilation mishaps, such as disconnections and obstructions of the breathing circuit. Monitoring these variables is also essential for setting and verifying parameters for effective ventilation. Respiratory system mechanics can be evaluated with the appropriate pressure and flow measurements. An understanding of the basic physics of gases is important to understand respiratory system mechanics and the principles of monitors used to evaluate the system.

Fig. 9-14. Examples of data available from combined side-stream gas analysis and Pitot tube flow technology as used in Datex Capnomac Ultima Monitor. **A,** Normal screen showing results of inspired and expired gas analysis; real-time tracings of carbon dioxide, airway pressure *(P),* and flow *(V̇); TV; MV;* peak pressure, PEEP, and respiratory rate. **B,** Zoom screen showing volume *(V)* versus pressure *(P_{aw})* loop, as well as additional measured and calculated numeric data, including compliance *(C),* which reads 107 ml/mm Hg. **C,** Zoom screen showing flow *(V̇)* versus volume *(V).* The loops in *B* and *C* can be stored for comparison with subsequent displays. **D,** Zoom screen showing volume-pressure loop stored from *B.* The same patient has been turned into the prone position, but no changes have been made to any of the ventilatory controls. Note the shift to the right of the new volume-pressure loop *(solid line)* and the decrease in compliance (now 54 ml/mm Hg). (Tracings courtesy of James B. Eisenkraft, M.D.)

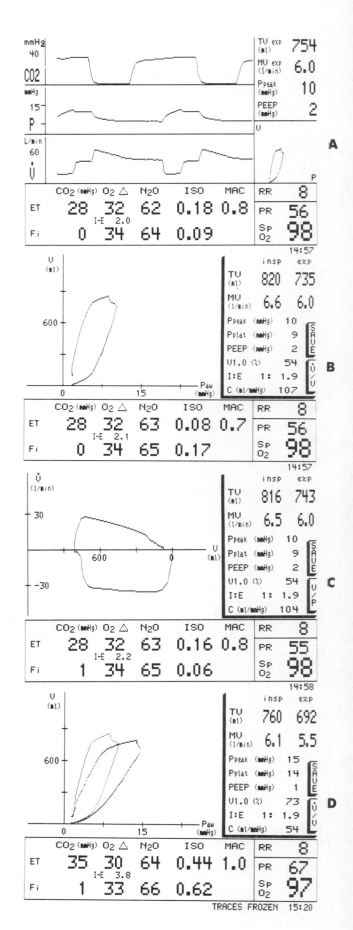

Pressure monitors commonly used during anesthesia include various mechanical manometers, such as Bourdon gauges, and bellows gauges, as well as calibrated fluid columns. Electromechanical manometers, such as metal wire and semiconductor strain gauges and membrane pressure switches, are commonly employed as respiratory system and breathing circuit monitors.

A variety of flow and volume meters for determining inspiratory and expiratory gas quantities are commonly used during anesthesia. Flow meters such as the vane anemometer and the Pitot tube work by responding to the kinetic energy losses of flowing gas as an obstruction is encountered. These devices are primarily influenced by the density of the respiratory gas. Problematic influences include the inertia of vane devices and viscous losses in the Pitot tube. Monitors such as the pneumotachometer operate by measuring the viscous losses of the flowing gas impeded by a resistance. These devices, primarily influenced by the viscosity of the gas, are inaccurate when flow is turbulent and kinetic losses occur.

New devices on the horizon for measuring flow in an anesthesia system utilize the gas analysis capability of new monitors to make appropriate corrections to the flow meter. Also, combinations of technology, such as pneumotachometer and Pitot tube designs, have the promise of improving accuracy and convenience.

REFERENCES

1. Elliott WR, Topulos GP: The influence of the mechanics of anesthesia breathing circuits on respiratory monitoring, *Biomed Instrum Technol* 24:260-265, 1990.
2. Sabo BA, Olinder PJ, Smith RB: Obstruction of a breathing circuit, *Anesth Rev* 10:28-30, 1983.
3. McIntyre WR, Knopes KD, Ossey KD: Anesthesia ventilators should have adjustable high-pressure alarms, *Anesthesiology* 63:231-232, 1985 (letter).
4. Pyles ST, Berman LS, Modell JH: Expiratory valve dysfunction in a semiclosed circle anesthesia circuit: verification by analysis of carbon dioxide waveform, *Anesth Analg* 63:536-537, 1984.
5. Anagnostou JM, Hults SL, Moorthy SS: PEEP valve barotrauma, *Anesth Analg* 70:668-676, 1990.
6. Famewo CE: A not-so-apparent cause of intraluminal tracheal tube obstruction, *Anesthesiology* 58:593, 1983 (letter).
7. Arai T, Kuzume K: Endotracheal tube obstruction possibly due to structural fault, *Anesthesiology* 59:480-481, 1983 (letter).
8. Arellano R, Ross D, Lee K: Inappropriate attachment of PEEP valve causing total obstruction of ventilation bag, *Anesth Analg* 66:1049-1050, 1987.
9. Marks JD, Schapera A, Kraemer RW, et al: Pressure and flow limitations of anesthesia ventilators, *Anesthesiology* 71:403-408, 1989.
10. Bendixen HH, Hedley Whyte J, Laver MB: Impaired oxygenation in surgical patients during general anesthesia with controlled ventilation, *N Engl J Med* 269:992-996, 1963.
11. Cooper EA: Physiological deadspace in passive ventilation: relationships with tidal volume, frequency, age, and minor upsets of respiratory health, *Anaesthesia* 22:199-219, 1967.
12. Campbell EJM, Nunn JF, Peckett BW: A comparison of artificial ventilation and spontaneous respiration with particular reference to ventilation-bloodflow relationships, *Br J Anaesth* 30:166-175, 1958.
13. Clarke AD: Potential deadspace in an anaesthetic mask and connectors, *Br J Anaesth* 30:176-181, 1958.
14. Coté CC, Petkau J, Ryan JF, et al: Wasted ventilation measured in vitro with eight anesthetic circuits with and without inline humidification, *Anesthesiology* 59:442-446, 1983.
15. Nunn JF: *Applied respiratory physiology,* London, 1977, Butterworths, p 180.
16. Wilson RS: Monitoring the lung: mechanics and volume, *Anesthesiology* 45:135-145, 1976.
17. Milic-Emili J, Mead J, Turner JM, et al: Improved technique for estimating pleural pressure from esophageal balloons, *J Appl Physiol* 19:207-211, 1964.
18. Rehder K, Marsh HM: *Respiratory mechanics during anesthesia and mechanical ventilation.* In *Handbook of physiology,* Bethesda, Md, 1986, American Physiological Society, Chapter 43.
19. Weast RC editor: *CRC handbook of chemistry and physics,* ed 65, Boca Raton, 1985, CRC Press, pp D192-193.
20. White FM: *Fluid mechanics.* New York, 1979, McGraw Hill, p 29.
21. Hill DW: *Properties of liquids gases and vapours.* In *Physics applied to anaesthesia,* ed 4, London, 1980, Butterworths, p 177.
22. Cobald RSC: *Displacement, force, and motion transducers.* In *Transducers for biomedical measurements: principles and applications,* New York, 1974, Wiley, p 120.
23. Wright BM: A respiratory anemometer, *J Physiol (Lond)* 127:25P, 1955.
24. Nunn JF, Ezi-Ashi TI: The accuracy of the respirometer and ventigrator, *Br J Anaesth* 34:422-432, 1962.
25. FitzGerald MX, Smith AA, Gaensler EA: Evaluation of electronic spirometers, *N Engl J Med* 289:1283-1288, 1973.
26. Fleish A: Der Pneumotachometer—ein Apparat zur Beischwindigkeitregistrierung der Atemluft, *Arch Ges Physiol* 209:713-722, 1925.
27. Farre R, Peslin R, Navajas D, et al: Analysis of the dynamic characteristics of pressure transducers for studying respiratory mechanics at high frequencies, *Med Biol Eng Comput* 27:531-537, 1989.
28. Finucane KE, Egan BA, Dawson SV: Linearity and frequency response of pneumotachographs, *J Appl Physiol* 32:121-126, 1972.
29. Yeh MP, Adams TD, Gardner RM et al: Effect of O_2, N_2, and CO_2 composition on nonlinearity of Fleisch pneumotachometer characteristics, *J Appl Physiol* 56:1423-1425, 1984.
30. Turney SZ, Blumenfeld W: Heated Fleish pneumotachometer: a calibration procedure, *J Appl Physiol* 34:117-121, 1973.
31. Sykes MK, Vickers MD, Hull CJ: *Measurement of gas flow and volume.* In *Principles of clinical measurement,* Oxford, 1981, Blackwell Scientific, p 198.

Part III

PATIENT MONITORS

Chapter 10

CAPNOGRAPHY

Michael L. Good, M.D.
Nikolaus Gravenstein, M.D.

The capnograph functions as an "electronic stethoscope," showing the cyclic appearance and disappearance of carbon dioxide when the lungs are being ventilated and no carbon dioxide when they are not. Confirming tracheal intubation is the most important clinical application of capnography. The American Society of Anesthesiologists' 1991 *Standards for Basic Intraoperative Monitoring* specifically includes the "identification of CO_2 in the expired gas" to confirm correct placement of a tracheal tube.[1] Yet the capnograph can and should be used as much more than just an electronic stethoscope. Carbon dioxide homeostasis involves many organ systems; the clinician skilled in capnography can interpret the capnogram to gain information about the patient's metabolism, cardiovascular system, and, most importantly, the adequacy of ventilation of the patient's lungs.

This chapter reviews the terms and definitions pertinent to capnography and then summarizes the different clinical applications of capnography. A systematic method for interpreting the capnogram and the factors that create a difference between arterial and expired carbon dioxide concentrations are discussed. Finally, a list is given of the pitfalls of capnography that can lead the clinician to misinterpret data from the capnograph and thus to misdiagnose a problem.

TERMS AND DEFINITIONS

The Greek root *kapnos*, meaning "smoke," is used to form the words *capnometry*, the practice of measuring carbon dioxide in respiratory gas, and *capnometer*, the instrument that does this. (Carbon dioxide can be thought of as the "smoke" of cellular metabolism.) The term *capnometer* is used to identify a simple instrument that provides only digital data—specifically, the minimum and maximum values of carbon dioxide during each respiratory cycle. This is in contrast to a *capnograph*, an instrument that displays, in addition to digital data, a capnogram. The capnogram is a plot of the airway carbon dioxide concentration as a function of time (Fig. 10-1). Both capnometers and capnographs digitally report carbon dioxide concentrations labeled "inspired" and "end-tidal." Actually, these instruments cannot determine the different phases of respiration but simply report the minimum and maximum carbon dioxide values detected during each carbon dioxide (i.e., respiratory) cycle. In certain instances (for example, an incompetent inspiratory unidirectional valve or an erratic breathing pattern), the minimum carbon dioxide concentration may not always equal the inspired carbon dioxide concentration; similarly, the maximum carbon dioxide concentration may not always be the end-tidal carbon dioxide

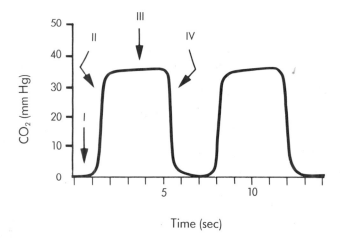

Fig. 10-1. A typical capnogram obtained during controlled mechanical ventilation through a circle anesthesia breathing system. The capnogram is divided into four phases: *(I)* inspiratory baseline, *(II)* expiratory upstroke, *(III)* expiratory plateau, and *(IV)* inspiratory downstroke. (Reproduced with permission from Good ML: *Capnography: uses, interpretation, and pitfalls.* In Barash PG, Deutsch S, Tinker J, editors: *ASA refresher courses in anesthesiology, vol 18,* Philadelphia, 1991, JB Lippincott.)

Table 10-1. Comparison of side-stream and main-stream capnographs

	Side-stream	Main-stream
Disconnection site	Yes	Yes
Sampling catheter leak	Yes	No
Calibration gas	Yes	No
Sensor damage	No	Some
Multiple gas analysis	Yes	No
Use on nonintubated patients	Yes	No

Reproduced in modified form with permission from Good ML: *Capnography: uses, interpretation, and pitfalls.* In Barash PG, Deutsch S, Tinker J, editors: *ASA refresher courses in anesthesiology, vol 18,* Philadelphia, 1991, JB Lippincott.

concentration. Thus the terms *minimum inspired* (P_ICO_2 min) and *maximum expired* ($P_ECO_2$max) partial pressure of carbon dioxide are more appropriate.

Side-stream, or sampling, capnographs aspirate respiratory gas from an airway sampling site and transport the gas sample through a tube to a remote carbon dioxide analyzer. Main-stream, or in-line, capnographs position the carbon dioxide analyzer on the airway, and respiratory gas is analyzed as it passes through a special adapter; no gas is removed from the airway. Each type of system has advantages and disadvantages (Table 10-1). Both increase the number of components and connection sites in the breathing circuit, each connection site being a potential disconnection site. Side-stream capnographs give falsely low carbon dioxide readings if the sampling catheter has a leak,

because room air is entrained through the leak and dilutes the carbon dioxide in the respiratory gas sample. Main-stream carbon dioxide analyzers add some bulk to the breathing system between the tracheal tube and the Y-piece. To calibrate a side-stream analyzer, calibration gas must be aspirated into the sampling catheter. The main-stream analyzer is simply snapped into a calibration cell on the capnograph (i.e., no calibration gas is needed). The sensitive electronics of some main-stream analyzers are vulnerable to mechanical damage. Multiple gases can be analyzed with the side-stream configuration because the respiratory gas sample can be passed through multiple gas analyzers. The respiratory gas from nonintubated, spontaneously breathing patients can be sampled and analyzed with a side-stream capnograph but not with a main-stream capnograph. Finally, the gas aspirated from a side-stream analyzer must eventually be disposed of via a scavenging system.

MEASUREMENT TECHNIQUES

Several analytical techniques can be used to measure respiratory carbon dioxide. Carbon dioxide strongly absorbs infrared light, particularly at wavelength 4.3 μm; thus, most stand-alone capnometers and capnographs use infrared light absorption, a relatively inexpensive technique, to measure respiratory carbon dioxide. Mass spectrometry, Raman spectroscopy, or photoacoustic spectroscopy can also be used. A chemical carbon dioxide indicator, the Fenem FEF* has also recently been introduced.[2] The chemical indicator is housed within an airway adapter, which is positioned between the tracheal tube and the breathing system. When respiratory carbon dioxide strikes the indicator paper, a pH-dependent dye changes color from purple to yellow. A color guide surrounding the indicator facilitates approximation of the exhaled carbon dioxide concentration into increments of 0.5%. (See also Chapter 8.)

SYSTEMATIC INTERPRETATION OF THE CAPNOGRAM

Similar to the electrocardiogram or chest radiogram, the capnogram, when systematically interpreted by the clinician, provides the maximum amount of information.[3] This analysis should include the following:

I. Verify presence of exhaled carbon dioxide
II. Identify and analyze
   A. Inspiratory baseline
   B. Expiratory upstroke
   C. Expiratory plateau
   D. Inspiratory downstroke
III. Check $P_ICO_2$min and $P_ECO_2$max
IV. Estimate or measure $PaCO_2 - P_ECO_2$max
V. Search for causes of hypercapnia or hypocapnia, if either is present

*Fenem, New York.

Exhaled carbon dioxide

Is there exhaled carbon dioxide? This is the fundamental question following placement of every tracheal tube. When the capnograph does not register exhaled carbon dioxide, failure to ventilate the patient's lungs must be assumed. The differential diagnosis includes esophageal intubation, accidental extubation, disconnection, or apnea. The important role of capnography in helping to detect esophageal intubation cannot be emphasized too strongly. In a review of 17 different methods for differentiating tracheal from esophageal intubation, only direct visualization of the tracheal tube between the vocal cords and the presence and persistence of exhaled carbon dioxide proved to be 100% reliable.[4] All other methods had one or more documented failures.

Some clinicians are concerned that, if carbon dioxide was forced into the stomach during bag and mask ventilation before attempted intubation, and if the esophagus was subsequently intubated, a normal, "tracheal" appearing capnogram would result. Indeed, when the stomachs of anesthetized patients are sampled for carbon dioxide following induction of general anesthesia and tracheal intubation, low concentrations of carbon dioxide are detected.[5,6] Data on tracheal and esophageal capnograms generated by a canine model and a mechanical lung model showed that even when the stomach is filled with 5% carbon dioxide, a subsequent "esophageal" capnogram is characterized by a stepwise decrease in carbon dioxide concentration with each successive ventilatory cycle; such an esophageal capnogram is easily distinguished from a normal tracheal capnogram[7] (Fig. 10-2).

In a similar study, also using a canine model, the stomach was filled with a carbonated beverage and, following esophageal intubation, the esophageal capnogram obtained was similarly characterized by the rapid washout of carbon dioxide from the stomach.[8] Clinicians should confirm tracheal intubation by the presence and persistent reappearance of carbon dioxide with each respiratory cycle. If the carbon dioxide concentration decreases with each successive ventilatory cycle and quickly becomes undetectable, esophageal intubation or circulatory collapse must be considered.

Disconnection within the breathing system is easily detected with capnography by a flat capnogram with a carbon dioxide reading of zero. A flat capnogram is also produced by other causes of apnea, such as complete obstruction to gas flow within the breathing or scavenging system, failure to turn on the mechanical ventilator, the bag-ventilator selector switch being in the bag position during mechanical ventilation, or failure of the mechanical ventilator. Spontaneously breathing patients (intubated or not) may become apneic from intravenous or inhaled anesthetic agents, and this too results in a flat capnogram. Not until all of the above mechanisms have been absolutely ruled out by clinical examination should failure of the capnograph be considered. If the capnograph itself is suspect, the anesthesiologist can

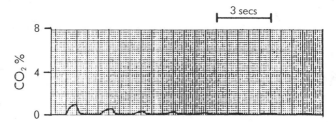

Fig. 10-2. A typical capnogram from an esophageal intubation. Note the rapid decline of the carbon dioxide to zero. Compare this capnogram to the normal capnogram in Figure 10-1.

quickly disconnect the sampling or sensing adapter and exhale into it to determine if the capnograph is working and if the sampling catheter is patent. If so, exhaled carbon dioxide will quickly register on the capnogram.

The four phases of the capnogram

The shape of a normal capnogram depends on the type of breathing system being used (for example, circle or Mapleson) and on the mode of ventilation (controlled, assisted, or spontaneous). When an anesthetized patient is receiving controlled mechanical ventilation of the lungs through a circle anesthesia breathing system, the normal capnogram has a rectangular appearance and is divided into four phases or segments, labeled I through IV, for analysis (Fig. 10-1).

Inspiratory baseline. During mechanical inspiration, fresh gas with no carbon dioxide rushes by the carbon dioxide sampling or sensing site, and the capnograph traces the inspiratory baseline (I). The carbon dioxide concentration during this phase is zero because there is no rebreathing of carbon dioxide with a normally functioning circle breathing system. If the inspiratory baseline is elevated $(CO_2 > 0)$, carbon dioxide is being rebreathed (Fig. 10-3, C). The differential diagnosis includes an incompetent expiratory valve, exhausted carbon dioxide absorbent, or gas channelling through the absorbent. The inspiratory baseline may or may not be elevated when the inspiratory valve is incompetent. A more characteristic effect on the capnogram of an incompetent inspiratory valve is a slanted inspiratory downstroke (see below).

With a Mapleson circuit, there is almost always carbon dioxide rebreathing, the degree of which depends on complex relationships between fresh-gas flow (FGF), minute ventilation, and respiratory rate and pattern (Fig. 10-4). If carbon dioxide rebreathing is excessive, the capnograph helps the clinician to select the appropriate rate of FGF for the patient's respiratory pattern.

Expiratory upstroke. Shortly after mechanical inspiration ends, the lungs recoil and gas quickly exits through the trachea. As fresh gas in the anatomic deadspace (no carbon dioxide) is quickly washed away and replaced by carbon dioxide–rich alveolar gas, the expiratory upstroke (II) appears on the capnogram. The upstroke, which should be steep, becomes slanted (Fig. 10-3, A) if gas flow

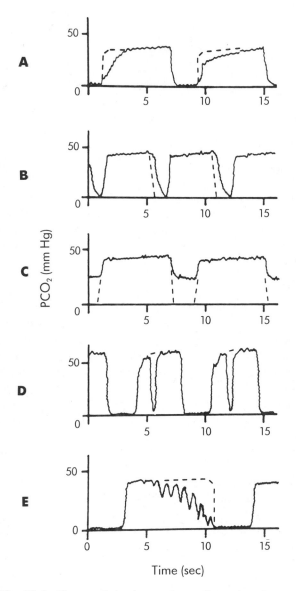

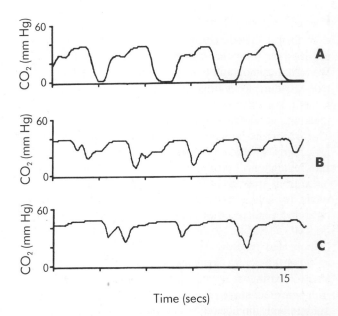

Fig. 10-4. Effect of rate of fresh gas flow (FGF) on P_ICO_2min and P_ECO_2max when a Mapleson D breathing system is used to ventilate the lungs of a healthy man weighing 70 kg. **A,** A FGF of 10 L/min results in a P_ICO_2min of zero and a P_ECO_2max of 37 mm Hg. **B,** An FGF of 5 L/min results in a P_ICO_2min of 10 mm Hg and a P_ECO_2max of 39 mm Hg. **C,** An FGF of 1 L/min results in a P_ICO_2min of 20 to 30 mm Hg, depending on the length of the expiratory pause, and a P_ECO_2max of 48 mm Hg.

Fig. 10-3. Characteristic abnormal waveforms *(continuous line)* superimposed on a a normal waveform *(dotted line).* **A,** Increased airway resistance caused by bronchospasm or a kinked tracheal tube; **B,** incompetent inspiratory valve, where part of the expired gas flows back into the inspiratory limb and is inspired with the next breath; **C,** incompetent expiratory valve, where expired gas is reinspired through the expiratory limb; **D,** patient taking breaths and overriding mechanical ventilation; **E,** cardiogenic oscillations caused by the rhythmic increase and decrease in intrathoracic volume with each cardiac cycle. *P_{CO_2},* partial pressure of carbon dioxide. (Reproduced with permission from van Genderingen HR, Gravenstein N, van der Aa JJ, et al: Computer-assisted capnogram analysis, *J Clin Monit* 3:198, 1987.)

is partially obstructed, if a side-stream analyzer is sampling gas too slowly, or if the response time of the capnograph is too slow for the patient's respiratory rate. Gas flow may be obstructed in the breathing system (for example, by a kinked tracheal tube) or in the patient's airway (for example, in the presence of chronic obstructive pulmonary disease or acute bronchospasm). Slow gas sampling allows each discrete sample of expired carbon dioxide to become diluted by the adjacent fresh gas, and artifactual carbon dioxide readings result.[9] The same effect is seen with long or wide-bore gas sampling tubing. When a capnograph with a choice of gas sampling flow rates is used, the highest sampling rate is best; there is no benefit or indication for using a slow sampling rate, even in pediatric patients.[10]

Expiratory plateau. As exhalation continues, the capnogram plateaus. If ventilation and perfusion were perfectly matched in all lung regions, alveolar gas would have a constant carbon dioxide concentration and the expiratory plateau (III) would be perfectly horizontal. However, ventilation and perfusion are not perfectly matched in all lung units, especially in patients who are supine and whose lungs are being mechanically ventilated with positive pressure. Therefore, as exhalation continues, carbon dioxide slowly increases as gas from lung units with a lower ratio of ventilation to perfusion *(V/Q)* reaches the sampling site, and even the normal expiratory plateau has a gentle upward slope.

With partial obstruction to gas flow, either in the breathing system or in the patient's airways, the capnogram continues to slope upward (Fig. 10-3, *A*) instead of plateauing and may still be rising when the next inspiratory downstroke begins. When this is observed, P_ECO_2 max may not correlate closely with $PaCO_2$. In some cases, inserting a long expiratory pause after a breath results in a higher P_ECO_2max that more closely approximates $PaCO_2$.

The normally smooth expiratory plateau can be interrupted by bumps and dips. If the surgeon pushes against the diaphragm, gas from the expiratory reserve, which has a high carbon dioxide content, may be forced into the upper airway, which creates a bump in the expiratory plateau. If a patient receiving controlled mechanical ventilation makes an inspiratory effort, fresh gas will be drawn over the carbon dioxide sampling or sensing site, which creates a dip in the capnogram (Fig. 10-3, *D*). Some refer to such dips as "curare clefts," implying that more muscle relaxant is indicated. This is unfortunate, because the patient who attempts to breathe spontaneously during mechanical ventilation may be hypoxic, hypercarbic, or too lightly anesthetized.[11] The administration of muscle relaxants should be guided by a neuromuscular blockade monitor, not the capnogram.

The expiratory plateau continues after active exhalation is completed because exhaled carbon dioxide remains at the carbon dioxide sampling or sensing site. In some patients, especially those with a slow respiratory rate, the pulsatile heart and the pulsing of blood in and out of the pulmonary vasculature causes a small volume of gas to move in and out of the lungs. This movement may draw fresh gas back and forth over the carbon dioxide sampling or sensing site and thus may create oscillations in the capnogram (Fig. 10-3, *E*). These are called cardiac oscillations and have no diagnostic significance. Some capnographs will misinterpret these oscillations as breaths and will incorrectly report high respiratory rates and high $PICO_2$min. When a patient's lungs are being ventilated at a slow respiratory rate, continued gas sampling during the expiratory pause by side-stream capnographs draws fresh gas over the carbon dioxide sampling site and thus the expiratory plateau gradually decays.

Inspiratory downstroke. Shortly after the mechanical ventilator initiates inspiration, fresh gas rapidly washes carbon dioxide away from the carbon dioxide sensing or sampling site, and the capnogram draws the inspiratory downstroke (IV). Normally it is steep. An incompetent inspiratory valve allows carbon dioxide to accumulate in the inspiratory hose and thus the inspiratory downstroke becomes slanted (Fig. 10-3, *B*) as the carbon dioxide in the inspiratory limb is washed away. Other causes of a slanted inspiratory downstroke include slow mechanical inspiration, slow gas sampling, and partial carbon dioxide rebreathing with a Mapleson breathing system, especially at low rates of FGF.

Minimum inspired and maximum expired carbon dioxide

As previously discussed, capnometers and capnographs report digital values for the minimum and maximum carbon dioxide concentrations measured during each ventilatory cycle. An erratic breathing pattern or other problems (for example, cardiogenic oscillation or spontaneous inspiratory effort) may make it difficult for the instrument to

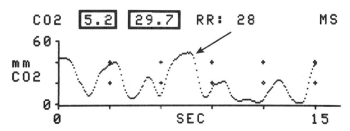

Fig. 10-5. Digitally reported inspired and end-tidal carbon dioxide values, respectively *(boxes)*, are incorrectly reported by the capnograph. The capnograph has difficulty determining these values because of the erratic respiratory pattern. The clinician, however, can easily determine the correct values by using the scale of the y-axis to measure the highest *(arrow)* and lowest points of the carbon dioxide waveform. Here, the actual minimum inspired carbon dioxide is clearly less than 5.2 mm Hg and the peak inspired carbon dioxide is approximately 45 mm Hg. *RR*, respiratory rate (breaths/min). (Reproduced with permission from Good ML: *Capnography: uses, interpretation, and pitfalls.* In Barash PG, Deutsch S, Tinker J, editors: *ASA refresher courses in anesthesiology, vol 18*, Philadelphia, 1991, JB Lippincott.)

correctly determine $PICO_2$min and $PECO_2$max (Fig. 10-5). The clinician, however, can compare the lowest and highest portions of the carbon dioxide waveform with the concentration scale on the y-axis and then visually determine whether the digitally reported $PICO_2$min and $PECO_2$max are correct. By examining the inspiratory downstroke, carbon dioxide rebreathing can be detected even if the reported $PICO_2$min is zero.

Difference between arterial and expired carbon dioxide

The best measure of the adequacy of ventilation of the lungs is $PaCO_2$. Typically, $PaCO_2$ and $PECO_2$max differ by 3 to 5 mm Hg in patients without significant lung dis-

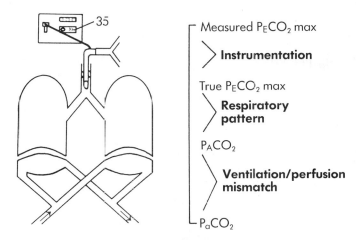

Fig. 10-6. Components of the difference between $PaCO_2$ and $PECO_2$max. *V/Q*, ratio of ventilation to perfusion. (Reproduced with permission from Good ML: *Capnography: uses, interpretation, and pitfalls.* In Barash PG, Deutsch S, Tinker J, editors: *ASA refresher courses in anesthesiology, vol 18*, Philadelphia, 1991, JB Lippincott.)

Table 10-2. Difference between $PaCO_2$ and $PECO_2max$ during general anesthesia

Investigator	Year	PaCO₂ − PₑCO₂max (mm Hg)		Comment
		Mean	**Range**	
Nunn and Hill[12]	1960	—	—	No cardiac or pulmonary disease
		4.5 ± 2.5	−0.4 to 7.7	During spontaneous respiration
		4.7 ± 2.5	1.7 to 9.1	During artificial respiration
Askrog et al.[13]	1964	3.6	1.5 to 6.1	After anesthesia induction with halothane
		5.5	2.6 to 10	After 90 to 150 min of halothane anesthesia
		0.9	0.6 to 1.9	No anesthesia
Takki et al.[14]	1972	3.5 ± 0.5	—	—
Whitesell et al.[15]	1981	0.8 ± 0.3	—	No lung disease
		3.3 ± 0.6	—	With lung disease
		—	—	Stable gradient on repeated measurement
Valentin et al.[16]	1982	5	−4 to 13	Pediatric patients
		—	—	During spontaneous respiration
Raemer et al.[17]	1983	4.1	0.8 to 13	Varying gradient on repeated measurement
Fletcher and Jonson[18]	1984	4.6	1.5 to 10.1	With small tidal volume
		2.3	−0.8 to 8.5	With large tidal volume
Shanker et al.[19]	1986	5.3 ± 2.9	3.5 ± 7.1	Nonpregnant patients
		0.8 ± 0.7	−4 to 6.8	Pregnant patients; 50% had negative difference

Reproduced with permission from Good ML: *Capnography: uses, interpretation, and pitfalls.* In: Barash PG, Deutsch S, Tinker JH, editors: *ASA refresher courses in anesthesiology, vol 18,* Philadelphia, 1991, JB Lippincott.

ease (Table 10-2). In some studies, this difference has varied during the course of anesthesia; in others, the difference has remained relatively constant. Closer examination of studies comparing $PECO_2max$ with $PaCO_2$ shows that *mean* $PaCO_2 − PECO_2max$ was reported for all patients in the study. The *range* of $PaCO_2 − PECO_2max$, however, was quite large, the difference being greater than 10 mm Hg in at least one patient in most studies. Thus, generally, the difference between $PaCO_2$ and $PECO_2max$, which is small in anesthetized patients without lung disease, can be large in some patients, especially those with lung disease and/or abnormal capnograms (for example, an upsloping plateau phase).

What factors cause the normally small difference between $PaCO_2$ and $PECO_2max$ to increase? The total difference can be divided into three components (Fig. 10-6):

1. $PaCO_2 − PACO_2$. The difference between $PaCO_2$ and the mixed alveolar partial pressure of carbon dioxide ($PACO_2$). Mismatching of ventilation and perfusion increases the difference between $PaCO_2$ and $PACO_2$. Examples are with pulmonary embolism and endobronchial intubation.
2. $PACO_2 − $ true $PECO_2max$. The difference between $PACO_2$ and the true partial pressure of carbon dioxide delivered to the upper airway, or actual carbon dioxide at the sensing or sampling site (true

$PECO_2max$). Breathing patterns that fail to deliver undiluted alveolar gas to the upper airway increase the difference between $PaCO_2$ and true $PECO_2max$. Examples are with high-frequency ventilation and as occurs in neonates and infants.
3. True $PECO_2max − $ measured $PECO_2max$. The difference between true $PECO_2max$ and measured $PECO_2max$ reported by the capnograph. Problems with the capnograph itself can increase this component of $PaCO_2 − PECO_2max$. Examples are with sampling catheter leaks, calibration error, and slow instrument response time.

$PaCO_2 − PACO_2$. Both increases and decreases in V/Q increase the difference between $PaCO_2$ and $PACO_2$. Consider a simplified, two-unit lung model (Fig. 10-7, *top*) with perfect matching of V and Q (i.e., V/Q in every lung unit is 1). Blood with a PCO_2 of 46 mm Hg returns to the lungs, and, after equilibration, both the pulmonary capillary blood and the alveolar gas have a PCO_2 of 40 mm Hg. The alveolar gas is exhaled, and the capnograph reports a $PECO_2max$ of 40 mm Hg. The $PaCO_2$ is also 40 mm Hg, and, in this simplified model, the difference between $PaCO_2$ and $PECO_2max$ is zero. Endobronchial intubation is an extreme example of V/Q less than 1 (Fig. 10-7, *middle*). All of the blood flow through the nonventilated lung represents shunt. As before, blood with PCO_2 of 46 mm Hg returns to the lungs. Gas is exchanged in the ventilated lung, and pulmonary blood and alveolar gas in this lung unit end up with a P_{CO_2} of 40 mm Hg. The non-ventilated lung unit allows no exchange of alveolar gas, so both pulmonary blood and alveolar gas eventually equilibrate at a P_{CO_2} of 46 mm Hg. Assuming equal distribution

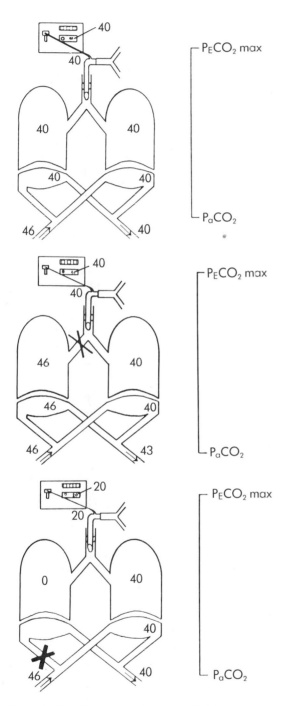

Fig. 10-7. An idealized two-unit lung model demonstrates how ventilation-to-perfusion mismatching increases the difference between $PaCO_2$ and $PECO_2$max. (Reproduced with permission from Good ML: *Capnography: uses, interpretation, and pitfalls.* In Barash PG, Deutsch S, Tinker J, editors: *ASA refresher courses in anesthesiology, vol 18,* Philadelphia, 1991, JB Lippincott.)

of blood flow, after pulmonary blood from the two lung units mixes, the resultant $PaCO_2$ is 43 mm Hg ([46 + 40]/2). Alveolar gas from the ventilated lung unit only is exhaled and reaches the capnograph, which reports a $PECO_2$max of 40 mm Hg. In this simplified lung model, a decreased V/Q increases the difference between $PaCO_2$ and $PECO_2$max from 0 to 3 mm Hg.

In contrast, the effect of a V/Q greater than 1 is illustrated by pulmonary embolism (Fig. 10-7, *bottom*). This is an example of increased dead space ventilation. Blood returning to the lungs has a P_{CO_2} of 46 mm Hg and can flow to only one lung unit because of the embolus. Alveolar gas in the nonperfused lung unit has a P_{CO_2} of zero. Pulmonary capillary blood and alveolar gas equilibrate in the perfused lung unit with a P_{CO_2} of 40 mm Hg. The resulting $PaCO_2$ is 40 mm Hg. Assuming equal ventilation of both lung units, the resultant $PECO_2$max is 20 mm Hg ([40 + 0]/2). In this simplified lung model, an increased V/Q, such as that caused by pulmonary embolism, increases the difference between $PaCO_2$ and $PECO_2$max from 0 to 20 mm Hg. This increase is consistent with the difference between $PaCO_2$ and $PECO_2$max measured in patients with acute pulmonary embolism. [20,21] The effect on $PaCO_2 - PECO_2$max is the same regardless of whether the embolus is composed of thrombus, air, fat, or amniotic fluid. Because $PECO_2$max drops so dramatically with an air embolism of just 0.07 ml/kg, capnography is a routine monitor when air embolism is possible (for example, during craniotomy with the patient in the sitting position).

$PaCO_2$ − true $PECO_2$max. If the patient has a rapid respiratory rate (for example, with high-frequency ventilation, or as occurs in infants and children), is breathing erratically, or is not exhaling completely (for example, with chronic obstructive pulmonary disease or bronchospasm), a mixed alveolar gas sample may not be delivered to the upper airway. The alveolar sample not only must be delivered to the upper airway but also must remain there long enough for the capnograph to measure it. Capnography in neonates and small children typically results in a larger $PaCO_2 - PECO_2$max gradient than in adults. Factors that contribute to this increase include low ratio of tidal volume to equipment deadspace, rapid ventilatory rate, high rate of FGF, and a rate of sampling by carbon dioxide analyzers higher than the expiratory flow rate of these small subjects. [22] Although intuitively appealing, use of a slow rate of sampling worsens the difference between $PaCO_2$ and $PECO_2$max by increasing the response time of the capnograph (see below). When a Mapleson breathing system is used, sampling as close as possible to the endotracheal tube connector decreases the dilution of the alveolar gas with fresh gas. [23]

The importance of the $PaCO_2$ − true $PECO_2$max component of $PaCO_2 - PECO_2$max was nicely demonstrated when $PECO_2$max sampled from the proximal connector was compared with that sampled from the distal tip of the tracheal tube. In subjects weighing greater than 12 kg, both proximal and distal $PECO_2max$ determinations correlated closely with $PaCO_2$. In subjects weighing less than 12 kg, only the gas sampled at the distal tip of the tracheal tube provided a $PECO_2max$ value that closely approximated $PaCO_2$.[24] In a relevant animal study (using rabbits weighing 2.7 to 3.6 kg), gas sampled from the 12-cm mark (which in newborns lies just outside the mouth) provided $PECO_2max$ values within 1 mm Hg of those obtained from sampling at the tip of the distal tracheal tube. Neither the FGF rate nor the mode of ventilation affected this small difference.[25] Uncuffed tracheal tubes, which are used in neonates and infants, compound the problem because exhaled gas escaping around the tube is not measured by the capnograph. (See also Chapter 26.)

True $PECO_2max$ − measured $PECO_2max$. Even if a mixed alveolar gas sample reaches the carbon dioxide sensing or sampling site, problems with the capnograph itself (i.e., a miscalibrated capnograph) may result in inaccurate carbon dioxide measurement. Small inaccuracies can arise if the processing algorithms in the capnograph do not accurately account for water vapor.[26] Infrared analyzers must also compensate for high concentrations of nitrous oxide and oxygen. A capnograph with a slow response time increases true $PECO_2max$ − measured $PECO_2max$. Response time refers to how fast the instrument can measure a step change in carbon dioxide concentration. For example, if the carbon dioxide sensing or sampling site is exposed to room air (no carbon dioxide) and then suddenly is flooded with 5% carbon dioxide, how long does it take for the capnograph to report a carbon dioxide value close to 5%? Note that manufacturers typically report only the time needed to register from 10% to 90% of the actual carbon dioxide concentration, which is significantly shorter than the clinically relevant response time for a 0% to 100% change to occur.

Why is response time clinically important? If the capnograph has a slow response time and the patient has a rapid respiratory rate, the respiratory gas may not remain at the carbon dioxide sensing or sampling site long enough to be completely measured. The more rapid the response time, the more likely it is that the capnograph accurately measures carbon dioxide when the respiratory rate is high.[27]

A subtle problem with side-stream capnographs that leads to a large increase in the value of true $PECO_2max$ − measured $PECO_2$ is partial obstruction of the sampling system. For example, if the water filter becomes saturated or extra filters are inserted, resistance to gas flow increases and the pressure within the carbon dioxide analyzing chamber may become subambient.

Attempting to protect a side-stream analyzer from moisture by routinely inserting an extra filter may thereby create a systematic error that increases the value of $PaCO_2$ − $PECO_2$ in all patients. A solution to this moisture problem is to interpose a heat-and-moisture exchanger between the tracheal tube and the carbon dioxide sampling site to eliminate the need for an extra filter.

Table 10-3. The relationship between $PECO_2max$ and $PaCO_2$

$PECO_2max$	$PaCO_2$
High	High
Normal	Normal or high
Low	Low, normal, or high

Reverse "gradient" ($PECO_2max > PaCO_2$). In most patients, $PECO_2max$ is less than $PaCO_2$. In some patients, however, $PECO_2max$ is greater than $PaCO_2$, and thus the value $PaCO_2 − PECO_2max$ is negative. In one study, negative $PaCO_2 − PECO_2max$ was noted in 50% of women receiving general anesthesia for cesarean section.[28] One explanation proposed is that some lung units have long time constants and a high $PaCO_2$. These lung units may continue to deliver carbon dioxide to the alveolar and exhaled gases even though $PaCO_2$ is low.[29] Factors that cause $PECO_2max$ to approach mixed venous carbon dioxide similarly cause $PECO_2max$ to exceed $PaCO_2$.[30] In many of these instances of $PECO_2max > PaCO_2$, we suspect miscalibration or some other problem with the capnograph or blood gas analyzer that affects accuracy. Consider also that $PaCO_2$, which fluctuates during the respiratory cycle, is lowest at end-inspiration and highest in blood traversing the pulmonary vasculature at end-expiration. If arterial blood that is sampled is representative of pulmonary capillary blood at end-inspiration, the sample will have a low $PaCO_2$ that may be exceeded by $PECO_2max$.

A number of problems and clinical circumstances increase the value of $PaCO_2 − PECO_2max$. In the clinical setting, when $PECO_2max$ is increased, $PaCO_2$ must also be increased, and increased ventilation of the patient's lungs is indicated. When $PECO_2max$ is normal, $PaCO_2$ may also be normal; but if $PaCO_2 − PECO_2max$ is greater than normal, $PaCO_2$ will be increased even though $PECO_2max$ is normal (Table 10-3). Finally, if $PECO_2max$ is low, $PaCO_2$ may be low, normal, or high, depending on $PaCO_2 − PECO_2max$. In certain patients—for example, those with lung disease or those weighing less than 12 kg—a larger than normal value of $PaCO_2 − PECO_2max$ should be anticipated. Whenever $PECO_2max$ does not seem consistent with the clinical situation, blood (arterial or venous) should be sampled for direct measurement of PCO_2.

Hypercapnia and hypocapnia

Clinicians are routinely confronted with hypercapnia ($PECO_2max > 45$ mm Hg) and hypocapnia ($PECO_2max < 30$ mm Hg). A systematic approach is best for searching for the cause. Causes of hypercapnia can be grouped into three categories: (1) alveolar hypoventilation, (2) carbon dioxide rebreathing, and (3) increased carbon dioxide output. There are many causes of alveolar hypoventilation during anesthesia, for example, a leak (as from a tear in a breathing hose or a partially open pop-off valve), an obstruction in the breathing system, or an inadequate minute ventilation setting on the ventilator. Rebreathing of carbon dioxide is readily detected by the associated abnormal capnograms outlined above. Increased carbon dioxide output may be due to endogenous or exogenous carbon dioxide. For example, during cases of malignant hyperthermia, extremely high values of $PECO_2max$ have been reported.[31,32] Capnography may be the best routine monitor for early identification of malignant hyperthermia. Carbon dioxide output and $PECO_2max$ also increase, though to a lesser degree, with fever, as from infection. The release of a limb tourniquet or a vascular clamp also increases carbon dioxide output of the lungs, with a corresponding, transient increase in $PECO_2max$. Exogenous carbon dioxide, such as that resulting from intravenous administration of bicarbonate ion (one ampule of which liberates more than 1 L of carbon dioxide) or abdominal insufflation of carbon dioxide during laparoscopy, also increases carbon dioxide output from the lungs and, if minute ventilation is held constant, $PECO_2max$ must increase.

The causes of hypocapnia can also be divided into three categories: (1) alveolar hyperventilation, (2) decreased carbon dioxide output, and (3) increased value of $PaCO_2 - PECO_2max$. During anesthesia, controlled mechanical ventilation of the patient's lungs may lead to passive hyperventilation, which depletes the body's stores of carbon dioxide and decreases $PECO_2max$. The patient's body temperature typically decreases during general anesthesia. This decreases metabolism and carbon dioxide output. Decreases in cardiac output, such as those accompanying hypovolemia and venous obstruction, also further decrease carbon dioxide output to the lungs. The value of $PaCO_2 - PECO_2$ has been thoroughly reviewed. Anything that increases or decreases V/Q from 1 increases the difference between $PaCO_2$ and $PECO_2max$.

CLINICAL APPLICATIONS OF CAPNOGRAPHY

Detection of untoward events

Clinicians use capnography intraoperatively to detect untoward events that, if undetected and uncorrected, might injure the anesthetized patient. A number of studies support the premise that capnography can detect the types of problems most likely to injure an anesthetized patient and can guide clinical management. For example, when the technique of critical-incident analysis was adapted to study human error and equipment failure in anesthesia, disconnection of the breathing circuit during mechanical ventilation was the most frequently identified critical incident.[33] Capnography readily detects disconnection within the breathing system. Of the 25 most frequent critical incidents identified in this study, more than 40% could have been identified with data from the capnograph.

Another study strongly supporting the intraoperative use of capnography is the American Society of Anesthesiologists' closed claims study.[34] In this study, experts reviewed closed malpractice claims against anesthesiologists. After reviewing 1541 cases, the experts identified "respiratory events" as the "single largest class" of problems resulting in litigation. Over one third (34%) of the adverse outcomes were associated with respiratory events. Of these, 35% were attributed to inadequate ventilation of the patient's lungs, 18% to esophageal intubation, and 17% to difficult tracheal intubation. Both inadequate ventilation of the patient's lungs and esophageal intubation are readily detected with capnography.

A similar case study analysis was conducted for the nine Harvard-affiliated hospitals.[35] Between 1972 and 1985, 11 claimants sought damages for anesthesia-related injuries. In 7 of these, inadequate ventilation of the patient's lungs was considered the underlying mechanism leading to injury of the patient. The investigator deemed capnography to be the most appropriate monitor of ventilation and thought it would have detected these problems. In another study, the cause of unexpected cardiac arrest during anesthesia was retrospectively studied over a 15-year period at a major university hospital.[36] Inadequate ventilation of the patient's lungs accounted for 11 of the 20 cardiac arrests.

Coté et al. prospectively studied capnography in a single-blind protocol involving 331 pediatric patients.[37] In 35 cases (>10%), capnography detected a critical incident. The authors judged 20 of these to have been life-threatening. Only 2 of the life-threatening incidents were detected simultaneously by the clinician's routine observation and other monitors. Thus capnography was deemed to be the best monitor of ventilation.

Maintenance of normocarbia

It is difficult to find scientific data supporting the notion that anesthesia is safer when, through controlled or assisted ventilation, $PaCO_2$ is kept in the normal range (35 to 45 mm Hg). An objective during virtually every routine administration of anesthesia, however, is to maintain the patient's vital signs and physiologic parameters as near as possible to preanesthetic values. This is certainly the goal for heart rate and blood pressure, and it makes sense to do this for carbon dioxide as well.

The physiologic consequences of hypercarbia and hypocarbia are well recognized. Increased $PaCO_2$ causes respiratory acidosis, increases cerebral blood flow and intracranial pressure in susceptible patients, increases pulmonary vascular resistance, and causes potassium to shift from the intracellular fluid into the serum. Conversely, hypocarbia caused by excessive mechanical ventilation of the lungs causes respiratory alkalosis, decreases cerebral blood flow, decreases pulmonary vascular resistance, and causes potassium to shift from the serum to the intracellular fluid. For certain patients, each of these situations can have hazardous effects.

The human body has the capacity to buffer 120 L of carbon dioxide.[38] During a prolonged anesthesia in which the lungs are hyperventilated, this carbon dioxide buffer becomes progressively depleted. Following emergence from anesthesia, metabolically produced carbon dioxide is sequestered into this buffer. Consequently, $PaCO_2$ increases at a rate slower than normal. In the same patients, the hypoxia-driven urge to breathe is blunted by residual anesthetics, which also shift the carbon dioxide ventilatory-drive curve to the right. Thus the patient can hypoventilate, or even become apneic, with neither a strong oxygen nor carbon dioxide stimulus to breathe. With capnography and an estimation of the difference between $PaCO_2$ and $PECO_2$max ($PaCO_2 - PECO_2$max), the parameters for mechanical ventilation can be adjusted to maintain normocapnia and to avoid the sequelae of either hyperventilation or hypoventilation.

Cardiopulmonary resuscitation

Capnography is emerging as an important monitor during cardiopulmonary resuscitation (CPR). During CPR, $PECO_2$max is low, which reflects the decreased pulmonary blood flow generated by chest compression when compared with that during normal cardiac contraction. Return of spontaneous circulation and increased pulmonary blood flow immediately and significantly increases $PECO_2$max,[39] which makes this one of the earliest signs of successful resuscitation. In one study of 10 patients who experienced out-of-hospital cardiac arrests, the mean $PECO_2$max, which was $1.7\% \pm 0.6\%$ (12.1 mm Hg $\pm$ 4.3 mm Hg) during chest compression, rose rapidly to $4.6\% \pm 1.4\%$ (32.8 mm Hg $\pm$ 10 mm Hg) following the return of spontaneous circulation.[40] Noting the difficulty in palpating peripheral arterial pulses during CPR, some investigators use $PECO_2$max to assess noninvasively the hemodynamic response to cardiopulmonary resuscitation.[41] Unlike the electrocardiograph, invasive pressure manometer, and pulse palpation, the capnograph neither requires interruption of chest compression nor is vulnerable to the mechanical artifacts of chest compression; therefore $PECO_2$max can be assessed without interrupting CPR.

Other studies have examined whether $PECO_2$max can be used to differentiate cardiac arrest patients likely to be resuscitated from those unlikely to be resuscitated. In one study, Callaham and Barton[42] found that following tracheal intubation, an initial $PECO_2$max greater than 15 mm Hg during CPR predicted the eventual return of pulsatile circulation with a sensitivity of 71% and a specificity of 98%. Similarly, Sanders et al.[43] demonstrated that a $PECO_2$max greater than 10 mm Hg predicted those patients who would eventually be resuscitated. The investigators in each study cautioned that a few patients with low $PECO_2$max were eventually resuscitated, so the clinician must incorporate all other available clinical data (e.g., cardiac rhythm of the patient) when deciding whether or not to continue CPR. A $PECO_2$max greater than 10 or 15 mm Hg, however, indicates that CPR is achieving some pulmonary blood flow. Because of a higher probability of re-

turn of pulsatile circulation, CPR should be continued in these patients.

A persistently low or progressive decrease in $PECO_2$max during CPR requires consideration of several, possibly concurrent, diagnoses:

> Esophageal intubation
> Cardiac tamponade
> Tension pneumothorax
> Massive pulmonary embolus
> Hypovolemia (severe)
> Hyperventilation (severe)
> Ineffective CPR

A low or absent $PECO_2$max is not necessarily diagnostic of esophageal intubation; during CPR, this possibility must be ruled out by clinical assessment (for example, direct visualization of the tracheal tube between the vocal cords). Hypovolemia, tamponade, pneumothorax, and pulmonary embolus can each create $V/Q > 1$ by interfering with cardiac filling or pulmonary blood flow and causing low $PECO_2$max. Similarly, ineffective CPR may do the same. Ineffective CPR may be a result of poor technique (compression location, compression depth, or compression/relaxation ratio) or fatigue of the resuscitator.[44] Alveolar hyperventilation is common during CPR as an enthusiastic resuscitator manually hyperventilates the lungs of a patient who already has a markedly decreased pulmonary blood flow. Constant and appropriate minute ventilation is essential to derive maximum benefit from carbon dioxide monitoring during CPR.

Weaning from mechanical ventilation

Intensivists have long sought a noninvasive method to guide the weaning of patients from mechanical ventilation. Can capnography be used in lieu of blood gas analysis? Two studies[45,46] show that, although changes in $PECO_2$max parallel changes in $PaCO_2$, the large and often variable difference between $PaCO_2$ and $PECO_2$max in patients in the intensive care unit (ICU) renders the capnograph relatively insensitive to hypercarbia in this setting. For example, in one case, a patient experienced a 10-mm Hg rise in $PaCO_2$ with no change in $PECO_2$max.[45] Thus, although capnography is useful for detecting many critical incidents in the ICU, at present, unless $PaCO_2 - PECO_2$max is known and stable, blood gas analysis still remains the method preferred by most intensivists for weaning patients from mechanical ventilation.

This insensitivity to hypercarbia in many ICU patients is also a shortcoming of capnography in the operating room. Therefore, regardless of the setting, if it is important to know a patient's precise $PaCO_2$, a blood gas analysis is still needed. Once the relationship between $PaCO_2$ and $PECO_2$max for a patient has been quantified, however, the value serves as a useful guide for future clinical management. Any time there is a significant change in blood pressure, tidal volume, continuous positive airway pressure, or any other parameter that can alter a patient's V/Q, its effect on $PaCO_2 - PECO_2max$ must be considered. Some investigators have actually used changes in $PaCO_2 - PECO_2max$ to define recovery from pulmonary disease and to guide therapy.[47] Even in patients with a large $PaCO_2 - PECO_2max$ gradient, if a maximal exhalation is actively or passively performed or if the peak $PECO_2max$ encountered over several minutes is used, $PaCO_2 - PECO_2max$ becomes very small.[48] Thus, although an imperfect predictor of $PaCO_2$, capnography has considerable applications for both monitoring and weaning intubated ICU patients.

Capnography is also used in the ICU or during transport to and from the ICU for the same purpose as in the operating room: to alert the clinician to such life-threatening problems as disconnection, failure of the mechanical ventilator, and severe hypercapnia. In those patients dependent on stable hyperventilation (for example, patients with increased intracranial pressure), the capnograph is an indispensable real-time monitor.

Monitoring the nonintubated patient

A spontaneously breathing patient who has not undergone intubation can be monitored with a side-stream capnograph. A variety of adaptations for face masks,[49] nasal airways,[50] and nasal cannulas[51,52] have been devised to facilitate capnography during regional anesthesia and monitored anesthesia care (see also Figs. 27-3 and 27-4). These systems allow not only the capnograph to serve as an apnea monitor but also, with proper application, $PaCO_2$ and $PECO_2max$ to correlate closely during nasal capnography.[51,53]

PITFALLS OF CAPNOGRAPHY

The clinician using capnography must avoid three pitfalls. First, capnography is not a substitute for maintaining sharp clinical skills (inspection, palpation, and auscultation). The capnograph is an electrical, optical, mechanical instrument; although reliable, it will eventually fail. Therefore, data from monitoring instruments and from clinical assessment should be combined to serve as a check-and-balance system. Thus, even in the event of instrument failure, competent monitoring will continue. Second, clinicians using capnography must interpret the capnogram. We have already pointed out the problems posed by reliance solely on digital inspired and end-tidal values reported by the monitor. Third, and most important, effective use of capnography depends on understanding the relationship between $PaCO_2$ and $PECO_2max$. Table 10-4 summarizes common problems that can be diagnosed completely or in part with the capnograph.

ACKNOWLEDGMENTS

The authors thank Kelly Spaulding for word processing and Lynn Dirk for editorial assistance in the preparation of this chapter.

Table 10-4. Untoward situations detected with capnography

Problem	Cause
No (or little) exhaled CO_2	Esophageal intubation
	Tracheal extubation
	Disconnection of capnograph or gas source
	Complete obstruction (equipment or pulmonary disease)
	Apnea
Elevated inspiratory baseline (phase I)	Open CO_2 bypass
	Partially exhausted CO_2 absorbent
	Channeling through CO_2 absorbent
	Incompetent expiratory valve
Prolonged expiratory upstroke (phase II)	Obstruction (equipment or pulmonary disease)
	Slow gas sampling or slow instrument response
Upsloping expiratory plateau (phase III)	Obstruction (equipment or pulmonary disease)
Prolonged inspiratory downstroke (phase IV)	Incompetent inspiratory valve
	Slow gas sampling or slow instrument response
Hypercapnia	Hypoventilation (leak, obstruction of air flow, inadequate ventilation)
	CO_2 rebreathing
	Increased CO_2 production or delivery (malignant hyperthermia, fever, CO_2 insufflation, bicarbonate administration, release of tourniquet or cross clamp)
Hypocapnia	Hyperventilation
	Decreased CO_2 production or delivery (hypothermia, decreased cardiac output)
	Increased gradient of arterial to maximum expired CO_2 (ventilation/perfusion mismatching, endobronchial intubation, pulmonary embolism [air, fat, thrombus, or amniotic fluid], shallow or rapid breathing, instrument or sampling problems, miscalibration)

Reproduced with permission from Good ML: *Capnography: uses, interpretation, and pitfalls.* In Barash PG, Deutsch S, Tinker J, editors: *ASA refresher courses in anesthesiology, vol 18*, Philadelphia, 1991, JB Lippincott.

REFERENCES

1. *Standards for basic intraoperative monitoring, directory of members*, Park Ridge, Ill, 1991, American Society of Anesthesiologists.
2. Goldberg JS, Rawle RP, Zehnder JL, et al: Colorimetric end tidal carbon dioxide monitoring for tracheal intubation, *Anesth Analg* 70:191-194, 1990.
3. Good ML: *Capnography: uses, interpretation, and pitfalls.* In Barash PG, Deutsch S, Tinker JH, editors: *ASA refresher courses in anesthesiology, vol 18*, Philadelphia, 1991, JB Lippincott.
4. Birmingham PK, Cheney FW, Ward RJ: Esophageal intubation: a review of detection techniques, *Anesth Analg* 65:886-891, 1986.
5. Linko K, Paloheimo M, Tammisto T: Capnography for detection of accidental oesophageal intubation, *Acta Anaesthesiol Scand* 27:199-202, 1983.

6. Sum-Ping ST, Mehta MP, Anderton JM: A comparative study of methods of detection of esophageal intubation, *Anesth Analg* 69:627-632, 1989.

7. Good ML, Modell JH, Rush W: Differentiating esophageal from tracheal capnograms, *Anesthesiology* 69:A266, 1988 (abstract).

8. Garnett AR, Gervin CA, Gervin AS: Capnographic waveforms in esophageal intubation: effect of carbonated beverages, *Ann Emerg Med* 18:387-390, 1989.

9. Gravenstein JS: *Gas monitoring and pulse oximetry,* Boston, 1990, Butterworths.

10. Gravenstein N: Capnometry in infants should not be done at lower sampling flow rates, *J Clin Monit* 5:63, 1989 (letter).

11. Martin RL, Stevens WC: Inspiratory effort is a sensitive guide to anesthetic depth, *Anesth Analg* 72:S171, 1991 (abstract).

12. Nunn JF, Hill DW: Respiratory deadspace and arterial to end-tidal CO_2 tension difference in anesthetized man, *J Appl Physiol* 15:383-389, 1960.

13. Askrog VF, Pender JW, Smith TC, et al: Changes in respiratory deadspace during halothane, cyclopropane, and nitrous oxide anesthesia, *Anesthesiology* 25:343-352, 1964.

14. Takki S, Aromaa U, Kauste A: The validity and usefulness of the end-tidal P_{CO_2} during anaesthesia, *Ann Clin Res* 4:278-284, 1972.

15. Whitesell R, Asiddao C, Gollman D, et al: Relationship between arterial and peak expired carbon dioxide pressure during anesthesia and factors influencing the difference, *Anesth Analg* 60:508-512, 1981.

16. Valentin N, Lomholt B, Thorup M: Arterial to end-tidal carbon dioxide tension difference in children under halothane anaesthesia. *Can Anaesth Soc J* 29:12-15, 1982.

17. Raemer DB, Francis D, Philip JH, et al: Variation in P_{CO_2} between arterial blood and peak expired gas during anesthesia, *Anesth Analg* 62:1065-1069, 1983.

18. Fletcher R, Jonson B: Deadspace and the single breath test for carbon dioxide during anaesthesia and artificial ventilation: effects of tidal volume and frequency of respiration, *Br J Anaesth* 56:109-119, 1984.

19. Shankar KB, Moseley H, Kumar Y, et al: Arterial to end-tidal carbon dioxide tension difference during caesarean section anaesthesia, *Anaesthesia* 41:698-702, 1986.

20. Hatle L, Rokseth R: The arterial to end-expiratory carbon dioxide tension gradient in acute pulmonary embolism and other cardiopulmonary disease, *Chest* 66:352-357, 1974.

21. Warwick WJ: The end-expiratory-to-arterial carbon dioxide tension ratio in acute pulmonary embolism, *Chest* 68:609-611, 1975.

22. Badgwell JM, Heavner JE, May WS, et al: End-tidal P_{CO_2} monitoring in infants and children ventilated with either a partial rebreathing or a non-rebreathing circuit, *Anesthesiology* 66:405-410, 1987.

23. Gravenstein N, Lampotang S, Beneken JEW: Factors influencing capnography in the Bain circuit, *J Clin Monit* 1:6-10, 1985.

24. Badgwell JM, McLeod ME, Lerman J, et al: End-tidal P_{CO_2} measurements sampled at the distal and proximal ends of the endotracheal tube in infants and children, *Anesth Analg* 66:959-964, 1987.

25. Rich GF, Sullivan MP, Adams MJM: Is distal sampling of end-tidal CO_2 necessary in small subjects? *Anesthesiology* 73:265-268, 1990.

26. Severinghaus JW: Water vapor calibration errors in some capnometers: respiratory conventions misunderstood by manufacturers? *Anesthesiology* 70:996-998, 1989.

27. Brunner JX, Westenskow DR: How carbon dioxide analyzer rise time affects the accuracy of carbon dioxide measurements, *J Clin Monit* 4:134, 1988 (abstract).

28. Shankar KB, Mosely H, Kumar Y, et al: Arterial to end-tidal carbon dioxide tension difference during cesarean section, *Anaesthesia* 41:698-702, 1986.

29. Jones NL, Robertson DG, Cain JW: Difference between end-tidal and arterial CO_2 and exercise, *J Appl Physiol* 47:954-960, 1979.

30. Sosis M: Arterial to end-tidal carbon dioxide gradients, *Anesth Analg* 67:486, 1988.

31. Dunn CM, Maltry DE, Eggers GWN: Value of mass spectrometry in early diagnosis of malignant hyperthermia, *Anesthesiology* 63:333, 1985.

32. Neubauer KR, Kaufman RD: Another use for mass spectrometry: detection and monitoring of malignant hyperthermia, *Anesth Analg* 64:837-839, 1985.

33. Cooper JB, Newbower RS, Kitz RJ: An analysis of major errors and equipment failures in anesthesia management: considerations for prevention and detection, *Anesthesiology* 60:34-42, 1984.

34. Caplan RA, Posner K, Ward RJ, et al: Adverse respiratory events in anesthesia: a closed claims analysis, *Anesthesiology* 72:828-833, 1990.

35. Eichhorn JH: Prevention of intraoperative anesthesia accidents and related severe injury through safety monitoring, *Anesthesiology* 70:572-577, 1989.

36. Keenan RL, Boyan CP: Cardiac arrest due to anesthesia, *JAMA* 253:2373-2377, 1985.

37. Coté CJ, Szyfelbein SK, Goudsouzian NB, et al: Intraoperative events diagnosed by expired carbon dioxide monitoring in children, *Can Anaesth Soc J* 33:315-320, 1986.

38. Nunn JF: *Applied respiratory physiology,* ed 3, London, 1987, Butterworths, p 226.

39. Falk JL, Rackow EC, Weil MH: End-tidal carbon dioxide concentration during cardiopulmonary resuscitation, *N Engl J Med* 318:607-611, 1988.

40. Garnett AR, Ornato JP, Gonzalez ER, et al: End-tidal carbon dioxide monitoring during cardiopulmonary resuscitation, *JAMA* 257:512-515, 1987.

41. Weil MH, Gazmuri RJ, Kette F, et al: End-tidal P_{CO_2} during cardiopulmonary resuscitation, *JAMA* 263:814-815, 1990 (letter).

42. Callaham M, Barton C: Prediction of outcome from cardiopulmonary resuscitation from end-tidal carbon dioxide concentration, *Crit Care Med* 18:358-362, 1990.

43. Sanders AB, Kern KB, Otto CW, et al: Carbon dioxide monitoring during cardiopulmonary resuscitation: a prognostic indicator for survival, *JAMA* 262:1347-1351, 1989.

44. Kalenda Z: The capnogram as a guide to the efficacy of cardiac massage, *Resuscitation* 6:259-263, 1978.

45. Healey CH, Fedullo AJ, Swinburne AJ, et al: Comparison of noninvasive measurement of carbon dioxide during withdrawal from mechanical ventilation, *Crit Care Med* 15:764-768, 1987.

46. Niehoff J, del Guercio C, LaMorte W, et al: Efficacy of pulse oximetry and capnometry in postoperative ventilatory weaning, *Crit Care Med* 16:701-705, 1988.

47. Chopin C, Fesard P, Mangalaboyi J, et al: Use of capnography in diagnosis of pulmonary embolism during acute respiratory failure of chronic obstructive pulmonary disease, *Crit Care Med* 18:353-357, 1990.

48. Weinger MB, Brimm JE: End-tidal carbon dioxide as a measure of arterial carbon dioxide during intermittent mandatory ventilation, *J Clin Monit* 3:73-79, 1987.

49. Pressman MA: A simple method for measuring end-tidal CO_2 during MAC and major regional anesthesia, *Anesth Analg* 67:900-906, 1988.

50. Norman EA, Zeig NJ, Ahmad I: Better designs for mass spectrometer monitoring of the awake patient, *Anesthesiology* 64:664, 1986 (letter).

51. Bowe EA, Boysen PG, Brome JA, et al: Accurate determination of end-tidal CO_2 during administration of oxygen by nasal cannulae, *J Clin Monit* 5:105-110, 1989.

52. Goldman JM: A simple, easy and inexpensive method for monitoring end-tidal CO_2 through nasal cannulae, *Anesthesiology* 67:606, 1987 (letter).

53. Roy J, McNulty S: An improved nasal prong apparatus for end-tidal carbon dioxide monitoring on awake sedated patients, *Anesthesiology* 71:A356, 1989 (abstract).

Chapter 11

PULSE OXIMETRY

Steven J. Barker, Ph.D., M.D.
Kevin K. Tremper, Ph.D., M.D.

No monitor of oxygen transport has had a greater impact on the practice of anesthesiology than the pulse oximeter. Unknown in the operating room before the 1980s, the pulse oximeter has rapidly become a minimum standard of anesthetic care. Its operation requires no special training or new skills on the part of the user. It is noninvasive and therefore almost free of risk. The pulse oximeter gives continuous, real-time estimates of arterial hemoglobin saturation, which can warn of hypoxemia from many causes, including loss of airway patency, loss of oxygen supply, and increases in venous admixture.

Figure 11-1 illustrates the stages of the oxygen transport system. It can be seen that the pulse oximeter monitors oxygen at the level of the arterial blood. Respired gas monitors can confirm only that oxygen is being delivered to the lungs, but the pulse oximeter also monitors the function of the lungs in transporting this oxygen to the arterial blood. However, this does not guarantee that oxygen is being delivered to or utilized by the tissues. This can be deter-mined only by monitors that function further down the oxygen transport chain.

In this chapter, the history and development of pulse oximetry are reviewed as well as its underlying physical and engineering principles. An understanding of these principles will enable the reader to predict the sources of measurement error. The pulse oximeter's accuracy, response, clinical applications, and limitations are also discussed.

HEMOGLOBIN SATURATION AND OXYGEN TRANSPORT

The pulse oximeter provides a noninvasive estimate of arterial hemoglobin saturation, a variable that is directly related to the oxygen content of arterial blood. Two definitions of hemoglobin saturation are currently in use. The older definition, referred to as *functional saturation*, or SaO_2, is related to the concentrations of oxyhemoglobin (O_2Hb) and deoxygenated (sometimes termed "reduced") hemoglobin (RHb) as follows:

$$SaO_2 = \frac{O_2Hb}{O_2Hb + RHb} \times 100\% \tag{1}$$

Additional species of hemoglobin are often present in adult blood, including carboxyhemoglobin (COHb) and methemoglobin (MetHb). This leads to the definition of *fractional hemoglobin saturation*, or $O_2Hb\%$, as the ratio of oxyhemoglobin to the total concentration of all hemoglobin species:

$$O_2Hb\% = \frac{O_2Hb}{O_2Hb + RHb + COHb + MetHb} \times 100\% \tag{2}$$

Fractional hemoglobin saturation is sometimes called *oxyhemoglobin fraction* or *oxyhemoglobin percent*.[1]

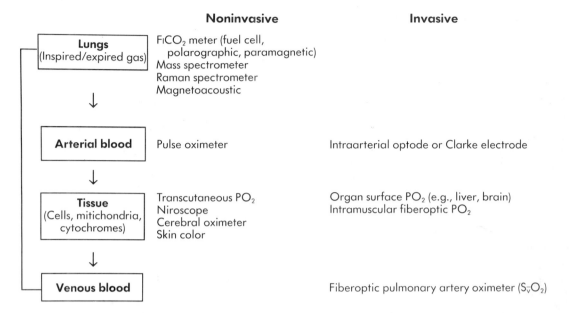

Fig. 11-1. Block diagram of the oxygen transport system. Both invasive and noninvasive monitors of oxygenation are listed for each level in the transport process.

Fractional arterial hemoglobin saturation is related to the arterial oxygen content, CaO_2, by the following formula:

$$CaO_2 = [1.37 \times Hb \times (O_2Hb\% / 100)] + (0.003 \times PaO_2) \quad (3)$$

where Hb is the total hemoglobin concentration in g/dl and PaO_2 is the arterial oxygen tension in mm Hg. The first term in Equation 3 represents the oxygen bound to hemoglobin, which under normal conditions (Hb = 15 g/dl; $O_2Hb\%$ = 98) equals 20 ml oxygen per 100 ml blood. The second term represents oxygen dissolved in plasma, which equals 0.3 ml/100 ml, for a PaO_2 of 100 mm Hg. Plasma-dissolved oxygen does not normally play a significant role in oxygen transport. Equation 3 shows that arterial oxygen content is directly proportional to both total hemoglobin (Hb) and fractional saturation ($O_2Hb\%$). $O_2Hb\%$ and PaO_2 are related by the oxyhemoglobin dissociation curve, shown in Fig. 11-2. For adults under normal conditions, this relationship predicts a saturation of 50% (P_{50}) at a PaO_2 of 27 mm Hg, 75% at a PaO_2 of 40 mm Hg, and 90% at a PaO_2 of 60 mm Hg. The normal dissociation curve is shifted to the right by acidosis, hypercarbia, hyperthermia, and increases in 2,3 diphosphoglycerate (DPG). For PaO_2 values greater than 90 mm Hg, $O_2Hb\%$ is nearly independent of PaO_2. This fact has important implications in the clinical interpretation of pulse oximeter data.

The amount of oxygen delivered to the tissues by the arterial blood (O_{2del}) is simply the product of the arterial oxygen content and the cardiac output, C.O., or

$$O_{2del} = CaO_2 \times C.O. \times 10 \quad (4)$$

The factor 10 appears in this equation because CaO_2 is usually measured in ml/100 ml and C.O. is measured in L/min. The quantity of oxygen consumed per minute ($\dot{V}O_2$) is then the difference between the arterial oxygen delivery (O_{2del}) and the venous oxygen return (O_{2ret}): $\quad$ (5)

$$\dot{V}O_2 = O_{2del} - O_{2ret} = (CaO_2 - C\bar{v}O_2) \times C.O. \times 10$$

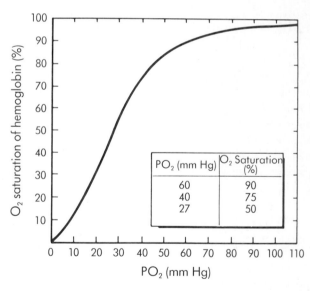

Fig. 11-2. The oxyhemoglobin dissociation curve. Hemoglobin saturation is plotted as a function of oxygen tension (PaO_2) in mm Hg. Under normal conditions for adults, a PaO_2 of 27 mm Hg yields a saturation of 50% (P_{50}). The curve is shifted to the right by acidosis, hypercarbia, increases in 2,3 diphosphoglycerate and hyperthermia.

The arterial oxygen content CaO_2 and the mixed venous oxygen content $C\overline{v}O_2$ in this so-called Fick equation can be replaced by corresponding expressions in terms of hemoglobin saturation from Equation 3: **(6)**

$$\dot{V}O_2 = 13.7 \times C.O. \times [(O_2Hb\%_a - O_2Hb\%_{\overline{v}})]/100$$

Subscripts a and $\overline{v}$ denote arterial and mixed venous hemoglobin saturations, and the small contributions of plasma-dissolved oxygen have been neglected in this form of the equation. Equation 6 shows clearly the relationship between oxygen consumption, arterial and mixed venous hemoglobin saturations, total hemoglobin, and cardiac output. This equation is very helpful in the interpretation of pulse oximeter or other oxygen monitoring data and their relationship to hemodynamic variables.

HISTORY OF PULSE OXIMETRY

Although the pulse oximeter became a standard of anesthetic care in the operating room in the 1980s, in vivo oximeters date back to the 1930s. In 1935 Carl Matthes developed the first instrument that measured hemoglobin oxygen saturation by transilluminating tissue. Matthes' device used two wavelengths of light, one visible and one infrared, much like the modern day pulse oximeter. This instrument could follow saturation trends but was difficult to calibrate. J. R. Squires developed a similar instrument that calibrated itself by compressing the tissue to eliminate blood, a technique that was used later in the first commercially marketed in vivo oximeters.

Glen Millikan created the first light-weight ear oximeter in the early 1940s for aviation research. Millikan first used the term *oximeter* to describe his device, which was used to measure hemoglobin saturation in pilots flying at high altitudes. Similar devices developed in the 1940s were used by Wood and others in the operating room. The first operating room application of an in vivo oximeter to appear in the anesthesiology literature was published in 1951.[2] Figure 11-3 shows a detailed record of the hemo-

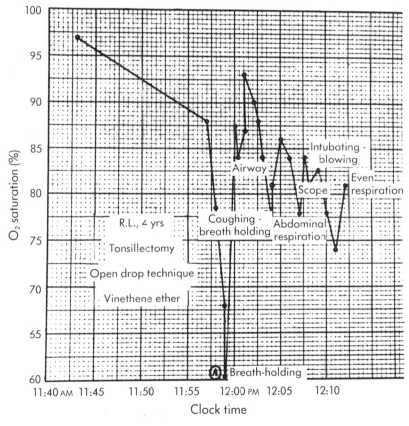

Fig. 11-3. Ear oximeter hemoglobin saturation plotted as a function of time for a four-year-old child undergoing general anesthesia for tonsillectomy. The anesthesia technique was open-drop ether with no supplemental oxygen. Note the significant desaturation associated with "breath holding" during induction of anesthesia. Saturation does not return to its preinduction baseline value at any time during the record. (Reproduced from Steven RC, Slater HM, Johnson AL, et al: The oximeter: a technical aid for the anesthesiologist, *Anesthesiology* 12:548, 1951, with permission.)

globin saturation (obtained from an ear oximeter) plotted versus time during a tonsillectomy. Even though this record shows a dramatic fall in saturation during the induction of anesthesia (described curiously as "breath holding" in the original figure), the device drew little attention from anesthesiologists until much later.

The lack of immediate acceptance of these early in vivo oximeters was partly due to their serious limitations. They were delicate instruments that required technicians for their calibration and operation. The ear-piece, generally large and cumbersome, produced enough heat to cause occasional burns. Hewlett-Packard made a major advance in ear oximetry in the 1970s, when they marketed their self-calibrating eight-wavelength ear oximeter. The Hewlett-Packard (HP) oximeter was shown to be reasonably accurate for intraoperative monitoring, but it was still burdened by the size and cumbersome nature of the sensor as well as the expense of the instrument.[3] Although the HP oximeter became a standard tool in pulmonary function laboratories, it had virtually no impact in the operating room.

The first pulse oximeter was invented by Takuo Aoyagi in the mid-1970s. While developing a method to measure intravenous dye wash-out curves using light transmission through the ear, Aoyagi discovered that his light-absorbance curves contained fluctuations caused by the arterial pulse. In dealing with this "artifact," he discovered that the relative amplitudes of the fluctuations at the two light wavelengths varied with arterial hemoglobin saturation. This fortuitous discovery soon led him to the creation of the first two-wavelength pulse oximeter, which was marketed by Nihon Kohden Corporation. Aoyagi's oximeter used filtered light sources and fiberoptic transmission cables between the instrument and the ear sensor, rendering the latter somewhat cumbersome for use in the operating room.

The next breakthrough in pulse oximetry came in the late 1970s, when Scott Wilbur of the Biox Corporation (now Ohmeda) developed the first ear sensor that used light emitting diodes (LEDs) and solid state photodetectors built into the sensor itself. The fiberoptic cables of previous ear oximeters were thereby replaced by a thin electrical cable.[4] The accuracy of the pulse oximeter was also improved by the incorporation of digital microprocessors into the instrument. Further electronic improvements were made by both Biox and Nellcor in the early 1980s, and the pulse oximeter was then ready to take its place as a standard operating room monitor. The success of Nellcor in marketing their N-100 pulse oximeter to anesthesiologists in the mid-1980s brought pulse oximeters into the operating room in large numbers. The instrument had now become reliable and easy to use as well as relatively inexpensive. It therefore gained rapid acceptance and quickly became a standard of care in the operating room by 1987. In the 1990s, no anesthesiologist would feel comfortable inducing general anesthesia without a functioning pulse

oximeter. An excellent and thorough review of the history of pulse oximetry and the development of blood gas analysis has been written by Severinghaus and Astrup.[5]

PHYSICS AND ENGINEERING OF PULSE OXIMETRY

Spectrophotometry

The science of spectrophotometry makes use of the measurement of light absorbance to determine the concentrations of various solutes in clear solutions. Matthes used this technique to determine hemoglobin oxygen saturation as early as the 1930s. The measurement is based on the Lambert-Beer law, which relates solute concentrations to the intensity of light transmitted through a solution:

$$I_{trans} = I_{in} e^{-\alpha} \quad (7a)$$
$$\alpha = dC_s\epsilon \quad (7b)$$

where:

I_{trans} = Intensity of transmitted light
I_{in} = Intensity of incident light
α = Absorbance
d = Distance light is transmitted through the solution (path length)
C_s = Concentration of solute
ϵ = Extinction coefficient of the solute

The extinction coefficient ϵ quantitates the tendency of a given solute to absorb light. As shown by Equations 7a and 7b, ϵ is the natural logarithm of the ratio I_{in}/I_{trans} for a solution whose concentration C and thickness d are both unity. The extinction coefficient is a known constant for a specific solute at a given wavelength. If a solute of known ϵ is in solution in a cuvette (transparent measurement chamber) of known dimensions, the solute concentration can then be calculated by Equation 7a from measurements of the intensities of incident and transmitted light. In a single-solute system, the absorbance α is simply the product of the path length, concentration, and extinction coefficient (Equation 7b). If multiple solutes are present, α is the sum of similar expressions for each solute; for example, $\alpha = d(C_1\epsilon_1 + C_2\epsilon_2)$ if there are two solutes. The extinction coefficients of the four common hemoglobin species in the red and infrared wavelength range are shown in Fig. 11-4.

Laboratory in vitro oximeters use this principle to determine the concentrations of several hemoglobin species by measuring light transmitted through a cuvette filled with a hemoglobin suspension produced from lysed red blood cells.[1] The analysis above assumes that both the solvent and the cuvette are transparent at the wavelengths used, the light path length is known exactly, and no unknown light-absorbing species are present in the solution. It is difficult to meet these requirements precisely in clinical devices. Therefore, instruments theoretically based on the Lambert-Beer law require empirical corrections to improve accuracy.

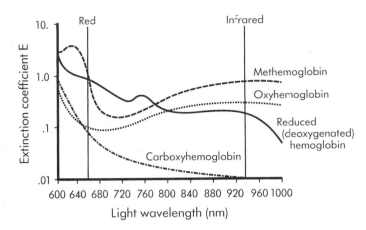

Fig. 11-4. Extinction coefficient plotted versus light wavelength in nanometers for four common hemoglobin species: oxyhemoglobin *(O₂Hb)*, reduced hemoglobin *(RHb)*, carboxyhemoglobin *(COHb)*, and methemoglobin *(MetHb)*. The absorbance of COHb is very similar to that of O₂Hb in the visible red wavelengths. MetHb has a high absorbance over a broad spectrum, giving it a characteristic brown color. (Adapted from Tremper KK and Barker SJ: Pulse oximetry: applications and limitations. In *Advances in Oxygen Monitoring, International Anesthesiology Clinics,* Boston, 1987, Little, Brown, pp 155-175.)

Engineering Principles

Pulse oximeters estimate arterial hemoglobin saturation by measuring the transmission of light at two wavelengths through a pulsatile vascular tissue bed. In principle, the pulse oximeter uses the finger, ear, or other tissue as a "cuvette" containing hemoglobin. However, living tissue contains many light absorbers other than arterial hemoglobin, including skin, soft tissue, bone, and venous and capillary blood. Early in vivo oximeters, such as Millikan's, compensated for this additional tissue absorbance by compressing the soft tissues during a calibration cycle to eliminate all blood. The absorbance of the bloodless tissue was then used as a baseline. These oximeters often heated the tissue during measurement to render it hyperemic and thus obtain an absorbance more dependent on arterial blood.

The pulse oximeter distinguishes the light absorbance of arterial blood from that of other absorbers in the tissue in a novel way. As shown in Fig. 11-5, light absorbance in tissue can be divided into a constant, or "direct current" (DC), component and a pulsating, or "alternating current" (AC), component. The AC component of absorbance is almost exclusively the result of arterial blood pulsations. These pulsations are caused by the systolic volume expansion of the arteriolar bed, which produces an increase in optical path length, thus increasing the absorbance (Equation 7b). Pulse oximetry is based on the assumption that arterial blood is the only pulsatile absorber; any other fluctuating light absorbers will therefore constitute sources of error.

The present generation of pulse oximeters uses two wavelengths of light: 660 nm (red) and 940 nm (near infrared). The pulse oximeter measures the AC component of the light absorbance at each wavelength and then divides it by the corresponding DC component (Fig. 11-5). The resulting *pulse-added absorbances* at the two wavelengths are independent of the intensity of incident light. The oximeter then calculates the ratio R of the two pulse-added absorbances:

$$(8)$$

$$R = \frac{AC_{660}/DC_{660}}{AC_{940}/DC_{940}}$$

It can be shown from the Lambert-Beer law that in the absence of dyshemoglobins (COHb, MetHb) the ratio R is uniquely related to the arterial hemoglobin saturation. Although the pulse oximeter saturation SpO_2 can be mathematically derived from the value of R via the theory described above, the oximeter actually uses an empirical calibration curve relating SpO_2 to R, such as the one shown in Fig. 11-6. The calibration curves used in all pulse oximeters are based on experimental data obtained from human volunteers. This empirical calibration is stored in the microprocessor memory of the pulse oximeter. The pulse oximeter does not require user calibration, but this does not imply that the instrument calibrates itself

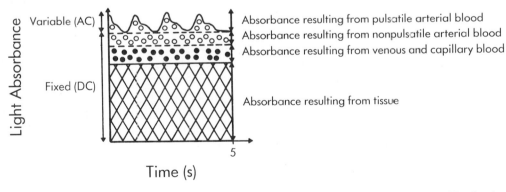

Fig. 11-5. A schematic of the light absorbancies of living tissue plotted versus time. The fixed (DC) absorbance results from solid tissues, venous and capillary blood, and the nonpulsatile arterial blood. The AC component is caused by pulsations in the arterial blood volume. (Adapted from *Ohmeda Pulse Oximeter Model 3700 service* manual, Ohmeda, 1986, Boulder, Colo, p 22.)

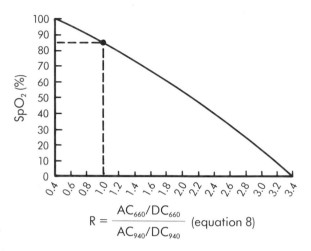

$$R = \frac{AC_{660}/DC_{660}}{AC_{940}/DC_{940}} \quad \text{(equation 8)}$$

Fig. 11-6. A typical pulse oximeter calibration algorithm, in which SpO_2 is plotted versus the ratio R (Equation 8). The value of R varies from roughly 0.4 at 100% saturation to 3.4 at 0% saturation. An R value of 1.0 corresponds to an SpO_2 reading of 85%. Although a similar curve can be derived from the Lambert-Beer law, this curve is actually a composite of experimental data obtained on healthy adult volunteers. (Adapted from Pologe JA: Pulse Oximetry: Technical aspects of machine design, In *Advances in Oxygen Monitoring.* International Anesthesiology Clinics, Edited by Tremper KK, Barker SJ. Boston, 1987, Little, Brown, p. 142.)

for each patient. In fact, the oximeter assumes the same calibration curve for every patient.

SOURCES OF ERROR

Given the physics and engineering design principles outlined above, the sources of error in SpO_2 readings are easily predictable. This section examines the most common sources of error in the operating room and intensive care settings, as well as some of the design approaches used to minimize these errors. The user must be well aware of these problems in order to know when to suspect erroneous data.

Dyshemoglobins and intravenous dyes

Because the pulse oximeter measures light absorbance at two wavelengths, it can deal with unknown concentrations of only two solutes, that is, two hemoglobin species (Equation 7). If any light-absorbing species other than O_2Hb and RHb is present, the pulse oximeter cannot accurately estimate saturation. As shown by the absorbance spectra in Fig. 11-4, both COHb and MetHb absorb light at one or both of the wavelengths used by the pulse oximeter. Significant concentrations of either of these dyshemoglobins can be expected to produce erroneous SpO_2 values. The fact that functional saturation (SaO_2) does not depend explicitly on dyshemoglobin concentrations (Equation 1) does not imply that SaO_2 can be determined by a two-wavelength oximeter. In the presence of these additional hemoglobins, an oximeter cannot measure the con-

centrations of any hemoglobin species with only two wavelengths of light (Equation 7).

The effects of carboxyhemoglobin on SpO_2 values have been determined experimentally in dogs.[6] Figure 11-7 shows SpO_2 as well as $O_2Hb\%$ determined by in vitro oximetry plotted as a function of COHb (expressed as a percentage of total hemoglobin, COHb%). Even when COHb% increases to levels greater than 70%, SpO_2 values remain greater than 90% at all times. The pulse oximeter interprets COHb as though it were composed mostly of O_2Hb, a fact that can be predicted from the absorbance spectra of Fig. 11-4. At the wavelength of 660 nm, COHb has roughly the same absorbance as O_2Hb; at 940 nm, COHb is relatively transparent. This is consistent with the clinical observation that patients with carboxyhemoglobinemia have a bright red skin color.

The effect of MetHb on SpO_2 values has been similarly evaluated in animal experiments.[7] Figure 11-8 shows SpO_2 and $O_2Hb\%$ determined by in vitro oximetry plotted as a function of MetHb%. As in the case of COHb (Fig. 11-7), the presence of MetHb causes the pulse oximeter to overestimate fractional hemoglobin saturation. However, the behavior of MetHb in Fig. 11-8 is significantly different in that the SpO_2 values tend to decrease with increasing MetHb until reaching a plateau at about 85%. For MetHb% values greater than about 30, there is no further decrease in SpO_2 (Fig. 11-8). When the O_2Hb concentration was further reduced by decreasing FIO_2 at fixed MetHb levels (i.e., increasing the RHb concentration), SpO_2 was shown to represent neither functional nor fractional saturation. This fact is again consistent with the light absorbance spectra of Fig. 11-4, which show that MetHb has a high absorbance value at both wavelengths of light used by the pulse oximeter. This high absorbance, which tends to give MetHb its characteristic brown color, adds to both the numerator and denominator of the ratio R given by Equation 8. Increasing both the numerator and denominator of this ratio by a fixed amount tends to drive the value of R toward 1.0. Reference to Fig. 11-6, shows that an R value of 1.0 corresponds to an SpO_2 value of 85%. This may explain why the pulse oximeter tends to read near 85% hemoglobin saturation in the presence of high MetHb levels.

Fetal hemoglobin (HbF) appears to have little effect upon the accuracy of pulse oximetry. This is because the extinction coefficients of HbF at the two wavelengths used by the pulse oximeter (660 and 940 nm) are not very different from the corresponding values for adult hemoglobin (HbA). This is fortunate because the percentage of Hb F present in neonatal blood varies with gestational age and is not accurately predictable. HbF produces small errors in multiwavelength in vitro oximeters. The oxygenated state of HbF is interpreted by these oximeters as consisting partially of COHb.[8] Theoretical considerations suggest that sickle hemoglobin (HbS) also has little effect

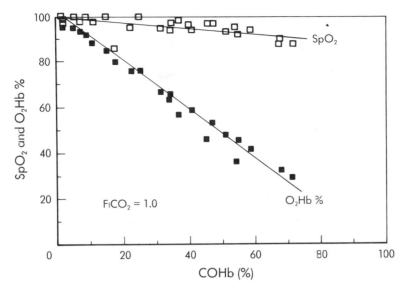

Fig. 11-7. SpO_2 and fractional saturation *(O₂Hb%)* plotted versus carboxyhemoglobin level *(COHb%)* for dogs inhaling carbon monoxide, 200 ppm. SpO_2 seriously overestimates arterial saturation in the presence of COHb and remains greater than 90% even for COHb% = 70. The pulse oximeter "sees" COHb as though it were mostly O_2Hb.

on pulse oximeter accuracy, but to date this has not been confirmed by clinical data.

The ratio *R,* and hence the SpO_2 value, can be affected by any substance present in the blood that absorbs light at 660 or 940 nm. Dyes injected intravenously for diagnostic purposes can have significant effects on SpO_2. Intravenous

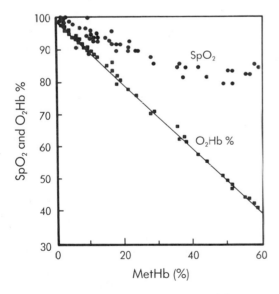

Fig. 11-8. SpO_2 and fractional saturation *(O₂Hb%)* versus methemoglobin level *(MetHb%)* for dogs with drug-induced (by benzocaine spray) methemoglobinemia. Although SpO_2 shows a downward trend with increasing MetHb%, MetHb% is consistently overestimated and it appears that a plateau is reached at $SpO_2 = 85\%$. When FIO_2 is decreased during this experiment, SpO_2 measures neither functional nor fractional saturation.

methylene blue has been shown to produce sudden large decreases in SpO_2 values.[9] Indigo carmine yields very small decreases in SpO_2, and indocyanine green has an intermediate effect. The extinction coefficients of these three dyes are shown plotted versus wavelength in the range 200 to 800 nm in Fig. 11-9.[9] A comparison of these absorbance spectra with those of hemoglobin (Fig. 11-4) clarifies the relative effects of the three dyes upon SpO_2 values. Bilirubin appears to have no significant effect at concentrations seen clinically.[10]

Nail polish has variable effects upon SpO_2 values, usually producing falsely low SpO_2 readings.[11] Relatively opaque, acrylic nail coverings can prevent the pulse oximeter from detecting any pulsatile absorbance at all. This problem can be averted by simply turning the sensor sideways so that the coated fingernail does not fall within the light path. Alternatively, an earlobe may be used as the site for sensor placement.

Wavelength uncertainty

The LED used as a light source by the pulse oximeter is not an ideal monochromatic (i.e., single wavelength of light) radiator. The LED emits light energy over a narrow but finite range of wavelengths. The center wavelength, or wavelength of peak energy radiation, varies measurably for diodes of the same specification. This variation can easily be ±15 nm. Figure 11-4 shows that a change in wavelength by this amount yields a significantly different extinction coefficient, particularly at the 660-nm wavelength. Pulse oximeter manufacturers have approached this problem in two ways. The simplest method is to determine the center wavelength of all LEDs and to reject those that

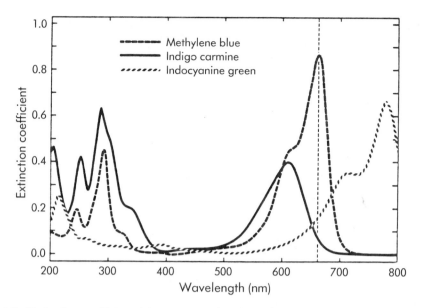

Fig. 11-9. Extinction coefficient *(ε)* versus wavelength *(λ)* in the range 200 nm to 800 nm for three dyes: methylene blue, indigo carmine, and indocyanine green. (Adapted from Scheller MS, et al: Effects of intravenously administered dyes on pulse oximetry readings, *Anesthesiology* 65:550-552, 1986.)

are outside of a specified wavelength range, for example, 660 ± 5 nm. This method is effective but expensive because of the large number of LEDs that must be discarded. The second method is to store multiple calibration algorithms in the pulse oximeter software, corresponding to several different LED center wavelengths. The electrical connector on the sensor cable is then pin-coded so that the appropriate algorithm is selected for a given sensor. Neither of these methods entirely eliminates the effects of variation in center frequency. This center wavelength variability does not affect the pulse oximeter's ability to follow changes in saturation, but it will produce between-sensor differences in the absolute value of SpO_2.[12]

Signal-to-noise ratio

The amplitude of the fluctuating, or AC, component of the light absorbance may be less than 1% of the amplitude of the DC component (Fig. 11-5). Any influence that either decreases the AC absorbance component, increases the DC component, or adds an artifactual AC component not related to arterial pulsations worsens the signal-to-noise ratio. The AC signal is decreased in low perfusion states; the DC signal is increased by ambient light reaching the detector; and artifactual AC signals are caused by motion of the patient (e.g., shivering) or venous pulsations (e.g., tricuspid regurgitation).

The photodiode light detector used in the pulse oximeter sensor cannot discriminate one wavelength of light from another; it is effectively "color-blind." The detector therefore responds to ambient room light as well as to light from either of the LEDs. In most pulse oximeters, this problem is approached by activating the red and infrared LEDs in an alternating sequence. During a part of this sequence, both LEDs are turned off and the photodetector determines the ambient background light. This sequence is repeated many times per second (480 Hz in the Ohmeda Biox 3700 pulse oximeter) in an attempt to eliminate light interference from rapidly changing ambient sources. Despite this ingenious design, ambient light artifact creates problems with the pulse oximeter's signal-to-noise ratio. This difficulty can be minimized by covering the sensor with an opaque shield of some sort, such as a surgical drape or towel.

If the peripheral pulse is weak, as during shock, the AC absorbance signal becomes extremely small compared with the DC signal. The pulse oximeter has an automatic gain control that adjusts either the LED intensity or the photodetector amplifier gain to compensate for changes in AC signal amplitude. When the pulsatile absorbance is small, the pulse oximeter maximizes its amplifier gain or LED brightness. Unfortunately, this process also amplifies background noise from all sources, including ambient light. At the highest amplifier gain, which may increase the signal as much as 10^9 times, the pulse oximeter may interpret components of the background noise as a pulsatile absorbance and generate an SpO_2 value from this artifact.[4] This phenomenon could be easily demonstrated in early pulse oximeters by placing a piece of paper between the photodetector and the LEDs in the sensor. Many oximeters would amplify the background noise and eventually display a pulse and SpO_2 value from it. This problem is also exemplified today by the so-called penumbra effect.[13] If a pulse oximeter finger sensor is partially dislodged in such a manner that the light passes through the fingertip at a grazing incidence, the oximeter may display a correct heart rate but an erroneous SpO_2 value. The SpO_2 value in this case is usually falsely low, which may be another example of the phenomenon $R = 1.0$ (Equation 8), discussed above and illustrated in Fig. 11-6.

All pulse oximeters display some sort of visual indicator of a pulsatile absorbance signal. This may be a simple one-dimensional LED laddergram display or a two-dimensional absorbance-versus-time plethysmogram. In most pulse oximeters, this displayed waveform represents the signal output after amplification and therefore does not correspond in any way to the actual amplitude of the absorbance pulsations. A few manufacturers have chosen to display a waveform whose height actually represents the pulsatile absorbance before amplification. It is the user's responsibility to determine what a particular pulse oximeter's waveform measures, but in general it cannot be assumed that waveform amplitude has any relation to pulse intensity. The pulse oximeter is not a quantitative monitor of peripheral perfusion, and it cannot be relied on to warn of impending ischemia or necrosis. The behavior of pulse oximeters during shock or low perfusion states has been examined in both humans and animals.[14-20] During hemorrhagic shock, the pulse oximeter may display no SpO_2 value at all or give a falsely low estimate. A study of patients in intensive care units showed that loss of signal was associated with low cardiac output states, extremes in systemic vascular resistance, hypothermia, and extreme anemia.[14] A recent study of failure rates of pulse oximeters in the operating room found that pulse oximeters (Nellcor N-100, Ohmeda 3700) failed in 1.12% of all patients.[15] Failure in this case was defined as the lack of an SpO_2 value for a cumulative period of 30 minutes or greater. If the original finger sensor failed to function in a particular patient, other probe sites (ear, nose) were tried before the patient was declared a failure. Higher failure rates were associated with poor preoperative physical status, long operations, and elderly patients.

Several studies have aimed at determining the thresholds for loss of signal during low perfusion states. Lawson, et al.[16] produced gradual occlusion of blood flow with a blood pressure cuff while monitoring flow at the fingertip using a laser-Doppler flow probe. They found in their healthy volunteers that the pulse oximeter lost the signal when blood flow had decreased to an average of 8.6% of its baseline value, which occurred at a cuff pressure of 96% of systolic pressure. Upon cuff deflation the signal returned at a blood flow of only 4% of baseline. Severinghaus, et al.[21] studied pulse oximeter behavior during several types of reduction in extremity blood flow, including via blood pressure cuff, brachial artery pressure clamp, and extremity elevation. Failure occurred at higher mean arterial pressures with the arterial clamp than with gravitational hypotension, showing the importance of pulsatility of the blood volume. These studies demonstrate that the pulse oximeter functions well over a wide range of blood flows and blood pressures in the extremity. Because it is designed to function independently of changes in flow or pressure, the pulse oximeter cannot be used to assess quantitatively the adequacy of peripheral perfusion, even though there have been attempts to do so.[17-19,22]

Artifacts caused by patient motion, particularly that caused by shivering, are difficult to deal with. Although it is rarely a serious problem in the operating room, shivering can make the pulse oximeter useless in the recovery room. The two current engineering approaches to this problem are (1) increased signal-averaging time and (2) ECG synchronization. In the first approach, the value of the ratio R is stored on a beat-to-beat basis for several seconds, and any discrepancies or sudden changes are rejected. The resulting running average is less sensitive to patient motion, but it is also slower to respond to sudden changes in saturation. In the second approach, developed by Nellcor, Inc., the pulse oximeter compares the pulsatile absorbance signal with a simultaneous ECG waveform to ensure that arterial pulsations are synchronous with the ECG.[23] When this C-Lock feature of the Nellcor N-200 is used, absorbance pulsations that are not correlated with an ECG R-wave are rejected and do not influence the SpO_2 value. This may be a useful refinement as long as a clean ECG waveform with unambiguous R-waves is available. Despite these improvements in low signal-to-noise ratio performance, shivering artifact remains a frustrating problem in the recovery room.[4]

The pulse oximeter is designed under the assumption that pulsations in light absorbance are caused by variations in arterial blood volume. However, it has been shown that venous blood is also pulsatile, and that the amplitude of these venous pulsations varies significantly between different parts of the body.[24] A study of human volunteers found that the mean SpO_2 value measured by a fingertip sensor decreased by 1.6% when the arm was moved from an elevated position to a dependent position. However, when the sensor was located on the hypothenar eminence during the same maneuver, SpO_2 decreased by 7.8%.[24] Earlobe sensors and reflectance pulse oximeter sensors placed on the forehead tend to exhibit the same behavior during changes of body position. Any increase in venous pulsations relative to arterial pulsations cause a decrease in SpO_2 toward venous values. The effect should be considered during any change in body position that varies the height of the pulse oximeter sensor with respect to the heart.

Another potent source of artifactual signal is the electrosurgical unit (ESU) or "Bovie". Although the ESU does not generate any light, the electromagnetic radiation from it is very intense and fills the operating room whenever the device is activated. The electrical cable leading from the pulse oximeter sensor to the instrument itself acts as an antenna, which responds to the electromagnetic radiation emitted by the ESU. This interference can be clearly seen on the ECG waveform, where it usually drowns the patient ECG tracing in a sea of artifact. The generation of pulse oximeters marketed in the mid-1980s was similarly affected: the SpO_2 value would disappear upon ESU activation, and a new value would not appear until 10 to 20 seconds after deactivation. The newer pulse oximeters have been greatly improved in this respect. In most clinical situations, they continue to display and update SpO_2 and heart rate values during ESU activation. However, most pulse oximeters continue to display their last "valid" SpO_2 value for some time during loss-of-signal periods. Therefore, the user can be certain that the pulse oximeter is actually following SpO_2 during ESU activation only if a reasonable plethysmograph waveform is displayed during these periods.

CLINICAL APPLICATIONS: ACCURACY AND RESPONSE

This section reviews the clinical applications of pulse oximetry, particularly in the operating room and recovery room. Also discussed are the physiologic limitations of pulse oximetry, that is, what clinical changes can and cannot be determined from saturation monitoring. In reviewing studies of pulse oximeter accuracy, some simple statistical considerations should be kept in mind. Clinical studies of pulse oximeter accuracy are an example of methods-comparison studies, in which two independent methods are used to measure the same variable simultaneously. One of the two methods is generally a new or unproven technique (in this case, pulse oximetry) and the other method is considered a "gold standard". The gold standard for pulse oximeter studies is invariably a laboratory multiwavelength in vitro cooximeter, such as the Instrumentation Laboratory model IL 482* or Radiometer OSM-3. Such devices claim an uncertainty on the order of ±1% (one standard deviation) for measurements of fractional saturation (Equation 2). Because the accuracy of today's pulse oximeters may be comparable to this figure, we must remember that both methods in such comparison studies have uncertainty. There is really no such thing as a gold standard for any monitor.

The recommended statistics for evaluating methods-comparison studies are the bias and precision as defined by Altman and Bland.[25,26] The bias is defined to be the mean difference between simultaneous measurements by the two methods, and the precision is the standard deviation of this difference. In this text the difference between measurements is defined as the pulse oximeter SpO_2 value minus the cooximeter $O_2Hb\%$ value. The value of the bias will demonstrate systematic error, that is, the tendency of one

of the two methods to overestimate or underestimate consistently relative to the other. The precision represents the variability or random error between the two methods. If both the systematic and random errors are clinically within acceptable limits, then the methods-comparison study can conclude that one method may be replaced by the other.

Unfortunately, many methods-comparison studies published in the medical literature have not included bias and precision values. Some do not even include a scattergram, or graphical representation of the data points. The reported statistics often include a correlation coefficient (r) and a linear regression slope and intercept of the data. Although useful, these statistics are not the most informative for evaluating methods-comparison data. The correlation coefficient is not a measure of the agreement between two variables; it is rather a measure of association. It is affected by the range of values covered by the data as well as by the agreement between the two methods.

Most pulse oximeter manufacturers claim an accuracy of ±2% (one standard deviation) for SpO_2 values between 70% and 100%. The uncertainty increases to ±3% for SpO_2 values between 50% and 70%, and no accuracy is specified for SpO_2 values below 50%. That is, for saturations above 70% the SpO_2 value should be within 2% of the actual saturation 68% of the time and within 4% (two standard deviations) 95% of the time. Table 11-1 summarizes the results from 12 studies of pulse oximeter accuracy: 5 in healthy volunteers, 3 in adult patients, and 2 each in pediatric and neonatal patients.[27] As shown in the table, the various authors have presented their data in different ways. The linear regression slope and intercept and the correlation coefficient are the most commonly given statistics. Some authors also provide standard error of the estimate ($S_{y \cdot x}$), which is the standard deviation of the y values about the linear regression line.

Two of the volunteer studies shown in Table 11-1 are of special interest in that they evaluated both accuracy and response times to relatively sudden changes in hemoglobin saturation.[28,29] Both studies discovered errors in pulse oximeter calibration algorithms, which were subsequently revised by some of the manufacturers. As a result of such after-market software revisions, seemingly identical pulse oximeters may actually function differently. Reports of experimental studies should therefore specify not only the pulse oximeter manufacturer and model number but also the software version installed.

The volunteer studies of Severinghaus and Naifeh[28,30] have compared the performance of a relatively large number of pulse oximeters during sudden, severe, transient desaturations. Subjects in one study[28] underwent very brief (45-second) desaturations to an $O_2Hb\%$ value of 40% to 70% (Fig. 11-10). The resulting bias values varied between +13% and −9%, with precision values as high as 16%. Finger sensors appeared to be less accurate than ear sensors, but this may have been a consequence of the unsteady nature of the experiment.

---

*Instrumentation Laboratory, Lexington, Mass.

Table 11-1. Pulse oximeter experimental and clinical accuracy data

Reference	Manufacturer	r	s	i	N	SEE% $(S_{y \cdot x})$	Range % high-low	Bias ± Prec.
Experimental studies in adult volunteers								
Yelderman[52]	N-100	0.98	1.03	−2.33	79	1.83	98-65	
Chapman[44]	Biox II	0.96	0.79	17.9	117	2.72	100-54	
Kagle[29]	Ohmeda 3700 (XJ1)	0.99	0.96	4.59	48	2.7*	99-60	
	N-100	0.99	0.96	5.34	48	2.7*	99-60	
Severinghaus[28]	N-100				60		70-40	6.6 ± 10.8
	N-200				60		70-40	−4.5 ± 8.2
	Ohmeda 3700				60		70-40	2.7 ± 5.8
	CR (.28)				60		70-40	1.4 ± 5.9
	PC (1600)				60		70-40	0.0 ± 3.5
	NO (3.3)				120		70-40	1.1 ± 5.4
	MQ (7)				36		70-40	−2.9 ± 5.2
	Datex				59		70-40	−1.6 ± 5.4
Nickerson[45]	Ohmeda 3700				165		100-65	−2.6 ± 2.1
	CR				165		100-65	−1.0 ± 2.8
	N-100				165		100-65	−0.4 ± 1.7
	NO				165		100-65	−1.0 ± 1.6
Clinical studies in adult patients								
Tremper[14]†	Biox III	0.57	0.93	5.22	383	3.09	100-81	1.4 ± 3.1
Mihm[46]	N-100	0.96	0.97	1.51	131		100-56	
Cecil[47]	Ohmeda 3700	0.83	0.95	0.42	333		100-62	−0.31 ± 2.44
	N-100	0.80	0.78	21.2	330		100-62	0.59 ± 3.02
Clinical studies in pediatric patients								
Fait[48]	N-100	0.89	1.05	−6.56	192		100-70	
Boxer[49]	N-100	0.95	1.01	0.15	108		95-35	−0.87 ± 3.7
Clinical studies in neonatal patients								
Mok[50]	N-100	0.84	0.65	27.8	27		100-43	1.4
Durand[51]		0.86	0.68	29.6	108	2	100-78	−0.2 ± 2.5

Modified from Tremper KK, Barker SJ: Pulse oximetry, *Anesthesiology* 70:98-108, 1989.

The values r, s, and i are linear regression correlation coefficients, slopes, and intercepts, respectively; N = number of data pairs; SEE (S_{yx}) is the standard error of the estimate. Bias is the mean difference between SpO_2 and SaO_2; Prec. is the standard deviation of the differences. All manufacturers' specified accuracies are similar, 1 SD = ±2%, 100% to 70-80%, 1 SD = ±3%, 70-80% to 50%, and unspecified <50%. Manufacturers: N-100 and N-200 (Nellcor); Biox II, Biox III, and Ohmeda 3700 (Ohmeda); CR (Critikon); PC 1600 (Physio Control); NO (Novametrix); MQ (Marquest); and Datex. The software revision is in parentheses following the manufacturer abbreviation when this information was provided in the referenced study. (*Nellcor N100 technical manual*, Nellcor Corporation, Hayward, Calif.; *Ohmeda 3700 pulse oximeter technical manual*, Ohmeda Division of BOC, Boulder, Colo.; *Novametrix 500 pulse oximeter technical manual*, Novametrix Medical Equipment, Wallingford, Conn.)

*These values of $S_{y \cdot x}$ are determined from the authors' 99% confidence intervals.

† The SpO_2 data were collected in patients with pulmonary artery catheters for simultaneous cardiac output determinations. Therefore, these patients were probably more critically ill than those in the other studies.

The pulse oximeter response times to the sudden change in saturation were much shorter for the ear probes, as shown in Fig. 11-10. The time for a 50% response to rapid desaturation or resaturation ranged from 10 to 20 seconds for the ear probe, whereas for the finger probes it varied between 24 and 50 seconds. A similar result was obtained in another study comparing response times of finger probes to those of both ear probes and reflectance sensors on the forehead.[31] Both studies showed a wide variation among subjects in response times for finger sensors, reflecting a wide range of lung-to-finger circulation times. These time delays and their variability among patients should be considered in the selection of sensor sites in clinical situations wherein SpO_2 can change rapidly, for example, in the op-

erating room. However, preliminary clinical studies also suggest that finger sensors are currently the most reliable in obtaining SpO_2 values during periods of hemodynamic instability.[32]

Pulse oximeter response to sudden SaO_2 changes is also affected by the signal averaging time of the instrument, which is generally user-selectable. For example, Novametrix allows the user to choose from four different averaging times ranging from 1 to 15 seconds. The displayed SpO_2 value represents a running average of data obtained over the most recent averaging time period. Therefore, the SpO_2 value will respond more quickly to a rapidly changing SaO_2 if a short averaging time is selected. On the other hand, if the signal-to-noise ratio is marginal or frequent ar-

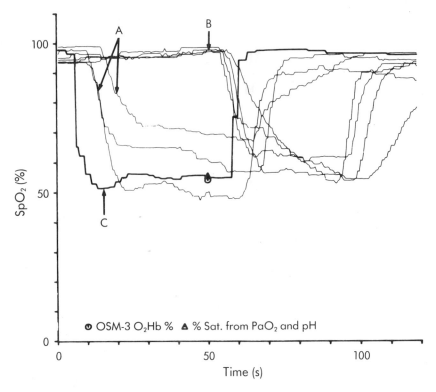

Fig. 11-10. Tracings of SpO_2 versus time for seven pulse oximeters during a rapid and brief desaturation in a healthy volunteer. Tracings labeled *A* represent three ear sensors; tracings *B* are four finger sensors; tracing *C* is the actual saturation calculated from expired oxygen tension measured by mass spectrometry. The ear sensors register the desaturation with a 10- to 15-second time lag, whereas the finger sensors show a nearly 50-second time lag in this volunteer. (Adapted from Severinghaus JW, Naifeh KH: Accuracy of response of six pulse oximeters to profound hypoxia, *Anesthesiology* 67:553, 1987, with permission.)

tifacts (e.g., electrocautery) are present, a longer averaging time will yield more accurate SpO_2 values. The user must determine the appropriate averaging time on the basis of the clinical setting. The default value of the averaging time, the value used when the instrument is first turned on, varies among manufacturers. It is important to know this default value for a particular instrument.

The accuracy of pulse oximetry found in clinical studies is comparable to the manufacturers' specifications, as shown in Table 11-1. However, the specified uncertainty of ±2% to ±3% refers to one standard deviation, or a confidence interval of 68%. That is, 68% of a large number of measurements made simultaneously by a "gold standard" would fall within 2% to 3% of the SpO_2 value. If it is desired to increase the confidence interval to 95%, the uncertainty becomes two standard deviations, or ±4%.

Clinical studies of accuracy consistently combine data from multiple patients to determine the uncertainty in SpO_2 values. This procedure yields a more pessimistic view of accuracy than would be obtained by studying results for individual patients. That is, if a pulse oximeter sensor is placed on a patient and the SpO_2 value is 95%, it is known that there is roughly a 68% probability that the patient's

true saturation lies between 93% and 97%. On the other hand, if the SpO_2 value on that same patient decreases from 95% to 93%, one can feel more certain that the patient's saturation is actually falling than one was of the original absolute SpO_2 value. This variability among patients is a price that must be paid for the convenience of having the pulse oximeter precalibrated with a universal algorithm. This calibration algorithm represents an average of data from a large number of healthy, adult volunteers. Alternatively, the manufacturers could have chosen to require user calibration on each individual patient. This would have yielded a more accurate pulse oximeter, but it would have destroyed some of the most attractive features of pulse oximetry, namely, the absence of user calibration and the immediate availability of SpO_2 data as soon as the sensor is placed on the patient.

The final question about the accuracy of any clinical measurement is what the user should do if the measured value is suspect. In the case of pulse oximetry, the answer depends on why the SpO_2 value is considered suspicious. The current gold standard for validation of SpO_2 is in vitro multiwavelength cooximetry. Laboratory cooximeters with four or more wavelengths (e.g., Instrumentation Laboratory IL-482 or Radiometer OSM-3) can determine either functional or fractional hemoglobin saturation even in the presence of MetHb or COHb. If the user suspects a significant dyshemoglobinemia—for example, in a patient with a smoke inhalation injury—cooximeter analysis of an arterial blood specimen should be considered mandatory. On the other hand, if the SpO_2 value is suspicious yet there is no possibility of a dyshemoglobinemia, an arterial blood gas analysis with calculation of SaO_2 will suffice. An example of this situation is the healthy patient with dark skin pigmentation whose SpO_2 values fall in the low 90s despite adequate ventilation with an adequate FIO_2. However, the clinician should remember that the arterial hemoglobin saturation value given by a blood gas analyzer is calculated from the measured PaO_2 and an assumed hemoglobin dissociation curve (Fig. 11-2).

Once the pulse oximeter was accepted as a minimum standard of anesthesia care in the operating room, it became unethical to perform randomized controlled studies of its clinical effectiveness.[33] Before pulse oximetry became a minimum standard, several such studies were attempted. Coté et al.[34] studied 152 pediatric patients during anesthesia and surgery. In one half of these patients, the SpO_2 data were unavailable to the anesthesiologist. They found that major events, defined as $SpO_2 \leq 85\%$ for more than 30 seconds, occurred significantly more often in those patients for whom the SpO_2 values were unavailable. Most of these major events occurred in patients under 2 years of age. A study of adult patients undergoing gynecologic surgery found SpO_2 values of less than 90% in 10% of all procedures and values of less than 85% in 5% of procedures. Clinical studies such as these, in which SpO_2 values were not available to the anesthesiologist, are no longer possible.

Since becoming a standard in the operating room, the pulse oximeter has also had a major clinical impact in other settings. Two studies in which SpO_2 was monitored during transport from the operating room to the recovery room found a high incidence of desaturation to SpO_2 values less than 90% in patients who did not receive supplemental oxygen.[35,36] These studies lend strong support to a uniform policy of transporting all patients from the operating room with supplemental oxygen. Clinical studies also suggest that SpO_2 should be continuously monitored in most patients in the recovery room. A study of pediatric patients showed no correlation between SpO_2 and a traditional postanesthesia recovery room score based on motor activity, respirations, blood pressure, mental status, and color.[37] The authors concluded that pediatric patients in the recovery room should be monitored continuously by pulse oximetry or given supplemental oxygen regardless of their apparent state of wakefulness. In another study, 14% of adult recovery room patients experienced SpO_2 values less than 90%.[38] A higher incidence of desaturation was associated with obesity, extensive surgery, advanced age,

and poor preoperative physical status. Many patients are more likely to experience hypoxemia in the recovery room than in the operating room. In general, patients in the recovery room no longer have a protected airway, nor are they receiving mechanically assisted ventilation. However, they have not recovered completely from the depressant effects of anesthesia and surgery.

The pulse oximeter, when functioning properly, provides warning of developing hypoxemia. However, at the elevated inspired oxygen fractions normally used in the operating room, SpO_2 does not provide an early warning of a decreasing arterial oxygen tension. As evident from the oxyhemoglobin dissociation curve (Fig. 11-2), PaO_2 must decrease to less than 90 mm Hg before saturation falls significantly. An excellent example of this limitation is the early detection of accidental endobronchial intubation. Figure 11-11 shows data from four different monitors of oxygenation plotted as a function of time for a dog undergoing general anesthesia at an FIO_2 of 0.5.[39] In addition to SpO_2, the plot shows PaO_2 values from sequential arterial blood samples, transcutaneous oxygen tension ($PtcO_2$), and the oxygen tension from an intraarterial fiberoptic optode blood-gas sensor ($OpPO_2$). At 0 minutes on the time axis, the endotracheal tube was guided from the trachea into the left mainstem bronchus via fiberoptic bronchoscopy. Within 3 minutes, the PaO_2 decreased from 360 mm Hg to 120 mm Hg, and the $PtcO_2$ and $OpPO_2$ values also fell significantly. However, the SpO_2 value never decreased below 98% during the entire experiment. In this situation, the pulse oximeter provided no indication that an endobronchial intubation had taken place, whereas the other monitoring techniques all showed significant changes. When this experiment was repeated for FIO_2 values of 0.3 or less, the pulse oximeter exhibited saturation decreases of 6% or more. This illustrates an important physiologic limitation of saturation monitoring: when an elevated FIO_2 is used, the PaO_2 value can decrease far below its baseline before the pulse oximeter will alert the clinician that something is amiss. Metaphorically speaking, the pulse oximeter is a sentry standing on the edge of the cliff of desaturation. It gives no warning when we are approaching the edge; it only tells us when we have fallen off.

Finally, no discussion of the clinical application of a monitor is complete without describing the risks and complications of the monitoring process. Because the pulse oximeter is a noninvasive device that does not (normally) produce heat or radiation, these risks might be expected to be nonexistent. Unfortunately, owing to the possibility of human error, this is not true. In a recent case report, a Physio-Control pulse oximeter sensor was mistakenly connected to an Ohmeda instrument.[40] The two oximeters use the same electrical connector, but the pin connections are entirely different. This resulted in severe thermal burns to both the finger and the earlobe of a newborn infant. The

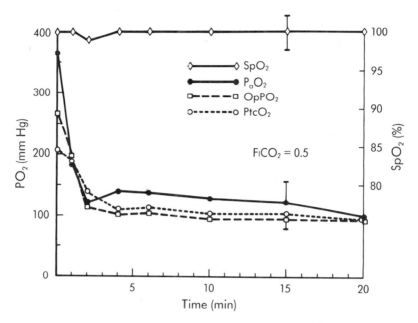

Fig. 11-11. Four oxygenation variables plotted versus time from the onset of endobronchial intu-bation *(Time 0)* in a dog at $FiO_2 = 0.5$. Arterial oxygen tension *(PaO$_2$)*, optode intraarterial oxy-gen tension *(OpPO$_2$)*, and transcutaneous oxygen tension *(PtcO$_2$)* all decreased rapidly during the first 2 minutes of endobronchial intubation, whereas the SpO$_2$ value did not change significantly at any time. (From Barker SJ, Tremper KK, Hyatt J, et al: Comparison of three oxygen monitors in detecting endobronchial intubation, *J Clin Monit* 4:241, 1988, with permission.)

lesson from this case is that compatibility between sensor and instrument must be ensured by the user before a sensor is placed on a patient. This is particularly important in view of the fact that many instruments are designed to use sensors of a different manufacturer.

Another risk of pulse oximetry is potential tissue is-chemia caused by disposable tape-on sensors. If these sen-sors are applied with caution, and it is remembered that soft tissue often swells during lengthy operations, the risk will be minimal. Remember that anything wrapped around the circumference of a digit can act as a tourniquet, partic-ularly if the extremity is dependent or if peripheral edema is likely.

The pulse oximeter is the most significant advance in oxygen monitoring since the development of the blood gas analyzer. It is the only oxygen monitor that provides con-tinuous, real-time, noninvasive data on arterial oxygen-ation. Because it is noninvasive and virtually risk free when used properly, the pulse oximeter should be used in all clinical settings in which there is a potential risk of ar-terial hypoxemia. It is already a minimum standard of care in the operating room, and it is rapidly becoming a stan-dard in other critical care settings. Hypoxia remains the most common cause of anesthesia-related preventable mor-tality.[41,42] The prudent use of pulse oximetry is therefore a fundamental responsibility of the anesthesiologist.

The pulse oximeter is not an ideal instrument because it is subject to measurement error as well as to physiologic limitations.[43] By understanding the physics and engineer-

ing principles of pulse oximetry as outlined in this chapter, the astute clinician can be aware of measurement errors and when they are likely to occur. The clinician can also minimize the impact of such errors by obtaining appropri-ate supportive data. For example, the smoke inhalation pa-tient should have a determination of carboxyhemoglobin level by in vitro cooximetry; the patient with heavy nail polish should have the polish removed or the sensor should be placed such that the light path does not pass through the fingernail. The pulse oximeter signal-to-noise ratio should always be optimized by careful sensor positioning, opaque coverings to prevent ambient light from reaching the sen-sor, and consideration of alternative sensor sites in patients who are shivering or have diminished peripheral pulses. The avoidance of hypoxia is a fundamental goal of every anesthesiologist, and an understanding of both the physics and physiology of continuous saturation monitoring by pulse oximetry can help the anesthesiologist to accomplish this task.

REFERENCES

1. Brown LJ: A new instrument for the simultaneous measurement of total hemoglobin, % oxyhemoglobin, % carboxyhemoglobin, % methemoglobin, and oxygen content in whole blood, *IEEE Trans Biomed Eng* 27:132-138, 1980.
2. Stephen CR, Slater HM, Johnson AL, et al: The oximeter: a techni-cal aid for the anesthesiologist, *Anesthesiology* 12:541-555, 1951.
3. Knill RL, Clement JL, Kieraszewicz HT, et al: Assessment of two noninvasive monitors of arterial oxygenation in anesthetized man, *Anesth Analg* 61:582-586, 1982.

4. Wukitsch MW, Tobler D, Pologe J, et al: Pulse oximetry: an analysis of theory, technology and practice, *J Clin Monit* 4:290-301, 1988.

5. Severinghaus JW, Astrup PB: History of blood gas analysis. VI. Oximetry, *J Clin Monit* 2:270-288, 1986.

6. Barker SJ, Tremper KK: The effect of carbon monoxide inhalation on pulse oximetry and transcutaneous PO_2, *Anesthesiology* 66:677-679, 1987.

7. Barker SJ, Tremper KK, Hyatt J: Effects of methemoglobinemia on pulse oximetry and mixed venous oximetry, *Anesthesiology* 70:112-117, 1989.

8. Cornelissen PJH, van Del WC, de Jong PA: Correction factors for hemoglobin derivatives in fetal blood as measured with the IL282 Co-Oximeter, *Clin Chem* 29:1555-1556, 1983.

9. Scheller MS, Unger RJ, Kelner MJ: Effects of intravenously administered dyes on pulse oximetry readings, *Anesthesiology* 65:550-552, 1986.

10. Veyckemans F, Baele P, Guillaume JE, et al: Hyperbilirubinemia does not interfere with hemoglobin saturation measured by pulse oximetry, *Anesthesiology* 70:118-122, 1989.

11. Coté CJ, Goldstein EA, Fuchsman WH, et al: The effect of nail polish on pulse oximetry, *Anesth Analg* 67:683-686, 1988.

12. Pologe JA: Pulse oximetry: technical aspects of machine design. *Int Anesthesiol Clin* 25:137-153, 1987.

13. Kelleher JF, Ruff RH: The penumbra effect: vasomotion-dependent pulse oximeter artifact due to probe malposition, *Anesthesiology* 71:787-791, 1989.

14. Tremper KK, Hufstedler S, Barker SJ, et al: Accuracy of a pulse oximeter in the critically ill adult: effect of temperature and hemodynamics, *Anesthesiology* 63:A175, 1985.

15. Freund PR, Overand PT, Cooper J, et al: A prospective study of intraoperative pulse oximetry failure, *J Clin Monit* 7:253-258, 1991.

16. Lawson D, Norley I, Korbon G, et al: Blood flow limits and pulse oximeter signal detection, *Anesthesiology* 67:599-603, 1987.

17. Narang VPS: Utility of the pulse oximeter during cardiopulmonary resuscitation, *Anesthesiology* 65:239-240, 1986.

18. Nowak GS, Moorthy SS, McNiece WL: Use of pulse oximetry for assessment of collateral arterial flow, *Anesthesiology* 64:527, 1986.

19. Skeehan TM, Hensley FA Jr: Axillary artery compression and the prone position, *Anesth Analg* 65:518-519, 1986.

20. Barrington KJ, Ryan CA, Finer NN: Pulse oximetry during hemorrhagic hypotension and cardiopulmonary resuscitation in the rabbit, *J Crit Care* 1:242-246, 1986.

21. Severinghaus JW, Spellman MJ Jr: Pulse oximeter failure thresholds in hypotension and vasoconstriction, *Anesthesiology* 73:532-537, 1990.

22. Graham B, Paulus DA, Caffee HH: Pulse oximetry for vascular monitoring in upper extremity replantation surgery, *J Hand Surg* 11A:687-692, 1986.

23. *Nellcor N-200 pulse oximetry note number 6. C-LOCK ECG synchronization principles of operation*, Hayward, Calif, 1988, Nellcor.

24. Kim JM, Arakawa K, Benson KT, et al: Pulse oximetry and circulatory kinetics associated with pulse volume amplitude measured by photoelectric plethysmography, *Anesth Analg* 65:1333-1339, 1986.

25. Altman DG, Bland JM: Measurement in medicine: the analysis of method comparison studies, *The Statistician* 32:307-317, 1983.

26. Bland JM, Altman DG: Statistical methods for assessing agreement between two methods of clinical measurement, *Lancet* 1:307-310, 1986.

27. Tremper KK, Barker SJ: Pulse oximetry, *Anesthesiology* 70:98-108, 1989.

28. Severinghaus JW, Naifeh KH: Accuracy of response of six pulse oximeters to profound hypoxia, *Anesthesiology* 67:551-558, 1987.

29. Kagle DM, Alexander CM, Berko RS, et al: Evaluation of the Ohmeda 3700 pulse oximeter: steady-state and transient response characteristics, *Anesthesiology* 66:376-380, 1987.

30. Severinghaus JW, Naifeh KH, Koh SO: Errors in 14 pulse oximeters during profound hypoxia, *J Clin Monit* 5:72-81, 1989.

31. Barker SJ, Hyatt J: Forehead reflectance pulse oximetry: time response to rapid saturation change, *Anesthesiology* 73(3A):A544, 1990.

32. Barker SJ, Le N, Hyatt J: Failure rates of transmission and reflectance pulse oximetry for various sensor sites, *J Clin Monit* 7:102-103, 1991.

33. Eichhorn JH, Cooper JB, Cullen DJ, et al: Standards for patient monitoring during anesthesia at Harvard Medical School, *JAMA* 256:1017-1020, 1986.

34. Coté CJ, Goldstein EA, Coté MA, et al: A single blind study of pulse oximetry in children, *Anesthesiology* 68:184-188, 1988.

35. Pullerits J, Burrows FA, Roy WL: Arterial desaturation in healthy children during transfer to the recovery room, *Can J Anaesth* 34:470-473, 1987.

36. Tyler IL, Tantisira B, Winter PM, et al: Continuous monitoring of arterial oxygen saturation with pulse oximetry during transfer to the recovery room, *Anesth Analg* 64:1108-1112, 1985.

37. Soliman IE, Patel RI, Ehrenpreis MB, et al: Recovery scores do not correlate with postoperative hypoxemia in children, *Anesth Analg* 67:53-56, 1988.

38. Morris RW, Buxchman A, Warren DL, et al: The prevalence of hypoxemia detected by pulse oximetry during recovery from anesthesia, *J Clin Monit* 4:16-20, 1988.

39. Barker SJ, Tremper KK, Hyatt J, et al: Comparison of three oxygen monitors in detecting endobronchial intubation, *J Clin Monit* 4:240-243, 1988.

40. Murphy KG, Segunda JA, Rockoff MA: Severe burns from a pulse oximeter, *Anesthesiology* 73:350-352, 1990.

41. Keenan RL, Boyan CP: Cardiac arrest due to anesthesia: a study of incidence and causes, *JAMA* 253:2373-2377, 1985.

42. Taylor G, Larson CP Jr, Prestwich R: Unexpected cardiac arrest during anesthesia and surgery: an environmental study, *JAMA* 236:2758-2760, 1976.

43. Severinghaus JW, Kelleher JF: Recent developments in pulse oximetry, *Anesthesiology* 76:1018-1038, 1992.

44. Chapman KR, Liu FLW, Watson RM, et al: Range of accuracy of two-wavelength oximetry, *Chest* 4:540-542, 1986.

45. Nickerson BG, Sakrison C, Tremper KK: Bias and precision of pulse oximeters and arterial oximeters, *Chest* 93:515-517, 1988.

46. Mihm FG, Halperin BD: Noninvasive detection of profound arterial desaturations using a pulse oximetry device, *Anesthesiology* 62:85-87, 1985.

47. Cecil WT, Thorpe KJ, Fibuch EE, et al: A clinical evaluation of the accuracy of the Nellcor N-100 and the Ohmeda 3700 pulse oximeters, *J Clin Monit* 4:31-36, 1988.

48. Fait CD, Wetzel RC, Dean JM, et al: Pulse oximetry in critically ill children, *J Clin Monit* 1:232-235, 1985.

49. Boxer RA, Gottesfeld I, Singh S, et al: Non-invasive pulse oximetry in children with cyanotic congenital heart disease. *Crit Care Med* 15:1062-1064, 1987.

50. Mok J, Pintar M, Benson L, et al: Evaluation of noninvasive measurements of oxygenation in stable infants. *Crit Care Med* 14:960-963, 1986.

51. Durand M, Ramanathan R: Pulse oximetry for continuous oxygen monitoring in six newborn infants. *J Pediatr* 109:1052-1055, 1986.

52. Yelderman M, New W: Evaluation of pulse oximetry, *Anesthesiology* 59:349-352, 1983.

Chapter 12

TEMPERATURE MONITORING

Ross H. Zoll, Ph.D., M.D.

The monitoring of temperature and body heat during anesthesia has sparked many controversies in spite of the (deceptively) simple concepts involved. Studies related to body heat began in ancient times, when heat was associated with life itself. Until fairly recently, the heart was thought to be the source of heat and life. With modern understanding of the mechanism of body-heat production and of the principles of heat transfer, most controversies should be resolved. Nevertheless, the complexity of body-heat management leaves many details still in question.

It is now known that body heat is produced primarily by metabolism. Basal metabolism amounts to approximately 100 W, or 4 J/kg/hr (or about 1600 kcal/day), but may increase as much as tenfold with vigorous activity. Certain physical principles are a useful aid to understanding heat exchange with the environment. With certain restrictions, heat and other forms of energy may be interchanged.

The first law of thermodynamics states that the energy of a closed system is constant, and the energy *(E)* of a system in contact with its environment changes with heat absorbed *(Q)* less any work done *(W)*:

$$\Delta E = \Delta Q + \Delta W$$

The energy *(E)* is a unique function of the temperature and parameters describing a system. In general, ΔW is insignificant in this discussion and the temperature changes discussed here are related to heat absorbed or lost (or produced as a result of metabolism). Two systems in equilibrium are at the same temperature and do not exchange heat or work.

The second law of thermodynamics states that the entropy *(S)* of the closed system (defined as that part of the internal energy of a body or substance which is not available for mechanical work but is used internally) always increases, but only for a reversible process:

$$\Delta S = \frac{\Delta Q}{T}$$

where Q = heat absorbed and T = temperature. In practice, the performance of work requires the generation of waste heat as well.

The third law of thermodynamics states that at $T = 0$ and $S = 0$ a temperature of absolute zero cannot be reached at all.[1]

The physical processes of heat exchange with the environment are well understood. However, the complex geometry of the human body and the complicated airflow near the skin do not lend themselves to precise calculations. Similarly, the distribution and transfer of heat within the body is understood, at least in principle, and is represented by the bioheat equation.[2]

PHYSIOLOGY OF TEMPERATURE REGULATION

When discussing temperature regulation, it is first important to consider that the body temperature varies significantly among various organs and considerably between the core and the periphery. These variations depend on various circumstances, and indeed, the importance of temperatures of various parts of the body may also vary. In ordinary situations, the core temperature of the blood in the great vessels of the chest, that perfuses the major organs and the brain, is uniform and well defined. The liver

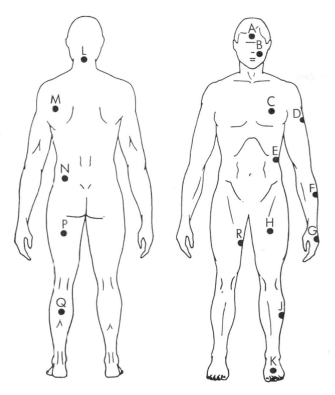

Fig. 12-1. Sites for measurement of skin temperature. (From Shanks CA: Mean surface temperature during anesthesia: an assessment of formulae in the supine surgical patient, *Br J Anaesth* 47:871, 1975.)

and other organs may be somewhat warmer because of their greater metabolic activity. Skeletal muscle may be cooler or warmer depending on activity level and environmental temperature. The hypothalamus has an important temperature-sensing function and normally is close to core temperature. It should be noted that some animals are capable of maintaining the brain at a temperature below that of the body, when body temperature is not as well controlled. This ability may persist to some small extent in humans.

Mean skin temperature *(MST)* is also important, both for its contribution to total body heat and for its sensory input to temperature-regulating activity. The contributions of skin and core temperatures to mean body temperature *(MBT)* and total body heat have been investigated with calorimetry, and the following estimates have been proposed:

$$MBT = 0.66T_{core} + 0.33T_{MST}$$

In awake individuals, the tympanic membrane temperature provides the most convenient and accurate measure of core temperature. Mean skin temperature is estimated most accurately by taking the average of up to 16 sites[3] (Fig. 12-1). For many purposes, however, four site approximations are sufficient.[4]

Consider the equation

Body heat (kJ) = MBT × 0.83 × 4.18 × Mass (kg)

The body's specific heat accounts for the factor 0.83. The

heat capacity of water is 1 kcal/kg, or 4.18 kJ/kg. Accurate calorimetry on living human subjects was facilitated by the development of the gradient-layer calorimeter, which allows measurement of steady-state heat flux.[5] This calorimeter consists of a large box covered with arrays of thermocouples that integrate the total heat flux through the box. Metabolic heat production can also be estimated from oxygen consumption or from carbon dioxide production.

Distinct peripheral receptors for cold and hot exist, and most sensory input is transmitted to the hypothalamus via the spinothalamic tracts. Temperature receptors have been identified throughout the core of the body and central nervous system. Although some spinal reflexes for temperature control exist, cerebral responses are predominant.

According to Benzinger's set-point theory (Fig. 12-2),[6] most peripheral temperature sensation is transmitted to the posterior hypothalamus, which responds to cold sensation (i.e., skin temperature below 33° C) by inducing increased metabolism and shivering. The anterior hypothalamus responds intrinsically to very slight increases in local temperature by inducing heat loss through sweating and vasodilation (independent of skin temperature), and by inhibiting posterior hypothalamic activity. Skin temperature is greatly affected by sweating and is therefore not suitable for directly regulating heat loss. Nevertheless, skin temperatures below 33° C inhibit the central response to increases in core temperature. An additional mechanism, not shown in Fig. 12-2, consists of a weak central response to local cold below 35.7° C.

More recently, there has been evidence to suggest that temperature responses may be subtly dependent on all body-temperature sensors in a way that approximates the relative importance of each portion of the body to total body heat,[7] although this may also be an oversimplification.[8] Total body heat is probably more closely related to stress during recovery and rewarming than to core temperature.

In awake individuals, the initial and most powerful response to environmental temperature changes is usually behavioral, perhaps involving changes in posture, dress, or shelter. Such responses, which are similar to the most primitive response mechanisms used by poikilotherms, are the most efficient metabolically. A great deal more energy is expended in raising basal metabolism and shivering. In fact, shivering actually increases heat loss by increasing peripheral blood flow and convective heat loss from the skin. Similarly, sweating requires metabolic energy and raises heat production.

EFFECTS OF ANESTHESIA

General anesthesia is associated with a decrease in core temperature of approximately 1° C in the first hour and by 0.3° C per hour thereafter. The initial temperature drop may be due in part to increased losses during prepping and draping but more likely reflects the redistribution of body heat from the core to the periphery with anesthesia-induced vasodilation.[9]

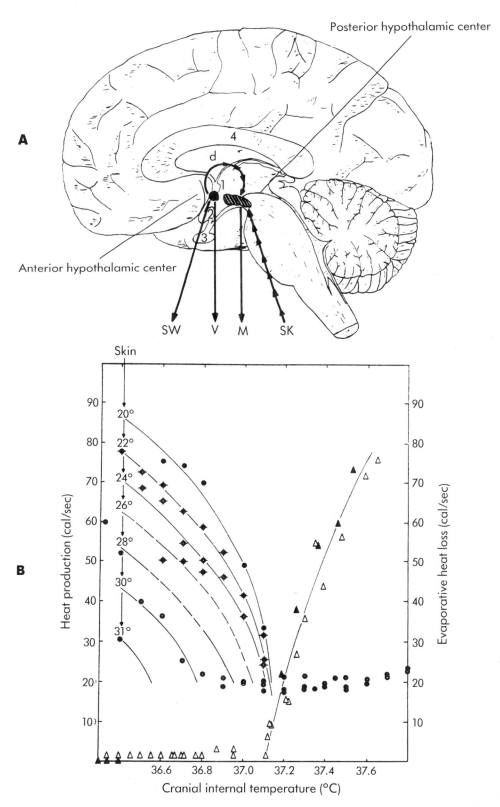

Fig. 12-2. A, Diagram of proposed mechanism for temperature regulation at setpoint. *SW,* efferent pathways to sweating mechanism; *V,* efferent pathways to control vasodilatation or vasoconstriction; *M,* efferent pathways for metabolic heat production; *SK,* afferent pathways for skin cold sensation; *d,* inhibition of cold response by central warmth perception; *1,* anterior commissure; *2,* optic chiasm; *3,* hypophysis; *4,* corpus callosum. **B,** Experimental evidence for set-point theory. *Left,* Metabolic heat production at decreased skin temperatures; *right,* evaporative heat loss at increased core temperature. (From Benzinger TH, Pratt AW, Kitzinger C: The thermostatic control of human metabolic heat production, *Proc Natl Acad Sci USA* 47, 730-739, 1961.)

Of course, general anesthesia completely eliminates any behavioral response to temperature change. Vasoconstriction is impaired by most anesthetic agents; muscle relaxants reduce heat production from resting tone in muscles and prevent shivering. Although central regulation of temperature is likely to be depressed, regulation still occurs, albeit at a lower temperature. Sessler[10,11,12] found that with potent inhaled agents, the threshold for the vasoconstrictive response to hypothermia decreases (to 34.4° C with halothane, 3° C per percent of isoflurane, and 34.2° C with nitrous oxide–fentanyl). Oxygen consumption increases only slightly, ruling out significant nonshivering thermogenesis (NST) in adults. However, infants do respond with NST under anesthesia.

Regional anesthesia inhibits cold sensation as well as shivering and vasoconstrictive responses in the anesthetized region. Central responses remain intact but may be insufficient to maintain temperature against increased losses. Metabolic heat production cannot be increased because catecholamine responses are inhibited. Rewarming during recovery is typically slower than the usually rapid recovery from general anesthesia.

Some specific effects of various agents are notable. Narcotics induce central hypothermia. Barbiturates cause peripheral vasodilation. Halothane produces ganglionic blockade and vasodilation. In combination, halothane and succinylcholine are associated with higher temperatures. Compared with other induction agents, ketamine is better able to maintain temperature during induction. Muscle relaxants prevent shivering and reduce heat production from tonic muscle activity.[13]

Shivering during and after general or regional anesthesia is often associated with hypothermia but may be caused by other obscure and controversial reasons. It is clear that, in some cases, shivering occurs from disinhibition of spinal reflexes and may be both inappropriate for the body temperature and different electrophysiologically from normal shivering.[14] Meperidine is specifically effective in controlling postanesthetic shivering.

IMPORTANCE OF MONITORING TEMPERATURE DURING ANESTHESIA

Temperature regulation is crucial to the survival of intact, awake animals and thus must be assisted during anesthesia in humans, when natural regulatory mechanisms are impaired and unusual heat loss or gain occurs. Under normal circumstances a temperature increase of 6° C or decrease of 9° C is fatal, although special support techniques can extend the lower range.

In fact, one of the early arguments for routine temperature monitoring was to detect malignant hyperthermia[15] in spite of temperature rise being a late change. Increased end-tidal carbon dioxide is the earliest metabolic change that is readily detected.

Because of the widespread use of air conditioning in operating rooms in the United States, accidental hyperther-

mia is no longer common. However, in tropical climates without air conditioned operating rooms, hyperthermia can still be of serious concern. Accidental hypothermia is by far the most common problem. Until recently, moderate hypothermia was not considered a problem. On the contrary, hypothermia decreases oxygen consumption and tissue damage in the presence of ischemia. It has since become clear that any heat loss during anesthesia must be restored during recovery. During recovery, shivering can increase oxygen demand 135% to 468%,[16] when respiratory and cardiovascular systems may be unable to respond normally to increased demand. Hemodynamic instability and discomfort are increased by hypothermia. Increased nitrogen loss has been observed.[17] Vasoconstriction may interfere with peripheral blood flow and jeopardize healing in the presence of peripheral vascular disease. Hypothermia increases sensitivity to anesthetic drugs, delays metabolism and excretion, depresses reflexes, delays awakening and discharge from the postanesthesia care unit,[18] and prolongs the need for mechanical ventilation. Coronary vasoconstriction may compromise myocardial oxygen balance. Hypothermia interferes with the function of the neuromuscular junction; and, as a result of lower peripheral temperature,[19] peripheral nerve stimulators may underestimate the strength of the diaphragm. Special requirements for temperature stability are associated with sickle cell disease or the presence of cold agglutinins. Elderly patients have decreased basal metabolism,[20] which increases the risk of hypothermia and concomitant disease, making them intolerant of additional stress.

Although uncommon, hypothermia below 32° C is ominous. Ventricular irritability increases, and if the temperature decreases to 28° C cardiac arrest is likely.[21] Cold irrigation or transfusion of large quantities of cold blood are common causes. Of course, with adequate support, deep hypothermia can be effective in preserving tissue subjected to ischemia. The level of support necessary ordinarily includes cardiopulmonary bypass for cooling and rewarming quickly and effectively.

Pediatric patients undergoing anesthesia are likely to require temperature monitoring and intervention, perhaps even more so than adults. In this population, malignant hyperthermia may arise more frequently. Accidental hypothermia is more likely with infants and small children, for whom the ratio of surface area to mass is large. In addition, infants and newborns are poorly insulated by subcutaneous fat, have less effective temperature regulation, and a smaller respiratory reserve for additional heat production. For newborns, who do not shiver, heat regulation depends on NST, which can increase heat production by only 100%.

MECHANISMS OF INTRAOPERATIVE HEAT LOSS

The four physical processes of heat transfer of interest here are radiation, conduction, convection, and evaporation. Radiation is probably the most significant route, but it is possible that any of these processes will overwhelm regulating mechanisms.

The radiation heat loss can be readily estimated from physical principles. All bodies emit electromagnetic radiation according to the law of black body radiation. By definition, a black body has a surface that is an ideal emitter and consequently that is also an ideal absorber. (An ideal absorber that was less efficient as an emitter would gain energy in violation of the second law of thermodynamics.) A black body appears black because all incident radiation is absorbed.*

The total radiation (q) integrated over all frequencies is

$$q = \epsilon \sigma T^4$$

where $\sigma = 5.67 \times 10^{-8}$ W/m^2/T^4 K.

For a nonideal emitter, the emissivity, ϵ, is included and depends on the surface of the body. For the human body, ϵ is very close to 1 at a wavelength of 9.3 μm, the peak of radiation at 37° C. Not all the surface area of the body "sees" room temperature, for example, the inner thigh. With some approximations, the total radiation loss from a naked adult in a room at 24° C (radiation loss minus radiation absorbed) is roughly 60 W or 216 kJ/hr. Clothing or draping reduces this loss substantially.

Conduction of heat from the body to a solid surface or to clothing follows a diffusion equation and can be expressed by Fourier's law:

$$Q = kA(T_s - T_{cl}) \, \Delta t/L$$

where

Q = Heat transfer
k = Conductivity constant
A = Surface area
T_s = Temperature of the skin
T_{cl} = Temperature of the clothing
Δt = Time interval
L = Conduction distance.

Application of this equation to the complicated surface contact of the patient with an OR mattress and drapes is difficult. However, measurements for clothing exist. For an individual in light clothing, conducted heat loss is approximately 15 W/m^2/°C. In the OR setting, conductive heat loss is probably small compared with other losses unless drapes and bedding are wet.

Convective heat loss is defined as heat loss due to moving fluid (air). Free convection is distinguished from forced air movement. The latter probably applies to OR conditions where ventilation is 10 or 20 air changes per hour. Velocity of air movement is included in the following equation in the constant h_{cv}, which also reflects posture and is probably in the range 2 to 10:

$$q = h_{cv}(T_s - T_a) \text{ W/m}^2$$
$$\cong 25 \text{ W/m}^2$$

where T_a is the temperature of the air. Clothing or drapes are very effective in decreasing convective loss by trapping air near the skin.

Considerable heat loss is attributed to latent heat of vaporization of water from open body cavities and from the respiratory tract. The latter is easily quantified and controlled. Without special provisions for heating and humidification, or very low flow or closed breathing systems, gases delivered by the anesthesia machine are cold and dry (see also Chapter 7). As a worst case scenario, consider the heat loss (Q) to a nonrebreathing system with dry gas at 20° C:

Q = Ventilation × Water content × Heat of vaporization
= 420 L/hr × 0.04 gH$_2$O/L × 0.58 kcal/gH$_2$O
× 4.18 kJ/kcal
= 40 kJ/hr

Up to 1600 kJ/hr may be lost through evaporation from the surgical field.[22] Additional heat is lost in warming the respiratory gases from room temperature to body temperature:*

Q = 420 L/hr × 0.409 cal/L × 17° C × 4.18
= 12 kJ/hr

where 0.409 is the heat capacity of the mixture of nitrous oxide and oxygen. Finally, heat may be lost to cold irrigation solutions, and temperature can be decreased by infusion of cold intravenous fluids.

CONTROLLING PATIENT HEAT LOSS

Avoiding hypothermia during anesthesia essentially means avoiding heat loss. Opportunities for rapid heat loss abound, and there are virtually no practical means of significant warming other than metabolic heat production. Heat may be lost rapidly to cold surroundings if there is a large temperature gradient. Rapid rewarming risks burns unless the cardiopulmonary bypass pump and heat exchanger[23] are used to ensure rapid equilibration. Other methods—such as microwave, short wave, or ultrasonic diathermy; warm irrigation; or radiant heaters— are theoretically possible but are usually impractical. The radiant heater, although uncomfortable for surgeons during surgery, is very useful in warming the skin to inhibit shivering postoperatively and for preparation and line placement in infants until draping is complete. Care is necessary to avoid burns.

Raising the OR temperature will control heat loss effectively. Although uncomfortable for the surgeon, this may be necessary if other methods are inadequate. OR temperatures above 21° C will generally prevent heat loss for adults.[24] However, much higher temperatures may be necessary for neonates.

Thermal contact with room temperature can be reduced by draping and blankets. Reflective blankets are helpful,[25] but water condensation inside impervious plastic sheets

---

*See the Appendix at the end of this chapter for further discussion of this subject.

*See also Chapter 7.

can increase conductive loss. Light clothing can extend tolerance to environmental temperature from 29° C to 21° C, and draping in the OR likely has a similar effect.[26]

Active warming mattresses and blankets can make a small contribution to thermal stability (2.7 to 5.2 kcal/hr/°C)[22] and are probably most effective if placed over the patient. Electric blankets may heat unevenly and cause burns. Even circulating water mattresses carry the risk of burns at pressure points if perfusion of the patient's skin is poor.[27]

Humidification of respiratory gases is most important in preventing airway drying and maintaining normal ciliary function[28] but may also conserve as much as 50 kJ/hr.[29] With active humidifiers, care must be taken to avoid airway burns.[30] Passive heat and moisture exchangers conserve approximately one half of the evaporative heat loss.[31] (See also Chapter 7.)

Whenever large volumes of blood or intravenous fluids are transfused or large volumes of irrigation are used, these fluids must be warmed. Each liter of fluid at room temperature lowers body temperature:

$$0.25° C \cong \frac{1}{70 \text{ kg}} \times 17° C$$

Similarly, each unit of blood at 4° C lowers body temperature approximately 0.25° C. Lethal hypothermia can result from failure to warm fluids.[21] With appropriate appli-cation of the aforementioned techniques, excessive heat loss can usually be prevented.

MONITORING TEMPERATURE DURING ANESTHESIA

Monitoring sites

The site for monitoring temperature during anesthesia depends on the surgical procedure, the type of anesthesia used, and the reason for temperature monitoring. When significant changes in body heat are expected, core temperature should be monitored. Although skin temperature contributes to total body heat, it reflects peripheral perfusion rather than core temperature.[32] For research purposes, total body heat can be calculated via estimates of mean skin temperature measured at multiple sites. However, this method is too cumbersome for routine use.

In most cases, the standard for measuring core temperature is now the temperature of pulmonary arterial blood. Exceptions are in thoracotomy and cardiopulmonary bypass, especially with cold cardioplegia, and during rapid transfusion. Otherwise, the temperature of pulmonary arterial blood correlates well with tympanic membrane temperature, distal esophageal temperature, and nasopharyngeal temperature. When a pulmonary arterial catheter is not otherwise necessary, any of these other sites usually suffices (Fig. 12-3).[33]

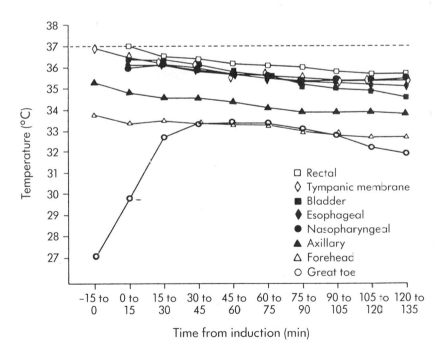

Fig. 12-3. Comparison of temperatures at various sites under general anesthesia. *Open squares,* rectal; *open diamonds,* tympanic membrane; *squares,* bladder; *diamonds,* esophageal; *circles,* nasopharyngeal; *triangles,* axillary; *open triangles,* forehead; *open circles,* great toe. (From Cork RC, Vaughan RW, Humphrey LS: Precision and accuracy of intraoperative temperature monitoring, *Anesth Analg* 62:211-214, 1962. With permission from the International Anesthesia Research Society.)

The temperature of the blood supplied to the tympanic membrane approximates that at the hypothalamus.[34] In some situations, the temperature of the tympanic membrane may be more meaningful to temperature regulation than other core temperatures. For example, fanning the face and panting can selectively cool the brain and produce a subjective sensation of normothermia during hyperthermia.[35] The placement of a temperature probe on or near the tympanic membrane risks perforation and bleeding, especially with heparinization.[36] The external auditory meatus is safer for this purpose but works well only if adequately insulated from outside temperature by a servo-controlled external heater.[37] Nasopharyngeal temperature may reflect the same blood supply as the hypothalamus but is more subject to error from displacement or leakage of respiratory gases and resulting cooling.[38]

The esophagus is a safe,[39] easily accessible, and accurate site for core temperature measurement during general anesthesia. A combination stethoscope and temperature probe is easily passed to a position near the heart. The temperature must be measured in the distal third or quarter of the esophagus to avoid cooling by respiratory gases in the trachea, even though this position may not be optimal for auscultation.[40]

Rectal temperature, though often convenient, is not particularly accurate as a measure of core temperature.[5] It is affected by heat-producing organisms in the bowel, cool blood returning from the legs, and insulation by the feces. Perforation is a small risk with this method. Rectal temperature changes too slowly to follow intraoperative changes in core temperature, particularly during cardiopulmonary bypass.

Bladder temperature correlates with core temperature when urine flow is high and is easily measured with combination Foley catheter–thermistor probe devices. During cardiopulmonary bypass, temperature changes too rapidly for the bladder temperature to follow core temperature. However, bladder temperature is influenced by blood returning from the legs through iliac veins and therefore reflects the temperature of muscle mass, which is intermediate between core and skin temperatures. Measurement of bladder temperature provides the best estimate of temperature drop after weaning from cardiopulmonary bypass. A bladder temperature over 36.2° C is associated with minimal temperature drop after bypass.[41]

Axillary temperature over the brachial artery with the arm adducted can give a reasonably accurate core temperature and is most reliable in infants and small children.[31] Similarly, sublingual temperature, although subject to error, is still useful, and awake patients tolerate the thermometer well.

Other sites may be of value in special situations. Myocardial temperature is readily measured with a needle probe during cardiopulmonary bypass. Skeletal muscle temperature provides the earliest indication of temperature change with malignant hyperthermia.[42]

Transducers and devices

Mercury thermometers. The mercury-in-glass thermometer is one of the oldest and simplest devices currently used for clinical thermometry. Neither the safest nor the fastest method, it is also very limited in its access to various remote sites of interest for thermometry in anesthesia. For most purposes, a telethermometer, which consists of a transducer probe connected by a cable to a monitor and a display, is an essential arrangement. The most commonly used transducers are thermistors and thermocouples.

Thermistors. Commonly used thermistors are metal-oxide semiconductors.[43] The electrical conductivity of semiconductors depends on thermally excited electrons and "holes" as charge carriers and therefore has a strong temperature dependence dominated by the concentration of charge carriers:

$$\sigma = \sigma_0 e^{-\Delta E/kT}$$

where the energy gap $\Delta E \approx 1$ electron volt (eV). In comparison, the thermal energy, kT, is approximately 1/40 eV. This equation yields a nonlinear resistance change with temperature, but the output can be linearized over a narrow range by the external circuit with some loss of sensitivity. For example, Yellow Springs Instruments 400* series probes have a resistance of about 1400 ohms at 37° C and about 3000 ohms at 20° C. Their simple battery-powered bridge circuit is shown in Fig. 12-4. Thermistor thermometers operate at reasonably low impedances and are relatively immune from interference. Although an outside power source is required, it can be as simple as a single battery cell. Power dissipation is rarely an issue. These transducers are inexpensive and stable, and their readings are reproducible at an accuracy of 0.1 or 0.2° C. They can be made small enough to fit inside a 25-gauge needle for measurement of muscle temperature.

One concern with the circuit in Fig. 12-4 is that, although it is battery-powered, it is not isolated from ground. If the case is set on a grounded metal surface, then the possibility exists of microshock or electrosurgical burns[44] at the probe site. Isolated circuits with electrosurgical protection are possible (see also Chapter 21). Obviously, more complicated circuits with digital displays and alarm capability are straightforward developments of this example.

Thermocouples. Thermocouples are junctions of two different metals. In a circuit consisting of two such junctions at different temperatures, a small voltage or current is generated. The voltage is known as the Seebeck effect. The temperature gradient produces a heat flux, carried largely by electrons, in each metal. According to the transport equations, an associated current (or voltage for an open circuit) is induced. Because of differences between metals, voltage gradients in each metal do not cancel precisely and the voltage difference can be measured with the arrangement shown in Fig. 12-5. The second law of ther-

*Yellow Springs Instruments, Yellow Springs, Ohio.

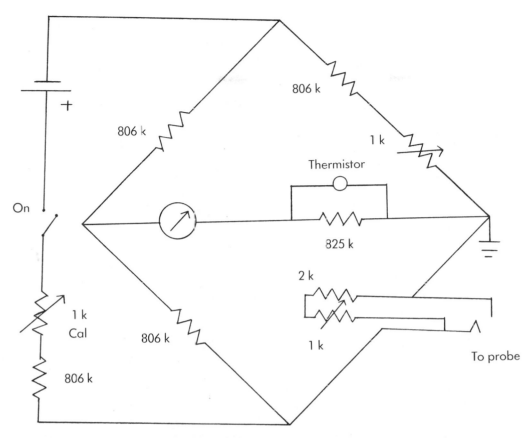

Fig. 12-4. Circuit for thermistor temperature monitor. This is a simple battery-powered bridge circuit.

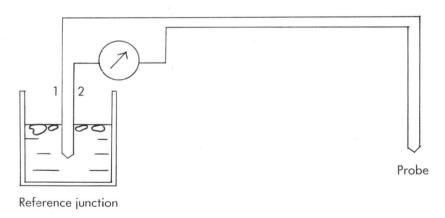

Fig. 12-5. Circuit for thermocouple thermometer. Probe consists of two different metals (*1* and *2*) that conduct heat differently, which results in the generation of a current that can be measured on the meter ⊙.

modynamics is not violated because heat is conducted along the wires from the hot junction to the cold junction. (By a related effect, refrigeration is produced when current is passed through the circuit from an external source.)

Thermocouples for clinical thermometry usually use copper-constantan (copper with 40% nickel) junctions. This combination produces 40 μV/° C. This small voltage is most easily measured with an amplifier; and although an outside power source is not required, in practice the apparatus is more complicated than the thermistor thermometer. The reference junction can be kept in a water-ice bath, in a heated or cooled oven, or even in contact with semiconductor circuits measuring its temperature and applying an appropriate compensation. Probes are less expensive

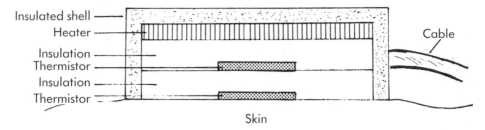

Insulated shell
Heater
Insulation
Thermistor
Insulation
Thermistor
Cable
Skin

Fig. 12-6. Diagram of zero-heat-flux double-thermistor skin probe. Skin is warmed to core temperature, so that there is no net heat exchange between the skin and the probe. Thermistor temperature then corresponds to core temperature. (From Lees DE, Kim YD: Noninvasive determination of core temperature during anesthesia, *South Med J* 73:1322-1324, 1980. By permission.)

and are available in very small sizes as well. Carefully made junctions are likely to be stable and accurate to 0.1° C.

Liquid crystal thermometers. Liquid crystals are liquids which have complicated structures with long-range order.[45] Liquid crystal thermometers use cholesteric liquid crystals, which have ordered layer structure with directional asymmetry in the plane of each layer. The orientation of this asymmetry rotates gradually with each succeeding layer, yielding a periodicity that may be the size of a wavelength of visible light or larger. This structure makes the substance optically active (it rotates the plane of polarized light). The optical properties are highly sensitive to temperature, and when liquid crystals are encapsulated in thin films or used with polarizers, the color changes with temperature. Optical changes with phase transitions between various structures can also be used for displaying temperature.

These devices are readily applied to measure skin surface temperature. Skin temperature does not correlate well with core temperature[46] but is often of interest itself for measurements of total body heat or for perfusion, as with regional blocks. Liquid crystal thermometers can be reasonably accurate for this purpose ($\pm$ 0.5° C); a correction factor, or offset, is often included, which purports to correct to core temperature.[47] Also, like more traditional thermometers, they do not lend themselves readily to remote viewing, although light-guide arrangements are used for special purposes such as measurements in microwave fields or magnetic resonance imaging (MRI) magnets.

Infrared tympanic thermometer. Another new thermometer that accurately measures core temperature even in awake subjects is the infrared tympanic membrane thermometer. A small probe covered with a disposable, transparent cover is inserted into the external auditory meatus, where the infrared detector can "see" the tympanic membrane. The thermopile detector (a series of thermocouples), which is thermally isolated from other sources of heat loss or gain, collects radiation from the tympanic membrane. After a few seconds, the data collected are converted to a temperature on the basis of an empirical

calibration. This method provides a prompt, accurate measure of core temperature if properly used with good visualization of the tympanic membrane and no leakage.[48] One should be aware that an offset may be set on the device so that the temperature corresponds to that at other sites of measurement, such as rectal or sublingual.[49]

Zero-heat-flux probe. Another method of core temperature measurement is the zero-heat-flux, insulated, double-thermistor skin probe (Fig. 12-6).[50] The principle is to warm the skin to core temperature with a heater. When this condition is reached, there will be no heat flux from the core to the skin or from the skin to the device heater. The temperatures of the skin and the device are then measured and compared. The problem with this device for clinical anesthesia is that the response time is too slow to track changes that might occur.[51]

APPENDIX

A cavity is an example of a black body. Inside the cavity, the distribution of radiation depends on the number of oscillators and the quantum mechanical energy of an oscilator at a temperature T:

$$I(\omega) = \frac{(h/2\pi)\omega}{\pi^3\,c^2\,e\{[(h/2\pi)\omega]/kT\}-1}$$

where:

$I(\omega)$ = Intensity of radiation at angular frequency ω
h = Planck's constant
c = Speed of light
k = Boltzmann constant.

This result was one of the first triumphs of quantum theory over classical physics. The derivation can be found in physics texts.[1] The wavelength of the peak of radiation emitted depends on the temperature as

$$\lambda = 2898/T \; \mu m$$

This relation is obtained by differentiating the black body law. At 37° C this occurs at 9.3 μm.

REFERENCES

1. Reif F: *Fundamentals of statistical and thermal physics*, New York, 1965, McGraw-Hill.
2. Chen MM: *The tissue energy balance equation*. In Shitzer A, Eberhart RC, editors: *Heat transfer in medicine and biology, vol 1*, New York, 1985, Plenum, pp 153-164.
3. Shanks CA: Mean surface temperature during anaesthesia: an assessment of formulae in the supine surgical patient, *Br J Anaesth* 47:871-875, 1975.
4. Ramanthan NL: A new weighting system for mean skin temperature, *J Appl Physiol* 19:531-533, 1964.
5. Benzinger TH: Heat regulation: homeostasis of central temperature in man, *Physiol Rev* 49:671-759, 1969.
6. Benzinger TH, Pratt AW, Kitzinger C: The thermostatic control of human metabolic heat production, *Proc Natl Acad Sci USA* 47:730-739, 1961.
7. Sessler DI, Moayeri A: Skin-surface warming: heat flux and central temperature, *Anesthesiology* 73:218-224, 1990.
8. Simon E, Pierau F-K, Taylor DCM: Central and peripheral thermal control of effectors in homeothermic temperature regulation, *Physiol Rev* 66:235-300, 1986.
9. Vale RJ: Cooling during vascular surgery, *Br J Anaesth* 44:1334, 1972.
10. Sessler DI, Olofsson CI, Rubinstein EH: The thermoregulatory threshold of humans during halothane anesthesia, *Anesthesiology* 68:836-842, 1988.
11. Sessler DI, Olofsson CI, Rubinstein EH, et al: The thermoregulatory threshold in humans during nitrous oxide-fentanyl anesthesia, *Anesthesiology* 69:357-364, 1988.
12. Sessler DI: *Temperature monitoring*. In Miller RD, editor: *Anesthesia*, ed 3, New York, 1990, Churchill Livingstone, pp 1227-1242.
13. Morley-Forster PK: Unintentional hypothermia in the operating room, *Can Anaesth Soc J* 33:515-527, 1986.
14. Sessler DI, Israel D, Pozos RS, et al: Spontaneous post-anesthetic tremor does not resemble thermoregulatory shivering, *Anesthesiology* 68:843-850, 1988.
15. Crocker BD, Okumura O, McCuaig DI, et al: Temperature monitoring during general anaesthesia, *Br J Anaesth* 50:1223-1228, 1980.
16. Bay J, Nunn JF, Prys-Roberts C: Factors influencing arterial PO_2 during recovery from anaesthesia, *Br J Anaesth* 40:398-407, 1968.
17. Carli F, Clark MM, Woollen JW: Investigation of the relationship between heat loss and nitrogen excretion in elderly patients undergoing major abdominal surgery under general anaesthesia, *Br J Anaesth* 54:1023-1028, 1982.
18. Conahan TJ, Wiliams GD, Apfelbaum JL, et al: Airway heating reduces recovery time (cost) in outpatients, *Anesthesiology* 67:128-130, 1987.
19. Heier T, Caldwell JE, Sessler DI, et al: The effect of local surface and central cooling on adductor pollicis twitch tension during nitrous oxide/isoflurance and nitrous oxide/fentanyl anesthesia in humans, *Anesthesiology* 72:807-811, 1989.
20. Goldberg MJ, Roe CF: Temperature changes during anesthesia and operations, *Arch Surg* 93:365-369, 1966.
21. Boyan CP, Howland WS: Blood temperature a critical factor in massive transfusion, *Anesthesiology* 22:559-563, 1961.
22. Hendrickx HHL: Paradoxical inhibition of decreases in body temperature by use of heated and humidified gases, *Anesth Analg* 61:393-394, 1982 (letter).
23. Curtis RM, Trezek GJ: *Analysis of heat exchange during cooling and rewarming in cardiopulmonary bypass procedures*. In Shitzer A, Eberhart RC, editors: *Heat transfer in medicine and biology, vol 2*, New York, 1985, Plenum, pp 261-286.
24. Morris RH, Wilkey BR: The effect of ambient temperature on patients monitored during surgery, not involving body cavities, *Anesthesiology* 32:102-107, 1970.
25. Bourke D, Wurm H: Intraoperative heat conservation using a reflective blanket, *Anesthesiology* 60:151-154, 1984.
26. Lilly RB, Jr: Inadvertent hypothermia: a real problem. In *ASA refresher courses in anesthesiology, vol. 15*, 93-107, 1986.
27. Crino MH, Nagel EL: Thermal burns caused by warming blankets in the operating room, *Anesthesiology* 29:149-150, 1968.
28. Chalon J, Patel C, Ali M, et al: Humidity and the anesthetized patient, *Anesthesiology* 50:195-198, 1979.
29. Shanks CA: Humidification and loss of heat during anaesthesia. II. Effects in surgical patients, *Br J Anaesth* 46:863-865, 1974.
30. Klein EF Jr, Graves SA: "Hot pot" tracheitis, *Chest* 65:225-226, 1974.
31. Bissonnette B, Sessler DI, LaFlamme P: Passive and active inspired gas humidification in infants and children, *Anesthesiology* 71:350-354, 1989.
32. Joly HR, Weil MH: Temperature of the great toe as an indication of the severity of shock, *Circulation* 39:131-138, 1969.
33. Cork RC, Vaughan RW, Humphrey LS: Precision and accuracy of intraoperative temperature monitoring, *Anesth Analg* 62:211-214, 1962.
34. Benzinger TH, Taylor GW: *Cranial measurements of internal temperature in man*. In Hardy JD, editor: *Temperature: its measurement and control in science and industry, vol 3*, New York, 1963, Reinhold, pp 111-120.
35. Cabanac M, Caputa M: Open loop increase in trunk temperature produced by face cooling in working humans, *J Physiol (Lond)* 289:163-174, 1979.
36. Wallace CT, Marks WE, Adkins WY, et al: Perforation of the tympanic membrane, a complication of tympanic thermometry during anesthesia, *Anesthesiology* 41:290-291, 1974.
37. Keatinge WR, Sloan REG: Measurement of deep body temperature from external auditory canal with servo-controlled heating around ear, *J Physiol* 234:8P, 1973.
38. Whitby JD, Duncan LJ: Cerebral, oesophageal and nasopharyngeal temperatures, *Br J Anaesth* 43:673-676, 1971.
39. Ritter DM, Rettke SR, Hughes RW, et al: Placement of nasogastric tubes and esophageal stethoscopes in patients with documented esophageal varices, *Anesth Analg* 67:283-285, 1988.
40. Freund PR, Brengelmann GL: Placement of esophageal stethoscope by acoustic criteria does not consistently yield an optimal location for the monitoring of core temperature, *J Clin Monit* 6:266-270, 1990.
41. Ramsay JG, Ralley FE, Whalley DG, et al: Site of temperature monitoring and prediction of afterdrop after open heart surgery, *Can Anaesth Soc J* 32:607-612, 1985.
42. Lucke JN, Hall GM, Lister D: Porcine malignant hyperthermia. I. Metabolic and physiologic changes, *Br J Anaesth* 48:297-302, 1976.
43. Cobbold RSC: *Transducers for biomedical measurements: principles and applications*, New York, 1974, Wiley.
44. Parker EO III: Electrosurgical burn at the site of an esophageal temperature probe, *Anesthesiology* 61:93-95, 1984.
45. Fergason JL: Liquid crystals, *Sci Am* 211:76-85, 1964.
46. Vaughan MS, Cork RC, Vaughan RW: Inaccuracy of liquid crystal thermometry to identify core temperature trends in postoperative adults, *Anesth Analg* 61:284-287, 1982.
47. Bjoraker DG: Liquid crystal temperature indicators, *Anesthesiology Review* 17:50-56, 1990.
48. Shinozaki T, Deane R, Perkins FM: Infrared tympanic thermometer: evaluation of a new clinical thermometer, *Crit Care Med* 16:148-150, 1988.
49. Intelligent Medical Systems: FirstTemp 2000A service manual. Intelligent Medical Systems, Carlsbad, Calif.
50. Lees DE, Kim YD: Noninvasive determination of core temperature during anesthesia, *South Med J* 73:1322-1324, 1980.
51. Muravchick S: Deep body thermometry during general anesthesia, *Anesthesiology* 58:271-275, 1983.

Chapter 13

BLOOD PRESSURE MONITORING

Timothy J. Quill, M.D.

What is blood pressure?
Invasive blood pressure monitoring
Manual (Riva-Rocci) technique
Oscillometric blood pressure devices
Peñaz (Finapres) technique
Arterial tonometry
Pulse transit time (Photometric method)

The frequent measurement of blood pressure during anesthetic administration is a standard practice throughout the world. Because of the significant blood pressure excursions that may be observed during surgery, and because of the presumed value of accurate, frequent, repeatable determinations in predicting certain intraoperative and postoperative problems, the tendency in recent years has been toward the use of automatic digital electromechanical instruments. Many of these devices function remarkably well, requiring little effort and special training of the user. This chapter discusses the various instruments and methods for measuring blood pressure currently in clinical use, including simple principles of operation, perceived advantages and disadvantages, relative accuracy, and factors that may affect operation. It is assumed that the reader is aware of recommended and reasonable limits for blood pressure and the medical implications of abnormal values. In this chapter is presented a brief, nontechnical explanation of the important points of modern blood pressure measurement technology.

WHAT IS BLOOD PRESSURE?

Nearly everyone is familiar with the originally reported measurement of blood pressure obtained by the Reverend Stephen Hales, who cannulated the femoral artery of a horse and measured the average height of the blood column at approximately 9 feet. Hales also described respiratory variation and pulsatile pressure, a remarkable achievement in the eighteenth century. Little further work was done until the late nineteenth century, when numerous investigators described noninvasive blood pressure determinations; notably, the auscultatory method of Korotkoff (1905) is still probably the most commonly used method of individual blood pressure determination throughout the world. On the other hand, the oscillometric technique originally described by Roy and Adami in 1890 is rapidly gaining popularity, because it is the theoretical basis for most automated noninvasive blood pressure measuring equipment manufactured today.

Accompanying the development of various methods of blood pressure determination was the controversy over the definition of systolic, diastolic, and mean blood pressures. For invasive methods producing a pulsatile waveform, the superficial definitions are simple: Systolic pressure is the maximum instantaneous pressure, diastolic pressure is the minimum, and mean pressure is the area under the waveform-time curve, divided by the time interval for one or more beats, a quantity that is easily determined electronically. Blood pressure determinations are highly dependent on the anatomic site of the determination;[1] usually there is an increase in systolic values and a decrease in diastolic values as blood pressure is measured more peripherally in the vascular tree of healthy subjects. This represents a typical systolic difference of approximately 20 mm Hg at a distance of 30 cm from the aortic root (in dogs). In patients with vascular disease and resultant poor arterial flow, further errors are introduced, usually producing decreases in systolic, diastolic, and mean flow at distal locations. Despite these well known predictable errors, the radial arterial pressure, determined by a small cannula inserted near the wrist, combined with an electronic transducer and display system, has become the de facto clinical standard of comparison for human blood pressure determinations. Nearly all published methodology comparisons and so-called accurate studies use the radial arterial pressure as the reference standard. This is done despite the fact that the choice of the radial artery is more one of safety and convenience rather than one of scientific validity. The central aortic root pressure, much less affected by arterial system variables, is probably a much more reliable standard, although measurement of this pressure in humans involves unacceptable risk.

Several different types and many commercial models of automated noninvasive blood pressure instruments have become available in the United States in recent years, and their use has become ubiquitous in anesthesia throughout the country and much of the world. Each method measures different physical quantities, from which values for systolic, diastolic, and mean blood pressure are derived. Noninvasive blood pressure readings never correlate exactly with measured invasive radial arterial blood pressure, no matter how carefully the instruments are constructed and calibrated or the methodology is validated. It is hoped, however, that the accuracy of any method is such that differences between readings are of little clinical consequence or significance. In general, this is true for most commercial oscillometric instruments, although other methodologies do not consistently seem to perform as well in all situations. Reliability of modern automated noninvasive oscillometric equipment has reached the point where it is basically unnecessary to back up the automated unit with an older (e.g. auscultatory) method, because the backup is less reliable than the automated method and most often represents a step downward in accuracy.

The standard unit of measure for blood pressure in the United States is millimeters of mercury (mm Hg), or torr, where 760 mm Hg = 1 standard atmosphere of pressure at sea level. Elsewhere in the world, kiloPascal (kPa) is often the standard unit of pressure measurement, where 1 kPa ≈ 7.5 mm Hg. Most commercial digital blood pressure instruments provide a readout with a resolution of 1 mm Hg, although this implied significance considerably exceeds the actual precision and repeatability of even the most accurate invasive units and certainly does not provide meaningful additional clinical information. The actual precision of the best devices is approximately 5 to 10 mm Hg. Calibration

accuracy of noninvasive blood pressure devices is commonly measured and adjusted by the manufacturer by comparison with radial arterial blood pressure in healthy human subjects.

As discussed above, radial arterial pressure correlates well with central aortic pressure,[1] but the two values may disagree by a considerable amount, especially in hypertensive and hyperdynamic patients and in patients with peripheral vasoconstriction or vascular disease.[2] In addition, every noninvasive method measures blood pressure indirectly, by inference from measured physical quantities,[3] such as cuff air pressure oscillations, so the correlation with invasive pressure is never perfect. Thus, when interpreting methods of comparison, it is important intuitively to consider the clinical implications of stated blood pressure differences, which are often inconsequential.

If the aortic root is taken as the desired reference point for blood pressure, all measurement techniques must take into account the effect of gravity and the water column hydrostatic pressure resulting from a difference of height between the aortic root and the location of the transducer. This amounts to a difference of approximately 7.5 mm Hg for every 10 cm difference in vertical height from the aortic root. The effect is always small for a brachial cuff, but it can be large (>100 mm Hg)—for example, if the pressure transducer is accidentally dropped on the floor or if an ankle cuff is used on an individual who is in the sitting position. Thus it is important either to consider this effect when the system is zeroed or to add or subtract a fixed amount to the measured blood pressure. This applies to both noninvasive and invasive instruments. Some novel and practical methods have been suggested to accomplish this compensation in the everyday clinical situation.[4]

INVASIVE BLOOD PRESSURE MONITORING

Invasive blood pressure monitoring is often the clinical method of choice if large hemodynamic transients are expected or encountered, frequent blood sampling is anticipated, or there is a need for continuous, accurate beat-to-beat blood pressure determination. The majority of continuous ECG monitoring units sold in the United States also have the capability of simultaneously measuring blood pressure. Besides the obvious advantage of allowing arterial blood sampling, the invasive method provides unsurpassed reliability and accuracy, especially when extremes of blood pressure are expected.

The usual method of invasive blood pressure monitoring consists of the percutaneous insertion of a small-bore (18- to 22-gauge) plastic catheter into a peripheral artery. The catheter is physically connected via plastic tubing to an electronic pressure transducer and display unit. The transducer is normally a sterile, miniature, self-contained assembly containing the electromechanical components within a clear plastic case. Most transducers incorporate an integral mechanism for providing a continuous, slow flush of sterile anticoagulant solution through the tubing and catheter in order to prevent clotting. In addition, a mechanism for rapid manual flushing is usually provided. The entire assembly is designed for single-patient use, at a cost of approximately $15 to $20 per patient. The use of solid-state, individually calibrated, and trimmed instruments has greatly improved the accuracy over previous partially disposable systems,[5] and in general an absolute accuracy of ±5 mm Hg or better throughout the measurement range can be expected. Identical transducer systems are normally used if central venous or pulmonary arterial pressures are to be monitored simultaneously.

Invasive arterial blood pressure monitoring is not without risk. Potential problems include symptomatic or asymptomatic arterial thrombosis, infection, accidental injection of intravenous drugs, nerve damage from trauma or hematoma, and exsanguination from accidental disconnection. All of these problems have been reported infrequently. Slogoff, et al.[6] studied arterial cannulation in a large series of surgical patients and concluded that the risks of radial artery cannulation are often exaggerated and that serious morbidity in adults is rare. They also found no evidence to support the long-held beliefs that the shape, size, and material of the catheter and duration of insertion are important predictors of complications. In addition, their study found no objective evidence that noninvasive determination of collateral flow before the catheter is inserted (e.g., Allen test) was of any value in predicting morbidity. Furthermore, there was no evidence that one cannulation site (e.g., radial, ulnar, brachial, axillary, femoral, dorsalis pedis) was safer than another. It is uncertain whether these conclusions can be extended to children and neonates, although the available evidence indicates that arterial cannulation in this population is a reasonably safe procedure.[7]

Arterial cannulation is often painful, and liberal local anesthesia combined with anxiolytic medication is highly recommended. Although many different insertion techniques have been described, most of these methods are successful in trained hands, and there is little to suggest that any technique is consistently safer or better than another. Realistically, a well trained clinician should expect a success rate of about 90% on the first attempt in a reasonably healthy patient with normal anatomy. Severe hypotension, vascular disease, or previous cannulation can make insertion difficult or impossible. In this case direct exposure of the artery via a surgical cutdown may be the only method to cannulate the artery successfully.

Common sense dictates that, to minimize possible complications, arterial catheters should be removed as soon as they are no longer needed. Continuous flushing with heparinized saline at a rate of 5 to 10 ml/hr to prevent clotting has become standard practice, and this capability is automatically incorporated in virtually all modern disposable transducer sets. In the intensive care unit, arterial catheters tend to stop functioning after 1 to 2 weeks, due to a combination of arterial inflammation, occlusion, and clot formation. This necessitates removal of the catheter and changing to an alternate site.

Ideally, an invasive blood pressure transducer should be small (i.e., incorporated in the catheter itself), reliable, free from nonlinearity and distortion, and inexpensive. Unfortunately, devices approaching this ideal are still experimental, although the introduction of disposable transducers has provided a technology with generally acceptable consistent performance in a reasonably sized package (Fig. 13-1). Many factors influence the accuracy of modern invasive arterial monitoring equipment, not the least of which is the ambiguity and disagreement over the exact quantitative definition of blood pressure.[3] Aortic root pressure is the accepted physiological standard, but safety considerations preclude routine measurement outside the laboratory. Radial arterial pressure reflects aortic pressure well in healthy, young individuals, but this is seldom the condition of patients requiring invasive monitoring. As previously mentioned, measured systolic pressure tends to increase and diastolic pressure to decrease as the location of the catheter becomes more peripheral,[1] due to resonance effects in the arterial tree, whereas mean pressure decreases only slightly. Vascular disease and vasoconstriction predictably decrease both systolic and diastolic measurements in proportion to the severity of the condition, but it is fairly common to note an error of 50 mm Hg or more in the cold, severely vasoconstricted patient.[2] In this situation, femoral invasive or brachial noninvasive oscillometric blood pressure readings often more accurately reflect aortic pressure than do radial invasive readings.

Modern electronic monitors are designed to interface reliably with electromechanical transducer systems without the need for extensive technical skills on the part of the clinician. A provision for static zeroing of the system is built into the monitor, and after the zeroing procedure is accomplished the system is ready for operation. As mentioned above, it is important to zero the system with the reference point at the approximate level of the aortic root in order to eliminate the effect of the fluid column of the transducer system. Most monitors display a waveform, preferably with a calibrated scale, as well as a digital numeric display of systolic, diastolic, and (often) mean pressures. Each manufacturer produces an electronic instrument with slightly different frequency response and filtering systems. The various techniques for extracting digital quantities vary from simple peak and valley detection to sophisticated algorithms incorporating digital noise filtering and compensation for artifact and ringing. Thus it is difficult to get two different monitors to read exactly the same numerical blood pressure, although the differences are likely to be small and clinically insignificant, especially with regard to the mean blood pressure value.

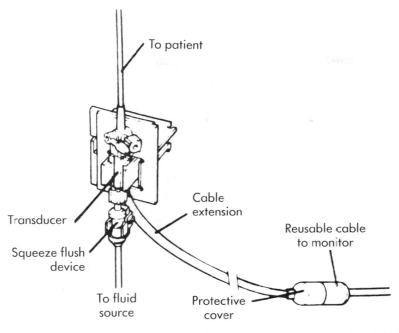

Fig. 13-1. Typical disposable hemodynamic pressure transducer. (By permission of Abbott Critical Care Systems, North Chicago, Ill.)

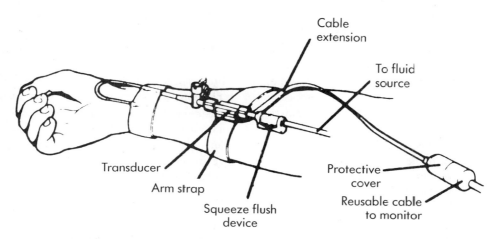

Fig. 13-2. Recommended setup of invasive disposable radial arterial transducer, including short length of connecting tubing.

Visualization of the pressure waveform, an important step in assuring the accuracy of digital readings, can be very useful in qualitatively inferring the inotropic and volume status of the patient. In general, a crisp upstroke implies a more hyperdynamic situation, and a broad peak or plateau of the blood pressure waveform implies adequate diastolic filling and venous volume.[3] Severely hypovolemic patients often demonstrate a sharp upstroke followed by an equally sharp descent nearly to baseline and a secondary, dicrotic, wave approximately half the height of the systolic ejection wave. Marked variation of systolic blood pressure with ventilation is often a sign of hypovolemia or

tamponade. A marked decrease in the systolic-diastolic difference with a normal mean pressure reading usually indicates a failing catheter or flush system or severe peripheral vasoconstriction.

The electromechanical assembly of catheter, transducer, and connecting tubing forms a less-than-ideal measuring system (Fig. 13-2) with the introduction of resonances and waveform distortion and resultant predictable errors in blood pressure determination.[8] Scaling errors have been all but eliminated with the introduction of disposable, individually calibrated transducers, but older systems require static calibration and comparison

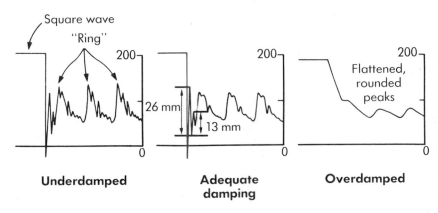

Fig. 13-3. Effect of damping coefficient upon arterial wave morphology. Note especially differences in systolic (peak) pressure.

with a reference manometer before use.[5] The inherent frequency response of the transducer itself is seldom a limiting factor with modern disposable units, but underdamping and ringing at a characteristic high frequency is the rule.[9] Underdamping increases systolic readings and simultaneously decreases diastolic readings, with little effect on the mean pressure (Fig. 13-3), generally exaggerating the effects of the vascular tree.[1] The fact that the catheter faces into the bloodstream likewise distorts the waveform and exaggerates systolic pressure readings. These errors are especially noticeable in the tachycardic, hyperdynamic patient. In practice, resonance errors are usually ignored, in which case mean pressure should be regarded as the value on the basis of which clinical decisions are made. Inexpensive, adjustable, disposable damping devices are available from many transducer manufacturers to eliminate the problem of ringing and overshoot and to enable the user to achieve adequate damping (Fig. 13-3). The use of connecting tubing that is as short as possible and careful attention to eliminating air bubbles throughout the system are also helpful in ensuring accuracy.[9]

Peripheral invasive blood pressure monitoring has become a standard technique in widespread clinical use where continuous, reliable blood pressure monitoring combined with the ability for convenient blood sampling is required. Modern disposable systems enable reasonable accuracy with a minimum of inconvenience. Arterial cannulation in the adult is a reasonably safe procedure to the best of our current knowledge, but it should nevertheless be used only when clinically indicated and appropriate.

MANUAL (RIVA-ROCCI) TECHNIQUE

The measurement of blood pressure with an air-inflatable cuff placed on the proximal arm and listening with a stethoscope over the brachial artery for Korotkoff sounds as cuff air pressure is slowly decreased remains the most common and inexpensive method of blood pressure deter-

mination. Systolic blood pressure is measured as the highest cuff pressure and diastolic blood pressure as the lowest pressure where regular Korotkoff sounds are heard. Mean blood pressure (BP) is not specifically measured, but it is often approximated as:

$$\text{Mean BP} = \text{Diastolic BP} + \frac{\text{Systolic BP} - \text{Diastolic BP}}{3}$$

The advantages of the Riva-Rocci (auscultatory) technique are numerous, including low cost, simplicity, lack of dependence on electricity, and ruggedness. The method represents a less-than-perfect correlation with invasive measurement of blood pressure because of numerous factors, including ambient noise, auditory acuity of the clinician, atherosclerotic vascular changes, obesity, and cuff size in relation to the limb.[10] In general, however, it is most accurate in the healthy patient. Riva-Rocci blood pressure is generally biased low (10 to 30 mm Hg) for systolic blood pressure and high (5 to 25 mm Hg) for diastolic pressure, especially in hypertensive patients.[11] Precision (scatter) is about ±20 mm Hg[12] when invasive radial arterial pressure is used as the standard. In critically ill hypotensive patients, it is often impossible to obtain a reliable auscultatory blood pressure without resorting to Doppler flow sensing devices in order to detect systolic arterial blood flow. With the increased use of pulse oximetry, systolic pressure can be reliably measured with a much improved sensitivity over manual palpation or Korotkoff sounds by noting the point of occlusion of pulsatile flow in the finger while observing the pulse (optical plethysmographic) waveform on the oximeter display.[13]

Despite a lack of accuracy and subjectivity compared with automated and invasive methods, manual auscultatory measurement of blood pressure remains in common use for patients who are not critically ill because the cost is unbeatable, and it is doubtful whether the observed errors in the healthy population are ever clinically meaningful. In patients who require frequent, objective measurement of blood pressure—for example, in the operating room—manual auscultatory methods have largely been replaced by automated oscillometric equipment.

During the 1970s, several automated devices were introduced (e.g., the Roche Arteriosonde), which utilized the Riva-Rocci technique to measure blood pressure automatically and noninvasively. They incorporated either a small microphone or a Doppler transducer into the cuff, which was placed over the brachial artery, and the cuff was inflated automatically by an air pump. These devices proved technically more complicated than oscillometric devices introduced later and gradually disappeared from clinical use. To the author's knowledge, no devices of this type are currently being manufactured.

OSCILLOMETRIC BLOOD PRESSURE DEVICES

It is common to observe pulsatile pressure variation in the gauge used to measure cuff air pressure during manual measurement of blood pressure using auscultation. Oscillometric cuff blood pressure methods all take advantage of this pulsatile variation in order to infer arterial blood pressure. The simplest technique is to deflate the cuff slowly from a pressure above the expected value. At a pressure roughly corresponding to systolic arterial pressure, the needle of the pressure gauge begins to oscillate slightly (1 to 5 mm Hg) with each cardiac stroke volume (Fig. 13-4). This value is assumed to be the systolic pressure, and for many years this was the standard method of measuring blood pressure in children, in whom Korotkoff sounds are difficult to hear. An enhancement of this technique is the oscillotonometer, a mechanical device equipped with two cuffs and a sensitive gauge, designed to amplify greatly the observed oscillations and thus increase the sensitivity. The mean pressure is usually assumed to be the cuff pressure that produces the maximum amplitude of oscillations. The diastolic pressure is difficult to measure directly by oscillometric methods because the oscillations decrease smoothly and gradually as cuff pressure decreases below the actual diastolic arterial value. The manual oscillotonometer has lost popularity since the development of automated devices.

Many different electronic oscillometric devices have been developed and commercially introduced, and they have become very widely used. Although the specific algorithms used to determine systolic, diastolic, and mean blood pressure values are proprietary with the individual manufacturer, in fact all of the devices probably function in a manner similar to the manual oscillometric techniques described above. Cuff pressure is first increased above the expected systolic blood pressure value; then it is slowly and automatically decreased while the pressure oscillations in the cuff are measured electronically. Computation of the diastolic blood pressure is inferred mathematically from the systolic and mean values, as well as from the characteristics of the "tail" of the oscillations at low pressures.

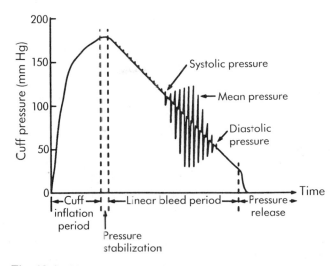

Fig. 13-4. Observed oscillations in cuff pressure during deflation (amplitude of oscillations greatly exaggerated).

Models manufactured since the mid-1980s utilize high-performance microprocessors and perform remarkably well.[14] They generally incorporate automatic repeated measurement at predetermined time intervals, automatic recording, serial data outputs, and sophisticated alarms.

Automatic oscillometric blood pressure devices offer distinct advantages over manual devices. They eliminate the clinician's subjectivity; and, for a noninvasive monitor, introduce an unprecedented degree of repeatability between subsequent readings. The algorithms are presumably optimized to correlate well with invasive blood pressure readings in the average healthy subject; and indeed, the precision and bias of a well designed unit are generally less than 10 mm Hg in this population.[14] The cuff is the same as the one used for manual auscultatory methods, and problems related to this methodology remain. In particular, atherosclerosis and chronic hypertension introduce errors in systolic (reading low) and diastolic (reading high) oscillometric blood pressures when the cuff is compared with invasive arterial pressure measurements.[15] Using the improper cuff size also introduces significant errors[10]: cuffs that are larger than needed produce erroneously low oscillometric readings and vice versa. Large cuffs read low especially if the cuff overrides itself into two layers, causing an increased transmission of air pressure to the arm and blood vessels. For similar reasons, relatively small cuffs produce erroneously high readings. Automatic, intermittent blood pressure monitoring also interferes with ipsilateral intravenous access and pulse oximetry.

Oscillometric units often function well for the obese patient and for children, for whom auscultatory methods usually fail. They also operate when used on either the calf or thigh if a cuff of appropriate size is used, a fact often overlooked by the clinician. Finally, the accuracy of an infant cuff used on the adult thumb seems to be adequate,[16] where brachial or lower extremity cuffs are precluded.

PEÑAZ (FINAPRES) TECHNIQUE

The continuous, beat-to-beat measurement of blood pressure is accurately accomplished using an intraarterial catheter, but this technique involves discomfort and risk for the patient and is not appropriate for use in healthy subjects on a routine basis. Nevertheless, it is desirable to measure blood pressure continuously and noninvasively under many circumstances, and this elusive goal was first reached in a practical form and reported by Peñaz[17] in 1973. The actual measuring element consists of a small air cuff designed to fit around the middle phalanx of the adult finger. The inner surface of the cuff contains a built-in light source that directs an infrared beam transversely through both digital arteries (Fig. 13-5). An infrared receiver on the opposite side of the finger then generates a signal proportional to the blood volume of the finger. The signal is used as a control signal in a feedback loop that causes rapid inflation or deflation of the cuff. Ideally, the feedback system instantaneously tracks pulsatile changes in the finger and inflates the cuff synchronously in order to maintain a constant infrared light absorbance (Fig. 13-6). This condition, known as volume clamping, produces an instantaneous cuff pressure very similar to the instantaneous arterial pressure in the finger. The cuff pressure is then sent to an amplifier and display system similar to that used for invasive pressure. This technology is used in the Finapres* blood pressure monitoring system.[18]

*Ohmeda, Madison, Wis.

The Peñaz method has several obvious limitations.[19] Low peripheral perfusion states reduce the useful signal to a point at which oscillation of the feedback system is difficult to prevent; thus accuracy suffers. When functioning perfectly, it accurately measures the blood pressure in the finger, which may or may not correlate with central arterial pressure. In the case of vascular disease or physiologic vasoconstriction (e.g., in hypothermia), blood pressure in the finger can be very low or even essentially absent, whereas the patient may actually be centrally hypertensive. Perfusion of the finger during continuous use is marginal,

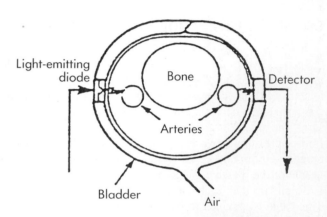

Fig. 13-5. Detail of the Finapres blood pressure cuff. LED = light-emitting diode.

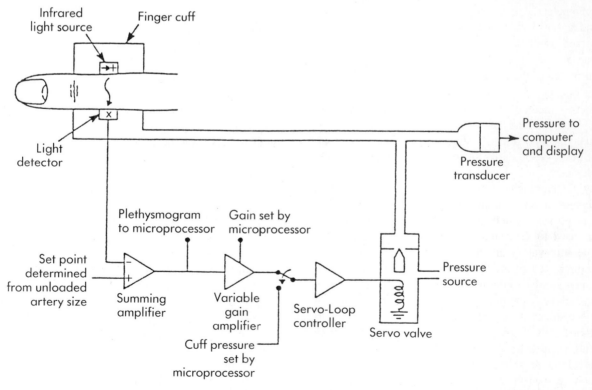

Fig. 13-6. Basic operation of the Ohmeda Finapres noninvasive blood pressure monitor. (By permission of Ohmeda, Inc., a Division of BOC Health Care, Inc., Madison, Wisc.)

although not apparently to a harmful extent, but fingertip cyanosis is often present.[20] Prolonged use in the conscious patient is sometimes accompanied by complaints of considerable ischemic pain. A recently implemented software "rest period" may help alleviate this problem, although the Peñaz device is probably contraindicated in such conditions as Raynaud's disease and sickle cell anemia.

Despite these problems, the Peñaz method, arguably the most successful implementation of beat-to-beat noninvasive blood pressure measurement, displays clinical accuracy in healthy subjects similar to that of the best oscillometric devices.[14] The pressure tracings produced by the Finapres often strikingly resemble those produced by simultaneous invasive radial artery catheters used during comparison studies.[18] The device has proven very useful where measurement of rapid blood pressure transients is desirable without the risk, discomfort, and expense of invasive arterial catheterization. By comparison, even the best oscillometric devices offer a blood pressure reading only approximately every 30 seconds.[21] In addition, confining the transducer system to one finger eliminates interference with intravenous infusions and pulse oximetry, which is often problematic with oscillometric monitors.

ARTERIAL TONOMETRY

Arterial tonometry, in this context, is the external application of a pressure transducer over an artery in order to infer blood pressure changes from changes in the amplitude of the transduced signal. This method, the oldest proposed for measurement of beat-to-beat blood pressure, until recently has been beset by the lack of a reliable transducer and support system and unacceptable sensitivity to uncompensated changes in dynamic arterial wall tension. A recently developed unit marketed by Nellcor (N-CAT) purports to have solved both of these problems.[22,23] A complex servo system applies a multi-element transducer over the radial artery at the wrist (Fig. 13-7). The perpendicular pressure is automatically adjusted in order to flatten the arterial wall and thus eliminate the radial (direction) component of arterial wall tension (Fig. 13-8), which

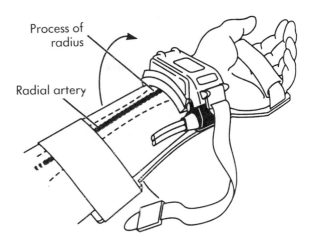

Fig. 13-7. Nellcor N-CAT arterial tonometer shown applied to the wrist. (By permission of Nellcor, Inc., Hayward, Ca.)

should enable changes in the transduced pulsatile signal to be roughly directly proportional to changes in beat-to-beat arterial blood pressure. The transducer in the multiple array with the strongest signal is automatically chosen for analysis. The method requires periodic calibration with a separate, built-in oscillometric monitor and brachial cuff placed on the contralateral arm.

This device as currently available has several obvious drawbacks. The requirement for a relatively clumsy machine to be applied to the wrist as well as a contralateral oscillometric cuff makes the monitor more awkward and inconvenient to use than simple oscillometric cuff units. It would take a dedicated clinician to use the device as currently offered on a routine basis. The wrist transducer assembly is so sensitive to motion artifact that it is impractical in the conscious, moving patient. Although an "arterial waveform" is displayed, it does not seem to necessarily resemble the actual arterial tracing in initial evaluations. Frequent calibration (every 3 to 10 minutes) with the oscillometric cuff seems to be required; thus the cuff is inflated much of the time. Accuracy has yet to be objectively evaluated.

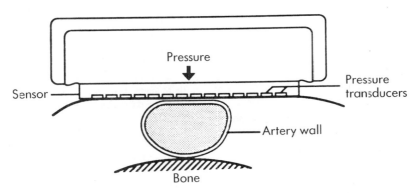

Fig. 13-8. Multiple sensors and arterial flattening as utilized by the Nellcor N-CAT arterial tonometer. (By permission of Nellcor, Inc., Hayward, Calif.)

There are some possible advantages to this method. It is theoretically less sensitive than the Peñaz method to inaccuracies caused by vascular disease and vasoconstriction, because the radial artery is so much larger than those of the finger. Discomfort in the cooperative, awake individual seems to be minimal, and cyanosis is not observed. Future innovations may lead to a more compact and less contraption-like realization of arterial tonometry.

PULSE TRANSIT TIME (PHOTOMETRIC METHOD)

The relationship between pulse wave velocity and blood pressure was first described in 1922 by Bramwell and Hill. Pulse transit times are measured using pulse transducers placed at two or more sites on the body. The transducers, located at different theoretical distances from the central circulation, measure the delay time between the sites (Fig. 13-9). Pulse transit time has long been used in psychiatric studies as a nonspecific index of cardiovascular activity, and it has long been noted that pulse transit time bears a roughly inverse relationship to systolic arterial blood pressure.[24] The relation to diastolic and mean pressure does not seem to be as clear. A commercial device recently introduced by Sentinel (Indianapolis, Ind.) purports to measure beat-to-beat arterial systolic, mean, and diastolic blood pressure on the basis of this principle. Pulses are measured by two optical transducers, most often located on the finger and the forehead. Calibration is periodically accomplished via a separate, built-in oscillometric monitor and brachial cuff placed on the arm. Changes in blood pulse transit time are transformed into blood pressure predictions using a proprietary algorithm.

The accuracy of this device has not been adequately evaluated in an objective fashion, and it depends to a large extent on the presumption of a relationship between blood pressure and transit time. The waveform provided on the integrated display does not resemble the actual arterial pressure profile but rather is a pulse profile similar to that provided by many pulse oximeters. The unit incorporates an integral pulse oximeter that also serves as one of the two pulse transducers.

The validity of this method remains unproven, although it theoretically eliminates most of the problems associated with the Peñaz and tonometric methods discussed above. If this methodology proves to be accurate, it will offer a beat-to-beat blood pressure technology only slightly more cumbersome than the now standard oscillometric unit combined with the similarly standard pulse oximetry.

Several methods of noninvasively measuring blood pressure have been developed into a practical working device. Thus far none of the continuous methods discussed consistently demonstrates the reliability and ease of use that have been realized by the oscillometric units. In addi-

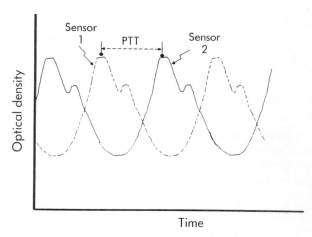

Fig. 13-9. Definition of pulse transit time *(PTT)* as measured by two optical sensors.

tion, the expense of the alternative technologies has largely limited their function to experimental protocols rather than regular everyday use.

Invasive measurement of blood pressure via a peripherally placed intraarterial cannula remains the method of choice when beat-to-beat blood pressure measurement is required for clinical care. Invasive monitoring is not without risk, but where continuous pressure monitoring and/or frequent blood sampling is required, the morbidity is quite acceptable.

REFERENCES

1. Hamilton WF, Dow P: An experimental study of the standing waves in the pulse propagated through the aorta, *Am J Physiol* 125:48-59, 1939.
2. Pauca AL, Hudspeth AS, Wallenhaupt SL, et al: Radial artery-to-aorta pressure difference after discontinuation of cardiopulmonary bypass, *Anesthesiology* 70:935-941, 1989.
3. Bruner JR: *Handbook of blood pressure monitoring,* Littleton, Mass. 1978, PSG.
4. Pennington LA, Smith C: Leveling when monitoring central blood pressures: an alternative method, *Heart Lung* 9:1053-1059, 1980.
5. Phillip JH, Phillip BK, Lehr JL: Accuracy of hydrostatic pressure measurement with a disposable dome transducer system, *Med Instrum* 19:273-274, 1985.
6. Slogoff S, Keats AS, Arlund C: On the safety of radial artery cannulation, *Anesthesiology* 59:42-47, 1983.
7. Selldèn H, Nilsson K, Larsson LE, et al: Radial arterial catheters in children and neonates: a prospective study, *Crit Care Med* 15:1106, 1987.
8. Gardner RM: Direct pressure measurement: dynamic response requirement, *Anesthesiology* 54:227-236, 1981.
9. Hunziker P: Accuracy and response of disposable pressure transducer-tubing systems, *Can Anaesth Soc J* 34:409-414, 1987.
10. Manning DM, Kuchirka C, Kaminski J: Miscuffing: inappropriate blood pressure cuff application, *Circulation* 68:763-766, 1983.
11. Finnie KJ, Watts DG, Armstrong PW: Biases in the measurement of arterial pressure, *Crit Care Med* 12:965-968, 1984.
12. Rutten AJ, Ilsley AH, Skowronski GA, et al: A comparative study of the measurement of mean arterial blood pressure using automatic oscillometers, arterial cannulation and auscultation, *Anaesth Intensive Care* 14:58-65, 1986.

13. Talke P, Nichols RJ, Traber DL: Does measurement of systolic blood pressure with a pulse oximeter correlate with conventional methods? *J Clin Monit* 6:5-9, 1990.

14. Gorback MS, Quill TJ: The relative accuracies of two automated noninvasive arterial pressure measurement devices, *J Clin Monit* 7:13-22, 1991.

15. Loubser PG: Comparison of intra-arterial and automated oscillometric blood pressure measurement methods in postoperative hypertensive patients, *Med Instrum* 20:255, 1986.

16. Gorback MS, Quill TJ, Block ES, et al: Non-invasive blood pressure measurement using an infant cuff applied to the thumb, *Anesth Analg* 69:668-670, 1989.

17. Peñaz J: Photoelectric measurement of blood pressure, volume, and flow in the finger, *Digest of the Tenth International Conference on Medical and Biological Engineering,* Dresden, 1973, p 104.

18. Boehmer RD: Continuous, real-time noninvasive monitor of blood pressure: Peñaz methodology applied to the finger, *J Clin Monit* 3:282-287, 1987.

19. Kurki T, Smith NT, Head N, et al: Noninvasive continuous blood pressure measurement from the finger: optimal measurement conditions and factors affecting reliability, *J Clin Monit* 3:6-13, 1987.

20. Gravenstein JS, Paulus DA, Feldman J, et al: Tissue hypoxia distal to a Peñaz finger blood pressure cuff, *J Clin Monit* 1:120-125, 1985.

21. Gorback MS, Quill TJ, Graubert DA: The accuracy of rapid oscillometric blood pressure determination, *Biomed Instrum Technol* 24:371-374, 1990.

22. Kemmotsu O, Yokota S, Yamamura T, et al: A non-invasive blood pressure monitor based on arterial tonometry, *Anesth Analg* 68:S145, 1989 (abstract).

23. Ekerle JS: *Tonometry, arterial.* In *Encyclopedia of medical devices and instrumentation, vol 4,* New York, 1988, John Wiley and Sons.

24. Lane JD, Greenstadt L, Shapiro D, et al: Pulse transit time and blood pressure: an intensive analysis, *Psychophysiology* 20:45-49, 1983.

Chapter 14

ELECTROCARDIOGRAPHIC MONITORING

Jolie Narang, M.D.
Daniel M. Thys, M.D.

ELECTROCARDIOGRAPHY

The intraoperative use of the electrocardiogram (ECG) has developed markedly over the last several decades.[1] Originally, this monitor was used during anesthesia for the detection of arrhythmias in high-risk patients. In recent years, however, its importance as a standard monitor has been recognized, and its use during the administration of all anesthetics is now recommended. Beyond its usefulness for the intraoperative recognition of arrhythmias, one of the major indications for ECG monitoring is the intraoperative diagnosis of myocardial ischemia.[2]

NORMAL ELECTRICAL ACTIVITY

Figure 14-1 shows the segments and intervals of the normal ECG. These elements are explained in the following subsections.

The P wave

Under normal circumstances, the sinoatrial (SA) node has the most rapid rate of spontaneous depolarization and is, therefore, the dominant cardiac pacemaker. From the SA node, the impulse spreads through the right and left atria. Specialized tracts can conduct the impulse to the atrioventricular (AV) node but are not essential. On the ECG, depolarization of the atria is represented by the P wave. The initial depolarization involves primarily the right atrium and occurs predominantly in an anterior, inferior, and leftward direction. Subsequently, it proceeds to the left atrium located in a more posterior position.

The PR interval

Once the wave of depolarization has reached the AV node, a delay is observed. The delay permits contraction of the atria and supplemental filling of the ventricular chambers. On the ECG, this delay is represented by the PR interval.

The QRS complex

After passage through the AV node, the electrical impulse is conducted along the ventricular conduction pathways consisting of the common bundle of His, the left and

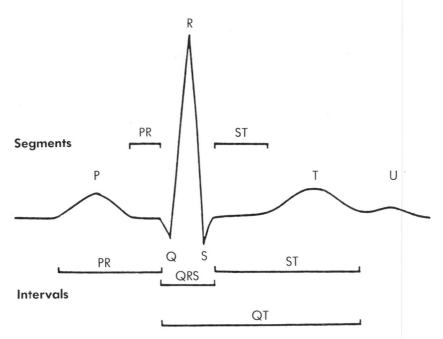

Fig. 14-1. Segments and intervals of the normal ECG.

right bundle branches, the distal bundle branches, and the Purkinje fibers. The QRS complex represents the progress of the depolarization wave through this conduction system. After terminal depolarization, the ECG normally returns to baseline.

The ST segment and T wave

Repolarization of the ventricles, which begins at the end of the QRS complex, consists of the ST segment and T wave. Ventricular depolarization occurs along established conducting pathways, but ventricular repolarization is a prolonged process occurring independently in every cell. The T wave represents the uncancelled potential differences of ventricular repolarization. The junction of the QRS complex and the ST segment is called the J junction. The T wave is sometimes followed by a small U wave, the origin of which is unclear. An inverted U wave has been associated with such clinically significant conditions as hypertension, coronary artery disease, valvular heart disease, and certain metabolic disorders. There may be an association between exercise-related or rest-related U wave inversion and significant stenosis of either the left anterior descending artery or the left main coronary artery.

LEAD SYSTEMS
Standard limb and precordial leads

The small electric currents produced by the electrical activity of the heart spread throughout the body, which behaves as a volume conductor, allowing the surface ECG to be recorded at any site. The standard leads are *bipolar leads* because they measure differences in potential between two electrodes. The electrodes are placed on the

right arm, the left arm, and the left leg. The leads are formed by the imaginary lines connecting the electrodes, and the polarities correspond to the conventions of Einthoven's triangle. They are labelled leads I, II, and III. By convention, lead I is formed by connecting the right arm and left arm electrodes, with the left arm being positive; lead II is formed by connecting the right arm and left leg, with the left leg being positive; and lead III is formed by connecting the left arm and left leg with the left leg being positive. If the three electrodes of the standard leads are connected through resistances of 5000 ohms each, a common central terminal with zero potential is obtained. When this common electrode is used with another active electrode, the potential difference between the two represents the actual potential. On a standard 12-lead ECG, three unipolar limb leads are usually recorded: aVR, aVL, and aVF. The *a*'s indicate that the limb leads are augmented and were obtained via Goldberger's modification. In this modification, the resistors are removed from the lead wires and the exploring electrode is disconnected from the central terminal. Goldberger's modification produces larger voltage deflections on the ECG.

Additional information on the heart's electrical activity is obtained when electrodes are placed closer to the heart or around the thorax. In the *precordial lead* system (Fig. 14-2), the neutral electrode is formed by the standard leads, and an exploring electrode is placed on the chest wall. The ECG is normally recorded with the exploring electrode in one or more of six precordial positions. Each lead is indicated by the letter *V* followed by a subscript numeral from 1 to 6, which indicates the location of the electrode on the chest wall.

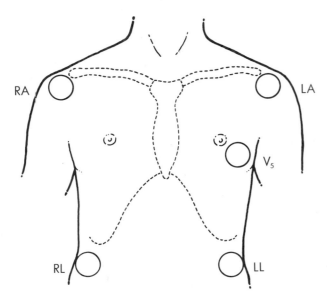

Fig. 14-2. Multiple lead ECG system consisting of four extremity electrodes: right arm *(RA)*, left arm *(LA)*, right leg *(RL)* and left leg *(LL)* and the V_5 lead.

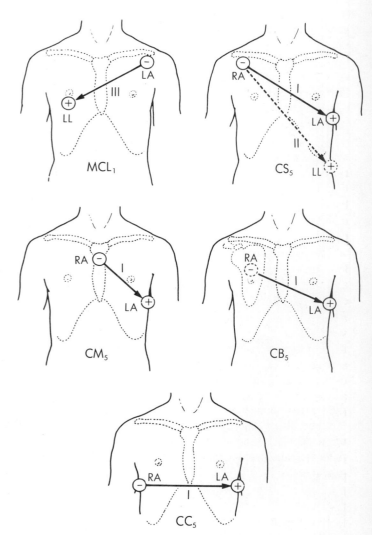

Fig. 14-3. Modified precordial lead arrangements. (From Thys DM, Kaplan JA, editors: *The ECG in anesthesia and critical care,* New York, 1987, Churchill Livingstone.)

Electrocardiographic monitoring systems

The three-electrode system. As the name implies, the three-electrode system utilizes only three electrodes to record the ECG. In such a system, the ECG is observed along one bipolar lead between two of the electrodes while the third electrode serves as a ground. A selector switch allows the user to alter the designation of the electrodes. Three ECG leads can be examined in sequence without changing the location of the electrodes. Although the three-electrode system has the advantage of simplicity, its use is limited in the detection of myocardial ischemia because it provides a narrow picture of myocardial electrical activity.

The modified three-electrode system. Numerous modifications of the standard bipolar limb lead system have been developed. Some of these are displayed in Fig. 14-3. They are used in an attempt to maximize P-wave height for the diagnosis of atrial arrhythmias or to increase the sensitivity of the ECG for the detection of anterior myocardial ischemia. In clinical studies, these modified three-electrode systems have been shown to be at least as sensitive as the standard V_5 lead system for the intraoperative diagnosis of ischemia.[3]

Central subclavicular lead. The central subclavicular (CS_5) lead (Fig. 14-3) is particularly well suited for the detection of anterior wall myocardial ischemia. The right arm (RA) electrode is placed under the right clavicle, the left arm (LA) electrode is placed in the V_5 position, and the left leg electrode is in its usual position to serve as a ground. Lead I is selected for detection of anterior wall ischemia, and lead II can be selected either for monitoring inferior wall ischemia or for the detection of arrhythmias.

If a unipolar precordial electrode is unavailable, this CS_5 bipolar lead is the best and easiest alternative to a true V_5 lead for monitoring myocardial ischemia.

Central back lead. The central back (CB_5) lead is useful for the detection of ischemia and supraventricular arrhythmias, as demonstrated in a study comparing CB_5 and V_5 in patients with closed and open chests.[4] The P wave was 90% larger in lead CB_5 than in lead V_5, and a good correlation between ventricular deflections of CB_5 and V_5 leads was noted. CB_5 is obtained by placing the RA electrode over the center of the right scapula and the LA electrode in the V_5 position. The lead selector switch should be on lead I. The CB_5 lead may be useful in patients with ischemic heart disease who are susceptible to the development of arrhythmias during the perioperative period.

When modified bipolar limb leads are used, the user should be aware that in certain aspects they differ significantly from true unipolar precordial leads. The modified precordial leads usually show a greater R-wave amplitude than standard precordial leads, and this can lead to amplification of the ST-segment response. The criteria for diagnosing myocardial ischemia (see the section on diagnosis of ischemia) may therefore need to be adjusted when modified bipolar leads are used. It has been shown during exercise stress-testing that normalization of the degree of ST-segment depression to the height of the R wave increases the sensitivity and specificity of the ECG for the recognition of myocardial ischemia.[5] Although similar corrections have not yet been tested during intraoperative monitoring, their possible importance should be kept in mind when intraoperative ECG recordings are examined.

The five-electrode system. The use of five electrodes allows the recording of the six standard limb leads (I, II, III, aV$_R$, aV$_L$, aV$_F$) as well as one precordial unipolar lead. Generally, the unipolar lead is placed in the V$_5$ position, along the anterior axillary line in the fifth intercostal space. With the addition of only two electrodes to the ECG system, up to seven different leads can be monitored simultaneously. Thus, this allows several areas of the myocardium to be monitored for ischemia or establishment of a differential diagnosis between atrial and ventricular arrhythmias.

In 1976, Kaplan and King[6] suggested monitoring lead V$_5$ as the best choice for the detection of intraoperative ischemia. London, et al.[7] demonstrated that, in high-risk patients undergoing non-cardiac surgery, when a single lead was used, the greatest sensitivity was obtained with lead V$_5$ (75%), followed by lead V$_4$ (61%). Combining leads V$_4$ and V$_5$ increased the sensitivity to 90%; whereas the standard combination of leads II and V$_5$ produced a sensitivity of only 80%. They also suggested that if three leads (II, V$_4$ and V$_5$) could be examined simultaneously, the sensitivity would rise to 98%.

Invasive ECG. The electrical potentials of the heart can be measured not only from a surface ECG but also from body cavities adjacent to the heart (esophagus or trachea) or from within the heart itself.

Esophageal ECG. The concept of esophageal electrocardiography is not new, and numerous studies have demonstrated the usefulness of this approach in the diagnosis of complicated arrhythmias. A prominent P wave is usually displayed in the presence of atrial depolarization, and its relationship to the ventricular electrical activity can be examined. The esophageal electrodes are incorporated into an esophageal stethoscope and welded to conventional ECG wires (Fig. 14-4). To record a bipolar esophageal ECG, the electrodes are connected to the right and left arm terminals and lead I is selected on the monitor. In one study of 20 cardiac patients,[8] 100% of atrial arrhythmias were correctly diagnosed with the esophageal lead (intracavitary ECG was used as the standard); lead II led to a correct diagnosis in 54% of the cases; and V$_5$ led to a cor-

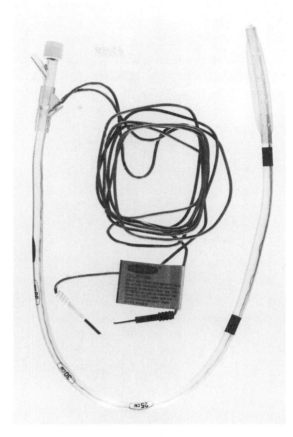

Fig. 14-4. The Cardioesophagoscope. The esophageal leads are made of plastic. The ECG wires are connected to the right arm and left arm leads and lead I is selected on the ECG monitor.

rect diagnosis in 42% of the cases. In addition, the esophageal ECG may be helpful in the detection of posterior wall ischemia due to its proximity to the posterior aspect of the left ventricle. To minimize the risk of esophageal burn injury, an electrocautery protection filter capable of filtering radio frequencies greater than 20 kHz should be inserted between the ECG cable and the esophageal lead.

Intracardiac ECG. For many years, long central venous catheters filled with saline have been used to record the intracardiac ECG. More recently, Chatterjee, et al.[9] have described the use of a modified balloon-tipped flotation catheter for recording intracavitary electrograms. The multipurpose pulmonary artery catheter that is presently available has all the features of a standard pulmonary artery catheter. In addition, three atrial and two ventricular electrodes have been incorporated into the catheter (Fig. 14-5). These electrodes allow the recording of intracavitary ECGs and the establishment of atrial or AV pacing. The diagnostic capabilities of this catheter are great, because atrial, ventricular, or AV nodal arrhythmias and conduction blocks can be demonstrated. The large voltages obtained from the intracardiac electrodes are relatively in-

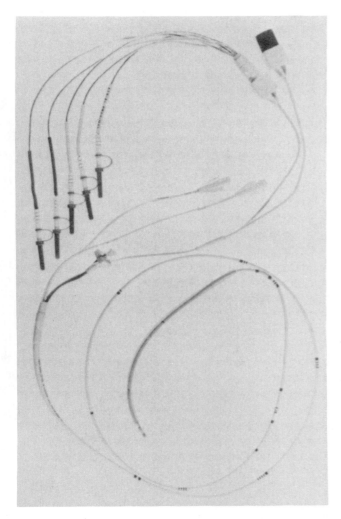

Fig. 14-5. The multipurpose pacing pulmonary artery catheter. Three atrial and two ventricular electrodes can be seen.

sensitive to electrocautery interference and are therefore useful for intraaortic balloon pump triggering.[10] Other pulmonary artery catheters have ventricular and atrial ports that allow passage of pacing wires. These catheters also can be used for diagnostic purposes or for therapeutic interventions (pacing).

Tracheal ECG. The tracheal ECG allows monitoring of the ECG when it is impractical or impossible to monitor the surface ECG. The tracheal ECG consists of a standard tracheal tube in which two electrodes have been embedded (Fig. 14-6). This device may be most useful in pediatric patients for the diagnosis of atrial arrhythmias.[11] The same safety precautions as for esophageal ECG should be followed.

DISPLAY, RECORDING, AND INTERPRETATION

The American Heart Association[12] has published instrumentation and practice standards for electrocardiographic monitoring in special care units. Because many of the principles enunciated in these standards are also applicable

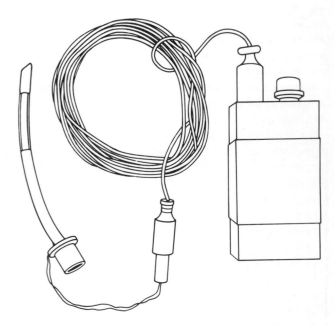

Fig. 14-6. Diagram of tracheal tube ECG system.

to intraoperative monitoring, they are often referred to in this chapter.

Basic requirements

The function of the ECG monitor is to detect, amplify, display, and record the ECG signal. The ECG signal is usually displayed on an oscilloscope, and most monitors now offer nonfade storage oscilloscopes to facilitate wave recognition. All ECG monitors for use in patients with cardiac disease should also have paper recording capabilities. The recorder is needed to make accurate diagnoses of complex arrhythmias, as well as to allow careful analysis of all the ECG waveforms. In addition, the recorder allows differentiation of real ECG changes from oscilloscope artifacts. The American Heart Association Special Report[12] defines a number of requirements that should be met by ECG monitoring equipment. (See Boxes 14-1 to 14-3.)

Oscilloscope displays. Most modern oscilloscopes are high-resolution monochrome or color monitors, similar to those used in computer technology. They frequently allow considerable flexibility in screen configuration, including waveform positions, colors, and sweep speeds. The norm in modern technology is to display two or three ECG channels simultaneously. These usually consist of two limb leads and one unipolar precordial lead. Average heart rates and optional arrhythmia and ST-segment information are displayed in alphanumeric format in addition to the waveforms.

Standard ECG recordings. The ECG is normally recorded on special paper containing a grid of horizontal and vertical lines. Distances between vertical lines represent time intervals, and distances between horizontal lines represent voltages. The lines are 1 mm apart, and every fifth

---

Box 14-1. Performance requirements

1. *Protection from overload:* Protection should be adequate (no damage) for 1 V (peak to peak), 60 Hz, applied for 10 seconds to any electrode connection. The device should recover within 8 seconds after a defibrillation shock of at least 5000 V, with a delivered energy of at least 360 joules.
2. *Isolated patient connection:* The system should include isolated patient connections to meet standards defined in American National Standards for Safe Current Limits for Electromedical Apparatus.[13]
3. *QRS detection:* Monitors should detect QRS complexes with amplitudes of 0.5 to 5.0 mV, slopes of 6 to 300 mV/sec, and durations of 70 to 140 msec for adult use or 40 to 120 msec for pediatric use. The system should not respond to signals with an amplitude of 0.15 mV or less or of a duration of 10 msec or less.
4. *Accuracy of heart rate meter:* The rate meter should be accurate to within the lesser of ±10% or ±5 beats/min over the range of 30 to 200 beats/min for adult use or 30 to 250 beats/min for pediatric use.
5. *Alarm range and accuracy:* Alarm rates should be accurate to within the lesser of ±10% or ±5 beats/min over the range of 30 to 100 beats/min for the lower limit, and 100 to 200 beats/min (adult) or 100 to 250 beats/min (pediatric) for the upper limit. Time to alarm after exceeding rate limits should not exceed 10 seconds.
6. *Noise tolerance:* Heart rate meters should remain accurate during application of a 60-Hz signal, 100 μV peak to peak, minimum. Their accuracy should not be affected when a triangular wave of 4 mV at 0.1 Hz is superimposed on a train of QRS signals of 0.5-mV amplitude and 100-msec duration.

From Mirvis DM, Berson AS, Goldberger AL, et al: Instrumentation and practice standards for electrocardiographic monitoring in special care units, *Circulation* 79:464-471, 1989.

Box 14-2. Performance standards

1. *Input dynamic range:* The device should display, without saturation, differential voltages of ±5 mV at rates up to 320 mV/sec; the output signal's amplitude shall not change more than ±10% over the range of DC offsets of ±300 mV applied to any lead.
2. *Input impedance:* Single-ended input impedance should be 2500 ohms minimum, at 10 Hz.
3. *System noise:* Noise due to all sources, including manufacturer-recommended patient cables should be less than 40 μV peak to peak.
4. *Overall system error:* Input signals with an amplitude limited to ±5 mV and varying at a rate up to 125 mV/sec should be reproduced with an error of less than ±20% or ±100 μV, whichever is greater.
5. *Upper cutoff frequency:* High frequency cutoff should be at least 40 Hz (−3 dB).
6. *Common mode rejection (CMR):* To test CMR, a 60-Hz signal, with a 200-pF source capacitance and a 10-V open circuit voltage, is applied from power ground to all patient electrode connections attached to a common node and with a parallel combination of a 5100-ohm resistor and 47-nF capacitor imbalance impedance in series with each patient lead (including RL, if supplied). Such a signal shall not produce an output signal exceeding 1 mV (peak to peak) with reference to the input over a 60-second period.
7. *Gain selections and accuracy:* Gains of 5 and 10 mm/mV should be provided, with a total allowable gain drift of ±0.66%/min and ±10% in 1 hour.
8. *Pacemaker pulse indication:* Unit shall visually indicate on the output display the presence of a pacemaker pulse of 0.2 mV, minimum, with reference to the input.
9. *Display during other monitoring function:* At least one ECG channel should be displayed continuously at all times, including entry and editing of data and procedures such as thermodilution cardiac output calculations.

From Mirvis DM, Berson AS, Goldberger AL, et al: Instrumentation and practice standards for electrocardiographic monitoring in special care units, *Circulation* 79:464-471, 1989.

---

line is heavier than the others. The speed of the paper is standardized to 25 mm/sec. Therefore on the horizontal axis 1 mm = 0.04 seconds and 0.5 cm = 0.20 seconds. On the vertical axis, 10 mm represents 1 mV. On every recording, a calibration mark of 1 cm = 1 mV indicates that the ECG is appropriately calibrated. The user should follow the manufacturer's recommended calibration procedure for each monitoring episode. Strip chart recorders that are part of an ECG monitoring system should meet all the standards for time-base accuracy, frequency response, linearity, and so forth, proposed for conventional ECG recording systems.[14,15]

Artifacts

Patient. The electrical signal that is generated by the heart and is monitored by the ECG is very weak, amounting to only 0.5 to 2 mV at the skin surface. To avoid signal loss at the interface of skin and electrode, the skin must be prepared properly. Hair should be removed from the electrode sites with scissors and razors. The skin should be cleaned with alcohol and free of all dirt. It is best to abrade the skin lightly to remove part of the stratum corneum, which can be a source of high resistance to the measured voltages. To avoid the problem of muscle artifact, electrodes should be placed over bony prominences whenever possible. Muscle movement, in the form of shivering, can produce significant ECG artifact.

Electrodes and leads. Loose electrodes and broken leads can produce a variety of artifacts that may simulate arrhythmias, Q waves, or inverted T waves. Pregelled, disposable electrodes made of silver metal and silver chloride electrolyte are usually used in the operating room.

Box 14-3. Disclosure requirements

1. Electrosurgery and diathermy protection, including disclosure if electrosurgery overload will cause damage
2. Respiration, leads-off sensing, and active noise-suppression methods, including disclosure of waveform type applied directly to the patient for detection
3. T-wave rejection capability, including disclosure of maximum T-wave amplitude for which heart rate indication is within error limits specified above
4. Heart rate averaging algorithm, including disclosure of type of algorithm used and frequency of display update
5. Heart rate meter accuracy and response to irregular rhythm for specified waveforms, including disclosure of meter time to indicate a change of ±40 beats/min from an initial indication of 80 beats/min
6. Time to alarm for tachycardia of specified waveforms
7. Pacemaker pulse rejection capability for specified pacemaker pulses with and without overshoots/undershoots
8. Service procedures and facilities, including name and location of acceptable repair facilities, recommendations for test methods to verify adequate performance, and frequency of recommended preventive maintenance

---

From Mirvis DM, Berson AS, Goldberger AL, et al: Instrumentation and practice standards for electrocardiographic monitoring in special care units, *Circulation* 79:464-471, 1989.

The technical standards for such electrodes have been published by the Association for the Advancement of Medical Instrumentation.[16] It is important that all the electrodes be moist, uniform, and not out of date. Needle electrodes should be avoided because of the risk of thermal injury. Some ECG monitors have built-in cable testers that enable a lead to be tested when the cable's distal (patient) end is connected to test terminals on the monitor. A high resistance causes a large voltage drop, indicating that the lead is faulty. The main source of artifact from ECG leads is loss of the integrity of the lead insulation. This subsequently leads to pick-up of other electric fields in the operating room, such as the 60-Hz alternating current from lights as well as currents from the electrocautery device. Any damaged ECG lead should be discarded for this reason. Movement of leads can also cause artifact.

Operating room environment. Many pieces of equipment found in the operating room emit electrical fields that can interfere with the ECG. These include the 60-Hz AC power lines for lights, electrosurgical equipment, cardiopulmonary equipment, and defibrillators. Most of this interference can be minimized by proper shielding of the cables and leads of the cardiogram, although to date the interference created by the electrosurgical equipment cannot be reliably filtered without distortion of the ECG. Electrocautery, the most important source of interference on the ECG in the operating room, frequently obliterates the ECG tracing. Analysis of the electrocautery equipment

has identified three component frequencies. Radiofrequency energy between 800 kHz and 2000 kHz accounts for most of the interference. Also contributing to electrocautery interference are the 60-Hz AC energy and the 0.1- to 10-Hz low-frequency noise from intermittent contact of the electrosurgical unit with the patient's tissues. Preamplifiers can be modified to suppress radiofrequency interference, but these filter circuits are still not widely available in the operating room.

Other causes of ECG artifacts in the operating room environment have been reported. Intraoperative monitoring of somatosensory-evoked potentials has been known to simulate pacemaker spikes.[17] These spikes are caused by the incorporation of a pacer enhancement circuit into certain ECG monitors. This problem can be eliminated by disabling the circuit. Recently, artifactual spikes have been noted to coincide with the drip rate in the drip chamber of a warming unit.[18] The spikes were probably related to the generation of static electricity from water droplets. Use of an automated percutaneous lumbar discetomy nucleotome has been reported to simulate supraventricular tachycardia, related to a mechanical interference.[19]

Monitoring system. All ECG monitors use filters to narrow the bandwidth in an attempt to reduce environmental artifacts. The high-frequency filters reduce distortions from muscle movement, 60-Hz electrical current, and electromagnetic interference from other electrical equipment.[20] The low-frequency filters ensure a more stable baseline by reducing respiratory and body movement artifacts as well as those resulting from poor electrode contact. The American Heart Association[12] recommends that a flat frequency response be obtained at a bandwidth of 0.05 to 100 Hz. The high-frequency limit of 100 Hz ensures that tracings are of sufficient fidelity to assess QRS morphology and accurately to evaluate rapid rhythms such as atrial flutter. The low-frequency limit of 0.05 Hz allows accurate representation of slower events such as P-wave and T-wave morphology and ST-segment excursion.

Most modern ECG monitors allow the operator a choice among several bandwidths. The actual filter frequencies tend to vary from manufacturer to manufacturer. One manufacturer (Hewlett-Packard, Andover, Mass.) allows a choice between a "diagnostic mode" with a bandwidth of 0.05 to 130 Hz for adults and 0.5 to 130 Hz for neonates, a "monitoring mode" with a bandwidth 0.5 to 40 Hz for adults and 0.5 to 60 Hz for neonates, and a "filter mode" with a bandwidth of 0.05 to 20 Hz.

The importance of bandwidth selection for the detection of perioperative myocardial ischemia was recently evaluated by Slogoff, et al.[21] They simultaneously used five ECG systems: a Spacelabs* Alpha 14 Model Series 3200 Cardule with bandwidth of 0.05 to 125 Hz and 0.5 to 30 Hz, a Marquette Electronics† MAC II ECG with a band-

*Redmond, Wash.
†Milwaukee, Wis.

width of 0.05 to 40 Hz and one with a bandwidth of 0.05 to 100 Hz, and a Del Mar‡ Holter recorder with a bandwidth of 0.1 to 100 Hz. The ST-segment positions with the three systems that used the lower filter limit (0.05 Hz) recommended by the American Heart Association were similar, whereas with the Spacelabs 0.5 to 30 Hz system they were consistently more negative. The ST-segment displacement on the Holter was consistently less negative and less positive. In at least one automated ST-segment analysis system (Hewlett-Packard, Andover, Mass.) the lower frequency filter (0.05 Hz) is automatically activated when the ST analyzer is turned on.

INDICATIONS
Diagnosis of arrhythmias

Arrhythmias are common during surgery, and their causes are numerous. They are most common during tracheal intubation or extubation and arise more frequently in patients with preexisting cardiac disease. The major contributing factors to the development of perioperative arrhythmias are:

1. *Anesthetic agents*. Halogenated hydrocarbons, such as halothane or enflurane, are known to produce arrhythmias, probably by a reentrant mechanism.[22] Halothane has also been shown to sensitize the myocardium to endogenous and exogenous catecholamines. Drugs that block the reuptake of norepinephrine, such as cocaine and ketamine, can facilitate the development of epinephrine-induced arrhythmias.
2. *Abnormal arterial blood gases or electrolytes*. Hyperventilation is known to reduce serum potassium concentration.[23] If the preoperative potassium is low, it is possible that serum potassium will decrease to the range of 2 mEq/L and thus precipitate severe cardiac arrhythmias.
3. *Tracheal intubation*. This may be the most common cause of arrhythmias during surgery and is often associated with hemodynamic alterations.
4. *Reflexes*. Vagal stimulation may produce sinus bradycardia and allow ventricular escape mechanisms to occur. In vascular surgery, these reflexes may be related to traction on the peritoneum or direct pressure on the vagus nerve during carotid artery surgery. Stimulation of the carotid sinus can also lead to arrhythmias.
5. *Central nervous system stimulation and dysfunction of the autonomic nervous system.*
6. *Preexisting cardiac disease*. Angelini, et al.[24] have shown that patients with known cardiac disease have a much higher incidence of arrhythmias during anesthesia than patients without known disease.

7. *Central venous cannulation*. The insertion of catheters or wires into the central circulation often leads to arrhythmias.

Once an arrhythmia is recognized, it is important to determine whether it produces a hemodynamic disturbance, what type of treatment is required, and how quickly treatment should be instituted. Treatment should be initiated promptly if the arrhythmia leads to marked hemodynamic impairment. Additionally, treatment should be instituted if the arrhythmia is a precursor of a more severe arrhythmia (e.g., frequent multifocal premature ventricular complexes [PVCs] with R-on-T phenomenon can lead to ventricular fibrillation) or if the arrhythmia could be detrimental to the patient's underlying cardiac disease (e.g., tachycardia in a patient with mitral stenosis). The standard limb lead II is preferred for the detection of rhythm disturbances because it usually displays large P waves.

Diagnosis of ischemia

Factors that predispose to the development of perioperative ischemia include perioperative events that affect the myocardial oxygen balance and the presence of preexisting coronary artery disease. A number of perioperative clinical studies[25,26] have found a high incidence of electrocardiographic evidence of ischemia (20% to 80%) in patients with coronary artery disease undergoing surgery, either cardiac or non-cardiac. In the anesthetized patient, the detection of ischemia by ECG becomes even more important because the hallmark symptom of angina is not available.

In recent years, it has also become evident that a significant number of patients suffer from asymptomatic or "silent" ischemia.[27] Silent ischemia is manifested by characteristic ECG signs of myocardial ischemia in the absence of angina and not necessarily associated with changes in hemodynamics or heart rate. Among patients with chronic, stable angina who have ST-segment depression during exercise, ambulatory ECG monitoring during daily life identifies transient ambulant ischemic episodes in approximately 40% to 50% of patients. In these patients, silent ischemic episodes account for about 75% of all ambulant ischemic episodes.[28] The ECG changes that arise during myocardial ischemia are often characteristic and will be detected with careful ECG monitoring. Although the ECG criteria for ischemia were established in patients undergoing exercise stress testing, they can also be applied to anesthetized patients (Box 14-4). These criteria are (1) horizontal or downsloping ST-segment depression of 0.1 mV (Fig. 14-7, *A and C*), (2) slowly upsloping ST-segment depression (Fig. 14-7, *B*) of 0.2 mV (all measured from 60 to 80 msec after the J point), and (3) ST-segment elevation of 0.1 mV in a non–Q-wave lead.[29]

It is commonly believed that monitoring for intraoperative myocardial ischemia is unnecessary in neonates. Whereas ECG lead monitoring for adults is concerned with

---

Box 14-4. ECG criteria for diagnosis of ischemia in anesthetized patients

Upsloping ST segment: 2 mm depression, 80 msec after J point

Horizontal ST segment: > 1 mm depression, 60 to 80 msec after J point

Downsloping ST segment: > 1 mm from top of curve to PQ junction

ST segment elevation

T wave inversion

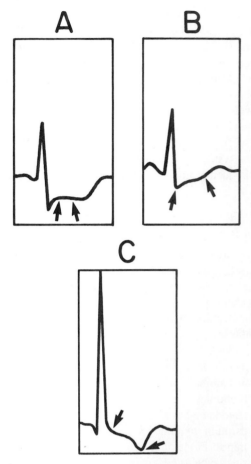

Fig. 14-7. Examples of ST-segment depression are shown between the arrows. **A,** horizontal ST segment; **B,** upsloping ST segment, **C,** downsloping ST segment.

the detection of ischemia as well as arrhythmias, neonatal ECG monitoring has focused on arrhythmia recognition alone. Recent studies, however, suggest that the neonatal heart is more susceptible to ischemia than the adult heart. Bell, et al.[30] have demonstrated the importance of calibrated ECG monitoring in neonates with congenital heart disease.

Although analysis of the ST segment provides sensitive information about myocardial ischemia, it should nonetheless be remembered that in about 10% of patients, underlying electrocardiographic abnormalities hinder the analysis. Some such abnormalities are caused by hypokalemia, administration of digitalis, left bundle branch block, Wolff-Parkinson-White syndrome, and left ventricular hypertrophy with strain. In patients with these problems, other diagnostic modalities, such as transesophageal echocardiography, should be considered.

Diagnosis of conduction defects

Conduction defects can also arise during surgery. They can result from the passage of a pulmonary artery catheter through the right ventricle, or they can be a manifestation of myocardial ischemia. Because high-grade (second- and third-degree AV blocks) conduction defects often have deleterious effects on hemodynamic performance, their intraoperative recognition is important.

AUTOMATED RECORDING

A number of anesthesiologists have used Holter monitoring to document the incidence of perioperative arrhythmias and ischemia. In Holter monitoring, ECG information from one or two bipolar leads is recorded by a miniature magnetic tape recorder. Up to 48 hours of ECG signals can be collected. The tape is processed subsequently by a playback system, and the ECG signals are analyzed. On most modern systems the playback unit includes a dedicated computer for rapid analysis of the data and automatic recognition of arrhythmias. A significant limitation of traditional Holter monitoring in the perioperative period is that recordings are usually analyzed and interpreted retrospectively. A real-time Holter monitor not only records specific ECG segments for later playback but

also analyzes the rhythm and ST segment in real time and alerts the user to acute perturbations.[31] The application of Holter monitoring is, as of yet, primarily limited to the research environment.

The Qmed device* (Fig. 14-8) is a small, continuous ECG recording device that has been used in patients undergoing either cardiac or non-cardiac surgery.[32,33] The device not only records the ECG signals but also performs an automatic analysis of the ECG tracing and sounds an alarm when ischemic changes are recognized. Abnormal events are selectively stored and are subsequently retrievable (Fig. 14-9).

COMPUTER-ASSISTED ELECTROCARDIOGRAM INTERPRETATION

Modern monitoring equipment is highly computerized, and most of the physiologic information is manipulated, analyzed, and stored in digital format. An early step in data collection, therefore, involves the conversion of ana-

---

*Qmed, Inc., Clark, N.J.

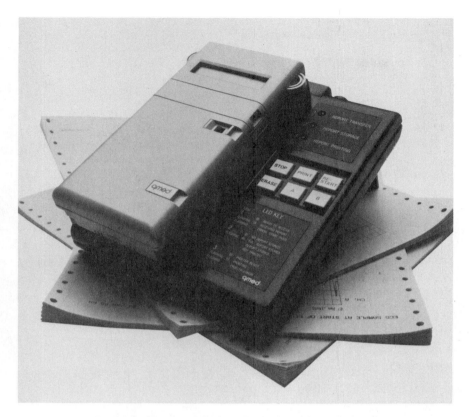

Fig. 14-8. The Qmed device. (From Qmed Inc, Clark, NJ.)

log signals (time-variable voltages or amplitudes) into digital format via an analog-to-digital converter. Once in digital format, the physiologic information can readily be subjected to a variety of analyses. In electrocardiography, the most common analyses, besides rate calculations, are related to the recognition of an arrhythmia and the detection of myocardial ischemia.

Arrhythmias

There is little doubt that during prolonged visual observation of the ECG on the oscilloscope, certain arrhythmias will go undetected. This was clearly demonstrated by Romhilt, et al.,[34] who showed that nurses in coronary care units failed to detect serious ventricular arrhythmias in 84% of their patients. Computers have, therefore, been designed for the automatic detection of arrhythmias in an attempt to increase the detection of abnormal rhythms. Using an early preprocessing algorithm called AZTEC, a computer accurately detected 78% of ventricular ectopic beats. It measured QRS width, offset, amplitude, and area to classify complexes in morphologic families.[35] In a prospective evaluation of such a system,[36] it was found that the computer accurately detected 95.4% of ventricular premature beats but only 82.4% of supraventricular premature beats. Other systems have depended on QRS recognition and cross-correlation with stored QRS complexes.[36] In

cross-correlation, each detected QRS complex is compared with a list of previously detected complexes. If a complex does not correlate ($r \leq 0.9$) with a previously stored complex, it is considered to have a new configuration and is added to the list. A number of points of the complex, such as the PR interval and ST segment, are stored as a template for future comparison. Whenever a new complex matches an existing template, it is averaged into that template so that each template represents a running average of all complexes of a particular configuration.[37] Each template is defined as normal, abnormal, or questionable, according to previously defined criteria. The American Heart Association[12] has published several parameters that need to be tested to permit a meaningful understanding of a system's values and limitations and to allow a reasonable comparison between systems.

Myocardial ischemia

Several computer programs for the on-line detection of ischemia and analysis of ST segments are now available commercially. Each manufacturer uses a different analysis technique, and not all the algorithms are in the public domain.

In one system (Marquette Electronics, Milwaukee, Wis.) an ST learning phase begins by looking at the first 16 beats, in all leads, for the dominant normal or paced

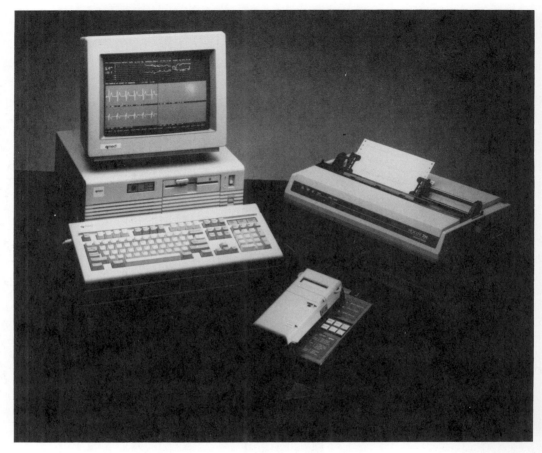

Fig. 14-9. Monitor I, Omni SI system: software for activity and analysis of ECG data in the Qmed. (From Qmed Inc, Clark, NJ.)

shape. The shapes are correlated via a selected number of points on each of the active, valid lead waveforms. An algorithm looks for leads in the fail or artifact mode to determine the number of valid leads used in the analysis. The algorithm also makes all leads positive to enable the sum of the points on the valid leads to be calculated. This sum is used in determining a peak or fiducial point. The fiducial point is used as a point of reference on the QRS complex. A template is formed from selected points around the fiducial point for each ECG lead. As each beat is analyzed, its template is compared to templates of previous beats. If the templates correlate within 75% of a previously stored shape, a match is declared and the template is classified as an existing shape. If there is no match, the template becomes a new shape. On the 17th beat the dominant QRS shape or paced shape is determined. The algorithm then searches for an additional 16 beats that correlate with the dominant template. With the 18th beat a process called incremental averaging is initiated.

Incremental averaging is a method of tracking positive or negative changes occurring on the waveform. These changes are tracked for each of the valid leads. The

changes may be either physiologic, such as ST-segment changes due to ischemia, or related to artifact caused by high-frequency noise. The changes are tracked by allowing an adjustment of only 0.1 mm, either positive or negative, from the prior shape of each beat. Upon the occurrence of the 32nd beat, the products of the incrementally averaged templates become the learned ST templates. Until ST is relearned, all changes in the QRS shape are tracked against this learned template. The isoelectric point and ST points are determined during the learning phase and are based on the width of the QRS shape. The isoelectric point is placed 40 msec before the onset of the QRS, and the ST point is placed 60 msec past the offset of the QRS measurement. The isoelectric point provides the point of reference for determining the measurement of the ST segment.

The technique of incremental averaging is well suited to a continuous input with slow changes. However, it links the speed at which changes occur in the template to the heart rate.[38] This system was recently evaluated intraoperatively in patients undergoing cardiac surgery.[39] The device monitored three selected leads and displayed the absolute values of the ST segment as a line. Upward deflection of the trend line indicated worsening ischemia, whereas a downward trend reflected return of the ST segment toward the isoelectric line. The authors concluded that once the device was clinically accepted, the awareness of ischemic changes increased among the participating anesthesiologists and therapeutic interventions were instituted more rapidly.

Other systems differ from the above in various ways. In the Hewlett-Packard system, a period of 15 seconds is analyzed first and the ST displacement is determined on five "good" beats. These displacements are ranked, and the median value is determined. This eliminates the influence of occasional PVCs and ensures that a representative beat is selected. The objective of this procedure is to obtain a representative beat rather than an average template. The measurement point for the ST segment can be selected as the R wave + 108 msec (default) or the J point + 60 or 80 msec. ST values and representative complexes are stored at a resolution of 1 minute for the most recent 30-minute trend and at a resolution of 5 minutes for the preceding 7.5-hour trend.

In a third system (Spacelabs, Redmond, Wash.) a composite ST segment waveform is developed every 30 seconds and compared to a reference tracing acquired during an initial learning period. The isoelectric and ST-segment points can be manually adjusted to any location on the ECG tracing, or they can be automatically set to predetermined values. To the authors' knowledge, the relative merits and shortcomings of each of these systems have not yet been compared in the clinical setting.

ELECTROCARDIOGRAM MONITORING DURING MAGNETIC RESONANCE IMAGING

Conventional ECG monitoring is not possible during magnetic resonance imaging (MRI) because the lead wires have to traverse magnetic fields, causing distortion of the electrical signal. The need for wires can be eliminated by use of telemetric ECG.[40] Another option consists of the fiberoptic transmission of ECG signals. In addition to ECG signals, capillary blood flow in the earlobe or lip measured by a laser Doppler system can be transmitted using fiberoptics.[41] With either transmission system, ECG artifacts are common with rapid pulse rates from the scanner.

The ECG should be monitored in all patients undergoing regional or general anesthesia. Although it does not provide information on the heart's mechanical function, it will allow the detection of electrical disturbances that can profoundly affect this function. Today, with the judicious use of selected lead combinations, most arrhythmias and ischemic events can be precisely diagnosed intraoperatively. This diagnostic activity is time consuming, however; and there is considerable evidence that many intraoperative ECG changes go undetected. There is little doubt that future technological developments will facilitate the intraoperative recognition of ECG disturbances and lead to better patient outcome.

REFERENCES

1. Thys DM, Kaplan JA, editors: *The ECG in anesthesia and critical care,* New York, 1987, Churchill Livingstone.
2. Skeehan TM, Thys DM: *Monitoring the cardiac surgical patient.* In Hensley FA, Martin DE, editors: *The practice of cardiac anesthesia,* Boston, 1990, Little, Brown.
3. Griffin RM, Kaplan JA: Myocardial ischaemia during noncardiac surgery: a comparison of different lead systems using computerized ST segment analysis, *Anaesthesia* 42:155-159, 1987.
4. Bazaral MG, Norfleet EA: Comparison of CB_5 and V_5 leads for intraoperative electrocardiographic monitoring, *Anesth Analg* 60:849-853, 1981.
5. Hollenberg M, Mateo G, Massie BM, et al: Influence of the R-wave amplitude on exercise-induced ST depression: need for a "gain factor" correction when interpreting a stress electrocardiogram, *Am J Cardiol* 56:13-17, 1985.
6. Kaplan JA, King SB: The precordial electrocardiographic lead (V_5) in patients who have coronary artery disease, *Anesthesiology* 45:570, 1976.
7. London MJ, Hollenberg M, Wong MG, et al: Intraoperative myocardial ischemia: localization by continuous 12 lead electrocardiography, *Anesthesiology* 69:232-241, 1988.
8. Kates RA, Zaidan JR, Kaplan JA: Esophageal lead for intraoperative electrocardiographic monitoring, *Anesth Analg* 61:781, 1982.
9. Chatterjee K, Swan HJC, Ganz W, et al: Use of a balloon-tipped flotation electrode catheter for cardiac monitoring, *Am J Cardiol* 36:56, 1975.
10. Lichtenthal PR: Multipurpose pulmonary artery catheter, *Ann Thorac Surg* 36:493, 1983.
11. Mylrea KC, Calkins JM, Carlson J, et al: ECG lead with the endotracheal tube, *Crit Care Med* 11:199, 1983.
12. Mirvis DM, Berson AS, Goldberger AL, et al: Instrumentation and practice standards for electrocardiographic monitoring in special care units, *Circulation* 79:464-471, 1989.
13. Association for the Advancement of Medical Instrumentation: American national standard for safe current limits for electromedical apparatus (ES-1/1985), Arlington, Va, 1985, ANSI/AAMI.
14. Pipberger HV, Arzbaecher RL, Berson AS, et al: Recommendations for standardization of leads and of specifications for instruments in electrocardiography and vectorcardiography. Report of the Committee on Electrocardiography, American Heart Association, *Circulation* 52:11-31, 1975.
15. Sheffield LT, Berson AS, Bragg-Remschel D, et al: Recommendations for standards of instrumentation and practice in the use of ambulatory electrocardiography. The task force of the Committee on Electrocardiography and Cardiac Electrophysiology of the Council on Clinical Cardiology, *Circulation* 71:626A-636A, 1985.
16. Association for the Advancement of Medical Instrumentation: American national standards for pregelled disposable electrodes, EC12-1983, Arlington, Va, 1984, ANSI/AAMI.
17. Legatt AD, Frost EAM: ECG artifacts during intraoperative evoked potential monitoring, *Anesthesiology* 70:559-560, 1989.
18. Paulsen AW, Pritchard DG: ECG artifact produced by crystalloid administration through blood/fluid warmer sets, *Anesthesiology* 69:803-804, 1988.
19. Lampert BA, Sundstrom FD: ECG artifacts simulating supraventricular tachycardia during automated percutaneous lumbar discectomy, *Anesth Analg* 67:1096-1098, 1988.
20. Arbeit SR, Rubin IL, Gross H: Dangers in interpreting the electrocardiogram from the oscilloscope monitor, *JAMA* 211:453-456, 1970.
21. Slogoff S, Keats AS, David Y, et al: Incidence of perioperative myocardial ischemia detected by different electrocardiographic systems, *Anesthesiology* 73:1074-1081, 1990.
22. Atlee JL, Rusy BF: Ventricular conduction times and AV nodal conductivity during enflurane anesthesia in dogs, *Anesthesiology* 47:498, 1977.

23. Edwards R, Winnie AP, Ramamurthy S: Acute hypocapneic hypokalemia: an iatrogenic anesthetic complication, *Anesth Analg* 56:786-792, 1977.
24. Angelini L, Feldman MI, Lufschonowski R, et al: Cardiac arrhythmias during and after heart surgery: diagnosis and management, *Prog Cardiovasc Dis* 16:469, 1974.
25. Sonntag H, Larsen R, Hilfiker O, et al: Myocardial blood flow and oxygen consumption during high-dose fentanyl anesthesia in patients with coronary artery disease, *Anesthesiology* 56:416-422, 1982.
26. Coriat P, Harari A, Daloz M, et al: Clinical predictors of intraoperative myocardial ischemia in patients with coronary artery disease undergoing non-cardiac surgery, *Acta Anaesthesiol Scand* 26:287, 1982.
27. Coy KM, Imperi GA, Lambert CR, et al: Silent myocardial ischemia during daily activities in asymptomatic men with positive exercise response, *Am J Cardiol* 59:45-49, 1987.
28. Pepine CJ: Is silent ischemia a treatable risk factor in patients with angina pectoris? *Circulation* 82(suppl II):135-142, 1990.
29. Chaitman BR, Hanson JS: Comparative sensitivity and specificity of exercise electrocardiographic lead systems, *Am J Cardiol* 47:1335-1349, 1981.
30. Bell C, Rimar S, Barash P: Intraoperative ST segment changes consistent with myocardial ischemia in the neonate: a report of three cases, *Anesthesiology* 71:601-604, 1989.
31. Dodds TM, Delphin E, Stone JG, et al: Detection of perioperative myocardial ischemia using Holter with real-time ST segment analysis, *Anesth Analg* 67:890-893, 1988.
32. Levin RI, Cohen D, Frisbie W, et al: Potential for real-time processing of the continuously monitored electrocardiogram in the detection, quantitation, and intervention of silent myocardial ischemia, *Cardiol Clin* 4:735-745, 1986.
33. Clements FM, McCann RL, Levin RI: Continuous ST-segment analysis for the detection of perioperative myocardial ischemia, *Crit Care Med* 16:710-711, 1988.
34. Romhilt DW, Bloomfield SS, Chai TC, et al: Unreliability of conventional electrocardiographic monitoring of arrhythmia detection in coronary care units, *Am J Cardiol* 31:457, 1973.
35. Oliver GE, Nolle FM, Wolff GA, et al: Detection of premature ventricular contractions with a clinical system for monitoring electrocardiographic rhythms, *Comput Biomed Res* 4:523, 1971.
36. Shah PM, Arnold JM, Haberen NA, et al: Automatic real-time arrhythmia monitoring in the intensive coronary care unit, *Am J Cardiol* 39:701, 1977.
37. Morganroth J: Ambulatory Holter electrocardiography: choice of technique and clinical uses, *Ann Intern Med* 102:73, 1985.
38. London MJ: *Monitoring for myocardial ischemia.* In Kaplan JA, editor: *Vascular anesthesia,* New York, 1991, Churchill Livingstone.
39. Kotter GS, Kotrly KJ, Kalbfleisch JH, et al: Myocardial ischemia during cardiovascular surgery as detected by an ST segment trend monitoring system, *J Cardiothorac and Vascular Anesth* 1:190-199, 1987.
40. Roth JL, Nugent M, Gray JE, et al: Patient monitoring during magnetic resonance imaging, *Anesthesiology* 62:80-83, 1985.
41. Higgins CB, Lanzer P, Stark D, et al: Imaging by nuclear magnetic resonance in patients with chronic ischemic heart disease, *Circulation* 69:523-531, 1984.

Chapter 15

NEUROMUSCULAR BLOCK MONITORING

Sorin J. Brull, M.D.
David G. Silverman, M.D.

In the 50 years since the introduction of curare into clinical anesthesia by Griffith and Johnson,[1] muscle relaxants have emerged as agents that are vital to the care and well-being of many patients undergoing anesthesia and surgery. However, there is still uncertainty as to the best means to administer muscle relaxants and monitor their effects. Patients vary widely in their response to relaxants,[2,3] necessitating careful titration of these agents for induction and maintenance of block and careful assessment of recov-

ery. As a result of this wide variability among patients, residual curarization has been documented following a variety of relaxant regimens,[4-9] despite the intraoperative use of nerve stimulators.[7,8,10]

NEUROMUSCULAR PHYSIOLOGY
Nerve conduction

The motor neuron is a single nerve cell whose body is located in the ventral horn of the spinal cord. From there, its axon extends to the muscle fibers that it innervates. When the membrane potential of the motor nerve is elevated to above threshold, an "all-or-none" action potential is generated and translated to each muscle fiber by means of a neuromuscular junction. The number of muscle fibers that are innervated by a single motor neuron (i.e., the innervation ratio of the motor unit) determines the functional intricacy of the particular muscle. For example, where fine movements are required, such as with the extraocular or digital muscles, the same neuron innervates only a few muscle fibers (low innervation ratio). This allows for very fine control of a single muscle group whose function is modulated by many neurons. In contrast, large muscle groups that do not require fine movement, such as the postural muscles of the back, have hundreds of muscle fibers innervated by only one neuron (high innervation ratio).[11,12]

Neuromuscular junction

The neuromuscular junction (NMJ) consists of the presynaptic region of the motor neuron, the motor end plate, and the intervening cleft (Fig. 15-1). The region is en-

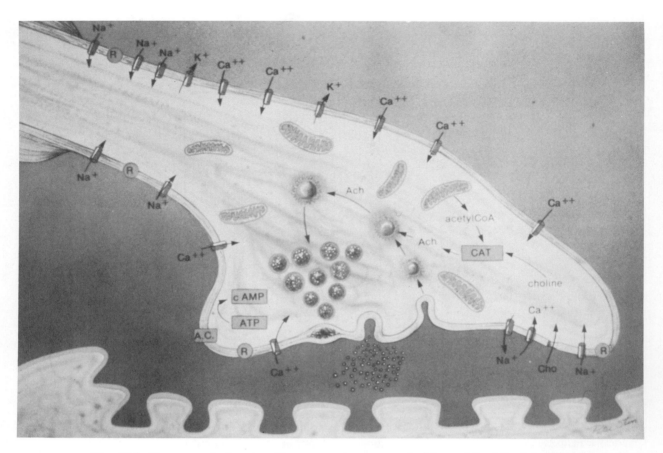

Fig. 15-1. Neuromuscular junction. The presynaptic nerve terminal is specialized for the synthesis, mobilization, and release of acetylcholine *(ACh)*. Its surface is lined with cation channels and cholinoceptors *(R)*. ACh is released into the cleft and binds at the postsynaptic end plate. (Sketch courtesy of Dr. Frank G. Standaert.)

closed by Schwann cells, which separate it from the surrounding tissues and extracellular fluid.[13] The presynaptic terminal is an unmyelinated portion of the axon that is designed for the synthesis of acetylcholine (ACh), its storage in specialized vesicles, and its release into the synaptic cleft. The membrane is folded into many closely interposed longitudinal gutters, which increase its surface area.[14] Each vesicle stored in the terminal contains a quantum of ACh that is capable of generating a miniature endplate potential (MEPP). Quanta are released continuously into the synaptic cleft by exocytosis. Excitation of the motor nerve (i.e., firing of the motor nerve) causes the synchronized release of multiple quanta, the effects of which sum at the end plate to generate a muscle action potential.

The postsynaptic membrane, much like the presynaptic membrane, is folded to increase its surface area. The postsynaptic end plate contains approximately 5 million receptor channels,[15] each of which consists of 5 subunits (2 alpha, 1 beta, 1 delta, and 1 epsilon) arranged in a rosette (Fig. 15-2). The recognition site of each of the two alpha subunits must be occupied by ACh or by an exogenous depolarizing agent for all-or-none opening of a given channel to occur. Each open channel then allows the entry of Na^+

and Ca^{++} into the cell, and the exit of K^+. The end-plate membrane serves as a resistor in such a way that the ion flux generates an end-plate potential (EPP). Individual EPPs may accumulate and thus sum to reach threshold. When approximately 250,000 to 500,000 channels (5% to 10%) of a given NMJ are open, the EPP typically reaches the threshold required to elicit a muscle action potential (MAP).[16] This usually occurs in response to a synchronized release of quanta from the nerve terminal. The end-plate response is short-lived because levels of ACh within the cleft are modulated by acetylcholinesterases arising from the postsynaptic membrane.

Beyond the end plate, a perijunctional rim of sodium channels (each containing two "gates") is responsible for propagation of the MAP.[17] In the resting state, the lower time-dependent gate is open and the voltage-dependent upper gate is closed.[16,18] Depolarization of the end plate opens the upper gate and permits all-or-none propagation of the MAP. The lower gate closes soon after the upper gate opens, thereby terminating the MAP. It remains closed until the upper gate closes and the cell resumes its resting state.

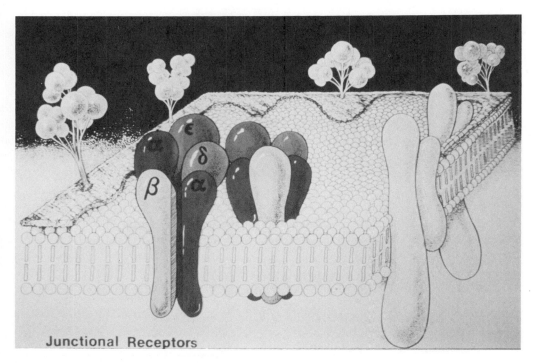

Fig. 15-2. Schematic of the postjunctional membrane. The two structures in the center represent receptors. Each member of the pair is made of five subunits (2α, 1β, 1δ, 1ϵ) arranged in a circle around a channel. The structure at the right represents Na-K-ATPase, another molecule that crosses from one side of the membrane to the other. The balloon-like structures at the periphery represent acetycholinesterase. (From Standaert FG: *Neuromuscular physiology*. In Miller RD, editor: *Anesthesia,* ed 3, New York, 1990 Churchill Livingstone.)

Muscle action potential and contraction

Once activated, the perijunctional rim of Na^+ channels initiates the MAP. This allows entry of Ca^{++} and its release from the sarcoplasmic reticulum. As the intracellular concentration of Ca^{++} increases, it opposes troponin inhibition of contraction and the muscle fibers contract through generation of actin-myosin bridges. Then rapid extrusion and reuptake of Ca^{++} return the muscle to its resting tension.

NEUROMUSCULAR BLOCK

Both nondepolarizing and depolarizing relaxants cause flaccid paralysis. The characteristic patterns of these types of block are illustrated in Fig. 15-3. Nondepolarizing agents compete with ACh by competitively binding to the alpha subunits of the receptor. They have a high affinity for the receptor but exhibit no appreciable agonist activity. Postsynaptic binding prevents the receptor channel from opening. Presynaptic binding may oppose the mobilization and release of ACh.[19,20]

Depolarizing agents bind with high activity to junctional receptors. In contrast to acetylcholine, neither succinylcholine nor decamethonium is hydrolyzed by acetylcholinesterases in the NMJ. Thus these agents increase the relative time during which the channels are open and hence cause prolonged end-plate depolarization. Initially, they cause generation of an MAP (which may be manifested by fasciculations); however, during persistent endplate depolarization, the lower Na^+ gate closes and prevents further ion exchange. A muscle action potential no longer can be propagated, and flaccid paralysis ensues.

In addition to the classic nondepolarizing and depolarizing forms of block, such phenomena as channel block and desensitization can inactivate the NMJ. Channel block entails direct occlusion of the receptor channel. Open-channel (use-dependent or voltage-dependent) block involves occlusion of an otherwise open receptor channel, typically by a charged molecule. Closed-channel block involves occlusion independent of channel opening. Desensitization occurs when the receptor and its channel are not responsive to the presence of agonists on both alpha subunits. This typically entails a reversible conformational change of variable duration[21,22] as a result of persistent binding of depolarizing agents to the receptor.[23,24] This persistent binding may change the typical (phase 1) block of a depolarizing relaxant to one that assumes the characteristics of a nondepolarizing block (phase 2). Long-term effects also may be a consequence of inactivation of cellular mechanisms by long, thin molecules, such as decamethonium, which may enter the cytoplasm through the open receptor channels. Barbiturates, potent volatile anesthetics, receptor agonists, cholinesterase inhibitors, local anesthetics, phenothiazines, calcium channel blockers, antibiotics, al-

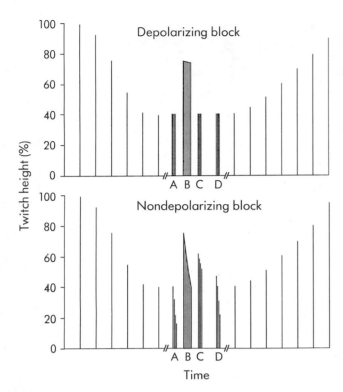

Fig. 15-3. Patterns of block. During depolarizing block, there is a progressive decrease of single-twitch height but no fade in response to rapid stimulation [train-of-four (A) or tetanus (B)], and there is no posttetanic facilitation of neuromuscular transmission (C and D). During nondepolarizing block, in addition to decline in single-twitch height, there is fade in response to train-of-four (A) and tetanus (B); and there is facilitation of subsequent (posttetanic) neuromuscular transmission (C and D).

---

cohol, naltrexone, and naloxone all may cause conformational changes of the receptor and/or occlude the channel.[16]

ESSENTIALS OF NEUROSTIMULATION

In the clinical setting, neurostimulation typically is delivered by a 9-V, adjustable-current stimulator via subcutaneous needles or surface electrodes (Box 15-1). The stimulus should be monophasic (i.e., square wave) because biphasic waves may produce repetitive stimulation. The other critical components of a stimulus are its pulse duration (in milliseconds) and intensity (in milliamperes) (Figs. 15-4 to 15-6).[25] Pulse duration must be less than 0.5 msec so as not to induce repetitive neural firing or direct muscle stimulation. The intensity of the stimulus should be sufficient to depolarize nerve fibers at the given pulse duration.[25]

When the effect of neuromuscular blocking agents on single-twitch responses is assessed over a period of time, the same number of nerve fibers must be stimulated. For this reason, anesthesiologists traditionally have relied on supramaximal current (i.e., a current 10% to 20% above

---

Box 15-1. Desirable features of a nerve stimulator

Essential

• Square-wave impulse, <0.5 msec duration
• Ability to maintain selected current for duration of impulse (i.e., constant current, variable voltage)
• Battery power
• Multiple patterns of stimulation: single twitch, train-of-four, double-burst, tetanus, posttetanic count

Optional

• Rheostat for adjustable current output
• Polarity output indicator
• Ability to calculate and display fade ratio and/or percent depression of single-twitch amplitude from control value
• High-output (up to 80 to 100 mA) and low-output (<5 mA) sockets
• Audible signal with each stimulus delivered
• Alarm for excessive impedance, lead disconnect, low battery
• Battery charge indicator

---

the current needed to stimulate all fibers in the nerve bundle). Use of a supramaximal current allows current to vary slightly over time without affecting the total number of nerve fibers stimulated. This is readily achieved with needle electrodes, typically at less than 10 mA. However, surface electrodes may fail to stimulate all fibers, especially when they are not in close proximity to the nerve (i.e., due to improper placement, or in obese patients), even at currents of 50 to 70 mA.

The current output of a stimulator must remain constant over time. However, as illustrated in Fig. 15-7, this, too, is not always the case. Although a constant current can be delivered most effectively with needle electrodes, their insertion into the skin may be painful to the awake patient. Therefore, surface electrodes are used most commonly in the clinical setting.[26] Skin resistance typically is decreased by use of an electrolyte solution (e.g., silver/silver chloride); several minutes are required to allow for this to attain optimal effectiveness. The time for this electrode "curing" may be accelerated by cleansing and degreasing the skin (e.g., with alcohol or acetone) and by abrading the skin with a preparation such as Omni Prep* (Fig. 15-8).

Although rare, complications associated with the use of nerve stimulators can arise. Needle electrodes may be a source of local irritation, infection, and nerve damage due to intraneural placement.[27,28] Needle electrodes are also more likely to be associated with local tissue burns from electrosurgical units because they provide good contact (with minimal resistance) for exit of high-frequency current over a small area of skin.

---

*D.O. Weaver & Co., Aurora, Colo.

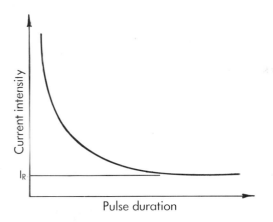

Fig. 15-4. Relationship between pulse duration and stimulating current. The magnitude of the stimulus *(curve)* required to initiate a nerve action potential is a function of the pulse duration and stimulating current. The rheobase current, I_R, is that stimulating current required to reach threshold at the longest pulse duration. The current intensity required to achieve nerve firing increases exponentially as the pulse duration decreases.

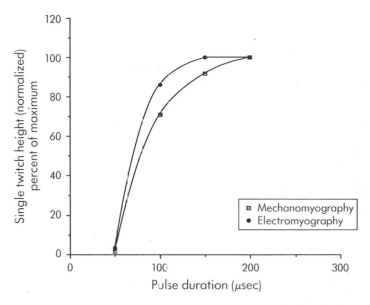

Fig. 15-5. Effect of pulse duration on the amplitude of the evoked response, as measured by electromyographic and mechanomyographic single-twitch heights, at a fixed stimulating current in a healthy volunteer. Little change is noted with pulse widths greater than 150 µsec.

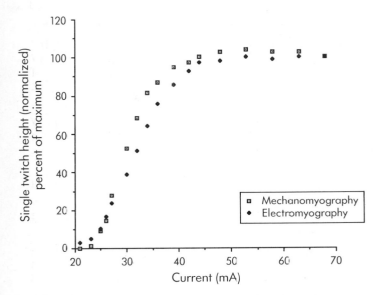

Fig. 15-6. Effect of stimulating current on the amplitude of the evoked response, as measured by electromyographic and mechanomyographic single-twitch heights, at a fixed pulse duration in a healthy volunteer. Little change is noted with currents greater than 35 mA.

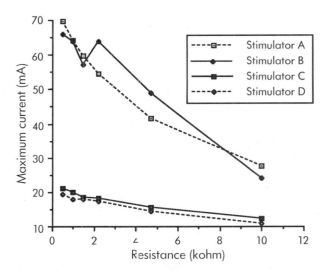

Fig. 15-7. Ability of four nerve stimulators (obtained from different manufacturers) to generate a constant current despite variations in resistance (in vitro). Note that two of the four tested stimulators were unable to deliver a supramaximal stimulus (typically >50 mA) even at the lowest resistance. The two stimulators capable of delivering a supramaximal current typically lost this ability at an external resistance greater than 3000 ohms.

Effect of stimulus frequency

In the setting of normal (unblocked) neuromuscular transmission, increasing the rate of stimulation from single stimuli at 0.1 Hz (one every 10 seconds) to brief tetanic stimulation at 50 to 100 Hz leads to repetitive muscle contractions without fade. At supraphysiologic rates of stimulation (e.g., above 70 to 200 Hz),[29,30] even normal neuromuscular transmission may fatigue. When a nondepolarizing block is present, such fatigue is noted at slower rates of neurostimulation. This constitutes the basis for assessments of response to tetanic (at 50 Hz) and train-of-four (at 2 Hz) stimulation.[31,32]

The rate of neurostimulation has pronounced effects on assessments of depth of block. In addition to promoting fatigue, frequent stimulation also leads to as much as a fivefold to sixfold increase in local blood flow. This may re-

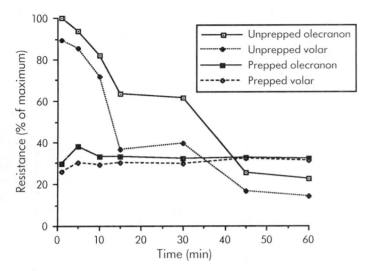

Fig. 15-8. Effect of cleansing and abrading the skin (with Omni Prep) on skin resistance. Without prior prepping, resistance at surface electrodes remains elevated over the olecranon groove and volar forearm for 10 to 30 minutes after electrode application.

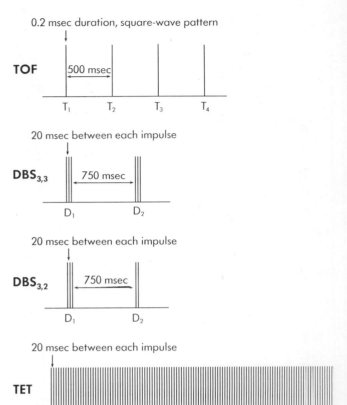

Fig. 15-9. Comparison of stimulating patterns for train-of-four, $DBS_{3,3}$, $DBS_{3,2}$, and tetanus at 50 Hz. The impulses comprising single-twitch, the four twitches of train-of-four, the two minitetanic bursts of double-burst stimulation, and the 5 seconds of tetanus are identical with respect to duration (e.g., 0.2 msec) and pattern (e.g., square-wave).

sult in more rapid delivery of relaxant to the stimulated muscle,[33,34] especially if neurostimulation is initiated prior to the administration of relaxant.[35] Ali and Savarese[36] reported that the apparent dose requirements for curare at the adductor pollicis muscle decreased by a factor of 3 as the stimulus frequency increased from 0.1 Hz to 1.0 Hz. Of perhaps even greater clinical significance is the effect of stimulus frequency on the apparent onset of block. Increasing the stimulus frequency results in a greater degree of neuromuscular depression at the site of stimulation for both depolarizing[35,37] and nondepolarizing block.[35,36,38,39]

PATTERNS OF STIMULATION

Currently, several patterns of stimulation are used to assess the degree of neuromuscular block. These include single stimuli, tetanic stimulation, train-of-four, and double-burst stimulation (Fig. 15-9). The newer nerve stimulators are capable of functioning in any of these modes, as well as in a posttetanic count mode (Fig. 15-10).

Single stimuli

The single-stimulus method consists of assessing the response to either an individual stimulus or serial stimuli, usually at frequencies between 0.1 Hz (1 stimulus every 10 seconds) and 1.0 Hz (1 stimulus per second). This is the least precise method of assessing partial neuromuscular block under clinical conditions, and it requires measurement of a baseline (no block) single-twitch amplitude for comparison with subsequent responses. In addition, the clinically useful range of block is limited because the re-

sponse to a single stimulus is not reduced until at least 75% to 80% of the receptors are occupied by relaxant, and the response disappears completely once 90% to 95% of the receptors are occupied.[40] Furthermore, single-twitch monitoring is highly sensitive to variations in stimulating current, temperature, and preload (i.e., resting muscle tension). As noted previously, it is imperative that the stimulating current remain constant over time in order to ensure that the same number of nerve fibers reach threshold with each stimulation. By applying a current that is 10% to 20% above that required to fire all fibers of the motor nerve (i.e., supramaximal), the impact of variables such as temperature, skin resistance, and changes in electrode conductance can be minimized. However, a supramaximal stimulus may not always be delivered when surface electrodes are used.

Tetanic stimulation

Tetanic stimulation consists of repetitive high-frequency (30 Hz or more) neurostimulation. This results in repetitive muscle action potentials and persistent muscular con-

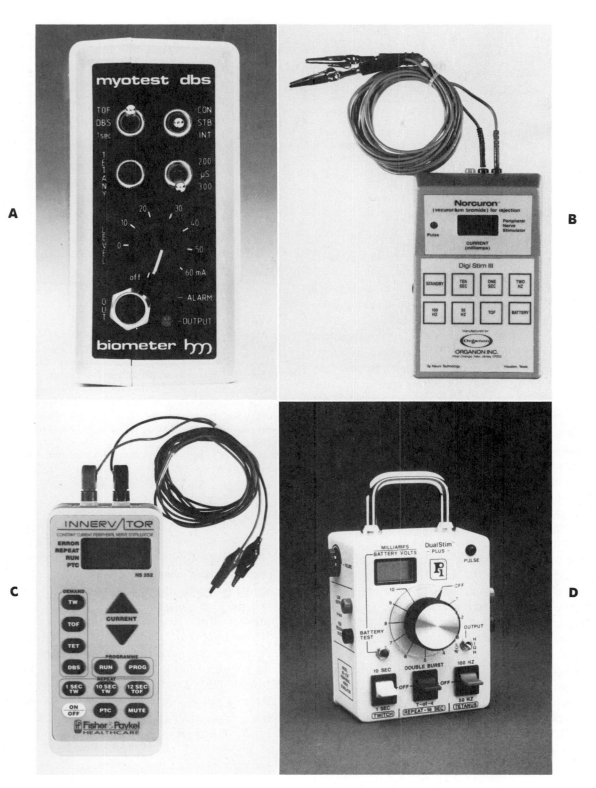

Fig. 15-10. Examples of newer model nerve stimulators. These devices typically are capable of delivering train-of-four, double burst, single-twitch, or tetanus at predetermined intervals or upon repeated triggering. The pulse duration may be set to 0.2 or 0.3 msec; stimulating current may be varied between 0 and 60 mA. **A,** Myotest DBS (Biometer, Copenhagen); **B,** Digi Stim III (Neuro Technology, Houston); **C,** Innervator (Fisher & Paykel, Auckland, New Zealand); **D,** DualStim Plus (Professional Instruments, Houston).

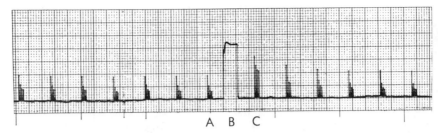

Fig. 15-11. Effect of tetanic stimulation (for 5 seconds at 50 Hz) on train-of-four monitoring at 12-second intervals during a vecuronium infusion. *(A)*, Baseline train-of-four ratio is 0.33. Following tetanus, *(B)*, T_4 is amplified to a greater degree than T_1; hence the T_4/T_1 ratio is increased transiently to as high as 0.70 *(C)*.

traction. In the unblocked NMJ, each contraction can be sustained for several seconds at frequencies as high as 70 to 100 Hz.[29] In clinical practice, a 5-second, 50-Hz tetanic stimulus is used most often because the evoked muscle tension approximates the tension developed during maximal voluntary effort.[29]

Although normal muscle responds to tetanic stimulation with summed contractions that overcome elastic forces and produce an augmented response, the tetanic response fades (i.e., fatigues) in the context of a nondepolarizing block (Fig. 15-3).[41,42] Tetanic fade most likely represents a presynaptic inability to mobilize ACh rapidly enough to maintain depolarization, despite repetitive nerve firing. It may be attributable to competition by nondepolarizing agents at presynaptic cholinergic receptors involved with Ca^{++} flux and ACh mobilization.[16] The consequences of the diminished release of ACh are magnified by binding of the nondepolarizing agent to the postsynaptic receptors, thereby decreasing the margin of safety. There also is evidence that fade in response to tetanic stimulation may occur during the use of potent inhaled anesthetics in the absence of nondepolarizing block.[30,43,44]

Another effect of a tetanic stimulus is the potential alteration of subsequent evoked neuromuscular responses. In the presence of a nondepolarizing muscle relaxant (or phase 2 block with a depolarizing relaxant), stimulation after a tetanus may result in posttetanic facilitation or potentiation. The magnitude of posttetanic effects on evoked twitch height is a function of depth of block.[45] Testing of neuromuscular function during this period can lead to overestimation of evoked responses (i.e., underestimation of depth of block) (Fig. 15-11). One theory to explain posttetanic facilitation is that the intense tetanic stimulus induces an increase in the mobilization and subsequent release of ACh quanta, which results in an increase in subsequent end-plate potentials.[46] Another theory has suggested that tetanus may have relatively long-term effects on the NMJ by "displacing" relaxant from the post-synaptic receptor.[47] In either case, posttetanic stimulation during nondepolarizing block leads to generation of a greater end-plate potential than obtained prior to tetanus.

Table 15-1. Minutes until detectable twitch response

Posttetanic counts*	Atracurium	Pancuronium
2	7	30
4	4	20
6	2	10
8	0-2	5

Data from Viby-Mogensen J, Howardy-Hansen P, Chraemmer-Jorgensen B, et al: Posttetanic count (PTC): a new method of evaluating an intense nondepolarizing neuromuscular blockade, *Anesthesiology* 55:458-461, 1981; and Bonsu AK, Viby-Mogensen J, Fernando PUE, et al: Relationship of post-tetanic count and train-of-four response during intense neuromuscular blockade caused by atracurium, *Br J Anaesth* 59:1089-1092, 1987.
*Number of responses to single-twitch stimuli at 1 Hz following 50-Hz tetanus for 5 seconds.

Posttetanic count

When the use of nondepolarizing blockers results in 100% twitch height depression, the potentiation that occurs following tetanic stimulation may enable detection of the response to single stimuli.[48,49] The number of twitches (the posttetanic count, PTC) elicited by serial stimulation at 1 Hz (beginning 3 seconds after a 5-second, 50-Hz tetanus) is inversely related to the depth of block: the greater the number of posttetanic responses, the less is the degree of block and the more rapid is the ensuing recovery (Table 15-1). This method of assessment also may be indicated if one wishes to ensure profound paralysis (i.e., ablation of PTC as well as response to twitch and tetanus). It also provides an indication as to when recovery of single twitch may be anticipated and thus provides a guide for planning reversal with anticholinesterases.

Train-of-four stimulation

Train-of-four (TOF) stimulation consists of four repetitive stimuli at a frequency of 2 Hz. As noted above, even this relatively slow rate of stimulation is associated with fade in the context of nondepolarizing block.

TOF is the most commonly employed method of neuromuscular assessment in clinical practice. It is far less painful to awake patients than tetanus and is not associated with prolonged posttetanic effects. In some cases, it may be more sensitive than tetanus to the presence of residual block.[31] In the context of nondepolarizing block, both TOF and tetanus result in fatigue, which is manifested by fade. However, in contrast to tetanus, TOF does not increase or facilitate neuromuscular responses during and after its application.[31,32,50]

Unlike single twitch, TOF does not require a prerelaxant baseline for comparison. It assesses the relationship among successive responses, thus serving as its own control. The relationship between the height of the fourth twitch (T_4) and that of the first twitch (T_1) is expressed as the T_4/T_1, or fade, ratio. In the absence of nondepolarizing block, the T_4/T_1 ratio is approximately 1.0. In the context of nondepolarizing block, declines in this ratio depend on such factors as the relaxant employed and whether monitoring is performed during onset or recovery. Typically at 70% to 75% receptor occupancy, T_4 starts to decrease selectively. At a T_4/T_1 ratio as low as 0.70, T_1 may still be close to its baseline height. When T_4 is no longer detectable either visually or mechanographically, T_1 is approximately 25% of its baseline height. This corresponds to a block of approximately 80% of the receptors. The third twitch (T_3) is lost when approximately 85% of receptors are blocked; the second twitch (T_2) is lost when approximately 85% to 90% of receptors are blocked.[51] During the remaining single-twitch monitoring, the height of T_1 progressively decreases, and T_1 is lost when 90% to 95% of receptors are blocked (Table 15-2).[40, 51]

Also in contrast to single-twitch monitoring, TOF may allow detection of a phase 2 block in response to a depolarizing agent. Normally, a depolarizing muscle relaxant causes a progressive decrease in the height of the single twitch or a symmetrical decrease in the height of all phases of the TOF or tetanus. Because there is no fade, the T_4/T_1 ratio is maintained near 1.0 until all twitches disappear. However, when a phase 2 block occurs, the depolarizing relaxant takes on features of a competitive (nondepolarizing) relaxant and fade develops in response to TOF or tetanic stimulation. This cannot be assessed by single-twitch monitoring.

Recently, another advantage of TOF has been noted. The T_4/T_1 ratio is consistent at submaximal as well as at supramaximal stimulating current intensities, so long as T_1 and T_4 responses are detectable[52,53] (Fig. 15-12, Table 15-3), especially at ≥10 mA above the T_4 threshold.[53]

Table 15-2. Approximate relationships among percent receptor block, single-twitch, and train-of-four during nondepolarizing block

Total receptors blocked (% of)	Twitch (T_1) (% normal)	T_4 (% normal)	T_4/T_1
100	0	0	—
90-95	0	0	T_1 lost
85-90	10	0	T_2 lost
	20	0	T_3 lost
80-85	25	0	T_4 lost
	80-90	48-58	0.60-0.70
	95	69-79	0.70-0.75
75	100	75-100	0.75-1.0
	100	100	0.9-1.0
50	100	100	1.0
25	100	100	1.0

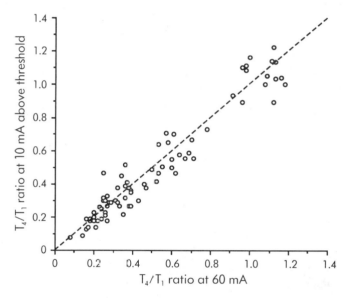

Fig. 15-12. Comparison of T_4/T_1 ratios at 10 mA above the T_4 threshold with those at 60 mA in patients undergoing general anesthesia and receiving a vecuronium infusion. The constancy of fade at these two currents was evidenced by their close correlation, $r = 0.94$. (From Silverman DG, Connelly NR, O'Connor TZ, et al: Accelerographic train-of-four at near-threshold currents, *Anesthesiology* 76:34-38, 1992.

Table 15-3. T_4/T_1 ratios at 20, 30, and 50 mA stimulating currents

Classification at 50 mA	20 mA	30 mA	50 mA
≤ 0.70 ($n = 28$)	0.500 ± 0.182	0.506 ± 0.169	0.513 ± 0.157
> 0.70, <0.95 ($n = 25$)	0.915 ± 0.104	0.916 ± 0.079	0.894 ± 0.067
≥ 0.95 ($n = 30$)	0.972 ± 0.060	0.972 ± 0.035	0.995 ± 0.022

From Brull SJ, Ehrenwerth J, Silverman DG: Stimulation with submaximal current for train-of-four monitoring, *Anesthesiology* 72:629-632, 1990.

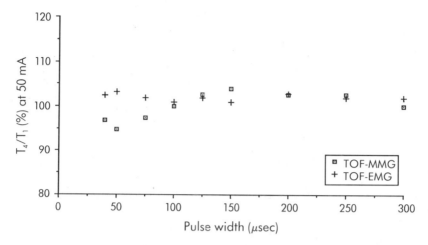

Fig. 15-13. Constancy of TOF ratio (EMG and MMG) at pulse widths ranging from 40 to 300 μsec in a healthy volunteer, in the absence of neuromuscular block.

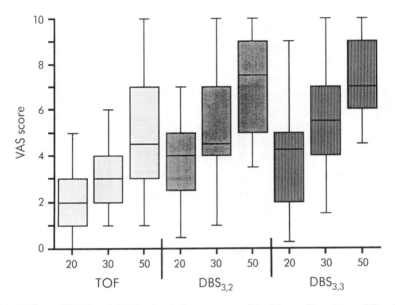

Fig. 15-14. Effect of TOF and DBS stimulating currents (20, 30, or 50 mA) on Visual Analog Scale (VAS) pain scores in unmedicated volunteers. *Shaded areas,* 25th to 75th percentiles; *horizontal lines within shaded areas,* medians; *extended bars,* 0 to 100th percentiles. (From Connelly NR, Silverman DG, O'Connor TZ, et al: Subjective responses to train-of-four and double-burst stimulation in awake patients, *Anesth Analg* 70:650-653, 1990.

Likewise, there is evidence that the ratio of the evoked responses is independent of stimulus duration (so long as the pulse width is <0.5 msec) (Fig. 15-13). The constancy of the T_4/T_1 ratio at varying current intensities and at varying stimulus durations facilitates testing of awake patients, because discomfort is directly related to the intensity of the stimulating current[54] (Fig. 15-14).

Double-burst stimulation

Double-burst stimulation (DBS) has been introduced as an alternative means of assessing neuromuscular block.[55-57] Although several different combinations of stimuli have been assessed, two patterns are used most commonly. $DBS_{3,3}$ consists of a minitetanic burst of three 0.2-msec impulses at a frequency of 50 Hz, followed 750 msec later by an identical burst. $DBS_{3,2}$ consists of a burst of three impulses at 50 Hz followed by a burst of two such impulses (Fig. 15-9). This pattern leads to responses of greater magnitude than those elicited by TOF (Fig. 15-15). DBS and TOF maintain a close relationship over a wide range in level of block (Fig. 15-16).[56-58]

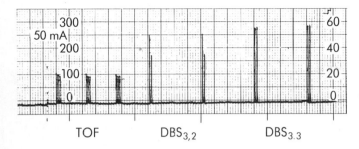

Fig. 15-15. Evoked responses of TOF (every 12 seconds), $DBS_{3,2}$, and $DBS_{3,3}$ (every 20 seconds) in an unmedicated volunteer. Although the magnitude of the individual responses is greater for DBS, the T_4/T_1 ratio of TOF and the D_2/D_1 ratio of $DBS_{3,3}$ are virtually equivalent; the D_2/D_1 ratio of $DBS_{3,2}$ is lower as a result of its second burst being of shorter duration than its first burst.

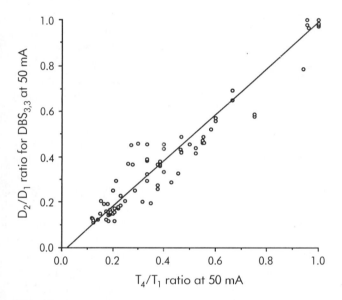

Fig. 15-16. Correlation of $DBS_{3,3}$ and TOF in response to 50-mA stimulation ($r = 0.98$). *Straight line,* line of best fit. Similar constancy was evidenced when TOF and $DBS_{3,2}$ were compared. Reproduced with permission from Brull SJ, Connelly NR, Silverman DG: Correlation of train-of-four and double burst stimulation ratios at varying amperages, *Anesth Analg* 71: 489-492, 1990.

SITES OF STIMULATION AND ASSESSMENT
Muscles of the extremities

Anesthesiologists most commonly monitor the response to ulnar nerve stimulation at the adductor pollicis muscle, even though this does not necessarily indicate the degree of block of either the diaphragm or the airway musculature. For ulnar nerve stimulation, one electrode is placed 1 cm proximal to the wrist on the radial side of the flexor carpi ulnaris, and the other is placed proximally either on the volar forearm or over the olecranon groove. Maximal effectiveness is obtained when the negative (depolarizing) electrode is placed distally over the nerve.[59,60]

Table 15-4. Measurable action potentials of four hand muscles in response to median and ulnar nerve stimulation

Muscle	Median nerve	Ulnar nerve
Adductor pollicis	79	73
Abductor pollicis brevis	93	54
First dorsal interosseous	54	91
Abductor digiti quinti	18	97

Data, obtained simultaneously on a four-channel EMG, identify the high degree of dual innervation of hand muscles. The adductor pollicis, the muscle monitored most commonly, has a high likelihood of dual innervation: it demonstrated a measurable action potential 79% of the time after median nerve stimulation and 73% of the time after ulnar nerve stimulation. (From Halevy J, Brull SJ, Booke J, et al: Dual innervation of hand muscles: potential influence on monitoring of neuromuscular blockade. *Anesthesiology* 75:3A:A814, 1991.)

The ulnar nerve primarily innervates the adductor pollicis, abductor digiti quinti and first dorsal interosseus muscles. Anesthesiologists typically monitor the force of contraction of the adductor pollicis muscle by visual or tactile means or by mechanographic force translation. Because this muscle is on the side of the arm opposite to the site of stimulation, there is little likelihood of direct muscle stimulation, which would falsely suggest incomplete block. Alternatively, the first dorsal interosseus and abductor digiti quinti muscles may be preferable for electromyography.[61-63] These muscles are less likely to receive dual innervation (by median as well as ulnar nerves), and the morphology of their electromyographic response is identified more readily (Table 15-4).[63] However, it should be noted that the abductor digiti quinti (minimi) muscle may be slightly more resistant to block than is the adductor pollicis muscle.[62,64]

In addition to the hand, other potential sites of stimulation and assessment on the extremities include the posterior tibial nerve behind the medial malleolus (plantar flexion) and the peroneal and lateral popliteal nerves (dorsiflexion) (Table 15-5).

Airway and facial muscles

Compared to peripheral muscles, the laryngeal and diaphragmatic muscles are less sensitive to nondepolarizing relaxants; that is, the dose required for 95% twitch height depression (ED_{95}) is approximately 1.5 to 2 times greater than that required for 95% twitch depression of the adductor pollicis.[65-69] Hence coughing, breathing, or vocal cord movement are still possible despite paralysis of the adductor pollicis muscle. The diaphragmatic muscles likewise evidence decreased sensitivity to depolarizing relaxants;[65] however, laryngeal muscles do not evidence such "sparing" in response to succinylcholine.[70]

Respiratory and airway muscles also differ from the adductor pollicis with respect to the time course of neuro-

Table 15-5. Sites of neurostimulation

Nerve	Location	Movement observed
Ulnar	Wrist or elbow	Thumb adduction, flexion of fourth and fifth fingers, abduction of fifth finger
Posterior tibial	Posterior to the medial malleolus	Plantar flexion of the big toe
Peroneal	Lateral to the neck of the fibula	Dorsiflexion of the foot
Facial	Near the tragus where the nerve emerges from the stylo-mastoid foramen, 2 to 3 cm posterior to the orbit	Contraction of orbicularis oculi or orbicularis oris

muscular block. Onset of, and recovery from, nondepolarizing and depolarizing relaxants are more rapid at the diaphragm and airway muscles.[67,70-73] This may be attributed to proximity to the central circulation, to better perfusion, and to different sensitivities to relaxants (i.e., quantity and quality of receptors). The adductor pollicis is predominantly a slow-twitch type muscle;[74] adult respiratory muscles are more a mixture of slow-twitch and fast-twitch types.[75]

In light of the relatively more rapid onset of block at the airway muscles, it may be argued that it is not necessary to wait for 95% to 100% adductor pollicis twitch depression in order to attain relaxation and intubating conditions.[76] However, monitoring the adductor pollicis at 0.1 Hz provides a desirable safety factor when a rapid sequence induction is performed in settings in which movement of the patient is unacceptable.[3,77] In support of this, it was noted[77] that excellent intubating conditions were not observed reliably until 30 seconds after 100% adductor pollicis depression (when stimulating at 0.1 Hz).

Monitoring of the response of the orbicularis oculi muscle to stimulation of the facial nerve may reflect the level of block at the airway musculature more closely than does monitoring of peripheral muscles.[78-80] However, the electrodes, which are placed over the nerve near the tragus (2 to 3 cm posterior to the lateral border of the orbit), may stimulate the muscle directly and thus may falsely indicate inadequate levels of block. In addition, this response is not readily quantified mechanographically.

MONITORING OF NEUROMUSCULAR BLOCK AND RECOVERY

Response to neurostimulation most commonly entails visual or tactile assessment of TOF fade. However, even in experienced hands (or under experienced eyes), this method typically underestimates the degree of fade. Precise assessment can be quantified only by electromyography (evoked muscle action potential) or mechanomyography (evoked muscle tension).

Force translation

The adductor pollicis force translation monitor is the device most commonly used to measure the evoked muscle response (Fig. 15-17). It consists of a force transducer and a ringed assemblage for appropriate orientation of the thumb. Isometric contraction of the adductor pollicis muscle in response to ulnar nerve stimulation is translated into an electrical signal that can be displayed on an interfaced pressure monitor and that can also be recorded. Currently available force transducers vary considerably in the range of force that they can withstand. Although a transducer with a range of 0 to 5 kg is suitable for most clinical applications in the context of nondepolarizing block, tetanic stimulation in the absence of block generates a force of 7.1 ± 2.2 kg.[30] This may overload (and possibly damage) transducers, which are not designed to withstand such forces.[81]

For optimal quantification of thumb adduction in response to ulnar nerve stimulation and for consistency when evaluation is performed over time, certain features are important: (1) keeping the arm and hand immobilized to attain consistent measurement; (2) orienting the ring/thumb complex to align thumb adduction with the axis of the force transducer; (3) abducting the thumb to a constant preload of 200 to 300 grams in order to optimize alignment of actin and myosin filaments; (4) ensuring unencumbered movement of the thumb/ring complex; (5) adjusting the monitor gain to account for the fact that, depending on the depth of block, the tension developed in response to tetanic stimulation may be 3 to 4 times higher than that achieved by a single twitch; (6) placing the patient's arm in a position that avoids nerve injury during prolonged immobilization; and (7) placing intravenous or intraarterial catheters and the blood pressure cuff on the opposite arm (when feasible).

Accelerography

The adductor pollicis force transducer is relatively cumbersome and must be interfaced with equipment that is not always readily available, especially in the recovery room. This has prompted the introduction of new monitoring techniques, such as accelerography. This utilizes a miniature transducer (piezoelectric wafer) to measure thumb acceleration (Fig. 15-18); when mass is constant, changes in force and acceleration are directly proportional (Force = Mass × Acceleration). As for force transduction, stimulation of the peripheral nerve (most commonly the ulnar) is achieved by indirect stimulation through surface elec-

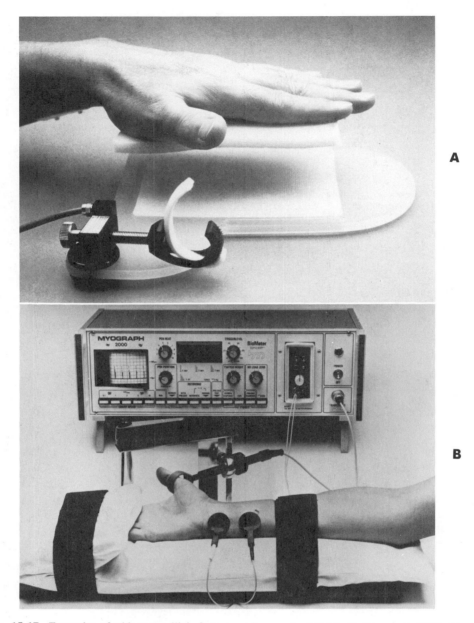

Fig. 15-17. Examples of adductor pollicis force transducers. **A,** APM-L; **B,** Myograph 2000. (**A,** From Professional Instruments, Houston; **B,** From Biometer, Copenhagen.)

trodes. Stimulating parameters may be adjusted similarly to those for assessment of force transduction with the exception that the accelerograph is not suitable for assessing the response to tetanic stimulation. During nondepolarizing block, the accelerograph provides a display and printout equivalent to that obtained by force transduction (Fig. 15-19).[82-84] However, T_4/T_1 may be greater than 1.0 in the absence of block. This may be attributable to thumb movement or to failure of the unsecured thumb (i.e., without preload) to return to its baseline position after the first of the four contractions in a train-of-four.[53]

Electromyography

The muscle action potential can be monitored in clinical as well as laboratory settings by electromyography (EMG). As illustrated for the muscles of the hand in Fig. 15-20, the EMG recording electrodes are placed over the mid-portion (motor-point) of the muscle and over its insertion. Significant data include the latency, amplitude, duration, and shape of the compound action potential (Fig. 15-21).

The motor latency (expressed in milliseconds) is the time interval between the onset of the stimulus and the ini-

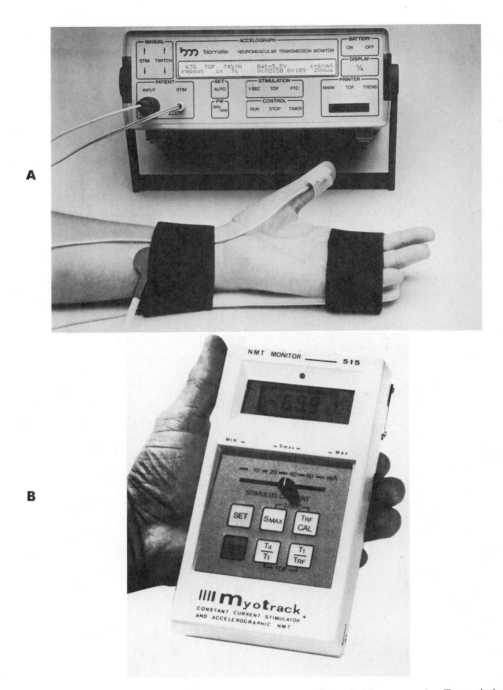

Fig. 15-18. Examples of acceleration monitors: **A,** Accelograph Neuromuscular Transmission Monitor. The digital information displayed on the screen can also be recorded graphically when interfaced with a printer. **B,** Model HH515. This hand-held device provides for stimulation as well as display of responses (e.g., T_4/T_1 ratio). (**A,** Biometer, Copenhagen; **B,** Myotrack Co., Van Nuys, Calif.)

tial deflection of the evoked motor response. It includes the nerve conduction time within the motor nerve fiber and the time required for neuromuscular transmission. The amplitude of the compound muscle action potential can be measured from the isoelectric line to the peak (baseline-to-

peak), from the negative peak to the positive peak (peak-to-peak), or as the area under the muscle action potential curve. It represents the sum of the amplitudes of the individual muscle fibers activated by the stimulus. The duration and morphology of the compound muscle action po-

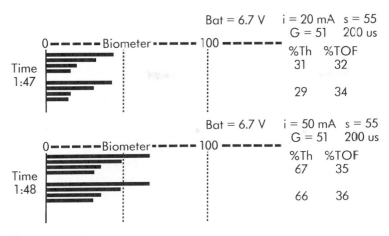

Fig. 15-19. Illustrative printout of accelerographic responses to two sets of train-of-four stimuli at 20 mA *(top)* and two sets at 50 mA *(bottom)*. Note the similar degree of fade despite different stimulating currents. In addition to printing lines that are proportional to twitch height, the device also displays battery voltage *(Bat)*, stimulating current *(i)*, supramaximal current established at onset *(s)*, gain *(G)*, pulse duration (in μsec), height of T_1 expressed as a percentage of baseline T_1 (in response to supramaximal stimulation at onset) *(%Th)*, and the T_4/T_1 ratio *(%TOF)*. (Accelerograph from Biometer, Copenhagen.)

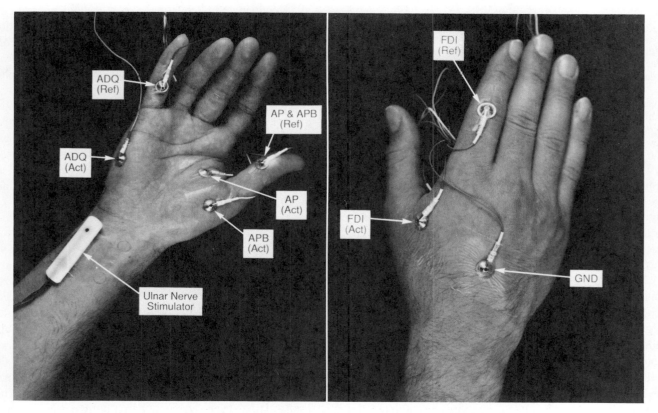

Fig. 15-20. Example of electrode placement for electromyographic monitoring of responses to stimulation of the ulnar nerve on the palmar (left) and dorsal (right) surfaces of the hand. *Act*, active electrode; *Ref*, reference electrode; *ADQ*, abductor digiti quinti; *AP*, adductor pollicis; *APB*, abductor pollicis brevis; *FDI*, first dorsal interosseous.

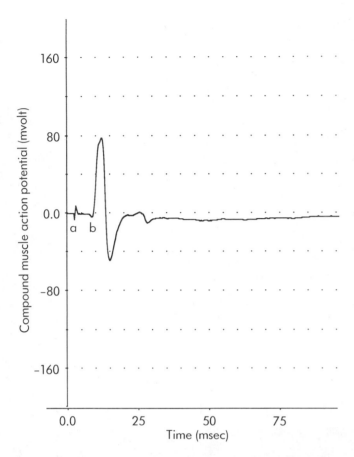

Fig. 15-21. EMG tracing obtained in a healthy volunteer with a Quantum 84 monitor. *x-axis,* time (in milliseconds); *y-axis,* compound muscle action potential (in millivolts); *a,* stimulus artifact; *b,* onset of EMG response. Motor latency is provided by $b - a$. Duration and morphology of the compound MAP are assessed from the first deflection to the time when the MAP returns to the isoelectric line (time epoch). (From Cadwell Laboratories, Kennewick, Wash.)

tential, which reflect the synchrony of contraction, are proportional to the distance from the stimulated site. For automated analysis of the electromyogram, either analog or digital techniques may be employed; they appear to produce results comparable to conventional manual measurement techniques.[85,86]

The EMG most commonly employed in the clinical setting is the Relaxograph integrated EMG monitor* (Fig. 15-22). This is a dedicated EMG instrument that measures a gated portion of the area under the EMG waveform. Other devices, such as the Quantum 84,† are multifunctional (i.e., they can evaluate auditory, visual, and somatosensory evoked potentials; conduction velocities; and spectral array). Their multichannel capabilities make them well suited for comparisons of responses at multiple sites.

*Datex, Shrewsbury, Mass.
†Cadwell Laboratories, Kennewick, Wash.

The mechanomyographic (MMG) and electromyographic responses do not always correlate with one another, nor do changes monitored with one technique necessarily parallel those monitored with the other technique. This may be attributable to the MMG's high sensitivity to factors that affect both muscle contraction and neuromuscular transmission. The EMG tends to be insensitive to mechanical events; however, it has been shown to be affected by preload.[87] In addition, the hypothenar muscles (which commonly are monitored for EMG) are less sensitive to nondepolarizing agents than the adductor pollicis muscle (which is monitored during force transduction).[62,64] These differences were noted in a recent study of seven volunteers receiving vecuronium.[88] Normal vital capacity, inspiratory pressure, and peak expiratory flow rate were achieved at an electromyographic T_4/T_1 ratio of 0.90. In contrast, the mechanomyographic T_4/T_1 ratio needed to perform normal respiratory tests was found to be only 0.50.

Two other examples may help to elucidate the differences between MMG and EMG monitoring. First, the MMG is affected by dantrolene, whereas the EMG is not; this is due to dantrolene's modulation of the calcium levels responsible for myofibril contraction. Second, the MMG and EMG respond differently to repetitive (tetanic) stimuli. Upon single-twitch stimulation at a supramaximal current, the muscle does not achieve maximal contraction because of the time required to overcome its elastic properties (a mechanical feature, not an electrical one). Over the course of a few repetitive stimuli, mechanomyographic responses gradually increase to a plateau (asymptote) as elastic forces are overcome. Furthermore, during tetanus, the contractile responses may sum despite a progressive decline in end-plate potentials. These phenomena also explain why, even in the absence of neuromuscular block, the MMG—but typically not the EMG—may show an augmented single twitch response following tetanic stimulation.

Visual and tactile assessment of evoked responses

In clinical practice, most anesthesiologists rely on visual or tactile means to assess responses to neurostimulation. For visual assessment, the observer should be positioned at an angle of 90° to the plane of movement. For tactile assessment, the observer's fingertips should be placed lightly over the distal phalanx of the thumb in the direction of movement (Fig. 15-23). Visual and tactile assessments are limited in that they often underestimate the depth of block, and significant degrees of block often may be missed even by experienced observers.[7,9,55,89-91] This limitation has been overcome partially by newer means of assessment, such as double-burst stimulation. Studies have reported that the fade of the sequential bursts of DBS is easier to detect than that between the first and fourth re-

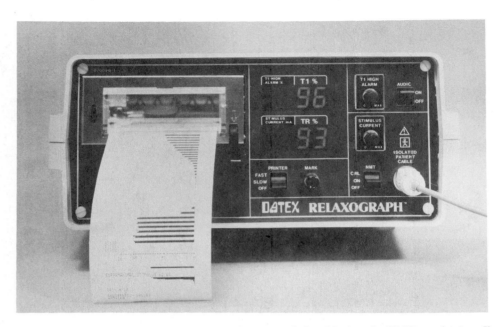

Fig. 15-22. Datex Relaxograph Neuromuscular Transmission Monitor for EMG monitoring. Illustrated are digital and graphic displays for both single twitch (T_1%) and train-of-four (TR%). (From Datex, Shrewsbury, Mass.)

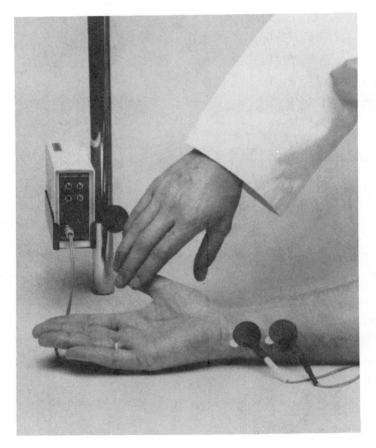

Fig. 15-23. Tactile assessment of thumb adduction in response to ulnar nerve stimulation. (Photograph courtesy of Biometer, Copenhagen.)

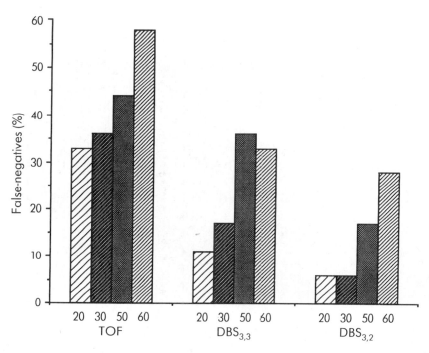

Fig. 15-24. Failure to identify an actual (mechanographic) TOF ratio <0.70 by visual inspection using TOF, $DBS_{3,3}$, and $DBS_{3,2}$ at 20, 30, 50, and 60 mA. TOF at 60 mA was associated with the highest incidence of false negative assessments. (From Brull SJ, Silverman, DG: Visual assessment of train-of-four and double burst stimulation fade at submaximal currents, *Anesth Analg* 73:627-632, 1991.)

Table 15-6. Ability to detect fade by visual or tactile methods at supramaximal stimulating current when actual TOF ratio is between 0.4 and 0.7

	True positives		
	TOF (%)	$DBS_{3,3}$ (%)	$DBS_{3,2}$ (%)
Engbaeck[56]		64	96
Drenck[55]	16	78	
Viby-Mogensen[89]	36		
Gill[90]	16	69	
Ueda[57]		73	96
Brull[91]	42	67	72

sponses of TOF (Table 15-6).[55-57,90,91] In addition, such testing may be performed just as reliably, as well as more comfortably, with submaximal stimulation (Figs. 15-24 to 15-26).[91]

Clinical applications

Despite increased understanding of the intricacy of neuromuscular function, there is still lack of a consensus as how best to monitor block during such critical times as onset and recovery. Routine clinical care entails a number of compromises. Although assessment of thumb adduction in response to ulnar nerve stimulation is not necessarily indicative of the degree of block at the airway musculature, it is still the method most commonly employed to measure neuromuscular block. Even though mechanographic assessment is more accurate than either visual or tactile assessment, the MMG and EMG rarely are applied in routine clinical settings because of their increased cost, lack of availability, and difficulty of use.

It is disturbing that investigators as well as clinicians lack a uniform approach to the pattern and rate of neurostimulation. Clearly, rate of stimulation can affect delivery of a drug and may promote neuromuscular fatigue. Furthermore, the nature of stimulation determines what information may be gained by assessment of thumb adduction.

In their own practice, the authors prefer to monitor onset of paralysis prior to intubation with single twitch at 0.1 Hz. While TOF at 10- to 12-second intervals might provide some additional information, it may accelerate apparent onset of block at the monitoring site. TOF stimulation at 20-second intervals, although not associated with marked acceleration of onset of block, may not be frequent enough to monitor effectively the rapid changes typically seen during onset of block. Alternatively, it may be argued that slow stimulation of the ulnar nerve underestimates the rate of onset of block at the airway musculature and that it may be less likely to identify minor differences among re-

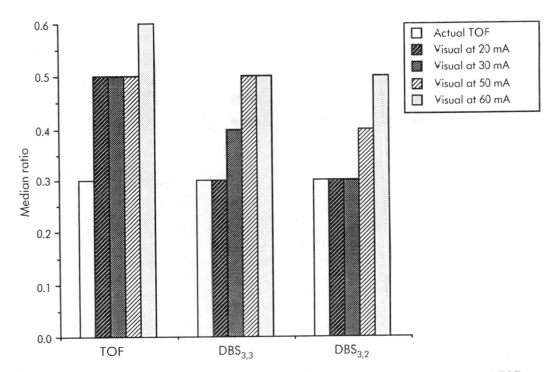

Fig. 15-25. Degree of overestimation of actual TOF ratio by visual inspection when actual TOF ratio was <0.70. Quantitative estimation by visual means significantly overestimated the actual ratio *(unshaded bar)* at all currents for TOF, at currents of 30, 50, and 60 mA for $DBS_{3,3}$, and at 50 and 60 mA for $DBS_{3,2}$. (From Brull SJ, Silverman DG: Visual assessment of train-of-four and double burst induced fade at submaximal currents, *Anesth Analg* 73:627-632, 1991.)

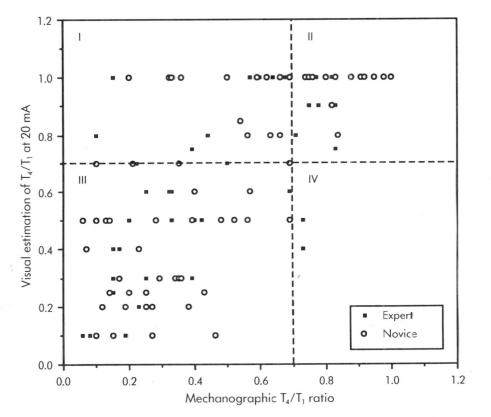

Fig. 15-26. Scattergram comparing the visual estimation of T_4/T_1 at 20 mA to the actual (mechanographic) ratio at 60 mA by experts *(filled squares)* and novices *(open circles)*. Quadrant I indicates incorrect estimation that $T_4/T_1 > 0.70$. Quadrant II indicates accurate estimation that $T_4/T_1 > 0.70$. Quadrant III indicates accurate estimation that $T_4/T_1 < 0.70$. Quadrant IV indicates incorrect estimation that $T_4/T_1 < 0.70$. (From Brull SJ, Silverman DG: Visual assessment of train-of-four and double burst-induced fade at submaximal currents, *Anesth Analg* 73:627-632, 1991.)

laxants. The aforementioned must be viewed in the context of the requirements of the given setting. If it is necessary to document the time at which there is adequate relaxation to permit intubation without coughing or movement, then it is preferable to wait for complete ablation of single twitch at 0.1 Hz. If it is not necessary to ensure "ideal" conditions, then a lesser degree of block may be acceptable.

In the patient who has already undergone tracheal intubation, the rate of onset is less critical. The authors prefer intermittent TOF monitoring in this setting, because it provides information about fade as well as twitch height depression. During maintenance of block, TOF at 10- to 12-second intervals may be used because there is less concern about the effect of rapid stimulation on delivery of relaxant. At depths of block during which there is loss of T_4, the number of responses to TOF stimulation can simply be counted. When all four responses to TOF stimulation are lost, depth of block is assessed by monitoring the posttetanic count (PTC). This is particularly helpful if it is desired to increase the likelihood of vocal cord paralysis, such as during laser surgery of the cords or airway; in those cases, PTC should be 0.

During emergence and recovery, the authors rely primarily upon TOF (or DBS) stimulation. When deciding whether extubation of the trachea is indicated, a T_4/T_1 ratio >0.70 is generally considered to be indicative of adequate recovery. Counting the number of twitches in response to TOF is helpful at relatively deep levels of block. Additional information may be gained by assessing response to tetanic stimulation and examining the degree of posttetanic facilitation. Specifically, if no twitch is attainable, the response to tetanus or the number of posttetanic counts provides valuable information about depth of block and degree of spontaneous recovery.

In the post anesthesia care unit (PACU), the authors rely on clinical signs and will evaluate response to TOF if neuromuscular block is suspected. Recent reports have documented that the T_4/T_1 of TOF and D_2/D_1 of DBS remain constant at submaximal stimulating currents.[52,53,58] Testing with submaximal stimulus currents not only decreases the discomfort associated with TOF monitoring but also may improve the quality of visual assessment.[91] If fade is not detected by visual assessment at low current, it is unlikely to be detected at a higher current. If residual neuromuscular block is a concern, mechanographic (MMG) quantification is preferable to qualitative evaluations.

In all cases, the data generated in response to local neurostimulation should be viewed in the context of clinical signs and symptoms. Once considered a valuable indicator of adequate recovery, a T_4/T_1 ratio >0.70 no longer is considered to be a guarantee of airway protection. Likewise, clinical criteria are not necessarily definitive, especially in the context of residual anesthesia. A study in

Table 15-7. The relationship among clinical signs in healthy, awake volunteers receiving low doses of curare

Parameter	Peak insp. force (cm H$_2$O)
Control (no relaxant)	−90
Five-second head lift	−53
Effective swallowing	−43
Patent airway without jaw lift	−39
Glottic closure against valsalva	−30
Vital capacity >33% of control	−20

Control subjects could generate a peak inspiratory force of −90 cm H$_2$O and perform all maneuvers. Following low-dose curare, the ability to maintain one's airway and swallow effectively was not assured even if the peak inspiratory force was −30 cm H$_2$O.[92]

awake volunteers[92] noted that even the ability to generate a vital capacity more than 33% of control and to maintain a patent airway without jaw lift does not guarantee effective swallowing or airway protection (Table 15-7).

Although the benefits of neuromuscular blocking agents are well recognized, a certain amount of morbidity is associated with their use. Appropriate dosing of relaxant and reversal drugs and appropriate monitoring of their effects can increase the utility and safety of these valuable agents.

REFERENCES

1. Griffith HR, Johnson GE: The use of curare in general anesthesia, *Anesthesiology* 3:418-420, 1942.
2. Katz RL: Neuromuscular effects of *d*-tubocurarine, edrophonium and neostigmine in man, *Anesthesiology* 28:327-336, 1967.
3. Silverman DG, Swift CA, Dubow HD, et al: Variability of onset times within and among relaxant regimens, *J Clin Anesth* 4:28-33, 1992.
4. Viby-Mogensen J, Jorgensen BC, Ording H: Residual curarization in the recovery room, *Anesthesiology* 50:539-541, 1979.
5. Lennmarken C, Lofstrom JB: Partial curarization in the postoperative period, *Acta Anaesthesiol Scand* 28:260-262, 1984.
6. Andersen BN, Madsen JV, Schurizek BA, et al: Residual curarization: a comparative study of atracurium and pancuronium, *Acta Anaesthesiol Scand* 32:79-81, 1988.
7. Bevan DR, Smith CE, Donati F: Postoperative neuromuscular blockade: a comparison between atracurium, vecuronium, and pancuronium, *Anesthesiology* 69:272-276, 1988.
8. Brull SJ, Ehrenwerth J, Connelly NR, et al: Assessment of residual curarization using low-current stimulation, *Can J Anaesth* 38:164-168, 1991.
9. Beemer GH, Rozental P: Postoperative neuromuscular function, *Anaesth Intensive Care* 14:41-45, 1986.
10. Pederson T, Viby-Mogensen J, Bang U, et al: Does perioperative tactile evaluation of the train-of-four response influence the frequency of postoperative residual neuromuscular blockade? *Anesthesiology* 73:835-839, 1990.
11. Feinstein B, Lindegård B, Nyman E, et al: Morphological studies of motor units in normal human muscles, *Acta Anat (Basel)* 23:127-142, 1955.
12. Carlsöö S: Motor units and action potentials in masticatory muscles, *Acta Morphol Neerl Scand* 2:13-19, 1958.
13. Birks R, Huxley HE, Katz B: The fine structure of the neuromuscular junction of the frog, *J Physiol (Lond)* 150:134-144, 1960.

14. Dunant Y: On the mechanism of acetylcholine release, *Prog Neurobiol* 26:55-92, 1984.

15. Peper K, Bradley RJ, Dreyer F: The acetylcholine receptor at the neuromuscular junction, *Physiol Rev* 62:1271-1340, 1982.

16. Standaert FG: *Neuromuscular physiology.* In Miller RD, editor: *Anesthesia,* New York, 1990, Churchill-Livingstone, pp 659-684.

17. Betz WJ, Caldwell JH, Kinnamon SC: Increased sodium conductance in the synaptic region of rat skeletal muscle fibres, *J Physiol (Lond)* 352:189-202, 1984.

18. Katz AM, Messinso FC, Herbette L: Ion channels in membranes, *Circulation* 65(suppl I):2-10, 1982.

19. Bowman WC: Prejunctional and postjunctional cholinoceptors at the neuromuscular junction, *Anesth Analg* 59:935-943, 1980.

20. Bowman WC, Marshall IG, Gigg AJ: Is there feedback control of transmitter release at the neuromuscular junction? *Semin Anesth* 3:275-283, 1984.

21. Standaert FG: Donuts and holes: molecules and muscle relaxants, *Semin Anesth* 3:251-261, 1984.

22. Gage PW, Hammill OP: Effects of anesthetics on ion channels in synapses, *Int Rev Physiol* 25 (*Neurophysiol* 4): 1-46, 1981.

23. Neubig RR, Boyd ND, Cohen JB: Conformations of Torpedo acetylcholine receptor associated with ion transport and desensitization, *Biochemistry* 21:3460-3467, 1982.

24. Sakmann B, Patlak J, Neher E: Single acetylcholine-activated channels show burst-kinetics in presence of desensitizing concentrations of agonist, *Nature* 286:71-73, 1980.

25. Mortimer JT: *Electrical excitation of nerve.* In: Agnew WF, McCreery DB, editors: *Neural prostheses,* Englewood Cliffs, NJ, 1990, Prentice-Hall, pp 67-83.

26. Kopman AF: A safe surface electrode for peripheral-nerve stimulation, *Anesthesiology* 44:343-345, 1976.

27. Gray JA: Nerve stimulators and burns, *Anesthesiology* 42:231-32, 1975.

28. Lippmann M, Fields WA: Burns of the skin caused by a peripheral nerve stimulator, *Anesthesiology* 40:82-84, 1974.

29. Merton PA: Voluntary strength and fatigue, *J Physiol (Lond)* 123:553-564, 1954.

30. Stanec A, Heyduk J, Stanec G, et al: Tetanic fade and posttetanic tension in the absence of neuromuscular blocking agents in anesthetized man, *Anesth Analg* 57:102-107, 1978.

31. Ali HH, Savarese JJ, Lebowitz PW, et al: Twitch, tetanus and train-of-four as indices of recovery from nondepolarizing neuromuscular blockade, *Anesthesiology* 54:294-297, 1981.

32. Lee C, Barnes A, Katz RL: Neuromuscular sensitivity to tubocurarine: a comparison of 10 parameters, *Br J Anaesth* 48:1045-1051, 1976.

33. Goat VA, Yeung ML, Blakeney C, et al: The effect of blood flow upon the activity of gallamine triethiodide, *Br J Anaesth* 48:69-73, 1976.

34. Saxena PR, Dhasmana KM, Prakash O: A comparison of systemic and regional hemodynamic effects of *d*-tubocurarine, pancuronium, and vecuronium, *Anesthesiology* 59:102-108, 1983.

35. Curran MJ, Donati F, Bevan DR: Onset and recovery of atracurium and suxamethonium-induced neuromuscular blockade with simultaneous train-of-four and single twitch stimulation, *Br J Anaesth* 59:989-994, 1987.

36. Ali HH, Savarese JJ: Stimulus frequency and dose-response curve to *d*-tubocurarine in man, *Anesthesiology* 52:36-39, 1980.

37. Connelly NR, Silverman DG, Brull SJ: Temporal correlation of succinylcholine-induced fasciculations to loss of twitch response at different stimulating frequencies, *J Clin Anesth* 4:190-193, 1992.

38. Ali HH, Savarese JJ: Stimulus frequency is essential information, *Anesthesiology* 50:76-77, 1979 (letter).

39. Blackman JG: Stimulus frequency and neuromuscular block, *Br J Pharmacol* 20:5-16, 1963.

40. Waud BE, Waud DR: The margin of safety of neuromuscular transmission in the muscle of the diaphragm, *Anesthesiology* 37:417-422, 1972.

41. Ali HH, Utting JE, Gray C: Stimulus frequency in the detection of neuromuscular block in humans, *Br J Anaesth* 42:967-978, 1970.

42. Lee C, Katz RL: Fade of neurally evoked compound electromyogram during neuromuscular block by *d*-tubocurarine, *Anesth Analg* 56:271-275, 1977.

43. Miller RD, Eger EI II, Way WL, et al: Comparative neuromuscular effects of Forane and halothane alone and in combination with *d*-tubocurarine in man, *Anesthesiology* 35:38-42, 1971.

44. Cohen PJ, Heisterkamp CV, Skovsted P: The effect of general anesthesia on the response to stimulus in man, *Br J Anaesth* 42:543-547, 1970.

45. Brull SJ, Connelly NR, Silverman DG: Effect of tetanus on train-of-four and double burst stimulation: potentiation and time to recovery, *Anesthesiology* 74:64-70, 1991.

46. Liley AW, North KAK: An electrical investigation of the effects of repetitive stimulation on mammalian neuromuscular junction, *J Neurophysiol* 16:509-527, 1953.

47. Feldman SA, Tyrrell MF: A new theory on the termination of action of the muscle relaxants, *Proc R Soc Med* 63:692-695, 1970.

48. Viby-Mogensen J, Howardy-Hansen P, Chraemmer-Jorgensen B, et al: Posttetanic count (PTC): a new method of evaluating an intense nondepolarizing neuromuscular blockade, *Anesthesiology* 55:458-461, 1981.

49. Bonsu AK, Viby-Mogensen J, Fernando PUE, et al: Relationship of posttetanic count and train-of-four response during intense neuromuscular blockade caused by atracurium, *Br J Anaesth* 59:1089-1092, 1987.

50. Ali HH, Kitz RJ: Evaluation of recovery from nondepolarizing neuromuscular block, using a digital neuromuscular transmission analyzer: preliminary report, *Anesth Analg* 52:740-745, 1973.

51. Lee C: Train-of-four quantitation of competitive neuromuscular block, *Anesth Analg* 54:649-653, 1975.

52. Brull SJ, Ehrenwerth J, Silverman DG: Stimulation with submaximal current for train-of-four monitoring, *Anesthesiology* 72:629-632, 1990.

53. Silverman DG, Connelly NR, O'Connor TZ, et al: Accelographic train-of-four at near-threshold currents, *Anesthesiology* 76:34-38, 1992.

54. Connelly NR, Silverman DG, O'Connor TZ, et al: Subjective responses to train-of-four and double burst stimulation in awake patients, *Anesth Analg* 70:650-653, 1990.

55. Drenck NE, Ueda N, Olsen NV, et al: Manual evaluation of residual curarization using double burst stimulation: a comparison with train-of-four, *Anesthesiology* 70:578-581, 1989.

56. Engbaek J, Ostergaard D, Viby-Mogensen J: Double burst stimulation (DBS): a new pattern of nerve stimulation to identify residual neuromuscular transmission, *Br J Anaesth* 62:274-278, 1989.

57. Ueda N, Viby-Mogensen J, V-Olsen N, et al: The best choice of double burst stimulation pattern for manual evaluation of neuromuscular transmission, *J Anesth* 3:94-99, 1989.

58. Brull SJ, Connelly NR, Silverman DG: Correlation of train-of-four and double burst stimulation ratios at varying amperages, *Anesth Analg* 71:489-492, 1990.

59. Rosenberg H, Greenhow DE: Peripheral nerve stimulator performance: the influence of output polarity and electrode placement, *Can Anaesth Soc J* 25:424-426, 1978.

60. Berger JJ, Gravenstein JS, Munson ES: Electrode polarity and peripheral nerve stimulation, *Anesthesiology* 56:402-404, 1982.

61. Kalli I: Optimal electrode site on the hand for evoked EMG monitoring, *Anesthesiology* 73:A911, 1990 (abstract).

62. Kalli I: Effect of surface electrode position on the compound action potential evoked by ulnar nerve stimulation during isoflurane anaesthesia, *Br J Anaesth* 65:494-499, 1990 (abstract).

63. Halevy J, Brull SJ, Booke J, et al: Dual innervation of hand muscles: potential influence on monitoring of neuromuscular blockade, *Anesthesiology* 75:A814, 1991 (abstract).

64. Kopman AF: The relationship of evoked electromyographic and mechanical responses following atracurium in humans, *Anesthesiology* 63:208-211, 1985.

65. Smith CE, Donati F, Bevan DR: Potency of succinylcholine at the diaphragm and adductor pollicis muscle in man, *Anesth Analg* 67:625-630, 1988.

66. Donati F, Antzaka C, Bevan DR: Potency of pancuronium at the diaphragm and the adductor pollicis muscle in humans, *Anesthesiology* 65:1-5, 1986.

67. Donati F, Plaud B, Meistelman C: Vecuronium neuromuscular blockade at the adductor muscles of the larynx and adductor pollicis, *Anesthesiology* 74:827-832, 1991.

68. Debaene B, Guesde R, Clergue F, et al: Plasma concentration response relationship of pancuronium for the diaphragm and the adductor pollicis in anesthetized man, *Anesthesiology* 73:A887, 1990 (abstract).

69. Laycock JRD, Donati F, Bevan DR: Potency of atracurium and vecuronium at the diaphragm and adductor pollicis muscle in humans, *Br J Anaesth* 59:1321P, 1987 (abstract).

70. Meistelman C, Plaud B, Donati F: Neuromuscular effects of succinylcholine on the vocal cords and adductor pollicis muscles, *Anesth Analg* 73:278-282, 1991.

71. Smith CE, Donati F, Bevan DR: Effects of succinylcholine at the masseter and adductor pollicis muscles in adults, *Anesth Analg* 69:158-162, 1989.

72. Chauvin M, Lebreault C, Duvaldestin P: The neuromuscular blocking effect of vecuronium on the human diaphragm, *Anesth Analg* 66:117-122, 1987.

73. Pansard JL, Chauvin M, Lebreault C, et al: Effect of an intubating dose of succinylcholine and atracurium on the diaphragm and adductor pollicis in humans, *Anesthesiology* 67:326-330, 1987.

74. Johnson MA, Polgar W, Weightman D, et al: Data on the distribution of fibre types in thirty-six human muscles: an autopsy study, *J Neurol Sci* 18:111-129, 1973.

75. Katz B, Miledi R: Estimates of quantal content during "chemical potentiation" of transmitter release, *Proc R Soc Lond* 205:369-378, 1979.

76. Hughes R, Payne JP: Clinical assessment of atracurium using the single twitch and tetanic responses of the adductor pollicis muscles, *Br J Anaesth* 55:47S-52S, 1983.

77. Bencini A, Newton DEF: Rate of good intubating conditions, respiratory depression and hand muscle paralysis after vecuronium, *Br J Anaesth* 56:959-965, 1984.

78. Ho LC, Crosby G, Sundaram P, et al: Ulnar train-of-four stimulation in predicting face movement during intracranial facial nerve stimulation, *Anesth Analg* 69:242-244, 1989.

79. Caffrey RR, Warren ML, Becker KE: Neuromuscular blockade monitoring comparing the orbicularis oculi and adductor pollicis muscles, *Anesthesiology* 65:95-97, 1986.

80. Stiffel P, Hameroff SR, Blitt CD, et al: Variability in assessment of neuromuscular blockade, *Anesthesiology* 52:436-437, 1980.

81. Freund FG, Merati JK: A source of errors in assessing neuromuscular blockade. *Anesthesiology* 39:540-542, 1973.

82. Werner MU: A methods-comparison study of acceleration, EMG and force responses during recovery from a non-depolarizing block in children, *Anesthesiology* 73:A911, 1990 (abstract).

83. May O, Kirkegaard-Nielson H, Werner MU: The acceleration transducer: an assessment of its precision in comparison with a force displacement transducer, *Acta Anaesthesiol Scand* 32:239-243, 1988.

84. Viby-Mogensen J, Jensen E, Werner M, et al: Measurement of acceleration: a new method of monitoring neuromuscular function. *Acta Anaesthesiol Scand* 32:45-48, 1988.

85. Bergmans J: Computer assisted online measurement of motor unit potential parameters of electromyograms in electrical diagnosis. *Electromyography* 11:161, 1971.

86. Kopec J, Hausmanowa-Petrusewicz I: Application of automatic analysis of electromyogram in clinical practice, *Riv Patol Nerv Ment* 99:65-74, 1978.

87. Kopman AF: The effect of resting muscle tension on the dose-effect relationship of *d*-tubocurarine: does preload influence the evoked EMG? *Anesthesiology* 69:1003-1005, 1988.

88. Dupuis JY, Martin R, Tétrault JP: Clinical, electrical and mechanical correlations during recovery from neuromuscular blockade with vecuronium, *Can J Anaesth* 37:192-196, 1990.

89. Viby-Mogensen J, Jensen NH, Engbaek J, et al: Tactile and visual evaluation of the response to train-of-four nerve stimulation, *Anesthesiology* 63:440-443, 1985.

90. Gill SS, Donati F, Bevan DR: Clinical evaluation of double-burst stimulation, *Anaesthesia* 45:543-548, 1990.

91. Brull SJ, Silverman DG: Visual assessment of train-of-four and double burst induced fade at submaximal currents, *Anesth Analg* 73:627-632, 1991.

92. Pavlin EG, Holle RH, Schoene RB: Recovery of airway protection compared with ventilation in humans after paralysis with curare, *Anesthesiology* 70:381-385, 1989.

Part IV

HAZARDS AND
SAFETY FEATURES

Chapter 16

HAZARDS OF THE ANESTHESIA DELIVERY SYSTEM

James B. Eisenkraft, M.D.
Richard M. Sommer, M.D.

Parts of this chapter are adapted from Eisenkraft JB, Sommer RM: *Equipment failure: anesthesia delivery systems.* In Benumof JL, Saidman LJ, editors: *Anesthesia and perioperative complications,* St Louis, 1992, Mosby–Year Book.

PERSPECTIVE

Failure of the anesthesia delivery system alone is a rare cause of anesthesia-related injury to or death of a patient. More commonly the delivery system is misused, the operator errs, or the delivery system fails in combination with the anesthesiologist being unaware that failure has taken place. In most cases of anesthesia machine failure, a temporal window of opportunity exists during which the anesthesiologist can detect the problem and correct it before the patient is harmed. Therefore, a sound understanding of the anesthesia delivery system and the ways in which it can fail or be misused provides the basis for safe anesthesia practice.

Cooper, et al.[1] collected 1089 descriptions of critical incidents during anesthesia, of which approximately 30% were related to equipment failure, including breathing circuit disconnection, gas flow-control errors, loss of gas supply, leaks, misconnections, and ventilator malfunctions. Seventy of the 1089 incidents resulted in a substantive negative outcome for the patient, and of these only 3 were attributable to equipment failure. This confirmed a previous impression that human error is the dominant problem in anesthesia mishaps.[2] Although equipment failure is rarely the cause of death during anesthesia, critical incidents related to equipment are not infrequent and have prompted improvements in machine design and construction.[3]

Buffington, et al.[4] intentionally created five faults in a standard anesthesia machine and then invited 190 attendees at a Postgraduate Assembly of the New York State Society of Anesthesiologists to identify them within 10 minutes. The average number of discovered faults was 2.2; 7.3% of participants found no faults and only 3.4% found all five. The authors concluded that greater emphasis was needed in educational programs on the fundamentals of anesthesia machine design and detection of hazards.[4]

In an effort to improve patient safety and proper use of the anesthesia machine, the American Society of Anesthesiologists (ASA), the Anesthesia Patient Safety Foundation (APSF), and others supported the use of checklists to enable the anesthesia practitioner to ensure that the anesthesia delivery system was functioning normally prior to the start of an anesthetic. In 1986, the United States Food and Drug Administration (FDA) in cooperation with the ASA, machine experts, and manufacturers published a generic apparatus checklist to enable the practitioner to check out anesthesia equipment thoroughly prior to its use (see Chapter 22).[5] March and Crowley[6] evaluated the FDA recommended checklist and individual practitioner checklists in order to determine whether the existence of the FDA checklist would improve detection of anesthesia machine faults. Participants in this study were given machines with four faults that were detectable if the FDA checklist was used properly. The results of the study revealed 25.8% of faults were found with the practitioner's checklist and 29.9% were found with the FDA checklist. In either case the results were poor and indicated that the mere introduction of the FDA checklist in 1986 did not improve the ability of these anesthesiologists to detect machine faults. However, it should be noted that in this study no attempt was made to ensure that the FDA checklist was used properly during the checkout procedure.

Kumar, et al.[7] conducted a random survey of 169 anesthesia machines and ancillary monitors in 45 hospitals in Iowa. The machines ranged in age between 1 and 28 years (the oldest being 1958 vintage). Five machines had no back-up source of oxygen, 60 had no functioning oxygen analyzer, 15 had gas leaks of greater than 500 ml/min (2 proximal to the common gas outlet and 13 in the patient circuit). Fourteen of the 383 vaporizers tested did not meet the manufacturer's calibration standards, and 20 had been added downstream of the machine common gas outlet. Of the 123 machines with ventilators, 16 had no alarm for low airway pressure and only 31 had a high-pressure alarm. Of the ventilators surveyed, 59% were of the hanging bellows design and 41% of the standing design; 95.5% had a scavenging system, but in 24.3% the scavenging circuit connectors were indistinguishable from the breathing circuit connectors, a potentially hazardous situation.[7] The use of these old machines increases the risk for development of problems related to the delivery system; in addition, equipment users may not be as educated as they should be in their ability to detect such problems.

With patient safety as the primary concern, over the past several years the basic gas machine has evolved into the present, more sophisticated anesthesia delivery system. Safety of the delivery system has been enhanced in two basic ways: (1) pneumatic and mechanical design features (such as proportioning systems and vaporizer interlock) have been incorporated into the systems, and (2) system monitors with alarms (such as volume, pressure, oxygen concentration) have been added to alert the user to system malfunctions.

The most current voluntary consensus standard describing the features of a modern machine is that published by the American Society for Testing and Materials (ASTM) in March 1989, which describes the minimum performance and safety requirements to be used in the design of anesthesia machines for human use.[8] This standard supersedes the Z79.8-1979 document published by the American National Standards Institute (ANSI) in 1979.[9] It is anticipated that the use of a state-of-the-art delivery system, which includes certain basic system monitors, together with adoption of the Standards for Basic Intraoperative Monitoring, as published by the ASA in 1986 and periodically updated,[10] will enhance patient safety. As in the case of monitoring standards; however, absolute confirmation may be difficult.[11]

Complications caused by the anesthesia delivery system may be operator induced (misuse) or attributable to failure of a component. The categories of oxygen delivery, carbon dioxide elimination, circuit pressure and volume problems, inhaled anesthetic agent doses, problems of humidification of inhaled gases, and electrical failure are discussed in detail. Delivery system checkouts and standards are discussed in Chapter 22. This chapter demonstrates the way in which a delivery system failure or operator error can lead to problems for the patient.

COMPLICATIONS
Hypoxemia

Hypoxemia, which for the purposes of this chapter is defined as a PaO_2 less than 60 mm Hg, may be caused by problems with the anesthesia delivery system or by problems within the patient. If the patient is adequately ventilated and the alveolar oxygen concentration is as expected, then a problem with the patient is the cause of hypoxemia. Pulmonary conditions that cause shunting, venous admixture, ventilation-perfusion mismatch, or, less likely, diffusion defects can cause hypoxemia. Examples of these conditions are pneumonia, atelectasis, pulmonary edema, pneumothorax, hemothorax, pyothorax, pulmonary embolism, alveolar proteinosis, and bronchospasm. In addition, conditions that decrease mixed venous oxygen, such as anemia and shock, may also cause or contribute to hypoxemia (Box 16-1).

The anesthesia delivery system may cause hypoxemia by failing to deliver sufficient oxygen to the lungs and thereby reducing the alveolar oxygen concentration (Box 16-2). Inadequate ventilation, caused by either apnea or low minute ventilation, are well described causes of alve-

---

Box 16-1. Causes of inadequate arterial oxygenation

Failure to deliver adequate oxygen to the alveoli

Inadequate alveolar ventilation
Low F_IO_2

Intrapulmonary pathology

Shunt
Ventilation/perfusion mismatch
Diffusion defects

Box 16-2. Causes of failure to deliver oxygen to the alveoli

Upstream of the machine

Liquid oxygen reservoir empty or filled with hypoxic gas (e.g., nitrogen)
Crossed hospital pipelines
Crossed hoses or adapters in the operating room
Closed pipeline valves
Disconnected oxygen hose
Failure of back-up hospital oxygen reserve

Within the machine or circuit

Cylinder filled with hypoxic gas
Empty oxygen cylinder
Incorrect cylinder on oxygen yoke
Crossed pipes within machine
Closed oxygen cylinder valve
Oxygen flowmeter off
Failure of proportioning system
Oxygen leak within the machine or flowmeter
Incompetent or absent circuit unidirectional valves
Breathing circuit leak
Closed system anesthesia with inadequate fresh oxygen supply
Inadequate ventilation

---

olar hypoxia. These problems can arise due to failure to initiate manual or mechanical ventilation or due to failure to recognize a major leak or disconnection in the breathing circuit even though ventilation is attempted. The anesthesia delivery system may also cause hypoxemia by delivering insufficient oxygen from the machine to the breathing circuit.[12]

Insufficient or low inspired oxygen concentrations can be definitively detected via the use of an oxygen analyzer. The oxygen analyzer is a critical monitor because although it may appear that pure oxygen is being delivered from the oxygen flowmeter, if the gas in the flowmeter is not in reality oxygen, then the patient will receive a hypoxic gas mixture.[13] Without the oxygen analyzer this condition would not be recognized.[12] The pulse oximeter, a valuable

patient monitor, does not replace the oxygen analyzer. A low reading on a properly functioning pulse oximeter merely indicates that the patient's hemoglobin is poorly saturated with oxygen.[14,15] However, only the oxygen analyzer in the breathing circuit would be able to determine that the cause was inadequate delivery of oxygen to the patient. Therefore, these two monitors are complementary and both should be employed to ensure patient safety.

The oxygen analyzer is not without limitations. In order to act as a valuable safety device it must have an adequate power source and be properly calibrated. In addition, it must be positioned such that it is sampling the gases that the patient will breathe. An analyzer placed at the inspiratory valve may indicate a normal oxygen concentration, but if there is a disconnection between that point and the patient, the patient will not receive that gas. For this reason it is critical that the anesthesiologist understand the equipment design and the limitations of this device. The analyzer must function normally, the circuit valves must be present, the circuit must be intact, and the patient must be ventilated if the reading on the oxygen analyzer is to reflect the oxygen that is being delivered to the alveoli. Vigilant observation of patient ventilation, the integrity of the breathing system, and the oxygen analyzer ensure proper delivery of oxygen to the patient.

The gas entering the anesthesia machine from the hospital piped gas supply system or the oxygen cylinders may contain a gas other than oxygen. The central liquid oxygen reservoir may be filled with liquid nitrogen instead.[15] The pipelines throughout the hospital may be crossed so that nitrous oxide or some other gas may be flowing through the oxygen pipeline. Placement of a nitrous oxide wall adapter on one end of an oxygen hose would allow that hose to be attached to the wall's nitrous oxide source and the anesthesia machine's oxygen inlet. Thus nitrous oxide would flow through the oxygen flowmeter on the machine.[16-19] (Fig. 16-1)

Because of these problems with the wall oxygen source some have recommended that only oxygen cylinders be used. However, this approach overlooks the possibility that an oxygen cylinder may contain a gas other than oxygen.[14,15] A nitrous oxide cylinder or another gas cylinder may be attached to the oxygen yoke if the pin index system were defeated by removal of a pin or by placement of more than one washer between the yoke and the cylinder. Finally, crossed pipes within the machine would allow a gas other than oxygen into the oxygen flowmeter.[20,21]

Turning on the oxygen flow control valve may result in no gas flow.[22] The hospital's central oxygen system may be empty, shut down, or otherwise unavailable to deliver oxygen.[23] The oxygen hose may be disconnected from the wall to the anesthesia machine. The back-up cylinders may be empty, absent, or turned off.[16] The oxygen flow control valve or oxygen piping in the machine may be obstructed, thereby preventing the flow of oxygen to the flowmeter.[24,25] The flowmeter bobbin or rotameter may become

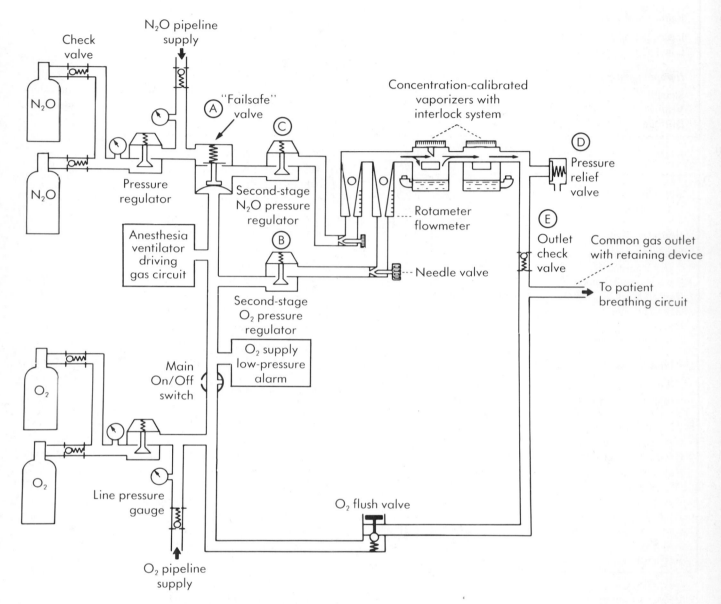

Fig. 16-1. Schematic of contemporary generic anesthesia delivery system. Although many safety features are employed to ensure that oxygen is flowing through the oxygen pipes of the anesthesia machine, none of these devices is foolproof. If a gas other than oxygen were delivered to the oxygen pipes within the machine, it would be detected only by a calibrated oxygen analyzer or equivalent gas analysis monitor. **A,** Pressure sensor shut-off valve (Ohmeda) or oxygen failure protection device (Dräger); **B,** second stage oxygen regulator used in Ohmeda but not Dräger machines; **C,** second stage nitrous oxide regulator used in Ohmeda Modulus machines with the Link 25 proportion limiting system; **D,** pressure relief valve used in certain Ohmeda machines (see Table 2-1), not used in Dräger machines; **E,** outlet check valve used in certain Ohmeda machines (see Table 2-1), not used in Dräger machines.(Adapted from *Check-out: a guide for preoperative inspection of an anesthesia machine* (1987) with permission of the American Society of Anesthesiologists, 520 N. Northwest Highway, Park Ridge, Ill. 60068-2573.)

stuck, and it may appear that gas is flowing from that flowmeter even when it is not.[12] Leaks in the oxygen flowmeter tube or the low-pressure portion of the anesthesia machine can permit loss of oxygen before it reaches the common gas outlet of the machine.[26-29]

Anesthesia machines that are currently manufactured by Ohmeda and North American Dräger are equipped with devices that help prevent the delivery of a hypoxic mixture. Machines of older vintage may not have these accessories. On the older machines the nitrous oxide flowmeter could be turned on without the oxygen flowmeter also being turned on. This could lead to the delivery of a hypoxic gas mixture in the breathing circuit; the oxygen analyzer would detect this problem and the anesthesiologist would have to recognize it and respond by adding oxygen to the mixture.

Although the controllers help prevent the delivery of hypoxic mixtures, they are not foolproof and cannot be relied on entirely as the only method to prevent a hypoxic mixture. The Ohmeda Link 25 proportion limiting system causes the oxygen flow control valve to increase flow if a hypoxic mixture would otherwise result when only oxygen and nitrous oxide are being used. This system can fail if the needle valve is broken in the closed position or if the linkage between the flowmeter controls does not work.[25,30,31] The Dräger oxygen ratio monitor controller on some machines is modified at the factory in order to permit use of closed-system anesthesia; this adjustment permits delivery of a hypoxic mixture. In addition, the limitation of all oxygen proportioning systems is that they do not analyze the gas that is flowing through the oxygen flowmeter; the oxygen analyzer addresses this function[12] (see Chapter 2).

Abnormalities in the anesthesia breathing circuit can lead to a hypoxic mixture. Absent or incompetent unidirectional valves in the circle system can permit rebreathing of exhaled gas, which, if insufficiently mixed with fresh gas, would present the patient with a hypoxic mixture. In the Mapleson circuits (Figs. 16-2 and 16-3) loss of the fresh gas supply from the machine leads to severe rebreathing of a hypoxic mixture as the patient uses up the oxygen and replaces it with carbon dioxide. Failure of the fresh gas supply in the circle system results in a breathing mixture that becomes progressively hypoxic as the oxygen is used up and nitrous oxide is left behind.[32-35]

Leaks in the breathing circuit lead to loss of gases. If a hanging bellows ventilator is used, the lost gas may be replaced with entrained room air as the bellows descends by gravity during exhalation.[36] A standing bellows collapses if a significant leak develops. In addition, system leaks can lead to severe hypoventilation. The sources of leaks may be valve housings, circuit hoses, pressure monitor hoses, connection sites, pressure relief valves, and carbon dioxide absorbers. Leaks can also be caused by subatmospheric pressure being applied to the system from a scavenger suction or by a catheter that has unintentionally been passed into the trachea alongside the tracheal tube.[12,18,37]

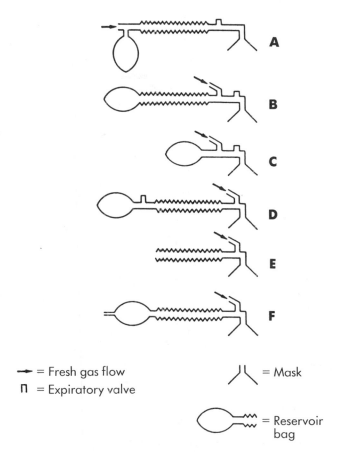

Fig. 16-2. Mapleson classification of rebreathing systems A through F. The Mapleson A circuit is also referred to as the Magill attachment. (From Conway CM: Anaesthetic breathing systems, *Br J Anaesth* 57:649, 1985.)

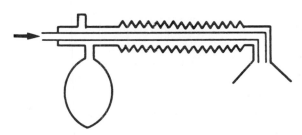

Fig. 16-3. Bain circuit. Coaxial Mapleson D. Arrow indicates fresh gasflow.

Leaks in the ventilator bellows allow the pressurizing gas in the ventilator bellows housing to enter the patient circuit. Depending on the gas used, this could affect the composition of the breathing mixture.[38]

Closed-system or low-flow anesthesia can lead to the delivery of a hypoxic mixture. The total flow of gas is adjusted to compensate for the uptake of nitrous oxide and oxygen. However, if the oxygen content of the circuit gases is not carefully monitored, the uptake of nitrous oxide may be low and that of oxygen may be high. The resultant mixture could be hypoxic.

Hyperoxia

Administration of a mixture that contains more oxygen than desired results in hyperoxia. This rarely presents a problem and can be detected with an oxygen analyzer. Insufficient nitrous oxide or air administered from the flowmeters can lead to hyperoxia. Flowmeter leaks and inaccurate flowmeters may cause gases to be lost, with resultant high oxygen concentrations. Finally, a leak in a ventilator bellows that allows injection of pressurizing oxygen (Ohmeda ventilator 7000, 7800 series) into the bellows may cause the inspired oxygen to increase.[38,39]

Hypercarbia

When carbon dioxide production exceeds elimination, the arterial carbon dioxide tension rises until equilibrium is achieved. During anesthesia, patient factors or delivery system conditions may cause hypercarbia.

Patients who are breathing spontaneously are prone to hypercarbia because of the depressant effects of anesthetics on the central respiratory center, weakness from muscle relaxants, and motor blockade during spinal or epidural anesthesia. Complete or partial airway obstruction can cause hypercarbia. Pulmonary conditions that cause a large shunt, and increased metabolic production of carbon dioxide without a concomitant increase in ventilation also cause hypercarbia (see also Chapter 10).

The anesthesia delivery system can be a source of hypercarbia. Apnea caused by failure to ventilate either manually or mechanically raises the carbon dioxide concentration. Ventilating with an inadequate tidal volume or respiratory rate reduces alveolar ventilation and creates hypercarbia. Leaks in the machine, circuit, and ventilator, and failure to fill the bellows may lead to hypoventilation[12] (Box 16-3).

The anesthesia breathing circuit may contain insufficient gas if the pipeline gas source fails. However, this type of problem can be overcome by use of the reserve gas cylinders on the anesthesia machine.[18,22,36] Inside the machine, leaks may develop either at the oxygen yoke or from a faulty check valve that permits gas to escape into the room. It is also possible for gas to leak from the pipes, flowmeters, vaporizers, vaporizer selector switches, and vaporizer mounts on the machine.[12,18,40-46]

The interface hose from the anesthesia machine to the breathing circuit and the breathing circuit itself may be the sources of a leak.[32-36] Disconnections and leaks of sufficient magnitude lead to hypercarbia. Flow of gas from the machine to the circuit may be obstructed either in the machine or in the interface hose.[47-50] Leaks in valve housings, tracheal tubes, ventilator hoses, reservoir bag, ventilator bellows, and system relief valves can reduce the volume in the breathing system and cause hypercarbia.[12,18,51-66] In addition, subatmospheric pressure applied to the breathing system can reduce the system volume and cause hypercarbia. Sources of subatmospheric pressure are

---

Box 16-3. Causes of hypercarbia

Patient factors during spontaneous breathing

Central respiratory depression
Muscle relaxants
Motor blockade (regional anesthesia)
Airway obstruction
Severe pulmonary shunting

Delivery system problems

Apnea (failure to initiate or continue controlled ventilation)
Inadequate minute ventilation (low tidal volume or respiratory rate)
Increased apparatus dead space
Missing or incompetent unidirectional valves
Incorrectly assembled circle system
Exhausted carbon dioxide absorbent or channeling
Carbon dioxide absorber by-pass open (certain older systems)
Unintended administration of carbon dioxide
Inadequate fresh gas flow in a system without carbon dioxide absorption

---

vacuum hoses on scavenger interfaces, nasogastric tubes that have been placed in the trachea and suctioned, and sampling catheters from side-stream gas analysis systems (see Chapter 8).[67]

The anesthesia ventilator can cause hypercarbia if the settings are such that inadequate alveolar ventilation is provided. Either the rate may be too low or the tidal volume may be too small. On ventilators that allow one to set the tidal volume, ventilatory rate, inspiratory-to-expiratory ratio, and flow of compressing gas independently of each other, smaller tidal volumes than desired may be delivered. The reason for this is that the ventilator may cycle to exhalation before the bellows empties completely and delivers the preset volume to the patient. Factors that can cause this problem are high respiratory rate, low I:E ratio, low rate of inflow of the ventilator driving gas, and decreased pulmonary compliance. This problem can be discovered by careful observation of the ventilator bellows and monitoring of the exhaled tidal volume.

Low pulmonary compliance also causes volume to be lost because some of the tidal volume expands the compliant breathing circuit tubing. This volume is measured by the circuit spirometer during exhalation, but it does not contribute to the alveolar ventilation. Pressure-preset ventilators may cycle to exhalation before an adequate tidal volume has been delivered. This also causes hypercarbia if it is unrecognized. Therefore it is important to monitor the tidal volume and minute ventilation and not to assume that the amount set on the ventilator will in fact be delivered to the patient. Under this circumstance it would be better to monitor arterial and end-tidal carbon dioxide.

Fresh gas from the anesthesia machine contributes to the ventilator tidal volume and minute ventilation that the

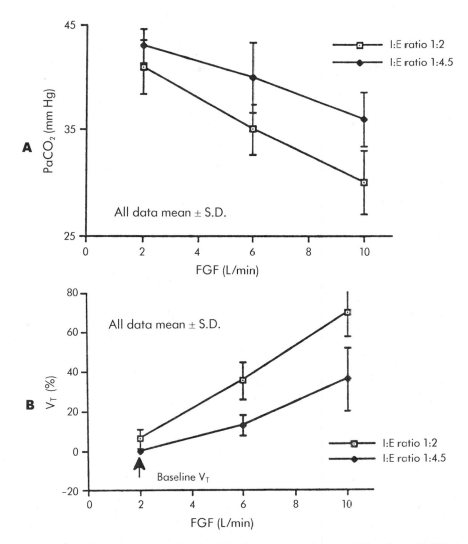

Fig. 16-4. A, Effect of fresh-gas flow and inspiratory-to-expiratory (*I:E*) ratio on $PaCO_2$ in patients during mechanical ventilation using an anesthesia ventilator with fixed rate and bellows tidal volume. Note that as fresh-gas flow increases, or the *I:E* ratio increases from 1:4.5 to 1:2, $PaCO_2$ decreases. This is due to an increase in alveolar ventilation caused by an increase in tidal volume. Conversely, a decrease in fresh-gas flow or *I:E* ratio results in a decrease in $PaCO_2$. The volume of gas added to the circuit during each inspiration is that exiting the ventilator bellows plus that fresh-gas flow entering the circuit during inspiration (when the ventilator relief valve is closed). The latter volume is $[I/(I+E)] \times [FGF/f]$, where f is the respiratory rate. Patient tidal volume, which determines alveolar ventilation and therefore $PaCO_2$ is determined by the above formula, less gas compressed in the circuit during inspiration. This volume is calculated as: Circuit compliance × Peak Inspiratory Pressure. **B,** Effect of fresh-gas flow and *I:E* ratio on measured tidal volume V_T during mechanical ventilation using an anesthesia ventilator at fixed rate and bellows tidal volume. As fresh-gas flow or *I:E* ratio increases, the measured V_T increases because during inspiration the fresh-gas inflow is added to the delivered bellows tidal volume. (From Scheller MS, Jones BR, Benumof JL: The influence of fresh gas flow and *I:E* ratio on tidal volume and $PaCO_2$ in ventilated patients, *J Cardiothoracic Anesth* 3:564, 1989.)

patient receives. This is because the fresh-gas flow entering the circuit during inspiration represents additional tidal volume. If the patient is normocarbic and the fresh-gas flow is reduced, or if the *I:E* ratio is changed such that exhalation is prolonged, the result is a decreased tidal volume and an increase in $PaCO_2$[68,69] (Fig. 16-4).

The carbon dioxide absorber may cause hypercarbia by acting as a source of leaks from the circuit or by failing to absorb the carbon dioxide produced by the patient. The absorber may not be closed and sealed properly. Improperly applied gaskets and absorbent granules on the gaskets can prevent the absorber canister from being sealed.

Failure to close the handle can also cause a huge leak.[70] Exhausted granules and channeling of gas through the absorber prevent the absorption of carbon dioxide. This causes rebreathing of exhaled gas and hypercarbia. Finally, machines equipped with absorber bypass switches allow the exhaled carbon dioxide to be rebreathed. If this is not monitored carefully, the patient may become hypercarbic.

The color of the dye in the carbon dioxide absorbent indicates whether or not the absorbent has been exhausted. However, it has been noted that the ethyl violet indicator can be photodeactivated by fluorescent lights and can thereby give the false impression that the absorbent is fresh when it is in fact exhausted.[71] On machines that have carbon dioxide flowmeters, their unintentional or improper use may act as a source of hypercarbia.[72,73]

The breathing circuit, by increasing apparatus dead space, can increase dead space ventilation and act as a cause of hypercarbia. Specifically, the unidirectional inspiratory and expiratory valves may be absent or broken, or they may malfunction in the open position. Large volume tubes (e.g., goosenecks) placed between the Y piece of the breathing circle and the tracheal tube increase dead space and may cause hypercarbia if compensatory ventilatory maneuvers are not employed.

The components of the breathing circuit must be arranged in such a way as to prevent rebreathing. Three arrangements of the circle system must be avoided:

1. The fresh-gas inlet must not be between the patient and the expiratory unidirectional valve.
2. The adjustable pressure limit (pop-off) valve must not be between the patient and the inspiratory unidirectional valve.
3. The reservoir bag must not be between the patient and the inspiratory or expiratory unidirectional valves.[74]

The Mapleson systems will permit the rebreathing of carbon dioxide and allow hypercarbia to develop if appropriate precautions are not taken. For example the Mapleson A circuit (the Magill attachment) should be used only with spontaneously breathing patients, and the fresh-gas flow must be at least 0.7 times the minute ventilation. In addition, the hose between the patient and the reservoir bag must be long enough so that exhaled carbon dioxide does not reach the reservoir bag[18,75] (Fig. 16-2).

The Mapleson B and C systems always permit the rebreathing of exhaled carbon dioxide because exhaled gas is directed into a blind pouch. In order to prevent hypercarbia with these systems fresh-gas flows of 1.5 to 2.5 times normal minute ventilation must be used and the patient must be hyperventilated. If the patient is breathing spontaneously the metabolic work performed increases. However, controlled ventilation with these circuits does not create this problem because the work of breathing is not being performed by the patient.[75]

The T-piece systems, Mapleson D, E, F, function similarly. Fresh-gas flows of 2.5 to 3 times minute ventilation prevent rebreathing at calculated normal minute ventilation. Alternatively, reduced fresh-gas flows can be employed, but hypercarbia is prevented by hyperventilation. If the fresh gas connection is disrupted, hypercarbia will occur. This may be an especially difficult problem with the Bain circuit (coaxial Mapleson D) because the disconnected or kinked inner hose may go unnoticed (see also Chapters 4 and 26).[41,76-79]

Some anesthesia machines have circle systems, which do not have carbon dioxide absorbers. As with the Mapleson D circuit, patients need fresh-gas flows of 2.5 to 3 times the calculated minute ventilation or hyperventilation at lower fresh-gas flows in order to avoid hypercarbia.

Hypocarbia

When carbon dioxide elimination exceeds production, $PaCO_2$ falls. When equilibrium between the two processes is achieved, a new steady state develops and $PaCO_2$ stabilizes. General anesthesia, muscle relaxants, and hypothermia reduce metabolic rate. If minute ventilation is not decreased the patient becomes hypocarbic. In addition, hyperventilation in general causes hypocarbia.

Hyperventilation and the resultant hypocarbia can be caused by simply having either the tidal volume, ventilatory rate, or both set too high. The fresh-gas flow, which contributes to the minute ventilation, will cause the patient to become hypocarbic if its contribution is not taken into account when the ventilator is set. In patients with very compliant lungs the contribution of the fresh-gas flow may be very significant.[68,69] The driving gas from the ventilator may increase ventilation if there is a leak in the bellows. Driving gas can enter the breathing circuit, increase the volume delivered to the patient, and also affect the composition of the circuit gases. The result is hyperventilation of the patient with an unintended gas mixture.[38,39,80]

Circuit pressure and volume problems

Essential to delivery of anesthesia to, and oxygenation and ventilation of, the patient is adequate movement of gases between the delivery system and the patient's lungs. Four basic causes of failure of this function have been described by Schreiber[12] as follows:

1. Occlusion in the ventilatory (inspiratory or expiratory) pathway
2. Insufficient amount of gas in the breathing system
3. Failure to initiate artificial ventilation when required
4. Disconnection in the breathing system during mechanical ventilation

Occlusions. The anesthesia system is composed of numerous tubes that may become occluded.[81] In general, such occlusions can be found outside the tube, within the wall, or within the lumen of the tube. Tubing misconnec-

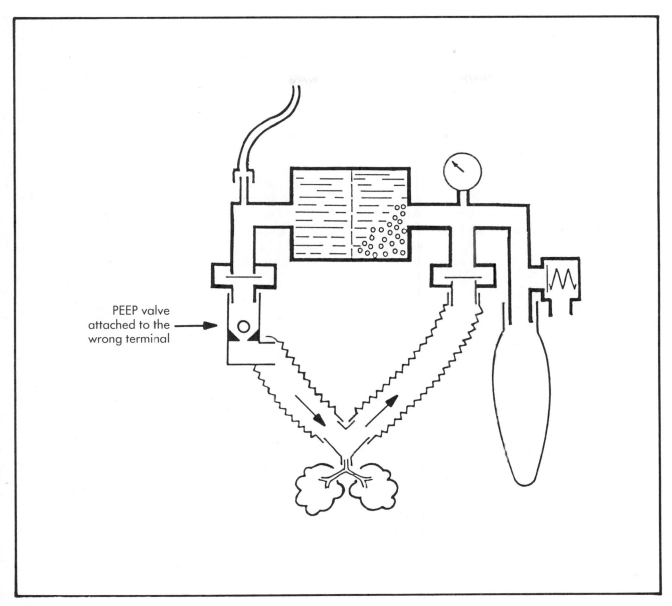

Fig. 16-5. A PEEP valve that permits flow in one direction only will block the inspiratory path if erroneously attached to the inspiratory limb. (From Schreiber P: *Safety guidelines for anesthesia systems,* Telford, Pa, 1985, North American Dräger.)

tions have become less common since the introduction of standard diameters. However, if adapters are used, misconnections are still possible. In general, circuit tubing connections are 22 mm in diameter, scavenging tubing is 19 mm in diameter, and the common gas outlet and tracheal tube connectors are 15 mm in diameter.[12] Accessories added to the circuit may cause an obstruction. Filters placed in the circuit, incorrectly connected humidifiers, and manufacturing defects in tubing have all been reported as causes of total occlusion of the breathing circuit.[18,82-84]

A freestanding positive end-expiratory pressure (PEEP) valve may cause obstruction if it is incorrectly placed in the inspiratory limb of a circle system.[11,12] The PEEP valves that use a weighted ball (such as those made by Boehringer Company, Wynnewood, Pa.) are designed to be mounted vertically on the expiratory side of a circle system. In one case, the weighted-ball PEEP valve was erroneously placed horizontally and reversed in the expiratory limb between the circuit and the exhalation unidirectional valve. When the oxygen flush was operated, the metal ball was driven downstream, totally obstructing the PEEP valve and circuit, preventing exhalation, and causing elevated intrathoracic pressure. In another case, the PEEP valve was placed on the inhalation side in reversed fashion; this caused total obstruction on the inhalation side of the circuit and prevented inspiration (Fig. 16-5). Because of such potential errors, many consider freestanding PEEP valves to be undesirable (see also Chapter 4).[85]

Although total occlusion of the breathing circuit should activate a pressure or volume alarm in most cases, depending on the system used, these alarms may be fooled when the tracheal tube is totally occluded.[11] Consider a breathing circuit with a pressure-monitoring system incorporating a fixed setting of +65 cm H_2O for the high-pressure alarm limit threshold, such as that used on the Dräger Narkomed 2A anesthesia machine. When the tracheal tube becomes totally obstructed (due to a kink or total intraluminal obstruction), the pressure rises in the circuit, which satisfies the low-pressure alarm. However, unless the pressure reaches +65 cm H_2O, the high-pressure alarm is not activated. The peak pressure achieved in the circuit during inspiration depends on the inspiratory flow control setting (which determines the driving pressure available to compress the bellows), the preset tidal volume, the inspiratory time, and the fresh-gas inflow rate from the anesthesia machine. At low ventilator inspiratory flow settings, the driving pressure of the ventilator may be 50 cm H_2O or less, which, when combined with normal rates of fresh-gas inflow from the machine, may result in failure of the peak inspiratory pressure to reach the high-pressure alarm threshold of +65 cm H_2O. During exhalation, excess gas is released normally from the patient circuit. The volume alarm may also be fooled in this situation, depending on its low-limit threshold setting. In the system described, the low-volume alarm threshold was fixed at 80 ml. This situation involved total failure to ventilate the patient and would be immediately detectable by continuous capnometry, by pressure and volume alarms whose thresholds can be set close to the normal values for that particular patient, or by continuous monitoring of breath sounds.

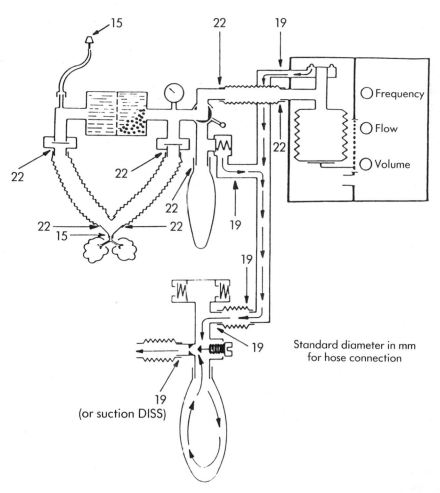

Fig. 16-6. The diagram illustrates the different diameters for hose terminals in the anesthesia breathing and scavenger systems. Unrelieved subatmospheric pressure from the scavenger system can be applied directly to the patient circuit through the adjustable pressure limiting (APL) valve. This creates subatmospheric pressure in the breathing circuit and consequently in the lungs. (From Schreiber P: *Safety guidelines for anesthesia systems,* Telford, Pa, 1985, North American Dräger.)

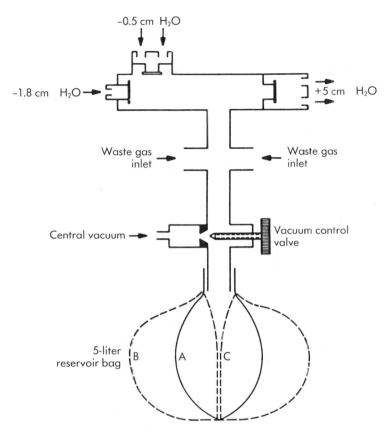

Fig. 16-7. Dräger closed scavenger interface. *A,* Normal state of scavenging reservoir bag; *B,* inadequate removal or excessive delivery rate of waste gas to interface. Bag is distended and excess gas is vented when pressure exceeds 5 cm H_2O; *C,* excessive suction or inadequate rate of delivery of waste gas to scavenger interface. Reservoir bag is collapsed, and room air is entrained via negative pressure relief valve(s). (Reproduced by permission of North American Dräger, Inc., Telford, Pa.).

Misconnections and obstructions can usually be prevented or detected by testing of the breathing circuit before use with all accessories in place and in spontaneous, assisted, and controlled ventilation modes. Occasionally an obstruction can develop because of failure of a component during the case.[86]

Inadequate amount of gas in the breathing system. An insufficient volume of gas in the breathing system may be attributable to inadequate delivery or excessive loss. Inadequate delivery may be caused by failure of gas delivery to the machine or from the common gas outlet.[37,81] A decrease in oxygen supply pressure to the machine may cause a decrease in gas flows set at the flowmeters. Flow setting errors may occur. A disconnection, misconnection, or obstruction between the machine's common gas outlet and the patient circuit have a similar effect.

Inadequate volume of gas in the circuit may be caused by excessive removal. An active scavenging system utilizes wall suction to remove the waste gases from the scavenging interface. Excess negative pressure may be applied to the circuit if the negative-pressure relief (pop-in) valve or valves on the interface should become occluded.[87] A similar situation can arise with an open-reservoir scavenging system if the relief ports become occluded while suction is applied to the interface. A high subatmospheric pressure in the scavenging system may open the circuit adjustable pressure-limiting (APL) valve, transmitting the subatmospheric pressure to the patient circuit. If a ventilator were being used, unrelieved excess negative pressure in the scavenging system would in most cases tend to hold the ventilator pressure-relief valve to its seat, preventing its opening on exhalation and causing a high pressure to develop in the circuit[67] (Figs. 16-6 and 16-7).

A side-stream gas analyzer (such as a multiplexed mass spectrometer) connected to the patient circuit has been reported as the cause of excessive negative pressure in a breathing circuit where the fresh-gas flow of 50 ml/min during cardiopulmonary bypass was less than the mass spectrometer's gas sampling rate of 250 ml/min.[67] Sampling rates of commonly used gas analyzers vary between less than 50 ml/min to as high as 800 ml/min; therefore, considerable potential exists for creating negative pressure in the circuit if low fresh-gas flow rates are being used.[67]

Excess gas removal by a sampling device during spontaneous ventilation creates a subatmospheric pressure in the circuit that in turn causes the APL valve to close. This prevents the scavenging system negative-pressure relief valve or valves from relieving the negative pressure in the circuit. Maximum circuit subatmospheric pressure achieved by side-stream sampling devices during testing ranged from -11 to -148 mm Hg.[67] Such low pressures, if transmitted to the patient's airway, can lead to barotrauma and cardiovascular dysfunction.

Excessive volume loss resulting in negative pressures in the breathing system may arise if hospital suction is applied through the working channel of a fiberoptic bronchoscope that has been inserted into the system through an airway diaphragm adapter or by a suction catheter that has been accidentally advanced alongside the tracheal tube into the trachea.

Inadequate circuit volume and negative pressure may occur during spontaneous ventilation in the presence of a low fresh-gas flow rate and inadequate size of reservoir bag (such as a pediatric size used with an adult patient). During inspiration, the reservoir bag will collapse and a negative pressure will arise in the circuit. Circuit APL valves usually have a minimum opening pressure that is slightly greater than that needed to distend the reservoir bag. If the bag were of correct size but noncompliant, or if the APL valve had a low opening pressure, during exhalation most of the gas would exit through the APL valve rather than fill the bag. The net result would be an inadequate reservoir volume for the next inspiration.[12] Modern circuit pressure monitors incorporate a subatmospheric-pressure alarm such that when pressure is less than -10 cm H_2O at any time, audible and visual alarms are triggered.[88,89]

Failure to initiate artificial ventilation. Failure to initiate artificial ventilation is usually attributable to an operator error. The error may be failure to turn on the ventilator (for example, after tracheal intubation or separation from cardiopulmonary bypass), setting a respiratory rate of zero breaths per minute, failure to select the "automatic" (ventilator) setting at the "manual/automatic" selector switch in the circuit, or failure to connect the ventilator circuit hose (either at the patient circuit connector by the selector switch or at the bag mount).[12] Because some older circuit volume and pressure alarms must be deliberately enabled or are enabled only when the ventilator is on, these monitors will not detect that the ventilator has not been turned on. In this respect, continuous capnography provides the most sensitive monitor of ventilation. If the delivery system incorporates a standing-bellows ventilator, failure to connect the ventilator tubing to the circuit will cause the bellows to collapse. With either bellows design, when a ventilator is turned on but the "manual" (bag) mode is selected at the selector switch, then during inspiration the bellows will attempt to empty against a total obstruction and its failure to empty will be readily observed. Failure to ventilate in this situation is annunciated by both low-pressure and volume alarms. Some older designs of

circle system lack a "manual/automatic" selector switch, and the APL valve must be closed to effect intermittent positive-pressure ventilation (IPPV) when the ventilator hose is connected to the bag mount. Failure to close the APL valve is yet another cause of failure to initiate IPPV.

Even if the breathing system incorporates a selector switch, there are occasions when the primary anesthesia ventilator fails and a free-standing ventilator is brought in to provide IPPV. The foregoing considerations then apply if the new ventilator is connected to the circuit via the bag mount connection; that is, the "manual" mode is selected and the APL valve is closed.

Leaks and disconnections in the breathing system. Breathing circuit disconnections and leaks are among the most common of anesthesia mishaps.[1,2,51,90] Anesthesia breathing systems contain numerous basic connections, and as more monitors, humidifiers, filters, and PEEP valves are added additional connections are needed (Fig. 16-8). Disconnections cannot be totally prevented; although some consider the 15-mm connector between the tracheal tube and the circuit a safety fuse to prevent unintentional extubation, most prefer a secure system that does not disconnect.[91] Circuit disconnections and their detection have been the subject of several reviews. Cooper, et al.[1] found that disconnections of the patient from the machine were responsible for 7.5% of critical incidents involving human error or equipment failure. Of these disconnections, about 70% occur at the Y piece.[1,2,11,51,90]

The risks of disconnection are reduced by secure locking of connecting components, use of disconnect (pressure, volume, capnography) alarms, and user education. Making secure friction connections, such as those between the tracheal tube and elbow adapter or between the adapter and the Y piece, requires that the user employ a pushing and twisting motion rather than merely pushing the two units together. When a disconnection occurs, the anesthesiologist must systematically trace the flow of gases through the breathing system, looking for the disconnection in the same way as would be done in the event of a no-gas-flow or obstruction situation.

Most disconnections are detectable by the basic breathing system monitors of pressure and volume. Pressure monitors annunciate an alarm if the peak inspiratory pressure in the circuit fails to reach the threshold low setting. The alarm setting on the monitor should be user adjustable; the user should be able to set it to a level just below the usual peak inspiratory pressure. Some monitors provide a continuous graphic display of the circuit pressure as well as of the alarm threshold or thresholds.[88] A response algorithm for the low-pressure alarm condition has been proposed[92] (Fig. 16-9).

The circuit low-pressure alarm can be fooled if it is not set at the correct sensitivity. Thus a circuit disconnection at the Y piece combined with sufficient resistance at the patient connector end may not trigger the low-pressure

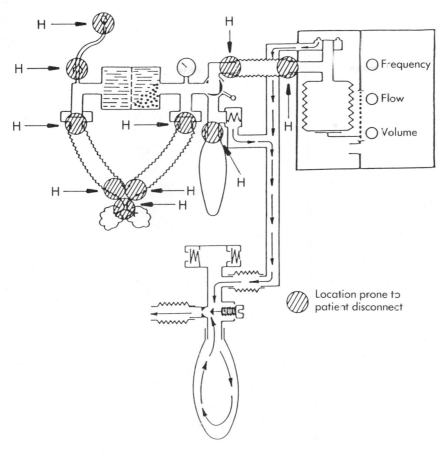

Fig. 16-8. A circle breathing system showing connecting points (indicated by *H*) with a potential for disconnects. (From Schreiber P: *Safety guidelines for anesthesia systems*, Telford, Pa, 1985, North American Dräger.)

alarm if inspiratory gas flow from the ventilator bellows is high enough and the low-pressure alarm threshold is crossed. Examples include unintended extubation of a patient who has a small-diameter tracheal tube where the tube connector offers a high resistance to gas flow, or occlusion of the open patient connector by the drapes.[12] A circuit low-pressure alarm sensing pressure in the absorber may be fooled if there is a high resistance between the inspiratory tubing connector and the Y piece, such as may be attributable to a cascade humidifier in the inspiratory limb of the circle.[93] Humidifiers may also represent the source of a detectable leak in the anesthesia circuit.[64]

A circuit low-pressure alarm is less likely to be fooled when a standing-bellows ventilator is being used, because failure of the bellows to fill adequately during exhalation will lead to lower peak pressures on the next inspiration (Fig. 16-10). With the hanging-bellows design, the peak inspiratory pressure with a disconnect tends to be higher than with a standing-bellows ventilator disconnect, the hanging bellows having filled completely during exhalation. A pressure alarm set to an inappropriately low threshold is therefore more likely to be fooled by a hanging-bellows ventilator (Fig. 16-11).

The common gas outlet of the anesthesia machine was a site of disconnections before the use of retaining devices.[32] The diameter of the tubing connecting the common gas outlet with the circuit is relatively narrow and offers relatively high resistance to gas flow compared with the 22-mm-diameter circuit tubing. If a hanging-bellows ventilator were being used with a large tidal volume setting, the machine-to-circuit connector-tubing resistance may be such that during inspiration the low-pressure alarm limit would be exceeded despite the leak.[32] During exhalation, room air would be entrained via the fresh-gas inflow tubing to refill the bellows (Fig. 16-11). A disconnection of this tubing may also lead to a hypoxic gas mixture in the circuit as air is entrained and oxygen is consumed. Detection of this type of disconnection, which is associated with air entrainment, is aided by an oxygen analyzer with an appropriately set concentration alarm threshold located in the patient circuit.

If, as is recommended, the circuit low-pressure alarm has been set to just below the peak inspiratory pressure, it should be recognized that more false-positive alarms will be generated. Thus, at a constant tidal volume setting, a decrease in fresh-gas flow, *I:E* ratio, or inspiratory flow

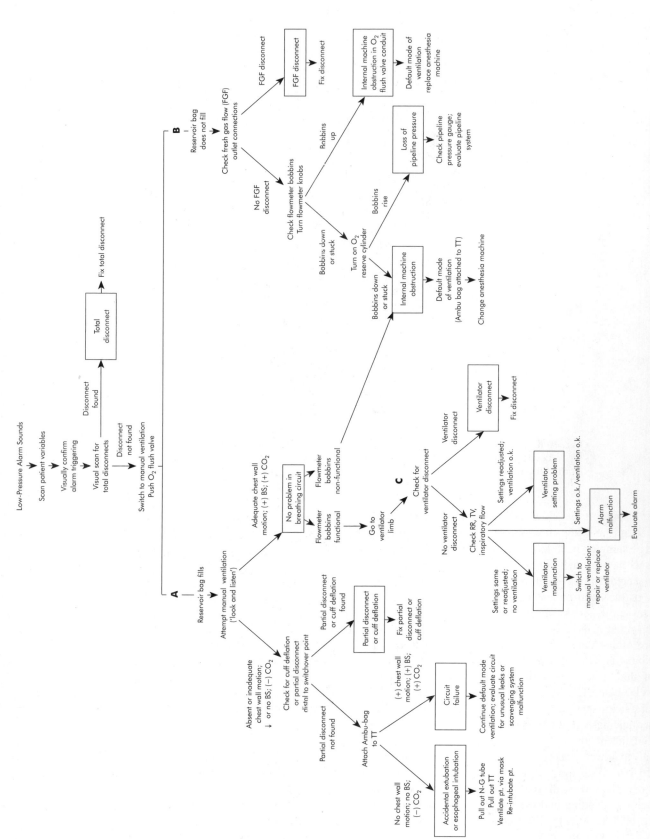

Fig. 16-9. Response algorithm for a low-pressure alarm condition. The three limbs of the algorithm are (*A*) the breathing circuit limb, (*B*) the fresh-gas flow limb, and (*C*) the ventilator limb. BS-breath sounds; TT tracheal tube. (From Raphael DT, Weller RS, Doran DJ: A response algorithm for the low-pressure alarm condition, *Anesth Analg* 67:876-883, 1988. Reproduced by permission of the International Anesthesia Research Society.)

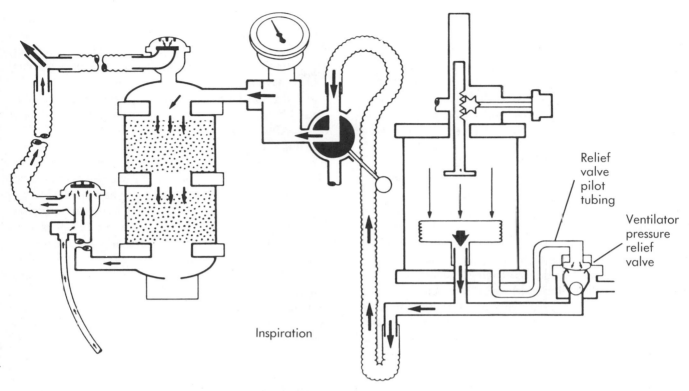

Relief
valve
pilot
tubing

Ventilator
pressure
relief
valve

Inspiration

Fig. 16-10. Dräger AV-E standing-bellows ventilator in inspiratory cycle. When a disconnect in the breathing circuit occurs with the standing-bellows ventilator, the bellows falls and does not re-expand until the circuit is made gas-tight again. (Reproduced by permission of North American Dräger, Inc., Telford, Pa.)

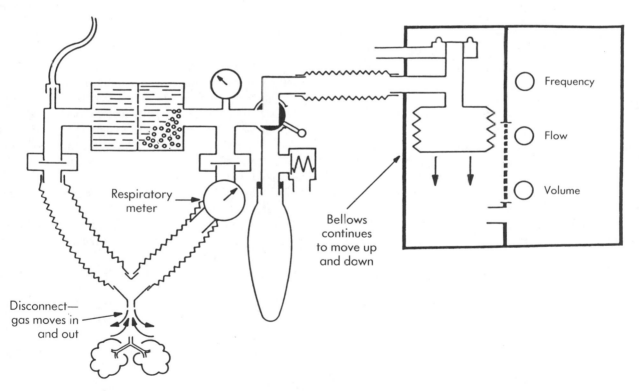

Frequency

Flow

Volume

Respiratory
meter

Bellows
continues
to move up
and down

Disconnect—
gas moves in
and out

Fig. 16-11. Safety limitation of descending (hanging) bellows design ventilator. In the event of a disconnect, the bellows continues its upward and downward movements. Room air is drawn into the circuit during exhalation as the bellows descends. During inspiration, gas flow may be sufficient to satisfy a low-threshold pressure alarm. (From Schreiber P: *Safety guidelines for anesthesia systems,* Telford, Pa, 1985, North American Dräger.)

rate, or an increase in respiratory rate will decrease the peak inspiratory pressure, thereby triggering the alarm. However a false-positive alarm, with an appropriate response, is preferable to failing to detect a potentially hazardous situation, provided that the user does not permanently silence the alarm (see Chapter 17).

Leaks from the circuit, other than those attributable to component disconnection, may also result in inadequate exchange of gas between system and patient. Leaks may arise in any component because of cracking, incorrect assembly, or malfunction of a system component, particularly the ventilator pressure-relief valve.[52,54,60,64,94]

During inspiration, the ventilator pressure-relief valve is normally held closed by the pressure of the driving gas from the bellows housing (Fig. 16-10). If this valve is not held closed during inspiration, then gas in the patient circuit may be vented to the scavenging system rather than going to the patient. Incompetence of the ventilator pressure-relief valve has been reported in connection with pilot-line disconnection or occlusion and valve damage.[52-54,95] In such a situation, the loss of volume from the circuit would be detected by appropriately set pressure and volume alarms, but the source of the leak might be less obvious. If a closed-reservoir scavenging system is in use, the diagnosis is made by observation of the scavenging system reservoir bag (Fig. 16-7).[53] The bag normally fills during exhalation, as gas is released from the patient circuit, and empties during inspiration, when the ventilator pressure-relief valve is closed. If the ventilator pressure-relief valve is incompetent, the scavenging system reservoir bag will be seen to fill during the inspiration, as the ventilator bellows empties its contained gas into the scavenging system.[53]

Leaks and malfunctions in the patient circuit are sometimes first detected by an airway gas monitor capable of measuring nitrogen.[96] Application of negative pressure to the circuit by a malfunctioning scavenging system, or intermittently by a hanging-bellows ventilator during exhalation, may cause entrainment of air into the breathing system through a small leak otherwise unrecognized by pressure, volume, or even carbon dioxide monitoring.[96] A leak of room air or other gases into the patient circuit may result in dilution of the anesthesia gas mixture and, potentially in an extreme case, awareness under anesthesia.[97] Leaks into the patient circuit may occur if there is a hole in the ventilator bellows. In this case, the high pressure in the driving gas circuit forces driving gas into the patient circuit during inspiration. With an Ohmeda ventilator the diluting gas is 100% oxygen, but with a Dräger AV-E it is a mixture of air and oxygen.[98,99] Such an event might be detected by a change in inspired oxygen fraction (FiO_2), peak inspiratory pressure, tidal or minute volume, end-tidal carbon dioxide, or a multigas or agent analyzer.

High pressure in the breathing system. The anesthesia machine provides a continuous flow of gas to the pa-

tient circuit. Whenever circuit gas inflow rate exceeds outflow rate, excessive pressures can develop. If these pressures are transmitted to the patient's lungs, severe cardiovascular compromise, barotrauma, and even pneumothorax may arise.[100,101]

During spontaneous ventilation, high pressure may be caused by inadequate opening (or even complete closure) of the APL valve, kinking or occlusion of the tubing between the APL valve and the scavenging interface, or malfunction of the interface positive-pressure relief valve. During spontaneous ventilation, the bag will distend to accommodate the excess gas. Reservoir bags are highly distensible and limit the maximum circuit pressure to approximately 45 cm H_2O. Nevertheless, such an airway pressure could produce hypotension by inhibiting venous return. Increases in circuit pressure will be more rapid when the fresh-gas inflow rate is high, for example, during prolonged use of the oxygen flush.[102]

Excessive pressure in the circuit may occur during use of an anesthesia ventilator. During inspiration the ventilator pressure-relief valve is normally held closed (Fig. 16-10). Thus a high inspiratory gas-flow rate will be associated with increased peak pressures in the circuit.

There are many reports of ventilator malfunctions causing excessive circuit pressures. Failure of the ventilator to cycle from inspiration to expiration results in driving gas continuing to enter (Dräger) or enter but not leave (Ohmeda) the bellows housing. This causes the ventilator pressure-relief valve to remain closed and excess pressure to build up within the circuit. The pressure increase is limited by the driving gas pressure prevailing in the bellows housing.[102] In Dräger ventilators, this pressure depends on the setting of the inspiratory flow-control knob.[12,94]

Other reported causes of the ventilator pressure-relief valve failing to open normally include mechanical obstruction of the driving gas exhaust system (Dräger AV-E muffler),[103] kinking of a Dräger AV-E ventilator pressure-relief valve pilot line during inspiration,[94] failure of a solenoid valve causing persistent inhalation, and diffusion of nitrous oxide into the space between the two pieces of rubber constituting the relief valve diaphragm, causing insidious PEEP.[104] Even with normal ventilator function, high pressures in the circuit may be caused by occlusion of the tubing between the ventilator pressure-relief valve outlet and the scavenging system (Fig. 16-12) or by obstruction of the scavenging interface pop-off valve. In such cases, as the pressure in the patient circuit rises, the ventilator bellows empties less completely and may even become distorted.

High pressures arising in the circuit are detected by the circuit pressure monitor, which incorporates two types of alarms.[12] A continuing-pressure alarm is annunciated usually when the circuit pressure remains in excess of +15 cm H_2O for more than 10 seconds. A high-pressure alarm is annunciated when the circuit pressure exceeds the

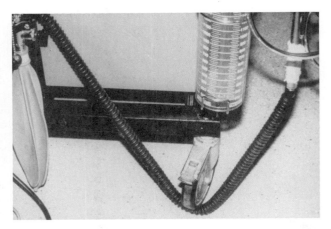

Fig. 16-12. High pressure in the patient circuit due to occlusion of the tubing between the circuit APL valve and the scavenging interface. Note that the scavenging interface reservoir bag is collapsed.

threshold limit, which, in modern monitors, is set by the user but has a default setting of 50 to 65 cm H_2O, depending on the unit. When either of these alarms is annunciated during mechanical ventilation, a problem should be suspected with the ventilator circuit. Circuit pressure can be immediately relieved by disconnection of the patient from the circuit at the Y piece, inspiratory hose, or expiratory hoses, or by selecting the manual (bag) mode and relieving pressure by opening the adjustable pressure-limiting valve. The incorporation of safety relief valves into the circuit as a protection against high pressures has not been popular, because these devices limit the ability to ventilate a patient with poor total thoracic compliance.[12]

As a protection against development of excessive pressures in the patient circuit during mechanical ventilation, pressure limiting devices are available from both Ohmeda and Dräger. The Ohmeda 7800 series ventilators incorporate an inspiratory high- pressure limit such that when the selected threshold (pressure measured in patient circuit downstream of the inspiratory unidirectional valve) is exceeded, the ventilator cycles to expiration, driving gas circuit pressure falls to zero, and excess patient circuit gas is discharged to the scavenging system via the ventilator pressure-relief valve. Basic Dräger AV-E ventilators are not pressure-limited, but a pressure-limit control is available and may be retrofitted to certain standing-bellows design AV-E units.[105] The Dräger pressure-limit control device senses the pressure in the patient circuit at the bellows, and whenever the threshold high-pressure limit is exceeded, a valve opens in the driving gas circuit (bellows housing) to release excess driving gas to the atmosphere, thereby limiting driving gas pressure such that patient circuit pressure does not exceed the set limit for the remainder of the inspiration. The time cycling (*I:E* ratio and set ventilatory rate) of the Dräger AV-E is thus maintained,[105]

in contrast to the Ohmeda 7800 series ventilators.[106] Both the Dräger and the Ohmeda approaches to limiting pressure in the patient circuit require a normally functioning ventilator pressure-relief valve, because it is through this valve (the opening pressure of which is controlled by the pressure in the driving gas circuit) that excess gas and pressure is relieved from the patient circuit. If the pressure-relief valve or its outflow path should become obstructed, neither the Dräger nor the Ohmeda pressure-limiting mechanisms would be effective in relieving pressure in the patient circuit.

Anesthetic agent dosage and administration problems

Patient complications may arise as a result of an anesthetic agent overdosage or underdosage or administration of an incorrect agent. Hazards of vaporizer malfunction causing anesthetic overdosage or underdosage are caused by incorrect handling, incorrect agent use, human error, and, rarely, internal breakdown of the vaporizer itself.

Liquid agent in the fresh-gas piping. Lethal anesthetic agent overdosage may occur when excessive amounts of saturated vapor or even liquid agent enter the bypass portion of the vaporizer, the machine piping between the vaporizer and the common gas outlet, the interface hose, or the breathing circuit.[107] The overdosage situation is more likely with a measured-flow type of vaporizer arrangement (Copper Kettle or Verni-Trol), because calculation or flow setting errors can easily arise. In addition, some older designs of vaporizers can be overfilled so that excess liquid could enter the fresh gas piping. Modern vaporizers are concentration-calibrated and are designed to prevent overfilling (see also Chapter 3).[8]

Tilting or tipping of a vaporizer may cause liquid agent to enter the bypass of the vaporizer or the machine piping. One milliliter of liquid potent volatile agent produces approximately 200 ml of vapor at 20° C.[108] If 1 ml of liquid halothane were to enter the common gas piping, it would require 20 L of fresh gas to dilute the resulting vapor to a concentration of 1%, or a minimum alveolar concentration (MAC) of approximately 1.3. It is easy to appreciate how a relatively small volume of liquid agent in the wrong place can have a profound effect on a patient.

If a vaporizer has been tilted or tipped and there is concern that liquid agent may have leaked into the piping of the machine, then with no patient connected to the system, the vaporizer should be drained and then flushed with a high flow rate of oxygen from the flowmeter (not the oxygen flush, which bypasses the vaporizer), the vaporizer dial should be set to a high concentration during this procedure. If any doubt still exists as to the safe function of the vaporizer, it should be withdrawn from clinical service until certified safe for use by an authorized service representative. Additional caution is needed with a halothane vaporizer that has been tipped. Liquid halothane contains thymol, a sticky preservative that does not evaporate. Thy-

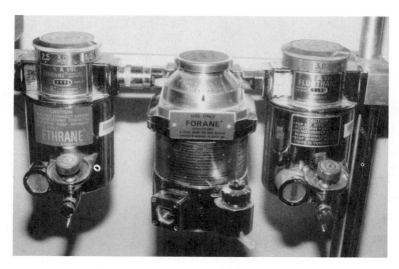

Fig. 16-13. Three concentration-calibrated vaporizers mounted in series. In the absence of an interlock device, all three are turned on and set to 3% output concentration so that vapor from the upstream vaporizers can enter the vaporizing chambers downstream. On the two outer vaporizers, concentration is increased by turning the dial clockwise, whereas in the center vaporizer, the modern convention is followed in that concentration is increased by turning the dial counterclockwise. (From Eisenkraft JB, Sommer RM: *Equipment failure: anesthesia delivery systems.* In Benumof JL, Saidman LJ, editors: *Anesthesia and perioperative complication,* St. Louis, 1992, Mosby–Year Book.)

mol entering the flow-control and temperature-compensating parts of a vaporizer could cause vaporizer malfunction even after the halothane has been flushed out of these parts.

Modern vaporizers are mounted on the back bar of the anesthesia machine. Ohmeda Tec 4 and Tec 5 vaporizers are designed to be easily mounted on or removed from Selectatec Series Mounted manifolds.[109,110] Because they are designed to be removable, Tec vaporizers incorporate an antispill mechanism that prevents liquid agent from entering the bypass sections. Dräger Vapor 19.1 vaporizers are not designed to be easily removed from the Narkomed machine.[111] These vaporizers should be removed by authorized service personnel only. These vaporizers do not incorporate an antispill mechanism; the risk of agent spillage is minimized by the "permanent" mounting. Nevertheless, liquid agent can spill in such vaporizers if the whole Dräger Narkomed anesthesia machine is tilted or even laid on its side, as may happen if the machine is too close to an electrically powered operating table that is being raised.

Design of the concentration dial. Anesthetic agent overdosage may also occur if a vaporizer delivers unexpectedly high concentrations. In modern vaporizers, output concentration increases when the dial is turned counterclockwise.[8] In some older vaporizers, turning the dial clockwise increases concentration. Some machines may still be equipped with the older design or even a combination of the two designs, which might therefore present a hazard if the dial is turned inappropriately (Fig. 16-13). It is therefore important that the anesthesiologist deliberately

observe the dial and calibration settings when changing a vaporizer dial concentration setting. In addition, it is desirable to uniformly equip machines with modern vaporizers which increase concentration by turning the dial counterclockwise.

Incorrect filling of vaporizers. Anesthetic agent overdosage or underdosage can occur if an agent-specific vaporizer is filled wholly or partially with an incorrect agent.[108,112] If an empty concentration-calibrated vaporizer designed for one agent is filled with an agent for which it was not designed, the vaporizer concentration output may be erroneous.[113,114] Because at room temperature the vaporizing characteristics of halothane and isoflurane are almost identical, this problem currently applies only to interchanging halothane or isoflurane with enflurane (see Chapter 3, Table 3-2).

A more dangerous situation would arise if a vaporizer designed for methoxyflurane (an agent with a saturated vapor pressure of 20.3 mm Hg at 20° C) were filled with halothane, enflurane, or isoflurane (see Chapter 3, Table 3-3). A methoxyflurane vaporizer filled with halothane and set to deliver 1% methoxyflurane (6 MAC of methoxyflurane) would deliver 14.8% (approximately 20 MAC) halothane. As the use of methoxyflurane has almost completely disappeared, such errors are now unlikely.

The outputs of erroneously filled vaporizers are shown in (Chapter 3, Table 3-4). Erroneous filling affects the output concentration and consequently the MAC or potency output of the vaporizer.[113] Thus an enflurane vaporizer set to 2% (1.19 MAC) but filled with halothane will deliver

3.21% (4.01 MAC) of halothane, that is, 3.3 times the anticipated anesthetic potency output (see Chapter 3, Table 3-5).[113]

Erroneous filling of vaporizers may be prevented by careful attention to the specific agent and the vaporizer when filling is performed. Agent-specific keyed filling mechanisms, analogous to the pin-index system for medical gases, are available as options on modern vaporizers.[18,109-11] Liquid anesthetic agents are available packaged in bottles that have agent-specific collars. An agent-specific filling device has one end that fits the collar on the agent bottle and another end that fits only the vaporizer designed for that agent. These filling devices, although well intentioned, have not gained much popularity. Thus agents are not always supplied in agent-specific collared bottles, and a problem with erroneous fitting of a collar to a bottle has even been reported.[115] The ASTM F1161-88 standard states that the vaporizer filling mechanism should be fitted with a permanently attached standard, agent-specific, keyed filling device to prevent accidental filling with the wrong agent.[8] Agent-specific filling devices will assume even greater importance if and when desflurane (see the section about desflurane Chapter 3) is introduced into general clinical use. Incorrectly filling a modern variable-bypass vaporizer (such as Tec 5) with desflurane could lead to very high concentration outputs of this agent. It can be calculated that an isoflurane variable-bypass vaporizer set to deliver 1% isoflurane (0.87 MAC) but filled with desflurane will deliver approximately 13% desflurane (2.6 AC) at 20° C. A small increase in temperature would lead to a drastically increased output concentration, and the situation could become uncontrolled and potentially lethal if the desflurane were to boil. The design features of a vaporizer for desflurane are discussed in Chapter 3.

Perhaps a more likely scenario is that an agent-specific vaporizer that is partially filled with a correct agent is topped up with an incorrect agent.[113] This situation is more complex and less easily predicted in terms of vaporizer output, and large errors can arise in delivered vapor administration. Halothane, enflurane, and isoflurane, when mixed, do not react chemically but do influence the extent of each other's ease of vaporization. Halothane facilitates the vaporization of both enflurane and isoflurane and in the process is itself more likely to vaporize.[116] The clinical consequences depend on the potencies of each of the mixed agents as well as on the delivered vapor concentrations. If a halothane vaporizer 25% full is refilled to 100% with isoflurane and set to deliver 1%, the halothane output is 0.41% (0.51 MAC) and the isoflurane output is 0.9% (0.78 MAC) (Chapter 3, Table 3-5).[113] In this case, the output potency of 1.29 MAC is not far from the 1.25 MAC (1% halothane) expected.

On the other hand, an enflurane vaporizer 25% full and set to deliver 2% (1.19 MAC) enflurane, that is filled to 100% with halothane has an output of 2.43% (3.03 MAC) halothane and 0.96% (0.57 MAC) enflurane.[113] This rep-

resents a total MAC of 3.6, or three times that intended. In any event, it is important that erroneous filling of vaporizers be avoided. If erroneous filling is suspected, the vaporizer should be emptied and, if necessary, serviced, flushed, and refilled with the correct agent.

Simultaneous use of more than one vaporizer. Modern anesthesia vaporizers incorporate an interlock system to prevent simultaneous use of more than one vaporizer and agent.[8] Older anesthesia machine designs had up to three variable-bypass vaporizers arranged in series such that fresh gas passed through each vaporizer (albeit the bypass flow) to reach the common gas outlet of the anesthesia machine. Without an interlock device, which would have permitted only one vaporizer to be in use at any time, it was possible to have all three vaporizers on simultaneously (Fig. 16-13). Apart from potentially overdosing the patient, the agent from the upstream vaporizer could contaminate the agent or agents in the downstream vaporizers.[2,117,118] During subsequent use, the output of the downstream vaporizer would be contaminated and the concentration of the emerging gas and vapor mixture would be indeterminate and might even be lethal. With such in-series arrangements, care must be taken to ensure that only one vaporizer is on at any time and, to minimize risk in case cross-contamination should occur, the sequence of vaporizers from upstream to downstream should be such that the agent that has the lowest saturated vapor pressure is upstream (that is, farthest from the patient). The correct series sequence is therefore methoxyflurane, enflurane, isoflurane, halothane, with halothane being closest to the common gas outlet of the anesthesia machine. As the use of safety interlocking devices increases, the foregoing may be of historical interest only.

Although vaporizer interlock systems represent a desirable (and now standard) safety feature on modern machines, failures of these systems have been reported.[8,119,120] Failure may result in more than one vaporizer being on at the same time.[119] Exclusion of the selected vaporizer has been described with a Selectatec system.[120] It is therefore important that the anesthesiologist check the interlock system periodically for correct function.

The safety features of the vaporizer interlock system can also be defeated if a free-standing vaporizer is used in series with the fresh-gas flow but downstream of the common gas outlet. Such arrangements, configured by the user, are potentially dangerous and should not be used.[121]

Pumping effect. Measured-flow and some other, older, designs of concentration-calibrated vaporizers were subject to the so-called pumping effect, which could result in increased output concentrations during mechanical ventilation when low fresh-gas flow rates were in use. The explanation for this effect is that, during positive-pressure ventilation, increased pressure in the vaporizer caused bypass gas to enter the vaporizing chamber of the vaporizer, thereby increasing output.[18] Recent vaporizing systems are designed to be compensated for or protected against the

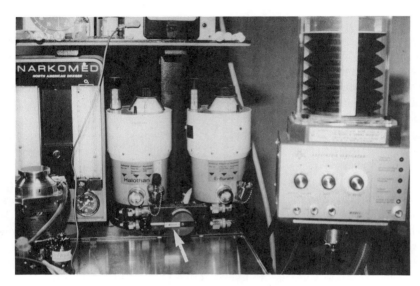

Fig. 16-14. The Dräger Vapor enflurane vaporizer *(right)* is turned on, but the selector switch *(arrow)* is pointing to the halothane vaporizer. Consequently, no anesthetic vapor is delivered to the breathing circuit.

pumping effect.[109-111] In older Ohmeda anesthesia machines, vaporizer protection is afforded by an outlet check valve located just upstream of the common gas outlet; this configuration prevents increases in pressure in the patient circuit from being transmitted back into the machine and thence to the vaporizer. Some older designs of vaporizer (such as the Ohio Ethane vaporizer) incorporated a check valve into the vaporizer outlet.[36] The most modern vaporizers (Ohmeda Tec 5 and Dräger Vapor 19.1) do not use check valves but use baffles or other design features to prevent the pumping effect.[109-111]

If an anesthesia machine is to be used for a patient who is susceptible to malignant hyperthermia, it has been recommended that the vaporizers be removed and that the machine be flushed with oxygen at 10 L/min for 5 minutes, with replacement of the fresh-gas outlet hose and use of a new disposable circle system that includes fresh carbon dioxide absorbent.[122] Others have disagreed with some of these recommendations.[123]

Anesthetic agent underdosage. Anesthetic agent underdosage may also occur, resulting in light anesthesia, patient movement, or even awareness. Perhaps the most common problem is forgetting to turn the vaporizer on. In some early vaporizer exclusion systems (Dräger Vapor, Ohio Selectatec), the vaporizer dial could be turned on while the vaporizer was excluded from the gas delivery system (Fig. 16-14). In recent systems the exclusion mechanism is activated only when the vaporizer is turned on; thus this potential problem is avoided.[88,109-111]

Miscellaneous malfunctions. The unintentional delivery of high concentrations of anesthetic vapor may be caused by any kind of internal malfunction of the vaporizer; regular checking of function and output calibration are essential. Such checking should ideally be performed in the usual-use environment of the vaporizer. Thus the output of Ohmeda Tec 4 vaporizers has been found to be accurate in the proximity of a 1.5-tesla magnet in a magnetic resonance imaging suite.[124,125]

Although numerous design features have helped to make modern vaporizing systems safer for the patient, ideally an agent-specific analyzer should be used in the patient circuit to monitor inhaled concentrations.[126] A variety of such units using various technologies are available, and all incorporate alarm features (see Chapter 8).

Humidification problems

Humidification of the inspired gases is desirable because it (1) prevents heat loss caused by evaporation of water from the tracheobronchial tree, (2) maintains moisture in the conducting airways and thereby facilitates ciliary function, and (3) prevents water loss from the patient by evaporation. Humidity can be provided by heat and moisture exchange devices that are connected to the tracheal tube and by moistening of the inside of the breathing tubes and reservoir bag with water before use.[127,128] In addition, unheated water vaporizers can be employed to provide moisture to the patient. However, the disadvantage of any system that does not employ heat is that it will cool as evaporation takes place and the amount of humidity generated will therefore be reduced.[18]

Heated humidifiers (vaporizers) are devices through which the inspired gases are passed in order to saturate the gases with water at the temperature of the humidifier. The dry gases either bubble through the humidifier or pass over the surface of the water. The heat is usually provided by electricity.

The advantage of this type of system is that the inspired gases become saturated with water at an elevated temperature. However, as the gas cools on leaving the humidifier, condensation occurs in the tubing and the amount of humidity delivered to the patient decreases. The condensation problem can be managed by heating the gases in the inspiratory hose either externally or internally with a heating wire. Keeping the distance from the humidifier to the patient as short as possible also decreases the amount of condensation (see also Chapter 7).

Another technique is to heat the humidifier to a temperature higher than body temperature so that as the inspired gases cool in the inspiratory tubing they enter the tracheal tube at the desired temperature. This technique must be used carefully in order to avoid burning the patient's tracheobronchial tree. It is therefore mandatory to monitor the temperature of the inspired gases at the tracheal tube to ensure that the gases are not too hot. Because the gases that are delivered to the patient have at most 100% relative humidity, there is little chance that the patient will experience fluid overload when a heated humidifier is employed.[18]

Hazards associated with the "artificial nose" (heat and moisture exchanger) include misconnection, obstruction, and disconnection.[129,130] A heated humidifier may cause bulk water delivery to the patient, thermal trauma to the airway, or obstruction of the breathing circuit, or it may become an electrical or fire hazard. These devices are electrically powered; thermostat failure may lead to superheating of the gases in the humidifier, causing the plastic inspiratory tubing to soften.[18,131] A soft inspiratory hose may become completely occluded or develop a hole (resulting in a large leak), thereby preventing ventilation of the patient. This problem can be avoided by making sure that the gas flow through the humidifier is initiated before the humidifier is turned on.[132]

Humidity can also be provided with a nebulizer technique. Nebulizers create droplets of water either by a jet of gas over the surface of the water or ultrasonically. Unlike the heated vaporizer, the nebulizer creates three hazards. It can act as a nidus for bacterial transmission; there may be increases in respiratory resistance; and the patient can become overhydrated. Therefore, extreme care should be taken in cleaning the nebulizer, sterile water must be used, and the amount of water delivered must be carefully monitored. In addition, because of the risk of increased respiratory resistance, nebulizers should probably not be used with patients who are breathing spontaneously.

When using heated humidifiers or nebulizers, the anesthesiologist should guard against (1) fluid overload, (2) thermal injury, (3) additional sites for disconnection within the breathing circuit, (4) obstruction to gas flow, (5) burning of the equipment because of electrical malfunction, (6) shock hazards, and (7) the risk of infection transmission via the nebulizer.

Electrical failure

Currently manufactured anesthesia machines rely on electrical and mechanical devices in order to function properly. The electrical system powers the ventilator, alarm system, and integral monitors. The power cord of the machine utilizes 90 to 130 V at 50 to 60 Hz alternating current (AC). On the machine itself there are usually four additional receptacles, which can provide electrical power for such additional equipment as monitors. There is a 12-V rechargeable battery that acts as a back-up power source if the external power fails.[133]

The preoperative check of such a machine includes a status review of the AC power and the reserve battery. Cases should not be started if either of these is not functioning. A discharged battery requires approximately 16 hours to recharge. The power switch on the machine mechanically activates the flow of gases through the flowmeter and turns on the electrical power. In the event of an electrical power failure, having the switch turned on allows the gases to flow to the flowmeters. The battery provides power to the electrical devices that are built into the machine; these include the ventilator, the alarm system, and the integral monitors. External electrical appliances that are plugged into the convenience receptacles are not powered by the battery.

The battery provides power for approximately 30 minutes. When its voltage drops to below 10 V, all power to the machine ceases in order to prevent a deep discharge of the battery. Failure of the battery would cause the monitors, the alarm system, and the ventilator on the machine to stop functioning. Manual ventilation would be required.[133]

Leaving the machine power on with the electrical cord disconnected from the wall is a common cause of battery discharge. This should be discovered on the pre-use check of the equipment, and the machine should not be used until the battery is recharged. Another source of trouble is accidentally plugging the power cord from the machine into one of the machine auxiliary receptacles. In essence, the machine is plugged into itself and has no external power supply. The anesthesiologist is alerted to this problem if the AC power failure indicator is activated and the "battery in use" light is on.

The electrical portion of the machine has several circuit breakers, which generally protect circuits for the AC power supply, the battery, and the auxiliary receptacles. When any of the electrical systems of the machine malfunction, the circuit breakers should be checked to determine if they have been tripped.[133]

The anesthesiologist has been responsible for anesthesia machine electrical failure. In one reported case, the anesthesiologist had intended to turn off the ventilator but instead turned off the main power switch to the machine. The effect was to turn off the gas flow, the alarm system, and the ventilator. In this situation, because the alarm system no longer functioned, it was up to the anesthesiologist, through vigilance, to recognize that the machine had been turned off and to intervene appropriately.[134]

Electromagnetic interference (EMI) is another potential cause of delivery system failure. Thus, extreme amounts of EMI or power line disturbances have been reported to lead to failure of the Ohmeda 7810 ventilator.[135] Because this model of ventilator incorporates pressure, volume, and oxygen monitors, these alarm functions, as well as ventilation, will all fail simultaneously. This emphasizes the need for continuous capnometry and observation of ventilation in all anesthetized patients. When function is interrupted, the Ohmeda 7810 ventilator can reset and resume normal function when the EMI has ceased. If normal function does not resume, manual ventilation should be commenced. In order to restore mechanical ventilation and monitoring functions, Ohmeda recommends turning the system master on/off switch to off, and after approximately 5 seconds returning this switch to the on position.[135] Cycling the mechanical ventilation on/off switch on the front panel of the ventilator module will not reset the ventilator. The alarm limit settings of all monitors controlled by the system monitor on/off switch should then be checked and adjusted as necessary. Because any electronic device can be adversely affected by extremes of EMI and power line disturbances, constant surveillance of all monitoring and life support equipment is mandatory.[135]

Total electrical failure in the operating room affects all equipment that does not have a battery back-up system. This includes all monitors, the anesthesia machine, the cardiopulmonary bypass machine, and the electric lights. All institutions should have an emergency plan, including battery-powered flashlights, for this type of utility failure.[136,137] The 1991 *Accreditation Manual for Hospitals,* which is published by The Joint Commission on Accreditation of Health Care Organizations, requires hospitals to have an emergency power system for the operating room in the event of loss of electrical power from outside the hospital.[138]

Hazards due to interactions with carbon dioxide absorbent

When carbon dioxide absorption is employed, as in most modern circle systems, the absorbent must be compatible with the anesthetic gases in use. Trichloroethylene may react with soda lime to produce dichloroacetylene, phosgene, and carbon monoxide, which are potentially neurotoxic gases. Trichloroethylene is not used in the United States but was commonly used in the United Kingdom. Sevoflurane, a new potent inhaled anesthetic, is unstable in the presence of soda lime,[139] but the products, although potentially toxic, do not seem to attain toxic concentrations.

Three cases have been reported in which excessive levels of carbon monoxide were discovered incidentally in the blood gas analysis obtained during anesthesia.[140] Because all three patients were the first cases anesthetized on Monday mornings, a slow chemical reaction within the machine or absorber circuit was suspected. In no case were there any intraoperative clinical indications to suggest carbon monoxide poisoning. A subsequent abstract[141] reported a total of 28 cases of unexplained carboxyhemoglobin (COHb) elevation in patients in three institutions. Most cases occurred following a 24 hour period of nonuse of an anesthesia machine. There was no particular association with particular anesthetics, although a possible interaction with the carbon dioxide absorbent (both Sodasorb* and Baralyme†) was suspected. Absorbent canisters that had been in service longer were found to be more likely to contain high concentrations of carbon monoxide. Used Sodasorb was found to contain formate, whereas unused Sodasorb contained no formate. When used Sodasorb that contained formate was heated, gaseous carbon monoxide was detected. The authors concluded that gaseous carbon monoxide may be produced in carbon dioxide absorbent following exposure to fluorinated anesthetics. Thus when isoflurane or enflurane is allowed to incubate with strong bases in carbon dioxide absorbent canisters, formate may be produced as an intermediate, with subsequent liberation of carbon monoxide. In this study, several anesthesia machines were reported to have dangerously high carbon monoxide concentrations potentially capable of producing clinically significant poisoning.[141] Further studies are needed to identify fully the mechanism of carbon monoxide production and the clinical significance of these observations. Meanwhile, it would seem advisable to avoid allowing potent inhaled agents to stagnate with carbon dioxide absorbent for prolonged periods.

Flushing the anesthesia circuit, and the absorbent canister in particular, with high flows of oxygen prior to clinical use should dilute any potentially toxic product down to clinically insignificant concentrations. Other measures that would tend to minimize any potential hazard from carbon monoxide include using fresh soda lime absorbent when a machine has not been used for some time and using high fresh-gas flows during administration of the anesthetic.

PREVENTION OF COMPLICATIONS
Preanesthetic checkout of the anesthesia delivery system

The purpose of the preanesthetic checkout is to determine that all the necessary equipment is present and functioning as expected before the induction of anesthesia. The usefulness of this is self-evident; moreover, its usefulness is supported in the anesthesia literature, which describes anesthesia machine malfunctions that could have been discovered before the case began had a thorough check of the equipment been performed. In August 1986, the FDA released its *Anesthesia Apparatus Checkout Recommenda-*

*WR Grace & Co., New York, N.Y.
†Chemetron, St. Louis, Mo.

tions,[5] which stated that "this checkout, or a reasonable equivalent, should be conducted before administering anesthesia. [see Chapter 22, Box 22-1.] This is a guideline which users are encouraged to modify to accommodate differences in equipment design and variations in local clinical practice. Such local modifications should have appropriate peer review. Users should refer to the operators manual for special procedures or precautions." Many anesthesia departments have adopted these recommendations without modification; others have modified them to suit their needs. Whichever approach is taken, it is absolutely critical that the machine be carefully inspected and checked before use.

When the delivery system is checked before the start of anesthesia, it is desirable to arrange it in the way it will be used during the case. Moving the machine after the case has begun, modifying the breathing circuit with a humidifier, or adding other components can affect the performance of the anesthesia delivery system. Inspecting the machine in the condition in which it will be used during the operation minimizes this type of problem.[94] However, the preoperative equipment check does not guard against the problem of intraoperative equipment failure. The anesthesiologist must be vigilant in the monitoring of equipment performance and ready to intervene in any hazardous situation.

The FDA 1986 generic guidelines for machine inspection are self-explanatory (see Chapter 22, Box 22-1). Steps 5, 7, 8, 10, 12, 13, 15, 16, 17, and 24 are set out in greater detail below.

Step 5: Check the oxygen cylinder supplies. First, the oxygen-pressure gauge should read zero. The pipeline oxygen source should be disconnected, and one of the reserve oxygen cylinders should be opened. The pressure should be noted, the cylinder valve closed, and the system depressurized by pressing the oxygen flush button. The second cylinder should be opened and its pressure noted. High-pressure gas leaks should be sought, the manifestation of which is a high-pitched hissing noise. When the pressure of each cylinder is tested, the pressure on the oxygen-pressure gauge must be zero before the cylinder is opened; otherwise, the residual pressure in the oxygen piping system will be displayed, and the anesthesiologist may be misled into believing that the cylinder contains more oxygen than it does. At least one of the cylinders should be nearly full, and cylinders that are one quarter full or less should be replaced. At the conclusion of the cylinder checks the cylinder valves should be closed. This prevents the use of the cylinder supply without the anesthesiologist's being aware of it (see also Chapter 2).

Step 7: Check the nitrous oxide and other cylinder gas supplies. The nitrous oxide test is performed similarly to the oxygen cylinder tests. However, the reading on the pressure gauge will remain at 745 psig until most of the liquid nitrous oxide has been used up. The cylinder must be weighed in order to find how much of this agent is in it (see Chapter 1).[112]

Step 8: Test the flowmeters. The floats should be at the bottom of the flow tubes. When the flow control valves are opened, the floats should move smoothly and not stick. Make certain that the floats are not stuck at the top of the flow tubes.

Step 10: Test the oxygen pressure failure system. The oxygen and other gas flows should be set to midrange. Next the oxygen cylinder is closed, and the pressure in the oxygen piping is released by pressing on the oxygen flush button. The flow of all gases must be seen to fall to zero, and if an oxygen pressure failure alarm is present it should sound when the oxygen pressure falls below the threshold. All other cylinders are then closed and the gases bled from the piping system. The oxygen cylinder is then closed and oxygen bled from the piping system. After the test is complete the flow-control valves are closed.

Step 12: Add any accessory equipment to the breathing system. It is very important to have the entire breathing system fully assembled *before* it is tested for leaks and proper function. This is because it is possible to modify the system with malfunctioning equipment after it has been checked. Under those circumstances, the circuit check would fail to detect the system malfunction.

Step 13: Calibrate the oxygen monitor. The oxygen monitor is absolutely critical and should be calibrated to read 21% when exposed to room air. The alarm should be tested for proper function at low oxygen concentrations. The sensor should then be exposed to the breathing circuit, and 100% oxygen should be flowing through the system. The monitor should read close to 100%. Slight inaccuracy at the 100% end of the scale can be tolerated, but the monitor must be accurately calibrated at the 21% end.

Step 15: Check the unidirectional valves. Each limb of the breathing circuit should be checked for valve function. One should not be able to exhale through the inspiratory hose or inhale through the expiratory hose of the circuit. After this test the circuit should be reassembled.

Step 16: Test for leaks in the machine and breathing system. The APL (pop-off) valve should be closed, and the patient end of the breathing circuit should be occluded. The system should be pressurized to 20 cm H_2O by oxygen flowing from the flowmeter. The circuit should maintain this pressure with no gas entering the breathing circuit and without the reservoir bag being squeezed. If there is a decrease in pressure, the amount of leak can be quantified by flowing oxygen until the pressure is held steady. On machines with a check valve proximal to the common gas outlet, a negative-pressure leak test at the common gas outlet must be performed to rule out a leak upstream from that valve. See Chapters 2 and 22 for more details.

Step 17: Test the exhaust valve and scavenger system. The APL valve must be opened, and the pressure should be seen to fall to zero. With the valve open, no positive or negative pressure should exist in the circuit when there is no flow of gas from the oxygen flush. Positive pressure in the circuit indicates that there is obstruction to flow at the APL valve or distal to it in the scavenging system. Negative pressure in the circuit probably is caused by a faulty negative pressure-relief system or valve within the scavenger interface (See Fig. 16-7.)

Step 24: Set airway pressure and/or volume monitor alarm limits. If the alarm limits are adjustable, the airway pressure limits should be set several cm H_2O below the peak airway pressure for the minimum ventilation-pressure alarm, and approximately 10 cm H_2O above the peak airway pressure for the continuing-pressure and high-pressure alarms. The minimum volume alarm should be set to a point close to but below the delivered minute volume. Setting the alarms in this way makes the system as sensitive as possible to changes in the patient or breathing system that may adversely affect the patient's ventilation. It is again emphasized that the operator's manual should be consulted for specific delivery system check-out procedures.

FDA anesthesia apparatus checkout recommendations, 1992

Data from the study by March and Crowley[6] suggest that the 1986 FDA checklist did not improve the ability of anesthesiologists to detect faults in the anesthesia machine. Although there are several possible explanations for this failure, including lack of formal training in machine checkout and use of a checklist, it was concluded that "rewriting of the FDA checklist may be required to improve its utility as a clinical tool."[6] At the time of writing, only a draft of the proposed FDA *Anesthesia Apparatus Checkout Recommendations* of 1992 was available (see Chapter 22, Box 22-2). The final version is due to be published in late 1992. The proposed checkout is simpler than the 1986 version. Noteworthy is that it begins with checking that emergency ventilation equipment is available and functioning. A backup source of oxygen and a self-inflating bag should be continuously available in the event that the delivery system fails.

Monitoring of circuit pressures and volumes

Pressures. The ATSM F1161-88 standard[8] requires the machine to have breathing system pressure monitoring as well as either exhaled volume or ventilatory carbon dioxide monitoring. The machine must have a means to monitor pressure continually in the breathing system, and the pressure monitor must be designed to trigger a visual and audible high-priority alarm when pressure in the system (1) exceeds a user-adjustable limit for high pressure or (2) exceeds a user-adjustable limit for continuing positive airway pressure for more than 15 seconds. The latter alarm threshold should be adjustable between 10 and 30 cm H_2O. The pressure monitor and alarm must be enabled and function-

ing automatically whenever the anesthesia machine is in use.

The ASA *Standards for Basic Intraoperative Monitoring*[10] require that when ventilation is controlled by a mechanical ventilator, there should be in continuous use a device that is capable of detecting disconnection of components of the breathing system. The device must emit an audible signal when its alarm threshold is exceeded. This is the circuit low-pressure alarm, sometimes loosely termed the "disconnect" alarm. If the pressure in the circuit does not exceed the user-set minimum within a set period (usually 15 seconds, but this may be set at 60 seconds to allow a slow respiratory rate to be deliberately set on the ventilator), the alarm is annunciated. Modern circuit pressure monitors also annunciate an alarm when the pressure in the breathing system falls below -10 cm H_2O at any time (subatmospheric pressure alarm).

Modern delivery systems incorporate a mechanical pressure gauge that is usually mounted on the absorber, and the circuit pressure can be measured at that point (Fig. 16-15). In addition, pressure can be sensed at almost any point in the circuit and be transmitted through pilot tubing to a remote electronic pressure monitor that incorporates audible and visual alarms. Ideally, pressure should be sensed at the patient connector, but water and sterilization problems make this site impractical.[12] Sensing pressure by the absorber may fail to detect abnormalities between the patient and the inspiratory and expiratory unidirectional valves. Thus, if a free-standing PEEP valve were correctly inserted between the expiratory limb of the circuit and the exhalation unidirectional valve, the PEEP would not be detectable by a pressure monitor sensing pressure by the absorber (Fig. 16-15). Although the circle system is the one most commonly used, other circuits, such as the Bain or Mapleson F, may be employed, and pressure-monitoring adapters are available for use in these situations.

The pressure monitoring and alarm connections in both the Dräger and Ohmeda absorber systems are self-sealing. If the pressure-monitoring sensor is disconnected from the absorber and the circle is then used, the low-pressure alarm is activated (senses atmospheric pressure), and yet the circuit pressure gauge displays normal pressures.

Monitoring of pressure at the absorber may also fail to detect a patient circuit disconnection during positive-pressure ventilation. Because the ventilator delivers its tidal volume in the proximity of the pressure alarm sensing point (Fig. 16-15), the low-pressure alarm limit may be satisfied if it is not set to be sensitive enough (that is, if it is not set to slightly below the usual peak inspiratory pressure). It therefore is important to recognize where in the circuit the pressure gauge senses pressure and where the pressure monitoring and the alarm system are sensing pressure, if the two differ.

Volumes. The ASTM F1161-88 standard[8] also requires monitoring of exhaled volume or ventilatory carbon dioxide. An alarm is activated if the patient's exhaled volume

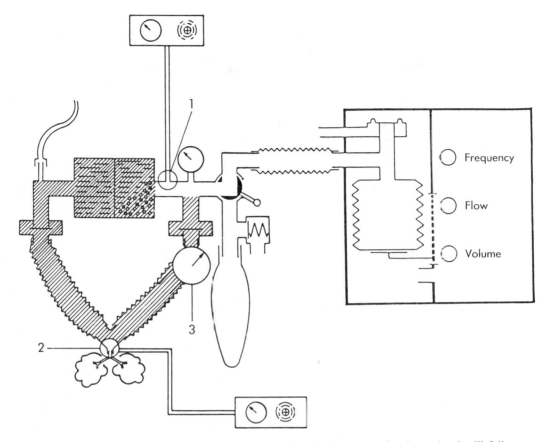

Fig. 16-15. Sensing locations for pressure alarms in a circle system. Sensing point *1* will fail to detect adverse pressure conditions or apnea in the event of an occlusion in the shaded area. Sensing pressure at point *2* would be preferable but would not recognize an occluded tracheal tube. 3, volume meter. (From Schreiber P: *Safety guidelines for anesthesia systems*, Telford, Pa, 1985, North American Dräger.)

falls below an operator-adjustable minimum. The monitor must be designed to be in an enabled condition and functioning automatically whenever the anesthesia machine is in use. When the volume monitor alarm is disabled, a low-priority alarm is to be annunciated.[8] Modern circle systems also incorporate a spirometer, which measures tidal and minute volumes, demonstrates reversal of gas flow if it should occur (e.g., because of incompetence of the exhalation unidirectional valve), and, if electronic, incorporates low and high alarm limits. Mechanical spirometers do not incorporate an alarm. In Dräger systems the spirometer is located on the absorber side (downstream) of the expiratory unidirectional valve. In Ohmeda systems it is usually placed just upstream of the expiratory valve. In both systems it is the gas volume flowing through the expiratory limb of the circuit (exhaled volume) that is measured.

Monitoring exhaled volumes is valuable when a low-volume alarm limit can be set to be sensitive, that is, to just less than the set ventilation parameters (including tidal volume, ventilatory rate, fresh-gas flow, *I:E* ratio). A disconnection in the patient circuit should result in a decrease in displayed tidal volume and minute volume (Fig. 16-15). Unlike the pressure gauge, which is sensing pressure usually at the absorber, the spirometer usually gives an indication of flow problems in the patient circuit.

In the event of a circuit disconnection, a spirometer in the expiratory limb may, however, be "fooled" if a hanging-bellows design of ventilator is being used. Thus during exhalation a weight in the hanging bellows causes it to descend, drawing room air in through the disconnection site, through the spirometer, and into the descending bellows (Fig. 16-11). With such a scenario, the decrease in the tidal volume reading compared with the tidal volume before the disconnection occurred is that attributable to the lost fresh gas from the flowmeters. Unless the low-volume alarm limits have been set to be very sensitive, a disconnection of the patient circuit with a hanging-bellows ventilator will likely go undetected by a spirometer in the expiratory limb of the circle. A disconnection of the tubing between the ventilator and the breathing circuit would, however, be detectable by both the spirometer and the pressure monitor.

It has been mentioned previously that the standing-bellows design of ventilator is preferred because a disconnection is more obvious since the bellows fails to fill on exhalation and that an expiratory limb spirometer is less likely to be fooled. It is also possible for an expired spirometer to be fooled by a standing-bellows ventilator when there is a patient circuit disconnection. The mechanism is as follows: When the disconnection occurs, the standing bellows empties, falling to its bottom resting position as if the largest possible tidal volume had been delivered (Fig. 16-10). At end-exhalation, the pressure in the driving gas circuit is zero, but the empty bellows contains a residual volume of patient circuit gas. On the next inspiration, driving gas pressure in the bellows housing rises and the bellows is actively compressed, discharging some of the contained residual gas volume. With the next exhalation cycle, the rubber bellows resumes its original unpressurized configuration and may aspirate gas from the patient circuit. Gas drawn into the bellows through the spirometer will cause the spirometer to record a volume of as much as 140 ml, depending on the size of the bellows.[142] An inappropriately set low-volume alarm thus might record an "adequate" tidal volume and be fooled in this circumstance.

Although monitoring of pressure and exhaled volume are now required in modern delivery systems, it is apparent from the above discussion that not all ventilation or pressure problems will be detectable when these monitors are used as presently configured. Detection is improved by "bracketing" the user-adjustable alarm-limit thresholds close to the patient's normal high and low pressures and volumes. Some older monitors had fixed alarm limits, and even some modern ones have default settings, which may not provide adequate warning of problems in the circuit. Problems associated with alarm limits being set too insensitive are discussed further in Chapter 17.

A disposable pneumotachometer head placed by the patient's airway might represent an improvement over the current monitors, because it can (with corrections for gas composition and humidity) provide instantaneous measurements of flow, volume, and pressure at this important site.[143] The Datex Capnomac Ultima with Spirometry, an example of such a system, is described in more detail in Chapter 9.

The anesthesia delivery system may cause complications to the patient because of misuse or component failure. Anesthesia equipment failure and misuse represent a small proportion (4%) of the national database of anesthesia-related malpractice claims (Closed Claims Study of the ASA Committee on Professional Liability), and among these cases misuse was more common than equipment failure.[144] The delivery system continues to evolve as more is learned about patient safety and as design and monitoring features are added. Clearly, a basic understanding of the structure and function of the delivery system will enhance patient safety by avoiding misuse and facilitating troubleshooting or alternative techniques if a component should fail. All anesthetizing locations should have immediately available a tank supply of oxygen and a resuscitation bag for use in the event of a total machine failure.

Although some states (in particular New York and New Jersey) have implemented regulations with regard to the practice of anesthesiology, as of April 1992 only the state of New Jersey has published regulations concerning requirements for anesthesia equipment, safety, maintenance, and inspection.[145] Other states may well follow (see also Chapter 25).

REFERENCES

1. Cooper JB, Newbower RS, Kitz RJ: An analysis of major errors and equipment failures in anesthesia management: considerations for prevention and detection, *Anesthesiology* 60:34-42, 1984.
2. Cooper JB, Newbower RS, Long CD, et al: Preventable anesthesia mishaps: a study of human factors, *Anesthesiology* 49:399-406, 1978.
3. Sykes MK: Incidence of mortality and morbidity due to anaesthetic equipment failure, *Eur J Anaesthesiol* 4:198-199, 1987.
4. Buffington CW, Ramanathan S, Turndorf H: Detection of anesthesia machine faults, *Anesth Analg* 63:79-82, 1984.
5. Anesthesia apparatus checkout recommendations, Rockville Md, 1986, United States Food and Drug Administration.
6. March MG, Crowley JJ: An evaluation of anesthesiologists' present checkout methods and the validity of the FDA checklist, *Anesthesiology* 75:724-729, 1991.
7. Kumar V, Hintze MS, Jacob AM: A random survey of anesthesia machines and ancillary monitors in 45 hospitals, *Anesth Analg* 67:644-649, 1988.
8. Minimum performance and safety requirements for components and systems of anesthesia gas machines, F1161-88, Philadelphia, 1989, American Society for Testing and Materials.
9. Minimum performance and safety requirements for components and systems of continuous flow anesthesia machines for human use, ANSI Z79.8-1979, New York, 1979, American National Standards Institute.
10. Standards for basic intraoperative monitoring (last amended October 1990; effective Jan 1, 1991), Park Ridge, Ill, 1986, American Society of Anesthesiologists.
11. Eichhorn JH: Prevention of intraoperative anesthesia accidents and related severe injury through safety monitoring, *Anesthesiology* 70:572-577, 1989.
12. Schreiber P: *Safety guidelines for anesthesia systems*, Telford, Pa, 1985, North American Dräger.
13. Abraham ZA, Basagoitia J: A potentially lethal anesthesia machine failure, *Anesthesiology* 66:589-590, 1987 (letter).
14. Jawan B, Lee JH: Cardiac arrest caused by an incorrectly filled oxygen cylinder: a case report, *Br J Anaesth* 64:749-751, 1990.
15. Holland R: Wrong gas disaster in Hong Kong, *Anesthesia Patient Safety Foundation Newsletter* 4:26, 1989.
16. Feeley TW, Hedley-Whyte J: Bulk oxygen and nitrous oxide delivery systems: design and dangers, *Anesthesiology* 44:301-305, 1976.
17. O'Connor CJ, Hobin KF: Bypassing the diameter-indexed safety system, *Anesthesiology* 71:318-319, 1989.
18. Dorsch JA, Dorsch SE: *Understanding anesthesia equipment construction, care, and complications*, Baltimore, 1984, Williams and Wilkins.
19. Anderson B, Chamley D: Wall outlet oxygen failure, *Anaesth Intensive Care* 15:468-469, 1987 (letter).
20. Bonsu AK, Stead AL: Accidental cross-connexion of oxygen and nitrous oxide in an anaesthetic machine, *Anaesthesia* 38:767-769, 1983.
21. Heath ML: Accidents associated with equipment. *Anaesthesia* 39:57-60, 1984.

22. Lacoumenta S, Hall GM: A burst oxygen pipeline, *Anaesthesia* 38:596-597, 1983 (letter).

23. Carley RH, Houghton IT, Park GR: A near disaster from piped gases, *Anaesthesia* 39:891-893, 1984.

24. Beudoin MG: Oxygen needle valve obstruction, *Anaesth Intensive Care* 16:130-131, 1988 (letter).

25. Khalil SN, Neuman J: Failure of an oxygen flow control valve, *Anesthesiology* 73:355-356, 1990.

26. Williams AR, Hilton PJ: Selective oxygen leak: a potential cause of patient hypoxia, *Anaesthesia* 41:1133-1134, 1986.

27. Hanning CD, Kruchek D, Chunara A: Preferential oxygen leak: an unusual case, *Anaesthesia* 42:1329-1330, 1987, (letter).

28. Moore JK, Railton R: Hypoxia caused by a leaking Rotameter: the value of an oxygen analyser, *Anaesthesia* 39:380-381, 1984 (letter).

29. Cole AG, Thompson JB, Fodor IM, et al: Anaesthetic machine hazard from the Selectatec block, *Anaesthesia* 38:175-177, 1983 (letter).

30. Richards C: Failure of a nitrous oxide-oxygen proportioning system, *Anesthesiology* 71:997-999, 1989.

31. Goodyear CM: Failure of nitrous oxide-oxygen proportioning device, *Anesthesiology* 72:397-398, 1990

32. Ghanooni S, Wilks DH, Finestone SC: A case report of an unusual disconnection, *Anesth Analg* 62:696-697, 1983.

33. Henshaw J: Circle system disconnection, *Anaesth Intensive Care* 16:240, 1988 (letter).

34. Horan BF: Unusual disconnection, *Anaesth Intensive Care* 15:466-467, 1987 (letter).

35. Rossiter SK: An unexpected disconnection of the gas supply to a Cape Waine 3 ventilator, *Anaesthesia* 38:180, 1983 (letter).

36. Capan L, Ramanathan S, Chalon J, et al: A possible hazard with use of Ohio Ethane vaporizer, *Anesth Analg* 59:65-68, 1980.

37. Lee O, Sommer RM: Pressure monitoring hose causes leak in anesthesia breathing circuit, *Anesth Analg* 73:365, 1991.

38. Ripp CH, Chapin JW: A bellows leak in an Ohio anesthesia ventilator, *Anesth Analg* 64:942, 1985 (letter).

39. Spoor J: Ventilator malfunction, *Anaesth Intensive Care* 14:329, 1986 (letter).

40. Heine JF, Adams PM: Another potential failure in an oxygen delivery system, *Anesthesiology* 63:335-336, 1985.

41. Berner MS: Profound hypercapnia due to disconnection within an anaesthetic machine, *Can J Anaesth* 34:622-626, 1987.

42. McQuillan PJ, Jackson IJ: Potential leaks from anaesthetic machines: potential leaks through open rotameter valves and empty cylinder yokes, *Anaesthesia* 42:1308-1312, 1987.

43. Bamber PA: Safety hazard with cylinder yoke on a Boyle's machine, *Anaesthesia* 41:1260-1262, 1986 (letter).

44. Jablonski J, Reynolds AC: A potential cause (and cure) of a major gas leak, *Anesthesiology* 62:842-843, 1985 (letter).

45. Jove F, Milliken RA: Loss of anesthetic gases due to defective safety equipment, *Anesth Analg* 62:369-370, 1983 (letter).

46. Pyles ST, Kaplan RF, Munson ES: Gas loss from Ohio Modulus vaporizer selector-interlock valve, *Anesth Analg* 62:1052, 1983 (letter).

47. Wan YL, Swan M: Exotic obstruction, *Anaesth Intensive Care* 18:274, 1990 (letter).

48. Boscoe MJ, Baxter RC: Failure of anaesthetic gas supply, *Anaesthesia* 38:997-998, 1983 (letter).

49. Hogan TS: Selectatec switch malfunction, *Anaesthesia* 40:66-69, 1985.

50. Milliken RA, Bizzarri DV: An unusual cause of failure of anesthetic gas delivery to a patient circuit, *Anesth Analg* 63:1047-1048, 1984 (letter).

51. Sara CA, Wark HJ: Disconnection: an appraisal, *Anaesth Intensive Care* 14:448-452, 1986.

52. Khalil SN, Gholston TK, Binderman J, et al: Flapper valve malfunction in an Ohio closed scavenging system, *Anesth Analg* 66:1334-1336, 1987.

53. Eisenkraft JB, Sommer RM: Flapper valve malfunction, *Anesth Analg* 67:1132, 1988 (letter).

54. Sommer RM, Bhalla GS, Jackson JM, et al: Hypoventilation caused by ventilator valve rupture, *Anesth Analg* 67:999-1001, 1988.

55. Poulton TJ: Unusual corrugated tubing leak, *Anesth Analg* 65:1365, 1986 (letter).

56. Nelson RA, Snowdon SL: Failure of an adjustable pressure limiting valve, *Anaesthesia* 44:788-789, 1989 (letter).

57. Cooper MG, Vouden J, Rigg D: Circuit leaks, *Anaesth Intensive Care* 15:359-360, 1987 (letter).

58. Hutchinson BR: An unusual leak, *Anaesth Intensive Care* 15:355, 1987 (letter).

59. Ferderbar PJ, Kettler RE, Jablonski J, et al: A cause of breathing system leak during closed circuit anesthesia, *Anesthesiology* 65:661-663, 1986.

60. Raja SN, Geller H: Another potential source of a major gas leak, *Anesthesiology* 64:297-298, 1986 (letter).

61. Brown MR, Burris WR, Hilley MD: Breathing circuit mishap resulting from Y-piece disintegration, *Anesthesiology* 69:436-437, 1988 (letter).

62. Herbst TJ: Preventing delivery of hypoxic gas mixtures, *Anesthesiology* 72:775, 1990 (letter).

63. Robblee JA, Crosby E, Keon WJ: Hypoxemia after intraluminal oxygen line obstruction during cardiopulmonary bypass, *Ann Thorac Surg* 48:575-576, 1989.

64. Lamarche Y: Anaesthetic breathing circuit leak from cracked oxygen analyzer sensor connector, *Can Anaesth Soc J* 32:682-683, 1985 (letter).

65. Miller DC, Collins JW, Wallace L: Failure of the expiratory valve on a Bain system, *Anaesthesia* 43:992, 1988 (letter)

66. Seow LT, Davis R: Circuit disconnections, *Anaesth Intensive Care* 16:242, 1988 (letter).

67. Mushlin PS, Mark JB, Elliott WR, et al: Inadvertent development of subatmospheric airway pressure during cardiopulmonary bypass, *Anesthesiology* 71:459-462, 1989.

68. Ghani GA: Fresh gas flow affects minute volume during mechanical ventilation, *Anesth Analg* 63:619, 1984.

69. Scheller MS, Jones BR, Benumof JL: The influence of fresh gas flow and *I:E* ratio on tidal volume and $PaCO_2$ in ventilated patients, *J Cardiothoracic Anesth* 3:564-567, 1989.

70. Birch AA, Fisher NA: Leak of soda lime seal after anesthesia machine check, *J Clin Anesth* 1:474-476, 1989 (letter).

71. Andrews JJ, Johnston RV, Bee DE, et al: Photodeactivation of ethyl violet: a potential hazard of sodasorb, *Anesthesiology* 72:59-64, 1990.

72. Nunn JF: Carbon dioxide cylinders on anaesthetic apparatus, *Br J Anaesth* 65:155-156, 1990.

73. Razis PA: Carbon dioxide: a survey of its use in anaesthesia in the U.K., *Anaesthesia* 44:348-351, 1989.

74. Eger EI II: *Anesthetic systems: construction and function*. In Eger EI, editor: *Anesthetic uptake and action*, Baltimore, 1974, Williams and Wilkins, pp 206-227.

75. Conway CM: *Anaesthesia breathing systems*. In Scurr CF, Feldman S, editors: *Scientific foundations of anaesthesia*, London, 1982, Heinemann, pp 557-566.

76. Sims C, Cullingford DW: Kinking of the Mera-F-Circuit, *Anaesth Intensive Care* 15:243, 1988 (letter).

77. Forrest PR: Defective anaesthetic breathing circuit, *Can J Anaesth* 34:541-542, 1987 (letter).

78. Jackson FJ: Tests for co-axial systems, *Anaesthesia* 43:1060-1061, 1988 (letter).

79. Hewitt AJ, Campbell W: Unusual damage to a Bain system, *Anaesthesia* 41:882-883, 1986 (letter).

80. Neufeld PD Walker EA, Johnson DL: Survey on breathing system disconnetions, *Anaesthesia* 41:438-439, 1986 (letter).

81. Goldman JM, Phelps RW: No flow anesthesia, *Anesth Analg* 66:1339, 1987 (letter).

82. Koga Y, Iwatsuki N, Takahashi M, et al: A hazardous defect in a humidifier, *Anesth Analg* 71:712, 1990.

83. Schroff PK, Skerman JH: Humidifier malfunction: a cause of anesthesia circuit occlusion, *Anesth Analg* 67:710-711, 1988.

84. Spurring PW, Small LF: Breathing system disconnexions and misconnexions: a review of some common causes and some suggestions for improved safety, *Anaesthesia* 38:683-688, 1983.

85. Arellano R, Ross D, Lee K: Inappropriate attachment of PEEP valve causing total obstruction of ventilation bag, *Anesth Analg* 67:1050-1051, 1987.

86. Anagnostou JM, Hults S, Moorthy SS: PEEP valve barotrauma, *Anesth Analg* 70:674-675, 1990.

87. Sharrock NE, Leith DE: Potential pulmonary barotrauma when venting anesthetic gases to suction, *Anesthesiology* 46:152-154, 1977.

88. Narkomed 3 anesthesia system, operator's instruction manual. Telford, Pa, 1986, North American Dräger.

89. Modulus II Plus Anesthesia Machine, preoperative checklists, operation and maintenance manual. Madison, Wisc, 1988, Ohmeda, The BOC Group, Inc.

90. McEwen JA, Small CF, Jenkins LC: Detection of interruptions in the breathing gas of ventilated anaesthetized patients, *Can J Anaesth* 35:549-561, 1988.

91. McIntyre JW, Nelson TM: Application of automated human voice delivery to warning devices in an intensive care unit: a laboratory study, *Int J Clin Monit Comput* 6:255-262, 1989.

92. Raphael DT, Weller RS, Doran DJ: A response algorithm for the low pressure alarm condition, *Anesth Analg* 67:876-883, 1988.

93. Slee TA, Pavlin EG: Failure of a low pressure alarm associated with use of a humidifier, *Anesthesiology* 69:791-793, 1988.

94. Eisenkraft JB: Potential for barotrauma or hypoventilation with the Dräger AV-E ventilator, *J Clin Anesth* 1:452-456, 1989.

95. Choi JJ, Guida J, Wu W-H: Hypoventilatory hazard of an anesthetic scavenging device, *Anesthesiology* 65:126-127, 1986.

96. Lanier WL: Intraoperative air entrainment with Ohio Modulus anesthesia machine, *Anesthesiology* 64:266-268, 1986.

97. Baraka A, Muallem M: Awareness during anaesthesia due to a ventilator malfunction, *Anaesthesia* 34:678-679, 1979.

98. Waterman PM, Pautler S, Smith RB: Accidental ventilator induced hyperventilation, *Anesthesiology* 48:141, 1978.

99. Longmuir J, Craig DB: Inadvertent increase in inspired oxygen concentration due to defect in ventilator bellows, *Can Anaesth Soc J* 23:327-329, 1976.

100. Dean HN, Parsons DE, Raphaely RC: Bilateral tension pneumothorax from mechanical failure of anesthesia machine due to misplaced expiratory valve, *Anesth Analg* 50:195-198, 1971.

101. Sears BE, Bocar ND: Pneumothorax resulting from a closed anesthesia ventilator port, *Anesthesiology* 47:311-313, 1977.

102. Sprung J, Samaan F, Hensler T, et al: Excessive airway pressure due to ventilator control valve malfunction during anesthesia for open heart surgery, *Anesthesiology* 73:1035-1038, 1990.

103. Roth S, Tweedie E, Sommer RM: Excessive airway pressure due to a malfunctioning anesthesia ventilator, *Anesthesiology* 65:532-534, 1986.

104. Henzig D: Insidious PEEP from a defective ventilator gas evacuation outlet valve, *Anesthesiology* 57:251-252, 1982.

105. Pressure limit control, operator's instruction manual, Telford, Pa, 1988, North American Dräger.

106. Ohmeda 7000 electronic anesthesia ventilator, service manual. Madison, Wisc 1985, Ohmeda, The BOC Group, Inc.

107. Kopriva CJ, Lowenstein E: An anesthetic accident: cardiovascular collapse from liquid halothane delivery, *Anesthesiology* 30:246, 1969.

108. Eisenkraft JB: *Vaporizers and vaporization of volatile anesthetics, vol 2, Progress in anesthesiology,* San Antonio, Tex, 1988, Dannemiller Memorial Educational Foundation.

109. Tec 5 continuous flow vaporizer, operation and maintenance manual. Steeton, UK, 1989, Ohmeda.

110. Tec 4 continuous flow vaporizer. Steeton, UK, 1987, Ohmeda.

111. Operator's manual, Dräger 19.1 Vaporizer. Lubeck, Germany, 1986, Drägerwerk, A.G.

112. Eisenkraft JB: *The anesthesia delivery system,* In Rogers MC, Tinker JH, Covino BG, Longnecker DE, editors: *Principles and practice of anesthesiology,* St. Louis, 1992, Mosby–Year Book.

113. Bruce DL, Linde HW: Vaporization of mixed anesthetic liquids, *Anesthesiology* 60:342-346, 1984.

114. Chilcoat RT: Hazards of mis-filled vaporizers: summary tables, *Anesthesiology* 63:726-727, 1985.

115. Riegle EV, Desertspring D: Failure of the agent-specific filling device, *Anesthesiology* 73:353-354, 1990.

116. Korman B, Ritchie IM: Chemistry of halothane-enflurane mixtures applied to anesthesia, *Anesthesiology* 63:152-156, 1985.

117. Murray WJ, Zsigmond EK, Fleming P: Contamination of in-series vaporizers with halothane-methoxyflurane, *Anesthesiology* 38:487, 1973.

118. Dorsch SE, Dorsch JA: Chemical cross-contamination between vaporizers in series, *Anesth Analg* 52:176-180, 1973.

119. Silvasi DL, Haynes A, Brown ACD: Potentially lethal failure of the vapor exclusion system, *Anesthesiology* 71:289-291, 1990.

120. Cudmore J, Keogh J: Another Selectatec switch malfunction, *Anaesthesia* 45:754-756, 1990.

121. Marks WE, Bullard JR: Another hazard of freestanding vaporizers: increased anesthetic concentration with reversed flow of vaporizing gas, *Anesthesiology* 45:445, 1976.

122. Beebe JJ, Sessler DI: Preparation of anesthesia machines for patients susceptible to malignant hyperthermia, *Anesthesiology* 69:395-400, 1988.

123. Cooper JB, Philip JH: More on anesthesia machines and malignant hyperthermia, *Anesthesiology* 70:561-562, 1989.

124. Rao CC, Brandl R, Mashak JN: Modification of Ohmeda Excel 210 anesthesia machine for use during MRI, *Anesthesiology* 71:A365, 1989 (abstract).

125. Rao CC, Krishna G, Emhardt J: Anesthesia machine for use during MRI, *Anesthesiology* 73:1054-1055, 1990 (abstract).

126. Munshi C, Dhamee S, Bardeen-Henschel A, et al: Recognition of mixed anesthetic agents by mass spectrometer during anesthesia, *J Clin Monit* 2:121-124, 1986 (abstract).

127. Bickler PE, Sessler DI: Efficiency of airway heat and moisture exchangers in anesthetized humans, *Anesth Analg* 71:415-418, 1990.

128. Turner DA, Wright EM: Efficiency of heat and moisture exchangers, *Anaesthesia* 42:1117-1119, 1987 (letter).

129. Bengtsson M, Johnson A: Failure of a heat and moisture exchanger as a cause of disconnection during anaesthesia, *Acta Anaesthesiol Scand* 33:522-523, 1989.

130. Prasad KK, Chen L: Complications related to the use of a heat and moisture exchanger, *Anesthesiology* 72:958, 1990.

131. Ward CF, Reisner LS, Zlott LS: Murphy's law and humidification, *Anesth Analg* 62:460-461, 1983.

132. Shroff PK, Skerman JH: Humidifier malfunction: a cause of anesthesia circuit occlusion, *Anesth Analg* 67:710-711, 1988 (letter).

133. Operators manual, North American Dräger Narkomed 2B, Telford, Pa, 1988, North American Dräger.

134. Maurer WG: A disadvantage of similar machine controls, *Anesthesiology* 75:167-168, 1991.

135. Urgent medical device safety alert. Madison, Wis, 1991, Ohmeda, A BOC Health Care Co.

136. Greenhalgh DL, Thomas WA: Blackout during cardiopulmonary bypass, *Anaesthesia* 45:175, 1990 (letter).

137. Welch RH, Feldman JM: Anesthesia during total electrical failure, or what would you do if the lights went out? *J Clin Anesth* 1:358-362, 1989.
138. *Accreditation manual for hospitals, the 1991 joint commission, vol 1,* Oakbrook Terrace, Ill, 1990, The Joint Commission on Accreditation of Healthcare Organizations, pp 205-206.
139. Tanifuji Y, Takagi MS, Kobayashi K, et al: The interaction between sevoflurane and soda lime or Baralyme, *Anesth Analg* 68:S285, 1989 (abstract).
140. Moon RE, Meyer AF, Scott D, et al: Intraoperative carbon monoxide toxicity, *Anesthesiology* 73:A1089, 1990 (abstract).
141. Moon RE, Ingram C, Brunner EA, et al: Spontaneous generation of carbon monoxide within anesthesia circuits, *Anesthesiology* 75:A873, 1991 (abstract).
142. Gravenstein JS, Nederstigt JA: Monitoring for disconnection: ventilators with bellows rising on expiration can deliver tidal volumes after disconnection, *J Clin Monit* 6:207-210, 1990.
143. Bardoczky GI, d'Hollander A: Continuous monitoring of the flow-volume loops and compliance during anesthesia. *J Clin Monit* 8:251-252, 1992 (letter).
144. Vistica MF, Posner KL, Caplan RA, et al: Role of equipment failure and misuse in anesthetic-related malpractice claims. *Anesthesiology* 73:A1008, 1990 (abstract).
145. New Jersey register, Subchapter 18: Anesthesia 21 N.J.R. 503-504, February 21, 1989.

Chapter 17

VIGILANCE, ALARMS, AND INTEGRATED MONITORING SYSTEMS

Matthew B. Weinger, M.D.
N. Ty Smith, M.D.

This chapter discusses several topics in which the interface between human and machine or, more accurately, the interface between anesthesiologist and anesthesia equipment, plays a crucial role. On the basis of the title of this chapter, some may think at first glance that the topics covered are unrelated. However, these three topics—vigilance, alarms, and integrated monitoring systems—are in fact closely interrelated.

The administration of anesthesia is predominantly a complex monitoring task and, as such, requires sustained vigilance. Unfortunately, humans are not very good at monitoring because they are error-prone and their vigilance is susceptible to degradation by a variety of human, environmental, and system or equipment factors. In fact, human error is the major cause of most anesthetic mishaps. Therefore, designers of anesthetic equipment have attempted to "aid" the anesthesiologist by incorporating devices and systems to augment vigilance and monitoring performance. Alarms, intended to notify the operator of potential critical situations, are effective only if properly designed and implemented. The recent promise of completely integrated anesthesia workstations (with "smart" alarms, monitoring aids, etc.) remains unfulfilled. However, such systems are on the horizon. Their successful implementation will require a more complete understanding of the task of administering anesthesia and of the factors that affect the performance of the anesthesiologist in this complex environment.

ANESTHETIC MISHAPS

As many as 3000 preventable instances of anesthesia-related death or brain damage occur in the United States each year.[1] Human error appears to be the major cause of these preventable mishaps.[2-5] Several studies[5,6] have demonstrated that human errors, such as "unintentional gas flow change" or "syringe swap", might account for up to 70% of anesthetic mishaps. In a study by Keenan and Boyan,[1] 75% of intraoperative cardiac arrests observed appeared to be caused by preventable anesthetic errors. In another study,[7] inadequate observation of patients was a contributing factor in one-third of deaths. Preventable anesthetic morbidity and mortality remains a major problem for our specialty. As the practice of anesthesia becomes more complex, with a proliferation of sophisticated devices and techniques that enable anesthesiologists to care for more critically ill patients, the risk associated with the occurrence of critical events increases.

Even under ideal conditions, performance on complicated tasks is rarely perfect.[8] In complex systems consisting of humans and machines, human error is almost always a factor.[9,10] For example, the percentage of accidents caused by aircrew error appears to be greater than 50%.[11,12] Accidents are usually caused by the cumulative effect of a number of events rather than by one isolated incident.[12] Why do highly trained and experienced individuals make errors, and what factors influence the occurrence of these errors? What can be done to decrease their incidence or to mitigate their negative outcomes? Unfortunately, research thus far has only begun to provide adequate answers to these questions.

HUMAN ERROR

Errors are a normal component of human cognitive function and play a major role in learning.[10] However, most errors do not result in damaging consequences. An error that results in an unacceptable outcome is often called an accident.[13] Errors are most likely to deteriorate into a damaging situation when conditions prevent the appropriate corrective responses. Errors committed by anesthesiologists can have catastrophic consequences if not corrected. Yet, Cooper and colleagues[6] showed that most critical events in anesthetic practice were discovered and corrected before a serious mishap occurred. It is crucial to understand the determinants of recovery from anesthetic errors. Factors such as sleep deprivation, miscommunication, and equipment problems not only can increase the potential for error but also may preclude effective recovery.

Two types of error are slips and mistakes (Box 17-1). Both of these can take the form of errors of omission (omitting a task step or even an entire task) or errors of commission (incorrect performance).[14] Slips are most likely to occur during activities for which one is highly trained and, therefore, are performed outside of active conscious thought. Drug syringe swaps, a commonly described anesthetic critical event,[6] are a form of slip. Errors of omission can occur when unexpected distractions interrupt a well-established behavioral sequence; errors of com-

---

Box 17-1. Types of human error

Type of error	*Description*
Mistake	Inappropriate intention or action, often due to lack of training or knowledge
Slips	Appropriate intention or action at inappropriate time
Mode error	Erroneous classification of the situation
Description error	Ambiguous or incomplete specification of intention
Capture error	Correct schemata at incorrect time, often due to task overlap
Faulty activation or triggering	Activation of inappropriate action or failure to activate appropriate action
Data driven error	Automatic actions inappropriate for the situation but called into play by ongoing action sequences
Fixation errors	Failure to revise actions with changing conditions, "cognitive lockup"
Confirmation bias	Tendency to seek confirming data for existing hypotheses
Representational errors	Faulty mental model of the system and its function or malfunction

Modified from Norman D: *The psychology of everyday things*, New York, 1988, Basic Books.

mission arise when automated schema (or preprogrammed subroutines) are inappropriately called into play by specific stimuli without conscious processing.[10] An individual, particularly when under stress, tends to revert to a high-frequency (well learned) response in such situations. Experts may in fact be more likely than novices to make these kinds of errors.

DeAnda and Gaba[15] found that during simulated anesthesia cases, anesthesia residents generated *unplanned* critical incidents at a rate of nearly two per simulated case. Eighty-six percent of the incidents were due to human error. Of these, nearly one quarter were due to fixation errors. Fixation errors occurred when the subject was unable to focus on the most critical problem at hand because of persistent, inappropriate attention or actions directed elsewhere.

In contrast to slips and fixation errors, mistakes are technical or judgmental errors. Thus, mistakes are caused by inadequate or incorrect information, inappropriate decision-making skills or strategies, inadequate training, lack of experience, or insufficient supervision or backup.

People are more likely to commit errors when they are mismatched to the task or when the system is not user friendly. Factors that can influence error commission include skill level, attitude, inexperience, stress,[14] poor supervision,[16] task complexity,[14] and inadequate system design (Box 17-2). The topic of human error in anesthesia has been covered in some detail by Gaba.[17,18]

At least some of what, at first glance, appears to be human error can often be traced back to poorly designed interfaces between human and machine.[19] In fact, Norman[20] suggests that "the real culprit in most errors or accidents involving complex systems is, almost always, poor design." Poor operational design can introduce great risk of system failure due to operator error. Factors related to system-induced error include boredom due to overautomation, overreliance on automated devices, and poor team coordi-

nation. Good operating practice is essential but not sufficient for minimizing system risk: First, the design of the system must be fundamentally sound; next, the system must be properly constructed and implemented; the operators must be thoroughly familiar with the system; and finally, ongoing quality control must assure that system use is appropriate over the full range of possible conditions. This applies to the anesthesia workspace and must be considered when introducing new anesthesia equipment to this unique environment.

VIGILANCE AND MONITORING PERFORMANCE

Vigilance has been equated to "sustained attention."[21] Attention requires alertness, selection of information, and conscious effort. Alertness indicates the receptivity of the individual to external information. Mackworth[22] defined vigilance as "a state of readiness to detect and respond to certain specified small changes occurring at random intervals in the environment." Thus, in its broadest sense, "anesthetic vigilance" can be viewed as a state of clinical awareness whereby dangerous conditions are anticipated or recognized and promptly corrected (Box 17-3). Monitoring is by definition a vigilance task, and the administration of anesthesia is a complex monitoring task. The anesthesiologist must continuously evaluate the patient's medical status while assessing the effects of anesthesia and surgical intervention. Complex memory, decision making, vigilance, and attention are the most vulnerable to compromise under the stressful work conditions often experienced in the operating room.

Psychologists and engineers have studied vigilance for many years. Investigators in fields outside of medicine, most notably in aviation, have applied this information to understanding performance on complex monitoring tasks. Studies have identified environmental factors and man-machine interface variables that can impair vigilance and performance in air traffic control,[23] train driving,[24,25] auto-

---

Box 17-2. Some typical causes of human error in anesthesia

Cause of error	*Example*
HUMAN FACTORS	
Task complexity	Not ventilating after coming off cardiopulmonary bypass
Lack of training or experience	Rapid administration of vancomycin or protamine
Stress	Swap of drug syringe or ampule during critical situation
Ill health	Under the influence of opiates or other substances
ENVIRONMENTAL FACTORS	
Noise or miscommunication	Misheard surgeon and wrong antibiotic administered
Workplace constraints	Circuit disconnect due to moving equipment or personnel
EQUIPMENT AND SYSTEM FACTORS	
Poor equipment design	Light bulb goes out on laryngoscope
False and/or noisy alarms	Failure to recognize critical situation after alarms are disabled
Mismatch of human-machine functions	Failure to detect ongoing event while vital signs are manually recorded onto record

---

Box 17-3. Definitions

Term	*Definition*
Perception	To attain awareness or understanding, usually via the senses
Attention	A conscious effort to remain alert and to perceive and select information
Vigilance	A state of readiness to detect and respond to changes in the monitored environment; a state of "sustained attention"
Monitoring	A vigilance task involving the observation of one or several data streams in order to detect specified changes often occurring at random intervals
Anesthesia vigilance	A state of clinical awareness whereby dangerous conditions are anticipated or recognized and promptly corrected
Judgment	The formation of an opinion or evaluation on the basis of available information
Cognition	The act or process of knowing, including both awareness and judgment
Decision making	The act of choosing between alternative diagnoses or possible actions, on the basis of judgment

---

Modified from Swain A, Weston L: *An approach to the diagnosis and misdiagnosis of abnormal conditions in post-accident sequences in complex man-machine systems.* In Goodstein L, Andersen H, Olsen S, editors: *Tasks, errors, and mental models,* London, 1988, Taylor and Francis, pp 209-229; Weinger M, Englund C: Ergonomic and human factors affecting anesthetic vigilance and monitoring performance in the operating room environment, *Anesthesiology* 73:995-1021, 1990; and Mackworth N: Vigilance, *The Advancement of Science* 53:389-393, 1957.

mobile driving,[26] and nuclear power plant control.[27] The armed forces now consider the potential impact of such factors at the earliest stages of the design of new weapons systems.[28]

In most complex monitoring tasks, increased task complexity or duration generally leads to impaired performance.[29,30] A major factor in the effect of additional tasks on performance appears to be what personal resources (perceptual or cognitive) are required for each new task and whether those resources are already taxed. Other factors known to impair vigilance include noise, environmental pollution, fatigue, sleep deprivation, and boredom[31] (Fig. 17-1). Performance can also be impaired if the individual is under stress, of ill health, or using drugs. Personality factors, training, and experience also affect performance. Jennings and Chiles[32] showed that, of all performance skills, complex monitoring tasks (like those in anesthesia or aviation) are the most likely to be influenced by environmental or task variables.

RESEARCH IN ANESTHETIC VIGILANCE

In one of the earliest ergonomic studies of anesthesia,[33] link analysis was used to examine how anesthesiologists used their time in the operating room. The practice of anesthesia was divided into a number of discrete activities, and the frequency and sequence of each activity was determined. The relationship (or link) between different activities was then analyzed. One principal finding was that anesthesiologists directed their attention away from the patient 42% of the time. Other time-motion studies[34-38] appeared to support these findings. In recent studies, the effects of level of experience on the workload and vigilance of residents administering anesthesia has been examined. In novice residents, visual vigilance was significantly im-

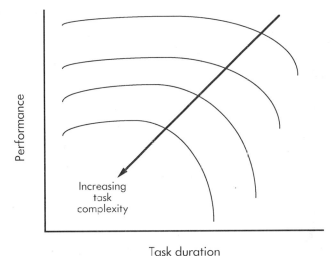

Fig. 17-1. There is a curvilinear relationship between task performance and task duration whereby increasing task duration leads to impaired performance. This curve shifts to the left as the complexity of the task increases.

paired during such manual tasks as airway manipulation.[39] Task density analysis[40] suggested that when activity level was high, the average amount of time spent per task was low. In contrast, when activity level was low, the average amount of time spent per task was high. These studies have provided important descriptive information about the task of administering anesthesia as well as demonstrating the potential usefulness of these kinds of studies for examining the effects of human, environmental, and equipment factors on vigilance and task performance. Chapter 18 provides additional discussion of task analysis studies in anesthesia.

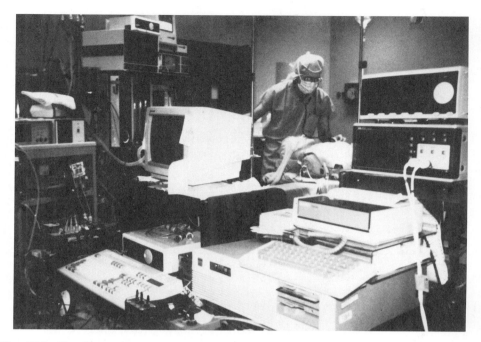

Fig. 17-2. The Comprehensive Anesthesia Simulation Environment (CASE) developed by Dr. David Gaba at Stanford University. The keyboard, computer, and other controls *(lower left)* permit the simulation director to orchestrate the simulation by adjusting the data presented on the anesthesia monitors and devices. A subject is seen *(upper right)* administering to the patient manikin. (Photograph courtesy of David Gaba, M.D.)

In the last few years there has been a marked increase in interest in the factors that impair anesthetic vigilance, and some preliminary studies have been undertaken. Well controlled studies are essential to understand the character of anesthesia vigilance and monitoring performance. Studies should be designed to utilize techniques and procedures that have been repeatedly validated by investigators in other fields. Some aspects of this human factors literature were introduced to anesthesiologists in a recent review article.[31]

Simulation in anesthesia

To investigate how anesthesiologists respond to critical incidents in real clinical settings, Gaba and DeAnda[41] have developed the Comprehensive Anesthesia Simulation Environment (CASE), which attempts to simulate the entire anesthesia environment in an actual operating room setting. The simulations are controlled by a clinically experienced simulation director who uses scenario scripts. CASE is currently being used to collect data on the response of both experienced and inexperienced anesthesiologists to critical incidents and as an educational tool[42] (Fig. 17-2). (See also Chapter 20.) In one study,[15] of the 132 unplanned incidents (36 considered critical) during 19 simulations with anesthesia residents used as subjects, human error accounted for 86% of the incidents whereas equipment failure accounted for only 3%. The incidence of human error during simulated anesthesia in this study is similar to that found by Cooper[6,43] among anesthesiologists in the operating room. These studies are important because they document the frequent occurrence of error in anesthesia and also because they validate the use of simulation to study the types and causes of critical incidents in anesthesia.

A number of anesthesia simulators are now under development. Some of these systems simulate only part of the anesthesia task;[44] others are more comprehensive.[18,45] Some are only computer (screen) based and are therefore portable[46,47] (Fig. 17-3, see color insert). Others are partial task trainers, primarily used for educational purposes, such as Philip's Gas Man, a computer model of uptake and distribution of anesthetic gases.[48] The Utah Anesthesia Workstation[44] consists of a central display that uses a Macintosh computer to control a combination of 17 sensors and monitors that provide detailed information about the anesthesia delivery system. The computer monitors the system via a set of preprogrammed rules. The system is capable of reliably identifying 26 different critical events with regard to the anesthesia machine and breathing circuit. Simulation and modeling are likely to gain an increasingly important role in the design and implementation of anesthesia monitoring systems.

FACTORS AFFECTING VIGILANCE

A wide range of factors can affect anesthetic vigilance and monitoring performance (Box 17-4). The following discussion provides a perspective on how everyday occur-

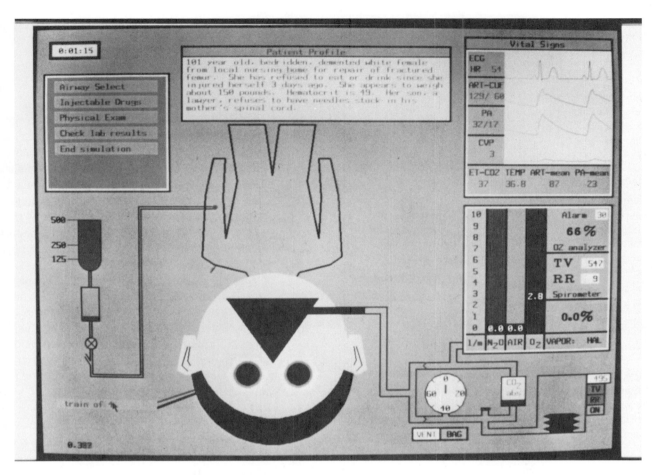

Fig. 17-3. Screen-based anesthesia simulators, such as SLEEPER, developed by Dr. N. Ty Smith at the University of California, San Diego, are useful tools for teaching the cognitive aspects of anesthesia care. These computer-based simulators can accurately depict the physiological responses of "patients" to a variety of pharmacological interventions or disease processes. (See color insert.) (Photograph courtesy of N. Ty Smith, M.D.)

rences can significantly impair vigilance, potentially leading to an increased risk of critical events and, as a result, anesthetic morbidity or mortality.

Noise

The noise level in the operating room can be quite high. Shapiro and Berland[49] measured noise levels associated with specific tasks in the operating room during several typical surgical procedures, finding that "the noise in the OR frequently exceeds that of a freeway." The effects of noise on performance depend on the type of noise and the task being performed.[50,51] In addition, other environmental and human factors can interact with noise to affect task performance.[52] Noise levels similar to those found in operating rooms detrimentally affect short-term memory tasks[51] and may also mask task-related cues and cause distractions during critical periods.[53] Difficult tasks that require high levels of perceptual and/or information processing are negatively affected by noise.[54] High noise levels (particularly with long-term exposure) produce physiological changes consistent with stress.[55] Exposure to loud noise also activates the sympathetic nervous system, a situation that may augment the effects of other factors and lead to impaired decision making during critical incidents.[31,52]

There is little doubt that background noise interferes with effective verbal communication. When multiple tasks are required, the presence of background noise may bias attention toward the dominant task.[56] The effects of noise and sleep deprivation interact; the former is an activator (or arouser), and the latter is a deactivator. When both factors are present, they often cancel each other's effects.[57] Time of day may play a differential role in the impact of each of these influences on task efficiency.[58]

Although loud noise is clearly disruptive and can impair auditory vigilance (e.g., ability to monitor the esophageal stethoscope) the presence of low levels of background (white) noise may have a beneficial effect on performance of complex tasks.[59] Several studies[60,61] have suggested that the presence of familiar background music may improve vigilance.

Box 17-4. Factors affecting intraoperative vigilance and performance

Environmental factors

Noise
Temperature and humidity
Environmental toxicity
Ambient lighting
Workspace constraints

Human factors

Human error
Fatigue
Sleep deprivation
Circadian effects and shiftwork
Breaks
Boredom
Substance use or abuse
State of health and stress
Training and experience
Psychosocial factors
Personality factors

Task and information factors

Primary task load
Secondary task intrusion
Misinformation or distracting information
Alarms and warnings
Interpersonal and team communication

System and equipment factors

System-induced errors
Equipment failure
Poor equipment design
Misunderstanding of equipment design or function
Automation

Temperature

Uncomfortable environmental temperatures, a common situation in many operating rooms, can impair vigilance.[62-64] Although there appears to be significant variability in the effects of temperature on performance depending on the experimental situation (i.e., other environmental, task, and subject variables), as a general rule, temperatures that promote general fatigue decrease performance.[62] Extremely cold temperatures have a deleterious effect on some cognitive tasks, primarily because of the distraction of the cold environment and the associated decrease in manual dexterity.[65] These effects often show up as increases in errors and memory deficits.[66] Studies in the industrial workplace[67] suggest that when temperatures fall outside a preferred range (17° C to 23° C), workers are more likely to exhibit unsafe behaviors (which could lead to occupational injury). Temperatures in some adult ORs can be as low as 7° C, and those in pediatric ORs may ap-

approach 30° C. The negative effects of temperature are probably augmented by other factors that enhance fatigue or impair performance.

Environmental toxicity (exposure to vapors)

There is voluminous literature on the effects of trace anesthetic vapors on the performance of anesthesiologists. The early studies of Bruce, et al.[68] reported that exposure to 550 ppm nitrous oxide and 14 ppm halothane led to a significant decrease in performance on complex vigilance tasks. However, their study used as subjects Mormon dental students, who may have been uniquely sensitive to the effects of the anesthetic gases. Smith and Shirley[69] subsequently showed that acute exposure to trace anesthetic gases in amounts commonly seen in an unscavenged operating room had no effect on performance in naive volunteers. It thus appears that impaired vigilance due solely to trace anesthetic gases is probably not a problem in the modern, well-scavenged operating room. This is supported by a recent well-controlled cross-over study[70] in which anesthesiologists showed no differences in either mood or cognitive ability between working in a scavenged operating theater compared with the intensive care unit (with no trace gases). (See also Chapter 5.)

Interpersonal and team factors

The anesthesiologist must function as an integral part of the operating room team. In other highly complex tasks involving teamwork (e.g., commercial aviation) the team has generally been together for a long time and is well-practiced. Team communication involves unspoken expectations, traditions, general assumptions regarding task distribution, and chain-of-command hierarchies, as well as individual emotional and behavioral components. Alterations in any of these factors can impair effective team function.[71] Extended to the OR, these findings suggest that the anesthesiologist who is confronted with a new surgeon, OR nurse, or anesthesia resident should be sensitive to the new interpersonal environment and should exercise extra vigilance by making a special effort to communicate clearly and unambiguously, particularly in stressful situations. Communication may prove even more difficult when some or all of the team members are subjected to such other stressors as fatigue or sleep deprivation.

Fatigue

Fatigue is the inability or unwillingness to continue effective performance of a mental or physical task. Fatigue is caused by hours of continuous work or work overload, whereas boredom is thought to be more a function of insufficient work challenge and understimulation.[72] Extreme fatigue leads to objectively measurable symptoms of exhaustion and psychological aversion to further work. There is a powerful psychological component to the continued ability to perform skilled physical or mental tasks in the

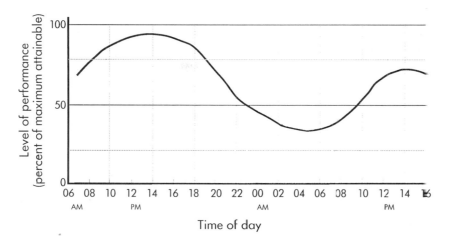

Fig. 17-4. Theoretical performance of a complex task as a function of the influences of sleep loss and disturbance of circadian rhythm over a 36-hour period. Note that performance is best at certain times of day, generally between 10 A.M. and 3 P.M., but decreases markedly during the early morning hours. After a sleepless night, the amplitude of circadian fluctuations is dampened and performance remains depressed below that seen the previous day. This figure is a composite based on multiple studies of sustained cognitive performance of different tasks by day-time workers who were not physicians. (Reprinted from Weinger MB, Englund CE: Ergonomic and human factors affecting anesthetic vigilance and monitoring performance in the operating room environment. *Anesthesiology* 73:995-1021, 1990.)

face of worsening fatigue. Although some extremely fatigued individuals can be induced to perform,[73] the quality and wisdom of continued work under these circumstances is questionable, and this is certainly so in situations where human lives may be at stake. Individuals, however, display marked differences in their response to factors or situations leading to fatigue or its amelioration.

Few studies of fatigue have used physicians as subjects. Those that have, have typically involved sleep loss and, primarily because of their poor methodology, have raised more questions than they answered. Fatigue and sleep loss are often covariants in studies examining continuous, long work schedules; and, in turn, both are modulated by circadian processes. Because the effects of these variables interact,[74] it is difficult to separate the relative contribution of each factor to performance decrement.

Individuals subjected to excessive work, fatigue, or inappropriate shift schedules show degraded performance, impaired learning and thought processes, irritability, memory deficits, and interpersonal dysfunction.[31,75] Fatigued subjects pay less attention to peripherally located instruments and are inconsistent in their responses to external stimuli. Fatigued subjects, when coping with task demands, exhibit less control over their own behavior and tend to select more risky alternatives (or short cuts).[73] If sufficiently motivated, fatigued subjects can attain relatively normal performance on tasks of short duration,[76] but they find it difficult to sustain performance on vigilance or monitoring tasks of long duration.[77,78] Adding sleep loss

or shiftwork accentuates fatigue-induced performance decrements.[79]

Sleep deprivation

Although they are similar in some of their performance-shaping effects and are certainly interactive, sleep deprivation and fatigue are different processes. A large body of research[76,80-84] supports the contention that sleep deprivation and disturbances in circadian rhythm can dramatically impair performance on monitoring tasks. A single night of sleep loss can produce decrements in performance, especially with regard to skilled cognitive tasks (Fig. 17-4). Impairment can be seen shortly after initiation of the task, and within 20 to 35 minutes for many tasks.[85] However, in most sustained work activities, major decrements usually occur after 4 hours and again after 18 hours.[86]

Studies involving one or more days without sleep reveal that subjects exhibit progressive decreases in reaction time and increases in response variability[87] (Box 17-5). Work rate is appreciably slowed, particularly when subjects are required to make choices.[88] In vigilance tasks, omission errors increase[89] whether visual or auditory signals are presented.[90,91] Sleep loss impairs active use of working memory,[87] particularly when the sleep loss precedes learning.[92] Sleep-deprived workers fail to appropriately allocate attention, set task priorities, and sample for sources of potential faulty information.[93,94] Because many of these skills are essential to the anesthesiologist for optimal performance, it is clear that sleep loss can be extremely detrimental. There

---

Box 17-5. Some potential effects of sleep deprivation on vigilance and performance

Decreases in reaction time
Increases in response variability
Decreases in work rate
Difficulties making choices
Increases in omission errors
Impaired working memory
Failure to allocate attention appropriately
Difficulty setting task priorities
Failure to evaluate potential faulty information

---

are, however, wide individual differences in the amount of daily sleep required.[95]

Haslam's field work[96] indicated that some sleep (2 to 3 hours in a 24-hour period) is better than none at all, at least for subjects involved in military exercises. For example, in studies of sleep-deprived military subjects, a 2-hour nap was insufficient, 3 hours permitted maintenance of previous levels of (already impaired) performance, and a full 4-hour nap was required before baseline performance was restored.[76,97,98] Taking a short nap (of less than 2 hours) at the circadian low point (see the section on circadian changes) produces greater cognitive impairment than does taking a nap of the same length at the peak of the circadian cycle.[99,100] Another problem of napping is that of sleep inertia. If a sleep-deprived subject is permitted to nap, then following the nap there will be a period of sleep inertia during which the subject will exhibit a low level of arousal and significantly impaired vigilance and performance. Sleep inertia can last as long as 2 hours.[76]

In one of the first studies of the effects of sleep loss on physician performance, Friedman, et al.[81] showed that the skill of sleep-deprived medical interns to detect cardiac dysrhythmias was significantly lower than that of interns with a normal amount of rest. Hart and colleagues,[101] in a well-designed study of 30 first-year medical residents, demonstrated mild but significant disturbances in memory, decision making, and motor execution in on-call residents deprived of normal sleep (2.7 ± 2.2 hours slept) compared with those getting a full night's rest (7.9 ± 1.3 hours). Unfortunately, other studies[102-107] designed to assess the impact of sleep deprivation on the ability of physicians (usually house staff) to perform clinical duties have generally had serious methodological flaws. In one recent relatively well-designed but small study, six volunteer anesthesia residents were trained to perform visual and auditory reaction-time tests as well as a test of fine-motor coordination.[108] The subjects were then tested in two morning sessions 24 hours apart; a cross-over design was used. There were no differences in baseline performance between the group on call and the group not on call. However, at the end of the 24-hour period, the on-call residents

showed worse performance than those not on call on the visual reaction-time and coordination-scanning tests but not on the auditory reaction-time test. Subjective fatigue was also significantly greater in the on-call residents. The authors noted that the performance decrements observed in the on-call residents were of the same order of magnitude as those observed after a moderate oral dose of alcohol when the same psychomotor tests were used.

These studies, as well as the large array of more theoretical work on sleep deprivation and performance, lend support to the contention that patient care can be compromised if a fatigued or sleep-deprived clinician is allowed to administer an anesthetic, to operate, or to perform other medical procedures. The issue of decreased clinical performance of house officers and other physicians as a result of overwork and sleep deprivation has recently gained national attention.[109] From the literature it can be concluded that the sleep schedule of the anesthesiologist is an important variable in determining capacity for intraoperative vigilance and performance. It thus appears reasonable to consider a discussion of restrictions on anesthesiologists' work schedules. Individuals must recognize that it is neither unprofessional nor weak to admit sleepiness or fatigue when on the job,[110] and they must attempt to either make time to recuperate or seek a clinical replacement. Individuals exhibit significant differences in their responses to acute or chronic sleep loss, and all anesthesiologists must be cognizant of their own limitations.

Circadian changes and shiftwork

Periodic, rhythmic fluctuations in bodily processes, including performance and work efficiency, have been well documented.[57,72] Over 50 neurophysiological and psychological rhythms that potentially influence human performance have been identified.[111] Most studies of rhythmic changes in efficiency have focused on cycles of about one day, called circadian processes. An individual's normal rhythm can be significantly influenced by environmental conditions, illness, time-zone changes, and altering shift schedules. During normal wake time, circadian-related fluctuations in performance can range from 14% to 43%[57] (Box 17-6).

In rapidly changing schedules of regular work hours (e.g., routinely and frequently changing from day shift to night shift), performance rhythm amplitudes show variations as great as 50%.[112] The rate and amount of adjustment to shift changes or extended work days is an individual matter.[113,114] However, several studies of shiftwork revealed that some individuals were never able to adjust[115] and continued to show greater sleep, social, and health problems.[116-118] Efficiency of permanent night-shift workers is at least 10% less than that of comparable day-shift coworkers,[119] and minor accidents[112] and errors in vigilance monitoring[120] arise most frequently during night shifts and the early morning hours. On the other hand, fully acclimated night-shift workers have a realigned circadian cycle such that their best performance occurs during their normal shift. Swing-shift workers seem to have the most difficulty establishing a normal diurnal rhythm.[80] Because adjustment to shiftwork takes at least several days, if shift rotations are required, the rotation should be clockwise and never less than two weeks per shift.[116]

Alterations in the normal circadian rhythms cause changes in arousal as well as other mental and physical functions and play a major role in the effects on task performance of acute sleep loss, napping, and recovery from disruptions in normal sleep schedule. Phase shifts are introduced by sleep interruption. Some circadian functions are altered and normal rhythms may be disrupted even after multiple brief interruptions in an otherwise full night's sleep.[121] The peak and minimal performance times normally expected by the individual are similarly shifted. This can lead to a false sense of competence during normal working hours following acute sleep loss. For example, an anesthesiologist who has been up working most of the previous night, after recovering from sleep inertia in the early part of the next morning, may feel remarkably awake, perhaps even euphoric. Yet studies have documented degraded performance on complex tasks in such situations[100] (Fig. 17-4). By midafternoon, dramatic decreases in arousal and feelings of well-being accompany parallel decrements in performance. That evening, the anesthesiologist probably has difficulty falling asleep, especially if an afternoon nap was taken. In fact, sleep-to-wake cycles can be disturbed for up to 36 hours, and the anesthesiologist may remain more prone to error during this recovery phase.[122,123]

Breaks

Common sense suggests that relief from a prolonged monitoring task should enhance subsequent performance. Both anecdotal reports and laboratory studies have indicated that people prefer self-paced tasks and will take a break when needed.[86] Short breaks have been shown to alleviate fatigue as well as to increase employee satisfaction and productivity in machine-paced jobs.[85] For worker-controlled sedentary jobs, short breaks or a change in activity

will increase performance and relieve boredom.[86,124] However, thus far there is little experimental evidence to support the widely held belief that performance will improve following a break from a prolonged, complex monitoring task such as administering anesthesia.

The optimal frequency and duration of breaks is still unknown for most occupations. Warm[125] has recommended that monitoring tasks be limited to sessions of less than 4 hours. Breaks have been required by many contracts (and legislation in some countries), particularly for occupations in which impaired worker performance could endanger worker or public safety (i.e., transportation workers).

Cooper, et al.,[126,127] in a study of critical incidents associated with intraoperative exchanges of anesthesia personnel, found 90 incidents occurring during a break. Twenty-eight of these incidences were said to be favorable (i.e., the relieving anesthesiologist discovered and corrected a potentially dangerous preexisting situation); only 10 incidents were cited as being unfavorable (i.e., the relieving anesthesiologist "caused" the critical incident). In the remainder of the incidents either the problem was perpetuated by the relieving anesthesiologist or the incident could not be classified. Unfortunately, because of the possibility of biased reporting, the relative frequency with which relief results in favorable versus unfavorable outcomes cannot be determined from this type of study. On the other hand, out of the 1089 total critical incidents studied, Cooper and colleagues failed to find a single incident due to relief which resulted in significant morbidity or mortality. However, the detection of problems during a break probably depends on a systematic and comprehensive review of the anesthetic course by the relieving anesthesiologist. It has been recommended that specific relief-exchange protocols be developed and strictly adhered to (Box 17-7).[126]

Boredom

Boredom generally occurs when tasks are repetitious, uninteresting (monotonous), and undemanding. Boredom is the result of a requirement to maintain attention in the absence of relevant task information[128] and is most likely to occur in semiautomatic tasks that prevent mind-wandering but are not fully mentally absorbing. Boredom is thus a problem of information underload.[72] Boredom appears to be a major problem in many complex real-life tasks, such as train driving[25,129] and aviation.[130] These results, as well as those from laboratory experiments, suggest that in the presence of boredom, increased effort is necessary to suppress distracting stimuli and a generalized feeling of fatigue.[131] Boredom can be minimized by altering the sequence of tasks in a busy job[132] or adding tasks to a monotonous job.[133] Dividing attention among several tasks (time-sharing) may not diminish monitoring performance and, in some circumstances, may improve it.[134,135]

Box 17-7. Recommended standard relief protocol

The relieving anesthesiologists must establish familiarity with
   The patient's preoperative status
   The course of the anesthetic
   The course of the surgical procedure
   The overall anesthetic plan
   The arrangement of the equipment, apparatus, drugs, and fluids.
The two anesthesiologists must communicate the relief plans with the surgeon(s).
The original anesthesiologist must not leave the room until the relieving anesthesiologist is in control of the situation and has all of the necessary information to continue with the anesthetic.
The original anesthesiologist should not leave the room if the patient is unstable or the anesthetic is not likely to remain in a steady-state condition for at least 5 to 10 minutes.
Care must be taken to communicate all special information that is not recorded or may not be readily evident.
Under normal circumstances, the relieving anesthesiologists should not appreciably alter the course of preexisting anesthetic management.
Before transfer of control, the original anesthesiologist should carefully go through these same steps with the relieving anesthesiologist.
If the relieving anesthesiologist is to finish the case, special care should be taken to explain the anesthetic plan.

Modified from Cooper J, Long C, Newbower R, et al: Critical incidents associated with intraoperative exchanges of anesthesia personnel, *Anesthesiology* 56:456-461, 1982.

Stress and performance

Sources of stress affecting performance can be found in the work environment (social and physical),[136,137] in the tasks involved (mental load and pacing), and in the individual (health related, job matching, and personality).[138,139] Stress is a broad term, and depending on its type and magnitude, it can result in either degraded or enhanced performance. A subject's performance will be significantly influenced by interaction with the environment and its associated stresses, the work to be performed in this environment, and the level of incentive for performing.

Many personal interactions in the operating room can affect performance adversely (e.g., dealing with the difficult surgeon or the uncooperative nurse). Other, outside factors can also influence an anesthesiologist's performance, for example, financial worries or a recent fight with a spouse. Such domestic stresses have been shown to increase the likelihood of accidents.[140]

Box 17-8. Some common physiological correlates of stress

Increased heart rate
Increased blood pressure
Decreased beat-to-beat variability in heart rate
Increased T-wave peak amplitude
Increased respiratory rate
Increased pupil diameter
Increased skin conductance
Altered voice characteristics

Stressful environmental conditions impair vigilance, especially in situations of conflict.[141] The level of stress can be assessed by measurement of either physiological or psychological parameters. The physiological correlates of stress generally correspond to sympathetic nervous system activity. Studies have used heart rate,[141,142] skin conductance,[143] respiratory rate,[144] beat-to-beat variability in heart rate,[130,145] T-wave peak amplitude on ECG,[130] changes in voice characteristics,[130] and catecholamine excretion[146] to assess stress levels during performance of complex tasks. With increasing workloads during simulated and real flights in high-performance aircraft, cosmonauts who exhibited physiological signs of stress had more false alarms and were more disorganized.[130] Thus increased workload or mental stress increases activity in the sympathetic nervous system, which can lead to deleterious physiological responses[147] (Box 17-8).

The physiologic response of the anesthesiologist to the stress of giving anesthesia may be a crucial variable, yet it has received little attention. Toung and colleagues[148] studied the change in the heart rates of anesthesiologists during induction and intubation. There was a 60% increase over baseline heart rate in first-year residents at the time of intubation (Fig. 17-5). More experienced clinicians had a smaller increase in rate. Subsequently, these investigators showed[149] that prior medical training, even if not related to anesthesia, was associated with a diminished stress response to the administration of anesthesia. Repeated exposures to a specific situation results in diminished endocrine (stress) responses if the subject has learned to cope with the situation.[146]

Substance use and abuse

Recent data from the American Medical Association[150] suggest that 1% to 2% of practicing physicians are addicted to drugs and up to 8% can be classified as alcoholics. Anesthesiologists may be at higher risk for drug abuse than other physicians.[151] Although the abuse of drugs and alcohol is obviously detrimental to job performance, a variety of other, ostensibly innocuous drugs, such as caffeine, antihistamines, and nicotine, can also influence vigilance and monitoring skills.

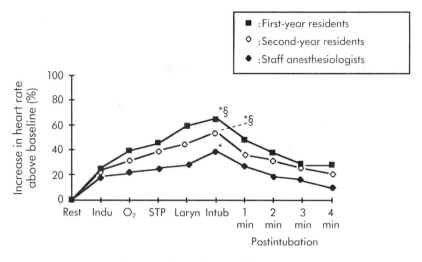

* P<0.05 when compared between groups
*§ P<0.001 when compared with pre-induction rates

Fig. 17-5. The heart rate of anesthesiologists increases above baseline during the induction of anesthesia. This increase in heart rate, a physiological correlate of stress and workload, is greatest in first-year anesthesia residents and diminishes with increasing experience. (From Toung T, Donhan R, Rogers M: The stress of giving anesthesia on the electrocardiogram of anesthesiologists, *Anesthesiology* 61:A465, 1984 [abstract].)

A small dose of caffeine, such as that found in a typical caffeinated soft drink, can have a positive effect on vigilance and performance.[152] Yet, a recent study[153] suggested that even among regular coffee drinkers, caffeine ingestion can magnify the physiological consequences of stress. Antihistamines have also been associated with performance decrements on simulated tasks.[154,155] However, the new "non-sedating" antihistamines, such as terfenadine (Seldane), may be without significant performance-degrading effects.[156] Phenothiazines and perhaps other antiemetics can also impair performance on complex tasks.[155]

There is little doubt that alcohol ingestion markedly impairs vigilance as well as psychomotor performance.[157-159] In fact, pilot simulator–based training studies[160] have documented significant impairment in performance at blood alcohol levels as low as 20 to 35 mg/dL, well below that considered legally drunk. Perhaps just as important, the effects of hangover from alcohol can also significantly affect performance,[161,162] even in the absence of the perception of impairment by the individual being tested.[161,163,164] Recent work on hangover effects suggests that individuals should wait *at least 14 hours* after alcohol consumption before performing such complex monitoring tasks as flying an aircraft or administering anesthesia.

It is well known that marijuana intoxication impairs performance,[165] and marijuana ingestion has been implicated as a causative factor in recent railroad and airline accidents.[166-168] What may not be appreciated is that, like alcohol, marijuana intoxication can be associated with a hangover condition that may impair performance,[169] even after 24 hours and in the absence of an appreciation by the subjects of their impairment.[170]

Personality factors

Subjects of different personality types perform differently on vigilance tasks.[145] In fact, individual psychological or physiological differences may be the most important confounding factors in performance of vigilance tasks.[171] For example, for some tasks, the incidence of error may be better predicted on the basis of individual personality traits (such as emotional stability) than on the basis of the nature of the particular task.[172] Individual preferences for particular living, working, and sleeping schedules may be related to biological profiles. Thus, working and/or sleeping at times diametrically opposed to an individual's biologically-rooted personality characteristics leads to performance inefficiency and fatigue. Important factors in predicting adjustment to on-call duties may include an individual's adaptability to changes in normal sleeping schedule and the ability to overcome drowsiness.[173]

Training and experience

Few people would argue that training and experience are important in ensuring a high level of performance of a complex task. Aviation accident rates directly correlate with flight experience[11] (Fig. 17-6). Individual clinical

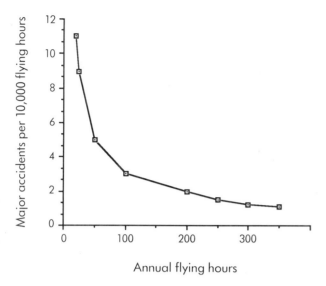

Fig. 17-6. In aviation, there is a strong correlation between flight experience and accident rate. Consistent with this finding, recent task analysis data support the hypothesis that the experience of the anesthesiologist may affect the incidence of anesthetic morbidity and mortality.

practice may significantly influence anesthetic morbidity.[174] Additional training and experience may obviate the negative effects on performance of stress or increased workload.[175] Gaba and DeAnda[42] showed that more experienced residents were better able to correct simulated untoward intraoperative events yet had no faster detection times than residents with one year less of training. However, individual differences, perhaps in experience or education, appeared to be much more important than amount of training.

Workload and task characteristics

Many factors influence the probability of continuous satisfactory job performance, including personal problems, excessive workload, and specific characteristics of the task itself.[27] An example of how workload or task requirements can influence performance comes from a recent study[176] of 12 relatively inexperienced private pilots asked to perform a series of flight maneuvers on a simulator under increasingly difficult conditions until performance failure occurred. Under high-workload conditions, the subjects tended to decompose maneuvers into smaller, more manageable tasks. The subjects also omitted portions of the tasks that were not essential to maintain a minimum level of performance (i.e., safely flying the aircraft). Often the omission of a task component is unintentional—such as a lapse of memory during a routine but important procedure.[177] Such behavior, resulting in dire consequences in real life, becomes more noticeable in sleep-deprived individuals.

In most complex monitoring tasks, performance is never perfect over time,[8] and increased task complexity (or duration) generally impairs performance.[29,30] Human

senses can be particularly inaccurate, especially in dynamic situations.[11,178] For instance, an individual can generally effectively process only one input channel at a time (called *resource allocation*). A major factor in the effect of an additional task on performance appears to be what personal resources (perceptual, cognitive, output modalities) are required for the new task and whether those resources are already taxed.[179] Researchers have thus proposed a theoretical curvilinear relationship among performance, workload, and skill which probably also applies to the task of administering anesthesia (Fig. 17-7).

In a study of pilot performance under different workload conditions,[175] it was shown that with increasing workload, subjects tended to stare longer at the primary (i.e., more important) instruments. In addition to fixating less frequently on their secondary instruments *(load shedding)*, when pilots did gaze at these instruments, it was for a longer time. The presumption was that with increasing workload the subjects required more processing time to perceive the information available from each instrument. The performance of more experienced pilots was less strongly influenced by workload. Thus, as task complexity increases in a busy anesthetic case, this same phenomenon may be manifested by poor recordkeeping, sloppy routine, or lapses of vigilance. This is supported by a study in which Lambert and Paget[180] examined the influence of intraoperative teaching on the time spent by residents in patient-oriented and equipment-oriented tasks. They suggested that tutoring during "inappropriate" times markedly detracted from patient monitoring. This suggestion is supported by recent task analysis data.[39]

Observation of practicing anesthesiologists reveals that, during times of low workload, many add an additional (often unrelated) task to their routine, presumably in order to prevent boredom. These secondary tasks can include clinically relevant (though perhaps unnecessary) functions,

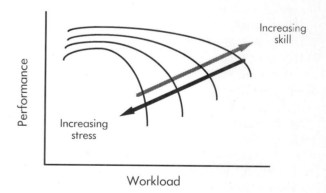

Fig. 17-7. For most complex tasks, including anesthesia, there is a curvilinear relationship between task performance and workload. Performance begins to deteriorate as workload increases. Skill in the task shifts this curve upward and to the right, and increased stress has opposing effects. (Reprinted from Weinger MB, Englund CE: Ergonomic and human factors affecting anesthetic vigilance and monitoring performance in the operating room environment. *Anesthesiology* 73:995-1021, 1990.)

such as rechecking the composition or organization of the anesthesia workspace. Alternatively, it is not uncommon to observe anesthesiologists reading, listening to music, attending to personal hygiene, or conversing with their colleagues about non-patient care matters. Whether these activities affect vigilance is difficult to assess. It is clear that during periods of low workload, to the extent that a low arousal state is avoided, these additional activities can have a beneficial effect. It is not known whether, in selected anesthetic cases that are long and impose minimal physical and cognitive demands, tasks unrelated to patient care (e.g., reading) improve or hinder vigilance. However, given the absence of formal training of anesthesiologists in proper time management and multitasking paradigms, there is likely to be tremendous individual variability in the impact of these unrelated activities on anesthetic vigilance. It is interesting to note that laboratory studies[181,182] have suggested that there is a discrete time-sharing ability that can be separated from other vigilance skills. It is thus likely that some anesthesiologists, during prolonged and uncomplicated anesthetics, actually enhance their overall vigilance by performing other tasks. This problem must be studied further before any definitive recommendations can be made. In any case, the conditions of the intraoperative environment, tasks, and equipment must be altered to minimize boredom and yet not be so continuously busy as to be stressful. This will yield the highest consistent levels of vigilance and optimal performance, regardless of the anesthesiologist involved.

EQUIPMENT AND SYSTEM FACTORS

Although the percentage of anesthesia mishaps that are caused primarily by equipment appears to be relatively small,[6] the contribution to error by the anesthesia provider caused by poor equipment design, maintenance, or performance may be significant. Thus, one wonders about the hidden factors that might have contributed to a catastrophe but were not elicited by the accident investigation. For example, did distracting alarms contribute to the end result? Or, more importantly, did poor equipment design more or less subtly influence the outcome?

At least one prominent author[20] has suggested that almost all human error is caused by inadequate or inappropriate equipment or system design. The equipment that the anesthesiologist encounters in the operating room is essentially of two types: the anesthesia machine—soon to become the anesthesia workstation—and the monitors. Yet, these two types of equipment increasingly share common problems. For example, both have developed over the decades in a haphazard way, and both currently present themselves in the operating room in an equally haphazard fashion.

Poor equipment design

Poor equipment can manifest itself in many ways, including design, performance, user and service manuals,

and maintenance. At least two factors make design of equipment for the operating room particularly difficult. First, the operating room is a hostile environment that does not treat equipment or personnel kindly. Second, it is difficult to elicit from the user precise or optimal equipment requirements for the OR setting. Block, et al.[183] describe the installation of one of the first computerized monitoring systems specifically designed for the operating room. Before designing this system, they carefully polled anesthesiologists to determine what they wanted. After the system was built, the users decided that they really wanted something different. This change may reflect capriciousness less than it does changing experience and evolving expectations. Nonetheless, it makes the designer's task more difficult. At the very least, in the design and manufacture of new equipment, continuous and direct contact between the designer and the user are essential.

Artifact, which remains a serious problem, can be caused by poor design of either hardware or software. Inadequate shielding of ECG cables can lead to the presence of motion artifact. If the software cannot handle this artifact, the heart rate calculator will give either no value or, worse yet, an incorrect value. Fortunately, artifact management has improved markedly over the past several years. For example, the incidence of pulse oximeter artifact has decreased considerably, such that it is no longer of significant concern to many who use automated anesthesia record-keeping devices.

Computing and displaying incorrect values can be particularly disastrous: the clinician could easily withhold or institute therapy inappropriately or be unable to follow the course of therapy. The impact of wrong numbers can be even more immediate. Many years ago, a slave display that showed the systolic and diastolic arterial pressures in large numbers for everyone in the room to see, was installed in the authors' institution. Unfortunately, the pressure values were 20 to 30 mm Hg too low, and the surgeons frequently became so upset with the blood pressure that they could not concentrate on the surgery.

Poor design can be particularly frustrating because it is often so difficult to deal with after the fact. Poor hardware design may show up as confusing displays, too many buttons, or inappropriate control mechanisms. Software related design problems include confusing displays and wrong numbers. Combined hardware and software problems include poor handling of artifact and irrational alarms. Chapter 18 gives a complete discussion of anesthesia system design and the ergonomics of the anesthesia workspace.

Optimal design of complex microprocessor-based equipment requires a delicate balance between a device that is too complicated for the operator to understand and one that is deceptively simple. If there are too many displays, or if the displays are confusing, performance may be suboptimal and errors can arise during crisis situations. The complexity of the Aegis radar display system and some inherent design flaws proved to be a major cause of the mistaken downing of a commercial airliner by the *USS Vincennes*. On the other hand, well intended attempts to simplify a device can produce equally poor results. Cook et al.[184] described a humidifier that had been redesigned from a manual device to an automatic one. The users at their hospital liked the newer device because it was simpler. Research showed, however, that they did not understand its underlying operation. For example, they did not know the procedure required to reactivate the device after an alarm; nor did they know that the heating elements were turned off after an alarm. To "reset" the device after an alarm had sounded, users simply turned it off and on again. In essence, the device was not intuitive in its design or functionality.

Each individual component of a system may be well thought out, but if the system design as a whole is faulty, the result will be unsatisfactory. Often the design is appropriate for one venue but is transferred to another without the unique attributes of the new environment being taken into account. For example, many companies make "integrated" monitors, with several devices incorporated into one large box, often with all of the monitored variables displayed on a single large screen. However, many of these monitors were originally designed for the ICU and provide trend displays that use a scale of 6 or more hours. For most anesthetic cases the resulting display is far too compressed.

The ultimate performance of the equipment is the most important consideration. Poor performance may be related to poor design, implementation, or construction; to inappropriate use; or to inadequate supporting equipment. As an example of inadequate supporting equipment, several older models of the Macintosh computer suffered breakdown because a less expensive (and subsequently found to be less reliable) power supply was used. If a piece of equipment does not do what it is supposed to, is frequently failing unexpectedly, or gives erroneous values, patient care will likely suffer.

The use of simulation may achieve many of the design goals required for safer and more user-friendly equipment. By testing several designs under almost real clinical situations, the manufacturer will be able to determine efficiently which design, if any, is the most useful. Simulation can also be used for training: the clinician will be able to learn safely and quickly how to use a device, even under the most demanding conditions.

User manuals and documentation

The user theoretically depends on the operator's manual for many purposes: becoming acquainted with the monitor during its initial use, learning its finer points, and troubleshooting. Unfortunately, documentation and manuals for medical monitors follow the same trend as other manuals: they are poorly written, confusing, and incomplete. All too often, the immediately essential or desired information is impossible to find. As a result of these shortcomings, most operator's manuals are simply not used by clinicians. The Anesthesia Patient Safety Foundation has recognized this problem and is working with industry to write better manuals. Currently, attempts are being made to compose readable manuals for a few selected devices, such as a capnograph and a pulse oximeter.

Another consideration is education of anesthesiologists on the equipment that they use. Is that education the responsibility of the manufacturer, the hospital, the FDA, the user, or some society, such as the Anesthesia Patient Safety Foundation or the Society for Technology in Anesthesia? Whatever the case may be, it is true that the technical education of the anesthesiologist is sadly deficient at all stages, from medical student to experienced clinician. Until this educational problem is addressed, the interaction between the user and complex machines will remain suboptimal, and equipment-induced or system-induced errors will occur that will be inappropriately blamed on the user.

Equipment maintenance

Anesthesia machines in particular require continual maintenance, and this must be provided by experienced personnel. Maintenance training, traditionally accomplished at the factory, usually requires several weeks. Optimally, maintenance should be performed by either a representative of the manufacturer itself or a well-trained independent sales and maintenance group. (See also Chapters 23 and 24.)

Maintenance errors can follow the same pattern as errors in any field: a chain of events, each link by itself not enough to cause a disaster, contributes to the outcome. One of the most notorious occurred over two decades ago in an episode in which the medical gases supplied to an anesthesia machine were switched.[185] A hospital maintenance worker repaired the oxygen hose during the night so that he would not disrupt the operating room routine. What he did, much of it in good faith, is a classic example of a chain of mishaps: (1) An oxygen connector was attached to one end of each of two hoses and a nitrous oxide connector to the other end; (2) both hoses were black, rather than color-coded; and (3) he carefully and neatly twisted the hoses around each other. In those days before the circuit oxygen analyzer and the pulse oximeter, the first patient to be anesthetized with this machine died. It was soon realized that the second patient was undergoing the same problem—the anesthesia machine was completely disconnected, and the patient was ventilated with an independent, portable source of oxygen.

This case achieved considerable notoriety and was responsible both for the increased awareness of the possibility of operating room gas switches and for the realization that continuous measurement of inspired oxygen is necessary. Sadly enough, gas switches still happen,[186] and the *Anesthesia Patient Safety Foundation Newsletter* recently reported that a second switching episode had occurred in the same hospital, with the same supply company involved.[187] (See also Chapters 1 and 16.)

Equipment obsolescence

Anesthesia machines are designed to be long-lasting and rugged, and their manufacturers have largely succeeded in this goal. Thus a large number of older machines are still in service and present a variety of problems: (1) Integral parts wear out and do not function as intended; (2) components do not perform up to today's standards (which can change relatively rapidly); (3) functions available on modern machines are absent; and (4) some components may actually be dangerous. Some examples of dangerous components include the Copper Kettle (Foregger, A Division of Puritan Bennett) (which can deliver a saturated vapor), in-circuit vaporizers, and vaporizers without an interlock mechanism. (See also Chapter 3.) What to do with these machines represents a major dilemma. There are so many out-of-date machines that it is not possible cost effectively to replace them all at once. Furthermore, some might argue that an experienced anesthesiologist is safer using customary equipment, instead of a technologically overwhelming, new workstation. On the other hand, a less experienced anesthesiologist, trained only on modern equipment and suddenly confronted with an old piece of equipment during an emergency represents to the patient a dangerous and potentially threatening situation.

ALARMS

The need to incorporate alarms into monitoring systems stems from several factors: The number of variables to be monitored has increased tremendously; the equipment used to collect and display these variables has become exceedingly sophisticated; and, as discussed above, with the complexity of the task and the stresses involved, the anesthesiologist is unlikely to be able to detect all out-of-range variables or conditions without the assistance of a machine. In fact, if displays were easy to comprehend and presented all of the relevant information (and no irrelevant information), and if all the required clinical information were in one easy-to-read location, then perhaps alarms would be less important.[188] Unfortunately, this situation does not yet exist. In fact, as in the aviation industry,[189] with the increasing sophistication of anesthesia monitors and equipment, the number of alarms has increased almost exponentially.

The objective of any alarm system is to optimize the probability of dealing successfully with the problem at hand.[190] Alarms actually serve several functions[188]: they assist the anesthesiologist in the detection of adverse or unanticipated conditions in either the patient or the equipment; they aid the fatigued or otherwise nonvigilant anesthesiologist; and they assist in situations where stress, workload, lack of training, or other factors negatively impact on the ability of the anesthesiologist to detect or respond to undesirable conditions.

Once an alarm sounds, the next step is to identify the source and the cause of the alarm. An alarm is of no benefit if it does not also provide the user with sufficient information to correct the alarm condition (either directly, or by indicating where to look to get the necessary data). In fact, an alarm tone that cannot be identified is extremely distracting and could exacerbate a potentially difficult clinical situation. Different conditions can cause an alarm condition, including an unexplained change in one or more of the monitored signals, an unexpected or undesirable response of the patient to an intervention, equipment failure, and the possibility of the display of false or misleading clinical information.[188]

An alarm should be more than just an indicator of an abnormal condition; it must provide some preliminary information about the condition that activated the alarm. However, too much information provided in the initial alarm state can confuse or mislead the operator, especially if the alarm is based on a single variable or if multiple alarms are simultaneously activated. The sounding (and subsequent identification) of a particular alarm narrows the focus of the user's attention to one aspect of the system. Some alarms (such as a circuit disconnect alarm) are very specific with respect to the area of the system that must be examined and the fund of knowledge that must be accessed to correct the problem. In fact, with these types of alarms, an experienced user can correct the condition with very little conscious effort. In contrast, other alarms (such as a high pulmonary arterial diastolic pressure alarm or a low right hemisphere EEG spectral edge frequency alarm) may require extensive examination of other clinical variables and significant conscious processing to determine the clinical condition that activated the alarm state.

The designer of an alarm system must consider the method as well as the consequences of the interruption produced by the alarm.[190] An alarm system should produce an alarm signal as soon as possible after an alarm condition has been detected.[191] It should be easy for the user to identify the source of the alarm. Accurate information about the cause of the alarm state must be provided. The user's attention must then be held long enough to ensure that the problem that caused the alarm has been corrected. Finally, interference from other, less important alarm conditions must be minimized during the response to the original alarm condition.

Human factors principles must be applied to the design of alarms. These principles include selection of physiological variables to be monitored, control of alarm limits, reliable detection of out-of-range events, intelligent decisions regarding states not requiring an alarm, provision of

---

Box 17-9. Some principles of good alarm design

Human factors principles must be applied (see Chapter 18).

The physiological variables to be followed and the alarm limits (with appropriate user control) must be carefully selected.

There must be reliable detection and device intelligence regarding states not requiring an alarm (good "artifact management").

Alarms must be prioritized (consider industry-wide standards).

Alarm states must correlate with clinical urgency.

The use of different alarm modalities (e.g., audio, visual) and their integration must be considered.

The user must be able to silence alarms, at least temporarily.

Output signals must be user-friendly and not produce a negative affective response ("turn it off!").

Designers must consider, on a case-by-case basis, the clinical usefulness of incorporating clinically relevant data into alarms.

Alarms should be standardized across all medical devices likely to be used in the same clinical environment.

---

user-friendly output signals to the operator, and standardization across medical systems[192] (Box 17-9).

False alarms

Little is known about the effects of false alarms on intraoperative vigilance and monitoring performance. Although alarms can be useful in terms of improving recognition of critical situations, if improperly designed, they will actually degrade performance.[192] Intraoperative alarms can give misleading information as well as being distracting. Porciello's[193] survey of critical care unit physicians revealed that many found dysrhythmia alarms to be inaccurate, misleading, and disturbing. O'Carroll[194] found that over a 3-week period in an ICU only 8 out of 1455 alarm soundings indicated potentially life-threatening problems. Forty-five percent of the false alarms were from ventilators; another 35% were from infusion pumps. In an operating room study by Meijler,[195] at least 80% of 731 warnings occurring during cardiac surgery were of no clinical utility. Kestin, et al.[196] showed that 75% of all audio alarms were spurious and only 3% indicated an actual patient risk. In this study, it was noted that an alarm sounded every 4.5 minutes (with an average of 10 per case).

The occurrence of a false alarm requires time and effort to verify the patient's actual condition. This may distract attention away from other tasks or conditions. The false alarm may also lead to an inappropriate action that will take additional time and also potentially pose a risk to patient safety. Many anesthesiologists disconnect or ignore alarms that sound falsely or are annoying.[197] Fifty-seven percent of Canadian anesthesiologists said they disabled auditory alarms, primarily because of the frequent occurrence of false or spurious alarms.[197] Also, many alarm tones are intentionally distracting or obnoxious and thereby elicit a "make it stop" response. In a recent study,[198] it was found that many common commercial clinical alarms induced a negative affective response. "Make it stop!" is the primary intrinsic response of individuals to such auditory stimuli.[190] This is undesirable in an alarm because it not only leads to an augmented sympathetic response to the alarm tone (increasing the stress associated with the situation) but also the subject's primary response will be to disable the alarm as promptly as possible, perhaps without adequately attending to the meaning or significance of the alarm state. Some pilots believe that all but the most critical alarms should be silenced during conditions of high workload.[199]

Alarm notification modality

No crucial alarm condition should be indicated via a single modality. Most experts believe that general information can be presented solely with a visual indication or message, whereas warnings should be indicated by both audio and visual alarm modalities. It is best if both auditory tones and a visual indication occur simultaneously. In a complex environment with many different alarms, a proper mix of alarm notification modalities is necessary to prevent confusion or decreased responsiveness.

Consistent with the widespread use of audio alarms in anesthesia equipment, studies have suggested that for critical information, auditory presentation leads to a quicker and more reliable response than does visual presentation.[200] However, the auditory mode of alarm notification presents several problems. Alarm tones from different devices may sound similar, making identification of the source of the alarm difficult or even stressful. Loeb and colleagues[201] demonstrated that in the absence of other cues, clinicians could identify the source of alarm tones only 34% of the time. In this study, the authors recorded alarm tones and then played them back to 44 clinicians outside of the operating room. The recognition of the alarm was greater for alarms heard more frequently. There was no relationship between the complexity of the alarm tone and the ability to recognize its meaning. Another problem with auditory alarms is that localization or recognition of specific alarm tones may require normal auditory acuity. Anesthesiologists with a hearing deficit may have difficulty determining the source of sounds in the operating room. Hearing acuity, especially above 1 kHz, decreases with age. Yet 50% of all alarm tones currently used have much of their sound energy above 2 kHz. Thus older clinicians may have additional difficulty identifying high-frequency alarms.[202] Higher pitched tones are also more difficult to localize.[203]

```
┌─────────────────────────────────────────────────────┐
│  Box 17-10.  Some common normal and                  │
│     alarm sounds in the OR                            │
│                                                       │
│  Sound                                          dB    │
│                                                       │
│  Jet ventilator                                120    │
│  Hewlett-Packard Merlin monitor (all alarms; at  91   │
│     highest setting)*                                 │
│  Fisher and Paykel humidifier (temperature probe  86  │
│     not plugged in)                                   │
│  Aspen Labs ATS tourniquet (disconnect)          84   │
│  Dräger Narkomed 2 anesthesia machine (loss of ox- 84 │
│     ygen supply)                                      │
│  Dräger Narkomed 2 anesthesia machine (circuit   78   │
│     disconnect)                                       │
│  IVAC 560 infusion pump (bottle clamp)           77   │
│  Surgical instruments against each other in sterile ba- 75 │
│     sin                                               │
│  Hewlett-Packard Merlin monitor (all alarms; at  74   │
│     standard setting)                                 │
│  Aspen Labs Electrocautery Unit (return fault)   74   │
│  Intercom                                        72   │
│  Tonsil tip suction                              70   │
│  Nellcor pulse oximeter (maximum volume)         66   │
│  Surgeon's conversation (at patient's ear)       66   │
│  Background music at patient's ear               65   │
└─────────────────────────────────────────────────────┘
```

*The noise levels produced by a variety of common, commercially available alarm sounds are presented in *italics*.

The high noise levels in the operating room may mask or obscure some alarm tones. With a sound meter* the peak noise level (dB) produced by a variety of common sounds and alarms in several operating rooms at the University of California San Diego Medical Center was recently measured. Readings were obtained at a distance of 1 foot from the source, and the median maximum value from three successive readings was used. The noise levels obtained for some common OR sounds (Box 17-10) correlated with those previously reported by others.[49,201,202]

*Scott Type 450B sound meter, Scott Instruments, Maynard, Mass.

Visual alarm lights can be coded by their color, brightness, size, location, and flashing frequency. Flashing lights are more noticeable and are traditionally used for more crucial information. Color codes have been standardized for instrument panels and alarm displays (Table 17-1). Red is used only for emergency or warning signals. Yellow indicates caution, and green indicates "power on" or device activation. It must be recognized, however, that a sizable percentage of the population is color-blind, and thus crucial alarm information must be coded simultaneously by other methods. In addition to lights, visual information can be presented as full or abbreviated text, icons, or other symbols. Coding of these visual messages should be consistent with the protocols used for simple display lights. Alarm tones and visual indications should be different for different levels of alarm priority.

Auditory tones can also be coded in several ways in addition to loudness, which is not effective because of its disruptive nature. The pattern, pitch, tone, and frequency of an alarm tone can be modified to provide distinguishing features ("Which alarm is this?") and other contextual information. A good example of information coding of auditory signals can be found in the frequency modulation of the Nellcor and Ohmeda pulse oximeters, in which the frequency of the tone decreases as the patient's oxygen saturation decreases. Recently, some human factors experts have advocated more extensive use of similar "earcons" in anesthesia. An example of an immediately understandable alarm sound used in some advanced fighter cockpit designs to indicate "low on fuel" is the sucking noise made by the last bit of sink water going down the drain. Some sophisticated forms of coding of auditory alarm tones can include melody (as advocated by Block[204]) or actual voice messages. Recent data suggest that synthesized-voice warning messages may be particularly effective when used sparingly and only for crucial alarms.[205] However, voice messages can be *extremely* disruptive if they are frequent, present information that is already known ("The car door is open."), or represent false alarms.

Some alarm designers have emphasized the importance of consistency of alarm tone.[203] That is, a particular alarm tone should have the same meaning regardless of where it

Table 17-1. Example of alarm hierarchy

Alarm priority	Meaning	Desired response from operator	Visual indication	Auditory indication
High priority	Emergency, warning	Immediate	Flashing red	Complex tone, continually repeated at fast pace
Medium priority	Caution	Prompt	Flashing yellow	Less complex tone, less frequently repeated
	Alert	Increased vigilance	Continuous yellow	No tone or simple tone, infrequently repeated
Low priority	Information, notice	Awareness, confidence	Green or other	None

is encountered throughout the work environment. Generally, within a single clinical care environment such as the operating room, no more than 10 (and preferably as few as 6) different tones should occur. Several approaches to allocating alarm tones have been proposed.[203] Currently, alarm tones are "equipment-based" in the sense that each device has a different tone. However, in a truly equipment-based approach, all pulse oximeters would produce identical alarm tones independent of manufacturer. Similarly, such equipment as ventilators, infusion pumps, and monitors would all have their own unique tones. Alternatively, in the "priority-based" approach, all devices would use the same three tones (warning, caution, and notice). Although this is practical for completely centralized alarm systems, with the distributed multiple device environment commonly seen in the present-day OR, utilizing the same alarm tones in all devices would make it difficult to identify the source and meaning of any given alarm. Another approach would be based on patient risk: conditions producing a given magnitude of risk would produce a particular tone. The perceived risk could be combined with the urgency of required response. The problem with such an approach is that patient risk and required response time can vary tremendously, depending on individual patient factors and the overall clinical situation. Thus in selected situations a "low risk–slow response" alarm tone may, in fact, represent a "high risk–rapid response" situation, and yet the anesthesiologist may be lulled into complacency about the importance of the alarm. Obviously, an integrated approach to alarms in the operating room must incorporate a combination of patient risk, required response time, and source (which type of equipment and what kind of physiological variable is generating the alarm) into a coherent prioritized system to optimize appropriate response. Any approach must be flexible enough to permit expansion with new technological and medical advances.

In an attempt to develop such a alarm system for civil aviation in Great Britain, Patterson[206] developed a series of general and context-specific alarm tones, which were subsequently modified for use in the medical environment. Patterson alarm sounds consisted of well-defined, complex sequences of tones producing distinctive auditory rhythms or signatures. Each tone was composed of at least four harmonics to improve its melodic character. As described by Kerr,[203] three "general" alarm sounds of increasing complexity (advisory, caution, and warning) were proposed. Six "specialized" alarm categories were also described (ventilation, oxygenation, cardiovascular, artificial perfusion, drug administration, and temperature), each with its own unique auditory signature. For each category, both a caution alarm and a warning alarm were specified. Urgency was indicated when the tone sounded more quickly rather than more loudly.

The use of the Patterson sounds in anesthesia remains controversial. The studies that led to the development of the Patterson sounds are now more than 10 years old and

may not be applicable to the OR setting, especially given recent advances in monitoring devices and technology. This approach requires individual devices to generate several complex tones, adding cost and complexity. More important, the use of Patterson alarms in individual (nonintegrated) devices will certainly worsen existing problems of noise and stress in the OR environment. The cockpit of an airplane is a different workspace than an operating room, and the task of flying an airplane is not entirely analogous to that of administering anesthesia. In the cockpit, only the flight crew must listen and attend to alarms. In the OR, surgeons, nurses, and awake patients are a captive audience who find extraneous sounds disturbing and without obvious meaning. At present there are no good data to support the use of any particular system of alarm tones in the OR environment. Scientific studies must be performed to evaluate the impact of different alarm modes and tones on the anesthesiologist's vigilance and on the performance of the whole OR team. The entire operating room environment must be considered, not just individual devices.

Alarm limits

It is generally better to anticipate a critical condition than to respond to it. Thus, alarms are most useful if they are activated before the deleterious condition arises. In order to prevent patient injury, when the values (or limits) at which a particular alarm sounds are set, the following must be taken into account: the rate at which the variable is likely to change (deteriorate), the response time of the measurement system, the response time of the alarm system, and the response (or correction) time of the anesthesiologist. This topic is covered in some detail by Kerr.[203] To ensure that alarms sound long before a dangerous condition has arisen without too frequently being spurious requires considerable "intelligence" on the part of both the system and the user. Systems that adjust alarm thresholds on the basis of the condition of the patient or the system could markedly reduce the stress and workload on the user as well as reduce the occurrence of spurious alarms. One of the major areas of interest for alarm designers is the development of automated alarm-limit setting. The Ohmeda Modulus CD (central display) anesthesia machine has implemented an "alert limit" approach in some of its display options (Fig. 17-8).

The criterion that determines whether or when a particular alarm sounds is called the *threshold value* or *alarm limit*. This limit can be set either by the equipment manufacturer or by the user. Except for a few alarm states such as "wall oxygen disconnect" or "oxygen tank pressure low," whose limits are virtually fixed and rarely if ever need to be changed, other alarm conditions must be adjusted on the basis of the particular clinical situation. The limits that are chosen will, in most situations, determine the incidence of false alarms. Thus it is important to permit the user easily to alter alarm limits. However, the frequent need to adjust limits in order to prevent the occur-

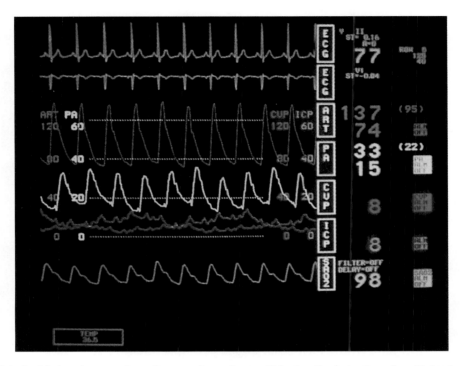

Plate 1. Modern integrated monitors employ color to aid in the discrimination of multiple physiological waveforms and digital values. On the SpaceLabs PC2, each of the waveforms can be displayed on a different scale and in a different color. The reliance on software rather than hardware has provided equipment manufacturers with greater power and flexibility of design. (Reprinted by permission of SpaceLabs, Inc., Redmond, WA.)

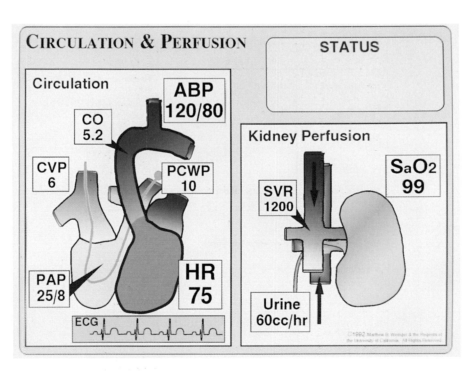

Plate 2. The integrated anesthesia workstation displays of the future will take advantage of powerful microprocessors and improved understanding of the human physiological response to anesthesia to present clinical data in a more intuitive and relevant manner. In this depiction, display integration, clinically relevant object displays, color signatures, and highlighting are employed to yield iconic representations that mirror the anesthesiologist's mental model of human physiological processes. Note the logical positioning of redundant information. Animation could be used (e.g., a beating heart) to provide increased information content; this would obviate the need for waveform displays. Trending of data (not shown) could also be readily incorporated into such a display. (Reprinted by permission of Matthew B. Weinger, M.D.)

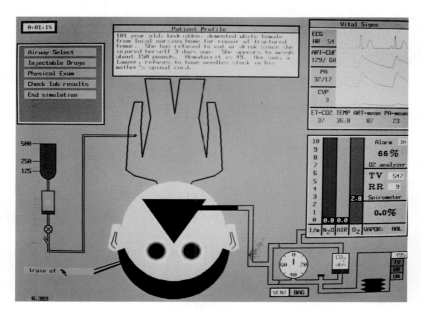

Plate 3. Screen-based anesthesia simulators, such as SLEEPER, developed by Dr. N. Ty Smith at the University of California, San Diego, are useful tools for teaching the cognitive aspects of anesthesia care. These computer-based simulators can accurately depict the physiological responses of "patients" to a variety of pharmacological interventions or disease processes. (Photograph courtesy of N. Ty Smith, M.D.)

Drug Class	Label color	Example
Induction agent	Yellow	Thiopental 2.5% Date
Tranquilizer	Orange	Midazolam mg/ml
Muscle relaxant	Fluorescent red	Curare mg/ml
		Succinylcholine mg/ml
Relaxant antagonist	Fluorescent red with white stripes	Neostigmine mg/ml
Narcotic	Blue	Morphine mg/ml
Narcotic antagonist	Blue with white stripes	Naloxone mg/ml
Major tranquilizer	Salmon	Droperidol mg/ml
Vasopressor	Violet	Ephedrine mg/ml
		Epinephrine mcg/ml
Hypotensive agent	Violet with white stripes	Nitroprusside mg/ml
Local anesthetic	Gray	Lidocaine mg/ml
Anticholinergic agent	Green	Atropine mg/ml

Plate 4. Standard color codes for user-applied syringe drug labels.

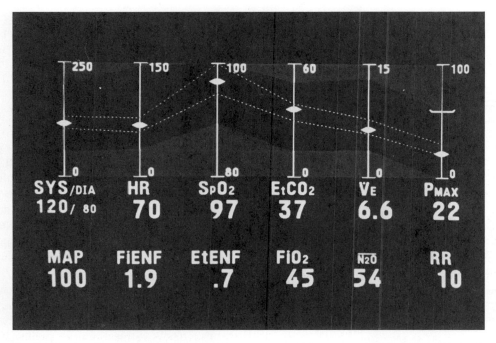

Fig. 17-8. The use of alert limits *(dashed lines)* may provide a more sensitive threshold for detecting adverse trends in patient vital signs, thus allowing intervention prior to the attainment of a full "alarm" condition. Such alert zones would be particularly useful if they were modified on the basis of the individual patient's actual ongoing physiological responses to surgery and anesthesia. (Reprinted by permission of Ohmeda, A Division of BOC Health Care, Inc. Madison Wis.)

rence of false or annoying alarms is undesirable and will undoubtedly lead the user to disable the alarm completely.

There are several ways to determine reasonable alarm limits for a particular variable.[188] For example, for factory default limits, a consensus of experienced users could be used. Most clinicians would agree that a diastolic blood pressure of over 110 mm Hg or less than 30 mm Hg is abnormal. Alternatively, device manufacturers might use previous or collected knowledge about a particular physiological variable, perhaps on the basis of statistical data from large numbers of similar patients. These two approaches would inevitably result in alarm limits for individual patients which are either too restrictive or not restrictive enough. A more sophisticated approach would be to design the device so that it dynamically adjusts its alarm limits on the basis of actual ongoing patient values. For instance, the system could keep track of blood pressure over the preceding 20 minutes and then set alarm limits at ±20% of the average of these values. Investigators are currently attempting to use simulation, computer modeling, and integrated alarm technology to develop "smart" alarms that can relate several variables together, diagnose spurious alarm states, and provide additional information to the user.

Control of alarms

If properly designed, visual alarms do not impair critical display information. Therefore, it should never be necessary to disable them. The system must promptly recognize that the alarm condition has been corrected and immediately silence the associated alarm tone or indication. Nevertheless, it is often necessary to silence or disable auditory alarms. However, there must be a visual indication that an auditory alarm has been silenced. High-priority alarm tones should be able to be only temporarily disabled, for 45 seconds to 2 minutes.

It is essential that the user be able to test the alarm to assure that it will produce the expected sound at the appropriate time. Two kinds of tests should be available: a power test and a limit test. For the power test, either at power-up or upon activation of a test switch, all modalities of the alarm should be activated. For the limit test, there should be a way for the user to adjust or modify the device and/or its alarms manually such that the ability of the alarm to trigger upon reaching the desired limit can be directly tested.

Integrated alarm systems

There is still some controversy over the value of centralized alarm displays, because they may make it more difficult for the user to localize quickly the precise source of the alarm, especially during situations of high workload. When a centralized display is used, the system must provide as much information as possible about the source and cause of the alarm condition. The clinically most important alarm must be indicated first and foremost. Other,

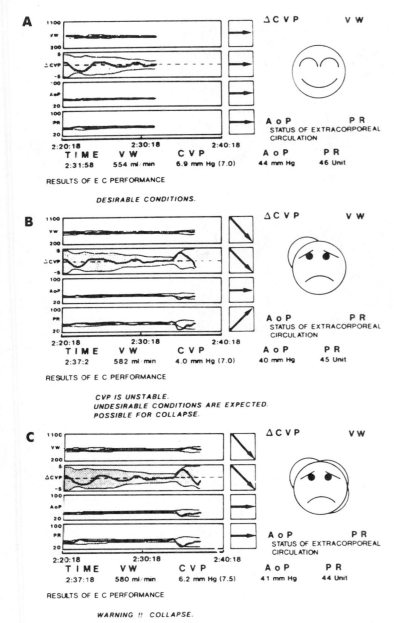

Fig. 17-9. Three examples of one proposed comprehensive display/alarm system which uses four different levels of information presentation. In addition to the usual digital and trend data, the system displays an arrow for each variable indicating the overall direction of the trend, a message area for both specific alarm states and general system status, and a global "face" display to indicate overall system performance. (From Fukui Y: *An expert alarm system.* In Gravenstein J, Newbower R, Ream A, et al, editors: *The automated anesthesia record and alarm systems,* Stoneham, Mass., 1987, Butterworth.)

less important alarms should be suppressed during the annunciation of the higher priority alarm. For example, Fukui[207] described an indicator and alarm status display that employed four different levels of information. In addition to the usual waveforms and digital values, the display included an arrow that indicated the direction of the trend

in values at the present time, a message area with both specific alarm states and general system status, and, finally, a "face" that indicated overall system performance (Fig. 17-9).

Smart alarms

Appreciable effort has been expended in recent years to make alarms "intelligent." Theoretically, these computer-based systems could provide interactive event recognition, reduce the incidence of false alarms, enhance vigilance, and aid in data manipulation.[208] Unfortunately, thus far, commercially available alarms are not particularly "smart." Part of the problem is that we do not understand very well the task of administering anesthesia: how do anesthesiologists make decisions and what information is important to those decisions? In addition, any given value of a monitored variable is "context-specific." It is difficult for the system to know, for a particular patient and under specific conditions, whether an isolated value is normal or abnormal.

Thus far, investigators have employed two approaches in their attempts to develop smart alarms: rule-based expert systems[208] and neural networks.[209] Rule-based expert systems use elaborate "if-then" programs to set contingencies for alarm conditions or limits. Rule-based alarm strategies work relatively well in straightforward (and foreseeable) situations, such as those that involve the integration of several different devices with known effects on each others' function. For example, a pulse oximeter monitor could be designed so that if a noninvasive blood pressure cuff is on the same arm as the oximeter probe and the cuff inflates, then the S_pO_2 alarm would be disabled during the blood pressure reading.

Pan, et al.[210] described a rule-based intelligent anesthesia monitoring system that incorporated the slope and minimum and maximum values of multiple monitored variables to make specific clinical diagnoses. The system was tested for its ability to diagnose problems of breathing circuit integrity and to assess adequacy of ventilation and oxygenation. The system correctly identified 91% of mechanical malfunctions within 30 seconds and 100% of adverse physiological conditions within 10 breaths.

A more sophisticated approach toward the development of intelligent alarms in anesthesia is represented by the A Logical Alarm Reduction Mechanism (ALARM) system described by Beinlich and Gaba.[211] They used a computerized representation of statistical-likelihood (probabilistic) reasoning to aid the clinician in developing clinical diagnoses during critical events. Their prototype system statistically related physiological variables with potential diseases or problems by using objective conditional probability equations (to compute the statistical likelihood that a given physiological state was caused by a particular event). In preliminary testing, ALARM made the correct diagnosis in 71% of the test cases presented. This approach could be considered a hybrid of the rule-based expert systems and neural networks.

A neural network is a parallel processor that consists of multiple, interconnected nodes. A node is a site in which incoming data are processed; the resultant outcome is presented to subsequent nodes via data-flow pathways. The conditions at all adjacent nodes influence each others' state. In this way, the information passes through the network in a wave whereby all relevant factors (including those that the programmer may not have anticipated) impact on the result. The neural network is much more like the human brain than is a traditional serial computer and, as such, may be particularly good at tasks requiring pattern recognition or associative processing. Theoretically, abnormalities in the state of a complex system (such as the anesthesia workspace) would be particularly amenable to detection by a neural network. The other advantages of these parallel systems are that they could provide information about the interrelationships between monitored variables and that they may be robust in diagnosing unanticipated or unusual alarm conditions. In one recent study[212] examining machine or circuit fault conditions, alarms generated by a neural network permitted a more rapid detection of the underlying problem than those generated by conventional systems. Neural networks may also provide important specific diagnostic information during complicated critical events in fully integrated monitoring systems.[209,213]

Design of alarms of the future

In order to design the anesthesia alarm systems of the future, a number of important factors must be considered. Most important, human factors principles must be applied. The physiological variables to be alarmed and the alarm limits chosen must be carefully selected. The clinical usefulness of alarms will be enhanced with reliable detection and device intelligence regarding states not requiring an alarm (artifact management). User-friendly output signals, both auditory and visual, must be provided. Designers must determine whether complete integration is always desirable. The anesthesiologist cannot always look up (e.g., during laryngoscopy), so that in the absence of sound discrimination, in a centralized alarm system the clinician may not be able to locate the device that is alarming.

Alarm prioritization remains important, especially in fully integrated systems. The alarm condition must correlate with clinical level of urgency. Some organizations advocate industry-wide categorization of alarm priorities (e.g., high/medium/low) as well as standardization across medical devices. However, if standards are too restrictive then innovation or new technology may be impeded. For example, the requirements for alarm annunciation used in a personal (ear-piece) audio system may be significantly different from those for general operating room broadcast. Ongoing deliberations of national and international standards organizations may represent a good forum for attaining a consensus on some of these issues. In any case, new alarm designs must undergo rigorous clinical testing in real or accurately simulated conditions (in conjunction with other alarms and sounds that will normally be present).

INTEGRATED MONITORING SYSTEMS
History and rationale

In 1902, Harvey Cushing[214] recommended that respiration and heart rate be monitored and recorded whenever anesthesia was administered. A few years later he introduced the measurement of blood pressure. It was soon recognized that the anesthetic techniques of the time were associated with labile hemodynamics. Since Cushing's time, more than two dozen clinical variables have been added to the anesthetic record. However, new variables have often been monitored as much because a new device or technique permitted their measurement as because any careful scientific study demonstrated that their use added significantly to safety of the patient. The most recent additions include the pulse oximeter, the end-tidal carbon dioxide monitor, the processed EEG, and the transesophageal echocardiograph. Unfortunately, research in anesthesia ergonomics has not kept pace with advances in clinical anesthesia and monitoring technology. As a result, the status quo in anesthesia monitoring is now a nonintegrated configuration in which the various monitors are arranged idiosyncratically. The most common arrangement is to stack as many of the displays on the anesthesia machine as possible. The location of a particular monitor is usually determined by its size or the date of acquisition: the smaller ones are stacked upon the larger ones or the newer ones on top of the older ones.

With more monitors—each having its own displays, sounds, alarm settings, cables, and methods of operation, —the anesthesiologist's workspace has become quite complex. The haphazard arrangement and types of monitors frequently hinder the acquisition of information on which decision-making depends and may impact on the safety of patients. Setting up, calibrating, connecting to the patient, and monitoring these devices requires additional attention, thereby further decreasing the amount of time spent directly observing or interacting with the patient.

A trend toward integrating the display of information from diverse clinical sources is just beginning in commercially available anesthesia monitoring systems. Anesthesia equipment increasingly incorporates microprocessor-based intelligent systems, and with these systems comes the capability to present large amounts of clinical information in new ways. However, as systems become more complicated and automated, they may become more susceptible to human error.[10,178] Little information exists on how monitored data are used by clinicians.[215,216] The effects of the type of information, the display mode, and the relationships between them on monitoring performance are as yet unknown.

The transition from the present, widely scattered, discrete devices to single integrated systems will be painful for several reasons. First, there is a large base of discrete devices already installed, and the process of replacing them will require many years. In addition, the integration process itself entails many difficulties, which relate to physical, electronic, and software problems. Integration implies connection, and unless the same company makes all the components of a monitoring system, there will be incompatibilities—in cabling, in connectors, in signals, and in the software that manipulates the data and transmits them from one component of the anesthesia workstation to another. The last process involves handshaking, a technique that sounds easier than it is because, at present, each company seems to have their own protocol. To connect to the presently available major monitors, the ARKIVE automated anesthetic recordkeeper must accommodate 75 different protocols. One full-time person in the company does little else but develop handshaking protocols. The problem of physical and electronic connections has been illustrated vividly by the recent reports of overheated pulse oximeter probes when the cable and probe from one manufacturer are connected to another's device (see Chapter 11). As the type and number of devices grow, more problems of this sort will arise.

The medical information bus

Bidirectional electronic data communication has been essential to enhancing labor effectiveness in manufacturing, commerce, banking, and other industries. The ability to interface medical devices to patient care computer systems has been hampered by the lack of an interface standard that meets the unique requirements of the acute patient care setting. A potential solution to many of these problems is the medical information bus (MIB). Although the final standards have not yet been adopted or implemented, the MIB promises to be a boon for both manufacturers and users. It will, in essence, allow any two or more pieces of equipment that adhere to the standard to communicate with each other more easily and at a more rapid rate than is currently possible.

The effort to set up these standards began in 1982, when a group of hospitals recognized the problems of medical device interconnection. To meet this challenge, a committee was formed consisting of device vendors, computer system vendors, clinical engineers, and clinicians. In 1984, the MIB Committee received a sanction from the Institute for Electronic and Electrical Engineers (IEEE) to work on a formal standard. The committee's mission was to develop an international standard for open systems communication in acute health care applications.

The MIB is a proposed international standard for bidirectional interconnection of medical devices and computing resources within a medical center or hospital. It speci-

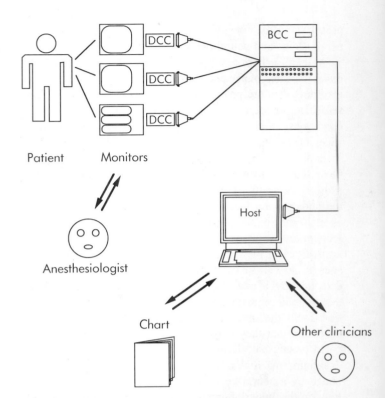

Fig. 17-10. The medical information bus (MIB) is a proposed international standard for hardware and software communication protocols for bidirectional interconnection of medical devices. Not only monitors but also computers, recordkeepers, laboratory equipment, and other devices could easily communicate by way of the MIB protocol. *BCC,* bedside communications controller; *DCC,* device communications controller. (Modified from Fiegler A, Stead S: The medical information bus, *Biomed Instrum Technol* 24:101-111, 1990.)

fies a local area network specifically designed to provide connection-oriented communication services between medical devices or between medical devices and computers (Fig. 17-10). The local area network that the MIB describes is distinguished from other types of data networks in that it is optimized for use in an acute patient care setting. It is intended to enable host computers to interface with medical devices in a hospital environment in a compatible, vendor-independent fashion, to be highly accurate and reliable, to accommodate the inevitable high frequency of network reconfiguration, to provide a simple user interface, and to support a wide range of topologies.

Implementation of these objectives has been through a family of standards that define the overall architecture, electrical characteristics, network characteristics, and language by which they communicate. Preexisting international standards have been used as much as possible. Where new standards have been defined, concepts have been used to facilitate future expansion of what is turning out to be a very complex system. For a detailed description of the MIB, including its uses and its potential, the reader is referred to a review by Fiegler and Stead.[217]

Computers in integrated monitoring systems

A major advance in anesthesia equipment has been the incorporation of microprocessor-based intelligent systems.[218,219] In particular, studies have shown[220] that the precise control of ventilators and measurement of many variables can best be performed with microprocessor-based systems. A number of institutions have developed modular computer-based anesthesia delivery systems (e.g., the Boston anesthesia system,[218] the Arizona program,[221] and the Utah Anesthesia Workstation[44]). These concepts are slowly being included in new commercial anesthesia workstations. An understanding of the ergonomic factors that affect anesthetic performance will enhance the ability to implement automated anesthesia tasks such as drug administration and recordkeeping, the development of smart alarms, and novel ways of presenting clinical information. However, if integration and computerization are done poorly, without careful thought and application of the principles of human factors design,[20] then performance and the incidence of human error may, in fact, increase.

Data management in integrated displays

One of the major problems with the current nonintegrated approach to monitoring is the need for the human mind to process a large amount of widely dispersed data. To pack a lot of information into a small space requires ingenious methods, and many integrated systems currently available do not incorporate appropriate methods to make "compressed" data easily understandable. Probably the first attempts to pack clinical information were used with the EEG and included the compressed spectral array (CSA),[222] the density-modulated spectral array (DSA),[223,224] and aperiodic analysis, which is still used in the Lifescan.[225] These techniques permit the compression of hundreds and thousands of pages of EEG data into just a few pages. More important, the information displayed is much more understandable than the original display. CSA EEG was included in one of the earliest truly integrated displays, called the Comprehensive Integrated Clinical/Research Anesthesia Monitor (CICRAM).[226] Fleming,[224] the originator of the DSA, stated that most displays were not packed tightly enough and that the human was capable of processing very tightly packed information. The DSA was designed to be used with the early integrated displays of the 1970s, simple oscilloscopes and strip-chart recorders. Another early integrated monitor, the Cerebrotrac, incorporated Fleming's idea into its display, which was the first to use color in the strip-chart format on a monitor screen. In all of these displays, especially the strip-chart style displays, the ability to scan down (Cerebrotrac) or across (Fleming) a display allowed the clinician to integrate information easily and thereby to assess cause and effect. An important principle learned from these early integrated displays was that the data must be packed or processed in a way that is intuitive, that is, in a way that corresponds to the "mental model" of the user about the source or etiology of the data presented.

Until recently, all of the commercial displays for the operating room have used time as a variable. Most cockpit displays in aircraft ignore time and simply present the continually changing data. Time-domain displays cannot pack as many variables together as can other types of displays. For example, Siegel[227] developed a complex polygon-based system for displaying 11 variables in the intensive care unit. The polygon showed one node for each variable, and the distance of the node from the center of the polygon was related to the value of the variable. The variables were arranged so that the shape of the polygon could assist the clinician in a quick interpretation of the state of the patient. The new Ohmeda Modulus Central Display (CD) anesthesia machine has incorporated a similar display that can be alternated on the same section of the screen with a conventional time-domain display (Fig. 17-11). The Ohmeda polygon contains fewer variables than Siegel's original implementation, and, it is important to note that the polygon can be reset at any time to its normal, symmetrical shape. Deneault[228] observed that even without training, under simulated conditions, anesthesiologists could detect certain critical events as well with the polygon system as with the conventional strip-chart (time) format. They speculated that performance would improve with training and experience. It should be noted, however, that the polygon display on the Ohmeda CD machine was not specifically designed in such a way that actual shape (rather than simply a deviation from symmetry) would provide diagnostic information.

Ikeda[229] has described a display that incorporates a model of inhaled anesthetic agent uptake and distribution as well as a system for continuously sampling mean inspired and expired gases. Using the continuously available concentrations of the inhaled agent, the model adapts itself to the patient. A trend display on a screen shows inhaled, exhaled, arterial, and brain concentrations of the agent. The model is connected to the vaporizer, so that any change in inhaled anesthetic concentration will be input directly into the model. Thus, the trend display includes a 20-minute projection of concentrations, so that the user can gradually adjust the delivered (vaporizer) concentration until a desired future concentration is achieved (e.g., brain concentration for emergence). The use of a model makes this a very tightly packed integrated display because many factors are taken into account: cardiac output, alveolar ventilation, and inspired and expired agent concentrations, among others.

Design considerations for integrated displays

There is now a large body of literature on methodologies that optimize complex visual displays.[230] Moray[231] enumerates several design priorities for complex display systems: for example, the number of displays and the time required to perceive information should be minimized. When the information provided by diverse sensors is integrated into a single coherent display, the user's workload

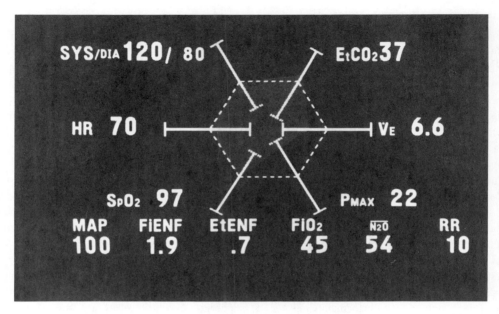

Fig. 17-11. The polygon display on the Ohmeda Modulus CD anesthesia machine is an example of an integrated configural display that graphically relates a number of key physiological variables. Deformation of the hexagon rapidly indicates a deviation from the predefined "normal" physiological state of the patient. While these kinds of displays appear useful in other fields, their value in the anesthesia environment remains to be demonstrated. (Reprinted by permission of Ohmeda, A Division of BOC Health Care, Inc., Madison Wis.)

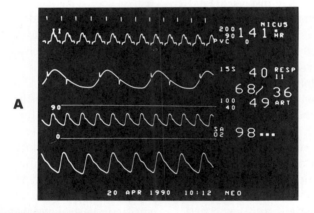

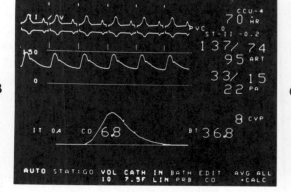

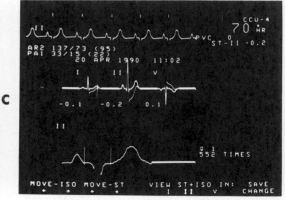

Fig. 17-12. A, Like a number of other currently available integrated devices, the Marquette 7010 monitor simultaneously displays multiple physiological waveforms and digital values. B, Cardiac output curves and calculations can be displayed directly on the monitor screen. However, due to limited screen space, other data disappear when cardiac output measurements are performed. C, Multilead automated ST-segment analysis is a potentially useful feature now available on many integrated monitors. (Reprinted by permission of Marquette Electronics, Inc., Milwaukee, Wis.)

may be reduced. The time required to perceive information can be shortened by use of display integration, analog or graphic rather than digital visual displays, sound and color signatures, highlighting,[232] and poignant visual or audible messages instead of vague, cryptic warnings.[233] Some data suggest that analog displays of information may be easier for the mind to process than digital displays of the same information, especially in situations of high workload.[234] Novel methods of displaying critical information, such as rate-of-change functions,[235] may also improve performance. Integrated displays may be most effective when the displayed variable represents a physiologically relevant interaction of the underlying inputs (e.g., the relationship between heart rate and ejection fraction).[236] The ultimate integrated display may be the line-drawing face developed by Fukui[207] (Fig. 17-9). A few simple lines indicate the patient's status in a format that incorporates everyday experience.

Until recently, these concepts have been applied only sporadically to anesthesia monitors.[237-239] However, monitors are now commercially available which incorporate all of the major physiological variables in a single integrated display (Figs. 17-11 through 17-17). These monitors incorporate such additional special features as cardiac output calculation (Fig. 17-12, B), ST-segment analysis (Fig. 17-12, C), real-time on-screen HELP (Fig. 17-13), and even on-screen diagnostics for equipment maintenance (Fig. 17-14). Ohmeda (Fig. 17-15) and North American Dräger

have recently introduced completely integrated anesthesia workstations that include gas and drug delivery systems as well as comprehensive clinical monitoring capabilities. Other manufacturers, such as Marquette (Fig. 17-12, A), Space Labs (Fig. 17-16; also see color insert), and Hewlett Packard (Fig. 17-17), have designed their clinical monitors to interface relatively smoothly with existing anesthesia machines. Unfortunately, although these devices are a major improvement over previously available nonintegrated monitors, they still have significant ergonomic shortcomings. Many of these displays are crowded and difficult to read, especially during situations of high workload. In the most common menu-driven schemes, crucial waveforms and other clinical data may disappear when the user is performing other, secondary tasks, such as cardiac output measurements or ST-segment analysis (Fig. 17-12). The human factors benefits of the color coding of waveforms and values may outweigh the cost disadvantage (compare Fig. 17-13 and color insert of 17-16) but this may not be fully appreciated by all clinicians or hospital purchasing representatives. Despite these criticisms, manufacturers of anesthesia equipment should be congratulated for their current generation of integrated monitors. For the next generation of monitors and equipment, more attention must be paid to the interface between human and device so that these systems will be user-friendly. Chapter 18 discusses the human factors issues in equipment design.

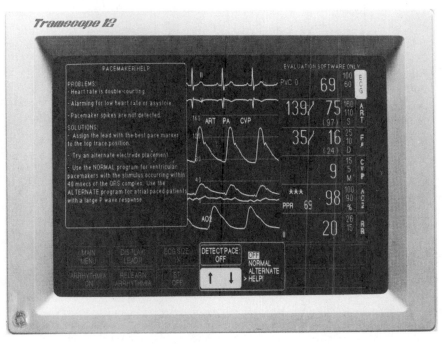

Fig. 17-13. The new integrated monitors provide real-time on-screen HELP. In this example, HELP is provided for a problem with pacemaker pulse detection. (Reprinted by permission of Marquette Electronics, Inc., Milwaukee, Wis.)

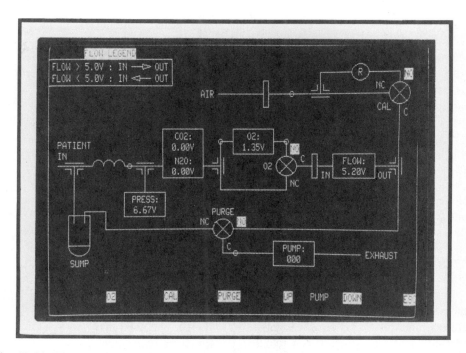

Fig. 17-14. The Datascope MULTINEX integrated gas analysis monitor provides on-screen diagnostics for enhanced troubleshooting and maintenance. (Reprinted by permission of Datascope Corp., Paramus, NJ.)

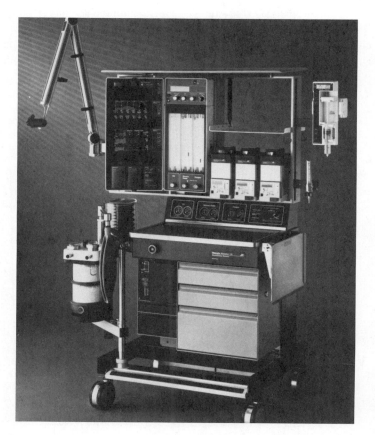

Fig. 17-15. Several manufacturers have recently marketed completely integrated anesthesia workstations that contain comprehensive monitoring capabilities as well as delivery systems for gases and potent inhaled anesthetics. The incorporation of computer-controlled, continuous intravenous infusions of short-acting anesthetic agents will probably be the next step in the evolution of the anesthesia workstation. Shown here is the Ohmeda Modulus CD. (Reprinted by permission of Ohmeda, a Division of BOC Health Care, Inc., Madison Wis.)

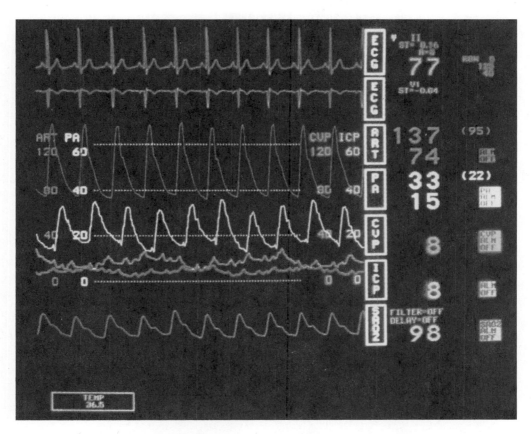

Fig. 17-16. Modern integrated monitors employ color to aid in the discrimination of multiple physiological waveforms and digital values. On the Space Labs PC2, each of the waveforms can be displayed on a different scale and in a different color. The reliance on software rather than hardware has provided equipment manufacturers with greater power and flexibility of design. (See color insert.) (Reprinted by permission of SpaceLabs, Inc., Redmond, Wash.)

Future issues in complex integrated systems. One advantage of fully computerized systems is that each piece of data can be presented in the context appropriate to the system's current state and the operator's immediate needs. However, when a fully computerized system is used, hundreds or thousands of different displays (or menus) are possible and a hierarchical organization may be inadequate to provide guidance to the operator attempting to navigate through the display system.[240] Unfortunately, design guidelines for the relationships between multiple interrelated computerized displays are generally lacking.

With the introduction of integrated displays, the critical design pitfalls are partially shifted from individual displays to the relationships and interactions among displays. Design errors at this level can lead to new kinds of problems, including having to navigate through too many useless or inefficient displays, getting lost in the display network, tunnel vision or "keyhole" effects (restricting oneself to a small subset of displays), and mental overload related to management of the data presented.[240] As stated by Woods et al.,[240] "Given that one of the problems in existing control centers is data overload in rapidly changing circumstances, the shift to more computer-based systems can ex-

acerbate this problem as well as mitigate it." The use of rapid prototyping by designers can lead to a proliferation of display screens ("We can do it, so why not include it?") without adequate consideration of the navigational requirements between displays. With rapid prototyping the same design mistake can be promulgated rapidly on a larger scale.

The amount of potentially displayable data is always much larger than the amount of physically available screen space; therefore, with poor design the risk of tunnel vision is significant. In complex integrated display systems, the user will thus have difficulty maintaining a broad overview of system status, especially when required to navigate frequently through multiple displays.[240] One commercially available operating room monitor has over 150 different menu display screens. It is, therefore, important to provide overview displays, which rapidly present crucial aspects of system status.

Unfortunately, there are as yet no data to support the benefits of integrated data display in the OR setting. "Heads-up" displays, in which the information is projected onto a visor worn by the operator, have been shown to improve performance by eliminating the need to refocus or

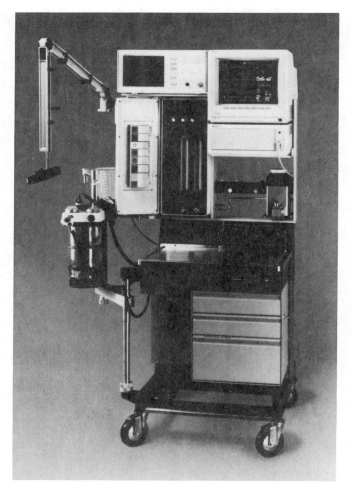

Fig. 17-17. Collaboration among different manufacturers, such as those making monitors and those making anesthesia machines, has led to unprecedented interconnectivity that produces well-integrated anesthesia workstations. Pictured here is the Hewlett-Packard Merlin system integrated into an Ohmeda Modulus anesthesia machine. Many manufacturers now recognize the potential value of the open architecture approach. (Reprinted by permission of Hewlett-Packard, North Hollywood, Calif.)

change eye position.[11] It is unclear whether such displays would play a useful role in the operating room. How the implementation of these concepts to anesthesia will affect monitoring performance remains to be seen but must be examined.

The ultimate goal of the integrated clinical monitors of the future will be to present only the data the anesthesiologist actually requires at precisely the time they are required. Information overload must be minimized. Clinical decision-making will be enhanced if the relationship between individual physiological variables is readily apparent. Thus, to accomplish these goals, future displays will employ a variety of techniques, including display integration, graphical rather than digital display, sound and color signatures, animation, highlighting, and poignant visual or audible messages. Novel methods of displaying such critical information as rate-of-change functions may also be

used. A promising approach, validated in the military setting, is the use of sophisticated object displays containing iconic representations that mirror the anesthesiologist's mental model of human physiological processes (Fig. 17-18; also see color insert).

This chapter has discussed ways in which the interface between the anesthesiologist and the anesthesia equipment can play a crucial role in influencing the outcome of the anesthetic administered. The administration of anesthesia is predominantly a complex monitoring task and, as such, requires sustained vigilance. Human error has been said to be the major cause of most anesthetic mishaps. However, poorly designed equipment certainly contributes to the occurrence of error in anesthesia practice. Humans are not very good at monitoring because their vigilance is susceptible to degradation by a variety of human, environmental, equipment, and system factors. Therefore, designers of an-

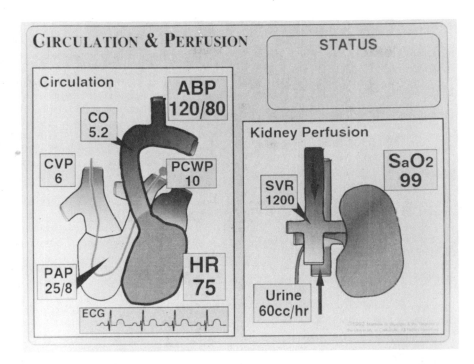

Fig. 17-18. The integrated anesthesia workstation displays of the future will take advantage of powerful microprocessors and improved understanding of the human physiological response to anesthesia to present clinical data in a more intuitive and relevant manner. In this depiction, display integration, clinically relevant object displays, color signatures, and highlighting are employed to yield iconic representations that mirror the anesthesiologist's mental model of human physiological processes. Note the logical positioning of redundant information. Animation could be used (e.g., a beating heart) to provide increased information content; this would obviate the need for waveform displays. Trending of data (not shown) could also be readily incorporated into such a display. (See color insert.) (Reprinted by permission of Matthew B. Weinger, M.D.)

esthetic equipment must assist the anesthesiologist by incorporating devices and systems to augment vigilance and monitoring performance. Alarms, intended to notify the operator of potential critical situations, are effective only if properly designed and implemented. The recent promise of completely integrated anesthesia workstations (with such features as "smart" alarms and monitoring aids) remains unfulfilled. However, such systems are on the horizon. Their successful implementation will require a more complete understanding of the task of administering anesthesia and of the factors that affect performance of the anesthesiologist in this complex environment.

ACKNOWLEDGMENTS

We gratefully acknowledge the advice and support of Dr. Carl E. Englund and Dr. Larry T. Dallen as well as the editorial assistance of Holly Forcier.

REFERENCES

1. Keenan R, Boyan P: Cardiac arrest due to anesthesia, *JAMA* 253:2373-2377, 1985.
2. Keenan R: Anesthesia disasters: incidence, causes, and preventability, *Semin Anesth* 5:175-179, 1986.
3. Olsson G, Hallen B: Cardiac arrest during anaesthesia: a computer-aided study in 250,543 anaesthetics, *Acta Anaesthesiol Scand* 32:653-664, 1988.
4. Utting J, Gray T, Shelley F: Human misadventure in anaesthesia, *Can Anaesth Soc J* 26:73-79, 1979.
5. Craig J, Wilson M: A survey of anaesthetic misadventures, *Anaesthesia* 36:933-936, 1981.
6. Cooper J, Newbower R, Long C, et al: Preventable anesthesia mishaps: a study of human factors, *Anesthesiology* 49:399-406, 1978.
7. Holland R: Special committee investigating deaths under anaesthesia: report on 745 classified cases, 1960-1968, *Med J Aust* 1:573-593, 1970.
8. Frankmann J, Adams J: Theories of vigilance, *Psychol Bull* 59:257-272, 1962.
9. Salvendy G: *Handbook of human factors*, New York, 1986, Wiley.
10. Allnutt M: Human factors in accidents, *Br J Anaesth* 59:856-864, 1987.
11. Rolfe J: Ergonomics and air safety, *Appl Ergonom* 3:75-81, 1972.
12. Billings C, Reynard W: Human factors in aircraft incidents: results of a 7 year study, *Aviat Space Environ Med* 55:960-965, 1984.
13. Cherns A: *Accidents at work.* In Welford A, editor: *Society: problems and methods of study*, London, 1962, Routledge and Kegan Paul, pp 247-267.
14. Miller D, Swain A: *Human error and human reliability.* In Salvendy G, editor: *Handbook of human factors*, New York, 1986, Wiley, pp 219-250.
15. DeAnda A, Gaba D: Unplanned incidents during comprehensive anesthesia simulation, *Anesth Analg* 71:77-82, 1990.
16. Meister D: Comparative analysis of human reliability models, Report #L0074-107, Westlake Village, Calif, 1971, Bunker-Ramo Electronics Systems Division.
17. Gaba D, Maxwell M, DeAnda A: Anesthetic mishaps: breaking the chain of accident evolution, *Anesthesiology* 66:670-676, 1987.

18. Gaba D: Human error in anesthetic mishaps, *Int Anesthesiol Clin* 27:137-147, 1989.

19. Bell T: The limits of risk analysis, *IEEE Spectrum* 26:51, 1989.

20. Norman D: *The psychology of everyday things,* New York, 1988, Basic Books.

21. Stroh C: *Vigilance: the problem of sustained attention,* Oxford, UK, 1971, Pergamon.

22. Mackworth N: Vigilance, *The Advancement of Science* 53:389-393, 1957.

23. Singleton W: *The analysis of practical skills,* Lancaster, UK, 1978, MTP. pp 209-235.

24. Sen R, Ganguli A: An ergonomic analysis of railway locomotive driver functions in India, *J Hum Ergol* 11:187-202, 1982.

25. Kogi K, Ohta T: Incidence of near accidental drowsing in locomotive driving during a period of rotation, *J Hum Ergol* 4:65-76, 1975.

26. Luoma J: Perception and eye movements in simulated traffic situations, *Acta Ophthalmol (suppl) (Copenh)* 161:128-134, 1984.

27. Woods D, Wise J, Hanes L: An evaluation of nuclear power plant safety parameter display systems, *Human Factors* 25:110-114, 1981.

28. Lowry J, Seaver D: Handbook for quantitative analysis of MAN-PRINT considerations in army systems, Research Product 88-15, Washington DC, 1988, United States Army.

29. Wilkinson R: Some factors influencing the effect of environmental stressors upon performance, *Psychol Bull* 72:262-270, 1969.

30. Thackray R, Bailey J, Touchstone R: The effect of increased monitoring load on vigilance performance using a simulated radar display, *Ergonomics* 22:529-539, 1979.

31. Weinger M, Englund C: Ergonomic and human factors affecting anesthetic vigilance and monitoring performance in the operating room environment, *Anesthesiology* 73:995-1021, 1990.

32. Chiles W: *Workload, task, and situational factors as modifiers of complex human performance.* In Alluisi E, Fleishman E, editors: *Human performance and productivity: stress and performance effectiveness,* Hillsdale, NJ, 1982, Lawrence Erlbaum Associates, pp 32-36.

33. Drui A, Behm R, Martin W: Predesign investigation of the anesthesia operational environment, *Anesth Analg* 52:584-591, 1973.

34. Boquet G, Bushman J, Davenport H: The anaesthetic machine: a study of function and design, *Br J Anaesth* 52:61-67, 1980.

35. Kennedy P, Fiengold F, Wiener E, et al: Analysis of tasks and human factors in anesthesia for coronary-artery bypass, *Anesth Analg* 55:374-377, 1976.

36. McDonald J, Dzwonczyk R: A time and motion study of the anaesthetist's intraoperative time, *Br J Anaesth* 61:738-742, 1988.

37. McDonald J, Dzwonczyk R, Gupta B, et al: A second time-study of the anaesthetist's intraoperative period, *Br J Anaesth* 64:582-585, 1990.

38. Dallen L, Nguyen L, Zornow M, et al: Task analysis/workload of anesthetists performing general anesthesia, *Anesthesiology* 73:A498, 1990 (abstract).

39. Gaba D, Herndon O, Zornow M, et al: Task analysis, vigilance, and workload in novice residents, *Anesthesiology* 75:A106, 1991.

40. Herndon O, Weinger M, Paulus M, et al: Analysis of the task of administering anesthesia: additional objective measures, *Anesthesiology* 75:A487, 1991 (abstract).

41. Gaba D, DeAnda A: A comprehensive anesthesia simulation environment: recreating the operating room for research and teaching, *Anesthesiology* 69:387-394, 1988.

42. Gaba D, DeAnda A: The response of anesthesia trainees to simulated critical incidents, *Anesth Analg* 68:444-451, 1989.

43. Cooper J, Newbower R, Kitz R: An analysis of major errors and equipment failures in anesthesia management: considerations for prevention and detection, *Anesthesiology* 60:34-42, 1984.

44. Loeb R, Brunner J, Westenskow D, et al: The Utah Anesthesia Workstation, *Anesthesiology* 70:999-1007, 1989.

45. Good M, Gravenstein J: Anesthesia simulators and training devices, *Int Anesthesiol Clin* 27:161-166, 1989.

46. Schwid H, O'Donnell D: The anesthesia simulator-recorder: a device to train and evaluate anesthesiologists' responses to critical incidents, *Anesthesiology* 72:191-197, 1990.

47. Smith N: *Mathematical model of uptake and distribution of inhalation anaesthetic agents.* In Viars P, editor: *Anesthesia par inhalation,* Paris, 1987, Arnette, pp 87-118.

48. Philip JH: *Gas man: understanding uptake and distribution in anesthesia and analgesia,* Chestnut Hill, Mass, 1991, Med Man Simulations.

49. Shapiro R, Berland T: Noise in the operating room, *N Engl J Med* 287:1236-1238, 1972.

50. Broadbent D: *Human performance and noise.* In Harris C, editor: *Handbook of noise control,* New York, 1979, McGraw-Hill, pp 17:1-17:2.

51. Hockey G: *Effects of noise on human work efficiency.* In May D, editor: *Handbook of noise assessment,* New York, 1978, Van Nostrand Reinhold, pp 335-372.

52. Jones D: *Noise,* Chichester, UK, 1983, Wiley, pp 61-95.

53. Poulton E: A new look at the effects of noise: a rejoiner, *Psychol Bull* 85:1068-1079, 1978.

54. Eschenbrenner A: Effects of intermittent noise on the performance of a complex psychomotor task, *Human Factors* 13:59-63, 1971.

55. Andren L, Hansson L, Bjorkman M, et al: Noise as a contributory factor in the development of arterial hypertension, *Acta Med Scand* 207:493-498, 1980.

56. Miles C, Auburn T, Jones D: Effects of loud noise and signal probability on visual vigilance, *Ergonomics* 27:855-862, 1984.

57. Englund C: *Human chronopsychology: an autorhythmic study of circadian periodicity in learning, mood and task performance,* San Diego, 1979, United States International University.

58. Blake M: *Temperature and time of day,* London, 1971, Academic Press, pp 109-148.

59. Hartley L, Williams T: Steady state noise and music and vigilance, *Ergonomics* 20:277-285, 1977.

60. Wolf R, Weiner E: Effects of four noise conditions on arithmetic performance, *Percept Mot Skills* 35:928-930, 1972.

61. Fontaine C, Schwalm N: Effects of familiarity of music on vigilant performance, *Percept Mot Skills* 49:71-74, 1979.

62. Ramsey J: *Heat and cold.* In Hockey G, editor: *Stress and fatigue in human performance,* Chichester, UK, 1983, Wiley, pp 33-60.

63. Fine B, Kobrick J: Effect of heat and chemical protective clothing on cognitive performance, *Aviat Space Environ Med* 58:149-154, 1987.

64. Epstein Y, Keren G, Moisseier J, et al: Psychomotor deterioration during exposure to heat, *Aviat Space Environ Med* 51:607-610, 1980.

65. Ellis H: The effects of cold on the performance of serial choice reaction time and various discrete tasks, *Human Factors* 24:589-598, 1982.

66. Baddeley A, Cuccuro W, Egstrom G, et al: Cognitive efficiency of divers working in cold water, *Human Factors* 17:446-454, 1975.

67. Ramsey J, Burford C, Beshir M, et al: Effects of workplace thermal conditions on safe work behavior, *J Safety Res* 14:105-114, 1983.

68. Bruce D, Bach M, Arbit J: Trace anesthetic effects on perceptual, cognitive, and motor skills. *Anesthesiology* 40:453-458, 1974.

69. Smith G, Shirley A: A review of the effects of trace concentrations of anaesthetics on performance, *Br J Anaesth* 50:701-712, 1978.

70. Stollery B, Broadbent D, Lee W, et al: Mood and cognitive functions in anaesthetists working in actively scavenged operating theatres, *Br J Anaesth* 61:446-455, 1988.

71. Kanki B, Lozito S, Foushee H: Communication indices of crew co-ordination, *Aviat Space Environ Med* 60:56-60, 1989.
72. Hockey G: *Changes in operator efficiency as a function of environmental stress, fatigue and circadian rhythms.* In Boff K, Kaufman L, Thomas J, editors: *Handbook of perception and human performance,* vol 2, *Cognitive processes and performance,* New York, 1986, Wiley, pp 44:1-44:49.
73. Holding D: *Fatigue,* New York, 1983, Wiley, pp 145-168.
74. Dodge R: Circadian rhythms and fatigue: a discrimination of their effects on performance, *Aviat Space Environ Med* 53:1131-1136, 1982.
75. Parker J: The effects of fatigue on physician performance: an underestimated cause of physician impairment and increased patient risk, *Can J Anaesth* 34:489-495, 1987.
76. Englund C, Ryman D, Naitoh P, et al: Cognitive performance during successive sustained physical work episodes, *Behav Res Meth Instru Comput* 17:75-85, 1985.
77. Englund C, Krueger G: Introduction to special section on methodological approaches to the study of sustained work/sustained operations, *Behav Res Meth Instru Comput* 17:3-5, 1985.
78. Krueger G, Englund C: Methodological approaches to the study of sustained work/sustained operations, *Behav Res Meth Instru Comput* 17:587-591, 1985.
79. Haslam D: Sleep loss, recovery sleep, and military performance, *Ergonomics* 25:163-178, 1982.
80. Åkerstedt T: Field studies of shiftwork. II. Temporal patterns in psychophysiological activation in workers alternating between night and day work, *Ergonomics* 20:621-631, 1977.
81. Friedman R, Bigger J, Kornfield D: The intern and sleep loss, *N Engl J Med* 285:201-203, 1971.
82. Haslam D: The military performance of soldiers in sustained operations, *Aviat Space Environ Med* 55:216-221, 1984.
83. Johnson L, Naitoh P: The operational consequences of sleep deprivation and sleep deficit, AGARD Rep. No. AG-192, London, 1974, North Atlantic Treaty Organization.
84. Morgan B, Brown B, Alluisi EA: Effects on sustained performance of 48 hours of continuous work and sleep loss, *Human Factors* 16:406-414, 1974.
85. Krueger G: Sustained work, fatigue, sleep loss and performance: a review of the issues, *Work Stress* 3:129-141, 1989.
86. Alluisi E, Morgan B: *Temporal factors in human performance and productivity.* In Alluisi E, Fleishman E, editors: *Human performance and productivity,* vol 3, *Stress and performance effectiveness,* Hillsdale, NJ, 1982, Lawrence Erlbaum Associates, pp 165-247.
87. Williams H, Lubin A, Goodnow J: Impaired performance with acute sleep loss, *Psychol Monogr* 73:1-26, 1959.
88. Wilkinson R: Interaction of lack of sleep with knowledge of results, repeated testing and individual differences, *J Exp Psychol* 62:263-271, 1961.
89. Williams H, Kearney O, Lubin A: Signal uncertainty and sleep loss, *J Exp Psychol* 69:401-407, 1965.
90. Wilkinson R: Rest pauses in a task affected by lack of sleep, *Ergonomics* 2:373-380, 1959.
91. Wilkinson R: The effect of lack of sleep on visual watchkeeping. *Q J Exp Psychol* 12:36-40:1960.
92. Williams H, Greseking C, Lubin A: Some effects of sleep loss on memory, *Percept Mot Skills* 23:1287-1293, 1966.
93. Hockey G: Changes in attention allocation in a multi-component task under loss of sleep, *Br J Psychol* 61:473-480, 1970.
94. Hockey G: Changes in information selection patterns in multisource monitoring as a function of induced arousal shifts, *J Exp Psychol* 101:35-42, 1973.
95. Webb W: *Sleep: the gentle tyrant,* Englewood Cliffs, NJ, 1975, Prentice-Hall.
96. Haslam D: The military performance of soldiers in continuous operations: exercise "Early Call" I and II. The twenty-four hour workday. Johnson L, Tepas D, Colquhoun, W, et al, editors: Proceedings of a symposium on variations in work-sleep schedules, Publication #81-127, Cincinnati, Ohio, 1981, US Dept of Health and Human Services (NIOSH), pp 549-580.
97. Naitoh P, Englund C, Ryman D: Sustained operations: research results, Report No. 87-17, San Diego, Calif, 1987. Naval Health Research Center.
98. Naitoh P, Angus R: *Napping and human functioning during prolonged work.* In Dinges D, Broughton R, editors: *Sleep and alertness: chronobiological behavior and medical aspects of napping,* New York, 1989, Raven Press, pp 221-246.
99. Dinges D, Orne M, Orne E: Assessing performance upon abrupt awakening from naps during quasi-continuous operations, *Behav Res Meth Instru Comput* 17:37-45, 1985.
100. Naitoh P: *Circadian cycles and restorative power of naps.* In Johnson L, Tepas D, Colquhoun W, et al: *Biological rhythms, sleep, and shiftwork,* New York, 1981, Spectrum, pp 553-580.
101. Hart R, Buchsbaum D, Wade J, et al: Effect of sleep deprivation on first-year residents' response times, memory, and mood, *J Med Educ* 62:940-942, 1987.
102. Beatty J, Ahern S, Katz R: *Sleep deprivation and the vigilance of anesthesiologists during simulated surgery.* In Mackie R, editor: *Vigilance: theory, operational performance, and physiological correlates,* New York, 1977, Plenum Press, pp 511-527.
103. Wallace-Barnhill G, Florez G, Turndorf H, et al: The effect of 24-hour duty on the performance of anesthesiology residents on vigilance, mood, and memory tasks, *Anesthesiology* 59:A460, 1983 (abstract).
104. Klose K, Wallace-Barnhill G, Craythorne N: Performance test results for anesthesia residents over a five day week including on-call duty, *Anesthesiology* 63:A485, 1985 (abstract).
105. Narang V, Laycock J: Psychomotor testing of on-call anaesthetists, *Anaesthesia* 41:868-869, 1986.
106. Denisco R, Drummond J, Gravenstein J: The effect of fatigue on the performance of a simulated anesthetic monitoring task, *J Clin Monit* 3:22-24, 1987.
107. Deaconson T, O'Hair D, Levy M, et al: Sleep deprivation and resident performance, *JAMA* 260:1721-1727, 1988.
108. Lichtor J, Nuotto E, Hendren M, et al: The effect of sleep deprivation on psychomotor performance in anesthesia personnel, *Anesth Analg* 68:S164, 1989 (abstract).
109. Lees D: New York state regulations to be implemented: work hours, resident supervision, anesthesia monitors mandated, *Anesth Patient Safety Found Newslett* 3:18-24, 1988.
110. Squires B: Fatigue and stress in medical students, interns, and residents: It's time to act! *Can Med Assoc J* 140:18-19, 1989.
111. Turnbull R: Diurnal cycles and work-rest scheduling in unusual environments, *Human Factors* 8:385-398, 1966.
112. Folkard S, Monk T: *Shiftwork and performance.* In Colquhoun W, Rutenfranz J, editors: *Studies of shiftwork,* London, 1980, Taylor and Francis, pp 263-272.
113. Blake M: Relationship between circadian rhythm of body temperature and introversion-extroversion, *Nature* 215:896-897, 1967.
114. Horne J, Ostberg O: Individual differences in human circadian rhythms, *Biol Psychol* 5:179-190, 1977.
115. Folkard S, Monk T, Lobban M: Short and long-term adjustment of circadian rhythms in "permanent" night nurses, *Ergonomics* 21:785-799, 1978.
116. Colquhoun W, Rutenfranz J: *Studies of shiftwork,* London, 1980, Taylor and Francis.
117. Reinberg A, Vieux N, Andlauer P: *Night and shift work: biological and social aspects,* Oxford, UK, 1981, Pergamon Press.

118. Verhaegan P, Maasen A, Meers A: Health problems in shiftworkers: the twenty-four hour workday. Johnson L, Tepas D, Colquhoun W, et al, editors: Proceedings of a symposium on variations in work-sleep schedules, Publication #81-127, Cincinnati, Ohio, 1981, US Dept. of Health and Human Services, pp 335-346.

119. Colquhoun W: *Biological rhythms and human performance*, London, 1971, Academic Press.

120. Bjerner B, Swensson A: Shiftwork and rhythm, *Acta Med Scand Suppl* 278:102-107, 1953.

121. Aschoff J, Giedke H, Poppel E, et al: *The influence of sleep interruption, and of sleep deprivation or circadian rhythms, in human performance*. In Colquhoun W, editor: *Aspects of human efficiency*, Oxford, UK, 1972, English Universities Press, pp 135-150.

122. Naitoh P, Englund C, Ryman D: Restorative power of naps in designing continuous work schedules, *J Hum Ergol* 11 (Suppl):259-278, 1982.

123. Naitoh P, Englund C, Ryman D: Extending human effectiveness during sustained operations through sleep management, Proceedings of the 24th DRG seminar on the human as the limiting element in military systems, Toronto, 1983, Defense Research Group, pp 113-138.

124. McCormick E, Tiffin J: *Industrial psychology*, Englewood Cliffs, NJ, 1974, Prentice-Hall.

125. Warm J: *Sustained attention in human performance*, New York, 1984, Wiley.

126. Cooper J, Long C, Newbower R, et al: Critical incidents associated with intraoperative exchanges of anesthesia personnel, *Anesthesiology* 56:456-461, 1982.

127. Cooper J: Do short breaks increase or decrease anesthetic risk? *J Clin Anesth* 1:228-231, 1989.

128. Welford A: *Fatigue and monotony*. In Edholm O, Bacharach A, editors: *The physiology of human survival*, London, 1965, Academic Press, pp 431-462.

129. Haga S: An experimental study of signal vigilance errors in train driving, *Ergonomics* 27:755-765, 1984.

130. Simonov P, Frolov M, Ivanov E: Psychophysiological monitoring of operator's emotional stress in aviation and astronautics, *Aviat Space Environ Med* 51:46-50, 1980.

131. Davies D, Shakleton V, Parasuraman R: *Monotony and boredom*. In Hockey G, editor: *Stress and fatigue in human performance*, Chichester, UK, 1983, Wiley, pp 1-32.

132. Wilkinson R, Edwards R: Stable hours and varied work as aids to efficiency. *Psychonomic Sci* 13:205-206, 1968.

133. Froberg J: *Sleep deprivation and prolonged work hours*. In Froberg J, Monk T, editors: *Hours of work: temporal factors in work scheduling*, Chichester, UK, 1985, Wiley, pp 67-76.

134. Gould J, Schaffer A: The effects of divided attention on visual monitoring of multi-channel displays, *Human Factors* 9:191-202, 1967.

135. Tyler D, Halcomb C: Monitoring performance with a time-shared encoding task, *Percept Mot Skills* 38:382-386, 1974.

136. Raymond C: Mental stress: "occupational injury" of 80's that even pilots can't rise above, *JAMA* 259:3097-3098, 1988.

137. Girodo M: The psychological health and stress of pilots in a labor dispute, *Aviat Space Environ Med* 59:505-510, 1988.

138. Smith M: *Occupational stress*, New York, 1986, Wiley, pp 844-860.

139. Dille J: Mental stress causes accidents, too, *Aviat Space Environ Med* 53:1137, 1982.

140. Bignell V, Fortune J: *Understanding system failures*, Manchester, UK, 1984, Manchester University Press, pp 190-204.

141. Smith B, Principato F: Effects of stress and conflict difficulty on arousal and conflict resolution, *Brit J Soc Psychol* 73:85-93, 1982.

142. Hart S, Hauser J: Inflight application of three pilot workload measurement techniques, *Aviat Space Environ Med* 58:402-410, 1987.

143. Barabasz A: Enhancement of military pilot reliability by hypnosis and psycho-physiological monitoring: preliminary inflight and simulator data, *Aviat Space Environ Med* 56:248-250, 1985.

144. Casali J, Wierwille W: On the measurement of pilot perceptual workload: a comparison of assessment techniques addressing sensitivity and intrusion issues, *Ergonomics* 27:1033-1050, 1984.

145. Thackray R, Jones K, Touchstone R: Personality and physiological correlates of performance decrement on a monotonous task requiring sustained attention, *Br J Soc Psychol* 351-358, 1974.

146. Svensson E, Thanderz M, Sjoberg L, et al: Military flight experience and sympathoadrenal activity, *Aviat Space Environ Med* 59:411-416, 1988.

147. Rozanski A, Bairey N, Krantz D, et al: Mental stress and the induction of silent myocardial ischemia in patients with coronary artery disease, *N Engl J Med* 318:1005-1012, 1988.

148. Toung T, Donham R, Rogers M: The stress of giving anesthesia on the electrocardiogram of anesthesiologists, *Anesthesiology* 61:A465, 1984 (abstract).

149. Toung T, Donham R, Rogers M: The effect of previous medical training on the stress of giving anesthesia, *Anesthesiology* 65:A473, 1986 (abstract).

150. Colford J, McPhee S: The ravelled sleeve of care: managing the stresses of residency training, *JAMA* 261:889-893, 1989.

151. Spiegelman W, Saunders L, Mazze R: Addiction and anesthesiology, *Anesthesiology* 60:335-341, 1984.

152. Leiberman H, Wurtman R, Emde G, et al: The effects of low-dose caffeine on human performance and mood, *Pyschopharmacol* 92:308-312, 1987.

153. Lane J, Williams R: Cardiovascular effects of caffeine and stress in regular coffee drinkers, *Psychopharmacol* 24:157-164, 1987.

154. Moskowitz H: Attention tasks as skills performance measures of drug effects, *Br J Clin Pharmacol* 18:51S-61S, 1984.

155. Hyman F, Collins W, Taylor H, et al: Instrument flight performance under the influence of certain combinations of antiemetic drugs, *Aviat Space Environ Med* 59:533-539, 1988.

156. Gaillard A, Gruisen A, deJong R: The influence of antihistamines on human performance, *Eur J Clin Pharmacol* 35:249-253, 1988.

157. Aksnes E: Effect of small dosages of alcohol upon performance in a Link trainer, *J Aviat Med* 25:680-688, 1954.

158. Collins W: Performance effects of alcohol intoxication and hangover at ground level and at simulated altitude, *Aviat Space Environ Med* 51:327-335, 1980.

159. Erwin C, Wiener E, Linnoila M, et al: Alcohol-induced drowsiness and vigilance performance, *J Stud Alcohol* 39:505-516, 1978.

160. Henry P, Davis T, Engelken E, et al: Alcohol-induced performance decrements assessed by two Link trainer tasks using experienced pilots, *Aerospace Med* 45:1180-1189, 1974.

161. Franck D: 'If you drink, don't drive' motto now applies to hangovers as well, *JAMA* 250:1657-1658, 1983.

162. Laurell H, Tornos J: Statens Vag-och trafikinstitut Rapport No. 222A, 1983.

163. Seppala T, Leino T, Linnoila M, et al: Effects of hangover on psychomotor skills related to driving: modification by fructose and glucose, *Acta Pharmacol Toxicol* 38:209-218, 1976.

164. Yesavage J, Leirer V: Hangover effects on aircraft pilots 14 hours after alcohol ingestion: a preliminary report, *Am J Psychiatry* 143:1546-1550, 1986.

165. Janowksy D, Meacham M, Blaine J, et al: Marijuana effects on simulated flying ability, *Am J Psychiatry* 133:384-388, 1976.

166. Lewis M, Ferraro D: *Flying high: the aeromedical aspects of marihuana*, Springfield, Va, 1973, National Technical Information Service.

167. National Transportation Safety Board: Central Airlines Flight 27, Newark Airport (March 30, 1983), 1983.

168. Engelberg S: Error by signal operator is called likely cause of Amtrak collision, *New York Times*, p 1, July 27, 1984.

169. Yesavage J, Leirer V, Denari M, et al: Carry-over effects of marijuana intoxication on aircraft pilot performance: a preliminary report, *Am J Psychiatry* 142:1325-1329, 1985.

170. Leirer V, Yesavage J, Morrow D: Marijuana carry-over effects on aircraft pilot performance, *Aviat Space Environ Med* 62:221-227, 1991.

171. Ware R, Baker R: *The effect of mental set and states of consciousness on vigilance decrement: a systematic exploration.* In Mackie R, editor: *Vigilance: theory, operational performance, and physiological correlates,* New York, 1976, Plenum Press, p 607.

172. Verhaegen P, Ryckaert R: Vigilance of train engineers, *Human Factors* 30:403-407, 1986.

173. Folkard S, Monk T, Lobban M: Towards a predictive test of adjustment to shift work, *Ergonomics* 22:79-91, 1979.

174. Slogoff S, Keats A: Does perioperative myocardial ischemia lead to postoperative myocardial infarction? *Anesthesiology* 62:107-114, 1985.

175. Harris R, Tole J, Stephens A, et al: Visual scanning behavior and pilot workload, *Aviat Space Environ Med* 53:1067-1072, 1982.

176. Haskell B, Reid G: The subjective perception of workload in low-time private pilots: a preliminary study, *Aviat Space Environ Med* 58:1230-1232, 1987.

177. Bandaret L, Stokes J, Francesconi R, et al: Artillery teams in simulated sustained combat: Performance and other measures, NIOSH Proceedings: The 24-hour workday, Publication #81-127, Cincinnati, Ohio, 1981, US Dept of Health and Human Services, pp 581-604.

178. Bergeron H, Hinton D: Aircraft automation: the problem of the pilot interface, *Aviat Space Environ Med* 56:144-148, 1985.

179. Wickens C: *The structure of attentional resources.* In Nickerson R, editor: *Attention and performance VIII,* Hillsdale, NJ, 1980, Lawrence Erlbaum, pp 239-257.

180. Lambert T, Paget N: Teaching and learning in the operating theatre, *Anaesth Intensive Care* 4:304-307, 1976.

181. Jennings A, Chiles W: An investigation of time-sharing ability as a factor in complex performance, *Human Factors* 19:535-547, 1977.

182. Siering G, Stone L: In search of a time-sharing ability in zero-input tracking analyzer scores, *Aviat Space Environ Med* 57:1194-1197, 1986.

183. Block FJ, Burton L, Rafal M, et al: Two computer-based anesthetic monitors: the Duke automatic monitoring equipment (DAME) system and the MICRODAME, *J Clin Monit* 1:30-51, 1985.

184. Cook R, Potter S, Woods D, et al: Evaluating the human engineering of microprocessor controlled operating room devices, *J Clin Monit* 7:217-226, 1991.

185. Mazze R: Therapeutic misadventures with O_2 delivery systems: the need for continuous in-line O_2 monitors, *Anesth Analg* 51:787-792, 1972.

186. Sato T: Fatal pipeline accidents spur Japanese standards, *Anesth Patient Safety Found Newslett* 6:14, 1991.

187. Holland R: Another "wrong gas" incident in Hong Kong, *Anesth Patient Safety Found Newslett* 6:9, 1991.

188. Beneken J, van der Aa J: Alarms and their limits in monitoring, *J Clin Monit* 5:205-210, 1989.

189. Federal Aviation Administration: Aircraft alerting systems criteria study, vol I: collation and analysis of aircraft alerting system data, FAA-RD-76-222, Springfield, Va, 1977, National Technical Information Service.

190. Quinn M: *A philosophy of alarms.* In Gravenstein J, Newbower R, Ream A, et al, editors: *The automated anesthesia record and alarm systems,* Stoneham, Mass, 1987, Butterworths, pp 169-173.

191. Schreiber P, Schreiber J: Structured alarm systems for the operating room, *J Clin Monit* 5:201-204, 1989.

192. Hyman W, Drinker P: Design of medical device alarm systems, *Med Instrum* 17:103-106, 1983.

193. Porciello P: Allarmi e unita' di cura coronarica, *G Ital Cardiol* 10:939-943, 1980.

194. O'Carroll T: Survey of alarms in an intensive therapy unit, *Anaesthesia* 41:742-744, 1986.

195. Meijler A: *Automation in anesthesia: a relief?* Berlin, 1987, Springer-Verlag.

196. Kestin I, Miller B, Lockhart C: Auditory alarms during anesthesia monitoring, *Anesthesiology* 69:106-109, 1988.

197. McIntyre J: Ergonomics: Anaesthetists' use of auditory alarms in the operating room, *Int J Clin Monit Comput* 2:47-55, 1985.

198. Stanford L, McIntyre J, Nelson T, et al: Affective responses to commercial and experimental auditory alarm signals for anesthesia delivery and physiological monitoring equipment, *Int J Clin Monit Comp* 5:111-118, 1988.

199. Veitergruber J, Doucek G, Smith W: *Aircraft alerting systems criteria study,* Washington, DC, 1977, Federal Aviation Authority.

200. Jones T, Kirk R: Monitoring performance on visual and auditory displays, *Percept Mot Skills* 30:235-238, 1970 (abstract).

201. Loeb R, Jones B, Behrman K, et al: Anesthetists can not identify audible alarms, *Anesthesiology* 73:A539, 1990 (abstract).

202. Wallace M, Ashman M: Volume and frequency of anesthetic alarms: are the current alarm systems appropriate for normal human ear aging? *J Clin Monit* 7:134, 1991.

203. Kerr J: Warning devices, *Br J Anaesth* 57:696-708, 1985.

204. Block FJ: Evaluation of users' ability to recognize musical alarm tones, *J Clin Monit* 8:285–290, 1992.

205. Hakkinen M, Williges B: Synthesized warning messages: effects of an alerting cue in single- and multiple-function voice synthesis systems, *Human Factors* 26 185-195, 1984.

206. Patterson R: Guidelines for auditory warning systems on civil aircraft, Paper No 82017, London, UK, 1982, Civil Aviation Authority.

207. Fukui Y: *An expert alarm system.* In Gravenstein J, Newbower R, Ream A, et al, editors: *The automated anesthesia record and alarm systems,* Stoneham Mass, 1987, Butterworths, pp 203-209.

208. Watt R, Navabi M, Mylrea K, et al: Integrated monitoring "smart alarms" can detect critical events and reduce false alarms, *Anesthesiology* 71:A338, 1989 (abstract).

209. Orr J, Westenskow D: A breathing circuit alarm system based on neural networks, *Anesthesiology* 71:A339, 1989 (abstract).

210. Pan P, van der Aa J, Gomez F, et al: Smart anesthesia monitoring system, *Anesthesiology* 73:A450, 1990 (abstract).

211. Beinlich I, Gaba D: The ALARM monitoring system: intelligent decision making under uncertainty, *Anesthesiology* 71:A337, 1989.

212. Orr J, Simon F, Ing D, et al: Response time with smart alarms, *Anesthesiology* 73:A447, 1990 (abstract).

213. Cohn A, Rosenbaum S, Miller P: An alternative parallel computing approach to intelligent hemodynamic monitoring, *Anesthesiology* 73:A541, 1990 (abstract).

214. Cushing H: On the avoidance of shock in major amputations by cocainization of large nerve trunks preliminary to their divisions. With observations on blood pressure changes in surgical cases, *Ann Surg* 36:321-345, 1902.

215. Gravenstein JS, Weinger MB: Why investigate vigilance? *J Clin Monit* 2:145-147, 1986.

216. Philip J, Raemer D: Selecting the optimal anesthesia monitoring array, *Med Instrum* 19:122-126, 1985.

217. Fiegler A, Stead S: The medical information bus, *Biomed Instrum Technol* 24:101-111, 1990.

218. Cooper J, Newbower R: The Boston anesthesia system, *Contemp Anesth Prac* 8:207-219, 1984.

219. Hankeln K, Michelsen H, Schipulle M, et al: Microprocessor-assisted monitoring system for measuring and processing cardiorespiratory variables: preliminary results of clinical trials, *Crit Care Med* 13:426-431, 1985.

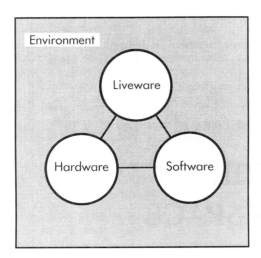

Fig. 18-1. The SHEL model of system resources.

ings, equipment, and materials used for the job. The second class, the *software,* consists of the rules, guidelines, policies, procedures, and customs involved in the job. People make up the third class of components, *liveware.* These components act together within a larger context, or *environment,* which is composed of external physical, economic, social, and political factors affecting the job. Ergonomics is concerned with improving the interactions between the liveware component and the other components.

Ergonomics is both a science and a profession. It encompasses both research and application. One goal of ergonomics research is to understand and describe the capabilities and limitations of human performance. Another is to develop principles of interaction between people and machines. Examples of ergonomics research are the measurement and compilation of anthropomorphic data and the investigation of visual perception in relation to a particular task. Application involves the use of these data in the development of equipment, systems, and jobs. For example, anthropomorphic data are used in the design of a chair, and the selection of colors for a display is based on an understanding of visual perception, information processing, and decision theory.

Some aspects of ergonomics focus on the worker and the human-to-human interfaces within the system. This may include task and workload analysis, examination of vigilance and fatigue, and analysis of worker interactions. The focus of this chapter is on the interface between the liveware and the hardware, or the interface between the human and the machine.

ERGONOMICS STUDIES IN ANESTHESIOLOGY

Only a few ergonomics studies in anesthesiology have been published. This section briefly reviews some of this work. The focus is to identify human-machine interface factors that affect the patient's safety and the anesthesiologist's job performance.

Task analysis studies

Task analysis is a basic ergonomics methodology for evaluating jobs or designing new human-machine systems. Several variants of this methodology are used, depending on the focus of the problem. Typically, task analysis methods involve the structured decomposition of work activities and the classification of these activities into a series of tasks. At least three interacting components can be identified and described for each task: the task's goals, constraints, and behaviors.[7] Time and motion studies are one method of determining task behavior.

One of the first formal time and motion studies ever was an analysis of surgeons' tasks in the operating room.[3] Frank and Lillian Gilbreth conducted time and motion studies of surgical teams during the early 1900s.[8] They discovered that surgeons spent an inordinate amount of time looking for instruments as they picked them off a tray. Their findings led to the current practice of the surgeon requesting instruments from a nurse, who places the instrument in the surgeon's hand.[3]

More recently, time and motion studies of the anesthesiologist have been performed. Drui, et al.[9] observed 43 operations, recording 8 with time-lapse photography. Their goal was to investigate factors that promoted dissatisfaction and inefficiency in the anesthesiologist. They found that the anesthesiologists were physically idle 40% of the time and that their attention was directed away from the patient-surgical field 42% of the time. The authors noted that filling out the anesthesia record occupied a large proportion of the anesthesiologist's time but was rated by the subjects as relatively unimportant and easy to perform. They observed that it took an average of 30 seconds to take the blood pressure and pulse. However, the time was increased when an esophageal stethoscope was used instead of a precordial stethoscope, when the pressure gauge was located on the anesthesia machine instead of at the head of the operating room table, or when the patient was hypotensive. On the basis of these and other findings, the authors recommended automating the anesthesia record and redesigning the anesthesia machine to increase productivity and decrease the amount of distraction away from the patient-surgical field.

Kennedy, et al.[10] performed a similar study during three coronary bypass procedures. They recorded each case using time-lapse cinematography and analyzed each frame to detect the types and sequences of activities performed by the anesthesiologists. They found that observing the patient and scanning the operative and monitoring field were the two most frequent activities. However, attention was directed away from the patient-surgical field 30% of the time. Logging data on the anesthesia record occupied 10% to 15% of the anesthesiologist's time, and this activity was tightly linked with observing instrument displays. Their analysis of the data indicated that the activity patterns were different during four distinct phases of the procedure: induction, pre-bypass, bypass, and post-bypass. Like Drui, et al., they recommended automation of the anesthesia record and a more structured arrangement of equipment around the patient-surgical field.

Neither of the above studies directly resulted in a redesign of anesthesia equipment. However, in 1976, the Fraser Harlake company produced a prototype line-of-sight anesthesia machine designed by Goodyear and Rendell-Baker.[11] With this machine, the user could see both the patient and the machine controls with minimal eye movement. The machine, never made commercially available, may have influenced the design of the Ohio Modulus-Wing anesthesia machine. An important feature of the Modulus-Wing machine was that the displays and controls could be positioned next to the patient.

Before redesigning an anesthesia system, Boquet et al.[12] collected 16 hours of time and motion data during general anesthetic procedures. They recorded and classified 31 manual activities and 26 visual activities. In their study, 40% of the anesthesiologist's visual attention was directed away from the patient or surgical field. The anesthesiologist was physically idle 72% of the time. Logging data on the anesthesia record occupied 6% of the anesthesiologist's time and was frequently linked to measurement of blood pressure. The patterns of activity were different during the four quarters of the anesthetic procedure. These authors then proposed an anesthesia machine design, changing the placement of displays and controls.

Recent studies have confirmed previous findings that the anesthesiologist spends significant amounts of time on indirect patient-related tasks and that the distribution of tasks is influenced by the stage of the anesthetic procedure.[13,14] For example, during induction there is a high density of tasks, with airway management accounting for approximately 40% of the time.[14] One new study suggests a beneficial effect of automation. McDonald and colleagues[15,16] at Ohio State University replicated their previous time-motion techniques on 30 cases in which automated blood pressure devices, ventilators, and disconnect alarms were employed. With newer technology, the time that anesthesiologists spent directly observing or monitoring the patient increased to nearly 60% of their total task time.

Investigators at the University of California San Diego Medical Center have performed comprehensive task analysis on both novice and experienced anesthesia care providers.[13,14,17] A trained observer in the operating room recorded the anesthesiologist's activity using 12 or 28 task categories. Record-keeping consumed 10% to 20% of total case time and was related to observing monitors (Fig. 18-2).[14,17] Task density analysis revealed that when activity level was high, the average amount of time spent per task was low. In contrast, when activity level was low, the amount of time spent per task increased (Fig. 18-3).[17]

The similarities of the results in these time and motion studies are striking, especially because they have been conducted over 20 years in a wide distribution of settings.

Although they are useful for describing the actions and activities of the anesthesiologist in the existing workspace, the above studies cannot be used to quantify mental workload because cognitive processing can occur while the worker is apparently idle. Workload assessments are important both for evaluating the cognitive requirements of new workplace designs and equipment and for predicting the cognitive capacity for additional tasks.

In a study of mental workload, Gaba and Lee[18] used the ability of anesthesia residents to perform an extra task during administration of anesthesia as a measure of cognitive workload on the primary task. They found that performance of the secondary task was compromised in 40% of the samples (i.e., secondary task was skipped or there was a greater than 30-s excess response time). Workload was highest during the induction and emergence phases of anesthesia. High workload occurred during performance of manual tasks, conversations with operating room personnel, and interactions with the attending anesthesiologist. Workload has also been objectively quantified by other types of secondary task probing.[13,14,17] During these studies, subjective workload was also assessed every 10 minutes by both the observer and the subject. Workload and stress were greatest during induction, decreased during maintenance, and increased again during the emergence phase of anesthesia (Fig. 18-4). These findings on cognitive workload, when reviewed in the context of earlier time and motion studies, indicate that during the course of a typical operating room procedure the anesthesiologist's workload is heavy 20% to 30% of the time, very low 30% to 40% of the time, and, the anesthesiologist is physically active but able to respond to an additional task the remainder of the time.

The above studies present a number of general implications for equipment design. Equipment can act to decrease workload and increase idle time through automation of certain tasks, such as record-keeping. Poorly designed equipment can increase workload, decrease idle time, and distract the anesthesiologist from the patient-surgical field. Equipment should aid rather than distract during the induction phase of anesthesia, which is a time of high task activity and mental workload for the anesthesiologist.

Critical incident studies

Critical incident analysis is an established method for investigating human error. It was first used in 1954 to study near-accidents in aviation.[19] The technique involves structured interviews of people who have been involved in, or observed, unsafe acts or actual accidents. Analysis of these interviews often provides evidence of behavior patterns and other recurrent factors that may contribute to accidents.

Cooper and colleagues first applied the critical incident technique to anesthesiology.[20,21] During the period from 1975 through 1984, they collected descriptions of 1089 critical incidents from 139 anesthesiologists, residents, and

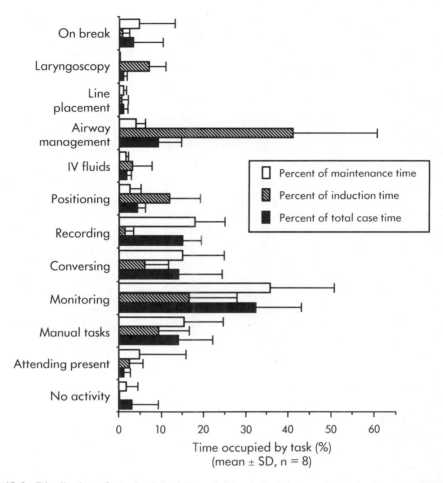

Fig. 18-2. Distribution of anesthesiologist's activities during 8 general anesthesia cases. The histogram presents the percent of time utilized in each of the 12 task categories during induction of anesthesia, during maintenance, and for the total case. Note that, as expected, airway management predominates during induction and that monitoring, recording, and conversing predominate during maintenance. Monitoring and record-keeping consume 30% and 15% of the total case time, respectively, which is consistent with previous studies.

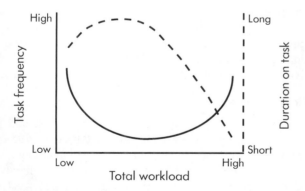

Fig. 18-3. Relationships among the anesthesiologist's workload, task frequency, and duration. At low workloads, the time spent on a particular task is high. In contrast, when workload is high, the average time spent per task is much lower. At both low and high workloads, a more limited subset of tasks is performed more frequently.

nurse anesthetists. The descriptions were obtained through a combination of retrospective interviews and contemporaneous reports. Critical incidents were defined as occurrences of "human error or equipment failure that could have led (if not discovered or corrected in time) or did lead to an undesirable outcome, ranging from increased length of hospital stay to death."[21] Their data indicate that human error was responsible for 65% to 70% of the incidents. Of the 67 incidents that resulted in substantive negative outcomes, there were 28 technical human errors, 23 judgmental errors, and 13 vigilance errors. A number of recurrent technical human errors were related to the design or organization of equipment. Examples of these included syringe swaps, gas-flow-control technical errors, vaporizers off unintentionally, drug ampule swaps, drug overdoses (technical), misuses of blood pressure monitors, breathing-circuit-control technical errors, and wrong intravenous lines

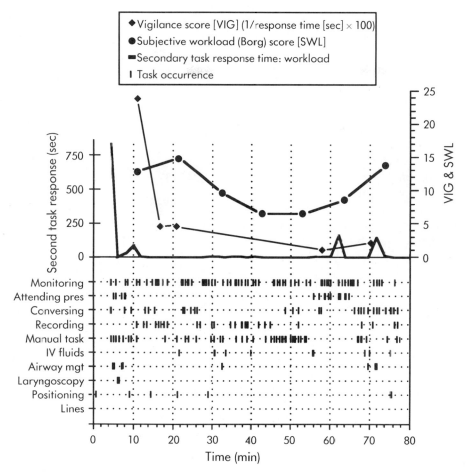

Fig. 18-4. Task analysis and measurements of workload for a single anesthetic procedure. Vigilance score was measured as the time required for the anesthesiologist to recognize the illumination of a small red light located adjacent to the ECG monitor. Subjective workload was self-reported on a scale from 6 (doing nothing at all) to 20 (extreme exertion). Secondary task response time was the latency (in seconds) for the anesthesiologist to answer a simple addition problem presented on a Macintosh computer located next to the anesthesia drug cart. An observer in the OR used accepted task analysis techniques to determine what tasks arose over time during the case. The individual manual and visual tasks were condensed into 10 categories for presentation. Each vertical tick mark represents a single occurrence of that task category.

used. On the basis of their findings, the authors recommended a standardized system of syringe labels and redesign of the breathing circuit to prevent disconnections.

A detailed description of one of their critical incidents, gas-flow-control technical error, illustrates the importance of evaluating equipment designs prior to implementation. At one of the hospitals where the studies were conducted, all of the anesthesia machines had been modified. On each machine, the oxygen flow-control knob had been replaced with a large, square knob in an attempt to distinguish it from the nitrous oxide knob. However, rather than preventing gas-flow-control errors, the knob was found to be a contributing factor. Half of the accidental decreases in oxygen flow occurred when the knob was bumped by an object as it was being placed on the surface of the anesthesia machine.

Subsequent critical incident studies[22,23] have been performed via contemporaneous reporting systems. In each, human error has been the predominant cause of mishaps, and the patterns of incident types and associated factors have been similar. Kumar, et al.[23] demonstrated that critical incidents decreased when an anesthesia equipment checklist was used, old anesthesia machines were replaced, and incidents were discussed at department conferences. They recommended critical incident surveillance as a method of identifying specific problems and assuring quality control.

Gaba and DeAnda[24] have created an anesthesia simulator to investigate factors of accident evolution and techniques used by clinicians to recognize and recover from critical events. The simulator recreates the operating room environment with real monitors and equipment as well as a patient mannequin. This simulated environment provides an additional opportunity to study the occurrence of critical events. In an initial study of behavior of residents in response to planned critical incidents, they noted problems and errors that arose in addition to the planned events. They documented 132 unplanned events during 19 simulated cases; 87 events were attributed to human error, and only 4 were equipment failures.[25] However, many of the human failures involved errors in the use of equipment, for example "failure to switch the ventilator power back on after hand-ventilating the patient,"[25] and neglecting to turn on the oxygen flow during preoxygenation. This study indicated that errors commonly occur, that many errors involve interactions with equipment, and that most errors are detected and corrected before they become hazardous to the patient.

Attention studies

Vigilance, the ability to sustain attention, has long been considered important to the anesthesiologist, as reflected in the word's inclusion on the official seal of the American Society of Anesthesiologists.[26] A substantial body of knowledge concerning vigilance has evolved in the psychology literature. This work was originally motivated by the problem of radar operators, who for extended periods performed the task of detecting barely perceptible events at sometimes infrequent intervals. However, the problem may be somewhat different for anesthesiologists, whose attention is distracted due to simultaneous demands, conflicting tasks, and poor equipment design. Selective attention is the ability to filter out distractions and concentrate on the signal.

Kay and Neal[27] investigated whether automation in anesthesia decreases vigilance. They studied whether the vigilance of a group of anesthesia residents using automated blood pressure monitoring devices (ABPDs) was reduced in comparison to a group who determined blood pressure manually. To assess vigilance, the resident's earpiece was clamped and the time that passed until this was recognized was noted. The authors concluded that using ABPDs may decrease vigilance because monitoring interruptions were less quickly detected when ABPDs were used. However, the results must be considered inconclusive, because the study had a number of methodological flaws.[26,28]

Cooper and Cullen[28] subsequently described a better method for investigating auditory vigilance. They used a computer-controlled device to occlude the stethoscope tubing silently at random intervals during routine general anesthesia cases. Study participants were instructed to press a button to restore function whenever they perceived the absence of stethoscope sounds. The elapsed time between the occlusion of the tubing and the press of the button was automatically recorded. They studied 320 stethoscope occlusions in 32 intubated patients. The interval from occlusion to detection ranged from 2 to 457 seconds with a mean of 34 seconds (Fig. 18-5). They concluded that au-

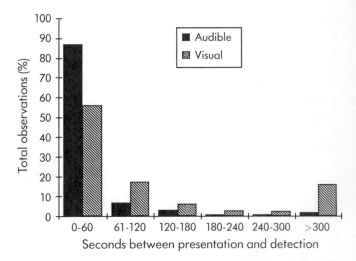

Fig. 18-5. Comparison of intraoperative vigilance of anesthesiologists from two different studies. Audible vigilance was assessed as response time to detect occlusion of the esophageal stethoscope. Visual vigilance was measured as response time to detect an abnormal value displayed on a physiologic monitor. (Modified from Cooper JO, Cullen BF: Observer reliability in detecting surreptitious random occlusions of the monaural esophageal stethoscope, *J Clin Monit* 6:271-275, 1990, and Loeb RG: Intraoperative vigilance toward a physiologic monitor, *Anesth Analg* 74:S190, 1990.)

ditory vigilance during general anesthesia was typically high but not infallible. Manual tasks and conversations interfered with auditory vigilance, because the subjects were involved in one of these activities in all instances of response times greater than 5 minutes.

Loeb[29] studied the vigilance of eight anesthesia residents by displaying numbers at random intervals on an operating room monitor during operative procedures. The residents were required to detect an "abnormal" value and respond by pressing a button on the anesthesia machine. During 60 minor operative procedures, the average response time was 61 ± 61 seconds (mean ± standard deviation) and 56% of the detections were made within 60 seconds. Thus, Loeb[29] and Gaba, et al.[13] both found that visual signal response times were longer during the periintubation phase than during the maintenance of the anesthetic. When related to Cooper's study, it appears that response times in the operating room are longer for visual than for auditory signals (Fig. 18-5).

Yablock, in a preliminary study[30] concluded that anesthesia residents were less vigilant during cases in which automated record-keeping devices were used than during cases in which records were maintained manually. However, caution must be employed in interpreting these data because the measure of vigilance may not have been valid.

ERGONOMICS GUIDELINES

An important step toward the development of ergonomically sound equipment and systems is that the equipment developer incorporate ergonomics principles and guidelines during the predesign phase. A number of ergonomics handbooks and guidelines have been published for equipment designers in fields outside of medicine.[31-34] More recently, the Association for the Advancement of Medical Instrumentation (AAMI) has published *Human Factors Engineering Guidelines and Preferred Practices for the Design of Medical Devices*.[35] The document includes recommendations regarding general design, controls, visual displays, audio signals, and consoles. Of note, the guidelines recognize some idiosyncracies of the medical environment: that users of medical equipment are often female, that medical devices are often moved, that medical devices must withstand common cleaning and disinfecting agents, and that safety for the patient and user are paramount. A major portion of the document contains tables and figures of specific design criteria, such as separation distances between controls and control movement specifications, based on anthropometry and population stereotypes. The AAMI is currently revising the document to stay abreast with changes in technology, especially the trend toward electronic controls and displays and embedded microprocessors.

Principles of good device design

User requirements need to be emphasized during the design of equipment and devices. The goal is to produce devices that are easily maintained, have a good user interface, and are tailored to the user's abilities. This is best accomplished during the early phases of system and equipment design, when the ergonomics and engineering specialists can work together with end users to produce a safe, reliable, and usable product.[36] Norman eloquently presents this principle of user-centered system design in *The Psychology of Everyday Things*.[37] This text is recommended for all engineers, programmers, and designers responsible for the development of new medical devices. Some of the key aspects of user interface design that Norman emphasizes are: (1) make things visible; (2) provide good mapping; (3) create appropriate constraints; (4) simplify tasks; and (5) design for error.

Make things visible. A well designed interface between human and machine conveys to the user the purpose, operational modes, and controlling actions for the device. If the design of the device or system is based on a good conceptual model, its purpose will be readily apparent to the user. Most devices have several operational modes. The user must be able to determine rapidly and accurately whether the system is in the desired mode and when the mode changes. With most devices, a number of user actions are possible at any given time; with complex systems, the allowable commands often depend on the current operational mode. The user should be able to tell what actions are possible at any given instant and what will be the consequences of those actions. *Feedback* must be provided after each user action; it should be readily understandable and match the user's intentions.

Knowledge about the function and operation of a device should be readily apparent to the user. The function and operation of many devices is generally known. People expect certain objects always to function in a particular manner (e.g., knobs are for turning, buttons are for pushing). With other devices, the function can and often should be implied by the device itself. That is, by design, the purpose of a particular control or operation should be readily apparent to the user (e.g., the large horizontal handle on the side of the anesthesia machine is for pulling the device from one location to another). Such intuitive operation may be difficult to attain with complex, microprocessor-controlled, multifunction devices. However, when the design requires of the user knowledge about the device's controls, actions, or responses (e.g., "To see the systolic blood pressure trend plot, I must push a particular sequence of soft buttons in a specific order"), then the need for training increases and there is a greater chance of user errors under stressful conditions or with high workloads.

Provide good mapping. Mapping is the relationship between an action and a response. Mapping may be natural or artificial. Natural mappings are intuitive; artificial mappings must be learned. Artificial mappings that have been learned so well that the relationship between action and effect is recognized at a subconscious or automatic level are called conventional mappings. On an anesthesia machine, squeezing the bag in order to inflate the lungs is a natural mapping. Turning the oxygen flow-control knob counterclockwise to increase gas flow is an artificial mapping. However, because this design follows the conventional mapping of valves, users do not typically have difficulty adjusting the flow of oxygen on the anesthesia machine. Unfortunately, on many medical devices, methods for adjusting alarm limits or for resetting alarms are via artificial, nonstandard mappings.

For any device, there are actually three different stages of mapping: between intentions and the required action; between actions and the resulting effects, and between the information provided about the system and the actual state of the system. Inappropriate mapping at any stage leads to delayed learning and poor user performance. If natural or well known artificial mappings are not used, then the designer should seek preexisting standards or perform tests to ascertain optimal mappings. Mappings should be consistent within any system.

Create appropriate constraints. Constraints are limitations to the user's available options or actions. Constraints can be physical, semantic, cultural, or logical. The provision of a control that can be oriented only in specific ways is a physical constraint (e.g., a switch can be either on or off). With a semantic constraint, the meaning of a particular situation controls the set of possible actions.[37] For example, the sounding of an alarm is meant to indicate the need to take some kind of action. Cultural constraints are a set of allowable actions in social situations (e.g., signs, labels, and messages are meant to be read). Natural mappings work by logical constraints. When a series of indicator lights are arranged in a row, each with a switch underneath, the logical constraint dictates that the switch underneath a particular indicator light controls or is associated with that light. Devices, particularly their human interface components, should be designed to be simple, logical, and intuitive.

Design for error. Human performance is never perfect. Most human errors arising from interactions between people and devices are *slips,* actions that do not occur as planned.[38] Accidentally pushing the wrong button is an example of a slip (see Chapter 17). It is the device designer's responsibility to anticipate user errors and to minimize the risk that these inevitable errors will produce ill effects. Actions with potentially undesirable consequences should be reversible. The designer can also implement forcing functions (a type of constraint). If an action is clearly undesirable, then the system should prevent the user from performing that action. An example of a forcing function is the oxygen/nitrous oxide interlock mechanism that prevents the delivery of a hypoxic gas mixture.

These principles of good design are not limited to the interface between user and machine. A well designed device is also easy to clean, maintain, and repair, and its documentation is organized and understandable.

Many currently available commercial devices violate these basic design principles. Potter and colleagues,[39] in an ergonomics evaluation of a new microprocessor-controlled respiratory gas humidifier, found that the device had hidden modes of operation, ambiguous alarm messages, inconsistent control actions, and complex resetting sequences. One clinically used respiratory gas analyzer issues arcane alarm messages and has multiple display formats that are difficult to access. Another gas analyzer has a hidden calibration mode that renders it unusable if the sampling tubing is not attached when the unit is initially powered up. We have noted that at least two brands of tourniquet controllers have no indicator that the cuff is inflated, although this impression is mistakenly given by a display of "cuff pressure" and a running timer on the front panel. At least some of what, on first glance, appears to be human error can often be traced back to poorly designed interfaces between human and machine.[40] Devices are often used inefficiently or incorrectly as a consequence of poor design.[39] When the device acts in unexpected ways, the user develops erroneous or inconsistent mental models of its operation.[41] This problem can be exacerbated when the user has not received adequate instruction before using the device.

Visual displays

Humans rely heavily on the visual sensory channel for communicating or obtaining information. The television, printed page, instrument dial, and line drawing are all examples of visual displays. An early application of ergonomics was the design of instrument displays for military applications.[42,43] Research continues on developing and improving visual displays for such diverse areas as the airplane cockpit, the nuclear power plant control room, and the office word processing workstation.[44,45] Although a complete description of this work is outside the realm of this chapter, a number of guidelines that have resulted from these studies are presented. Much of the specific information presented stems directly from the general considerations already discussed.

Properties of displays. Three criteria are fundamental to the performance of a display: visibility, legibility, and readability.[3] Visibility refers to the degree to which the individual characters or symbols on a display are detectable against the background. Visibility depends on display features, such as symbol size and background color. It is also influenced by such environmental factors as ambient light levels as well as by the limitations of human perception, such as color blindness and deficiencies of refractive index. Legibility pertains to the degree to which displayed numerals, characters, and symbols can be differentiated from one another. This is primarily influenced by features of the individual symbols, including size, simplicity of form, and stroke width. Readability is a quality that makes possible the quick and unambiguous interpretation of the information intended to be conveyed. For text displays, this is a function of semantics and letter spacing; for symbol displays, simplicity and organization are important.

The preferred size of display components depends on the viewing distance, ambient illumination, and the importance of the information. The perceived size of a symbol is a function of the visual angle. Numerals and letters on a cathode ray tube (CRT) should be large enough to be easily legible.[3] For visual search tasks, larger characters are required.[46] Tightly packed letters are preferable when text must be read and comprehended quickly, probably because fewer eye fixations are required.[3]

Displays of magnitude. Displays of magnitude can be either numerical or graphical. Digital displays, such as a digital watch or the odometer of a car, are numerical. Analog displays, such as the capnogram or the dial of a pressure gauge, are graphical. Dials are classified as either moving pointer on a fixed scale or moving scale with fixed pointers. Each display has advantages for particular tasks. Numerical displays require less space and are preferable when a precise numeric value is required, because they minimize errors and reading time. However, numerical displays are difficult to read if the value is changing rapidly. For instance, pilots are better at performing basic flight maneuvers in a simulator with analog displays than one with digital displays.[47] Moving pointers are preferable as indicators of control settings, because they provide the simplest relationship to the control motion. When qualitative information is sufficient—for example, for detecting the direction or rate of change of a value—a graphic display or moving pointer dial is preferred.[46] Reading a dial to extract quantitative information takes significantly longer (>400 msec) than does a qualitative reading to affirm that the pointer is in the right general location (125 to 200 msec).[48] Graphical displays of recent data are especially useful for trend detection and tracking.

The design of scales and pointers can dramatically affect the speed and accuracy of dial readings. When markers are not present for each value, people are able to interpolate but the time required to obtain the reading is prolonged.[3] It also takes longer to read a dial when the characters are rotated.[49] Therefore, all characters should be in a vertical orientation. To decrease parallax error, the pointer should be placed close to the surface of the scale.[3] To reduce the incidence of errors, the pointer should be single-ended or the end opposite the indicator should be the same color as the dial face.[50]

Grouping of displays. Displays should be grouped for optimal performance. Perceptual studies[46] support the grouping of important displays within the central 30° of the visual field. The normal visual field extends up to ± 30° vertically and ± 80° horizontally. Three areas of attention have been described, based on response time to visual stimuli.[51] The stationary field occupies the central 30° and is the area of foveal vision. Within this field, multiple displays can be viewed simultaneously without eye movements. The visual field between 30° and 80° is the eye field—the area of peripheral vision. Even when foveal vision is fixed on a display, information can still be extracted from the periphery. Peripheral vision is especially sensitive to motion, and it can act reflexively to guide the eye to the target information. Targets within the eye field can be brought into foveal view by eye movements; head movements are not required. The head field lies outside the central 80°. Displays in this area are outside of the peripheral visual field. To view displays in this area, the head must be moved under conscious control.

The relative importance of particular displays can be deduced from the frequency of readings during task analysis studies. Similarly, link analysis[7] can identify recurrent sequences of display readings. Optimally, important displays should be located in the most convenient positions and displays that are commonly viewed in sequence should be arranged adjacent to each other. To perform a task, a number of displays are often interpreted concurrently. When multiple channels of information must be mentally integrated, performance is often improved when the information is grouped. In contrast, when information from multiple channels must be kept distinct—for example, during focused attention on a single channel—then grouped presentation may be deleterious.[52] Most grouping methods are based on Gestalt theory, which describes the ways in which people identify boundaries and groups. Accepted Gestalt laws of grouping include proximity, similarity, closure, and continuity; newly proposed laws in-

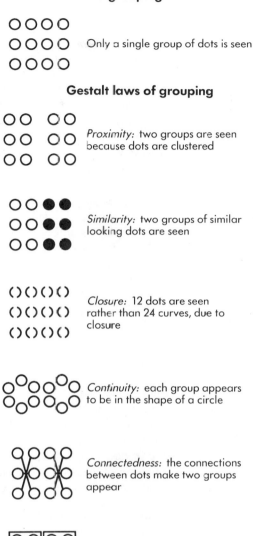

Fig. 18-6. Laws of grouping from Gestalt theory.

clude common region and connectedness.[53] These concepts are illustrated in Fig. 18-6.

Object displays. Dials and numerical displays are typically read sequentially. Clustering of displays can encourage parallel processing. However, placing displays close together in space does not guarantee parallel input of information and may actually interfere with focused attention on a particular display. One way of ensuring some parallel processing is with object displays, where multiple data elements are represented as attributes of a single object. When a single object is viewed, its multiple attributes, such as color, shape, and size, are perceived in parallel. In some nuclear reactor control rooms, polygon displays of safety parameter data have replaced banks of separate instrument dials. In these polygon displays, eight values are represented by the lengths of eight spokes that form the axes of an octagon. This type of display has also been incorporated into the Ohmeda Modulus CD anesthesia machine (see Chapter 17). Although object displays might seem implicitly superior to multiple dials, early studies have demonstrated some disadvantages to this approach. Petersen, Banks, and Gertman[54] compared object displays with multiple bar-graph displays in a task of monitoring for changes in the state of a system. They found that the object display was superior when subjects had to detect whether *any* parameter was out of tolerance, but that multiple bar-graphs were better for detecting the number and identities of the out-of-bound parameters.[55] Wickens and Andre[56] performed an experiment in which subjects viewed either a bar-graph display or an object display of three values for 1.5 seconds. The subject was then asked either to make a judgment on the basis of an integration of the values or to recall a single value. Performance was better on the integration task with the object display, but single values were more accurately recalled with the bar-graph display. These two studies are consistent with many others that support the principle of proximity compatibility. The principle states that combined displays are best suited to tasks that require information integration, whereas tasks that require independent information processing will benefit from more separate displays.[56] The validity of this principle has been challenged by Sanderson, et al[57], who claim that object displays are superior only when a simple geometric feature of the object directly correlates with the goal parameter of the task. For instance, to support judgments about systemic vascular resistance (SVR), an object display of cardiac output and blood pressure might be used instead of two individual bar-graph displays. The combined display would be expected to be superior only if a simple geometric feature of the object, such as area, correlated with the goal parameter, in this case SVR.

Siegel[58] has described the use of object displays to represent the physiologic status of critically ill patients. His display, called a circle diagram, maps 11 cardiovascular and pulmonary indices onto the axes of a polygon. The shape of the polygon can be compared with prototypical shapes to diagnose one of four shock states in an individual patient. The four states he has defined include a compensatory hyperdynamic state, two different deteriorating septic states, and a cardiogenic shock state. Because the display presents the physiologic state of the patient, rather than a collection of indices that must be interpreted by the clinician, it is more likely that physiologically significant trends will be detected early. However, testing of these novel displays must be performed in a real or simulated clinical setting before their routine use can be recommended.

Coding. Coding methods can be used to highlight targets of visual search tasks and to provide similarities for grouping. Common coding methods for display elements include color, alphanumeric symbols, geometric shapes, size, brightness, location, and flash rate. In a comparison of coding methods, Hitt[59] coded objects on a map with color, numerals, letters, and geometric shapes. Performance was then assessed on tasks of identification, counting, location, comparison, and verification. Color and numeric codes were superior in most tasks. Color is the most effective coding method for search tasks, where the subject must locate and count items in variable positions on a display. Search times can decrease by as much as 70% with color coding.[60] In a study of color coding to organize instruments on a simulated aircraft display,[55] common color coding of relevant instruments was found to facilitate integration of information, and distinct color coding improved the ability to focus attention on each instrument. Subjects commonly respond to color codes faster than to shape or alphanumeric codes. This may be because color is perceived earlier than other codes in the sequence of information processing. Another reason that color coding may be advantageous is that short-term memory is better for colors than for shapes or numbers.[55] Multiple coding methods can be combined, and there is evidence that the presence of color as a redundant coding dimension can lead to performance improvements over the use of either method alone.[55] Color coding may be most effective when the display is unformatted, the symbol density is high, or the operator must search for specified information. Color is less useful for identification tasks, where letters and numbers are preferable.[3] Combinations of hue, saturation, and lightness can be chosen so that, with training, 24 colors can be reliably discriminated. However, without training, subjects can reliably discriminate only 5 to 9 colors.[3] Color coding is most effective when the colors are consistent with prevailing population stereotypes. In the general population, red indicates danger and green indicates safety. To American anesthesiologists, green indicates oxygen, blue indicates nitrous oxide, and yellow indicates air.

One disadvantage of color coding is that it cannot be discriminated by the person who is color blind. Therefore, redundant coding must always be used when selection of the wrong object could have adverse consequences. Although color coding can improve complex displays, the indiscriminate use of color can be detrimental. A number of studies,[55,61] offer evidence that irrelevant color coding can interfere with cognitive processing of visual information. The overuse of color for coding purposes also increases the visual clutter of a display. Alternative or multiple coding methods should be considered when more than six codes must be discriminated on a single display.

Auditory displays

Most displays utilize the visual sensory channel, although auditory displays may sometimes be appropriate. Situations in which the auditory modality is preferable to the visual modality are listed in Table 18-1. A primary advantage of the human auditory system is that it can simultaneously detect signals from multiple locations. This makes auditory displays particularly useful for displaying alarms and warnings that require immediate response (alarms are discussed in Chapter 17). Signals that must be monitored continuously can be presented on auditory displays, because humans can process visual and auditory signals simultaneously.

Auditory displays should also take advantage of learned or natural relationships. For instance, the pitch should increase as the value increases. In general, the same signal should designate the same information in all situations. Because the number of recognizable auditory signals may be limited, auditory displays should not provide more information than is necessary. Complex messages may best be transmitted in two stages. The first stage should be an alerting signal to identify the general category of information. The second stage may then transmit more specific information. Auditory displays must be carefully designed to prevent masking of the signal by the noise of the environment.[62] A number of methods may be used to improve the signal-to-noise ratio: The signal intensity may be increased; a signal frequency can be selected at which the noise intensity is low; the signal can be presented for at least 0.5 seconds; or the signal can be presented to only one ear.[3] Extremely loud signals and signals with an abrupt onset should be avoided, because they tend to startle the operator. Continuous signals can also be disruptive, and perceptual adaption may limit their effectiveness. Variable or interrupted signals are thus preferable.

Manual controls

The user transmits information to the device via controls, just as the equipment transmits information to the user through displays. Many types of control exist for a variety of tasks. Switches or buttons are used to transmit binary, or on-off, information. Continuous information is usually conveyed with knobs, cranks, wheels, levers, or pedals. Keyboards are frequently used to enter numerical or alphabetic information. Cursor position on computer displays may be controlled with a mouse, joystick, trackball, digitizing tablet, or light pen.

The control's design influences the speed and error rate of user actions. Factors such as control type, control "feel" or resistance, control feedback (visual, audible, and tactile), control placement, and keyboard layout are all important considerations for the equipment designer. This section focuses on the concepts of compatibility and coding of controls.

Compatibility. The degree to which relationships between a stimulus and a response are consistent with human expectations, or compatibility, is paramount in the design of controls. This concept was introduced previously in the section on mappings. There are a number of advantages to conforming to expectations: Learning is faster; reaction time is decreased; fewer errors are made; and user satisfaction is enhanced.

Four types of compatibility have been identified: conceptual, spatial, movement, and modality.[3] Conceptual compatibility refers to the degree to which codes and symbols are understood by people who must use them. Spatial compatibility deals with the physical arrangement of controls and their associated displays. Movement compatibility relates to expectations that people have regarding the relationship between control or display movements and system responses. Modality compatibility has recently been proposed to explain the finding that the performance of certain tasks improves when the sensory modalities of the displays and controls match the conceptual nature of the task. For example, a verbal task, such as following a command, is performed more rapidly when the command is spoken rather than written.[3] Spatial and movement compatibility are discussed in more detail in the following paragraphs.

In general, for optimal performance, each control should be located directly below its corresponding display. Controls can be located above the related display, but the user's hand may block the view of the display while adjusting the control. Where the controls are grouped apart from the displays, the controls and their corresponding dis-

Table 18-1. Selection criteria for auditory versus visual presentation of information

Auditory presentation is appropriate when	Visual presentation is appropriate when
The message is simple	The message is complex
The message is short	The message is long
The message will not be referred to later	The message will be referred to later
The message deals with events in time	The message deals with location in space
The message must be responded to immediately	The message does not call for immediate action
The visual system of the person is overburdened	The auditory system of the person is overburdened
The receiving location is too bright	The receiving location is too noisy
The person moves about continually to perform the job	The person performs the job from one position

Adapted from Deathridge BH: *Auditory and other sensory forms of information processing.* In Van Cott HP, Kinkade RG, editors: *Human engineering guide to equipment design,* Washington, DC, 1972, American Institutes for Research.

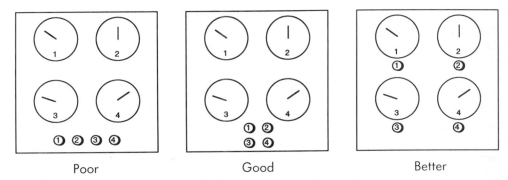

Fig. 18-7. Controls should be positioned directly below their corresponding displays whenever possible. Laws of spatial compatibility should be followed when controls are grouped apart from their displays.

plays should be arranged in similar patterns (Fig. 18-7). Controls should also be arranged to conform to the physical layout of the system. For instance, the throttles on a jet should conform left-to-right to the spatial relationship of the engines. Spacial conformity also refers to the physical similarity between controls and displays. Thus a round dial is a more appropriate display for a knob and a linear display is more appropriate for a slide control.

People's expectations regarding movement relationships are often based on population stereotypes. For example, moving a light switch up generally turns a light on in the United States, but the same action turns a light off in the United Kingdom.[63] Therefore, it is imperative that the designer consider the population that will use the device. Some guidelines for direction of control movements are listed in Table 18-2.

Coding. Mistaking one critical control for another has led to serious accidents in aviation (i.e., confusing the landing gear and flap controls), ground transportation (i.e., mistaking the accelerator for the brake pedal), and medicine (i.e., syringe swaps). Unambiguous identification of controls can decrease the incidence of such errors. Primary coding methods for controls include type, shape, texture, size, location, color, and labels. As with coding of display elements, the success of the coding method depends on detectability, discriminability, compatibility, meaningfulness, and standardization.

Shape is an effective method for coding of controls. It provides tactile feedback to the user, which is especially useful when the user does not routinely observe the operation of the control. Shape coding is used on most keyboards, where special keys are of different shapes and the F and J keys are often identified by raised dots. The Federal Aviation Administration[63] requires unique, standardized shapes for cockpit controls. Besides being easily distinguishable, some of these knobs have symbolic meaning. For example, the landing gear control resembles a wheel and the flap control is shaped like a wing.

Table 18-2. Control movement stereotypes in the United States

Function	Direction of control movement
On	Clockwise, up, right, forward
Off	Counterclockwise, down, left, backward
Increase	Clockwise, up, right, forward
Decrease	Counterclockwise, down, left, backward
Open valve	Counterclockwise
Close valve	Clockwise

Surface texture is another useful coding dimension. The textured rims of the dime, quarter, and half dollar provide a common example. Smooth, knurled, and fluted knobs can be reliably discriminated, even by the gloved hand.[50]

Color coding of displays was discussed previously. Similarly, color coding of controls can be effective if a small number of coding categories exist and if the colors are meaningful. Color can also be used to associate a control with a display. One disadvantage of color coding is that the user must look at the control during use.

The most effective way of identifying controls is with labels. The advantage of labels is that large numbers of meaningful codes can be developed. The disadvantages include the time required to read the label, the influence of lighting conditions and label position on legibility, and the possibility of reading errors in stressful situations and with high workloads. Therefore, additional coding methods are indicated when poor lighting or stressful conditions are present and when controls are cluttered or positioned out of the line of sight.

ERGONOMICS IN THE DESIGN OF THE ANESTHESIA COCKPIT

The number of monitors and devices in the typical operating room has increased rapidly in the last decade. Each year brings another new and complicated device that seems "necessary" to provide quality care. The most recent additions include the pulse oximeter, the capnometer, the processed electroencephalograph, and the transesophageal echocardiogram. As each device is introduced, the problem becomes finding the floor or shelf space to place it as well as an available electrical outlet.

The ergonomic problems of today's operating room include poor physical layout of displays, poor physical layout of controls, cluttered workspace, and information overload. These cannot be solved at the level of the individual monitors. Integration is the solution, and it must occur on two levels: physical and functional.[64] The topic of integration is covered in Chapter 17.

The anesthesia machine

The anesthesia machine probably has the best ergonomic design of any complex piece of equipment in the operating room. This is primarily a result of the development of comprehensive standards, such as those published by the American National Standards Institute (ANSI)[65] in 1979 and the American Society for Testing and Materials (ASTM)[66] in 1989. Equipment users and representatives from anesthesia machine manufacturers served on the committees that drafted these standards. The standards were based, in part, on user experiences reported in specialty journals and on relevant portions of the *Human Engineering Design Criteria for Military Systems, Equipment, and Facilities.*[34]

This section reviews the ergonomic design features of the anesthesia machine with reference to the requirements and rationale of selected specifications from the ASTM standard. This standard covers the design of continuous-flow anesthesia machines for human use. The anesthesia machine includes the gas piping and flow-control systems between the pressurized gas sources and the common gas outlet, the vaporizers, and the integrated oxygen concentration and ventilation monitors. Specifications for breathing circuits, ventilators, and such optional devices as humidifiers and positive end-expiratory pressure (PEEP) valves are not included in the standard. However, in light of the current evolution of integrated, microprocessor-controlled anesthesia delivery and monitoring systems, efforts are under way to set standards for the anesthesia workstation as a unified entity.

The current standard takes into account several idiosyncrasies of the anesthesia work environment: (1) that the operator may be positioned away from the machine; (2) that the anesthesiologist may stand or sit; and (3) that care is sometimes provided in remote locations, such as the radiology suite, where the ambient lighting is poor. This is exemplified by the general specification concerning placement and legibility of controls and displays.[66]

4.1.3 The faces of all scales and gauges shall be legible and all controls and indicators shall be visible at a distance of 1 meter

(3.3 feet) and at a light level of 215 lux (20 footcandles) to an operator with 6-6 (20-20) vision (corrected), seated or standing in front of the anesthesia machine. . . .

Another general requirement is that the manufacturer attach a pre-use checkout procedure to the anesthesia machine. This is important because the details of operation of anesthesia machines may differ. Clinicians cannot reliably detect faults in anesthesia machines, especially when faults are concealed and do not render the machine inoperative.[67] Cooper[21] identified failure to perform a preuse check as an important factor in critical events. Preoperative "preparation and check of equipment, drugs, fluids, and gas supplies"[68] is an important part of the anesthesia provider's responsibility.

Gas systems. A major intention of the specifications regarding anesthesia machine gas piping systems is the deterrence of cross-connections. Cross-connections can occur when the anesthesia machine is accidentally connected to the wrong cylinder or hospital central gas supply outlet. To prevent this, the ASTM standard requires pin index safety system (PISS) and diameter index safety system (DISS) fittings. The PISS is designed to prevent the attachment of a cylinder of one gas to the hanger yoke of another, the DISS is designed to prevent crossovers when equipment or flexible hoses are attached to a central pipeline system. Each hanger yoke and pipeline inlet must be permanently marked with the name or chemical symbol of the gas it accommodates, and color coding of each inlet is recommended. Cross-connections can also arise during construction or maintenance of the anesthesia machine or central piping system.[1,69] To deter these hidden crossovers by service personnel, the ASTM standard requires that piping be labeled with the gas content at each junction or where the piping joins the component, and the National Fire Protection Association[70] requires labels on all medical gas piping at 20-foot intervals. Even recently, fatalities have resulted from cross-connections in countries where such standards have not been adopted.[71]

A poorly designed analog pressure gauge may give the illusion that a gas cylinder is full when it is actually empty.[72] To prevent this, the ASTM standard specifies design criteria for anesthesia machine pressure gauges (Fig. 18-8). The pointer must be designed so that the indicator end is immediately distinguishable from the tail end; and circular pressure gauges must have the lowest pressure reading located in a standard position, between 6 and 9 o'clock. Each gauge must be clearly labeled with the name or chemical symbol of the gas it monitors. Most manufacturers also code the gauge by color. In the United States the color standards[73] for oxygen, nitrous oxide, and air are green, blue, and yellow, respectively, and those for helium, nitrogen, and carbon dioxide are brown, black, and gray, respectively.

Flow-control systems. There are three classes of primary gas controls on an anesthesia machine, the flow con-

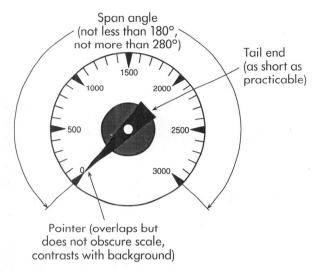

Span angle
(not less than 180°,
not more than 280°)

Tail end
(as short as
practicable)

Pointer (overlaps but
does not obscure scale,
contrasts with background)

Fig. 18-8. Recommended pressure gauge features. (From *Minimum performance and safety requirements for components and systems of continuous-flow anesthesia machines for human use,* Z79.8-1979, New York, 1979, American National Standards Institute.)

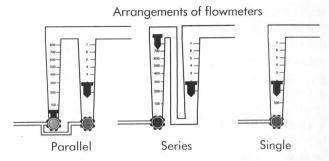

Arrangements of flowmeters

Parallel   Series   Single

Fig. 18-9. Arrangements of flowmeters. Serious mishaps have resulted with the parallel arrangement when the low-flow control knob was mistaken for the high-flow one. The series arrangement is less dangerous, but one flowmeter may still be mistaken for the other. (From Loeb RG: Preventing anesthesia machine-induced hypoxemia, *Wellcome Trends in Anesthesiology* 8:2-10, 1990.)

trols, the oxygen-flush control, and the vaporizer controls (which are discussed later). Each flow control is associated with a flow indicator, or flowmeter. Together these components form a flow-control system. The primary hazard that occurs with flow controls is unintentional and unrecognized dispensing of a hypoxic gas mixture.[74-76] The ASTM standard includes a number of ergonomic design specifications to discourage this event. Each flow-control knob is coded by label and color; the oxygen knob is additionally coded by shape and location. By convention, the oxygen control is located on the right-hand end of the group of flowmeters. To avoid confusion between machines, a counterclockwise turn always increases flow and a clockwise turn decreases it. This convention is also used for vaporizer concentration dials. Flow controls must also be designed to minimize their unintentional change from a preset position. The parallel arrangement of flowmeters, where more than one knob controls the flow rate of a single gas, has been a factor in patient deaths[1] (Fig. 18-9). The ASTM standard requires that each gas delivered to the machine's common gas outlet be controlled by no more than one knob, and a single flowmeter tube for each gas is recommended. The Thorpe flowmeter, which is commonly used on anesthesia machines, is calibrated for a single gas. If the flowmeter tubes are interchanged, their readings are no longer accurate. Thus, to comply with the ASTM standard, the manufacturer must ensure that flowmeters are not interchangeable.

The above discussion demonstrates that equipment can be designed to decrease the likelihood of user error. Equipment can also be constrained to prevent dangerous settings by the user. All new anesthesia machines pro-

duced for human use in the United States have flow-control systems that prevent the administration of hypoxic mixtures of oxygen and nitrous oxide, although the ASTM standard does not require this. Ohmeda anesthesia machines use the Link-25 Proportion Limiting Control System, a mechanical interlock between the nitrous oxide and oxygen flow controls, which prevents adjustment of nitrous oxide flow to greater than three times the oxygen flow. North American Dräger uses the Oxygen Ratio Monitor Controller (ORMC) system. This pneumatic electromechanical linkage between the nitrous oxide and oxygen flow-control systems measures the ratio of back pressures in the flowmeters and prevents oxygen concentration settings below 25%.

Proportioning devices offer an alternative way of controlling gas flows.[77] They are designed to dispense mixtures of oxygen and nitrous oxide. Proportioners have two controls, one for total gas flow and the other for percent oxygen, rather than the usual flow-rate controls for each gas. Hypoxic gas mixtures cannot be administered with these devices, and the dialed oxygen concentration is directly displayed. Two commercial devices, the Quantiflex Monitored Dial Mixer and the Ohio 30/70 proportioner were produced in the 1970s and 1980s. They are not currently being manufactured, due to problems with their internal complexity, their inability to set very low flow rates, and potential user confusion when switching between machines.

A limitation of the Ohmeda Link-25 and Dräger ORMC proportioning systems is that the ratio of only two gases can be controlled. Hypoxic settings of three or more gases, dispensed together or at different times, may be prevented with electronic flow-control systems.[78] Such systems are already being designed for use in future anesthesia machines.

Vaporizers. Inhaled anesthetic agents are potent drugs that may cause death due to overdosage.[79] Underdosage of these agents can result in undesirable cardiovascular response to surgical stimulation as well as awareness during surgery.[80] Thus accurate administration of these agents is critical. The variable-bypass vaporizer provides a major ergonomics improvement over the flowmeter-controlled vaporizer (i.e., Copper Kettle). Calculation errors by the user are avoided, and devices that reduce or prevent filling errors can be fitted to the agent-specific vaporizers.

The ASTM standard specifies a number of ergonomic requirements that reduce user errors. The vaporizer must be equipped with a clearly visible liquid-level indicator to prevent underdosage due to lack of liquid agent. To prevent delivery of liquid anesthetic into the breathing circuit, the vaporizer must be constructed so that overfilling is impossible.[75] To prevent an incorrect agent from being added to a single-agent vaporizer, each should be fitted with an agent-specific keyed filling device.[75] Vaporizer knobs must open in a counterclockwise direction, the same way as flow-control knobs.

Most manufacturers color code their vaporizers. The color standards for halothane, isoflurane, enflurane, and desflurane are red, purple, orange, and blue, respectively. All new anesthesia machines produced for human use in the United States have a vaporizer interlock mechanism that prevents the simultaneous administration of volatile agent from more than one vaporizer. Vaporizers are also mounted on the machine to prevent tipping, which could otherwise lead to overdosage.

A special agent-specific vaporizer is required for the administration of desflurane, a volatile anesthetic with a low boiling point and a high minimum alveolar concentration. No carrier gas enters the vaporizer. Rather, the vaporizer is electrically heated so that the agent can be dispensed under pressure in its gaseous state. A special one-way filling system is used to prevent backflow and vapor spray, because the pressure within the vaporizer reaches approximately 14 psig. The traditional glass sight window cannot be used because accidental breakage would result in a pressurized spray of desflurane into the operating room (see also Chapter 3).

Automation and future anesthesia machines. The technology of anesthesia machines is changing rapidly. Until now the flowmeters, vaporizers, and pressure regulators were all mechanical devices. Electronics were added only for monitoring purposes. However, anesthesia machines with electronic flowmeters and vaporizers are now being commercially produced, although they are not currently being marketed in the United States (see Chapter 33). New standards will need to be drafted for this generation of machines.

Experimental systems can automatically control delivery of inhaled anesthetics,[81,82] delivery of intravenous anesthetics,[83,84] depth of neuromuscular blockade,[85] and degree of ventilation.[86] Commercial systems are available that can automatically control a sodium nitroprusside infusion or generate an anesthetic record. The advent of electronic controls, reliable monitors, and small but powerful computers makes all of this possible. Automation can enhance system performance, increase safety, and decrease human workload.[87] However, automation will not necessarily lead to improved system performance in every situation. In fact, as systems become more automated, they may become more subject to human error. This has been clearly shown with regard to the interface between pilot and aircraft.[88] For example, inappropriate or excessive automation may result in low workload conditions leading to boredom and inattention.[89] A number of individuals[30,90,91] have expressed concerns about the potential negative impact of automation on vigilance. Unless equipment is designed and implemented properly, automation in anesthesia may not prove to be advantageous.

As automation is introduced into the anesthesia workplace, clinicians will need additional training. Otherwise, experienced clinicians may continue to practice the "old way" in the face of new devices providing different data or requiring different control strategies. Conversely, clinicians may fail to understand the underlying complexity of the system and the methods for resuming control when automation fails. Therefore, before a new technology is introduced into the operating room, all anesthesiologists must be retrained to optimize performance and avoid tragedies.[26]

Intravenous administration systems

The ergonomics problems of intravenous administration systems are all too familiar to the anesthesia practitioner. Tangled lines, inaccessible injection ports, and misidentified tubing are common problems, especially while a patient is being transported. Most of the complications that arise are not documented. However, there are multiple case reports in the literature of accidental injections of intravenous medications into arterial or epidural catheters.[92-95] Although no national standards address these issues, institutions, departments, and individual clinicians can adopt procedures to minimize problems.

The authors recommend that different types of tubing be used for intravenous, intraarterial, and epidural systems. Tubing and injection ports should be clearly labeled; color-coded tubing and stopcocks are commercially available. Tubing used for epidural infusions and arterial pressure monitoring should not have injection ports.[96] Transport racks may help keep tubing organized while the patient is moved; alternatively, superfluous tubing can be converted to heparin locks to prevent tangling during transport. The use of smaller, more user-friendly intravenous infusion devices specifically designed for administration of drugs rather than fluids may reduce the incidence of medication errors while critically ill patients are transported to and from the operating room.

Medication errors. Drug errors that result in the administration of the wrong drug or wrong dose are among

Drug class	Label color	Example
Induction agent	Yellow	**Thiopental 2.5%** Date
Tranquilizer	Orange	**Midazolam** mg/ml
Muscle relaxant	Fluorescent red	**Curare** mg/ml
		Succinylcholine mg/ml
Relaxant antagonist	Fluorescent red with white stripes	**Neostigmine** mg/ml
Narcotic	Blue	**Morphine** mg/ml
Narcotic antagonist	Blue with white stripes	**Naloxone** mg/ml
Major tranquilizer	Salmon	**Droperidol** mg/ml
Vasopressor	Violet	**Ephedrine** mg/ml
		Epinephrine mg/ml
Hypotensive agent	Violet with white stripes	**Nitroprusside** mg/ml
Local anesthetic	Gray	**Lidocaine** mg/ml
Anticholinergic agent	Green	**Atropine** mg/ml

Fig. 18-10. Standard color codes for user-applied syringe drug labels. (See color insert.)

the most frequent errors reported in critical incident studies of anesthesiologists.[21-23,97] The human error involved in these incidents should not be discounted; the anesthesiologist is ultimately responsible for ensuring the identity of a medication prior to administering it. However, a number of ergonomic deficiencies contribute to the problem. Labels on vials and ampules are often illegible, especially when they are printed directly on the glass. Similarities in packaging (i.e., vial shape, proprietary drug name, lettering style, and company logo) serve to code the medication by manufacturer rather than by drug type.[98] Prefilled syringes for emergency use tend to look alike, and their labels often become hidden within the syringe barrel as they are used. Standards to address some of these problems have been published by the ASTM.[99,100] They require that the name and concentration of the drug and the volume of the container be legible at 20 inches in dim hospital lighting. For prefilled emergency syringes, the label must be legible at 5 feet, even after the contents are dispensed. The United States Pharmacopoeia (USP) has federally mandated jurisdiction over the packaging and labeling of all drugs used by anesthesiologists in the United States and has begun to express interest in improving the current situation.

There is evidence that the risk of drug errors increases following intraoperative exchanges of personnel.[101] The incidence of these errors may be increased due to unlabeled or incompletely labeled syringes. A label containing the name and concentration of the drug should be affixed to the syringe at the time it is filled. The concentration is especially important when a nonstandard dilution is used. Although colored, preprinted labels have been available for some time, only recently has a national standard for syringe labels been promulgated.[102] Legibility and color codes are specified. Induction agents are yellow, muscle relaxants are fluorescent red, and narcotics are blue (Fig. 18-10; also see color insert). Special formats are reserved for succinylcholine, epinephrine, and antagonist agents.

Needlestick injuries. The danger of needlestick injuries to health care workers has received a great deal of attention. This is largely due to the epidemic of acquired immunodeficiency syndrome (AIDS), although only 13 cases of occupationally contracted AIDS transmitted via needles had been documented as of 1991. In contrast, up to 300 health care workers die each year from occupationally acquired hepatitis B.[103,104] Anesthesiologists are at higher risk for needlestick injuries than are other physicians. Needlesticks most frequently occur during or after disposal, rather than during use of the needle; between 20% to 40% occur during recapping.[103]

Improvements in the design of intravenous administration systems could reduce or eliminate the risk of needlestick injuries. This can be accomplished by designs that allow safer recapping of needles following use, provide protection of the needle during use, or allow elimination of needles from intravenous therapy. Devices in each class are commercially available.[105] Items that provide safer recapping include resheathing devices that hold the cap during insertion of the needle and retractable sheaths that extend over the needle from behind after use. These are especially useful when the needle must be exposed during use, such as during catheter placement, intramuscular injection, and venipuncture. Shielded needles are useful for intravenous injections and intravenous tubing/needle assemblies. Here, the needle is protected at all times within a plastic cylinder designed to fit over an injection port. A disadvantage of these devices is that, without an adapter, they cannot be used to withdraw medications from vials. The elimination of needles from intravenous therapy has been advocated.[106] This can be accomplished by using intravenous tubing with (Luer) injection sites rather than standard latex Y ports or flashbulbs. Luer ports with integrated antireflux valves are particularly useful during anesthesia because they allow intermittent injections to be administered with one hand. A device is also available to permit needle-free drug aspiration from multiple-dose vials; single-dose ampules still present a problem.

The operating room environment

The work environment has a pervasive influence on people's ability to perform their jobs. Diverse factors, such as the loudness of the ventilation system, the size of a doorway, or the glare from a light fixture, can hamper the ability to perform specific tasks. The operating room is a workplace for surgeons, anesthesiologists, nurses, technicians, orderlies, and radiographers. Ideally it should be designed to support the variety of tasks performed by each of these individuals. This section briefly reviews some of the implications of operating room design on the tasks performed by anesthesiologists. The topic of noise is discussed in Chapter 17.

Ambient lighting. Most of the clinical information that the anesthesiologist gathers is collected visually. The impact of illumination on task performance has received much attention from ergonomics and lighting specialists.[3] Illumination requirements depend on the characteristics of a given task, such as visibility and speed. In general, the more difficult the psychomotor task, the greater is the level of illumination required for optimal performance. For example, the suggested level of illumination for the surgical field is very high (10,000 to 20,000 lux), whereas monitoring in the anesthesia workspace may require only the

levels suggested for performance of visual tasks of medium contrast or small size (500 to 1000 lux).[3,107] Studies have indicated that brighter illumination is more satisfying and may improve performance,[3] decrease reaction time,[108] and increase social interaction.[109]

Other factors, such as color, glare, shadows, and heat production, must also be considered in design of operating room lighting. The spectral distributions of available light sources differ markedly, and these differences can affect people's ability to discriminate colors. Anesthesiologists must discriminate colors when evaluating the patient for cyanosis or jaundice and when using color-coded equipment. Therefore, minimizing color distortion by use of lights with a high color rendering index must be a priority.[3] Overhead lighting must also be diffused to decrease the glare and shadows that interfere with the anesthesiologist's ability to see monitor displays or to perform invasive procedures.[91]

Facility layout. The layout of the physical facility plays a role in user efficiency and satisfaction with the workplace. Factors to be considered with regard to space management for surgical facilities include the total quantity of space required, allocation of space for specific purposes, layout of the operating rooms, traffic patterns, and accessibility of ancillary and support services.[107] All of these factors have a direct impact on the tasks that the anesthesiologist performs.

The layout of the facility is especially important during the turnover time between surgical cases. A well planned facility encourages a smooth flow of people and materials. For instance, in an ambulatory surgical facility, patients should proceed in an orderly fashion from the reception area, through the changing and preoperative holding areas, to the operating room. At the conclusion of the procedure, the patient should be transported to the recovery room without crossing paths with the preoperative patients. The preoperative holding area and recovery room should be in the immediate vicinity of the operating rooms, so that the anesthesiologist does not need to change clothes and can be immediately available if required.[110] An example of a facility with a well designed traffic flow pattern is the Shock Trauma Center in Baltimore. There, the trauma patient is directly transported by elevator from the helicopter landing pad on the roof to the triage unit. Immediately adjacent to the triage unit are the operating rooms and a computerized tomography (CT) scanner facility. This provides an opportunity for the anesthesiologist to be involved in the initial resuscitation. Also, secondary resuscitation is not impaired during radiologic diagnostic procedures.

Efficiency is enhanced when the distances that must be traversed are minimized. If the anesthesiologist must travel outside of the operating rooms to procure drugs and equipment between cases, then turnover times will be prolonged. One approach to this problem is to provide centrally located operating room satellite pharmacies and anesthesia workrooms.[111] Alternatively, controlled substances can be dispensed in a pack to be worn on the anesthesiologist's body,[112] and carts within the room can be restocked with supplies by an anesthesia assistant. A common problem in operating room design is the lack of sufficient storage space. This can lead to cluttered hallways, which can be a hazard both to patients during transport and to personnel.

The anesthesiologist performs a complex job in a poorly designed workplace. Ergonomic "malpractice" is pervasive. The simplest pieces of equipment have hidden modes of operation and incomprehensible alarm messages. Displays and controls are scattered throughout the workplace. Medications come in poorly labeled containers, and needles threaten the safety of every health care worker. Facilities are noisy and poorly designed overall.

These problems cannot be addressed at a single level.[113] Research must continue to investigate the tasks of anesthesiologists and the equipment-related factors that influence their performance. Standard design specifications, authored by equipment producers and users, such as those by ASTM, ANSI, and AAMI, must continue to be developed. Equipment manufacturers must strengthen their commitment to ergonomics throughout the design phase. Anesthesiologists, as individuals and as a group, must demand better ergonomics in their equipment and should refuse to purchase devices with suboptimal designs. Finally, multidisciplinary groups, including anesthesiologists, surgeons, nurses, ergonomics specialists, biomedical engineers, and architects, must be assembled to address the problem at a systems level. The solutions will be found only when there is a comprehensive approach to improve the ergonomics of the anesthesia workspace.

REFERENCES

1. Mazze RI: Therapeutic misadventures with O_2 delivery systems: the need for continuous in-line O_2 monitors, *Anesth Analg* 51:787-792, 1972.
2. Epstein RM, Rackow H, Lee ASJ, et al: Prevention of accidental breathing of anoxic gas mixtures during anesthesia, *Anesthesiology* 23:1-4, 1962.
3. Sanders MS, McCormick EJ: *Human factors in engineering and design,* ed 6, New York, 1987, McGraw-Hill.
4. Meister D: *Conceptual aspects of human factors,* Baltimore, 1986, The Johns Hopkins University Press.
5. Wilson JR: *A framework and a context for ergonomics methodology.* In Wilson JR, Corlett EN, editors: *Evaluation of human work: a practical ergonomics methodology,* London, 1990, Taylor & Francis.
6. Edwards E: *Introductory overview.* In Wiener EL, Nagel DC, editors: *Human factors in aviation,* San Diego, 1988, Academic Press.
7. Stammers RB, Carey MS, Astley JA: *Task analysis.* In Wilson JR, Corlett EN, editors: *Evaluation of human work: a practical ergonomics methodology,* New York, 1990, Taylor & Francis.
8. Gilbreth FB: Motion study in surgery. *Can J Med Surg* 40:22-31, 1916.
9. Drui AB, Behm RJ, Martin WE: Predesign investigation of the anesthesia operational environment, *Anesth Analg* 52:584-591, 1973.
10. Kennedy PJ, Feingold A, Wiener EL, et al: Analysis of tasks and human factors in anesthesia for coronary artery bypass, *Anesth Analg* 55:374-377, 1976.
11. Rendell-Baker L: Problems with anesthetic gas machines and their solutions, *Int Anesthesiol Clin* 20:1-82, 1982.
12. Boquet G, Bushman JA, Davenport HT: The anesthesia machine: a study of function and design, *Br J Anaesth* 52:61-67, 1980.
13. Gaba DM, Herndon OW, Zornow M, et al: Task analysis, vigilance, and workload in novice residents, *Anesthesiology* 75:A1060, 1991 (abstract).
14. Dallen L, Nguyen L, Zornow M, et al: Task analysis/workload of anesthetists performing general anesthesia, *Anesthesiology* 73:A498, 1990 (abstract).
15. McDonald JS, Dzwonczyk RR: A time and motion study of the anaesthetist's intraoperative time, *Br J Anaesth* 61:738-742, 1988.
16. McDonald JS, Peterson SF, Hansell J: Operating room event analysis, *Med Instrum* 17:107-108, 1983.
17. Herndon OW, Weinger MB, Paulus M, et al: Analysis of the task of administering anesthesia: additional objective measures, *Anesthesiology* 75:A487, 1991 (abstract).
18. Gaba DM, Lee T: Measuring the workload of the anesthesiologist, *Anesth Analg* 71:354-361, 1990.
19. Flanagan JC: The critical incident technique, *Psychol Bull* 51:327-386, 1954.
20. Cooper JB, Newbower RS, Kitz RJ: An analysis of major errors and equipment failures in anesthesia management: considerations for prevention and detection, *Anesthesiology* 60:34-42, 1984.
21. Cooper JB, Newbower RS, Long CD, et al: Preventable anesthesia mishaps: a study of human factors, *Anesthesiology* 49:399-406, 1978.
22. Craig J, Wilson ME: A survey of anaesthetic misadventures, *Anaesthesia* 36:933-936, 1981.
23. Kumar V, Barcellos WA, Menta MP, et al: An analysis of critical incidents in a teaching department for quality assurance: a survey of mishaps during anaesthesia, *Anaesthesia* 43:879-883, 1988.
24. Gaba DM, DeAnda A: A comprehensive anesthesia simulation environment: re-creating the operating room for research and training, *Anesthesiology* 69:387-394, 1988.
25. DeAnda A, Gaba DM: Unplanned incidents during comprehensive anesthesia simulation, *Anesth Analg* 71:77-82, 1990.
26. Gravenstein JS, Weinger MG: Why study vigilance? *J Clin Monit* 2:145-147, 1986.
27. Kay J, Neal M: Effect of automatic blood pressure devices on vigilance of anesthesia residents, *J Clin Monit* 2:148-150, 1986.
28. Cooper JO, Cullen BF: Observer reliability in detecting surreptitious random occlusions of the monaural esophageal stethoscope, *J Clin Monit* 6:271-275, 1990.
29. Loeb RG: Intraoperative vigilance toward a physiologic monitor, *Anesth Analg,* 74:S190, 1992 (abstract).
30. Yablock DO: A comparison of vigilance using automated and handwritten records, *Anesthesiology* 73:A416, 1990 (abstract).
31. *Air Force systems command design handbook, human factors engineering,* AFSC DH 1-3, Wright-Patterson Air Force Base, Ohio, 1977, United States Air Force.
32. Brown CM: *Human-computer interface design guidelines,* Norwood, 1988, Ablex.
33. Gilmore WE: *Human engineering guidelines for the evaluation and assessment of video display units,* NUREG-CR-4227, Washington, DC, 1985, United States Nuclear Regulatory Commission.
34. *Human engineering design criteria for military systems, equipment, and facilities,* MIL-STD-1472C, Washington, DC, 1981, United States Department of Defense.
35. *Human factors engineering guidelines and preferred practices for the design of medical devices,* AAMI HE-1988, Arlington, Va, 1988, Association for the Advancement of Medical Instrumentation.

36. Bock FM: Considering human factors in the initial design of a medical computer system, *J Med Syst* 6:61-76, 1982.

37. Norman DA: *The psychology of everyday things,* New York, 1988, Basic Books.

38. Gaba DM: Human error in anesthetic mishaps, *Int Anesthesiol Clin* 27:137-147, 1989.

39. Potter SS, Cook RI, Woods DD, et al: The role of human factors guidelines in designing usable systems: a case study of operating room equipment, *Proc Human Factors Soc* 34:391-395, 1990.

40. Bell TE: The limits of risk analysis, *IEEE Spectrum* 26:51, 1989.

41. Cook RI, Potter SS, Woods DD, et al: Evaluating the human engineering of microprocessor-controlled operating room devices, *J Clin Monit* 7:217-226, 1991.

42. Elkin EH: *Effect of scale shape, exposure time, and display complexity on scale reading efficiency,* TR 58-472, Wright-Patterson Air Force Base, Ohio, 1959, United States Air Force.

43. Fitts PM, Jones E: *Psychological aspects of instrument display: analysis of 270 "pilot error" experiences in reading and interpreting aircraft instruments,* TSEAA-694-12A, Wright-Patterson Air Force Base, Ohio, 1947, United States Air Force.

44. Stokes AF, Wickens, CD: *Aviation displays,* In Wiener EL, Nagel DC, editors: *Human factors in aviation,* San Diego, 1988, Academic Press.

45. Ivergård T: *Handbook of control room design and ergonomics,* New York, 1989, Taylor & Francis.

46. Helander MR: *Design of visual displays,* In Salvendy G, editor: *Handbook of human factors,* New York, 1987, Wiley.

47. Koonce JM, Gold M, Moroze M: Comparison of novice and experienced pilots using analog and digital flight displays, *Aviat Space Environ Med* 57:1181-1184, 1986.

48. Allen RW, Clement WF, Jex HR: *Research on display scanning, sampling, and reconstruction using separate, main, and secondary tracking tasks,* NASA CR-1569, Hampton, Va, 1970, NASA.

49. Diffrient N, Tilley AR, Harman D: *Humanscale 4/5/6,* Cambridge, Mass, 1981, MIT Press.

50. Westhorpe RN: Ergonomics and monitoring, *Anaesth Intensive Care* 16:71-75, 1988.

51. Sanders AF: Some aspects of the selective process in the functional visual field, *Ergonomics* 13:101-117, 1970.

52. Barnett BJ, Wickens CD: Display proximity in multicue information integration: the benefits of boxes, *Human Factors* 30:15-24, 1988.

53. Rock I, Palmer S: The legacy of gestalt psychology, *Scientific American* 3:84-90, 1990.

54. Petersen PJ, Banks WW, Gertman DI: Performance-based evaluation of graphic displays from a nuclear power plant control room, *Proceedings of the Conference on Human Factors in Computer Systems,* New York, 1981, Association for Computing Machinery.

55. Stokes AF, Wickens C, Kite K: *Display technology: human factors concepts,* Warrendale, Pa, 1990, Society of Automotive Engineers.

56. Wickens CD, Andre AD: Proximity compatibility and information display: effects of color, space, and object display on information integration, *Human Factors* 32:61-77, 1990.

57. Sanderson PM, Flach JM, Buttigieg MA, et al: Object displays do not always support better integrated task performance, *Human Factors* 31:183-198, 1989.

58. Siegel JH: *Integrated approaches to physiologic monitoring of the critically ill.* In Gravenstein JS, Newbower RS, Ream AK, et al, editors: *An integrated approach to monitoring,* Boston, 1983, Butterworths.

59. Hitt WD: An evaluation of five different coding methods, *Human Factors* 3:120-130, 1961.

60. Christ RE: Review and analysis of color coding research for visual displays, *Human Factors* 17:542-570, 1975.

61. McDonald WA, Cole BL: Evaluating the role of colour in a flight information cockpit display, *Ergonomics* 31:13-37, 1988.

62. Sorkin RD: *Design of auditory and tactile displays,* In Salvendy G, editor: *Handbook of human factors,* New York, 1987, Wiley.

63. O'Hare D, Roscoe S: *Flightdeck performance: the human factor,* Ames, Iowa, 1990, Iowa State University Press.

64. Waterson CK, Calkins JM: Development directions for monitoring in anesthesia. *Semin Anesth* 5:225-236, 1986.

65. *Minimum performance and safety requirements for components and systems of continuous-flow anesthesia machines for human use,* Z79.8-1979, New York, 1979, American National Standards Institute.

66. *Minimum performance and safety requirements for components and systems of anesthesia gas machines,* F 1161-88, Philadelphia, 1989, American Society for Testing and Materials.

67. Buffington CW, Ramanathan S, Turndorf H: Detection of anesthesia machine faults, *Anesth Analg* 63:79-82, 1984.

68. *Guidelines for patient care in anesthesiology.* In *Directory of Members,* ed 56, Park Ridge, Ill, 1991, American Society of Anesthesiologists.

69. Ward CS: The prevention of accidents associated with anaesthetic apparatus, *Br J Anaesth* 40:692-701, 1968.

70. *Nonflammable medical gas systems,* NFPA 56F, Quincy, Mass, 1983, National Fire Protection Association.

71. Sato T: Fatal pipeline accidents spur Japanese standards, *APSF Newsletter* 6:14, 1991.

72. Blum LR: Equipment design and human limitations, *Anesthesiology* 35:101-102, 1971.

73. *Standard color-marking of compressed gas cylinders intended for medical use in the United States,* Pamphlet C-9, New York, 1982, Compressed Gas Association.

74. Katz D: Increasing the safety of anesthesia machines: 1) further modifications of the Dräger machine; 2) considerations for the standardization of certain basic components, *Anesth Analg* 48:242-245, 1969.

75. Rendell-Baker L: Some gas machine hazards and their elimination, *Anesth Analg* 55:26-33, 1976.

76. Schreiber P: *Safety guidelines for anesthesia systems,* Telford, Pa, 1984, North American Dräger.

77. Heath JR, Anderson MM, Nunn JF: Performance of the quantiflex monitored dial mixer, *Br J Anaesth* 45:216-220, 1973.

78. Loeb RG, Brunner JX, Westenskow DR, et al: The Utah Anesthesia Workstation, *Anesthesiology* 70:999-1007, 1989.

79. Keenan RI, Boyan CB: Cardiac arrest due to anesthesia, *JAMA* 2153:2373-2377, 1985.

80. Guerra F: Awareness and recall, *Int Anesthesiol Clin* 24:75-99, 1986.

81. Smith NT, Quinn ML, Flick J, et al: Automatic control in anesthesia: a comparison between the anesthetist and the machine, *Anesth Analg* 63:715-722, 1984.

82. Westenskow DR, Wallroth CF: Closed-loop control for anesthesia breathing systems, *J Clin Monit* 6:249-256, 1990.

83. Kern FH, Jacobs JR, Ungerleider RM, et al: Computerized continuous infusion of intravenous anesthetic drugs during pediatric cardiac surgery, *Anesth Analg* 72:487-492, 1991.

84. Raemer DB, Buschman A, Varvel JR, et al: The prospective use of population pharmacokinetics in a computer-driven infusion system for alfentanil, *Anesthesiology* 73:66-72, 1990.

85. Jaklitsch RR, Westenskow DR, Pace NL, et al: A comparison of computer-controlled versus manual administration of vecuronium in humans, *J Clin Monit* 3:269-276, 1987.

86. Lampard DG, Coles JR, Brown WA: Computer control of respiration and anaesthesia, *Anaesth Intensive Care* 1:382-392, 1973.

87. Tsang PS, Johnson WW: Cognitive demands in automation, *Aviat Space Environ Med* 60:130-135, 1989.

88. Bergeron HS, Hinton DA: Aircraft automation: the problem of the pilot interface, *Aviat Space Environ Med* 56:144-148, 1985.

89. Wiener EL: Controlled flight into terrain accidents: system-induced errors, *Human Factors* 19:171-181, 1977.

90. Goodman NW: A second time-motion study of the anaesthetist's intraoperative period, *Br J Anaesth* 65:841, 1990 (letter).

91. Weinger MB, Englund CE: Ergonomic and human factors affecting anesthetic vigilance and monitoring performance in the operating room environment, *Anesthesiology* 73:995-1021, 1990.

92. Dror A, Henriksen E: Accidental epidural magnesium sulfate injection, *Anesth Analg* 66:1020-1021, 1987.

93. Forestner JE, Raj PP: Inadvertent epidural injection of thiopental: a case report, *Anesth Analg* 54:406-407, 1975.

94. Gabrielczyk MR, Forensky J: Inadvertent intra-arterial injection of vecuronium, *Anesthesiology* 68:656-657, 1988 (letter).

95. Holley HS, Cuthrell L: Intraarterial injection of propofol, *Anesthesiology* 73:183-184, 1990.

96. Fromme GA, Atchison SR: Safety of continuous epidural infusions. *Anesthesiology* 66:94, 1987.

97. Chopra V, Bovill JG, Spierdijk J: Accidents, near accidents and complications during anaesthesia: a retrospective analysis of a 10-year period in a teaching hospital, *Anaesthesia* 45:3-6, 1990.

98. Murphy JL Jr: Endrate or Amidate *Anesth Analg* 73:237, 1991 (letter).

99. *Specification for identification and configuration of prefilled syringes and delivery systems for drugs (excluding pharmacy bulk packages), D4775,* Philadelphia, 1988, American Society for Testing and Materials.

100. *Specification for labels for small volume (less than 100 ml) parenteral drug containers, D4267,* Philadelphia, 1989, American Society for Testing and Materials.

101. Cooper JB, Long CD, Newbower RS, et al: Critical incidents associated with intraoperative exchanges of anesthesia personnel, *Anesthesiology* 56:456-461, 1982.

102. *Specification for user applied drug labels in anesthesiology, D4774,* Philadelphia, 1988, American Society for Testing and Materials.

103. Anderson DC, Blower AL, Packer JM, et al: Preventing needlestick injuries, *Br Med J* 302:769-770, 1991.

104. Jagger J, Hunt EH, Brand-Elnagger J, et al: Rates of needle-stick injury caused by various devices in a university hospital, *N Engl J Med* 319:284-288, 1988.

105. Needlestick prevention devices, *Health Devices* 20:154-180, 1991.

106. Kempen PM: Eliminating needle stick injuries, *Can Anaesth Soc J* 36:361, 1989 (letter).

107. Hejna WF, Gutman CM: *Management of surgical facilities,* Rockville, Md, 1984, Aspen.

108. Zahn J, Haines R: The influence of central search task luminance upon peripheral visual detection time, *Psychonomic Sci* 24:271-273, 1971.

109. Sanders M, Gustanki J, Lawton M: Effects of ambient illumination on noise level of groups, *J Appl Psychol* 59:527-528, 1974.

110. Burn JMB: Facility design for outpatient surgery and anesthesia, *Int Anesthesiol Clin* 20:135-151, 1982.

111. Ziter CA, Dennis BW, Shoup LK: Justification of an operating-room satellite pharmacy, *Am J Hosp Pharm* 46:1353-1361, 1989.

112. Partridge BL, Weinger MB, Sanford TJ: Preventing unauthorized access to narcotics in the operating room, *Anesth Analg* 71:566-567, 1990 (letter).

113. Gaba DM, Maxwell M, DeAnda A: Anesthetic mishaps: breaking the chain of accident evolution, *Anesthesiology* 66:670-676, 1987.

Chapter 19

RECORD-KEEPING AND AUTOMATED RECORD-KEEPERS

Jeffrey M. Feldman, M.D.
Michael L. Good, M.D.

Handwritten versus automated anesthesia records
    Clerical tasks
    Accuracy
    Completeness
    Legibility
    Vigilance
    Cost
    Controversy
    Criteria for acceptance of AARK technology
Current technology
    Design considerations
    Commercial systems
The future

The anesthesia record serves a number of important functions in anesthesia practice. Not only an important clinical tool, the record provides fundamental information for medicolegal purposes and supports such administrative aspects of practice as billing.[1] The first known anesthesia record[2] was created in 1894 by E.A. Codman as part of a study to document the course of an anesthetic case.* That first record noted heart and respiratory rates at 5-minute in-

*Cushing claims that a wager between Codman and himself concerning who was the best "etherizer" was the motivation for creation of the first anesthesia records. Codman, noting Cushing's flair for the dramatic, explained that F.B. Harrington, Codman's chief when he was a house officer, suggested that anesthesia records be kept.

tervals. Current handwritten records are subjected to much more intense scrutiny than was that first anesthesia record; and although the records now contain more information, the basic approach to record-keeping has changed very little.

Anesthesiologists and anesthetists often think of the anesthesia record as "their record," when in fact it is used by many other medical and nonmedical personnel (Box 19-1).[1] Postoperative users include the physicians and nurses who care for the patient in the postanesthesia care unit (PACU), on the postoperative surgical ward, and in the intensive care unit. These physicians and nurses consult the anesthesia record for such information as intraoperative blood loss, fluids and drugs administered, and overall hemodynamic stability. A patient's anesthesia

---

Box 19-1. Users of the anesthesia record

Anesthesiologists and anesthetists
Postoperative physicians and nurses
Future anesthesiologists and anesthetists
Administrators
Accountants
Quality assurance and peer review personnel
Attorneys

Adapted from Gravenstein JS: The automated anesthesia record, *Int J Clin Monit Comput* 3:131-134, 1986.

record is also important to anesthesiologists and anesthetists who consult it when preparing to administer a subsequent anesthetic to the same patient.

Administrators use the anesthesia record as a source of information concerning utilization of hospital facilities, personnel, equipment, and supplies. Accountants use the anesthesia record to obtain information necessary for accurate billing (e.g., name of the anesthesiologist, anesthesia-related procedures, beginning and ending times of anesthesia and surgery). Quality assurance and peer review auditors examine the anesthesia record to fulfill their responsibilities. Finally, attorneys use the anesthesia record as evidence both to defend and to prosecute anesthesiologists accused of malpractice.

For the provider of intraoperative anesthesia care, the anesthesia record has the following six primary functions or uses (Box 19-2): (1) as a log book, (2) as a clinical management tool, (3) as a trend and pattern plotter, (4) as a medicolegal document, (5) as a vigilance aid, and (6) as an information management tool.[3] The clinician uses the anesthesia record as a log book to record such data as demographic information about the patient; operating room location; time; identification numbers for the anesthesia machine, and other equipment, and drugs (e.g., lot number of spinal tray); and the number of intubation attempts. The anesthesia record is an important clinical management tool with which the clinician examines the relationship between a clinical intervention and the intended response. For example, the record helps the clinician track the relationships between doses and responses for the many drugs given during the course of an anesthetic.

The familiar markings of heart rate, blood pressure, and other physiologic variables as a function of time transform the anesthesia record into a trend and pattern plotter. Evolving trends are recognized more easily from graphs than from lists of numbers (Fig. 19-1). Such trends, particularly when two or more parameters are plotted together, often yield important clues about the patient's condition. Decreasing blood pressure with a slowing heart rate suggests a different clinical picture than does decreasing blood pressure with an increasing heart rate. Other clues are less subtle but just as important clinically. For example, decreasing central venous pressure and falling peak expired carbon dioxide suggest diminished cardiac output secondary to hypovolemia. Furthermore, when numbers are plotted rather than listed in a table (Fig. 19-1), both the direction and rate of change become readily apparent.

Finally, the anesthesia record is an important medicolegal document. It is the document most scrutinized during anesthesia-related legal proceedings. "If it isn't recorded, it didn't happen," describes how the anesthesia record is often regarded by a plaintiff's attorney. Because most clinicians are engaged in patient care activities during anesthetic induction, emergence, and emergencies, often little information is recorded on the anesthesia record during these times. It is during these times, however, that events

---

Box 19-2. Uses of the anesthesia record
Log book
Clinical management tool
Trend and pattern plotter
Medicolegal document
Vigilance aid
Information management tool

Adapted from Gravenstein JS: The uses of the anesthesia record, *J Clin Monit* 5:256-265, 1989.

---

leading to malpractice claims often arise and when complete documentation is most important.[4] An incomplete anesthesia record generated from memory may not adequately reflect the often heroic efforts made on the patient's behalf.

Considering the importance of the modern anesthesia record, the question is whether or not traditional methods of record-keeping are adequate to meet the demands now placed on the record. Technology now exists to automate much of the record-keeping process. Some practitioners have embraced this new technology as a means to improve the record; others assert that automated record-keeping is just another device to come between the clinician and the patient. (See also Chapter 17.)

The first part of this chapter addresses the controversies surrounding automated anesthesia record-keepers (AARKs). The current AARK technology is then reviewed. After gaining an understanding of the controversies and technology, the anesthesiologist can make an informed judgment about whether or not to adopt an AARK into clinical practice and which AARK to select.

HANDWRITTEN VERSUS AUTOMATED ANESTHESIA RECORDS

For the anesthesia record to meet all its requirements and satisfy users, it must be accurate, complete, and legible. Furthermore, because most anesthetics are given by the individual who keeps the record, that person must have sufficient clerical time available to generate a quality record. How do the automated and handwritten approaches compare with regard to this type of record (Table 19-1)?

Clerical tasks

The first anesthesia record included only a notation of heart and respiratory rates and a few written remarks. The modern record includes many additional items, such as vascular and airway pressures, gas concentrations and flows, temperature, dosages of pharmacologic agents, and intravenous fluids used. The time required to maintain the record has therefore increased significantly and often exceeds the time available.

The clerical activities of the anesthesiologist have been studied during coronary bypass[5] and general surgical[6] pro-

Time	Variable 1	Variable 2	Variable 3
1	10	13	11
2	25	10	12
3	41	17	12
4	56	20	12
5	60	22	12
6	62	23	14
7	60	24	19
8	58	25	36
9	54	26	51
10	52	27	64
11	49	28	60
12	47	29	53
13	45	30	47
14	43	34	39
15	41	45	32

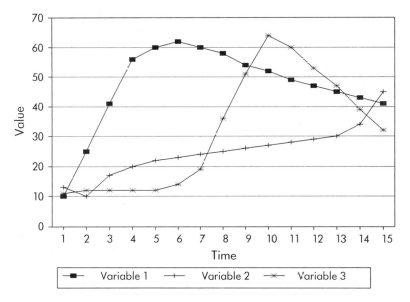

Fig. 19-1. Comparison of a series of numbers presented as a table and as a graph. The trends of the three variables are more easily ascertained when the data are presented in graphical form. Both direction of change and rate of change are easily visualized from the graph but not from the table.

Table 19-1. Handwritten versus automated anesthesia records

	Automated	Handwritten
Clerical time[8,9,10]	+/−*	+/−
Accuracy	+	−
Completeness	+	−
Legibility[1]	+	−
Vigilance[13]	−	+
Cost	−	+

*+ indicates an advantage of the technique; − indicates either no advantage or possible disadvantage.

cedures by examining videotapes of these procedures. Meijler[7] compared these studies by equating the tasks and plotting the results on a graph (Fig. 19-2). The task of logging data on the chart consumed 6% of the anesthesiologists' time during general surgery and 12% during coro-

nary artery bypass surgery. Proponents of automated record-keeping contend that the anesthesiologist spends less time keeping a record on an automated system and therefore has additional time to care for the anesthetized patient. For this contention to be true, keeping a record using an AARK should take less time than keeping it by hand. Because an AARK records monitored data automatically, the user saves the time usually required to transcribe data from the monitors. Time savings may be offset, however, by the increase in time spent entering notations into the AARK, which may be more awkward than with handwritten notation.

Although it is interesting to note the overall time devoted to record-keeping during anesthesia, this does not reflect those situations that require that 100% of the anesthesiologist's attention be directed to the patient, leaving no time for record-keeping. Thorough documentation is of particular importance when a significant adverse event occurs during anesthesia. Yet, typically, the anesthesiologist

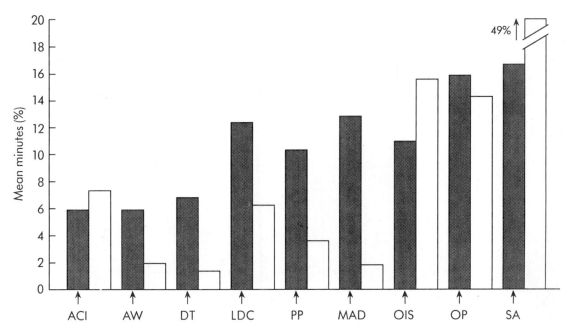

Fig. 19-2. The only available quantitative material on anesthesia workload is presented here. The time spent on nine subtasks in percentage of work-minutes is plotted for cardiac surgical procedures *(solid columns)* and for general procedures *(open columns)*. Arrow, cardiac procedure; *ACI*, adjust/calibrate instrument; *AW*, arrange equipment; *DT*, data transfer; *LDC*, log data; *PP*, prepare patient; *MAD*, mix/administer drugs; *OIS*, observe monitors; *OP*, observe patient; *SA*, scan area. (Solid columns after Kennedy, et al[5]; open colums after Boquet, et al.[6]) From Meijler AP: *Automation in anesthesia: a relief? A systematic approach to computers in patient monitoring,* New York, 1987, Springer-Verlag, p 23. Reproduced by permission.)

must complete the record from memory, and this may lead to an incomplete rendition of events. An AARK will faithfully record monitored information in much greater detail than a human recorder ever could.

Accuracy

The accuracy of automated record-keepers has been examined by comparison of the data obtained by the AARK to that on handwritten records. One early study[8] found major discrepancies between manual and computer-recorded values in 43 out of 100 records. These discrepancies often arose during induction of and emergence from anesthesia, when the clinician was occupied and had to make retrospective entries into the record from memory.

In a more recent study, Lerou, et al.[9] compared the handwritten records of 30 patients undergoing eye surgery with the records generated by a commercially available AARK. The users made entries on the handwritten record from values displayed by the record-keeper, and this allowed direct comparison of the record-keepers entries and the handwritten ones. Eight variables were collected by both the human and the machine. The fractions of missing and erroneous data were calculated by dividing the minutes of missing or erroneous data by the total minutes of anesthesia. These fractions were calculated for induction

(first 15 minutes), end of case or emergence (last 10 minutes), and maintenance (time in between) (Fig. 19-3). From these figures it is clear that the error fractions were greater during induction and emergence, when the clinician was occupied with patient care and delayed making entries on the record. Given that this study was limited to eye surgery, during which intraoperative events are not likely to alter homeostasis significantly, it is not surprising that the error rates were lower during maintenance. For other types of surgery that are likely to involve significant intraoperative changes demanding the anesthesiologist's time, it is possible that the maintenance error rates would be higher than those observed here.

The accuracy of recording blood pressure measurements has been examined, and interesting discrepancies have been found between handwritten values and those recorded automatically.[10] Fifty patients undergoing a variety of surgical procedures were studied. The authors found a tendency toward eliminating extreme blood pressure values in the handwritten record. The highest and lowest measured blood pressure did not appear on the handwritten record. Although there were 33 instances of automatically recorded diastolic blood pressure greater than 110 mm Hg, no handwritten record contained a diastolic blood pressure greater than 110 mm Hg. Because extremes in blood pres-

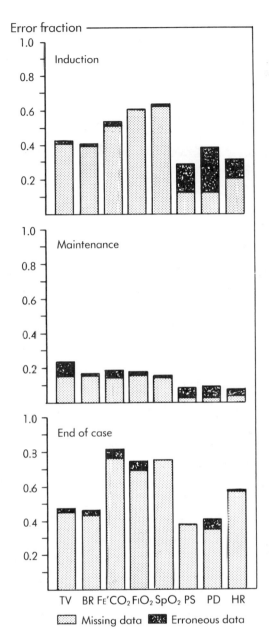

Fig. 19-3. The amount of missing and erroneous data on handwritten records is shown for the three major periods of anesthesia: induction (first 15 minutes), end of case (last 10 minutes), and maintenance (period in between). *TV*, Tidal volume; *BR*, breathing rate; $FE'CO_2$, end-tidal CO_2 fraction; FIO_2, inspired oxygen fraction in the anesthetic circuit; SpO_2, oxygen saturation by pulse oximetry; *PS*, systolic blood pressure; *PD*, diastolic blood pressure; *HR*, heart rate. (From Lerou JGC, Dirksen R, van Daele M, et al: Automated charting of physiological variables in anesthesia: a quantitative comparison of automated versus handwritten anesthesia records, *J Clin Monit* 4:37-47, 1988. Reproduced by permission.)

sure may be construed by some to represent suboptimal anesthetic management, these findings likely represent a bias toward recording less controversial values.

Three conclusions can be drawn from these studies: (1) The clinician is often occupied, especially during induc-

tion and emergence, and unable to make timely notations on the record; (2) entries made from memory are often inaccurate; and (3) there is likely a bias, conscious or unconscious, in the creation of the handwritten record.

The handwritten record may be inaccurate for a number of reasons, but the automated record may also be inaccurate. Artifact in monitored signals is a common problem in the operating room. Current AARK technology is designed to record exactly what is displayed on the monitor. If an artifactual value is displayed, the clinician can often identify it as such and will not record the value on the handwritten record. The AARK, however, faithfully records the artifactual information.

Studies of the incidence of artifact with an AARK[11,12] demonstrate that a small percentage of data—between 0.1% and 6%, depending on the parameter of interest—are artifactual. It is interesting to note that both of these studies demonstrated that the incidence of artifact decreased as AARK technology matured. This decrease is related to the use of newer monitors, which are more resistant to environmental influences, and also to improved artifact detection capability. In addition, artifactual data usually appear on the record as markedly different from the other values recorded. Therefore, they are unlikely to be regarded as a manifestation of poor anesthetic management.

Every practicing anesthesiologist has from time to time been occupied with other tasks and unable to keep an accurate record. In such situations, automated data collection is clearly useful. Often, more than enough time is available to maintain an accurate record by hand. However, there is more to keeping a good record than making timely marks on the paper.

Completeness

For most handwritten records, the most frequently recorded data are, by tradition, recorded every 5 minutes. This rate of recording, although well accepted, is probably not rational. If the choice of rate of recording were made on the basis of the need to capture significant changes in physiologic data, the interval would need to be more often than every 5 minutes. Significant changes in blood pressure and heart rate can occur within seconds. This is not a practical interval for a human recording handwritten data. However, most clinicians make an effort to represent dramatic physiologic changes on the record, regardless of the interval. Given today's computer technology, automated record-keepers can acquire data well within the frequency of physiologic changes. To avoid logging large amounts of normal data, the automated record-keeper can be programmed to increase the rate of recording when indicated.

The printed record generated by an AARK typically displays data at the intervals customary on handwritten records. AARK systems that record data to magnetic disk actually record the information more frequently than it is

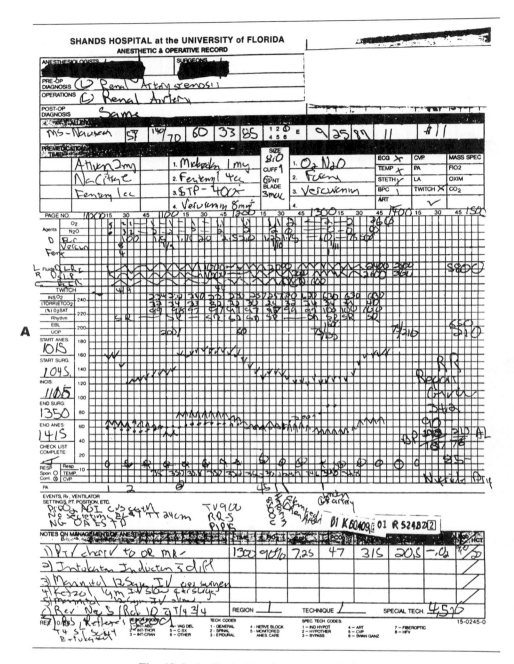

Fig. 19-4. **A,** Typical handwritten anesthesia record.

displayed on the handwritten record. If these magnetic records are retained, events can be reviewed in much greater detail than with either the printed or the handwritten records.

Legibility

The light-hearted comment often made to someone with illegible handwriting that, that person would make a good physician has an unfortunate ring of truth. In fact, many health care professionals have poor handwriting, or, in their effort to record rapidly changing events, the legibility

of their handwriting deteriorates. Figure 19-4, *A* shows a typical handwritten record, and Fig. 19-4, *B* shows a representative automated record. The automated record is clearly the more legible of the two.

Why is legibility important? From the most obvious point of view, an illegible record fails to serve the function for which it was created—that is, documentation of the course of anesthesia. Furthermore, an illegible anesthetic record may have serious medicolegal implications if it fails to document appropriate care.

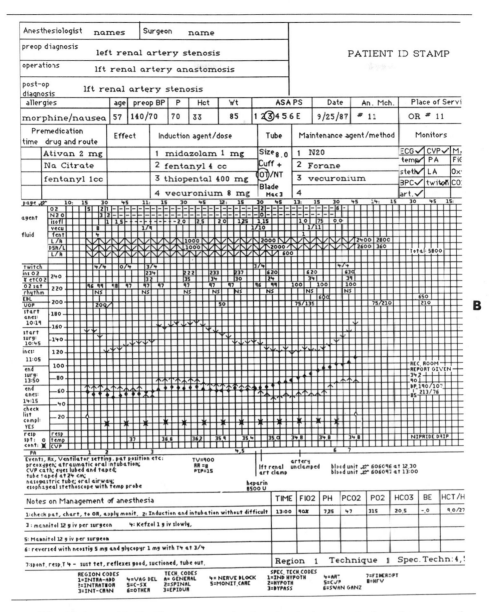

Fig. 19-4, cont'd. B, The same record, where handwritten entries have been retyped.

Vigilance

One purported advantage of the handwritten record is that the act of entering data on the record will make the clinician aware of physiologic trends. Does the clinician using an AARK suffer a decrement in vigilance by having monitored data charted automatically? Unfortunately, there is little objective data that assess the impact of an AARK on vigilance.

One study[13] suggests that vigilance may not be as well maintained when an AARK is used. Twelve anesthesia providers, experienced with both manual and automated record-keeping, were asked to use each method of record-keeping during 5 cases (10 cases total per clinician). During each case, an investigator entered the room and asked the anesthesiologist the current values of several monitored

parameters. The responses were compared to the current values on the monitors. For each parameter, a value was set to determine the clinically relevant error. The percentage of reported values that exceeded the clinically relevant error range were determined for each method of record-keeping (Table 19-2). Overall, when the AARK was used, 23% of values were not known within the defined relevant error range, whereas for manual record-keeping, 5% of values were not known. It would be interesting to note to what extent the clinically relevant error range would need to be changed to demonstrate no difference between the methods. These data suggest, however, that there may indeed be cause for concern regarding the impact on vigilance of an AARK. Perhaps clinicians who use an AARK need to modify their practice patterns to ensure continued vigilance.

Table 19-2. Comparison of the anesthesiologist's knowledge of current data using automated and manual record-keepers

Parameter	RE*	Percent of cases with relevant error		
		AR†	MR‡	P<
Blood pressure systolic	>2mm Hg	16	16	
Blood pressure diastolic	>9mm Hg	36	16	0.035
Temperature	>0.4°C	31	8	0.016
Heart rate	>9 beats/min	14	7	
ETCO$_2$§	>3 mm Hg	10	8	
F$_1$O$_2$	>4%	20	5	
Pip¶	>4cm H$_2$O	33	11	0.033
O$_2$ saturation	>2%	8	0	
One value or more not known		23	5	0.0007

*Clinically relevant error.
†Automated record.
‡Manual record.
§End-tidal carbon dioxide.
¶Peak inflation pressure.

Cost

With soaring costs of medical care, the cost of any new technology is a factor in its acceptance. This is likely a major factor in the rather slow acceptance of AARKs. The only costs associated with the handwritten record are those incurred by printing forms and buying pens. The cost of one AARK (which can function in only one location) may vary from several thousand to $20,000, not including the monitors that must be connected to it. The decision to purchase an AARK must therefore involve a cost/benefit analysis.

The cost savings associated with AARKs have yet to be documented, but AARKs may in fact pay for themselves. If the premise is accepted that the quality of the documentation provided by an AARK might help to avoid malpractice proceedings, then the cost of the AARK is clearly minimal. Because the AARK is used to record information necessary for billing purposes, it may help to improve collections. In the future, it will be possible to link AARKs electronically to billing services; this would eliminate the clerical processing of billing information. Bills would therefore be generated more quickly and with fewer errors.

AARKs can also facilitate tasks that now consume the resources of an anesthesia practice. Quality assurance analysis, required of all anesthesia practices, is increasingly scrutinized by hospital accreditation agencies. A busy anesthesia practice generates a large amount of quality assurance information that must be processed and analyzed. The AARK stores most of the information necessary to support quality assurance. That information can be transferred automatically to quality assurance software to generate the appropriate reports. In addition, because the

data are more complete and accurate than the handwritten record, quality assurance reports should be better when data that have been collected by an AARK are used.

Although no one to date has evaluated the cost effectiveness of AARKs, they potentially offer some major advantages that translate into significant cost savings that offset the cost of the device. As the technology matures, their cost may decrease. It is likely that these devices will mature into sophisticated data management systems that justify themselves by improving the quality and efficiency not only of record-keeping but also of billing and quality assurance.

Controversy

The proponents of AARKs assert that this technology provides an anesthesia record that is of a better quality and that is more complete, accurate, and legible than one that is handwritten. Opponents of AARKs believe that reduced vigilance is a problem and that recording of artifactual data may open the possibility of medicolegal exposure. The foregoing information suggests that there are elements of truth to both of these assertions. How can these opposing views be resolved? Will AARK technology ultimately fade away, or will it become an integral part of the anesthesia workplace?

Criteria for acceptance of AARK technology

In order to gain acceptance into routine clinical practice, a new device must satisfy one or more of the following criteria: (1) improve patient care, (2) reduce clinician workload, (3) decrease cost, (4) be medicolegally compelling, and (5) perform one important task or more that would otherwise not be done.[14] Does AARK technology satisfy any of these criteria?

Improved patient care. No data are available to document that AARKs improve patient care. Furthermore, it is unlikely that a conclusive study to collect such data is feasible given the low incidence of injury to patients due to anesthesia. AARKs may improve care by increasing the amount of time available to observe the patient, or they may be detrimental to care by reducing the awareness of monitored data. Each user must make a personal judgment in this regard. In any event, AARKs are unlikely to gain acceptance by improving patient care.

Reduced clinician workload. Clearly, AARKs reduce the clinician's workload associated with entering physiologic data on the record because these data are recorded automatically. The clinician using an AARK is not freed from all record-keeping activities because demographic, procedural, and drug information must still be entered manually. The AARK may not provide a method for entering information manually that is more convenient than handwritten entry. The workload advantages of the AARK are apparent during those situations in which all attention must be directed to the patient, although such situations are probably not frequent enough to stimulate acceptance of the technology.[15]

Decreased cost. Decreasing the cost of care is another dubious benefit of AARKs. The high cost of these devices relative to other equipment needed in the operating room has already been discussed. Although AARKs may reduce the cost of other information management tasks, this advantage remains to be documented.

Medicolegal aspects. When viewed from a medicolegal perspective, AARK technology begins to look more compelling. Incomplete anesthesia records may have serious medicolegal ramifications. One physicians' insurance trust fund has paid approximately $5 million in settlements over 10 years for all physicians (anesthesiologists included) solely due to poor record-keeping. In all of these cases, the physicians acted correctly, but their actions were not documented adequately in the medical record.*

It would seem, therefore, that a legible, complete, and credible ("unsmoothed") record generated automatically should vindicate the anesthesiologist in frivolous and nuisance lawsuits and should facilitate just settlement when a plaintiff deserves compensation.[14] Lawyers who defend anesthesiologists in malpractice cases agree that the "poor or incomplete anesthesia record" is the greatest obstacle to a successful defense against a malpractice claim.[16] Crawford Morris, an attorney experienced at defending physicians in malpractice litigation, writes about AARKs[17]:

Charting . . . is a "two-way street." Good charting helps, and bad charting hurts. With the use of such devices, each side is going to lose some malpractice cases it might have won with poorly decipherable records, and vice versa, but on balance, the presentation of actual facts should not only promote justice but also lead to more reasonable settlements. At least defense counsel won't have to meet the favorite arguments of plaintiff's counsel to the jury: "If the defendant didn't chart it, he didn't do it."

The value of a legible, accurate record to malpractice defense cannot be disputed. However, current AARKs record artifactual data, and there is great concern about the legal implications of these data. In most instances, experienced clinicians have no difficulty distinguishing real data from artifact. Artifact typically appears as a sudden change in the value of a parameter, distinct from the trend of other values of the same parameter. Scenarios can be imagined in which artifactual data might be used to incriminate an innocent anesthesiologist (e.g., a postoperative stroke entirely unrelated to the anesthetic could be attributed to a momentary artifactual hypotension recorded from an automated noninvasive blood pressure monitor). To date, no malpractice claims have been won or lost because of an AARK. As these devices proliferate, it is certain that malpractice litigation will ultimately involve data collected by an AARK. The role of the AARK in that setting will al-

most certainly have a major impact on the acceptance of this technology.

Information management. AARKs have the potential to perform information management functions that are not currently possible, and it is this potential that may ultimately drive their acceptance. The 1990s will bring an increasing demand on the anesthesia record for information. This new information management task for the anesthesia record is the result of several trends in anesthesia practice: (1) increased amount of information available from the record, (2) increased prevalence of quality assurance programs, and (3) the demand for anesthesia data by individuals outside the anesthesia department.

During the 1980s, the number of patient and machine parameters measured by the anesthesiologist greatly increased. Innovative devices that use advanced technology now allow noninvasive measurement of such important variables as oxyhemoglobin saturation by pulse oximetry, respiratory carbon dioxide by capnography, and myocardial contractility by transesophageal echocardiography. Now, even during the course of the most "simple" anesthetic, some 25 variables are tracked by the clinician; and during the course of a "complicated" anesthetic, approximately 75 variables can be directly measured or calculated.*

The 1980s also saw the widespread application of quality assurance principles to medicine in general, including anesthesiology. Most programs utilize self-reporting systems by which each clinician reports the untoward events that occur while patients are cared for. The quality assurance process typically requires an additional form in the anesthesia record, and the additional data must later be entered manually into a departmental computerized database for analysis. Enormous volumes of data and numerous reports are generated. The manpower required to perform quality assurance is so significant that automation of the process by using an AARK is appealing.

Because medical care is deemed too expensive by the public, the government, and commercial health insurance companies, many hospitals and medical departments have instituted cost accounting policies. Effective cost accounting requires large amounts of data concerning utilization of both human and material resources. For example, the use of a new, more expensive muscle relaxant must be evaluated against the benefits to the patient. This analysis can be completed only when an accurate assessment of the use of the current muscle relaxant is available. Correctly charging patients for disposable supplies (e.g., a central venous catheter or a pulse oximeter probe) depends on accurately identifying those patients in whom the products were used. Because many disposable supplies are used

---

*Martin Smith, Director, University of Florida College of Medicine Risk Management Fund, personal communication, 1988.

*Calkins JM. What variables should we measure? Presentation at the Annual Meeting of The Arizona Society of Anesthesiologists, February 1982, Scottsdale, Arizona.

during anesthesia, the anesthesia record becomes important for documenting that appropriate charges are added to the patient's bill.

Administrators of anesthesiology departments may choose to hire additional personnel to audit anesthesia records and extract the data necessary to satisfy administrative and accreditation needs. It is well known that computers have the ability to perform data manipulation better and faster than humans. Automatically generated anesthesia records capture much of the pertinent data in an electronic format and can readily transmit these data into a departmental information management system.

CURRENT TECHNOLOGY

To produce a useful automated record-keeping system requires design specifications that both address the user's needs and consider existing technology. This section discusses the challenges of designing an automated record-keeper and the technological solutions currently available to address these challenges.

Design considerations

The design considerations can be divided into three areas: input, output, and other applications (Table 19-3). Input capabilities include automatic acquisition of information and provisions for manual entry. Output capabilities include the generation of a printed record, storage of data on magnetic media, and integration with a computer network. Other applications include such additional capabilities of computerized systems as database management.

Input capabilities. The anesthesia record must include information on patient demographics, physiology, drugs and drug dosages, infusions, ventilator settings, anesthesia machine function, and the occurrence of significant events. Only some of this information can be recorded automatically; the clinician must still enter many items manually. Infusion pumps, ventilators, and anesthesia machines all have the potential to interface directly to the AARK, which would further reduce the amount of manual entry. Annotations constitute an important part of the record and will always require some method of manual entry—handwritten or otherwise. When the input capabilities of an AARK are considered, the flexibility of the automated input and the ease of entering items that are not recorded automatically should be taken into account.

Automated data entry. All AARK systems can interface to one or more patient monitors to record data. Most devices provide the capability to interface to monitors from different vendors. This feature is essential because anesthesia departments often purchase individual monitors at different times and rarely replace a complete set of monitors at one time. The AARK manufacturer should have the capability to interface with a large number of different monitors and should be willing to support the installation and maintenance of these interfaces.

Table 19-3. Design considerations for automated record-keepers

Record-keeping characteristic	Design consideration
Data input	
Automated	Proprietary versus communication with devices from several manufacturers
Manual	Handwritten (semiautomated systems) Keyboard: standard or special touch screen
Printed record	Continuous (real-time) versus print on demand
Other applications	Permanent storage: magnetic media; Networking to other computer systems

The importance of artifact detection deserves mention here because it is a primary shortcoming of automated data recording. Most monitors provide an interface, either analog or digital, which transmits the values displayed on the monitor to the record-keeper. Artifact detection software may be built into the monitor, but typically, if an artifactual value is displayed, it is transmitted via the data interface to the AARK. For example, consider electrocautery artifact in an ECG signal. It is quite common to see widely varying heart rates displayed on an ECG monitor during the use of electrocautery. The clinician is easily able to recognize the interference in the ECG tracing and disregard the heart rate value on the monitor. On the other hand, a data interface faithfully transmits the artifactual heart rate data for incorporation into the automated record.

Currently available AARK systems record arterial blood pressure, heart rate, temperature, inspired oxygen, oxygen saturation, and peak expired carbon dioxide. Additional vascular pressures are not always available, nor are additional temperature channels or partial pressures of gases and vapors. If the record-keeper cannot record all of the desired physiologic data, the remainder will have to be entered manually. The methods for manually entering data to the record-keeper vary considerably and have a major effect on the utility of the system to the clinician.

Manual data entry. Manual data entry is facilitated in a variety of ways by automated systems, none of which offers the same convenience as handwritten data entry. For this reason, some manufacturers have produced semiautomated systems, record-keepers that allow for easy handwritten entry of information in addition to automated recording of physiologic data. For a variety of reasons, these semiautomated systems have been relatively less successful than the fully automated systems, and the current trend is clearly in the direction of entering all information into the computer.

The operating room presents a number of challenges to the design of an input device. Space is limited, and users are typically not facile with a keyboard and have limited time and attention to devote to data entry. At the same time, capturing data as it is generated in the operating room is the goal of any automated record-keeping system. Some systems provide standard typewriter (QWERTY) keyboards, but these often prove unwieldy. Alternative input methods, such as dedicated keypads, barcode readers, digitizing tablets, and light pens have been tried with limited success.[18-21] Voice recognition technology is an option on one commercially available AARK. Although flawless word identification continues to be hampered by several problems, voice recognition will perhaps be more useful in the future. The most useful input technology currently available for the operating room is the touch screen, which is used in several commercial systems.

The touch screen. A touch screen is a computer monitor with a touch-sensitive surface that can sense the location of a finger on the screen. The user makes selections by touching the surface. Selections can be made from a list (e.g., of drug names); numbers can be selected (e.g., to enter dosages); and a keyboard can even be displayed for "typing" text. Text entry via a keyboard represented on the screen is unwieldy and even more cumbersome than via a standard keyboard (unless the amount of text entry is quite limited). Pointing to items on the screen is intuitive and therefore appealing to the naive user, but extensive touch selections can be tiresome. A well-designed touch screen minimizes the number of touches necessary to make a selection and can allow for rapid entry of large amounts of information. A potential problem with touch screens is that more than one screen is usually required to present all available options. If the method for selecting different screens is not carefully designed, the user will be frustrated by excessive touches required to find a selection or the inability to find a selection at all. Furthermore, the time required to display a new screen should be minimal so that users do not feel as if they are waiting for the screen to change.

Output capabilities

The printed record. A major advantage of automated systems over the handwritten record is that the printed record is highly legible. Any printing device capable of printing both graphics and text can be used to produce a legible record once the data have been acquired.

One important design consideration is whether the printed record is generated as data become available or at the completion of the case. Generating the record after the case has been completed requires that all data be stored during the operation, which also means that the data can be lost to a malfunction. The advantage of a real-time printed copy is that the record can be removed from the printer and completed by hand should the automated system fail.

Because all currently available record-keeping systems require some amount of manual entry, and because the user may be otherwise occupied at the time an event occurs, generation of the printed record in real time requires that the printing device be able to back up to print events entered after the fact. Pen plotters can move to any point on the record at any time, so they function well for retrospective entries. Dot matrix and laser printers are not readily adaptable to retrospective entry. All AARK systems can produce a record on demand, although it is typically generated at the end of the case.

Magnetic storage. Data can be stored locally on either hard or floppy disks, or they can be passed over a computer network to a central storage location. The main advantage of electronic data storage over the printed record is that electronic information can be stored at a much higher resolution. Commercially available AARK systems typically print an average of the data on the record at regular intervals, whereas the actual data received from the monitors can be recorded to disk as frequently as they are received.

The potential disadvantages of electronic data storage are loss of data due to equipment failure and problems concerning the security of patient information. The ability to store recorded data at regular intervals on a floppy disk is a very desirable feature of an AARK. The floppy disk provides the user with a current version of the record that can be removed and generated on another system should the AARK fail for any reason during a case. If data are stored only to a hard disk prior to printing, then a system failure may lead to a complete loss of the record or, at the very least, make the record inaccessible.

Most of the currently available AARK systems have the capability to transfer information onto a computer network. This is often implemented to allow the printing of a high-quality record on a central printer located, for example, in the PACU. Network capability has the potential to support many more features, such as integration with hospital information systems.

Commercial systems

Feldman previously described four features by which AARKs can be evaluated and compared.[22] These are the AARKSs (1) interface with monitoring instruments (e.g., generic or proprietary), (2) procedure for manual entry of drugs, procedures, and other nontransduced information, (3) printing characteristics (i.e., continuous or on demand), and (4) magnetic storage capabilities (e.g., computer floppy disk or computer network). To this original list is now added a fifth feature: algorithms for data processing and artifact rejection. These features are used in the following discussion to describe the AARK systems that are currently available (Table 19-4).

Arkive. The Arkive Patient Information Management System* consists of a touch-screen monitor for displaying an image of the anesthesia record, a cabinet housing the computer, and a printer (Fig. 19-5). Through an interface

---

*Diatek, San Diego, Cal.

Table 19-4. Comparison of commercial automated anesthesia record-keepers

Device Name	Interface	Input	Printing	Output	Data Processing
Arkive	Generic	Touch screen	On demand	Network, disk	Median filter, database macros
Co-Writer	Proprietary	Handwriting	Continuous	None	None
Compu-Record	Generic	Touch screen, keyboard	On demand	Network, disk	?
LifeLog	Generic	Touch screen, keyboard	On demand	Network, disk	Median filter
OR Data Manager	Proprietary (Vital Link)	Keyboard	On demand	Network, disk	?

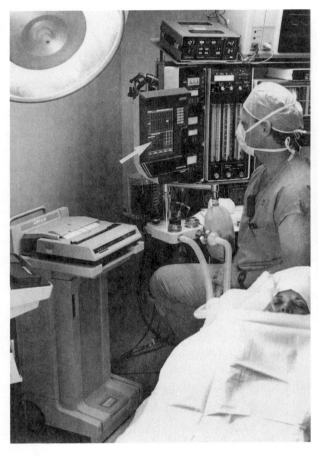

Fig. 19-5. The Arkive record-keeper is indicated by the white arrow. (Photograph courtesy of Diatek, San Diego, Cal.)

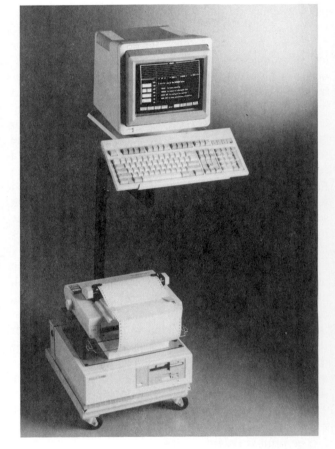

Fig. 19-6. The Compu-Record. (Photograph courtesy of PPG, Lenexa, Kan.)

box, this system can be configured to communicate with most of the commercially available physiologic monitors. Events, drugs, and procedural information are entered via the touch screen. Frequently used text entries (e.g., "direct laryngoscopy, atraumatic oral intubation on the first attempt, vocal cords visualized and clear, bilateral breath sounds present, expired CO_2 on capnograph") can be preconfigured using the touch screen and then retrieved and entered to the current anesthesia record with a few keystrokes. Continuous data (heart rate, invasive blood pressure) are sampled every 2 seconds, with the median value of 30 samples being recorded each minute (median filter).

Data are stored onto a floppy disk every minute. Although it can be printed on demand, the anesthesia record is typically printed at the end of a case. In the event of an electrical power failure, a battery back-up system allows Arkive to continue operating for 20 minutes. The system is sold in a stand-alone configuration or integrated into Ohmeda anesthesia machines.

Compu-Record. Compu-Record* utilizes a Hewlett-Packard VECTRA ES/12 microcomputer and a VGA color monitor with touch screen to display the anesthesia record

*PPG, Lenexa, Kan.

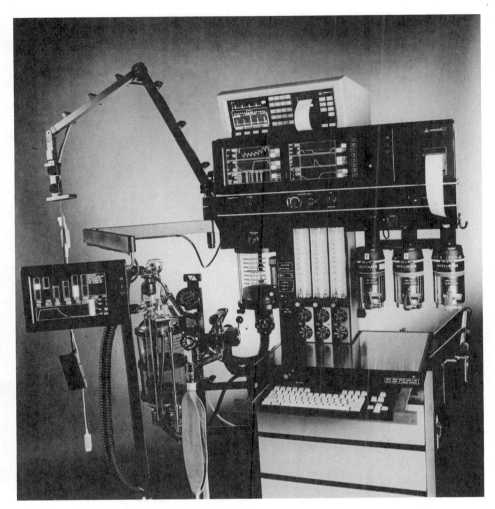

Fig. 19-7. The OR Data Manager record-keeper integrated with a Dräger Narkomed 4 anesthesia system. (Photograph courtesy of North American Dräger, Inc., Telford, Pa.)

(Fig. 19-6). The anesthesia record can be printed on a local dot matrix printer or can be transmitted through a computer network to a central laser printer (i.e., in the PACU). Magnetic disk storage is also possible. The system interfaces with most brands of physiologic monitors. Data are recorded from monitoring instruments every 15 seconds and stored to the computer hard disk every 2 minutes (which is the maximum time of lost data if electrical power is lost).

Nontransduced data, such as drug entries, procedural information, and other text entries, are manually entered via the touch screen, a standard (QWERTY) keyboard, or a combination of the two. For clinicians who can type, the standard typewriter keyboard facilitates easy data entry. Each CompuRecord operates as a stand-alone unit or can be networked to a centrally located file server that stores all anesthesia case files. The networked system allows automatic generation of charge vouchers, quality assurance reports, and other reports.

OR Data Manager. OR Data Manager* is designed to be part of the North American Dräger Narkomed anesthesia machine (Fig. 19-7). Its "in-board" version comes integrated into the Narkomed 4 anesthesia system; and its "out-board" version can be retrofitted to Narkomed 2B and 3 machines. The components of this AARK include a video display, keyboard, the computer processing unit, disk drives, and printer output port. With the in-board version of the system, the keyboard is built-in to the first drawer of the Narkomed 4 anesthesia machine. The drawer is conveniently opened for keyboard entry, then closed to conserve precious space in the anesthesia workstation. Customized function keys on the keyboard enable the user to mark artifactual data, indicate drug entries, change to a graphical display, and perform other record-keeping tasks. The OR Data Manager uses Dräger's Vital Link or OR Link data communications protocol. Only monitoring instruments that support this protocol can be used. Data are

*North American Dräger, Telford, Pa.

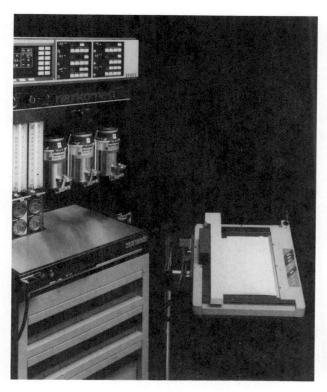

Fig. 19-8. The Co-Writer record-keeper. (Photograph courtesy of North American Dräger Inc., Telford, Pa.)

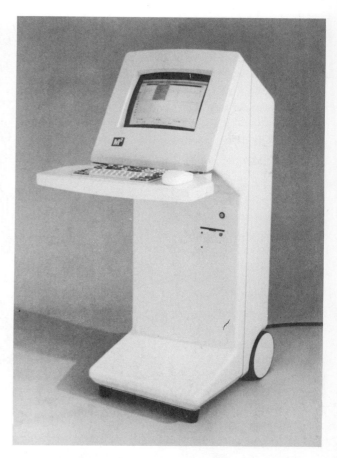

Fig. 19-9. The LifeLog record-keeper. (Photograph courtesy of Modular Instruments, Malvern, Pa.)

stored to disk every 30 seconds and plotted on the display and record every 5 to 15 minutes, depending on the parameter. Data are entered manually via the keyboard, and preconfigured text templates decrease the number of keystrokes necessary to enter commonly repeated text entries. The anesthesia record is printed on a laser printer or stored on floppy disk in an MS-DOS–compatible format. Data points can be edited both on-line and off-line. The system does not yet support network communications, although this feature is planned.

Co-Writer. Co-Writer* is a pen plotter designed to be used with Narkomed anesthesia systems, manufactured by North American Dräger (Fig. 19-8). It is a semiautomated anesthesia record-keeper. Physiologic data from monitoring instruments are recorded automatically, but nontransduced information, such as events, drug dosages, and procedure notes, must be handwritten on the record with a pen. There are, however, "drug" and "event" keys with which the anesthesiologist can mark the time line of the anesthesia record, but data relating to the drug administration or event must be handwritten. An ingenious feature is a pen well with a hidden switch. When the user withdraws the pen to write on the record, the plotter arm is recalled to the edge of the record so as not to obstruct the clinician. When the clinician returns the pen to its well, the plotter

continues recording monitored data. Data to be recorded appear on the Narkomed 3 anesthesia machine display for 20 seconds before they are recorded by Co-Writer. During this 20-second period, the user can block the recording of an artifactual value by pushing a button labeled "reject." The Co-Writer can be configured to write any anesthesia record format.

LifeLog. LifeLog* consists of a display monitor for presenting an image of the record, a keyboard and mouse for data entry, and a housing for the computer processing unit (Fig. 19-9). These components are assembled in two configurations. One is a single, free-standing workstation on lockable wheels. The other is a modular design, that encases the electronics, the computer processor, and the input/output connectors in one housing that can be positioned remotely from the workstation and enables the keyboard, mouse, and display screen to reside on the anesthesia machine. Data from physiological monitors are fed into the system through an interface box. The system connects to a computer network for printing the record on a central laser printer. The monitoring instruments are queried for data every 10 seconds. The user selects whether data

*North American Dräger, Telford, Pa.

*Modular Instruments, Malvern, Pa.

points are plotted every 30 seconds or every 60 seconds. A median filter algorithm is used to reject artifact. A unique feature of this AARK is its capability to edit data both numerically, by "tagging" suspect or artifactual data points, and graphically, by adjusting the curves on the graphics screen. An audit trail of all editing is maintained, and the record can be displayed with and without editing information by depression of a single key.

THE FUTURE

Currently available AARK systems are slowly gaining acceptance, although it will likely be many years before they become a standard component of the anesthesia workstation. Future advances that solve existing problems and ultimately drive the acceptance of these systems will be in the following areas: (1) increased automated data logging, (2) improved artifact detection, (3) enhanced methods for manual entry of information, and (4) integration with other practice management applications.

The trends in anesthesia workstation design are toward increasing the integration of monitoring equipment and electronic rather than mechanical design of the anesthesia machine. These trends increase the opportunity for gathering information automatically and including it in the record. For example, changes in gas flow are now entered manually, but future machines with electronic flow controllers will be able to report flow selections to an AARK. In addition, the Association for the Advancement of Medical Instrumentation (AAMI) and the Institute of Electrical and Electronics Engineers (IEEE) have been developing a standard for data communication between medical devices, called the medical information bus (MIB).[23] Acceptance of this standard, once defined, will enable intercommunication between all electronic medical equipment.

Artifact detection has already been improved in patient monitors, although many signals are still readily affected by the operating room environment. The trend toward integration is likely to help immensely with this problem because multiple signals with similar information can be used to identify artifact. For example, the ECG, SpO_2, and oscillometric blood pressure monitors all contain heart rate information, and combining data from each should enable a reliable assessment of heart rate despite interference disrupting the signal from one of the instruments.

Manual entry of information to the record that is not recorded automatically will be facilitated in several ways. Improved AARK design will enable easy storage and retrieval of large amounts of commonly entered text. For example, notes about induction of anesthesia made available at the beginning of the record could be eliminated from the choices once they have been selected. Although voice recognition technology will likely improve, the ability automatically to recognize natural language from a variety of speakers will not be available in the near future. One technology that will be readily available in the near future is automated handwriting recognition. This involves a pen or stylus for writing directly onto a touch-sensitive screen. Computers can now match printed characters with previously stored templates of the user's handwriting. The templates are created when the letters of the alphabet and numerals from 0 to 9 are written on the screen. Handwriting recognition is an exciting development because it offers the potential to interact with an AARK in a natural fashion. At present, software manufacturers have made great strides in developing handwriting recognition systems, although one has yet to be incorporated into a commercially available AARK.

Other applications that can be supported by an AARK, such as billing and quality assurance, have been described. AARK systems are already being integrated with these applications. Nevertheless, implementing a network of AARK systems in the operating room, connected to a central computer and configured with the software necessary to drive these other applications, is a considerable investment. The cost of such a system will most likely decrease over time. Operating rooms of the future will be constructed with computer network capabilities already in place. Hardware and software costs will also diminish, and the availability of sophisticated information management systems is likely in the near future.

The handwritten anesthesia record has served anesthesia care providers well for many years. The demands on the anesthesia record continue to increase, however; and accompanying them is the need for a legible, accurate, and complete anesthesia record. It is questionable whether even the most diligent clinician can maintain an adequate anesthesia record, especially during a crisis, when an accurate record is vital.

The process of anesthesia record-keeping has been automated, but the solutions present their own set of problems. AARK technology is currently in an intermediate phase of development. There is little doubt that an AARK will ultimately become a standard part of the anesthesia workstation. A survey of anesthesia practitioners at the 1990 Annual Meeting of the American Society of Anesthesiologists[24] revealed that 34% of those surveyed (104/306) rated AARKs as the technique they would most like to adopt in the future.

Given the complexity of AARK systems, the overall cost will probably not diminish greatly. The capabilities of these systems are certain to improve. Acceptance into clinical practice will be driven by improvements in technology, integration of the AARK with other equipment, and addressing the many information management problems facing modern anesthesia practice.

REFERENCES

1. Gravenstein JS: The uses of the anesthesia record, *J Clin Monit* 5:256-265, 1989.
2. Beecher HK: The first anesthesia records, *Surg Gynecol Obstet* 71:689-693, 1940.

3. Gravenstein JS: The automated anesthesia record, *Int J Clin Monit Comput* 3:131-134, 1986.

4. Whitcher C: *Advantages of automated record keeping*. In Gravenstein JS, Newbower RA, Ream AK, et al, editors: *The automated anesthesia record and alarm systems*, Boston, 1987, Butterworths.

5. Kennedy PJ, Feingold A, Wiener EL, et al: Analysis of tasks and human factors in anesthesia for coronary artery bypass, *Anesth Analg* 55:374-377, 1976.

6. Boquet G, Bushman JA, Davenport HT: The anaesthetic machine: a study of function and design, *Br J Anaesth* 52:61-67, 1980.

7. Meijler AP: *Automation in anesthesia: a relief? a systematic approach to computers in patient monitoring*, New York, 1987, Springer-Verlag, p 23.

8. Zollinger RM, Kreul JF, Schneider AJL: Man-made versus computer-generated anesthesia records, *J Surg Res* 22:419-424, 1977.

9. Lerou JGC, Dirksen R, van Daele M, et al: Automated charting of physiological variables in anesthesia: a quantitative comparison of automated versus handwritten anesthesia records, *J Clin Monit* 4:37-47, 1988.

10. Cock RI, McDonald JD, Nunziata E: Differences between handwritten and automatic blood pressure records, *Anesthesiology* 71:385-390, 1989

11. Edsall DW: Analysis and frequency of artifacts generated by anesthesia information management systems, *Anesthesiology* 73:A481, 1990 (abstract).

12. Stanley TE, Smith LR, White WD, et al: Incidence of vital sign artifact in automated anesthesia records, *Anesthesiology* 73:A483, 1990 (abstract).

13. Yablok DO: Comparison of vigilance using automated versus handwritten records, *Anesthesiology* 73:A416, 1990 (abstract).

14. Gravenstein N, Feldman JM: Anesthesia records and automation, *Semin Anesth* 8:119-129, 1989.

15. Drui AB, Behm RJ, Martin WE: Predesign investigation of the anesthesia operational environment, *Anesth Analg* 52:584-591, 1973.

16. Gibbs RF: The present and future medicolegal importance of record keeping in anesthesia and intensive care: the case for automation, *J Clin Monit* 5:251-255, 1989.

17. Morris C: *Legal aspects of monitoring*, In Gravenstein JS, Newbower RS, Ream AK, et al, editors: *The automated anesthesia record and alarm systems*, Boston, 1987, Butterworths, pp 270-271.

18. Apple HP, Schneider AJL, Fadel J: Design and evaluation of a semiautomatic anesthesia record system, *Med Instrum* 16:69-71, 1982.

19. Newbower RS, Cooper JB, Martin PJ: *A digitizing tablet for data entry in computer-assisted anesthesia record keeping*. In Gravenstein JS, Newbower RS, Ream AK, et al, editors: *The automated anesthesia record and alarm systems*, Boston, 1987, Butterworths, pp 99-107.

20. Klocke H, Inform D, Trispel S, et al: An anesthesia information system for monitoring and record keeping during surgical anesthesia, *J Clin Monit* 2:246-261, 1986.

21. Prakash O, van der Borden SG, Meij SH, et al: A microcomputer based charting system for documentation of circulatory, respiratory and pharmacological data during anesthesia, *Int J Clin Monit Comput* 1:155-160, 1984.

22. Feldman JM: Computerized anesthesia recording systems, *Adv Anesth* 6:325-354, 1989.

23. Figler AA, Stead SW: The medical information bus, *Biomed Instrum Technol* 24:101-111, 1990.

24. Profile of Anesthesiologists, *Anesthesiology News* 17(1):30, 1991.

Chapter 20

COMPUTERS AND SIMULATORS IN ANESTHESIA

Part I: Computers
Jan J. van der Aa, Ph.D.

Part II: Simulators
Joachim S. Gravenstein, M.D.

Part I: Computers in anesthesia

The proverbial computer revolution is history. We now take computers for granted, but it has been only 50 years since the first electronic computer (ENIAC) was operational. This computer weighed 30 tons, required more than 1500 square feet of floor space, and contained well over 18,000 vacuum tubes. Today's computers have undergone revolutionary changes in size, speed, power consumption, design, cost, and capabilities. As a result, their application is widespread, pervading almost every aspect of medicine. This chapter gives an overview of the basic functions of computers and some of their applications in anesthesiology. Although still in the early stages of development, people have made some imaginative uses of computers in order to create training devices and simulators for anesthesiologists.

WHAT IS A COMPUTER?

A computer is predominantly an electronic device that executes at high speed a sequence of operations according to a set of instructions. The two types of computer in current use are analog and digital. They differ primarily in the manner in which they perform computations and comparisons. Analog computers are circuits designed to process electronic signals to achieve a particular result. A simple example of an analog computer is the circuit built into an invasive blood pressure monitor that will electronically derive a mean blood pressure from the arterial waveform signal. Generally, analog computers are not programmable.

Most of the computers with which anesthesiologists are familiar are digital, a typical example being the common personal computer. The digital computer can understand and manipulate only symbols that consist of a series of digits. A digital computer responds to a series of yes or no (0 or 1) instructions. Because it can manipulate these 0's and 1's at blinding speed, the digital computer can outperform any human being when it comes to large numbers of calculations. The trick is to arrange the series of 0's and 1's so that they represent whatever needs to be symbolized. For example, the 0's and 1's could be arranged to designate a special code (instructions) that actually tells the computer what to do next and with what data. In contrast to the analog computer, the digital computer is programmable and these instructions are what make the computer programmable.

Programmability is the most important aspect of the digital computer and what distinguishes it from being just an extremely fast calculator. The computer can change the sequence in which the instructions are executed depending on the outcome of decisions made within the machine or on data from the outside world. A program (i.e., a structured sequence of instructions) tells the computer to store symbols made out of many rows of mixed 0's and 1's that are kept in an electronic storage system until needed.

In computer language, a bit (*bi*nary digi*t*) is used to refer to a 0 or a 1. A nibble is a series of 4 bits and a byte is a series of 8 bits. Finally, words are used to describe multiple bytes such as kilo and mega. Because the bits and bytes can be manipulated in many different ways, the computer can be adapted to perform a variety of tasks. The programmers devise specific rules that arrange and shuffle the bits, nibbles, and bytes so that one can use the computer to do word-processing, make complex calculations, or record variables from a monitor during anesthesia.

HOW DOES A DIGITAL COMPUTER WORK?

A computer consists of two main ingredients: hardware and software. The hardware includes such components as the electronic circuit boards, storage devices, keyboard, and display screen. These are generally the physical pieces of equipment. Software, on the other hand, consists of the series of instructions that enables the computer to execute its many functions.

Hardware

The computer's main component is the microprocessor, which is essentially the computer. Modern microprocessors are built onto a single silicon chip that is referred to as a "computer chip" (Fig. 20-1). The most important part of a microprocessor is the central processing unit (CPU), which consists of a number of electrical circuits. The CPU coordinates all of the computer's activities. The CPU contains areas called *registers* that are capable of temporary data storage. The CPU can assign special functions to specific registers. For example, one register (program counter) may be designated to hold the next instruction, while another register (accumulator) may be designated to receive only the results of the last operation performed.

Directly attached to the CPU is the computer's main memory. The memory is the computer's method of storing data. The computer memory is divided into two categories: random access memory (RAM) and read only memory (ROM). RAM and ROM differ in that in RAM the data can be changed and are stored only as long as there is a continuous power supply, whereas in ROM the data have been programmed ("burned in ROM"), cannot be changed, and are not dependent on electrical power to maintain memory.[1,2] The capacity of the ROM and RAM is determined by the number of bytes of data that can be stored in the specific memory chip or set of chips. The units are bytes, kilobytes (1 kbyte = 1024 bytes), megabytes (1 mbyte = 1024 × 1024 bytes), and gigabytes (1 gbyte = 1024 × 1 mbyte). The computer can obtain and manipulate data from both RAM and ROM memory; however, results can be stored only in RAM.

Other pieces of hardware include devices capable of bulk data storage as well as input/output (I/O) devices. Data can be stored in a variety of forms. These include magnetic (floppy and hard) disks, optical disks (CD-ROM disks), cassettes, and reels of tape. Data in RAM can be stored permanently on a magnetic disk, where they can be retrieved or modified and are no longer sensitive to power interruptions.

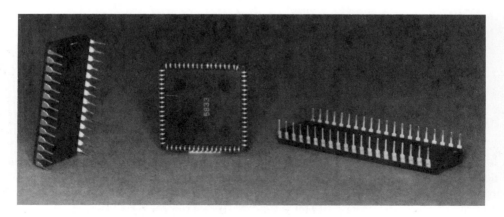

Fig. 20-1. Computer chips. The square chip in the center measures 1 cm × 1 cm.

The most familiar I/O devices include the keyboard, video display terminal (also called a cathode ray tube or CRT), and the popular mouse device. Input/output devices can also connect the computer to sensors that monitor pressure, temperature, and gas concentration in the operating room. Systems for voice recognition, voice synthesis, and even printers also fall into this category.

Software

The most important aspect of a digital computer is its programmability. Software refers to programs that control the operation of the computer. These are the step-by-step sequences of commands that instruct the computer to perform various functions. The program is actually a pattern of 0's and 1's (an algorithm) that is stored in the computer's main memory for subsequent execution. Programming is then the process of designing step-by-step algorithms that are useable by the computer. Today, the computer programmer no longer lists series of 0's and 1's but uses symbolic notations, known as assembly (machine) language. However, assembly language is still dependent on the machine's hardware design. High level languages were thus developed in order to achieve machine independence and to ease the writing of algorithms.

The program must first be decoded (inside the CPU) before it can be used, and this is the task of a series of programs that make up the operating system (OS). The functions of the operating system include loading the program into the main memory of the computer from one of the bulk storage devices; defining the way in which the user accesses the program, either with a keyboard or mouse; and ensuring that data to be printed are in fact sent to the printer. The OS echoes the keystrokes onto the computer screen for visual inspection. Pressing the "Enter" or the "Return" key then prompts the operating system to execute the command that has been entered by the user. Alternatively, a mouse can be moved across a flat surface to position a cursor at a specific place on the computer screen. A button is then clicked to indicate the desired position and that the particular command is to be executed. In many microcomputers, the OS is stored partly in ROM and partly loaded from the disk. Some examples of popular operating systems include MS-DOS, OS/2, VMS, Macintosh Operating System and Finder and UNIX.

To develop software that works well with the hardware to accomplish a specific task requires the services of a computer programmer. Programmers must work with clinicians when designing applications for computers in medicine. For example, it is relatively easy to write a program to keep track of blood pressure values on an anesthesia record. However, in order to make it truly useful, an integrated anesthesia record-keeper requires a coordinated effort between the programmer and the anesthesiologist.

MICROPROCESSORS

A microprocessor can be viewed as an inexpensive miniaturized version of a computer. Modern powerful microprocessors are built onto a single tiny piece of silicon and fitted into a plastic package as small as 2 square centimeters. Typically, this package has many electrical connections that accept inputs and provide outputs for other electrical components and communicate with the microprocessor's internal circuitry. In computer language this package is referred to as a "computer chip" (Fig. 20-1). When the appropriate RAM and ROM components, input and output devices (e.g., keyboard and CRT), and a data storage device (e.g., hard or floppy disk) are added to the microprocessor, a general purpose computer system has been assembled.

COMPUTER CATEGORIES

Today's computers are of three main types: mainframe, minicomputer, and microcomputer. They differ in size, speed of operation, amount of data that can be stored, and the number of simultaneous users. The mainframe will allow more than 100 people to use the system at the same time, while the minicomputer can support 20 to 40 users. The microcomputer is essentially a personal or desktop computer.

The speed at which a microprocessor is able to process information is determined by the *clock-speed*. The faster the clock-speed, the more rapidly the computer is able to execute functions. Thus, a modern microcomputer with a clock-speed of 25 MHz is approximately five times faster than the original IBM-PC with a clock-speed of 4.77 MHz.

A *coprocessor* is a piece of hardware that can be added to a computer to augment the speed of its functions. The coprocessor can relieve the main microprocessor of tasks it was not specifically designed to perform. It can also allow multiple processors to be connected in parallel and cooperate in the execution of programs. Many computers incorporate a math coprocessor, which is useful when it is necessary to perform extensive mathematical calculations such as in a large spread-sheet program.

Intercomputer communication

With information routinely being stored in a large variety of computer systems and with many of these data banks being of interest to physicians, accessing that material has become a vital part of the clinician's practice. For example, a hospital information system contains demographic information about the patient, the results of all the clinical tests that were ordered, and even computerized ECG readings. On a larger scale, nationally maintained data banks exist such as the National Library of Medicine's MEDLINE, which contains over 20 years of biomedical literature. Historically, access to particular computer systems was only possible if one possessed a terminal (a combination of a CRT and keyboard) which was directly connected to a particular computer system through an electrical cable extending from the computer to the terminal. Intercomputer communication today uses a wide variety of techniques, ranging from satellite links to fiber optic links, but also to a great extent, the existing telephone system. The device that connects computer systems to telephone lines for information interchange is the modem (short for modulator-demodulator).

For communication with the outside world the computer can employ a number of schemes. Most of the time this communication involves an exchange of letters and numbers as they appear in a typewritten text. The American Standard Committee for Information Interchange (ASCII) has devised a standard for the sequence of bits for such alphanumerical characters. In this standard, each character is represented by a specific eight-bit code. Using specialized electrical circuits acting as an intermediary called an interface, these character codes can be transferred to and from other computers and peripherals. There are two basic methods whereby these eight-bit character codes can move across the interface: either one bit at a time or all eight bits traverse the interface at the same time. The first mode is referred to as serial, and the second mode as parallel communication.

Modems typically connect to a computer using the Electronics Industries Association standard for serial communications RS-232. This standard describes in terms of hardware how characters are transferred along the serial communication interface and allows for two different devices to exchange information. The speed at which a modem transfers data (in bits of data per second, BPS) is often referred to as the baud rate. For example, a 2400-baud modem is capable of sending and receiving 2400 bits of information per second. Although many use the baud rate to refer to the speed of data transfer, the baud rate actually refers to the number of state changes per second on the serial communication line.[3,4]

For parallel communications no real standard has emerged. For connecting printers to computers, the Centronics parallel interface has become popular, while data communication between computer and laboratory equipment is frequently accomplished by using the IEEE-488 standard.

In addition to the hardware, communication by the modem requires special software packages that enable micro-, mini-, and mainframe computers to communicate with each other. These software packages manage the communication between computer and modem and between modems. They also allow the user to transfer information between computers typically using a well-defined protocol such as X-MODEM or KERMIT.[5,6]

COMPUTERS AND ANESTHESIA

In the days when computers were expensive and occupied much space, the prevailing applications consisted of establishing and analyzing administrative data. For example, a system that has been in service for almost 20 years at the Karolinska Hospital in Stockholm, Sweden, has been described by Olsson.[7] In the early 1970s with the ap-

pearance of minicomputers which were the size of multidrawer file cabinets, a number of investigators began using the computer during anesthesia for monitoring purposes, record-keeping, and decision support. Typically, data from physiologic monitors were automatically transmitted from a number of operating rooms to a centrally located computer where the data were analyzed, stored, and prepared for an intraoperative alphanumeric and trend display. In many instances, an automated or semiautomated version of an anesthesia record-keeping system was also incorporated.[8-11] The DAME system at Duke University was one of the first large-scale systems that installed a network of interconnected, computer-based, integrated monitoring systems into each monitoring location. These monitoring stations were connected to a centrally located minicomputer.[12] In the area of gas monitoring, Severinghaus and his group developed a centrally placed mass-spectrometer system that, under computer control, analyzed respiratory gases from a number of operating rooms on a time-share basis.[13] Computers also played an important role in computer-assisted teaching and instruction.

FUTURE TRENDS

Even though computers are already used extensively in clinical practice, the development of schemes for the simultaneous assessment of multiple signals, the integration of information, and the provision of differential diagnoses is now the focus of many research projects. Alarm technology and artifact rejection are other areas currently under intensive investigation. Both voice and handwriting recognition are promising technologies. Artificial intelligence (AI) applications in medicine have been developed to assist the clinician primarily in the area of consultation. The best known of these is MYCIN, a program that provides advice for the diagnosis and treatment of sepsis and meningitis.[14] A consultant's opinions developed by Miller and called "Attending," is a computer program that offers a critique of anesthesia plans proposed by a clinician.[15]

Intraoperative applications include the automated detection of breathing system malfunctions, for example a leak, an obstruction, or an incompetent valve. A computer can monitor pressure, flow, and PCO_2 in the system and recognize if patterns of these variables suggest a failure in the anesthesia circle. Two approaches have been used for this. Van der Aa and his coworkers have developed a real-time expert system, and Westenskow and his coworkers use a neural network approach to obtain similar results.[16-19] It is quite likely that there will be steady growth in the application of artificial intelligence to anesthesia.

Other applications for computers include rapid, repeated calculations. For example the moment-by-moment concentration of carbon dioxide in a Mapleson breathing system can be determined by computer. To study this system a model is constructed that defines the components of the system in mathematical terms. For a breathing system this would include the volume, the resistance, and the compliance of the tubing. To bring the system alive, one has to specify where fresh gas is admitted to the system, what the total flow would be, the patient's carbon dioxide production, and the patient's compliance, lung volumes, respiratory rate, and inspired-to-expired ratio. With this information, it is possible to perform a continuous calculation of carbon dioxide values at any point in the system, which in turn makes it possible to draw capnograms.[20]

It is also possible to model the cardiovascular system and calculate hemodynamic variables on a moment-to-moment basis. Modeling is now used extensively in the developments of training devices and simulators, which are covered in the next section. For intraoperative management, computer-based models will become indispensable.

REFERENCES

1. Millman J, Grabel A: *Microelectronics,* New York, 1937, McGraw-Hill.
2. Horowitz P, Hill W: *The art of electronics,* Cambridge. Mass, 1989, Cambridge University Press.
3. Sherman K: *DATA communications: a user's guide,* Reston, Va, 1981, Reston Publishing Company.
4. McNamara J: *Technical aspects of data communication,* Bedford, Mass, 1982, Digital Press.
5. Campbell J: *"C" programmer's guide to serial communication,* Indianapolis, Ind, 1988, Howard W. Sams.
6. *KERMIT protocol manual,* New York, 1984, Columbia University Center for Computing Activities.
7. Olsson GL: An interactive information system for anesthesia, *Computing Anesth Intensive Care* 10:183, 1982.
8. Apple H, Schneider A, Fadel J: Design and evaluation of a semiautomatic anesthesia record system, *Med Instrum* 16:69-71, 1982.
9. Mitchell M: Automated anesthesia data management and record keeping, *Med Instrum* 16:279, 1982.
10. Meijler A: Automation in anesthesia-a relief, Berlin, 1987, Springer Verlag.
11. Gravenstein JS, Newbower R, Ream AK, et al: *The automated anesthesia record and alarm systems,* Stoneham, Mass, 1987, Butterworths.
12. Block F, Jr, Burton L, Rafal M, et al: Two computer-based anesthetic monitors: the Duke automatic monitoring equipment (DAME) and the microdome, *J Clin Monit* 1:30-51, 1985.
13. Severinghaus J, Ozanne G: Multi-operating room monitoring with one mass spectrometer, *Acta Anaesthesiol Scand* 70:186-187, 1978 (Suppl).
14. Shortliffe EH: *Computer-based medical consulting: MYCIN,* New York, 1976, Elsevier.
15. Miller PL: Critiquing anesthetic management: the ATTENDING computer system, *Anesthesiology* 58:362-369, 1983.
16. Orr JA, Westenskow DR: A breathing circuit alarm system based on neural networks, *Anesthesiology* 71:A339, 1989 (abstract).
17. Orr J: *An anesthesia alarm system based on neural networks,* Ph.D. dissertation, Department of Bioengineering, University of Utah, December, 1990.
18. van Oostrom JH, van der Aa JJ, Nederstigt JA, et al: Intelligent alarms in the anesthesia circle breathing system, *Anesthesiology* 71:A335, 1989 (abstract).
19. van der Aa JJ: *Intelligent alarms in anesthesia: a real time expert system application,* Ph.D. thesis, Department of Electrical Engineering, Eindhoven University of Technology, 1990.
20. Beneken JEW, Gravenstein N, Gravenstein JS, et al: Capnography and the Bain circuit I: a computer model, *J Clin Monit* 1:103-113, 1985.

Part II: Simulators in anesthesia

Many comparisons have been drawn between anesthesia and aviation, because in both fields complex machines are employed, in both numerous controls must be operated, and both pilots and anesthesiologists must respond rapidly when the circumstances call for action. The comparison falls short, however, for two reasons. First, pilots are not expected to fly sick airplanes and second, the mechanics of an aircraft are understood far better than the physiology of a patient. Despite these shortcomings in the comparison, anesthesiologists should learn as much from pilots and their education as possible. Enter the flight simulator.

In the early days of aviation the problem arose of how to demonstrate to fledgling pilots the operation of controls, and how to make them aware of the possible problems to be encountered (two-seater airplanes had yet to be built). The first, simple flight simulators were built for this purpose.

In the intervening decades these simulators have grown tremendously in size, complexity, and cost. From the outside, modern flight simulators do not look like an airplane, but on the inside, students can soon forget that they are not in a real cockpit. All instruments are computer-driven and show faithfully all functions ordinarily monitored in a cockpit. An integral part of the simulator is the hydraulically operated stilts that support the "cockpit" and enable it to tilt, shake, and vibrate the entire system. In the cockpit the pilots look out through windows that show them an airport as long as they are on the ground, and once airborne, a view of the landscape below, inclusive of clouds passing by as if the plane itself were in fact moving. The simulator also obeys all commands of the controls, or if called for by the simulated scenario, disobeys the controls simulating an emergency and thus challenging the pilot to control the situation. The airline industry has concluded that the use of simulators is quite cost-effective.[1] Pilots who can fly the simulator need fewer hours in real planes, which not only saves money, but also reduces the training period and risks to the pilots as well. Some of the emergency protocols that need to be exercised would put pilot and plane at risk if practiced in the air instead of in a simulator.

Pilots practice both routine operation and emergencies in the simulator, which can be repeated as often as necessary to reach a desired level of proficiency. Since emergencies are rare, the simulator offers an ideal opportunity to become acquainted with the symptoms of an emergency and to practice the optimal management of the situation according to a detailed protocol.

Clearly, anesthesiologists face similar challenges. They must be proficient with routine care, which is a challenge for the novice in the field. They must stay attuned to the symptoms of the rare complication and act quickly to get the patient out of trouble. In the past, anesthesia personnel and students learned both anesthetic routines and emergency protocols in the operating room, sometimes to the discomfort of the patient. Certain emergencies could be discussed only in theory, because it would be unthinkable to put the patient into danger only to demonstrate a particular situation.

The potential use of simulators in anesthesia was recognized early by Abrahamson and Denson, who built SIM I, the first full-fledged anesthesia simulator, in the late 1960s.[2] Because the system was bulky and expensive, and perhaps because the profession was not ready to embrace something controlled by a computer, SIM II never saw the light of day, and SIM I slipped into obscurity.

In the meantime, the use of computers in anesthesia has become more and more accepted. A number of investigators have introduced software packages that enable the user to study specific phases of anesthesia using a personal computer (PC). These were originally called simulators but now are best referred to as training devices.[3] This distinguishes them from the full-bodied simulators that consist of an anesthesia workstation with an anesthesia machine, monitors, and a mannequin. Training devices fulfill an important function that may be incorporated in a simulator, but need not be. Training devices for anesthesia and anesthesia simulators will be discussed separately.

ANESTHESIA TRAINING DEVICES

A wonderful training device that can show complex interactions of ventilation and circulation, without making use of ongoing mathematical computation, is exemplified by a plexiglass model that contains water or oil in compartments representing the functional residual capacity (FRC), the lung tissue group, the muscle group, and the vessel-rich group.[4] Each compartment is filled with either gas and water (the lung) or oil (vessel-rich group and muscle group) in amounts fit to embody the respective compartments of a 70-kg man. Cardiac output is mimicked by blowing gas through the interconnected system. This model can be ventilated and anesthetic agents added to the inspired gas and their concentrations can be analyzed in the inspired and expired gases (Fig. 20-2). This ingenious model serves as a splendid introduction to the complexities of uptake and distribution of gases because the student can watch the bubbles (representing blood flow) course through the compartments on their way back to the lungs where the gas will be exhaled and sampled. The student can feel the lung compliance and airway resistance and can see the effects of changing the FRC and cardiac output. The authors of this model have based its construction on data generated from biological experiments and mathematical calculations.

It is, of course, possible to represent in a computer program the various compartments, blood flow through the compartments, and gas uptake and distribution in the compartments based on electrical analogies. One of the earliest of such models was Gas Man prepared by Philip.[5,6] Gas Man can be run on a PC and enables the user to select the fresh gas flow with which to administer the desired con-

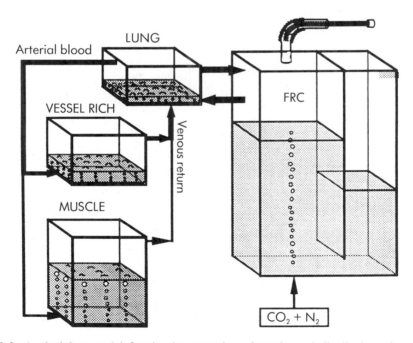

Fig. 20-2. A plexiglass model for the demonstration of uptake and distribution of anesthetic agents. A water-filled compartment (FRC) accepts mechanical ventilation from which gas is taken up and bubbled through boxes representing tissue compartments. (From Loughlin PA, Bowes WA, Westenskow DR: An oil-based model of inhalation anesthetic uptake and elimination, *Anesthesiology* 71:278-282, 1989.)

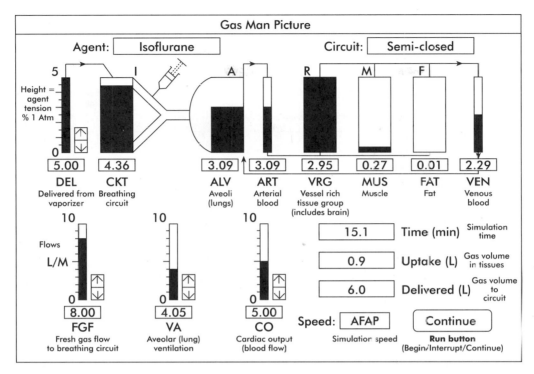

Fig. 20-3. Gas Man Picture display on the computer screen during operation of Gas Man. The user can select the type of circuit, agent, and concentrations of agent and can adjust fresh gas flow, alveolar ventilation, and cardiac output. (From Philip JH: *Gas Man: understanding anesthesia uptake and distribution,* Menlo Park, Calif, 1984, Addison-Wesley.)

centration of an anesthetic agent to a simulated person whose cardiac output and effective alveolar ventilation can be adjusted (Fig. 20-3). The system also allows a closed or semiclosed system configuration. It shows pictorially, numerically, and graphically the partial pressure of anesthetic in the breathing circuit, the alveoli, the arteries, the vessel-rich group, muscle, fat, and mixed venous blood, as well as the total gas volume taken up by the body and the total gas volume delivered to the breathing circuit. The user can also view the evolving partial pressures in the compartments in a graph with time on the abscissa and anesthetic partial pressure on the ordinate (Fig. 20-4). (See also Chapter 30.)

Calkins and coworkers have presented GUS, the acronym for a Gas Uptake Simulation program that also runs on a PC.[7] GUS calculates and displays gas concentrations in connective tissue, muscle, heart, brain, liver, kidney, fat, veins, lungs, and arteries, as well as inspired and expired concentrations of the different anesthetic agents and respiratory gases. The user can run the program for two different patients or two different agents at the same time. In this manner, the effects of different body size, ventilation settings, physiologic variables including cardiac output, and various shunts or different solubility constants can be demonstrated. The data can be displayed either with the help of a display of icons or a time vs. concentration graph (Fig. 20-5). A tutorial instructs the user on how to operate

the program. End-tidal and alveolar carbon dioxide concentrations can be demonstrated or the rate of elimination of the agent from a compartment or the anesthesia breathing circuit can be depicted.

Smith, et al. have taken a computer model that was originally analog and then hybrid* and converted it into a digital format.[8] This model is a complex physiologic and pharmacologic multiple transport model. Multiple means that it is actually several models working together. Transport means that it can carry anything in the blood or air, including gases and drugs. The gases, drugs, circulation, and respiration interact with each other. The digital model also incorporates injected drugs.

To the digital model, I/O devices (i.e., mouse and color monitor) have been added that allow access to the model. The monitor displayed a sketch of an operating room scene, complete with a patient, anesthesia machine and ventilator, monitors, infusions, and drugs. With the mouse, the user can place a mask, change the flowmeter settings, inject a drug, or control an infusion rate (Fig. 20-6).

Schwid and O'Donnell have developed an Anesthesia Simulator/Recorder (ASR) that, once again, runs on a PC.[9] It is designed to enable the anesthesiologist to practice the management of anesthetic incidents; for example,

---

*A hybrid computer is a combination of an analog and a digital computer. Although powerful, they are complex and temperamental.

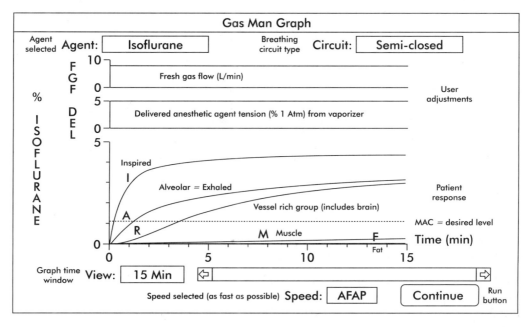

Fig. 20-4. Gas Man Graph showing the time course of the uptake and distribution exercise. (From Philip JH: *Gas Man: understanding anesthesia uptake and distribution,* Menlo Park, Calif, 1984, Addison-Wesley.)

the recognition of an esophageal intubation, anaphylaxis, or ST segment depression. The computer screen displays a patient surrounded by the usual instruments of the anesthesiologist's workplace (Fig. 20-7). Read-outs shown include a mass spectrometer, noninvasive sphygmomanometer, and pulse oximeter. Intravenous fluids, ventilator settings, and gas flowmeter controls are also displayed. Pharmacodynamic and pharmacokinetic as well as respiratory and cardiovascular physiologic models stand ready to respond to user input. The plasma concentration of more than 50 drugs can be estimated, and the effects of cardiovascular or respiratory insufficiency on the performance of the entire system can be demonstrated. At the end of the simulation run, or upon request, the system prints a summary for the user or an instructor for evaluation. The system has a "help" button that calls up clinical information to assist the user in the diagnosis and management of the simulated patient (Fig. 20-8).

ANESTHESIA SIMULATORS

The electronic training devices display the patient, instruments, and controls on computer screens. Whatever the user wished to administer or whatever control is to be changed must be conveyed to the system via a computer input (mouse, trackball, or keyboard). Anesthesia simulators also make extensive use of pharmacokinetic and pharmacodynamic models, as well as respiratory and cardiovascular models. Here, however, the user is confronted with a normal anesthesia workplace, including a functioning anesthesia machine with compressed gases, flowmeters, vaporizers, breathing circuit, valves, ventilator,

and the common anesthesia and physiologic monitors. The only deviation from reality is the patient, which is a plastic mannequin. The lungs, however, can breathe spontaneously or submit to manual or mechanical ventilation with the help of the anesthesia machine and its ventilator. Should the machine malfunction, the clinician can apply mouth-to-mouth or mouth-to-airway ventilation.

By 1992, two well-developed simulators had been exhibited. The Gainesville Anesthesia Simulator (presented by Good, et al.) contains a hybrid lung model (Fig. 20-9) that consumes oxygen, takes up or eliminates anesthetic agents, and exhales carbon dioxide. The mannequin can "breathe spontaneously" or the artificial lungs can be ventilated manually or mechanically.[10] A computer model of uptake and distribution receives the alveolar gas tensions in the mechanical lung gas blender to effect this exchange.[11-14] A mannequin challenges the anesthesiologist to manage the airway, auscultate the lungs and heart, and monitor the instruments for evidence of any developing problems.

While using the simulator, an instructor can initiate one of many clinical scenarios. Each scenario involves an active change in the function of one or another component of the simulator. For example, in one scenario a mechanical malfunction causes the FiO_2 to decrease. This is followed by falling levels of SpO_2, by cyanosis, and by tachycardia. The student is thus challenged to diagnose the source of the trouble and take appropriate actions to correct the problem. Sensors incorporated in the mannequin, the breathing circuit, and the controls of the anesthesia machine recognize what steps have been taken by the student.

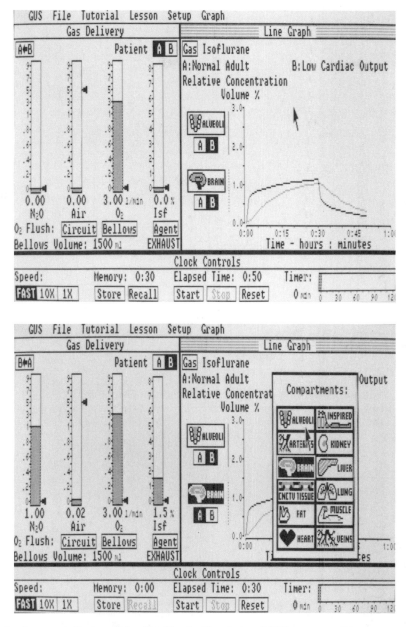

Fig. 20-5. Computer display of the Gas Uptake Simulation (GUS) program. The top panel shows an example of isoflurane washout from alveoli and brain. The bottom panel shows the compartments for which data are calculated.

If these steps are appropriate, the simulator control display will indicate that the source of the problem was correctly identified (for example a leak in the vaporizer). If the student does not find the origin of the problem, the instructor can explain the mechanisms that led to trouble using animated computer graphic displays that show the flow of gas through the anesthesia machine, breathing circuit, the ventilator, tracheal tube, and the patient's lungs and circulation (Fig. 20-10).

Gaba and his coworkers have developed CASE (Comprehensive Anesthesia Simulation Environment), a simulator including physiologic and pharmacologic models that also consists of an anesthesia machine, ventilator, and a sophisticated mannequin (Fig. 20-11).[15] The mannequin can be intubated, mechanically ventilated (by mask or tube), or auscultated, and it can regurgitate. An advanced feature of this current mannequin is that heart sounds are generated electronically and presented via four speakers

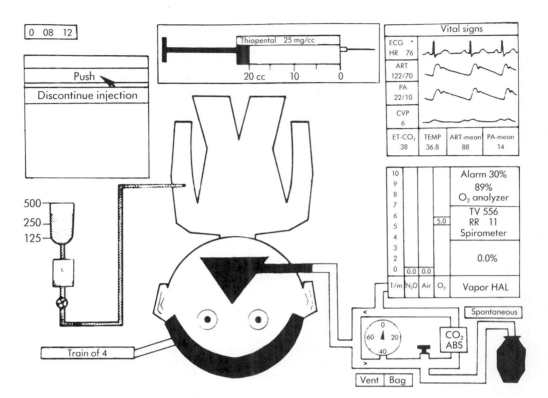

Fig. 20-6. Computer display of a training device that enables the user to inject, for example, thiopental and observe the simulated vital signs. (From Smith NT: *Mathematical model of uptake and distribution of inhalation anesthetic agents*. In Balagny E, Coseiller C, Cousin MT: *Anesthesia par inhalation,* Paris, 1987, Arnette Publishers, pp 87-118.)

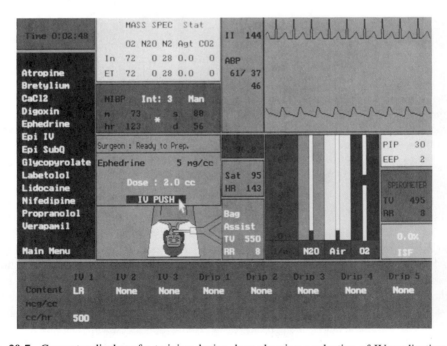

Fig. 20-7. Computer display of a training device, here showing a selection of IV medications. (From Schwid HA, O'Donnell D: The anesthesia simulator-recorder: a device to train and evaluate anesthesiologists' responses to critical incidents, *Anesthesiology* 72:191-197, 1990.)

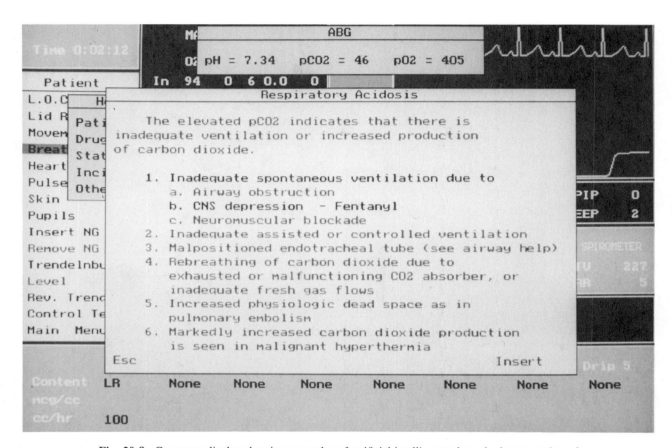

Fig. 20-8. Computer display showing examples of artificial intelligence; here the interpretation of clinical data. (From Schwid HA, O'Donnell D: The anesthesia simulator-recorder: a device to train and evaluate anesthesiologists' responses to critical incidents, *Anesthesiology* 72:191-197, 1990.)

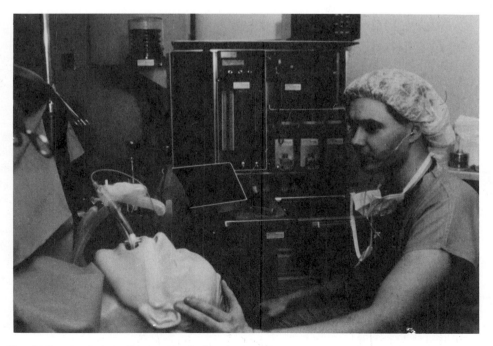

Fig. 20-9. The Gainesville Anesthesia Simulator. The computers are hidden. The anesthesia machine has been modified but this is not visible. Ventilator and monitors are standard instruments accepting input from the "patient's" respired gases or from computers.

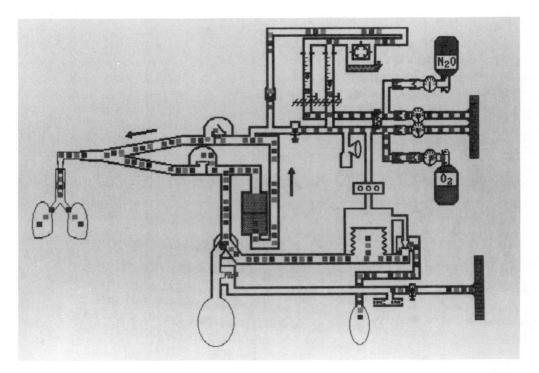

Fig. 20-10. Animated computer graphics of an anesthesia machine and breathing circuit used during didactic exercises after completion of a simulator run in the Gainesville Anesthesia Simulator.

CASE 1.2

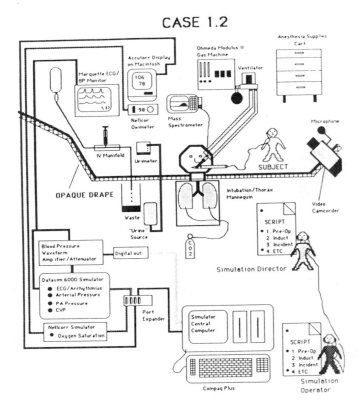

Fig. 20-11. Schematic diagram of the Comprehensive Anesthesia Simulation Environment (CASE) 1.2 system. The simulator provides input to all significant patient monitors. A mannequin allows tracheal intubation and provides certain clinical signs. The system is coordinated by a central computer that is controlled by a simulation operator and an anesthesiologist simulator director working from a script.

mounted on the chest. The software executes physiologic and pharmacologic models in parallel and in real-time using parallel processors called transputers. An instructor's workstation facilitates the conduct of the training exercise. In the use of CASE, the role of a surgeon can be played by an impatient instructor, to add tension to the simulation (Fig. 20-12).

A LOOK INTO THE FUTURE

Training devices and simulators have come of age in anesthesia. What role they will play in the future remains to be seen. Some expectations are as follows.

Training devices in education

Training devices require no more than a PC and a diskette with the necessary software and, thus, can be acquired by individual clinicians and made available in every department. This includes not only academic institutions with residency training programs, but also private practices. With computers becoming ubiquitous, several clinicians can make use of training programs simultaneously in classroom settings, lounges, offices, or wherever a suitable PC can be found.

Some new drugs have already been introduced with the help of a training program that enables the clinician to explore the pharmacokinetics and dynamics of the new agent. The program includes exercises that present patients with certain problems targeted by the new agent. The same could be done with new electronic monitoring devices. For example, the complex physics of the transesophageal

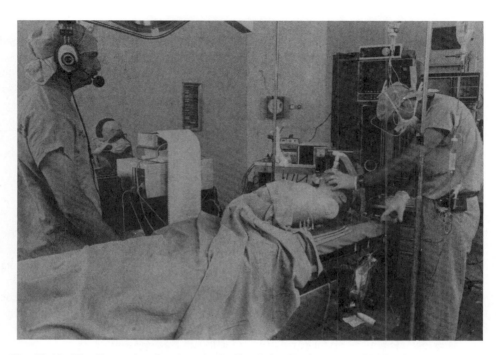

Fig. 20-12. The Comprehensive Anesthesia Simulation Environment (CASE) showing the anesthesiologist on the right and two instructors, one of whom is playing the role of a surgeon in a training exercise.

echocardiograph (TEE), the anatomical relationships of the various projections, and the appearance of different clinical entities in the TEE can all be demonstrated with the help of training programs. Tutorials addressing particular issues, such as a new management protocol for the immunologically suppressed patient, could be presented in a training program. A great advantage of such programs is their 24-hour availability. They enable clinicians to interact with the program and to analyze their performance, and it can be rerun until the user feels in command of all the material. Services would probably be developed that would offer updates of these training diskettes to subscribers and, thus, provide clinicians very flexible opportunities for continuing medical education.

Training devices as emulators

Despite the sophistication of current training programs, they currently cannot be used for a "trial run," to see how a certain patient might react to a specific amount of a drug or a hemorrhage of 1000 ml. Our limited knowledge of the complexities of human physiology, genetic differences, unknown aspects of a patient's disease, and the uptake and distribution of drugs make it impossible to prepare mathematical models that would predict how a *specific* patient would respond to anesthesia and surgery. However, if the data on an individual patient's response to the injection of a drug or the inhalation of an anesthetic are collected, it is then possible to predict (at least for a matter of minutes) how that patient would respond to another injection of the drug, change of dose, or change in the concentration

of the anesthetic. In the future, it may be possible to collect comprehensive data from a patient during anesthesia and then estimate after the fact how that patient might have fared with different anesthetic management. Such an exercise would be of great value. A computer performing these functions might be called an emulator, even though it would still fit into the larger category of a training device.

Simulators and education

The limited experience with the two existing anesthesia simulators in the United States make future predictions difficult. At this time, there are no scientific data to support the claim that simulators actually improve patient care. Such improvements in care could come either by permitting novices to practice their skills on inanimate systems rather than on patients, or by enabling training programs to graduate anesthesiologists who commit fewer errors than their predecessors who had learned their profession without the benefit of simulators. Also, at this time it is not possible to demonstrate that simulators shorten the training period for clinical personnel or render it less expensive than in the past. A potential drawback of simulator exercises is that students might learn rote responses to certain problems rather than an in-depth analysis of the problem as a whole. The analysis of two problems that are basically different but superficially similar might require entirely different responses from those taught in a typical simulator scenario. When more simulators are in use, prospective studies assessing their value in anesthesia should be forthcoming. The investigators have observed that those individuals who have been exposed to training sessions in the simulator have found them to be a positive experience.

Considerable obstacles will have to be overcome, however, before simulators can become universal aids in the education and training of anesthesia personnel. The biggest is the current cost of simulation. Even without the cost of software development, the cost of an anesthesia simulator alone exceeds $100,000 (1992 estimate). This price includes the cost of a modern anesthesia machine, full complement of monitors, a mannequin, a mechanical lung, and the computers required to run the system. Added to this is the recurring cost of instructors who run the simulation and personnel to maintain the system. Finally, simulators are bulky. Storing them where they would be readily accessible to anesthesia personnel, namely in the vicinity of an operating room, increases the cost. Consequently, simulators must be run with great efficiency as is true for the flight simulators in the aviation industry.

Many flight simulators of modern commercial jets are operated for 22 hours every day, leaving 2 hours per day for upgrading and preventive maintenance. It is probably not possible for even large departments to use the simulator with the same degree of efficiency as the airlines. Assuming that there are 2000 routine working hours in a year, if each resident were to spend 16 hours per year in the simulator and every faculty member would spend 8 hours per year, then a department with 100 residents and 50 faculty would occupy the simulator for these 2000 hours. For smaller departments regional centers could be established or simulators could be housed in a van so that they could be taken to individual hospitals or various medical meetings.

An alternative would be to develop component parts that could be attached to clinical anesthesia equipment to enable it to run a simulator exercise. It would be absolutely crucial to ensure that the simulator components could not be used in patient care. Regional instructors would be required to conduct the simulator exercises.

Although these difficulties are well recognized and the benefits of simulation have yet to be proven, the apparent advantages of the simulator have induced a number of educators to actively search for a means of establishing local or regional simulation capabilities. Indeed, suggestions have been made that anesthesia training programs in the future would include training devices and simulation integrated into the program. Training devices would be utilized to teach residents such things as the fundamentals of uptake and distribution of anesthetic agents, the anatomy of anesthesia machines and ventilators, the pharmacodynamics and pharmacokinetics of drugs in patients with different diseases, and the underlying engineering principles of modern monitors. Once these subjects have been mastered, the resident would be moved into the simulator. In 1991 an experiment in education by simulation was conducted at the Department of Anesthesiology of the University of Florida. To half of the new residents, a 10-hour curriculum was taught with the simulator, and to the other half, the traditional curriculum.[16] The simulator exercises were so well received by residents and faculty that the following year the department began using simulator exercises for all incoming residents during the first 6 weeks of their residency. Routine general anesthesia (induction, maintenance, and emergence) and anesthesia-related problems (airway, hypoxemia, hypotension) are the key experiences practiced with the simulator.

Simulators and certification

Over the years two types of certification have been established: one on the local level and the other on the national level. On the local level, the hospital, in response to requirements of the Joint Commission on Accreditation of Healthcare Organizations, lists the procedures that a physician is authorized to perform in the institution. At this time, it is rare to actually check whether physicians are capable of carrying out the procedures listed by them on their application for privileges. As more and more complex equipment is introduced into clinical practice, the question arises as to whether the practitioner should demonstrate competence in the use of the equipment. Training devices provide the opportunity to learn about the equipment while skill with the equipment can be gained by using simulators.

On the national level, simulators may some day play a role in specialty certifying examinations. Much work needs to be done before this can be recommended or introduced. Once a sufficient number of clinical scenarios have been incorporated into the repertoire of simulators, scenarios could be tested and the validity of examining candidates in the simulator could be established or rejected. Before adoption of simulation in the examination process, it would be necessary to show that the anticipated benefits (improved examination) justify the cost (equipment and personnel).

Simulators and technology

Simulators can be used to test the performance of new anesthesia machines, ventilators, and monitors. These tests can assess the clinical adequacy of the function of the new device, as well as design features. For example, under certain specific conditions, the flaw in the algorithm of a capnograph may cause the capnogram to obscure an important clinical feature. While such a flaw might not be discovered by the manufacturer, it might come to light when the instrument is tested in the simulator.

Similarly, the simulator can be used by clinicians to test prototypes of new devices and comment on the advantages or shortcomings in the human engineering of these devices. This would help manufacturers to develop a clinically more useful piece of equipment. The simulator could potentially decrease the manufacturers' cost of developing and marketing a new product, since design errors could be discovered and corrected before the product was marketed.

Research in human factors

Gaba's discussion of the use of simulators in the study of human performance in anesthesia points out that people will make both slips and mistakes.[17] A slip occurs when one mistakenly injects a drug other than the intended one by picking up the wrong syringe. A mistake occurs when a decision is made that can harm the patient. Gaba and co-workers used a simulator to expose clinicians to the stresses of an anesthesia disaster and then analyzed the factors that contributed to slips and mistakes. Preventable anesthesia disasters are usually multifactorial in origin and, thus, are difficult to study in life where analysis after the fact usually leaves many questions unanswered. In the simulator, it is possible to recreate identical circumstances for the testing of different clinicians, or for the testing of one variable that can be studied by keeping all but one factor constant. Contributing factors can be tested, such as equipment design, environment, organization of the team, education of personnel, effect of fatigue or drugs, as well as the personality of individuals involved in the case.

While candidates for anesthesia residencies are selected on the basis of many different factors, simulators may someday be useful in screening applicants for specific abilities. The potential uses for training devices and simulators in anesthesiology are just beginning to be appreciated. Further development and refinement of these devices will undoubtedly ensure their role in the education of every anesthesiologist.

Current simulators are too bulky and too costly to be cost effective if used by only the members even of a single large department. Yet, simulators offer unique training opportunities that should be made available to large numbers of clinicians who wish to practice the management of scenarios that cannot be created in the operating room without putting the patient at risk, or without causing delays in the schedule or inconveniences to the patient and clinical team. As long as simulators are as bulky and costly as is presently the case, simulators must either travel, perhaps in a van, from one meeting or institution to the next, or centers must be established that make simulator training available. Simulators are new to anesthesia and the profession will have to learn what they can offer. Gaba and De-Anda have examined the responses of anesthesiologists to challenges in the operating room.[15,17] Such studies can further the understanding of human factors that lead to problems in the operating room.

REFERENCES

1. Beach EB: *A case for simulation in cost-effective training.* In Gravenstein JS, Holzer JF, editors: *Safety and cost containment in anesthesia,* Boston, 1988, Butterworths, pp 201-205.
2. Denson JS, Abrahamson S: A computer-controlled patient simulator, *JAMA* 208:504-508, 1969.
3. Andrews DH: Relationships among simulators, training devices, and learning: a behavioral view, *Educ Tech* 28:48-54, 1988.
4. Loughlin PJ, Bowes WA, Westenskow DR: An oil-based model of inhalation anesthetic uptake and elimination, *Anesthesiology* 71:278-282, 1989.
5. Philip JH: *Gas Man: understanding anesthesia uptake and distribution,* Menlo Park, Calif, 1984, Addison-Wesley.
6. Garfield JM, Paskin S, Philip JH: An evaluation of the effectiveness of a computer simulation of anaesthetic uptake and distribution as a teaching tool, *Med Educ* 23:457-462, 1989.
7. *Gas Uptake Simulation (GUS) User reference,* No 18602-002 A, Release 3.0, Phoenix, 1987, Medical Education Inc.
8. Smith NT: *Mathematical model of uptake and distribution of inhalation anaesthetic agents.* In Balagny E, Coseiller C, Cousin MT: *Anesthesia par inhalation,* Paris, 1987, Arnette, pp 87-118.
9. Schwid HA, O'Donnell D: The anesthesia simulator-recorder: a device to train and evaluate anesthesiologists' responses to critical incidents, *Anesthesiology* 72:191-197, 1990.
10. Lampotang S, Gravenstein N, Banner MJ, et al: A lung model of carbon dioxide concentrations with mechanical or spontaneous ventilation, *Crit Care Med* 14:1055-1057, 1986.
11. Good ML, Gravenstein JS: Anesthesia simulators and training devices. In Pierce EC Jr, editor: *Risk management in anesthesia,* vol 27, *International anesthesiology clinics,* Boston, Fall 1989, Little, Brown, pp 161-166.
12. Good ML, Lampotang S, Gibby GL, et al: Critical events simulation for training in anesthesiology, *J Clin Monit* 4:140, 1988.
13. Good ML, Lampotang S, Ritchie G, et al: Hybrid lung model for use in anesthesia research and education, *Anesthesiology* 71:A982, 1989 (abstract).
14. Heffels JJM: A patient simulator for anesthesia training: a mechanical lung model and a physiological software model, Eindhoven University of Technology Research Reports, January 1990.
15. Gaba DM, DeAnda A: A comprehensive anesthesia simulation environment: recreating the operating room for research and training, *Anesthesiology* 69:387-394, 1988.
16. Good ML, Gravenstein JS, Mahla ME, et al: Can simulation accelerate the learning of basic anesthesia skills by beginning anesthesia residents? *Anesthesiology* 77:A1133, 1992 (abstract).
17. Gaba DM: Human error in anesthesia mishaps. *Int Anesthesiol Clin* 27:137-147, Fall 1989.

Chapter 21

LASERS AND ELECTRICAL SAFETY IN THE OPERATING ROOM

Part I: Lasers
Annette G. Pashayan, M.D.

Part II: Electrical Safety
Jan Ehrenwerth, M.D.

Part I: Lasers

The increasingly widespread use of lasers during surgery requires that all operating room personnel become familiar with the potential hazards associated with this product of modern science. This chapter will introduce clinicians to the major risks and safety precautions associated with laser use and emphasizes those risks with laser surgery of the airway.

MEDICAL LASERS AND THEIR APPLICATIONS

The word "laser" is an acronym for Light Amplification of the Stimulated Emission of Radiation. Laser light is produced when energy is directed at a "lasing medium." The lasing medium lends its name to the laser, for instance in the case of the CO_2 laser, electrical energy is aimed at carbon dioxide molecules. The lasing medium also determines the wavelength of light that will be produced by the instrument. When the lasing medium is stimulated by electricity, the electrons in the molecular orbit are excited and change orbital patterns in such a way as to emit energy in the form of light. Light produced in this fashion is known as "coherent radiation" because it is spatially and tempo-

Table 21-1. Lasers commonly used in the operating room

Laser	Wavelength (nanometers)	General considerations
Argon	488-515 (blue/green)	Absorbed selectively by hemoglobin and melanin or other similar pigments Transmitted through clear substances Tissue penetration: 0.5 to 2 mm
KTP* (frequency-doubled YAG)	532(green)	Strongly absorbed by hemoglobin, melanin, and similar pigments Transmitted through clear substances Tissue penetration: 0.5 to 2 mm
Dye laser	Variable with dyes	Wavelength can be tuned to suit application; e.g., 585 nm (yellow) for hemoglobin absorption and 630 nm (red) for photodynamic therapy
Nd:YAG†	1064 (near infrared)	More readily absorbed by dark tissue Transmitted through clear fluids Tissue penetration: 2 to 6 mm
CO_2	10,600 (far infrared)	Strongly absorbed by water and thus by all tissue, pigmented or not Tissue penetration: <0.5 mm
He-Ne‡	633 (red)	Used as a low-power coaxial aiming beam for nonvisible lasers (CO_2 and Nd:YAG) Has no significant tissue interaction

*Potassium titanyl phosphate
†Neodymium-doped yttrium-aluminum-garnet.
‡Helium-neon.

rally coherent,* collimated,† and monochromatic.‡ Coherent light can be focused into spots in which the power density is so great that the concentrated light can cut and vaporize tissue.

The way in which a particular laser interacts with tissue depends on the laser's wavelength as well as on its power density (Table 21-1). The CO_2 laser produces wavelenths of 10,600 nm, which is in the far infrared portion of the electromagnetic spectrum. This long wavelength is strongly absorbed by water, blood, and all biological tissue within a very shallow depth of penetration. Scatter and reflection of the CO_2 laser beam is negligible, and therefore little heat is dissipated to surrounding tissue. For this reason, the CO_2 laser is favored for procedures in which a precise incision is important, particularly operations involving the airway as well as neurosurgery and general, plastic, and gynecologic surgery.

The tunable dye laser beam uses as the lasing medium a liquid organic dye dissolved in an alcoholic solvent. An intense light source, such as another laser, is used to excite the dye solution, which then emits light over a range of wavelengths. Special tuning elements inserted into the laser produce each specific wavelength. Such lasers are used

for treatment of such dermatological conditions as portwine stains, in which case they are tuned either for 577 nm (yellow-green) or 585 nm (yellow) in order to be selectively absorbed by hemoglobin.[1] The tunable dye laser can also be used for photodynamic therapy when its wavelength is tuned to 630 nm (red); certain light-sensitive chemotherapeutic agents, when applied topically or injected, react when exposed to this wavelength and selectively destroy malignant tissue.

The neodymium-doped yttrium-aluminum-garnet (Nd:YAG) laser produces a wavelength of 1064 nm, which is in the near infrared portion of the spectrum (Table 21-1). This wavelength is considerably shorter than that of the CO_2 laser. The Nd:YAG laser light is weakly absorbed by water, and the beam is more scattered through tissue. Of the commonly used lasers, this particular instrument provides the deepest penetration, from 2 to 6 mm, and has a greater thermal effect. It is therefore well suited for tissue coagulation and debulking of tumors. Because the Nd:YAG laser's wavelength can be transmitted through fiberoptic cables, the laser can be passed through an endoscope to various sites within the body, including the tracheobronchial tree.

The potassium titanyl phosphate (KTP) laser produces wavelengths (532 nm) in the visible emerald-green portion of the electromagnetic spectrum (Table 21-1). The KTP laser is also called the frequency doubled YAG because its beam is produced by passing an Nd:YAG (1064 nm) beam through a potassium titanyl phosphate crystal to result in a

*Light where the photons are all of the same wavelength and maintain a relationship that is constantly in phase with each other.
†The property of a beam of light describing to what extent its photons move in a single direction. Thus, a highly collimated beam does not disperse in diameter as it gets farther away from its source.
‡Light that consists of a single wavelength or color.

532-nm wavelength. These wavelengths are weakly absorbed by water and highly absorbed by blood. The depth of tissue of penetration is between that of the CO_2 and the Nd:YAG lasers. The KTP laser therefore shares properties with both, being relatively precise for incision and providing good coagulation. It has applications in otolaryngology, for operations on the upper airway, and in neurosurgery.

The argon laser produces a short wavelength (488 to 515 nm) in the visible blue-green portion of the electromagnetic spectrum. The short wavelength allows for a very small beam, which, because it is visible, obviates problems of misalignment that can occur with the CO_2 and Nd:YAG lasers. The absorbent, diffusive, and reflective properties of the argon laser vary with various tissues. It is highly absorbed by hemoglobin and pigmented tissues, transmitted through watery tissues, and scattered by inhomogeneous tissue. For this reason the argon laser is used for ophthalmological operations on the retina and posterior parts of the globe. The argon laser is also highly useful for photocoagulation in dermatology and plastic surgery, to coagulate gastrointestinal bleeding, and for some applications in otolaryngology and neurosurgery.

Helium-neon (He-Ne) lasers, which produce a visible red light, are incorporated into CO_2 and Nd:YAG lasers and function as an aiming beam for the invisible wavelengths. The alignment of the He-Ne beam with the active beam must be checked prior to surgical procedures to assure the active beam can be accurately directed.

HAZARDS ASSOCIATED WITH MEDICAL LASERS

The American National Standards Institute (ANSI)[2] has classified lasers by their potential hazards on the basis of their optical emissions (Table 21-2). Each classification specifies control measures commensurate with its relative hazard. Generally speaking, the higher the class, the more hazardous is the laser; thus class 4 lasers are the most haz-ardous: specular or diffuse reflection as well as direct contact may damage eyes or skin. These lasers are also fire hazards. Most medical lasers are class 4 lasers, and therefore health care workers must know the risks of and safety measures appropriate to these instruments. The laser is a source of collimated monochromatic radiation, which can directly injure the eyes and skin. Lasers can also produce respiratory injury from inhalation of chemical toxins emitted when tissue is vaporized or from fires. The high electrical output of the instrument can also cause electrocution.

The part of the eye damaged by a laser depends on the laser's wavelength. Light emitted from lasers in the far infrared portion of the electromagnetic spectrum (3 to 1 mm), such as the CO_2 laser, is highly absorbed by all surfaces. Exposure to a CO_2 laser beam can damage the outer layers of the eye and thus cause corneal ulceration and opacification. Laser light in the near ultraviolet portion of the electromagnetic spectrum (320 to 390 nm) is absorbed primarily by the lens; near ultraviolet laser light is not commonly used in the operating room. Light from the argon, KTP, and Nd:YAG lasers, in the wavelength range of 400 to 1400 nm, is transmitted through the cornea and lens and can thus damage the retina. Such lasers are particularly dangerous because as the light is transmitted through the lens it is actually superfocused, so that a beam of extremely high power density reaches the retina and choroid structures. The extent of eye injury, however, depends not only on the wavelength of the laser but also on how the beam is viewed. Direct intrabeam viewing (Fig. 21-1, *A*) is considered to be the most hazardous form of exposure, specular reflection (Fig. 21-1, *B*) is the next most hazardous, and diffuse reflection (Fig. 21-1, *C*) the least hazardous.

The best way to protect the eye from the laser is to avoid exposure to the laser. So that patients and health care personnel do not accidentally come into contact with the laser, a warning of laser use should be posted on the outside of the operating room in which a laser is being

Table 21-2. Classification established by the American National Standards Institute for Lasers and Laser Hazards

Class	Description	Examples	Control measures
1	Beam is totally contained and device cannot emit accessible laser radiation.	Lasers used in laboratories for diagnostic work	No
2	Low-power visible lasers that are not intended for prolonged viewing; the normal blink reflex will protect the eye.	He-Ne aiming beam for CO_2 and Nd:YAG lasers	Yes
3a	Normally would not pose a hazard if viewed momentarily with the unaided eye.	Some ophthalmologic lasers are higher class 3	Yes
3b	May produce a hazard if viewed directly (intrabeam viewing and specular reflection).		
4	Hazardous if viewed directly or from diffuse reflection. Also produces fire hazards and skin hazards.	Most medical lasers including CO_2, Nd:YAG, argon, and KTP	Yes

Reproduced with permission from American National Standards Institute: *American national standard for the safe use of lasers*, ANSI Z136.1, New York, 1986.

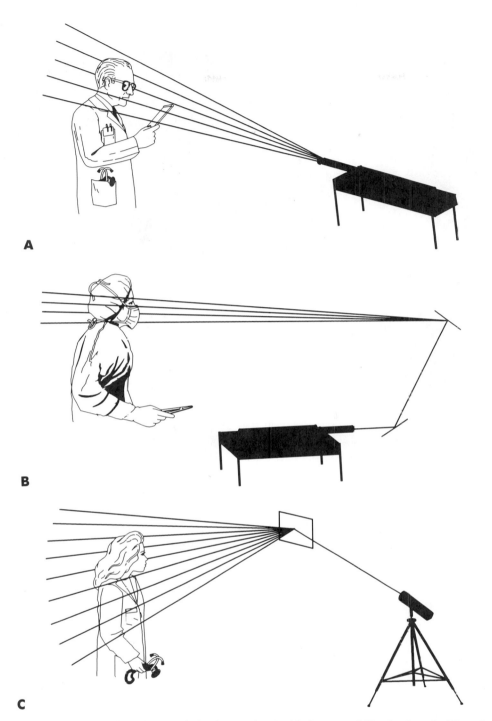

Fig. 21-1. The risk from laser radiation is associated with the type of illumination: **A,** Direct intrabeam viewing; **B,** specular reflection, where the angle of incidence equals or nearly equals the angle of reflection; **C,** diffuse reflection, where radiation is reflected over a wide range of angles.

used (Fig. 21-2). The sign should meet ANSI standards,[2] including specification of the laser wavelength in use, because only if the wavelength is known can the eyes be properly protected from the laser. Because far infrared radiation is absorbed by most surfaces, eyes can be protected from CO_2 laser radiation by any glasses or goggles. Laser beams of shorter wavelengths, however, including the argon, KTP, and Nd:YAG, require goggles of specific colors in order for the laser light to be absorbed. Such goggles should be appropriately labeled with the wavelength and power density for which they are protective. Tinted goggles may impair the anesthesiologist's ability to perceive subtle changes in the patient's skin color; therefore he/she depends on pulse oximetry to assess the patient's oxygenation.

Of less concern than eye damage is skin damage asso-

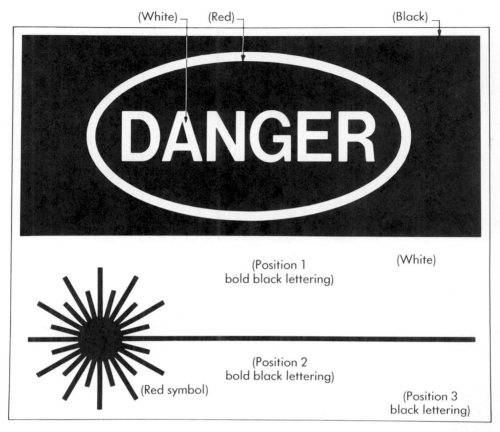

Fig. 21-2. Sample warning sign, with color requirements indicated, for certain class 3 and class 4 lasers. Numbered positions, always in bold lettering, correspond to specifications for wavelength of laser, class of laser, and eyewear requirements.

ciated with lasers,[2] which ranges from slight erythema to a full-thickness skin burn. Small, inconsequential burns of the surgeon's hands are a frequent problem accompanying laser use for surgery. More severe and extensive burns to the patient's skin near the surgical site can occur if drapes and flammable materials in the operating field ignite. Laser light, like other forms of electromagnetic radiation, may be mutagenic and thus may cause skin cancer. In order to prevent burns and accidental exposure during laser use the patient's skin around the operative field should be covered with wet towels.

Eye and skin damage can be further minimized by use of the appropriate type of surgical instrumentation. Routine surgical instruments for use in nonlaser surgery may have highly reflective, mirrorlike surfaces. Instruments with matte surfaces have been developed for use with lasers in order to diffuse reflected beams.

Vaporization of tissue by laser light produces smoke known as the *laser plume*. The laser plume, much like any smoke, can cause bronchial inflammation, and thus bronchospasm, in susceptible persons. Other reactions to the laser plume include lacrimation, nausea, and vomiting. The plume may contain mutagenic chemicals, much like cigarette smoke,[3] and also may carry such infectious agents as viral DNA.[4] For these reasons, laser plume should be removed from the operating room environment during such surgery by way of an evacuation system. In addition, personnel in the operating room should wear special laser masks, which prevent small particles from being inhaled into the tracheobronchial tree.

The laser hazard that is of greatest concern to the anesthesiologist is that of fires of the tracheal tube and breathing circuit, which can arise when lasers are used during airway operations. This particular topic is covered in greater detail in the following section.

CONSIDERATIONS DURING LASER SUGERY OF THE AIRWAY

Lasers are favored for resecting tumors and other obstructions of the airway because the laser enables very precise excision, which minimizes edema. Because the laser is an intense light that could provide an ignition source, laser surgery is associated with risk of fire[5,6] when flammable materials are used in the airway. This is especially true in the oxygen-rich or oxygen plus nitrous oxide–enriched atmosphere often used during general anesthesia. Although there is no absolute way to prevent a fire when a laser is used for airway surgery, guidelines and protocols have been developed to minimize the risk. The upper airway is considered separately from the trachea and bronchi because these areas require different approaches to airway management.

The upper airway

The CO_2 laser is most often used for operations on and around the larynx. Its beam is delivered through the operating microscope and directed by a micromanipulator. One approach to preventing fires when a laser is used during procedures at or above the larynx is avoiding the use of a tracheal tube altogether. When a tracheal tube is not used for laser laryngoscopies, a metal needle mounted in the operating laryngoscope can be used for jet ventilation.[7] With the tip of the needle either above or below the glottis, the surgeon directs a high-velocity jet of oxygen into the airway lumen. The lungs are ventilated with a large volume of oxygen and entrained room air. Because there is no flammable material in the airway, a fire is unlikely. Jet ventilation is favored by many surgeons because it allows excellent visibility of the surgical field. The airway, however, is not protected from other risks. Hypoventilation can be a problem with the jet ventilation technique. Patients who are at particular risk for hypoventilation include those with a highly obstructive airway lesion or decreased pulmonary compliance such as with bronchospasm, obesity, or chronic obstructive pulmonary disease. Spirometry is not possible and capnography is difficult and inaccurate during jet ventilation; thus hypoventilation may go undetected. The surgeon may be unable to direct the jet accurately, which may not only lead to hypoventilation but also may cause gastric distension or barotrauma, including pneumothorax and pneumomediastinum. Other risks to the unprotected airway include aspiration of gastric contents, surgical debris, and laser plume, as well as accidental burn and perforation of the trachea.

Another method of airway management that does not require tracheal intubation is insufflation.[8] With the patient breathing spontaneously, a potent inhaled agent is insufflated through a side port of the operating laryngoscope, a metal hook, or a catheter. As with jet ventilation, absence of flammable material in the airway minimizes the risk of fire and allows excellent visibility of the surgical field. As with any technique not requiring tracheal intubation, hypoventilation and aspiration are possible, and these may go undetected because capnography is difficult and inaccurate without a tracheal tube. Ventilation cannot be assisted or controlled with the insufflation technique. Depth of anesthesia may fluctuate with this technique; and because muscle relaxants cannot be used for spontaneously breathing patients, movement of the patient may lead to accidental contact between the laser beam and healthy tissue or flammable materials such as drapes and catheters. Insufflation also contaminates the ambient air with anesthetic gases and, in doing so, exposes operating room personnel to associated risks. If a catheter is used as the insufflation device, the risk of fire substantially increases.

The alternative to these techniques is intubation. Tracheal intubation secures the airway and thus protects it from aspiration of gastric contents, laser plume, and accidental laser burn to the trachea as well as providing a means of monitoring and controlling ventilation. With intubation, both inhalation and intravenous agents, including muscle relaxants, can be administered safely. All conventional tracheal tubes, however, are composed of materials that are readily ignitable and flammable (Table 21-3).

Polyvinylchloride (PVC) tracheal tubes, which are the tubes most commonly used in the operating room, are favored for most nonlaser operations because these tubes are clear and soft, they retain a patent lumen and a shape that conforms to the natural curves of the airway anatomy, and thus they are nontraumatic. Under well-controlled conditions, such as the helium protocol (Table 21-4), PVC will not ignite even when it is in contact with the laser beam; thus PVC tubes have been used successfully for airway laser surgery.[10] PVC tracheal tubes neither reflect laser light nor retain and transfer heat, and so they are not associated with injury of nontargeted tissue. Because PVC is transparent, condensation of airway vapor as well as evidence of combustion within the lumen can be monitored visually. PVC has a higher oxygen index of flammability than other readily available conventional tracheal tubes (Table 21-3). Despite these advantages of PVC, however, the fact that these tubes can ignite and maintain combustion in an oxygen-enriched atmosphere has caused them to fall into disfavor during laser procedures. If such tubes are used during airway laser procedures, strict adherence to a protective protocol is required to prevent a tracheal tube fire.

Presently available studies[9] indicate that red rubber and silicone tubes sustain combustion more readily than PVC tubes in room air (Table 21-3). Red rubber is thus susceptible to extraluminal fires; but because it is more resistant to puncture by CO_2 laser energy than is PVC (Table 21-3), intraluminal fires are less likely to occur with red rubber.[11] If an extraluminal fire arises, the surgeon and anesthesiologist may have time to extinguish the fire before it spreads to the high-oxygen environment inside of the tube. A problem with red rubber tubes, however, is that they are not transparent. If an intraluminal fire should develop, it might go undetected for a longer period of time than with PVC and therefore cause more extensive damage. Red rubber tubes may have an advantage in that, if ignited, they are less likely than PVC to soften and deform or to allow fragments into the tracheobronchial tree. Silicone, much like red rubber, can ignite in room air and, if ignited, rapidly becomes a brittle ash that easily crumbles; also, silicone tubes can separate and allow retained segments. Because of this, silicone is the least favored of all three of the conventional tracheal tube materials.

Table 21-3. Combustion properties of materials composing conventional tracheal tubes

Material	O_2 Index of flammability*†	Times with a 10-W laser beam and 50% O_2 and 50% N_2	
		Penetration time (sec)‡	Mean time to ignition (sec)‡
Polyvinylchloride	0.263	0.77	3.06
Silicone	0.189	Not tested	Not tested
Red rubber	0.176	41.48	33

*Fractional concentration of oxygen that sustains a candlelike flame.
†Wolf GL, Simpson JI: Flammability of tracheal tubes in oxygen and nitrous oxide enriched atmosphere, *Anesthesiology* 67:236-239, 1987.
‡Ossoff RG: Laser safety in otolaryngology—head and neck surgery: anesthetic and educational considerations for laryngeal surgery, *Laryngoscope* 99(suppl 48):1-26, 1989.

Table 21-4. Helium protocol for laryngotracheal CO_2 laser operations

Protocol consideration	Limitation
Gases	
Helium	Fraction of inspired helium>0.6
Oxygen	Fraction of inspired oxygen≤0.4
Inhalational anesthetics	Enflurane, halothane, or isoflurane
Nitrous oxide	Cannot be used for anesthetic maintenance
Tracheal tube	Unmarked, unwrapped polyvinylchloride
CO_2 laser	
Power density	≤10 W at 0.8-mm spot size (1992 W/cm²)
Exposure	Repeated bursts (<10 seconds of 0.5-second pulsed beam)
Monitoring	Standard monitors, oxygen analyzer, and pulse oximeter

Reproduced with permission from Pashayan AG, Gravenstein JS, Cassisi NJ, et al: The helium protocol for laryngotracheal operations with CO_2 laser: a retrospective review of 523 cases, *Anesthesiology* 68:801-804, 1988.

Combustion byproducts of PVC, red rubber, and silicone can all be highly toxic to the respiratory tract and thus are of obvious concern in this clinical setting.[11] Experience, however, indicates that thermal injury from a tracheal tube fire is of greater immediate concern and significance to a patient's outcome than is inhalation of a toxic byproduct.[12]

In order to use a conventional tracheal tube and at the same time prevent a laser fire, practitioners can wrap the tracheal tube with metallic tape or metallic-backed surgical sponges to shield the tube from the laser. Although this may keep the laser from igniting the tube, metallic tape has not been specially designed for this use. Metallic tape may reflect the laser beam onto nontargeted tissues, may have rough edges that can abrade mucosa, may cause the tube to kink, or may become dislodged and thus occlude the airway. Gaps in the wrapping may leave part of the tube exposed, and because a tube cannot be wrapped at or below the cuff, this area remains exposed and vulnerable. The adhesive backing or surface coating of some tapes can

be ignited by the laser. Not all metallic tapes can protect all types of tubes from all types of lasers at every power setting (Table 21-5).[13-15] Metallic wrapping confers no advantage when the site of operation is distal to the tube and/or the laser beam is delivered through the lumen of the tube. Sterility is difficult to maintain when tubes are prepared in this manner.

A recently marketed, metallic-based surgical sponge (Merocel*) has the advantage of being specifically designed for use on tracheal tubes during airway laser surgery. This preparation provides a much smoother surface against the tracheal mucosa than does metallic tape. Because the sponge is wetted with saline when in use, this diffuses any beam reflection. The wetted sponge, however, thickens the tube and thus makes it less useful for small children and patients with highly stenotic airways. The sponge must be kept wet throughout the operation in order to prevent thermal injury, fire, and tissue abrasion. Like tape wrapping, the sponge wrapping may occlude the airway should it become dislodged, may cause tube kinking, and does not protect the distal portion of the tracheal tube, including the tracheal tube's cuff.

Ready-to-use laser-resistant tubes are commercially available for airway laser operations (Table 21-6). Although these products are specifically designed to resist damage from laser energy, most of these tubes contain flammable components so that strict adherence to the manufacturer's warnings, precautions, and directions is essential. Most laser-resistant tubes have properties that are quite different from standard PVC tubes, and so the practitioner must be aware of the advantages and disadvantages of each tube (Table 21-6).[13]

Additional protective measures should be taken to prevent fires when flammable material is in the surgical field during airway laser operations. The use of oxidizers should be strictly limited to the minimum concentration of oxygen needed to support a clinically acceptable arterial oxygen saturation. The balance of fresh gas flow should be helium or nitrogen, with potent nonflammable inhaled agents added as clinically indicated. Nitrous oxide should

*Merocel Corp., Mystic, Conn.

Table 21-5. Ratings for commercially available laser-resistant wrapping for conventional tracheal tubes

Laser-resistant wrapping	Applicable laser
Copper (3M)	CO_2, Nd:YAG, KTP
Aluminum (3M)	CO_2, Nd:YAG, KTP
Sensing foil (Radio Shack)	CO_2
Metal-backed sponge (Merocel)	CO_2, KTP

not be used because it is an oxidizer and thus can support ignition and sustain combustion of flammable materials. Studies have shown that helium reduces the risk of ignition of tracheal tubes made with either PVC or red rubber.[16,17] Helium may have the additional advantage of facilitating gas flow through an area of obstruction in the airway and therefore may be especially useful for operations within the airway.

Limitation of the laser to the lowest clinically acceptable power density also helps prevent airway fires[16,17] and will, in turn, limit the depth of burn and the extent of tissue damage. Filling a tracheal tube's cuff with saline rather than air is another precautionary measure, but it also prolongs cuff deflation. The addition of methylene blue or some other biocompatible dye to the saline may be useful to help detect cuff perforation. In order to protect the cuff further, saline-soaked pledgets should be applied above the cuff. The pledgets should be layered and carefully placed to reduce the possibility of penetration. If not kept wet, pledgets may ignite. Strings attached to the pledget, if nonmetallic, can be severed and ignited by the laser. Other nonreflective operating platforms and protective devices should be used whenever possible during airway laser operations.

The lower airway

For lesions below the larynx but above the carina, the CO_2 or Nd:YAG laser may be used. Because the depth of burn is shallowest with the CO_2 laser, its wavelength is favored by many surgeons because tracheal perforation may be less likely than with the more deeply penetrating Nd:YAG beam. With either beam, surgical access may be obtained with a rigid, metal bronchoscope, and ventilation may be maintained through the side arm of the broncho-scope. The risk of fire is low with a metal bronchoscope, as long as a flammable cuff is not used to seal the airway.[18] Saline-soaked gauze applied around the broncho-scope in the upper airway may be used instead of a cuff to maintain a seal during ventilation. Although the fraction of inspired oxygen (FIO_2) is not of great importance to fire safety if only metal is in the airway, a high FIO_2 may cause dessicated tissues to spark as they are resected, which could lead to a fire. Helium added to the inspired gases not only decreases the risk of fire but also improves gas flow past the obstructive airway lesion. Special metal bronchoscopes with a matte finish are available for laser bronchoscopy; these reflect a laser beam in a diffuse manner, which is less likely to damage untargeted tissue. Although it is difficult to keep the patient from inhaling laser plume during bronchoscopy, maintaining apnea during laser firing minimizes this possibility. After brief periods of resection, the field should be suctioned, the airway sealed, and the lungs ventilated. The effect of the apnea on arterial oxygen saturation during such intermittent ventilation can be monitored by pulse oximetry.

For lesions below the carina, the Nd:YAG beam is most often used because it can be transmitted by fiberoptic cable. The surgeon can therefore access the field with either a rigid (metal) or flexible bronchoscope. The use of a metal bronchoscope with general anesthesia is preferred by most bronchoscopists because the rigid bronchoscope provides better access for biopsy, suctioning, and ventilation.[19,20] Ventilation may be maintained by any one of several techniques, including side arm-bag ventilation or jet ventilation through either the side arm or a tracheal catheter.[19] A metal bronchoscope reduces the risk of fire, but suction catheters and the fiberoptic cable carrying the laser beam are potential sources of ignition. The risk of fire increases as the cable becomes soiled with darkened, charred tissue, because the Nd:YAG's wavelength is

Table 21-6. Advantages and disadvantages of commercially available laser-resistant tracheal tubes

Description of resistant tube	Applicable laser	Advantages	Disadvantages
Aluminum/silicone spiral with self-inflating foam cuff (Fome-Cuf, Bivona, Inc., Gary, Ind.)	CO_2	Atraumatic external surface; cuff maintains seal even if punctured by laser; nonflammable inner surface	Contains flammable material (silicone); cuff difficult to deflate if punctured
Airtight, stainless steel, corrugated spiral with PVC tip and double cuff (Laser Flex, Mallinckrodt, St. Louis, Mo.)	CO_2, KTP	Tube maintains shape well; double cuff maintains seal after proximal cuff puncture; body of tube is nonflammable; noncuffed version available	Cuffed version contains flammable material (PVC); tubes are thick walled; metal may reflect beam onto nontargeted tissue
Silicone tubes wrapped with aluminum and Teflon, with methylene blue in cuff (Laser-Shield, Xomed, Inc., Jacksonville, Fla.)	CO_2, KTP	Wrapping protects flammable material and is smoother than manual tape wrapping; methylene blue aids in detection of cuff perforation	Contains flammable material (silicone); single cuff is vulnerable to laser damage

highly absorbed by darkly pigmented materials. For this reason, care must be taken to keep the fiberoptic tip clean throughout the laser procedure.

Small, distal airway lesions may be inaccessible with a rigid bronchoscope; in such cases a fiberoptic bronchoscope may be used for Nd:YAG laser resection. When a fiberoptic endoscope is used, anesthesia may consist of topical anesthesia with intravenous sedation, but this requires a very cooperative patient because the trachea can be easily perforated if the patient moves and displaces the targeted tissue. Ventilation and oxygenation may be difficult to control without tracheal intubation, and smoke inhalation is highly likely in a conscious, spontaneously breathing patient. When general anesthesia is used, the fiberoptic bronchoscope can be inserted through a large-diameter tracheal tube. Clear plastic tracheal tubes with no markings are less vulnerable to damage from the Nd:YAG laser than are standard PVC tubes with markings and radiopaque stripe or red rubber tubes.[21] If the PVC tube is soiled with blood or mucus, however, ignitability is greatly increased. Wrapping the tube with metallic tape does not protect it during laser bronchoscopy. Activating the laser during a held inhalation and suctioning laser smoke in the proximal airway during exhalation can minimize the volume of inhaled smoke and debris. In addition to the tracheal tube, the flexible endoscope may also ignite.[22] Ventilation with the lowest clinically acceptable FIO_2 in helium is likely to further decrease the risk of fire, but safe limits for FIO_2 and power density have not been determined for this system. Therefore, metal bronchoscopes are preferred over flexible bronchoscopes for lower airway laser operations whenever possible.

Management of airway fires

Because there is no way to eliminate totally the risk of fire when a laser is used in the airway, the operating room team should prepare and rehearse for an airway fire and must be constantly on the alert.[23,24] If immediate steps are followed to prevent fire from extending down the tracheobronchial tree (Table 21-7), and if appropriate secondary steps are taken in evaluation and treatment, the morbidity and mortality from a laser fire in the airway may be minimized.

If a fire occurs, disconnecting the breathing circuit from the tracheal tube is the quickest method of stopping the gas flow; this reduces the fire intensity by cutting off the oxygen. Simultaneously, because the intense heat from the fire lingers in the tracheal tube, the tube should be removed from the trachea to minimize thermal and chemical damage to the airway. Any smoldering materials should be irrigated with water immediately. If there are no obvious tube fragments or other foreign material in the airway, the trachea may be reintubated or ventilated by mask. Ventilation should initially be resumed with as low an FIO_2 as clinically acceptable to avoid rekindling undetected smol-

Table 21-7. Response to fires during laser operations on the airway

Steps	Measure
Immediate	
First	Disconnect oxygen source at Y piece and remove burning objects from the airway.
Second	Irrigate site with water if fire is still smoldering.
Third	Ventilate the patient by mask or reintubate the trachea and ventilate with as low an FIO_2 as possible.
Secondary	
Fourth	Evaluate extent of injury by bronchoscopy and laryngoscopy.
Fifth	Reintubate the trachea or perform a tracheostomy if needed.
Sixth	Monitor with oximetry, arterial blood gas analysis, or both, and chest radiograms for at least 24 hours.
Seventh	Use ventilatory support, steroids, and antibiotics as needed.

dering material. After these immediate steps, the airway must be evaluated more thoroughly by bronchoscopy and laryngoscopy to determine the extent and severity of injury (Table 21-7). Decisions regarding duration of monitoring and need for respiratory support and treatment will be made on the basis of this evaluation.

SAFETY PROGRAM

Every hospital and health care facility that uses lasers should have a formal safety program for administering and maintaining laser safety.[25] Such a program should be directed by a committee headed by a laser safety officer (LSO). The LSO should have the authority and responsibility for supervising the evaluation and control of laser hazards. The LSO can be a biomedical engineer, physician, nurse, or other health care worker who is knowledgeable and has had special training in monitoring and enforcing standards in the use of lasers. The LSO assures that prescribed safety measures are in effect throughout the health care facility. All operating procedures, alignment procedures, and checklists involved with laser use must be approved by the laser safety committee. Such a committee approves the wording of signs for use outside of all rooms in which a laser is used and provides such signs and labels to the personnel responsible for clinical care throughout the health care facility. The LSO must approve all incoming laser equipment before it is used. The LSO ensures adequate training of personnel and determines the level of credentialing necessary for surgeons and their assistants in the operation of the laser. In addition, the LSO and the laser safety committee must determine the categories of personnel who require medical surveillance during laser use to monitor for eye and skin injury. The laser safety committee should also be responsible for continuing education on and an in service program for laser safety and equipment maintenance.

REFERENCES

1. Epstein RH, Brummett RR Jr, Lask GP: Incendiary potential of the flash-lamp pumped 585-nm tunable dye laser, *Anesth Analg* 71:171-175, 1990.
2. American National Standards Institute: *American national standard for the safe use of lasers*, ANSI Z136.1, New York, 1986.
3. Tomita Y, Mihashi S, Nagata K, et al: Mutagenicity of smoke condensates induced by CO_2 laser irradiation and electrocauterization, *Mutat Res* 89:145-149, 1981.
4. Garden JM, O'Banion MK, Shelnitz LS, et al: Papilloma virus in the vapor of carbon dioxide-treated verrucae, *JAMA* 259:1199-1202, 1988.
5. Snow JC, Norton ML, Saluja TS, et al: Fire hazard during CO_2 laser microsurgery on the larynx and trachea, *Anesth Analg* 55:146-147, 1976.
6. Hirshman CA, Smith J: Indirect ignition of the endotracheal tube during carbon dioxide laser surgery, *Arch Otolaryngol* 106:639-641, 1980.
7. Rontal E, Rontal M, Wenokur ME: Jet insufflation anesthesia for endolaryngeal laser surgery: a review of 318 consecutive cases, *Laryngoscope* 95:990-992, 1985.
8. Johans TG, Reichart TJ: An insufflation device for anesthesia during subglottic carbon dioxide laser microsurgery in children, *Anesth Analg* 63:368-370, 1984.
9. Wolf GL, Simpson JI: Flammability of endotracheal tubes in oxygen and nitrous oxide enriched atmosphere, *Anesthesiology* 67:236-239, 1987.
10. Pashayan AG, Gravenstein JS, Cassisi NJ, et al: The helium protocol for laryngotracheal operations with CO_2 laser: a retrospective review of 523 cases, *Anesthesiology* 68:801-804, 1988.
11. Ossoff RH, Eisenmann TS, Duncavage JA, et al: Comparison of tracheal damage from laser-ignited endotracheal tube fires, *Ann Otol Rhinol Laryngol* 92:333-336, 1983.
12. Bingham HG, Gallagher TJ, Singleton GT, et al: Carbon dioxide laser burn of laryngotracheobronchial mucosa, *J Burn Care Rehab* 11:64-66, 1990.
13. ECRI: Laser resistant endotracheal tubes and wraps, *Health Dev* 19:107-139, 1990.
14. Sosis MB: Evaluation of five metallic tapes for protection of endotracheal tubes during CO_2 laser surgery, *Anesth Analg* 68:392-393, 1989.
15. Sosis MB, Dillon F: What is the safest foil tape for endotracheal tube protection during Nd:YAG laser surgery? A comparative study, *Anesthesiology* 72:553-555, 1990.
16. Pashayan AG, Gravenstein JS: Helium retards endotracheal tube fires from carbon dioxide lasers, *Anesthesiology* 62:274-277, 1985.
17. Ossoff RG: Laser safety in otolaryngology—head and neck surgery: anesthetic and educational considerations for laryngeal surgery, *Laryngoscope* 99(suppl 48):1-26, 1989.
18. Healy GB, Strong MS, Shapshay S, et al: Complications of CO_2 laser surgery of the aerodigestive tract: experience of 4416 cases, *Otolaryngol Head Neck Surg* 92:13-17, 1984.
19. Van der Spek AFL, Spargo PM, Norton ML: The physics of lasers and implications for their use during airway surgery, *Br J Anaesth* 60:709-729, 1988.
20. Brutinel WM, Cortese DA, Edell LES, et al: Complications of Nd:YAG laser surgery, *Chest* 94:902-903, 1988, (editorial).
21. Geffin B, Shapshay SM, Bellack GS, et al: Flammability of endotracheal tubes during Nd:YAG laser application in the airway, *Anesthesiology* 65:511-515, 1986.
22. Casey KR, Fairfax WR, Smith SJ, et al: Intratracheal fire ignited by the Nd:YAG laser during treatment of tracheal stenosis, *Chest* 84:295-296, 1983.
23. Schramm VL Jr, Mattox DE, Stool SE: Acute management of laser-ignited intratracheal explosion, *Laryngoscope* 91:1417-1426, 1981.
24. Rampil, IJ: Anesthetic considerations for laser surgery, *Anesth Analg* 74:424-435, 1992.
25. American National Standard Institute: *American National Standard for the safe use of lasers in health care facilities*, ANSI Z136.3, New York, 1988.

Part II: Electrical safety*

The myriad of electrical and electronic devices in the modern operating room greatly improve patient care and safety. However, these devices also have the potential to expose both the patient and operating room personnel to increased risks. To reduce this risk, the electrical system used in the operating room includes specific safety features designed to reduce the risk of electrical shock. Nevertheless, it is incumbent on the anesthesiologist to have a thorough understanding of the basic principles of electricity and an appreciation of the concepts of electrical safety applicable to the operating room environment.

PRINCIPLES OF ELECTRICITY

A basic principle of electricity is Ohm's Law, represented by the equation

$$E = I \times R$$

where E = electromotive force (volts), I = current (amperes), and R = resistance (ohms). Ohm's Law forms the basis for the physiologic equation where blood pressure is equal to cardiac output times systemic vascular resistance ($BP = CO \times SVR$). In this case, the blood pressure of the vascular system is analogous to voltage, the cardiac output to current, and systemic vascular resistance to the forces opposing the flow of electrons.

Electrical power is measured in units called *watts* (W). A watt is equal to the product of the voltage (E) and the current (I), and is defined by the formula

$$W = E \times I$$

The amount of electrical work done is measured in watts consumed per unit of time. The watt-second (a joule, J) is a common designation for electrical energy expended in doing work. The energy produced by a defibrillator is measured in watt-seconds (or joules), and the kilowatt-hour is used to measure larger quantities of electrical energy consumed. For example, an electrical power company charges consumers on the basis of kilowatt-hours of electricity used.

Wattage can be thought of not only as a measure of

Adapted in part from Ehrenwerth J: *Electrical safety*. In Barash PG, Cullen BF, Stoelting RK, editors: *Clinical anesthesia*, ed 2, Philadelphia, 1992, J.B. Lippincott. Reprinted with permission.

work done, but also as heat produced in any electrical circuit. Substituting Ohm's Law in the formula

$$W = E \times I$$

yields

$$W = (I \times R) \times I$$

or

$$W = I^2 \times R$$

Thus, wattage is equal to the square of the current (amperage) times the resistance. Using these formulas, it is possible to calculate the number of amperes and the resistance of a given device if the wattage and the voltage are known. For example, a 60-watt light bulb operating on a household 120-volt circuit would require 0.5 ampere of current for operation. Rearranging the formula so that

$$I = \frac{W}{E}$$
$$I = \frac{60 \text{ watts}}{120 \text{ volts}}$$
$$I = 0.5 \text{ ampere}$$

Using this in Ohm's Law,

$$R = E/I$$

the resistance of the bulb can be calculated to be 240 ohms. Thus,

$$R = \frac{120 \text{ volts}}{0.5 \text{ ampere}}$$
$$R = 240 \text{ ohms}$$

It is obvious from the above discussion that 1 volt of electromotive force applied across a 1-ohm resistance will cause 1 ampere of current to flow. Similarly, flow of 1 ampere of current induced by 1 volt of potential difference will generate 1 watt of power.

Direct and alternating currents

Any substance that permits the flow of electrons is called a *conductor*. Current is characterized by electrons flowing through a conductor. If the electron flow is always in the same direction, it is called *direct current* (DC). If the electron flow reverses direction at a regular intervals, it is termed *alternating current* (AC). Either of these types of current can be pulsed or continuous.[1]

The previous discussion of Ohm's Law is accurate when applied to DC circuits. However, when dealing with AC circuits, the situation is more complex because the flow of the current is opposed by a more complicated form of resistance, known as *impedance*.

Impedance

Impedance is defined as the sum of the forces that oppose electron movement in an AC circuit, and is designated by the letter Z. Impedance consists of resistance (ohms) but also takes into account capacitance as well as inductance. In actuality, when referring to AC circuits, Ohm's Law is defined as

$$E = I \times Z$$

An insulator is a substance that opposes the flow of electrons and therefore has a high impedance to electron flow, whereas a conductor has a low impedance to electron flow.

In AC circuits, the capacitance and inductance can be important factors in determining the total impedance. Both capacitance and inductance are influenced by the frequency (cycles per second, or Hertz, Hz) at which the AC reverses direction. The impedance is directly proportional to the frequency (*f*) times the inductance (IND),

$$Z \propto (f \times IND)$$

and the impedance is inversely proportional to the product of the frequency (*f*) and the capacitance (CAP):

$$Z \propto \frac{1}{f \times CAP}$$

As the AC increases in frequency, the net effect of both capacitance and inductance will increase. However, since impedance and capacitance are inversely related, total impedance will decrease as the product of the frequency and the capacitance increases. Thus, as frequency increases, impedance will decrease and more current will be allowed to flow.[2]

Capacitance

A capacitor consists of any two parallel conductors that are separated by an insulator (Fig. 21-3). A capacitor has the ability to store a charge, and capacitance is the measure of the ability to store a charge. In a DC circuit, the capacitor plates are charged by a voltage source (i.e., a battery), and the flow of current is only momentary. The circuit is not completed, and there can be no further flow of current unless a resistance is connected between the two plates and the capacitor is discharged.[3]

In contrast to DC circuits, a capacitor in an AC circuit permits current to flow even when the circuit is not completed by a resistance. This is attributable to the nature of AC circuits, in which the current flow is constantly being reversed. Since current flow results from the movement of electrons, the capacitor plates are alternately charged, first positive and then negative with each reversal of the current direction. The consequence of this is an effective flow of current as far as the remainder of the circuit is concerned, even though the circuit is not completed.[4]

Since the effect of capacitance on impedance varies directly with the AC frequency (in Hz), the greater the AC frequency, the lower the impedance. Therefore, high-frequency currents (0.5 to 2 million Hz), such as those used by electrosurgical units, will cause a marked decrease in impedance. As an example, a 20-million-ohm impedance

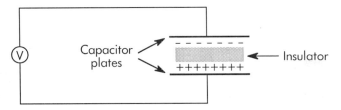

Fig. 21-3. A capacitor consists of two parallel conductors separated by an insulator. The capacitor is capable of storing charge supplied by a voltage source. (Used with permission from Ehrenwerth J: *Electrical safety.* In Barash PG, Cullen BF, Stoelting RK, editors: *Clinical anesthesia,* ed 2, Philadelphia, 1992, J.B. Lippincott.)

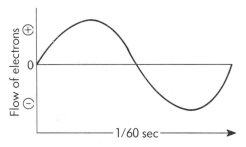

Fig. 21-4. Sine wave flow of electrons in a 60-Hz AC circuit. (Used with permission from Ehrenwerth J: *Electrical safety.* In Barash PG, Cullen BF, Stoelting RK, editors: *Clinical anesthesia,* ed 2, Philadelphia, 1992, J.B. Lippincott.)

in a 60-Hz AC circuit will be reduced to an impedance of only a few hundred ohms when the frequency is increased to 1 million Hz.[5]

Electrical devices use capacitors for various purposes. There is, however, a phenomenon known as *stray capacitance,* which is defined as capacitance that was not designed into the system but is incidental to the construction of the equipment.[6] All AC-powered equipment produces stray capacitance. An ordinary power cord, for example, consisting of two insulated wires running next to each other, will generate significant capacitance simply by being plugged into a 120-volt circuit outlet, even though the piece of equipment is not turned on. Another example of stray capacitance is found in electric motors. The circuit wiring in electric motors generates stray capacitance to the metal housing of the motor.[7] The clinical importance of capacitance is emphasized later in this chapter.

Inductance

Whenever electrons flow in a wire, a magnetic field is induced around the wire. If the wire is coiled repeatedly around an iron core, as in a transformer, the magnetic field can be very powerful. Inductance is a property of AC circuits in which an opposing electromotive force (EMF) can be generated electromagnetically in the circuit. The net effect of inductance is to increase impedance. Since the effect of inductance on impedance also depends on AC frequency (in Hz), increases in frequency will increase the total impedance. Therefore, the total impedance of a coil to electron flow will be much greater than its simple resistance.[4]

ELECTRICAL SHOCK HAZARDS

Alternating and direct currents

Whenever an individual contacts an external source of electricity, an electric shock is possible. An electrical current can stimulate contraction of muscle cells and thus can be used therapeutically in devices such as pacemakers or defibrillators. However, casual contact with an electrical current, whether AC or DC, can lead to injury or even death. Although it requires approximately three times as

much DC as AC to cause ventricular fibrillation,[3] this by no means renders DC harmless. Devices such as an automobile battery or a DC defibrillator can be sources of DC shocks.

In the United States, utility companies supply electrical energy in the form of alternating currents of 120 volts potential difference at a frequency of 60 Hz.* (The 60 Hz refers to the number of times in 1 second that the direction of current flow is reversed.[8]) Both the voltage and current waveforms form a sinusoidal pattern (Fig. 21-4).

To have the completed circuit necessary for current flow, a closed loop must exist, and there must be a voltage source to drive the current through the impedance. If current is to flow in the electrical circuit, a voltage differential or a drop in the driving pressure across the impedance is required. According to Ohm's Law, if the resistance is held constant, then the greater the current flow, the larger the voltage drop must be.[9]

The power company attempts to maintain the voltage in the electrical line constant at 120 volts. Therefore, by Ohm's Law, the current flow is inversely proportional to the impedance. A typical power cord consists of two conductors. One, designated the "hot," carries the current to the impedance; the other, the "neutral," returns the current to the source. The potential difference between the two is effectively 120 volts (Fig. 21-5). The amount of current flowing through a given device is frequently referred to as the "load." The load of the circuit is dependent on the impedance. A very high-impedance circuit allows only a small current to flow and thus will have a small load. A very low-impedance circuit will draw a large current and is said to be a large load. A *short circuit* occurs when there is a zero impedance load with a very high current flow.[10]

---

*The 120 volts of EMF and 1 ampere of current are the effective voltage and amperage in an AC circuit. This is also referred to as "RMS," which stands for "root-mean-square." In fact, it takes 1.414 amperes (amps) of peak amperage in the sinusoidal curve to give an effective amperage of 1 ampere. Similarly, it takes 170 volts (120 × 1.414) at the peak of the AC curve to produce an effective voltage of 120 volts.[8]

Source of shocks

To practice electrical safety, it is important for the anesthesiologist to understand the basic principles of electricity and to be aware of how accidents can occur. Electrical accidents or shocks occur when a person becomes part of or completes an electrical circuit. Thus, in order to receive a shock, one must contact the electrical circuit at two points, and there must be a voltage source (potential difference) to cause the current to flow through the person (Fig. 21-6).

When an individual contacts a source of electricity, damage can be produced in two ways. First, the electric current can disrupt the normal electrical function of cells. Depending upon its magnitude, the current can cause contraction of muscles, alter cerebral function, paralyze respiration, or disrupt normal cardiac function and lead to ventricular fibrillation. The second mechanism involves the dissipation of electrical energy throughout all the tissues of the body. An electric current passing through any resistance raises the temperature of that substance. If enough thermal energy is released, the temperature will rise sufficiently to produce a burn. Accidents involving household currents usually do not result in severe burns. On the other hand, in accidents involving very high voltages (i.e., power transmission lines), severe burns are common.

The severity of the shock that an individual receives depends upon the size of the current (number of amperes) and the duration of the contact. For the purposes of this discussion, electrical shocks are divided into two categories. *Macroshock* refers to large amounts of current flowing through a person, which can cause harm or death. *Mi-*

Table 21-8. Effects of 60-Hz AC on an average human for a 1-second duration of contact

Current	Effect
Macroshock	
1 mA (0.001 A)	Threshold of perception
5 mA (0.005 A)	Accepted as maximum harmless current intensity
10-20 mA (0.01-0.02 A)	"Let-go" current before sustained muscle contraction
50 mA (0.05 A)	Pain, possible fainting, mechanical injury; heart and respiratory functions continue
100-300 mA (0.1-0.3 A)	Ventricular fibrillation will start, but respiratory center remains intact
6000 mA (6 A)	Sustained myocardial contractions, followed by normal heart rhythm; temporary respiratory paralysis; burns if current density is high
Microshock	
100 μA (0.1 mA)	Ventricular fibrillation
10 μA (0.01 mA)	Recommended maximum allowable 60-Hz leakage current

A = amperes; mA = milliamperes; μA = microamperes.

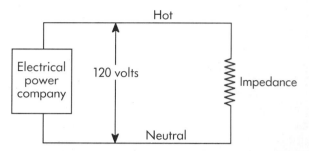

Fig. 21-5. A typical AC circuit where there is a potential difference of 120 volts between the hot and neutral sides of the circuit. The current flows through a resistance, which in AC circuits is more accurately referred to as *impedance,* and then returns to the electrical power company. (Used with permission from Ehrenwerth J: *Electrical safety.* In Barash PG, Cullen BF, Stoelting RK, editors: *Clinical anesthesia,* ed 2, Philadelphia, 1992, J.B Lippincott.)

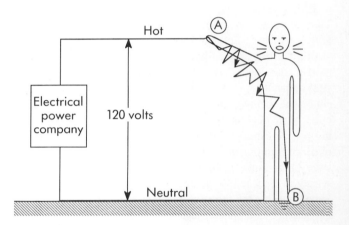

Fig. 21-6. An individual can complete an electrical circuit and receive a shock by coming into contact with the "hot" side of the circuit (Point A). This is because he or she is standing on the ground (Point B) and the contact Point A and the ground Point B provide the two contact points necessary for a completed circuit. The severity of the shock that the individual receives depends on skin resistance. (Used with permission from Ehrenwerth J: *Electrical safety.* In Barash PG, Cullen BF, Stoelting RK, editors: *Clinical anesthesia,* ed 2, Philadelphia, 1992, J.B. Lippincott.)

croshock refers to very small amounts of current, and applies only to the electrically susceptible patient who has an external conductor that is in direct contact with the heart. This may be a pacing wire or a saline-filled catheter such as a central venous or pulmonary arterial catheter. In the case of the electrically susceptible patient, even minute amounts of current (microshock) may cause ventricular fibrillation.

Table 21-8 shows the effects typically produced by various sized currents following a 1-second contact with a 60-Hz source. When an individual contacts a 120-volt household current, the severity of the shock will depend on their skin resistance, the duration of the contact, and the current density. Skin resistance can vary from a few thousand to more than one million ohms. If a person with a skin resistance of 1000 ohms contacts a 120-volt circuit, they would receive 120 mA (milliamperes) of current, which would probably be lethal. However, if that same person's skin resistance was 100,000 ohms, the current flowing would be 1.2 mA, which would be barely perceptible (see Table 21-8).

$$I = \frac{E}{R} = \frac{120 \text{ volts}}{1000 \text{ ohms}} = 120 \text{ mA} \quad \frac{120 \text{ volts}}{100,000 \text{ ohms}} = 1.2 \text{ mA}$$

The longer an individual is in contact with the electrical source, the more dire the consequences, since more energy will be released and more tissue damaged. Also, there will be a greater chance of ventricular fibrillation from excitation of the heart during the vulnerable period of the electrocardiographic cycle.

The term *current density* is merely a way of expressing the amount of current that is applied per unit area of tissue. The diffusion of current in the body tends to be in all directions. The larger the current or the smaller the area over which it is applied, the higher the current density. In relation to the heart, a current of 100 mA (100,000 μA) is generally required to induce ventricular fibrillation when applied to the surface of the body. However, only 100 μA (0.1 mA) is required to induce ventricular fibrillation when that minute current is applied directly to the myocardium through an instrument having a very small contact area, such as a pacing wire electrode. In this case, the current density is 1000 times greater when applied directly to the heart and therefore only 1/1000 as much energy is required to cause ventricular fibrillation. Therefore, the electrically susceptible patient can be electrocuted with currents well below 1 mA, which is the threshold of perception for normal humans.

The frequency at which the current reverses is also an important factor in determining the amount of current with which an individual can safely come into contact. Utility companies in the United States generate electricity at a frequency of 60 Hz because higher frequencies cause greater power loss through transmission lines, and low-

er frequencies result in a detectable flicker from light sources.[11]

The "let-go" current is defined as that current above which sustained muscular contraction occurs so that an individual would be unable to let go of an energized wire. The let-go current for 60-Hz AC power is 10 to 20 mA,[10,12,13] whereas at a frequency of 1 million Hz, a current of up to 3 amperes (3000 mA) is generally regarded as safe.[3] It should be noted that very high frequency currents do not excite contractile tissue; consequently, they do not cause cardiac arrhythmias.

It can be seen that for a completed circuit to exist, there must be a closed loop with a driving pressure (potential difference) to force a current to flow through a resistance in accordance with Ohm's Law, just as in the cardiovascular system there must be a blood pressure to drive the cardiac output through the systemic vascular resistance. Figure 21-7 illustrates that a hot wire carrying a 120-volt "pressure" through the resistance of a 60-watt light bulb produces a current flow of 0.5 ampere. The voltage in the neutral wire is approximately 0 volts, while the current in the neutral wire remains at 0.5 ampere. This correlates with the cardiovascular analogy in which a mean blood pressure difference of 80 mm Hg between the aortic root to the right atrium forces a cardiac output of 6 L/min through a systemic vascular resistance of 13.3 resistance units. However, the flow (in this case, the cardiac output, or in the case of the electrical model, the current) is still the same everywhere in the circuit. That is, the cardiac output on the arterial side is the same as the venous return to the right atrium.

Grounding

To understand fully electrical shock hazards and their prevention, one must have a thorough knowledge of the concepts of grounding. These concepts probably constitute the most confusing aspects of electrical safety, because the same term is used to describe several different principles.

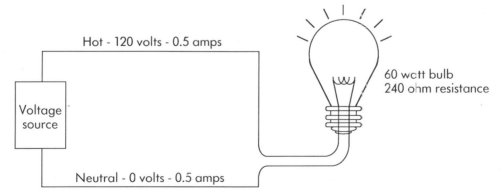

Fig. 21-7. A 60-watt light bulb has an internal resistance of 240 ohms and draws 0.5 amps of current. The voltage drop in the circuit is from 120 in the hot wire to 0 in the neutral wire, but the current is 0.5 amps in both the hot and the neutral wires. (Used with permission from Ehrenwerth J: *Electrical safety.* In Barash PG, Cullen BF, Stoelting RK, editors: *Clinical anesthesia,* ed 2, Philadelphia, 1992, J.B. Lippincott.)

In electrical terminology, *grounding* is applied to two separate concepts: the grounding of electrical *power,* and the grounding of electrical *equipment*. Thus, the concepts that power can be grounded *or* ungrounded, and that it may supply electrical devices that are themselves grounded or ungrounded, are not mutually exclusive. It is vital to understand this point as the basis of electrical safety (Table 21-9). While electrical *power* is grounded in the home, it is ungrounded in the operating room. In the home, electrical *equipment* may be grounded or ungrounded, but it should always be grounded in the operating room.

ELECTRICAL POWER—GROUNDED

Electrical utility companies universally provide power that is grounded (by convention, the earth ground potential is zero, and all voltages represent a difference between potentials). That is, one of the wires supplying the power to a home is intentionally connected to the earth. The utility companies do this as a safety measure to prevent electrical charges from building up in their wiring during electrical storms. This also prevents the very high voltages used in transmitting power by the utility from entering the home in the event of an equipment failure in their high-voltage system.[3]

The power enters the typical home via two wires that are connected to the main fuse or circuit breaker box (these two terms are used interchangeably in this chapter) at the service entrance. The "hot" wire supplies power to the "hot" distribution strip. The neutral is connected to the neutral distribution strip and to a service entrance ground (i.e., a metal pipe buried in the earth) (Fig. 21-8). From

Table 21-9. Differences between power and equipment grounding in the home and in the operating room[*]

	Power	Equipment
Home	+	±
Operating room	−	+

[*]+ = grounded; − = ungrounded; ± may or may not be grounded.

the fuse box, three wires leave to supply the electrical outlets in the house. In the United States the "hot" wire is color-coded black and carries an above-ground potential of 120 volts. The second wire is the neutral wire, which is color-coded white; and the third wire is the ground wire, which is either color-coded green or is uninsulated (bare wire). The ground and the neutral wires are connected at the same point in the fuse or circuit breaker box and are subsequently connected to a metal cold water pipe (Figs. 21-9 and 21-10). This system is also described as a "neutral grounded power system." The black wire is not connected to the ground, as this would create a short circuit. Rather it is attached to the "hot" (i.e., 120 volts above ground) distribution strip on which the circuit breakers or fuses are located. From there, numerous branch circuits supply electrical power to outlets in the house. Each branch circuit is protected by a circuit breaker or fuse that limits current to a specific maximum amperage. Most electrical circuits in the house are rated as 15- or 20-amp circuits. These typically supply power to the electrical outlets and lights in the house. Several higher-amperage circuits are also provided for appliances such as an electric stove

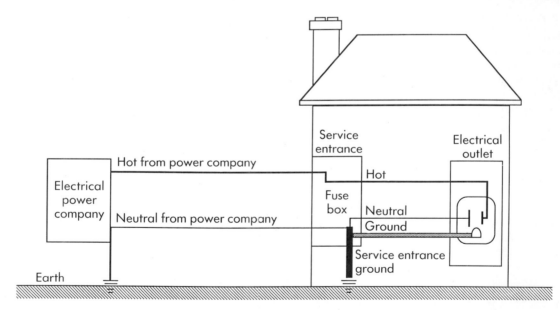

Fig. 21-8. In a neutral grounded power system, the utility company supplies two lines to the typical home. The neutral is connected to ground by the power company and is again connected to a service entrance ground where it enters the fuse box. The neutral and the ground wires are connected in the fuse box at the neutral bus bar, which is also connected to the service entrance ground. (Used with permission from Ehrenwerth J: *Electrical safety*. In Barash PG, Cullen BF, Stoelting RK, editors: *Clinical anesthesia*, ed 2, Philadelphia, 1992, J.B. Lippincott.)

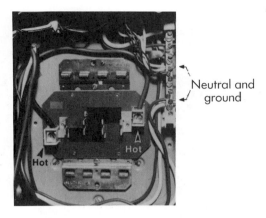

Fig. 21-9. Inside a fuse box with the circuit breakers removed. The *arrowheads* indicate the hot wires energizing the strips where the circuit breakers are located. The *arrows* point to the neutral bus bar where the neutral and ground wires are connected. (Used with permission from Ehrenwerth J: *Electrical safety.* In Barash PG, Cullen BF, Stoelting RK, editors: *Clinical anesthesia,* ed 2, Philadelphia, 1992, J.B. Lippincott.)

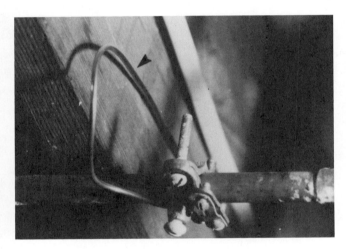

Fig. 21-10. The *arrow* indicates the ground wire from the fuse box connected to a metal cold water pipe. (Used with permission from Ehrenwerth J: *Electrical safety.* In Barash PG, Cullen BF, Stoelting RK, editors: *Clinical anesthesia,* ed 2, Philadelphia, 1992, J.B. Lippincott.)

or an electric clothes dryer, which can draw between 30 amps to 50 amps of current. The circuit breaker or fuse will interrupt the flow of current on the hot side of the circuit in the event of a short circuit, or if the demand placed on that circuit exceeds its threshold. For example, a 15-amp branch circuit will be capable of supplying 1800 watts of power.

$$W = E \times I$$
$$W = 120 \text{ volts} \times 15 \text{ amperes}$$
$$W = 1800 \text{ watts}$$

Therefore, if two 1500-watt hair dryers were simultaneously plugged into one outlet, the load would be too great for a 15-amp circuit, and the circuit breaker would open (trip) or the fuse would melt. This is done to prevent the circuit supply wires from melting and starting a fire.

The amperage of the circuit breaker on the branch circuit is determined by the thickness of the wire that it supplies. If a 20-amp breaker is used with wire rated for only 15 amps, the wire could melt and start a fire before the circuit breaker would be tripped. It is important to note that a 15-amp circuit breaker does not protect an individual from lethal electric shocks. The 15 amps of current that will trip the circuit breaker far exceed the 100 to 200 mA that will produce ventricular fibrillation.

The wires that leave the circuit breaker supply the electrical outlets and lighting for the rest of the house. In older homes, the electrical cable consists of two wires, a hot and a neutral, which supply power to the electrical outlets (Fig. 21-11). In newer homes, there is a third wire in the electrical cable (Fig. 21-12). This third wire is either green or uninsulated (bare) and serves as a ground wire for the power receptacle (Fig. 21-13). On one end, the ground wire is attached to the electrical outlet (Fig. 21-14); at the other, it is connected to the neutral distribution strip in the circuit breaker box along with the neutral (white) wires (Fig. 21-15).

It should be realized that in both the old and new situations the power is grounded. That is, a 120-volt potential exists between the hot (black) and the neutral (white) wires and between the hot wire and ground. In this case, the ground is the earth (Fig. 21-16). In modern home construction, there is still a 120-volt potential difference between the hot (black) and the neutral (white) wires, as well as between the hot wire and the equipment ground wire (which is the third wire) and between the hot wire and the earth (Fig. 21-17).

A 60-watt light bulb can be used as an example to fur-

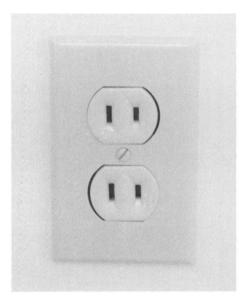

Fig. 21-11. An older-style electrical outlet supplied by only two wires (a hot and a neutral). There is no ground wire. (Used with permission from Ehrenwerth J: *Electrical safety.* In Barash PG, Cullen BF, Stoelting RK, editors: *Clinical anesthesia,* ed 2, Philadelphia, 1992, J.B. Lippincott.)

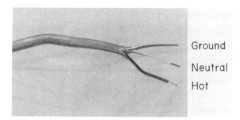

Fig. 21-12. A modern electrical cable in which a third, or ground, wire has been added. (Used with permission from Ehrenwerth J: *Electrical safety*. In Barash PG, Cullen BF, Stoelting RK, editors: *Clinical anesthesia*, ed 2, Philadelphia, 1992, J.B. Lippincott.)

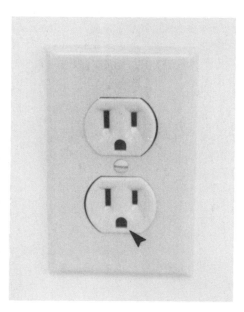

Fig. 21-13. A modern electrical outlet in which a ground wire is present. The arrow points to the part of the receptacle where the ground wire connects. (Used with permission from Ehrenwerth J: *Electrical safety*. In Barash PG, Cullen BF, Stoelting RK, editors: *Clinical anesthesia,* ed 2, Philadelphia, 1992, J.B. Lippincott.)

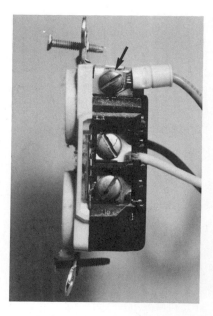

Fig. 21-14. Detail of a modern electrical power receptacle. The *arrow* points to the ground wire, which is connected to the grounding screw terminal. (Used with permission from Ehrenwerth J: *Electrical safety*. In Barash PG, Cullen BF, Stoelting RK, editors: *Clinical anesthesia,* ed 2, Philadelphia, 1992, J.B. Lippincott.)

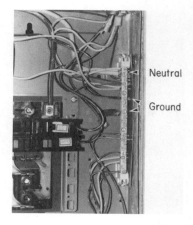

Fig. 21-15. The ground wires from the power outlets are run to the neutral bus bar, where they are connected with the neutral wires *(arrowheads)*. (Used with permission from Ehrenwerth J: *Electrical safety*. In Barash PG, Cullen BF, Stoelting RK, editors: *Clinical anesthesia,* ed 2, Philadelphia, 1992, J.B. Lippincott.)

ther illustrate this point. Normally, the hot and neutral wires are connected to the two wires of the light bulb socket, and throwing the light switch will cause the bulb to illuminate (Fig. 21-18). Similarly, if the hot wire is connected to one side of the bulb socket and the other wire from the light bulb is connected to the equipment ground wire, the bulb will still illuminate. If there is no equipment ground wire, the bulb will still light if the second wire is connected to any grounded metal object such as a water pipe or a faucet. This illustrates the fact that the 120-volt potential difference exists, not only between the hot and the neutral wires, but also between the hot wire and any grounded object. Thus, in a grounded power system, the current will flow between the hot wire and any conductor with an earth ground.

As previously stated, current flow requires a closed loop with a source of voltage. For an individual to receive an electric shock, they must contact the loop at two points. Since that person may be standing on the ground or be in contact with an object that is referenced to ground, only *one* additional contact point is necessary to complete the circuit and thus receive an electric shock. This is an unfortunate and inherently dangerous consequence of grounded power systems. Modern wiring systems have added a third wire, the equipment ground wire, as a safety measure to reduce the severity of a potential electric shock. This is accomplished by providing an alternate, low-resistance path-

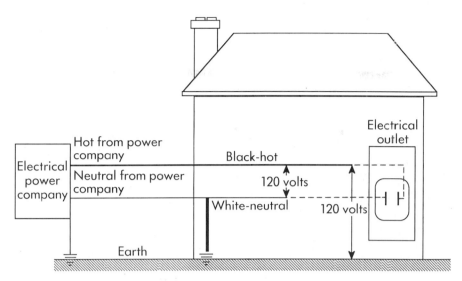

Fig. 21-16. A diagram of a house with older-style wiring that does not include a ground wire. A 120-volt potential difference exists between the hot and the neutral wires, as well as between the hot wire and the earth. (Used with permission from Ehrenwerth J: *Electrical safety*. In Barash PG, Cullen BF, Stoelting RK, editors: *Clinical anesthesia*, ed 2, Philadelphia, 1992, J.B. Lippincott.)

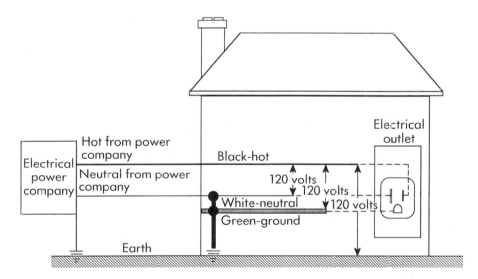

Fig. 21-17. A diagram of a house with modern wiring in which a third, or ground, wire has been added. The 120-volt potential difference exists between the hot and neutral wires, the hot and the ground wires, and the hot wire and the earth. (Used with permission from Ehrenwerth J: *Electrical safety*. In Barash PG, Cullen BF, Stoelting RK, editors: *Clinical anesthesia*, ed 2, Philadelphia, 1992, J.B. Lippincott.)

way through which the current can flow to ground.

Over time, the insulation covering wires may deteriorate. It is then possible for a bare, hot wire to contact the metal case or frame of an electrical device. The case would then become energized and constitute a shock hazard to someone coming in contact with it. Figure 21-19 illustrates a typical short circuit, where the individual has come in contact with the hot case of an instrument. This diagram illustrates the type of wiring found in older homes. There is no outlet ground wire, nor is the electrical

apparatus equipped with a ground wire. Here, the individual completes the circuit and receives a severe shock. Figure 21-20 illustrates a similar example, except that now a ground wire is part of the electrical distribution system. In this example, the equipment ground wire provides a pathway of low resistance through which the current can flow to ground. Therefore, most of the current would flow through the ground wire, and, although the person may receive a shock, it is unlikely to be fatal.

The electrical power supplied to homes is always

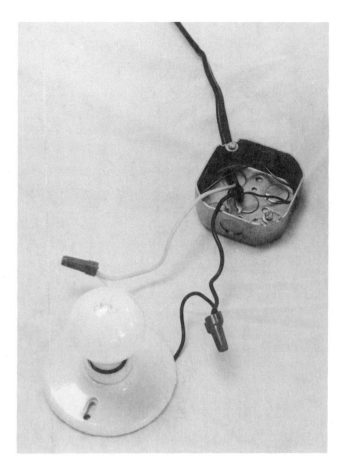

Fig. 21-18. A simple light bulb circuit in which the hot (black) and neutral (white) wires are connected with the corresponding wires from the light bulb fixture. (Used with permission from Ehrenwerth J: *Electrical safety.* In Barash PG, Cullen BF, Stoelting RK, editors: *Clinical anesthesia,* ed 2, Philadelphia, 1992, J.B. Lippincott.)

grounded. A 120-volt potential always exists between the hot conductor and the ground or earth. The third, or equipment ground, wire used in modern electrical wiring systems does not normally have current flowing through it. In the event of a short circuit, an electrical device with a three-prong plug (i.e., a ground wire connected to its case) will conduct most of the short-circuited or "fault" current through the ground wire and away from the individual. This provides a significant safety benefit to someone accidentally contacting the defective device. If a large enough fault current exists, the ground wire will also provide a means to complete the short circuit back to the circuit breaker or fuse, and will either melt the fuse or trip the circuit breaker. Thus, in a grounded power system, it is possible to have either grounded or ungrounded equipment, depending upon when the wiring was installed and whether the electrical device is equipped with a three-prong plug incorporating a ground wire. Obviously, attempts to bypass the safety system of the equipment ground should be avoided. Devices such as a "cheater plug" (Fig. 21-21) should not be used, because they defeat the safety feature of the equipment ground wire.

ELECTRICAL POWER—UNGROUNDED

The numerous electrically powered devices, along with their power cords, and puddles of saline solutions on the floor tend to make the operating room an electrically hazardous environment for both patients and personnel. Bruner and colleagues[14] found that 40% of electrical accidents in hospitals occurred in the operating room. The complexity of electrical equipment in the modern operating room demands that electrical safety be of paramount importance. In order to provide an extra measure of safety

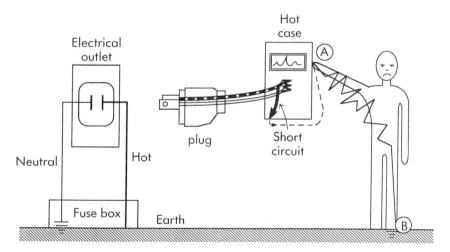

Fig. 21-19. When a faulty piece of equipment without an equipment ground wire is plugged into an electrical outlet not incorporating a ground wire, the case of the instrument will become hot. If an individual touches the hot case (Point A) he or she will receive a shock, because standing on the earth (Point B) completes the circuit. The current (dotted line) will flow from the instrument through the individual touching the hot case. (Used with permission from Ehrenwerth J: *Electrical safety.* In Barash PG, Cullen BF, Stoelting RK, editors: *Clinical anesthesia,* ed 2, Philadelphia, 1992, J.B. Lippincott.)

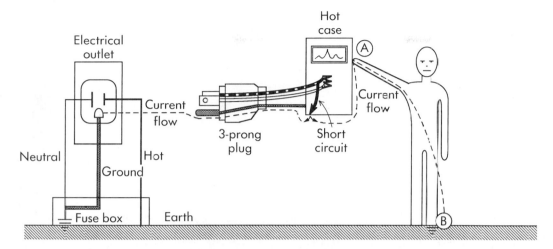

Fig. 21-20. When a faulty piece of equipment that incorporates an equipment ground wire is properly connected to an electrical outlet with a grounding connection, the current (dotted line) will preferentially flow through the low-resistance ground wire. An individual touching the case (Point A) and standing on the ground (Point B) will still complete the circuit; however, only a small part of the current will flow through the individual. (Used with permission from Ehrenwerth J: *Electrical safety*. In Barash PG, Cullen BF, Stoelting RK, editors: *Clinical anesthesia*, ed 2, Philadelphia, 1992, J.B. Lippincott.)

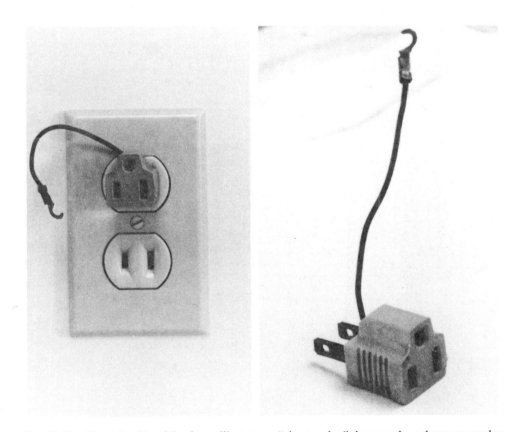

Fig. 21-21. The right side of the figure illustrates a "cheater plug" that permits a three-prong plug to be inserted into a two-prong outlet. The left side of the picture illustrates that the wire attached to the cheater plug is rarely connected to the screw in the middle of the outlet. This totally defeats the purpose of the equipment ground wire. (Used with permission from Ehrenwerth J: *Electrical safety*. In Barash PG, Cullen BF, Stoelting RK, editors: *Clinical anesthesia*, ed 2, Philadelphia, 1992, J.B. Lippincott.)

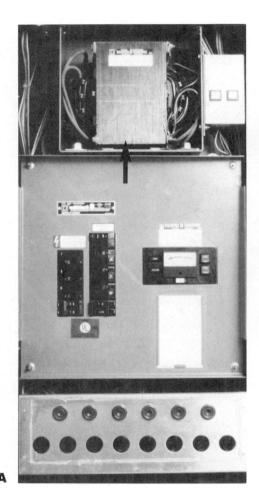

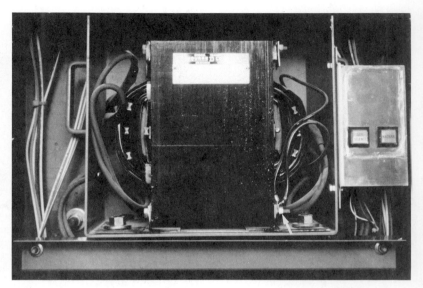

B

Fig. 21-22. A, An isolated power panel showing circuit breakers, line isolation monitor (LIM), and isolation transformer *(arrow)*. **B,** Detail of an isolation transformer with the attached warning lights. The *arrow* points to the ground wire connection on the primary side of the transformer. Note that no similar connection exists on the secondary side of the transformer. (Used with permission from Ehrenwerth J: *Electrical safety.* In Barash PG, Cullen BF, Stoelting RK, editors: *Clinical anesthesia,* ed 2, Philadelphia, 1992, J.B. Lippincott.)

A

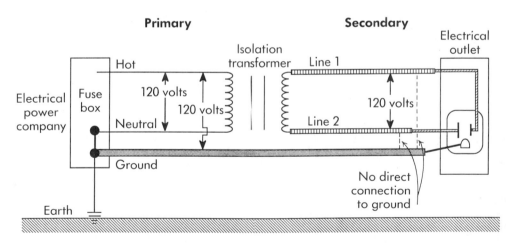

Fig. 21-23. In the operating room, the isolation transformer converts the grounded power on the primary side to an ungrounded power system on the secondary side of the transformer. A 120-volt potential difference exists only between line 1 and line 2. There is no direct connection between the power on the secondary side and ground. The equipment ground wire is, however, still present. (Used with permission from Ehrenwerth J: *Electrical safety.* In Barash PG, Cullen BF, Stoelting RK, editors: *Clinical anesthesia,* ed 2, Philadelphia, 1992, J.B. Lippincott.)

from gross electric shock (macroshock), the *power* supplied to most operating rooms is ungrounded. In this ungrounded power system, the current is isolated from ground potential. The 120-volt potential difference exists only between the two wires of the isolated power system, but no circuit exists between the ground and either of the isolated power lines.

Supplying ungrounded power to the operating room requires the use of an isolation transformer (Fig. 21-22). This device uses electromagnetic induction to induce a current in the ungrounded or secondary winding of the transformer from energy supplied to the primary winding. There is no direct electrical connection between the power supplied by the utility company on the primary side and the power induced by the transformer on the ungrounded or secondary side. Thus, the power supplied to the operating room is isolated from ground (Fig. 21-23). Since the 120-volt potential exists only between the two wires of the isolated circuit, neither wire is hot or neutral with reference to ground. In this case, they are simply referred to as line 1 and line 2 (Fig. 21-24). Using the example of the light bulb, if one connects the two wires of the bulb socket to the two wires of the isolated power system, the bulb will illuminate. However, if one connects one of the wires to one side of the isolated power and the other wire to ground, the bulb will not illuminate. If the wires of the isolated power system are connected, the short circuit will trip the circuit breaker. In comparing the two systems, the standard grounded power has a direct connection to ground, whereas the isolated system imposes a very high impedance to any current flow to ground.

The added safety of this system can be seen in Fig. 21-25. In this case, a person has come in contact with one side of the isolated power system (Point A). Since standing on ground (Point B) does not constitute a part of the isolated circuit, the individual does not complete the loop and will not receive a shock. This is because the ground is part of the primary circuit *(solid lines),* and the person is contacting only one side of the isolated secondary circuit *(cross-hatched lines).* The person does not complete either circuit (i.e., have two contact points); therefore, this situation does not pose an electric shock hazard. Of course, if that person contacts both lines of the isolated power system (an unlikely event) then they will receive a shock.

If a faulty electrical appliance which has an intact equipment ground wire is plugged into a standard household outlet, and the home wiring has a properly connected ground wire, then the amount of electrical current that will flow through the individual is considerably less than what will flow through the low-resistance ground wire. Here, an individual would be fairly well protected from a serious shock. However, if that ground wire was broken, the individual might well receive a lethal shock. No shock would occur if the same faulty piece of equipment were plugged into the isolated power system, even if the equipment

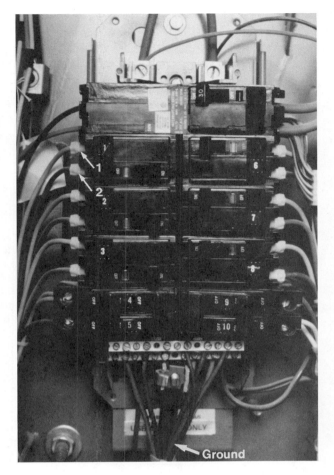

Fig. 21-24. Detail of the inside of a circuit breaker box in an isolated power system. The bottom *arrow* points to ground wires meeting at the common ground terminal. *Arrows* 1 and 2 indicate line 1 and line 2 from the isolated power circuit breaker. Neither line 1 nor line 2 is connected to the same terminals as the ground wires. This is in marked contrast to Fig. 21-15, where the neutral and ground wires are connected at the same point. (Used with permission from Ehrenwerth J: *Electrical safety.* In Barash PG, Cullen BF, Stoelting RK, editors: *Clinical anesthesia,* ed 2, Philadelphia, 1992, J.B. Lippincott.)

ground wire were broken. Thus, the isolated power system provides significant protection from macroshock. Another feature of the isolated power system is that the faulty piece of equipment, even though it may be partially short-circuited, will not usually trip the circuit breaker. This is an important feature, because the faulty piece of equipment may be part of a life-support system for a patient.

It is important to note that even though the power is isolated from ground, the case or frame of all electrical equipment is still connected to an equipment ground. The third wire (equipment ground wire) is necessary for a total electrical safety program.

Figure 21-26 illustrates a scenario involving a faulty piece of equipment connected to the isolated power system. This does not represent a hazard, but merely converts the isolated power back to a grounded power system as ex-

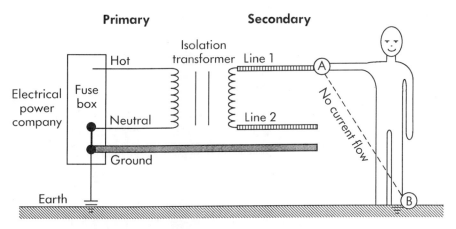

Fig. 21-25. A safety feature of the isolated power system is illustrated. An individual contacting one side of the isolated power system (Point A) and standing on the ground (Point B) will not receive a shock. In this instance, the individual is not contacting the circuit at two points and thus is not completing the circuit. Point A *(cross-hatched lines)* is part of the isolated power system, and Point B is part of the primary or grounded side of the circuit *(solid lines)*. (Used with permission from Ehrenwerth J: *Electrical safety.* In Barash PG, Cullen BF, Stoelting RK, editors: *Clinical anesthesia,* ed 2, Philadelphia, 1992, J.B. Lippincott.)

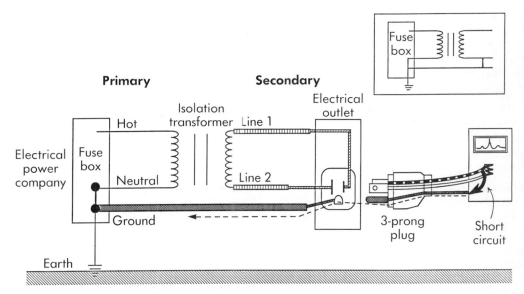

Fig. 21-26. A faulty piece of equipment plugged into the isolated power system does not present a shock hazard. It merely converts the isolated power system into a grounded power system. The figure insert illustrates that the isolated power system is now identical to the grounded power system. The dotted line indicates current flow in the ground wire. (Used with permission from Ehrenwerth J: *Electrical safety.* In Barash PG, Cullen BF, Stoelting RK, editors: *Clinical anesthesia,* ed 2, Philadelphia, 1992, J.B. Lippincott.)

ists outside the operating room. In fact, a *second* fault is necessary to create a hazard.

The previous discussion assumes that the isolated power system is perfectly isolated from ground. Actually, perfect isolation is impossible to achieve. All AC power systems and electrical devices manifest some degree of capacitance. As previously discussed, electrical power cords, wires, and electric motors exhibit capacitive coupling to the ground wire and metal conduits and "leak"

small amounts of current to ground (Fig. 21-27). This so-called *leakage current* partially ungrounds the isolated power system. This leakage current does not usually amount to more than a few milliamperes in an operating room, so that an individual coming in contact with one side of the isolated power system would receive only a very small shock (1 to 2 mA). Although this amount of current would be perceptible, it would not be dangerous.

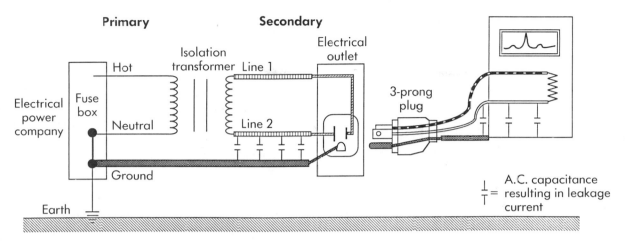

Fig. 21-27. The capacitance that exists in AC-powered lines and AC-operated equipment results in small "leakage currents" that partially degrade the isolation of the power system. (Used with permission from Ehrenwerth J: *Electrical safety*. In Barash PG, Cullen BF, Stoelting RK, editors: *Clinical anesthesia,* ed 2, Philadelphia, 1992, J.B. Lippincott.)

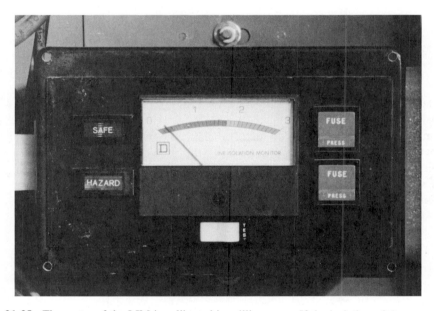

Fig. 21-28. The meter of the LIM is calibrated in milliamperes. If the isolation of the power system is degraded such that more than 2 mA (5 mA in newer systems) of current could flow, the hazard light will illuminate and a warning buzzer will sound. Note the button for testing the hazard warning system. (Used with permission from Ehrenwerth J: *Electrical safety*. In Barash PG, Cullen BF, Stoelting RK, editors: *Clinical anesthesia,* ed 2, Philadelphia, 1992, J.B. Lippincott.)

The line isolation monitor

The line isolation monitor (LIM) is a device that continuously monitors the integrity of an isolated power system. If a faulty piece of equipment is connected to the isolated power system, this will, in effect, change the system back to a conventional grounded system. The faulty piece of equipment will continue to function normally. Therefore, it is essential that a warning system be in place to alert the personnel that the power is no longer ungrounded. The LIM continuously monitors the isolated power to ensure that it is indeed isolated from ground, and the device has a

meter that displays a continuous indication of the integrity of the system (Fig. 21-28). In actuality, the LIM is continuously measuring the impedance to ground from each side of the isolated power circuit. As previously discussed, with perfect isolation, impedance would be infinitely high and there would be no current flow in the event of a first fault situation ($Z = E/I$, if $I = 0$, then $Z =$ infinity). Since all AC wiring and all AC powered electrical devices have some capacitance, small "leakage currents" are present that partially degrade the isolation of the system. The meter of the LIM will indicate (in milliamperes) the *total* amount of leakage in the system resulting from capacitance, electrical wiring, and any devices plugged into the isolated power system.

The reading on the LIM meter does *not* mean that current is actually flowing, but merely indicates how much current would flow in the event of a first fault. The LIM is set to sound an alarm at 2 mA or 5 mA, depending on the age and brand of the system. Once this preset limit is exceeded, visual and audible alarms are triggered to indicate that the isolation from ground has been degraded beyond a predetermined limit (Fig. 21-29). This alarm does not necessarily mean that a hazardous situation is present, but rather that the system is no longer totally isolated from ground. It would, in fact, require a second fault to create a dangerous situation.

For example, if the LIM was set to trigger an alarm at 2 mA, by Ohm's Law the impedance for either side (line 1 or line 2) of the isolated power system would be 60,000 ohms:

$$Z = \frac{E}{I}$$

$$Z = \frac{120 \text{ volts}}{0.002 \text{ amperes}}$$

$$Z = 60,000 \text{ ohms}$$

Therefore, if either side of the isolated power system had less than 60,000 ohms impedance to ground, the LIM would trigger an alarm. This might occur in two situations. The first is when a faulty piece of equipment is plugged into the isolated power system. In this case, a true fault to ground exists with a short circuit of essentially zero impedance from one line to ground. Now the system

would be converted to the equivalent of a grounded power system. This faulty piece of equipment should be removed and serviced as soon as possible. However, it could still be used safely if it was essential for the care of the patient. It should be remembered, however, that continuing to use this faulty piece of equipment would create the *potential* for a serious electric shock. This would occur if a *second* faulty piece of equipment were simultaneously connected to the isolated power system.

The second situation involves connecting many perfectly normal pieces of equipment to the isolated power system. Although each piece of equipment has only a small amount of leakage current, if the total leakage exceeds 2 mA, the LIM will trigger an alarm. Assume that in the same operating room there are 30 electrical devices each having 100 μA of leakage current. The total leakage current (30 × 100 μA) would be 3 mA. The impedance to ground would still be 40,000 ohms (120/0.003). The LIM alarm would sound, because the 2-mA set point has been violated. However, the system is still safe and represents a significantly different state than the first situation. For this reason, the newer LIMs are set to alarm at 5 mA instead of 2 mA.

The newest LIMs are referred to as third-generation monitors. The first-generation monitor, or static LIM, was unable to detect balanced faults (i.e., a situation in which there are equal faults to ground from both line 1 and line 2). The second-generation, or dynamic, LIM did not have this problem, but could interfere with physiologic monitoring. Both of these monitors would trigger an alarm at 2 mA, which led to annoying "false" alarms. The third-generation LIM corrects the problems of its predecessors and

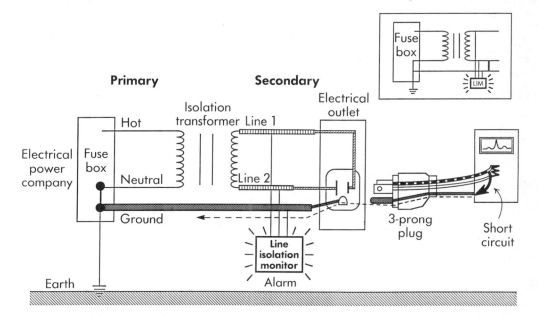

Fig. 21-29. When a faulty piece of equipment is plugged into the isolated power system, it will markedly decrease the impedance from line 1 or line 2 to ground. This will be detected by the LIM, which will sound an alarm. (Used with permission from Ehrenwerth J: *Electrical safety*. In Barash PG, Cullen BF, Stoelting RK, editors: *Clinical anesthesia*, ed 2, Philadelphia, 1992, J.B. Lippincott.)

has the alarm threshold set at 5 mA.[15] Proper functioning of the LIM depends on having both intact equipment ground wires as well as its own connection to ground. First- and second-generation LIMs could not detect the loss of the LIM ground connection. The third-generation LIM can detect this loss of ground to the monitor. In this case, the LIM alarm would sound and the red hazard light would illuminate, but the LIM meter would read zero. This condition will alert the staff that the LIM needs to be repaired. However, the LIM still cannot detect broken equipment ground wires. An example of a third-generation LIM is the Iso-Gard made by The Square D Company.

The equipment ground wire is a very important part of the safety system. If this wire is broken, a faulty piece of equipment that is plugged into an outlet will operate normally, but the LIM will not sound an alarm. A second fault could therefore cause a shock, without any alarm from the LIM. Also, in the event of a second fault, the equipment ground wire provides a low-resistance path to ground for most of the fault current (see Fig. 21-26). The LIM will only be able to register leakage currents from pieces of equipment that are connected to the isolated power system and have intact ground wires.

Ground fault circuit interrupter

The ground fault circuit interrupter (GFCI) is another popular device used to prevent individuals from receiving an electric shock from a grounded power system. Electrical codes for most new construction require that a GFCI circuit be present in potentially hazardous (e.g., wet) areas such as bathrooms, kitchens, or outdoor electrical outlets. The GFCI may be installed as an individual power outlet (Fig. 21-30) or may be a special circuit breaker to which all the individual protected outlets are connected at a single point. The special GFCI circuit breaker is located in the main fuse/circuit breaker box and can be distinguished by its red test button (Fig. 21-31).

Figure 21-7 demonstrates that the current flowing in both the hot and neutral wires is usually equal. The GFCI monitors both sides of the circuit for the equality of current flow, and if a difference is detected, the power is immediately interrupted. If an individual were to contact a faulty piece of equipment such that current flowed through the individual, an imbalance between the two sides of the circuit would be created, which would be detected by the GFCI. Because the GFCI can detect very small current differences (in the range of 5 mA), the GFCI will open the circuit within a few milliseconds, thereby interrupting the current flow before a significant shock occurs. Thus, the GFCI provides a high level of protection at a very modest cost.

The disadvantage of using a GFCI in the operating room is that it totally interrupts the power without warning. A defective piece of equipment could no longer be used, which might be a problem if it was of a life-support nature. If, however, the same faulty piece of equipment

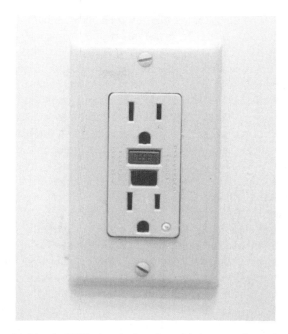

Fig. 21-30. A GFCI electrical outlet with integrated test and reset buttons. (Used with permission from Ehrenwerth J: *Electrical safety.* In Barash PG, Cullen BF, Stoelting RK, editors: *Clinical anesthesia,* ed 2, Philadelphia, 1992, J.B. Lippincott.)

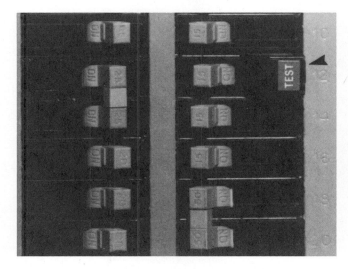

Fig. 21-31. Special GFCI circuit breaker. The *arrowhead* points to the distinguishing red test button. (Used with permission from Ehrenwerth J: *Electrical safety.* In Barash PG, Cullen BF, Stoelting RK, editors: *Clinical anesthesia,* ed 2, Philadelphia, 1992, J.B. Lippincott.)

was plugged into an isolated power system, the LIM would respond with an alarm, but the equipment could still continue to be used.

MICROSHOCK

As previously discussed, the concept of macroshock concerns relatively large amounts of current applied to the surface of the body. The current is conducted through all the tissues in proportion to their conductivity and area in a plane perpendicular to the current. Consequently, the "density" of the current (amps per square meter) that reaches the heart is considerably less than what is applied to the body surface. However, an electrically susceptible patient (i.e., one who has a direct external connection to the heart) may be at risk from very small currents; this is called *microshock*.[16] The catheter orifice or electrical wire with a very small surface area in contact with the heart results in a relatively large current density at that site.[17] Stated another way, even very small amounts of current applied directly to the myocardium will cause ventricular fibrillation. Microshock is a particularly difficult problem because of the insidious nature of the hazard.

In the electrically susceptible patient, ventricular fibrillation can be produced by a current that is below the threshold of human perception, although the exact amount of current necessary to cause ventricular fibrillation is unknown. Whalen and colleagues[18] were able to produce fibrillation with 20 µA of current applied directly to the myocardium of dogs. Raftery and associates[19] produced fibrillation with 80 µA of current in some patients. Hull[20] used data obtained by Watson and colleagues[21] to show that 50% of patients would fibrillate at current of 200 µA. Because 1000 µA (1 mA) is generally regarded as the threshold of human perception with 60-Hz AC current, the electrically susceptible patient can be electrocuted with one-tenth of normally perceptible currents. This is not only of academic interest, but also of practical concern, because many cases of ventricular fibrillation due to microshock have been reported.[22-27]

The stray capacitance that is part of any AC-powered electrical instrument may result in significant amounts of charge build-up on the case of that instrument. An individual who simultaneously touches the case of an instrument where this has occurred and the electrically susceptible pa-

tient may unknowingly cause a discharge to the patient that results in ventricular fibrillation. Once again, the equipment ground wire constitutes the principal protection against microshock for the electrically susceptible patient. In this case, the equipment ground wire provides a low resistance path by which most of the leakage current is dissipated instead of being stored as a charge.

Figure 21-32 illustrates a situation involving a patient who has a saline-filled catheter in the heart, with a resistance of approximately 500 ohms. The ground wire with a resistance of 1 ohm is connected to the instrument case. A leakage current of 100 µA will divide according to the relative resistances of the two paths. In this case, 99.8 µA will flow through the equipment ground wire, and only 0.2 µA will flow through the fluid-filled catheter. This extremely small current does not endanger the patient. However, if the equipment ground wire was broken, the electrically susceptible patient would be at great risk, because all 100 µA of leakage current could flow through the catheter and cause ventricular fibrillation (Fig. 21-33).

Modern patient monitors incorporate another method to reduce the risk of microshock for electrically susceptible patients. This method involves electrically isolating all patient connections from the power supply of the monitor by placing a very high impedance between the patient and any device. This limits the amount of internal leakage of current through the patient connection to a very small value. At present, the standard is less than 10 µA. For example, the output of an ECG monitor's power supply is electrically isolated from the patient by placing a very high impedance between the monitor and the patient's ECG leads.[6,28] Isolation techniques are designed to inhibit hazardous electrical pathways between the patient and the monitor while allowing the passage of the physiologic signal.

It must be remembered that the line isolation monitor is

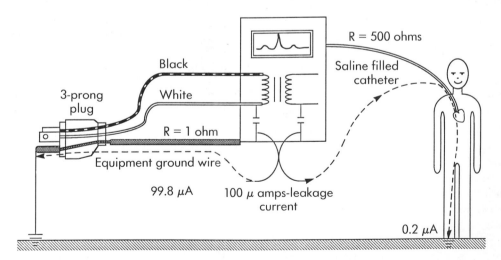

Fig. 21-32. The electrically susceptible patient is protected from microshock by the presence of an intact equipment ground wire. The equipment ground wire provides a low-impedance path in which the majority of the leakage current *(dotted lines)* can flow. (Used with permission from Ehrenwerth J: *Electrical safety*. In Barash PG, Cullen BF, Stoelting RK, editors: *Clinical anesthesia*, ed 2, Philadelphia, 1992, J.B. Lippincott.)

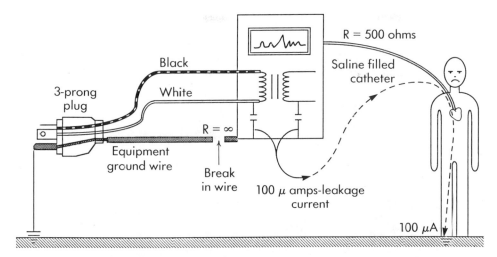

Fig. 21-33. A broken equipment ground wire results in a significant hazard to the electrically susceptible patient. In this case, the entire leakage current can be conducted to the heart and may result in ventricular fibrillation. (Used with permission from Ehrenwerth J: *Electrical safety.* In Barash PG, Cullen BF, Stoelting RK, editors: *Clinical anesthesia,* ed 2, Philadelphia, 1992, J.B. Lippincott.)

not designed to provide protection from microshock. The microampere currents involved in microshock are far below the LIM's threshold of protection. In addition, the LIM does not register the leakage of individual monitors, but rather it indicates the status of the total system. The LIM reading indicates the total amount of leakage current resulting from the entire capacitance of the system. This is the amount of current that would flow to ground in the event of a first-fault situation.

The essence of electrical safety is a thorough understanding of all the principles of grounding. As Bruner states, "Grounding is neither safe nor unsafe. Its significance is dependent on what is grounded and in what context."[9] The objective of electrical safety is to make it difficult for electrical current to pass through people. For this reason, both the patient and the anesthesiologist should be isolated from ground as much as possible. That is, their impedance to current flow should be as high as is technologically feasible. In the inherently unsafe electrical environment of an operating room, several measures can be taken to help ensure against contacting hazardous current flows. First, the grounded power provided by the utility company can be converted to ungrounded power by means of an isolation transformer. The LIM will continuously monitor the status of this isolation from ground, and warn that the isolation of the power (from ground) has been lost in the event a defective piece of equipment is plugged into one of the isolated circuit outlets. In addition, the shock that an individual could receive from a faulty piece of equipment is determined by the capacitance of the system and is limited to a few milliamperes. Second, all equipment plugged into the isolated power system has an equipment ground wire that is connected to the case of the instrument. This equipment ground wire provides an alternative low-resistance pathway enabling potentially

dangerous currents to flow to ground. Thus, the patient and the anesthesiologist should be as insulated from ground as possible and all electrical equipment should be grounded.

The equipment ground wire serves three functions. First, it provides a low-resistance path for fault currents, to reduce the risk of macroshock. Second, it dissipates leakage currents that are potentially harmful to the electrically susceptible patient. Third, it provides information to the LIM on the status of the ungrounded power system. If the equipment ground wire is broken, a significant factor in the prevention of electric shock is lost. Additionally, the isolated power system will appear safer than it actually is because the LIM is unable to detect broken equipment ground wires.

Because power cord plugs and receptacles are subjected to greater abuse in the hospital than in the home, the Underwriters Laboratories have issued a strict specification for special hospital-grade plugs and receptacles (Fig. 21-34), which are marked by green dots.[29] The hospital-grade plug is one that can be visually inspected or easily disassembled to ensure the integrity of the ground wire connection. Molded opaque plugs are not acceptable. Edwards[30] reported that out of 3000 non-hospital-grade receptacles installed in a new hospital building, 1800 (60%) were defective after 3 years. When 2000 of the non-hospital-grade receptacles were replaced with ones of hospital grade, no failures were reported after 18 months of use.

ELECTROSURGERY

On that fateful day in October 1926 when Harvey W. Cushing first used an electrosurgical machine invented by Professor William T. Bovie to resect a brain tumor, the course of modern surgery and anesthesia was forever altered.[31] The ubiquitous use of electrosurgery today attests

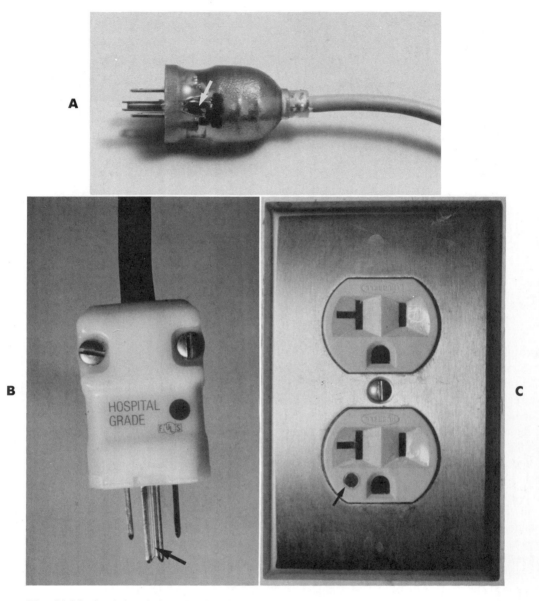

Fig. 21-34. A, A hospital-grade plug that can be visually inspected. The *arrow* points to the equipment ground wire, whose integrity can be readily verified. **B,** A hospital-grade plug that can be easily disassembled for inspection. Note that the prong for the ground wire *(arrow)* is longer than the hot or neutral prong, so that it is the first to enter the receptacle. **C,** The *arrow* points to the green dot denoting a hospital-grade power outlet. (Used with permission from Ehrenwerth J: *Electrical safety.* In Barash PG, Cullen BF, Stoelting RK, editors: *Clinical anesthesia,* ed 2, Philadelphia, 1992, J.B. Lippincott.)

to the success of Professor Bovie's invention. However, this technology was not adopted without some cost. The widespread use of electrocautery has, at the very least, hastened the elimination of explosive anesthetic agents from the operating room. In addition, as every anesthesiologist is aware, few things in the operating room are immune to interference from the "Bovie." The high-frequency electrical energy generated by the electrosurgery unit (ESU) interferes with everything from the ECG signal to cardiac output computers, pulse oximeters, and even implanted cardiac pacemakers.[32]

The ESU operates by generating very high-frequency currents (radiofrequency range) of anywhere from 500,000 to more than 1 million Hz. Heat is generated whenever a current passes through a resistance. The amount of heat (H) produced is proportional to the square of the current (I) and inversely proportional to the area (A) through which the current passes ($H = I^2/A$).[33] By concentrating the energy at the tip of the "Bovie pencil," the surgeon can produce either a cut or a coagulation at any given spot. This very high-frequency current behaves quite differently from the standard 60-Hz AC current, and can pass directly

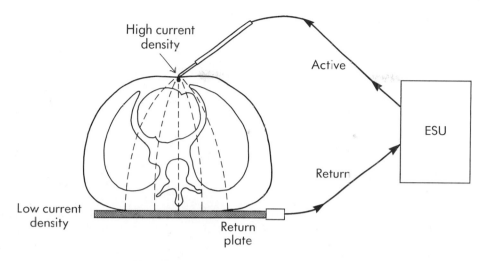

Fig. 21-35. A properly applied ESU return plate. The current density at the return plate is low, resulting in no danger to the patient. (Used with permission from Ehrenwerth J: *Electrical safety*. In Barash PG, Cullen BF, Stoelting RK, editors: *Clinical anesthesia*, ed 2, Philadelphia, 1992, J.B. Lippincott.)

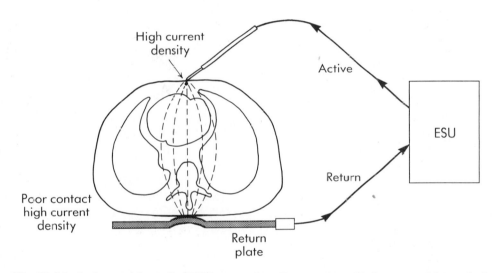

Fig. 21-36. An improperly applied ESU return plate. Poor contact with the return plate results in a high current density and a possible burn to the patient. (Used with permission from Ehrenwerth J: *Electrical safety*. In Barash PG, Cullen BF, Stoelting RK, editors: *Clinical anesthesia*, ed 2, Philadelphia, 1992, J.B. Lippincott.)

across the precordium without causing ventricular fibrillation.[33] This is possible because high-frequency currents have a low tissue penetration, and do not excite contractile cells.

The large amount of energy generated by the ESU can pose other problems to the operator and the patient. Cushing became aware of one such problem. He wrote, "once the operator received a shock which passed through a metal retractor to his arm and out by a wire from his headlight, which was unpleasant to say the least."[34] The ESU cannot be safely operated unless the energy is properly routed from the ESU through the patient and back to the unit. Ideally, the current generated by the active electrode

is concentrated at the ESU tip, constituting a very small surface area. This energy has a high current density and is able to generate enough heat to produce a therapeutic cut or coagulation. The energy then passes through the patient to a dispersive electrode of large surface area that returns the energy safely to the ESU (Fig. 21-35).

One unfortunate quirk in terminology concerns the return (dispersive) plate of the ESU. This plate, often incorrectly referred to as a "ground plate," is actually a dispersive electrode of large surface area that safely returns the generated energy to the ESU via a low-current density pathway. When enquiring whether the dispersive electrode has been applied to the patient, operating room personnel frequently ask "is the patient grounded?" Since the aim of electrical safety is to isolate the patient from ground, this expression is not only erroneous, but also leads to confusion.

Because the area of the return plate is large, the current density is low; therefore, no harmful heat is generated, and no tissue destruction occurs. In a properly functioning system, the only tissue effect is at the site of the active electrode that is held by the surgeon. Problems can arise if the electrosurgical return plate is improperly applied to the patient, or if the cord connecting the return plate to the ESU is damaged or broken. In these instances, the high-frequency current generated by the ESU will seek an alternate return pathway. Anything attached to the patient, such as ECG leads or a temperature probe, can provide this alternate return pathway. The current density at an ECG pad will be considerably higher than normal because its surface area is much less than that of the ESU return plate. This may result in a serious burn at the alternate return site. Similarly, a burn may occur at the site of the ESU return plate if it is not properly applied to the patient or if it becomes partially dislodged during the operation (Fig. 21-36). That this is not merely a theoretical possibility is evidenced by the numerous case reports involving patients who have received ESU burns.[35-40]

The original ESUs were manufactured with the power supply connected directly to ground by the equipment ground wire. These devices made it extremely easy for ESU current to return by alternate pathways. In fact, the ESU would continue to operate normally even without the return plate being connected to the patient. In most modern ESUs the power supply is isolated from ground to protect the patient from burns. It was hoped that by isolating the return pathway from ground, the only route for current flow would be via the return electrode. Theoretically, this would eliminate alternate return pathways and greatly reduce the incidence of burns.[5] However, Mitchell[41] found two situations in which the current could return via alternate pathways, even with the isolated ESU circuit. If the return plate were left either on top of an uninsulated ESU cabinet or in contact with the bottom of the operating room table, the ESU could operate fairly normally, and the current would return via alternate pathways. It will be recalled that the impedance is inversely proportional to the capacitance times the current frequency. The ESU operates at 500,000 to more than 1 million Hz, which greatly enhances the effect of capacitive coupling and causes a marked reduction in impedance. Therefore, even with isolated ESUs, the decrease in impedance allows the current to return to the ESU by alternate pathways. In addition, the isolated ESU does not protect the patient from burns if the return electrode does not make proper contact with the patient. Although the isolated ESU does provide additional patient safety, it is by no means foolproof protection against the patient receiving a burn.

Preventing patient burns from the ESU is a concern of all professional staff in the operating room. Not only the circulating nurse, but also the surgeon and the anesthesiologist must be aware of proper techniques and be vigilant to potential problems. The most important factor is the proper application of the return plate. It is essential that the return plate have the appropriate amount of electrolyte gel and an intact return wire. Reusable return plates must be properly cleaned after each use and disposable plates must be checked to be certain that the electrolyte has not dried out during storage. In addition, it is prudent to place the return plate as close as possible to the site of the operation. Electrocardiographic pads should be placed as far from the site of the operation as is feasible. Operating room personnel must be alert to the possibility that pools of flammable "prep" solutions, such as ether and acetone, can be ignited when the ESU is used. If the ESU must be used on a patient with a demand pacemaker, the return electrode should be located below the thorax, and preparations for treating potential arrhythmias should be available, including a magnet to convert the pacemaker to a fixed rate, a defibrillator, and an external pacemaker. The ESU has also caused other problems in patients with pacemakers, including reprogramming and microshock.[42,43] If the surgeon requests higher-than-normal power settings on the ESU, both the circulating nurse and the anesthesiologist should be alert to a potential problem. The return plate and cable should be inspected immediately to ensure that they are functioning and properly positioned. If this does not correct the problem, the return plate should be replaced. If the problem remains, the entire ESU unit should be taken out of service. Finally, an ESU that is dropped or damaged must be removed immediately from the operating room and thoroughly tested by a qualified biomedical engineer. Following these simple safety steps will prevent most patient burns from the ESU.

The previous discussion concerned only unipolar ESUs. There is a second type of ESU, in which the current passes only between the two blades of a pair of forceps. This type of device is referred to as a *bipolar* ESU. Because the active and return electrodes are the two blades of the forceps, it is not necessary to attach another dispersive electrode to the patient, unless a unipolar ESU is also being used. The bipolar ESU generates considerably less power than the unipolar, and is mainly used for ophthalmic and neurologic surgery.[2]

In 1980 Mirowski and colleagues[44] reported the first human implantation of a device to treat intractable ventricular tachyarrhythmias. This device, known as the *automatic implantable cardioverter-defibrillator* (AICD), is capable of sensing ventricular tachycardia and ventricular fibrillation and then automatically defibrillating the heart. Since 1980, thousands of patients have received AICD implants.[45,46] Because some of these patients may now present for noncardiac surgery, it is important that the anesthesiologist be aware of potential problems.[47] The use of a unipolar ESU may cause electrical interference that could be interpreted by the AICD as a ventricular tachyarrhythmia. This would trigger a defibrillation pulse to be delivered to the heart and would likely cause an actual episode of tachycardia or fibrillation. The patient with an AICD is also at risk for fibrillation during electroconvulsive therapy (ECT).[47] In both cases, the AICD should be disabled by placing a magnet over it. Also, an external defibrillator and a noninvasive pacemaker must be in the operating room whenever a patient with an AICD is anesthetized. If the anesthesiologist is unfamiliar with the operation of the AICD, then someone who is experienced with the device should be available.

Electrical safety in the operating room is a matter of combining common sense with some basic principles of electricity. Once operating room personnel understand the importance of safe electrical practice, they are able to develop a heightened awareness to potential problems. All electrical equipment must undergo routine maintenance, service, and inspection to ensure that it conforms to designated electrical safety standards. Records of these test results must be kept for future inspection because human error can easily compound electrical hazards. Starmer and associates[48] cite a case concerning a newly constructed laboratory where the ground wire was not attached to a receptacle. In another study Albisser and colleagues[49] found a 14% (198/1424) incidence of improperly or incorrectly wired outlets. Furthermore, potentially hazardous situations should be recognized and corrected before they become a problem. For instance, electrical power cords are frequently placed on the floor, where they can be crushed by various carts or the anesthesia machine. These cords should be relocated overhead or in an area of low traffic flow. Multiple-plug extension boxes should not be left on the floor where they can come into contact with electrolyte solutions. These boxes could easily be mounted on a cart or on the anesthesia machine. Pieces of equipment that have been damaged or have obvious defects in the power cord must not be used until they have been properly repaired. If everyone is aware of what constitutes a potential hazard, then dangerous situations can be prevented with minimal effort.

CONDUCTIVE FLOORING

Conductive flooring was mandated for operating rooms where flammable anesthetic agents were being administered. The conductive floor was specified to have a resistance of between 25,000 and 1 million ohms. This would minimize the build-up of static charges, which could cause a flammable anesthetic agent to ignite. The standards have been changed to eliminate the necessity for conductive flooring in anesthetizing areas where flammable agents are no longer used.

CONSTRUCTION OF NEW OPERATING ROOMS

A final area of electrical safety that is of concern to the anesthesiologist is in the design of new operating room facilities. Frequently, an anesthesiologist is asked to consult with hospital administrators and architects in designing new operating rooms. In the past, a very strict electrical code was enforced because of the use of flammable anesthetic agents. This code included a requirement for isolated power systems and LIMs. In recent years, the National Fire Protection Association (NFPA) has revised its standard for health-care facilities (NFPA 99-1984). These new standards no longer require isolated power systems or LIMs in areas designated for use of only nonflammable anesthetic agents.[50,51] Although they are not mandatory, NFPA standards are usually adopted by local authorities when revising their electrical codes.

This change in the standard creates a dilemma. The NFPA 99-Standard for Health Care Facilities-1990 edition mandates that "wet location patient care areas be provided with special protection against electric shock . . ." Section 3-4.1.2.6 further states, "this special protection shall be provided by a power distribution system that inherently limits the possible ground fault current due to a first fault to a low value, without interrupting the power supply; or by a power distribution system in which the power supply is interrupted if the ground fault current does, in fact, exceed a value of 6 milliamperes."

The decision of whether to install isolated power hinges on two factors. The first is whether the operating room is considered a *wet location;* and, if so, whether an interruption of the power supply is tolerable. Where power interruption is tolerable, a ground fault circuit interrupter (GFCI) is permitted as the protective means. However, the Standard also states that "the use of an isolated power system (IPS) shall be permitted as a protective means capable of limiting ground fault current without power interruption."

Most personnel who have worked in an operating room would attest to it being a wet location. The presence of blood, body fluids, and electrolyte solutions spilled on the floor all contribute to making it a wet environment.[52] The cystoscopy suite serves as a good example.

Once the premise that the operating room is a wet location is accepted, then it must be determined if a GFCI can provide the means of protection. The argument against using GFCIs in the operating room is illustrated by the following example. Assume that during an open-heart procedure, the cardiopulmonary bypass pump and the patient monitors are plugged into outlets on the same branch circuit. Also assume that during bypass, the circulating nurse now plugs in a faulty headlight. If there is a GFCI protecting the circuit, the fault will be detected, and the GFCI will interrupt all power to the pump and the monitors. This undoubtedly would cause a great deal of confusion and consternation among the operating room personnel and may place the patient at risk for injury. The pump would have to be manually operated while the problem was being resolved. In addition, the GFCI could not be reset (and power restored) until the headlight was identified as the cause of the fault and unplugged from the outlet. On the other hand, if the operating room was protected with an isolated power system and a LIM, then the same scenario would cause the LIM to trigger an alarm, but the pump and patient monitors would continue to operate normally. There would be no interruption of power, and the problem could be resolved without risk to the patient.

It should be realized that a GFCI is an active system. That is, a potentially hazardous current is already flowing and must be actively interrupted, whereas the isolated power system with a LIM is designed to be safe during a first-fault situation, and thus is a passive system.[53]

It is likely that hospital administrators may want to eliminate isolated power systems in new operating room construction as a cost-saving measure. However, Matjasko and Ashman,[52] Bruner and Leonard,[53] and Lennon and Leonard[54] all advocate the retention of isolated power systems, and it is this author's opinion that not to do so would be a short-sighted and foolhardy measure. This is especially true because the cost of adding isolated power is estimated to be less than 1% of the cost of constructing an operating room.[53] Although not perfect,[55] the isolated power system and LIM do provide both the patient and operating room personnel with a significant amount of protection in an electrically hazardous environment. Anesthesiologists need to be aware of this change and strongly encourage that new operating rooms be constructed *with* isolated power systems. The relatively small cost savings that the alternative would represent does not justify the elimination of such a useful safety system, and the use of GFCIs is not practical in the operating room environment.

REFERENCES

1. Bruner JMR: Hazards of electrical apparatus, *Anesthesiology* 28:396-425, 1967.
2. Hull CJ: Electrical hazards in monitoring, *Int Anesthesiol Clin* 19:177-195, 1981.
3. Leonard PF, Gould AB: Dynamics of electrical hazards of particular concern to operating-room personnel, *Surg Clin North Am* 45:817-828, 1965.
4. Miller F: *College physics*, ed 2, New York, 1967, Harcourt Brace and World, pp 457-459.
5. Uyttendaele K, Grobstein S, Svetz P: Monitoring instrumentation— isolated inputs, electrosurgery filtering, burns protection: What does it mean? *Acta Anaesthesiol Belg* 29:317-329, 1978.
6. Leonard PF: Characteristics of electrical hazards; *Anesth Analg* 51:797-809, 1972.
7. Taylor KW, Desmond J: Electrical hazards in the operating room, with special reference to electrosurgery, *Can J Surg* 13:362-374, 1970.
8. Leonard PF: Apparatus and appliances . . . current thinking. III. Alternating current, the isolation transformer, and the differential-transformer pressure transducer, *Anesth Analg* 45:814-817, 1966.
9. Bruner JMR: *Fundamental concepts of electrical safety.* In Hershey SG, editor: *ASA refresher courses in anesthesiology*, Philadelphia, 1974, J.B. Lippincott.
10. Harpell TR: Electrical shock hazards in the hospital environment: Their causes and cures, *Can Hosp* 47:48-53, 1970.
11. Buczko GB, McKay WPS: Electrical safety in the operating room, *Can J Anaesth* 34:315-322, 1987.
12. Wald A: *Electrical safety in medicine.* In Skalak R, Chien S, editors: *Handbook of bioengineering*, New York, 1987, McGraw-Hill.
13. Dalziel CF, Massoglia FP: Let-go currents and voltages, *AIEE Trans* 75:49, 1956.
14. Bruner JMR, Aronow S, Cavicchi RV: Electrical incidents in a large hospital: A 42 month register, *JAAMI* 6:222-230, 1972.
15. Bernstein MS: Isolated power and line isolation monitors, *Biomed Instrum Technol* 24:221-223, 1990.
16. Weinberg DI, Artley JL, Whalen RE, et al: Electric shock hazards in cardiac catheterization, *Circ Res* 11:1004-1009, 1962.
17. Starmer CF, Whalen RE: Current density and electrically induced ventricular fibrillation, *Med Instrum* 7:158-161, 1973.
18. Whalen RE, Starmer CF, McIntosh HD: Electrical hazards associated with cardiac pacemaking, *Ann NY Acad Sci* 111:922-931, 1964.
19. Raftery EB, Green HL, Yacoub MH: Disturbances of heart rhythm produced by 50-Hz leakage currents in human subjects, *Cardiovasc Res* 9:263-265, 1975.
20. Hull CJ: Electrocution hazards in the operating theatre, *Br J Anaesth* 50:647-657, 1978.
21. Watson AB, Wright JS, Loughman J: Electrical thresholds for ventricular fibrillation in man, *Med J Aust* 1:1179-1182, 1973.
22. Furman S, Schwedel JB, Robinson G, et al: Use of an intracardiac pacemaker in the control of heart block, *Surgery* 49:98-108, 1961.
23. Noordijk JA, Oey FJI, Tebra W: Myocardial electrodes and the danger of ventricular fibrillation, *Lancet* I:975-977, 1961.
24. Pengelly LD, Klassen GA: Myocardial electrodes and the danger of ventricular fibrillation, *Lancet* I:1234, 1961 (letter).
25. Rowe GG, Zarnstorff WC: Ventricular fibrillation during selective angiocardiography, *JAMA* 192:947-950, 1965.
26. Hopps JA, Roy OS: Electrical hazards in cardiac diagnosis and treatment, *Med Electr Biol Eng* 1:133, 1963.
27. Mody SM, Richings M: Ventricular fibrillation resulting from electrocution during cardiac catheterization, *Lancet* II:698-699, 1962.
28. Leeming MN: Protection of the electrically susceptible patient: A discussion of systems and methods, *Anesthesiology* 38:370-383, 1973.
29. Cromwell L, Weibell FJ, Pfeiffer EA: *Biomedical instrumentation and measurements*, (ed 2), Englewood Cliffs, NJ, 1980, Prentice-Hall, pp 430-446.
30. Edwards NK: Specialized electrical grounding needs, *Clin Perinatol* 3:367-374, 1976.
31. Goldwyn RM: Bovie: The man and the machine, *Ann Plast Surg* 2:135-153, 1979.
32. Lichter I, Borrie J, Miller WM: Radio-frequency hazards with cardiac pacemakers, *BMJ* 1:1513-1518, 1965.
33. Dornette WHL: An electrically safe surgical environment, *Arch Surg* 107:567-573, 1973.
34. Cushing H: Electro-surgery as an aid to the removal of intracranial tumors: With a preliminary note on a new surgical-current generator by W.T. Bovie, *Surg Gynecol Obstet* 47:751-784, 1928.
35. Meathe EA: Electrical safety for patients and anesthetists. In Saidman LJ, Smith NT, *Monitoring in anesthesia*, ed 2, Boston, 1984, Butterworths.
36. Rolly G: Two cases of burns caused by misuse of coagulation unit and monitoring, *Acta Anaesthesiol Belg* 29:313-316, 1978.
37. Parker EO: Electrosurgical burn at the site of an esophageal temperature probe, *Anesthesiology* 61:93-95, 1984.
38. Schneider AJL, Apple HP, Braun RT: Electrosurgical burns at skin temperature probes, *Anesthesiology* 47:72-74, 1977.
39. Bloch EC, Burton LW: Electrosurgical burn while using a battery-operated Doppler monitor, *Anesth Analg* 58:339-342, 1979.
40. Becker CM, Malhotra IV, Hedley-Whyte J: The distribution of radiofrequency current and burns, *Anesthesiology* 38:106-122, 1973.

41. Mitchell JP: The isolated circuit diathermy, *Ann R Coll Surg Engl* 61:287-290, 1979.
42. Titel JH, El Etr AA: Fibrillation resulting from pacemaker electrodes and electrocautery during surgery, *Anesthesiology* 29:845-846, 1968.
43. Domino KB, Smith TC: Electrocautery-induced reprogramming of a pacemaker using a precordial magnet, *Anesth Analg* 62:609-612, 1983.
44. Mirowski M, Reid PR, Mower MM, et al: Termination of malignant ventricular arrhythmias with an implanted automatic defibrillator in human beings, *N Engl J Med* 303:322-324, 1980.
45. Crozier IG, Ward DE: Automatic implantable defibrillators, *Br J Hosp Med* 40:136-139, 1988.
46. Elefteriades JA, Biblo LA, Batsford WP, et al: Evolving patterns in the surgical treatment of malignant ventricular tachyarrhythmias, *Ann Thorac Surg* 49:94-100, 1990.
47. Carr CME, Whiteley SM: The automatic implantable cardioverter-defibrillator, *Anaesthesia* 46:737-740, 1991.
48. Starmer CF, McIntosh HD, Whalen RE: Electrical hazards and cardiovascular function, *N Engl J Med* 284:181-186, 1971.
49. Albisser AM, Parson ID, Pask BA: A survey of the grounding systems in several large hospitals, *Med Instrum* 7:297-302, 1973.
50. Kermit E, Staewen WS: Isolated power systems: Historical perspective and update on regulations, *Biomed Tech Today* 1:86-89, 1986.
51. NFPA: National electric code (ANSI/NFPA 70-1984). Quincy, MA, 1984, National Fire Protection Association.
52. Matjasko MJ, Ashman MN: *All you need to know about electrical safety in the operating room*. In Barash PG, Deutsch S, Tinker J (editors): *ASA refresher courses in anesthesiology, vol 18*, Philadelphia, 1990, J.B. Lippincott.
53. Bruner JMR, Leonard PF: *Electricity, safety and the patient*, Chicago, 1989, Year Book Medical Publishers, p 300.
54. Lennon RL, Leonard PF: A hitherto unreported virtue of the isolated power system, *Anesth Analg* 66:1056-1057, 1987 (letter).
55. Gilbert TB, Shaffer M, Matthews M: Electrical shock by dislodged spark gap in bipolar electrosurgical device, *Anesth Analg* 73:355-357, 1991.

Part V

MAINTENANCE AND QUALITY ASSURANCE

Chapter 22

ANESTHESIA EQUIPMENT: CHECKOUT AND QUALITY ASSURANCE

John H. Eichhorn, M.D.

The analogy between administering general anesthesia and piloting a commercial jet may be somewhat overused, but it is singularly relevant in this context. The aviation industry has developed extraordinarily thorough plans involving acute and chronic interactions with its principal equipment, the commercial passenger jetliner. The acute component is the immediate preflight check to verify that a particular aircraft should fly safely that day on a given trip. The chronic component is the elaborate scheme of scheduled preventive maintenance, repair, exchange of old parts for new, and safety inspections of structural components. These are all oriented toward assuring that the aircraft will fly safely for the designated interval of weeks or months covered by that particular activity. In anesthesia practice, the analogy is obviously appropriate to an anesthesia equipment quality assurance (QA) program. The acute effort is the preanesthetic equipment check, and the chronic component is the vital and ongoing QA mechanism involving preventive maintenance, testing for safe function, and the detection of expected wear prior to the failure of a piece of equipment.

BACKGROUND

Because the practice of anesthesia is heavily dependent on the correct functioning of a large number of diverse pieces of equipment, and because anesthesia providers usually have technical and mechanical proclivities, reports of problems with anesthesia equipment have been prominent in the anesthesia literature virtually since its inception. A great many of the traditional problems that had

Although the majority of anesthesia critical incidents and overt catastrophes involve human error, some events involve overt equipment failure or failure of the anesthesia provider to discover an equipment problem. Most equipment problems in anesthesia practice are preventable, and this chapter is intended to help practitioners achieve that goal.

been common since recognizable anesthesia machines came into use—such as fresh gas rotameter leaks, ventilator leaks, and disconnections of poorly designed hose or tubing connectors—have been largely eliminated by the adoption and implementation of rigorous so-called voluntary design and fabrication standards by anesthesia machine manufacturers.[1] By no means does this suggest that equipment problems do not arise today. On the contrary, some problems, such as absent, broken, or stuck unidirectional breathing system valves or failure to remove the wrapper on prepackaged carbon dioxide absorbent inner canisters, are still of concern today. Also, because of the increasing complexity of anesthesia delivery systems, scrupulous attention to acute and chronic QA of anesthesia equipment is more important than ever. However, many of the details and the specific problems have changed. Although historical perspectives are valuable with regard to anesthesia equipment, this chapter focuses mainly on current concerns rather than on a litany of hundreds of problems that have been identified with anesthesia equipment over the years (see Chapter 16).

Prior treatises on anesthesia equipment provide useful references for reviewing the spectrum of defects and problems that have been reported with anesthesia equipment.[2,3] Rendell-Baker[4] edited a classic monograph that described 48 specific safety-related problems with anesthesia machines. Among these (in order of frequency) were problems with the vaporizer, the breathing system, the gas flowmeters, the mechanical functions of the machine, and human engineering. Spooner and Kirby[5] have outlined some of the data collected by the ECRI (formerly known as the Emergency Care Research Institute) regarding the role of equipment in anesthesia accidents. These data again suggest that a combination of the occasional overt device failure along with a large component of various types of human error led to the types of mishaps outlined in Table 22-1.

Further, pioneering work by Cooper and associates[6] suggested that among anesthesia critical incidents, 82% involved human error and only 14% overt equipment failure. Of course, many of the human errors involved unrecognized problems with the equipment, such as breathing system disconnection, that were not classic equipment failures (and that would not necessarily have been prevented or mitigated by the preanesthetic checkout of the anesthesia equipment). Among the equipment failures, 20% involved the breathing circuit, 18% the airway components, 12% laryngoscopes, and 12% the anesthesia machine. Failure to perform a normal check was cited 22 times among a list of 481 factors associated with 359 incidents. Follow-up studies[7] of 1089 preventable critical incidents found that only 4% of incidents with substantive negative outcomes involved equipment failure. Eleven percent to 19% of all incidents reported in the various parts of the study involved

Table 22-1. Types of equipment problems and incidents reported to the ECRI

Elements of incidents	Number (total = 179)	%
Part of anesthesia system implicated		
Scavenging system	52	29
Vaporizer	37	21
Breathing circuit	33	18
Absorber/pop-off/directional valve	15	8
Ventilator	15	8
Gas system/fail-safe/flush valve	13	7
Flow control and meter	14	8
Type of problem discussed		
Inadequacy or lack of component	53	30
Failure to function properly	55	31
Leaks and disconnects	30	17
Improper use	21	12
Misassembly	19	11
Sepsis	1	1
Resulting hazard		
Hypoxia	61	34
Pollution of operating room	48	27
Arrhythmia or cardiac arrest	30	17
Barotrauma	28	16
Lightened anesthesia	10	6
Infection	1	1
Explosion	1	1

Adapted from Spooner RB, Kirby RR: *Int Anesth Clin* 22(2):133-147, 1984.

equipment failure. However, 129 of 583 instances of human error involved anesthesia machine use, indicating that the interaction of the anesthesiologist with normally functioning equipment accounts for many problems. Minimizing this type of problem, by eliminating defects in the delivery system prior to the start of any anesthetic, is the goal of a thorough preuse anesthesia equipment checkout. Many other studies have also implicated the failure to perform an adequate preanesthetic checkout of the equipment as a factor in critical incidents and accidents. Heath[8] investigated serious anesthesia accidents in Great Britain and found the "principal cause of catastrophe . . . was user error involving disconnection or misconnection. Faulty systems of equipment management, combined in some cases with inadequate preanesthetic checking of apparatus, were responsible for the other instances."[8] Another study[9] in Great Britain found that the anesthesia equipment problems implicated in critical incidents were disconnections, leaks, disruption of gas supply, vaporizer misadventure, valve failure, and obstructions. They similarly concluded that, "Human error was more frequently responsible than equipment failure, and failure to perform a normal check was the factor most frequently associated."[9] More recently 1 of the 11 cases reported in the analysis of severe anesthesia injuries at the Harvard teaching hospitals[10] was caused by a misconnection of a vaporizer that had just been returned from servicing, a condition that would have been detected by a thorough preuse checkout of the anesthesia equipment.

PREANESTHESIA CHECKOUT

General acceptance by anesthesia providers that a preanesthetic checkout of the equipment should be done indicates that most anesthesiologists believe that this will help prevent untoward events during anesthesia administration. Studies in the early 1980s suggested that, in a test situation, practitioners consistently failed to find most of the intentionally created anesthesia machine faults.[11] On average, fewer than half of five major problems were discovered by a group of anesthesia practitioners. Among residents, the level of training was correlated with the ability to detect machine problems; third-year trainees were found to be more skilled than second-year or first-year trainees.[12] Both groups of investigators concluded that considerably more emphasis on education for machine checkout was needed in training programs. Because the subjects consistently checked items related to airway and hemodynamic maintenance while missing problems with the machine itself, they also concluded that consistent use of printed checklists would aid in the detection of machine faults.

Checkout procedures specific to individual models of anesthesia machines were provided and promoted by the machine manufacturers before the malpractice liability crises of the 1970s and 1980s. However, these developments focused intense emphasis on the liability implications of anesthesia equipment malfunction owing to the manufacturers having so-called "deep pockets" due to their perceived significant financial resources. This made the manufacturer an automatic target for inclusion as a defendant in a lawsuit whenever a major accident caused injury to a patient during general anesthesia. As a result, anesthesia machine manufacturers became more interested in being as sure as possible that practitioners would use their equipment in a safe manner.

Acknowledging the widely held belief that a thorough, well organized preanesthetic checkout of the anesthesia machine would help detect and correct potentially dangerous conditions, the manufacturers devised and promulgated detailed checklists for each model of anesthesia machine. Different makes and models have specific features that require individualization of the mechanics of the checkout procedure. Sales representatives and installers now take great pains to be certain that all anesthesia providers are given sufficient in-service education sessions on how to check out a new anesthesia machine.

It is worth remembering this true story from the early 1980s: A large teaching hospital phased out its old pneumatically powered anesthesia machines and replaced them with state-of-the-art machines that were both pneumatic and electronic. In these machines fresh gas would not flow unless the master pneumatic/electrical power on/off switch was turned on. A senior faculty member who had not attended any of the in-service sessions was called to administer general anesthesia for a stat cesarean section for fetal distress. Because this was his first encounter with the new anesthesia machine, he was unaware that there was an electric switch to turn on, and he could not make the machine function. Fortunately, a circulating nurse who had seen other anesthesiologists activate the machine turned it on. However, the implications of anesthesiologists understanding, learning, and performing a preanesthetic machine checkout are obvious.

The strong emphasis placed by the British on the technology of anesthesia practice shows in this area as well. Stimulated in part by accidents thought to be preventable, a simple generic checklist intended for any model of anesthesia machine was published.[13] It was suggested that it would take about 3 minutes to perform, a sharp contrast to the almost 15 minutes associated with the quite comprehensive checklist published by one anesthesia machine manufacturer. This contrast was an important harbinger of things to come in the United States.

In the United States, there was no generic preanesthesia checklist until 1986. Before that, emphasis was placed on the manufacturer's recommended checkout procedures, which often varied significantly between brands and models. In 1983, developments were stimulated by a series of anesthesia machine accidents that involved unintentional overdoses of volatile anesthetic due to the failure of an O ring on a turret that held three vaporizers and that rotated to select the volatile anesthetic to be delivered. These accidents received considerable publicity in the lay press, and the company involved ultimately stopped manufacturing anesthesia machines. Congressional hearings were held in 1984; one of the results was a charge to the United States Food and Drug Administration (FDA) to devise strategies to make anesthesia safer by helping to prevent a recurrence of such accidents. Accordingly, with some input from experts in anesthesia equipment and anesthesia practitioners, in August of 1986 the FDA published a generic preanesthesia checklist entitled Anesthesia Apparatus Checkout Recommendations, which is reproduced in Box 22-1.[14]

The 1986 FDA anesthesia apparatus checkout is extensive. There are 24 steps, some with as many as six substeps. There is a distinction placed on the steps (approximately half of the number and about two-thirds of the effort) intended for completion prior to the first anesthetic of the day. It was intended that these be omitted on successive cases in which the same anesthesiologist used the same machine. The full first-of-the-day procedure, if followed religiously, took almost 25 minutes. The interim

Box 22-1. FDA anesthesia apparatus checkout recommendations, 1986

This checkout, or a reasonable equivalent, should be conducted before administering anesthesia. This is a guideline which users are encouraged to modify to accommodate differences in equipment design and variations in local clinical practice. Such local modifications should have appropriate peer review. Users should refer to the operators manual for special procedures or precautions.

* 1. **Inspect anesthesia machine for**
   Machine identification number
   Valid inspection sticker
   Undamaged flowmeters, vaporizers, gauges, supply hoses
   Complete, undamaged breathing system with adequate CO_2 absorbent
   Correct mounting of cylinders in yokes
   Presence of cylinder wrench

* 2. **Inspect and turn on**
   Electrical equipment requiring warm-up (ECG/pressure monitor, oxygen monitor, etc.)

* 3. **Connect waste gas scavenging system**
   Adjust vacuum as required

* 4. **Check that**
   Flow-control valves are off
   Vaporizers are off
   Vaporizers are filled (not overfilled)
   Filler caps are sealed tightly
   CO_2 absorber by-pass (if any) is off

* 5. **Check oxygen (O_2) cylinder supplies**
   a. Disconnect pipeline supply (if connected) and return cylinder and pipeline pressure gauges to zero with O_2 flush valve.
   b. Open O_2 cylinder; check pressure; close cylinder and observe gauge for evidence of high pressure leak.
   c. With the O_2 flush valve, flush to empty piping.
   d. Repeat as in b. and c. above for second O_2 cylinder, if present.
   e. Replace any cylinder less than about 600 psig. At least one should be nearly full.
   f. Open less full cylinder.

* 6. **Turn on master switch (if present).**

* 7. **Check nitrous oxide (N_2O) and other gas cylinder supplies**
   Use same procedure as described in 5a. & b. above, but open and CLOSE flow-control valve to empty piping. Note: N_2O pressure below 745 psig indicates that the cylinder is less than ¼ full.

* 8. **Test flowmeters**
   a. Check that float is at bottom of tube with flow-control valves closed (or at min. O_2 flow if so equipped).
   b. Adjust flow of all gases through their full range and check for erratic movements of floats.

9. **Test ratio protection/warning system (if present).**
   Attempt to create hypoxic O_2/N_2O mixture, and verify correct change in gas flows and/or alarm.

*10. **Test O_2 pressure failure system**
   a. Set O_2 and other gas flows to mid-range.
   b. Close O_2 cylinder and flush to release O_2 pressure.
   c. Verify that all flows fall to zero. Open O_2 cylinder.
   d. Close all other cylinders and bleed piping pressures.
   e. Close O_2 cylinder and bleed piping pressure.
   f. CLOSE FLOW-CONTROL VALVES.

*11. **Test central pipeline gas supplies**
   a. Inspect supply hoses (should not be cracked or worn).
   b. Connect supply hoses, verifying correct color coding.
   c. Adjust all flows to at least mid-range.
   d. Verify that supply pressures hold (45-55 psig).
   e. Shut off flow-control valves.

*12. **Add any accessory equipment to the breathing system.**
   Add PEEP valve, humidifier, etc., if they might be used (if necessary remove after step 18 until needed).

13. **Calibrate O_2 monitor**
   *a. Calibrate O_2 monitor to read 21% in room air.
   *b. Test low alarm.
   c. Occlude breathing system at patient end; fill and empty system several times with 100% O_2.
   d. Check that monitor reading is nearly 100%

14. **Sniff inspiratory gas**
   There should be no odor.

*15. **Check unidirectional valves**
   a. Inhale and exhale through a surgical mask into the breathing system (each limb individually, if possible).
   b. Verify unidirectional flow in each limb.
   c. Reconnect tubing firmly.

From Anesthesia apparatus checkout draft recommendations, CRF 51, 60, 10673, March 28, 1986.
*If an anesthetist uses the same machine in successive cases, the steps marked with an asterisk (*) need not be repeated or may be abbreviated after the initial checkout.
†A vaporizer leak can only be detected if the vaporizer is turned on during this test. Even then, a relatively small but clinically significant leak may still be obscured.

Box 22-1, cont'd. FDA anesthesia checkout recommendations, 1986

†16. *Test for leaks in machine and breathing system*

a. Close APL (pop-off) valve and occlude system at patient end.

b. Fill system via O_2 flush until bag just full, but negligible pressure in system. Set O_2 flow to 5 L/min.

c. Slowly decrease O_2 flow until pressure *no longer rises* above about 20 cm H_2O. This approximates total leak rate, which should be no greater than a few hundred ml/min (less for closed circuit techniques). CAUTION: Check valves in some machines make it imperative to measure flow in step c. above when pressure *just stops rising*.

d. Squeeze bag to pressure of about 50 cm H_2O and verify that system is tight.

17. *Exhaust valve and scavenger system*

a. Open APL valve and observe release of pressure.

b. Occlude breathing system at patient end and verify that negligible positive or negative pressure appears with either zero or 5 L/min flow and exhaust relief valve (if present) opens with flush flow.

18. *Test ventilator*

a. If switching valve is present, test function in both bag and ventilator mode.

b. Close APL valve if necessary and occlude system at patient end.

c. Test for leaks and pressure relief by appropriate cycling (exact procedure will vary with type of ventilator).

d. Attach reservoir bag at mask fitting, fill system and cycle ventilator. Assure filling/emptying of bag.

19. *Check for appropriate level of patient suction.*

20. *Check, connect, and calibrate other electronic monitors.*

21. *Check final position of all controls.*

22. *Turn on and set other appropriate alarms for equipment to be used.*

(Perform next two steps as soon as is practical.)

23. *Set O_2 monitor alarm limits.*

24. *Set airway pressure and/or volume monitor alarm limits (if adjustable).*

*25. *Add any accessory equipment to the breathing system.*

Add PEEP valve, humidifier, etc., if they might be used (if necessary remove after step 18 until needed).

---

procedure before each subsequent case took 6 to 8 minutes. Although the 1986 FDA checkout was very well received as a reference and teaching tool, there was significant concern by both the FDA and anesthesia practitioners that it was too extensive to be practical in daily use, particularly in operating room environments that experienced rapid turnover. Informal surveys suggested that, as a result, the FDA checklist was not extensively used. Further, one study of 180 anesthesiologists in various settings[15] suggested that even having the FDA checklist in hand was not much of an aid in finding machine faults. Practitioners tended to rely on their own schemes of preanesthesia checkout rather than use the FDA checklist. Of additional interest is a 1990 FDA study[16] of 125 hospitals in four states, which showed that although 77% of the facilities in one of the states had some sort of checkout procedure, only 27% were using it and that, overall, only 26% of facilities actually used the FDA checklist in daily practice. Attention was turned to revising the 1986 version to make it more practical, more straightforward, and thus more likely to be accepted and used. A draft of the revised FDA apparatus checkout recommendations is shown in Box 22-2. A final version is due to be published late in 1992.

For further information on the checklist, please contact Jay Crowley or Robert Cangelosi at Food and Drug Administration, Center for Devices and Radiological Health, HFZ-240, Room 228, 1901 Chapman Avenue, Rockville, MD 20857; (301) 443-2436, (301) 443-8810 (fax).

CHECKOUT PROCEDURES

The relationship of the generic preanesthesia checklist to the model-specific procedures prescribed by the manufacturer need not be confusing. The core of the checkout procedure should be the FDA generic checklist because learning and using it will promote safe, efficient practice. At the same time, the practitioner must make the effort to become familiar with the manufacturer's suggested checkout procedures for a particular anesthesia machine and then integrate into the generic checklist any manufacturer-specific points. This is unnecessary with currently available equipment because the generic checklist is oriented toward precisely these machines. It is precisely because the generic FDA checklist is universally applicable that it is so valuable. Trainees or practitioners who become accustomed to using it will be able to incorporate new or different equipment into their practice. This checklist is not a substitute for appropriate in-service education, but it does make it possible for any anesthesia delivery system to be

Box 22-2. FDA draft anesthesia apparatus checkout recommendations, 1992

This checkout, or a reasonable equivalent, should be conducted before administration of anesthesia. These recommendations are only valid for an anesthesia system that conforms to current and relevant standards and includes an ascending bellows ventilator and at least the following monitors: capnograph, pulse oximeter, oxygen analyzer, respiratory volume monitor (spirometer) and breathing system pressure monitor with high and low pressure alarms. This is a guideline which users are encouraged to modify to accommodate differences in equipment design and variations in local clinical practice. Such local modifications should have appropriate peer review. Users should refer to the operators manual for specific procedures and precautions.

Emergency ventilation equipment

* 1. Verify Back-up Ventilation Equipment is Available and Functioning

High-pressure system

* 2. Check Oxygen Cylinder Supply
    a. Open O_2 cylinder and verify at least half full (about 1000 psig).
    b. Close cylinder.
* 3. Check Central Pipeline Supplies
    a. Check that hoses are connected and pipeline gauges read 45-55 psig.

Low-pressure system

* 4. Check Initial Status of Low-Pressure System
    a. Close flow-control valves and turn vaporizers off.
    b. Check fill level and tighten vaporizers' filler caps.
    c. Remove O_2 monitor sensor from circuit.
* 5. Perform Leak Check of Machine Low Pressure System
    a. Verify that the machine master switch and flow-control valves are OFF.
    b. Attach "suction bulb" to common (fresh) gas outlet.
    c. Squeeze bulb repeatedly until fully collapsed.
    d. Verify bulb stays *fully* collapsed for at least 10 seconds.
    e. Open one vaporizer at a time and repeat 'c' and 'd' as above.
    f. Remove suction bulb, and reconnect fresh gas hose.
* 6. Turn On Machine Master Switch and all other necessary electrical equipment
* 7. Test Flowmeters
    a. Adjust flow of all gases through their full range, checking for smooth operation of floats and undamaged flowtubes.
    b. Attempt to create a hypoxic O_2/N_2O mixture and verify correct changes in flow and/or alarm.

Breathing system

* 8. Calibrate O_2 Monitor
    a. Calibrate to read 21% in room air.
    b. Reinstall sensor in circuit and flush breathing system with O_2.
    c. Verify that monitor now reads greater than 90%.
9. Check Initial Status of Breathing System
    a. Set selector switch is in "bag" mode.
    b. Check that breathing circuit is complete, undamaged and unobstructed.

    c. Verify that CO_2 absorbent is adequate.
    d. Install breathing circuit accessory equipment to be used during the case.
10. Perform Leak Check of the Breathing System
    a. Set all gas flows to zero (or minimum).
    b. Close APL valve and occlude Y-piece.
    c. Pressurize breathing system to 30 cm H_2O with O_2 flush.
    d. Ensure that pressure remains at 30 cm H_2O for at least 10 seconds.

Scavenging system

11. Check APL Valve and Scavenging System
    a. Pressurize breathing system to 50 cm H_2O and ensure its integrity.
    b. Open APL valve and ensure that pressure decreases.
    c. Ensure proper scavenging connections and waste gas vacuum.
    d. Fully open APL valve and occlude Y-piece.
    e. Ensure absorber pressure gauge reads zero when:
        minimum O_2 is flowing.
        O_2 flush is activated.

Manual and automatic ventilation systems

12. Test Ventilation Systems and Unidirectional Valves
    a. Place a second breathing bag on Y-piece.
    b. Set appropriate ventilator parameters for next patient.
    c. Set O_2 flow to 250 ml/min, other gas flows to zero.
    d. Switch to automatic ventilation (ventilator) mode.
    e. Turn ventilator ON and fill bellows and breathing bag with O_2 flush.
    f. Verify that during inspiration bellows delivers correct tidal volume and that during expiration bellows fills completely.
    g. Check that volume monitor is consistent with ventilator parameters.
    h. *Check for proper action of unidirectional valves.*
    i. Exercise breathing circuit accessories to ensure proper function.
    j. Turn ventilator OFF and switch to manual ventilation (bag/APL)) mode.
    k. Ventilate manually and assure inflation and deflation of artificial lungs and appropriate feel of system resistance and compliance.
    l. Remove second breathing bag from Y-piece.

FDA DRAFT ver2.9, 4/2/92
*If an anesthetist uses the same machine in successive cases, these steps need not be repeated or may be abbreviated after the initial checkout.

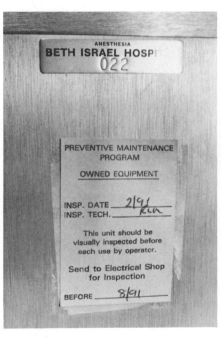

Fig. 22-1. Part of the general checkout regime, particularly of an anesthesia machine with which the practitioner is not closely familiar, should include verification of the machine's identification number and of the presence of a valid inspection sticker. The sticker is evidence of appropriate preventive maintenance and is more of a concern in the chronic quality assurance program that mandates periodic servicing and repair of equipment.

safely checked by a practitioner who follows it.

The FDA generic 1986 preanesthesia checklist began with a visual inspection that included verification of the presence of a valid inspection sticker, machine identification number (Fig. 22-1), and the overall absence of any obvious external damage. This inspection was dropped from the checklist revision largely because the spirit of it is incorporated by definition into the checkout process. Also, there was a point about the correct mounting of gas cylinders and the presence of a tank wrench, but these

items have been incorporated into point 2 of the new FDA checklist (see also Chapters 2 and 16).

Back-up ventilation equipment

A new element in the revised checklist is the need to verify the presence and correct function of back-up ventilation equipment (Fig. 22-2). Although it is true that a patient dependent on mechanical ventilation can be kept alive by a practitioner blowing into a tracheal tube, it is reasonable to insist that back-up ventilation equipment be immediately available in the OR. Back-up equipment can be life-saving following several types of mechanical failure of anesthesia equipment and can provide a temporary method to ventilate the patient while a major problem with the delivery system is being diagnosed and corrected.

High-pressure system

Reserve oxygen cylinders must be checked for correct mounting and the presence of adequate content (there should be at least one full cylinder with a pressure of approximately 1900 psig) (Fig. 22-3). In newly installed cylinders, leaks from an inadequately tightened yoke screw or a worn gasket are frequently detected at this time. Another controversy is whether one oxygen cylinder should be left open when the pipeline oxygen is in use. The argument in favor of this is that the check valve will keep the cylinder closed as long as pipeline pressure is normal, and the cylinder will be brought instantly on line if there is pipeline failure. The argument against this is that a pipeline failure could go unnoticed until the cylinder is exhausted. This is a potentially dangerous situation if there is only one reserve oxygen cylinder. Accordingly, the new FDA draft checklist states that reserve cylinders should be opened, checked, and then closed.

The integrity and correct, firm connection of central gas pipeline hoses must be verified each time a new practitioner approaches an anesthesia machine (Fig. 22-4). Normal pipeline pressure is about 50 to 55 psig for both oxygen and nitrous oxide (see Chapters 1 and 2).

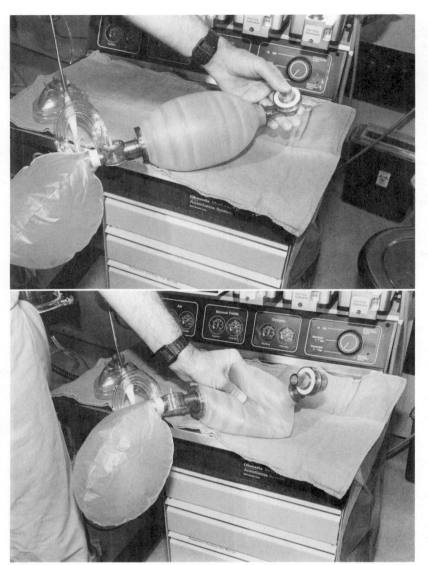

Fig. 22-2. A, Some form of back-up positive-pressure ventilation equipment must be available. The self-inflating resuscitator bag shown is supplied with its own mask and has an attached reservoir bag that should fill with oxygen and then vent when full while the 22-mm connector is occluded as shown. B, The bag functions correctly in that oxygen is delivered through the one-way valve and the reservoir starts to collapse as the bag starts to reinflate.

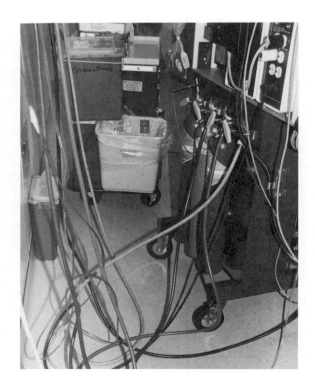

Fig. 22-3. Reserve oxygen cylinders are mounted on the rear or the side of the anesthesia machine. Their correct mounting in the tank yoke must be verified, and then each must be opened in sequence (with subsequent venting of the high-pressure side of the anesthesia machine) to check pressure. Central gas pipeline connection hoses must be checked for correct, tight connections at both the wall and the machine. Hoses should be inspected each day for damage that may be caused by heavy objects rolling over them. This is also a good time to try to organize the hoses and electric cables in a manner more orderly than shown in this picture.

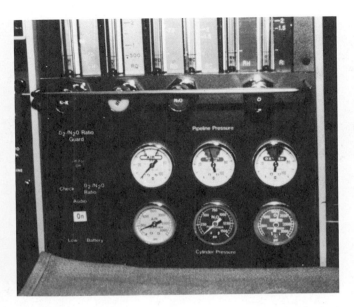

Fig. 22-4. Both cylinder and pipeline pressures must be checked before the start of each case. Reserve E cylinders of oxygen have a pressure of approximately 1900 psig when full.

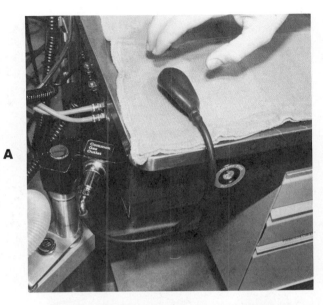

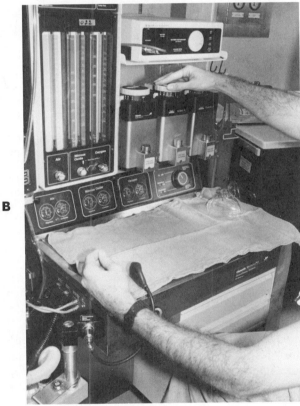

Low-pressure system

Before starting a check of the low-pressure system, all gas flow and vaporizers should be turned off, vaporizers filled and filler caps tightened, and the oxygen monitor sensor removed from the breathing system. A low-pressure side leak test should be performed (Fig. 22-5). This maneuver is very often neglected. With many personnel manipulating flow-control knobs, possibly in a rough manner, and filling and even exchanging vaporizers, the appearance of a low-pressure leak on a given day is a definite possibility. With the machine turned off and the flow control valves fully closed, a negative pressure is applied to the low-pressure side downstream from the flow control valves using a specially designed suction bulb that attaches to the fresh-gas outlet. If the bulb does not stay collapsed for a specified period, then air is being sucked by the bulb into the machine via a leak that will allow gas to escape when the machine is pressurized. The same maneuver is carried out, with each vaporizer opened in turn to check for leaks (which are comparatively common) associated with the vaporizer. This leak check as applied to the Ohmeda machines is described in further detail in Chapter 2.

The machine's master on/off switch is then turned on. On modern anesthesia machines, this usually causes a continuous low flow of oxygen, usually 200 to 300 ml/min, and the presence of this should be verified. If other electrical components, such as the oxygen monitor, are not automatically enabled when the master switch is turned on they should be activated at this time. Different models vary significantly in their electrical systems, and this is one area in which the manufacturer's protocols for initiation and checkout must be followed.

Fig. 22-5. The low-pressure leak test. **A,** With the machine off and the flow control valves fully closed, the special suction bulb that is supplied with the machine is connected to the common (fresh) gas outlet, pumped until it is fully collapsed, and then observed to verify that it stays collapsed, indicating that the low-pressure side of the machine is gas-tight. **B,** Then each vaporizer is opened in turn, and the maneuver is repeated to establish that there is no leak associated with that vaporizer. (See also Chapter 2.)

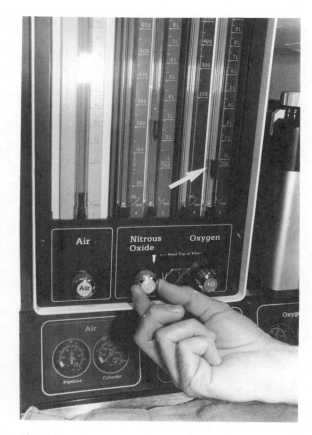

Fig. 22-6. An attempt to create a hypoxic fresh gas mixture is made by opening the nitrous oxide flow control valve. Either the oxygen flow should increase automatically (as indicated for this particular Ohmeda machine by the *arrow*) or the nitrous oxide flow should not increase and an alarm should sound when the mixture would exceed 72% nitrous oxide (Dräger).

Flowmeters should be checked by being opened and closed throughout their range of operation to verify smooth, correct function. Then, an attempt to create a hypoxic fresh gas mixture should be made by opening the nitrous oxide flow control valve (Fig. 22-6). Different models of machine have different mechanisms to prevent the creation of a hypoxic mixture, but either the oxygen flow should increase automatically to keep the oxygen percentage at 25% or more, or the nitrous oxide control knob should stop at that point, or despite further opening of the nitrous oxide flow control valve, the flow of nitrous oxide should not increase. (See Chapter 2, Proportioning Systems.) Certain machines may employ an alarm that sounds when the proportioning system is acting to prevent a hypoxic mixture.

Breathing system

With the selector switch in the "bag" mode, the breathing system must be inspected for integrity and the presence of adequate fresh carbon dioxide absorbent. The oxygen

monitor should be calibrated to 21% in room air and reinstalled; then it should read over 90% after 100% oxygen is flushed through the breathing system. The breathing system leak check (Fig. 22-7) is extremely important. This is because the system may have just been installed and is often made of plastic that is more prone to leaks than the traditional heavy rubber variety. The breathing system must be occluded at the adjustable pressure limiting (APL or pop-off valve) and at the patient connector. The oxygen flush valve is used to pressurize the circuit and reservoir

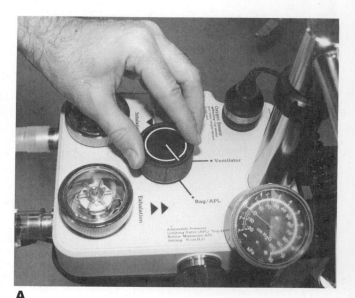

A

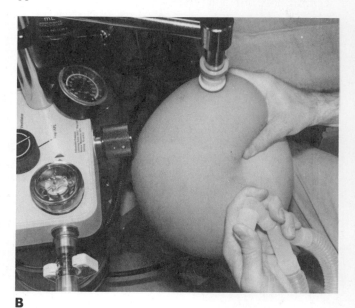

B

Fig. 22-7. The breathing system leak check. **A,** With the selector switch in the "bag" mode and the adjustable pressure limiting (APL or pop-off) valve closed, the breathing system connector is occluded and the system pressurized with the oxygen flush until the reservoir bag is inflated. **B,** The bag is then compressed to create a constant positive pressure of at least 30 cm water, which should not decrease over an interval of at least 10 seconds.

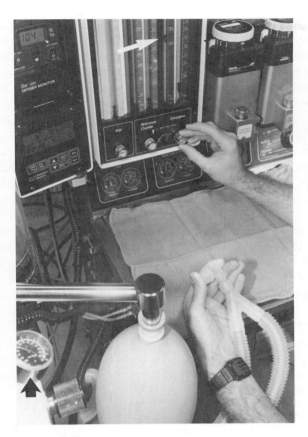

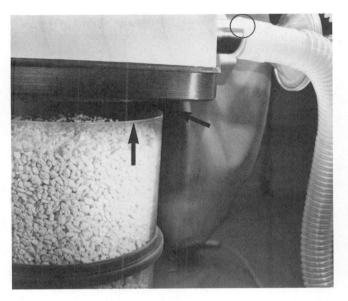

Fig. 22-9. Breathing system leaks. In this example, reconstructed for emphasis, the absorber canister has not been reseated at all *(arrows)* after an exchange of absorbent. Much more commonly, an effort is made to close the canister and seat the plastic rim in the rubber gasket, but there is either insufficient upward force to make a gas-tight seal or a misalignment so that the rim is not fully in contact with the gasket. Also, circuit tubing that is not firmly pushed onto the absorber head connectors *(circle)* can be loose enough to allow a leak without actually coming off.

Fig. 22-8. Alternative breathing system leak check. Again with the system occluded, oxygen flow is increased until the circuit pressure manometer just reads 20 cm water *(black arrow)* and holds that value. The flow *(white arrow* pointing to 260 ml/min on this machine) should be less than a few hundred ml per minute, indicating an acceptably low leak rate for the breathing system.

bag. The bag is then compressed to a pressure of at least 30 cm water and held to verify that there is no decrease in circuit pressure or deflation of the reservoir bag. This verifies that the breathing system is gas-tight. In the original 1986 FDA generic checklist,[14] an alternative method that is still favored by some practitioners was recommended (Fig. 22-8). With the patient connector occluded and the APL valve closed, the oxygen flow is adjusted until the pressure in the breathing system just holds at 20 cm water. If the flow needed for this is under a "few hundred" ml per minute, the breathing system is acceptably gas-tight.

Probably the most common cause of breathing system leaks is failure to reseal the carbon dioxide absorbent canister properly after the absorbent has been changed. Failure to attach the breathing circuit's corrugated tubing firmly to the absorber head connectors also accounts for a significant fraction of breathing system leaks that are discovered via the leak tests described here (Fig. 22-9).

Scavenger system

Waste gas scavenger systems vary significantly among the various models of anesthesia machines, making a

greatly detailed generic checkout difficult to create. This is another instance in which attention must be paid to the manufacturer's specified protocols, which come with the anesthesia machine. In general, there is a connection between the scavenging system and a vacuum source, usually the wall suction. Because wall suction is of sufficient magnitude to remove all the gas rapidly from the breathing system, there must be assurance that the interposed scavenging system functions correctly to prevent any direct connection of the vacuum to the breathing system.

The generic checklist calls for the breathing system to be occluded as before and pressurized. Then the APL (pop-off) valve is slowly opened to verify that the pressure decreases and the bag deflates slowly without becoming empty from negative pressure. Furthermore, with the APL valve fully open, the patient connector fully occluded, and only the minimum oxygen flow, no perceptible negative pressure should be measured on the circuit pressure manometer. Likewise, in the same circumstance activation of the oxygen flush should cause minimal positive pressure in the breathing system because all the gas should go out through the APL valve into the scavenging system.

In systems that have an additional rubber reservoir bag in the scavenging system, setting the fresh-gas flow to the anticipated total flow during the upcoming case allows adjustment of the scavenging system vacuum so that reservoir bag is slightly inflated—neither completely flat from negative pressure nor distended from positive pressure. This indicates that the vacuum is easily removing approximately the volume of the anticipated fresh-gas flow but not a great deal more. However, all scavenging systems are constructed so that if the vacuum becomes excessive they should entrain room air rather than aspirate gas from the breathing system (see also Chapter 5). This function is verified in the routine preventive maintenance check done periodically by service personnel.

Ventilators

Many different types of anesthesia ventilators are in use today. There is a strong movement in the anesthesia equipment field to encourage replacement of older descending (or hanging) bellows ventilators with the ascending bellows type because the bellows will not refill in expiration if the breathing system has become disconnected from the patient (see also Chapter 16). Accordingly, the new draft 1992 generic FDA preanesthetic checklist will deal only with maneuvers appropriate to the ascending bellows types of ventilators.

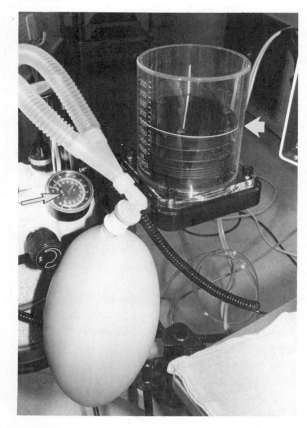

Fig. 22-10. Functional test of the ventilator. The reservoir bag should be attached to the breathing system patient connector, the oxygen flow set at 3 L/min, and the ventilator turned on. When it cycles and the bellows descend *(white arrow),* the bag should expand and the pressure in the breathing system *(black arrow)* should be within the expected normal range. The compliance of the bag should mimic exhalation and refill the bellows. It has been suggested that successful completion of this maneuver is an adequate test of the function of the unidirectional valves on the absorber head, but this is not universally accepted.

The ventilator leak check is simple. With the flow control valves fully closed, the circuit bag/ventilator selector switch should be turned to "ventilator," and the patient connector of the breathing system occluded. The ventilator bellows is then filled via the oxygen flush valve. The bellows should not perceptibly fall in 10 seconds, indicating that this portion of the breathing system is acceptably gas-tight.

A functional test of the ventilator must also be performed (Fig. 22-10). The circuit reservoir bag can be used as the equivalent of a test lung and attached to the patient connector of the breathing system. With an intermediate fresh gas flow, such as 3 L/min, the ventilator should cycle in the normal manner, with the compliance of the rubber bag mimicking exhalation and thus refilling the bellows during the expiratory phase.

During the functional test of the ventilator, the unidirectional valves on the absorber head can be observed to verify normal function. The new version of the generic checklist indicates this is a sufficient checkout of these valves. However, because these valves still may wear and break or become wet and stick, some experts recommend a separate, deliberate check of the function of the unidirectional valves.

Unidirectional valves

The original 1986 FDA checklist recommended that the person checking the anesthesia machine inhale and exhale into the patient connector while closely observing the unidirectional valves for free gas flow in the correct direction and no flow in the opposite direction (Fig. 22-11, *A*). A more definitive test is to disconnect and occlude each limb of the circuit and then breathe in and out of the other limb; the operator should be able to blow freely down the expiratory limb and meet total resistance when attempting to inspire (Fig. 22-11, *B*) and vice versa for the inspiratory limb (Fig. 22-11, *C*). These maneuvers have become controversial in recent years. Some anesthesia practitioners are concerned that these maneuvers may expose those performing them to trace concentrations of anesthetic gases from the absorber or rubber internal components or even (in spite of an apparent lack of objective evidence of this possibility) to residual infectious material that may have been exhaled by a patient previously anesthetized using that system. This, plus the fact that the manufacturers state generally that there are fewer failures of unidirectional valves with current design and fabrication, has contributed to the elimination of this maneuver from the revised 1992 generic checklist.

Monitors

Each monitor has its own proprietary checkout procedure, and the manufacturer's protocols should be followed. Most general anesthetics today involve the use of an ECG monitor, an inspired oxygen monitor, a capnograph, a pulse oximeter, a spirometer, and a pressure mon-

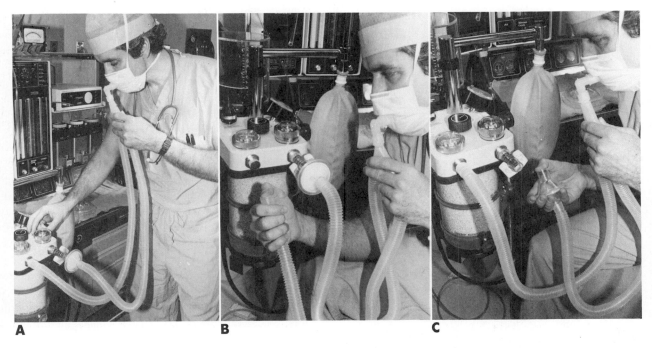

A   **B**   **C**

Fig. 22-11. Specific checkout of the breathing circuit unidirectional valves. **A,** The operator can inhale and exhale through a mask into the patient connector of the breathing circuit and observe the appearance of correct function of the unidirectional valves. However, isolating each limb allows full functional testing of each valve. **B,** With the inspiratory limb removed and occluded, the operator should be able to blow freely down the expiratory limb and should meet absolute resistance when attempting to inspire. **C,** With the expiratory limb disconnected and occluded, the operator should be able to inspire freely and should meet total resistance to forced expiration.

itor with high and low limit alarms. Each should be checked for correct function, normal calibration where applicable, and appropriate settings for the alarm limits. Probably the equipment in which the alarm limits are the most important is the inspired oxygen monitor (Fig. 22-12). Many have default settings (such as 18% oxygen) below which the lower-limit alarm cannot be set, and the alarm should be set routinely to an oxygen percentage high enough above that of room air so that any significant entrainment of air into the breathing system will trigger the lower-limit alarm.

Suction

The draft of the 1992 FDA generic preanesthesia checklist continues the need to check the availability and function of wall suction. Suction is critically important to anesthesia care because it is the only major piece of equipment used routinely by anesthesiologists whose function cannot be replaced in a life-threatening crisis by the anesthesiologist's own body. An anesthesiologist can monitor, ventilate, and even intubate if necessary without any equipment at all. An anesthesiologist cannot, however, adequately clear a pharynx full of secretions or vomitus without an adequately functioning suction; thus suction is a genuinely vital piece of anesthesia equipment. One simple way to check the suction (Fig. 22-13) is to determine whether there is enough negative pressure for the tubing to attach to the operator's finger and support its own weight while suspended in the air.

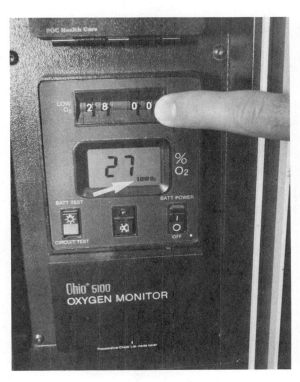

Fig. 22-12. Oxygen monitor alarm limit settings. Probably the most important monitor alarm to test is the lower-limit setting of the oxygen monitor, shown here set at 28%. The sensor should be removed and exposed to room air so that the oxygen percentage falls below the threshold and activates the alarm, auditory and visual *(arrow)*.

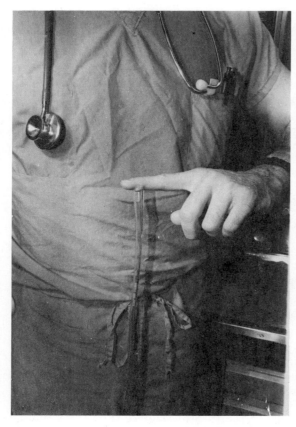

Fig. 22-13. Checking the negative pressure of the suction. The force of the suction is adequate if this maneuver can be performed.

Final position

Upon successful completion of the preanesthesia checklist, the anesthesia machine should be left ready for use. Flowmeters and vaporizers should be turned completely off, the selector switch set to the "bag" mode, the APL valve left open, and the breathing system firmly attached and prepared for use.

ALTERNATIVE PREANESTHESIA CHECKOUT PROTOCOLS

Several other generic preanesthesia checklists have been published, ranging from one much simpler[2] than the draft 1992 FDA generic checklist to another even more elaborate.[3] Some focus specifically on the anesthesia delivery system, and others encompass all equipment used in anesthesia care. The American Society of Anesthesiologists (ASA) in the late 1980s sponsored and distributed as part of its Patient Safety Video Series a videotape entitled "Check-Out: A Guide for Preoperative Inspection of an Anesthesia Machine." It essentially presented the original 1986 FDA theme, and included specific checks of the nitrous oxide sources, the oxygen pressure failure system (fail-safe), and the absorber bypass valve—points that were eliminated in the draft 1992 FDA version. Although

the ASA unofficially endorses the FDA efforts in the United States, other societies have generated their own versions of a checklist.

The Canadian Anaesthetists' Society checklist[17] is straightforward in that it lists the points to be covered without any accompanying instructions on how to perform the check (as do most other generic checklists). This checklist mentions that vaporizer filling ports should be keyed, or indexed, to prevent filling with an incorrect volatile anesthetic. This is one of the checklists that covers the broader range of materials and equipment used in anesthesia care. Significant emphasis is given to routine equipment, which includes verifying the presence of airways, multiple functioning laryngoscopes, tracheal tubes (that have been checked for patency and cuff function), stylet, intubating (Magill) forceps, IV supplies, blood pressure cuffs of various sizes, and various monitors. Also included are drugs, both stock and drawn up in syringes, and, finally, the location of special equipment such as defibrillators, emergency drugs, and a kit for managing difficult intubations.

Several other societies, including those in Germany, Australia, and Singapore, have published specific guidelines or protocols for preanesthesia checkout. The British have various checklists[13] and also have wrestled with the question of whether or not a specific checklist should be mandatory.[18] The consensus is, of course, that some checkout procedure must be done, but some of the issues of concern are the associated administrative organization, assignment of duties to support personnel, and record-keeping.

Partly because of a belief that the 1986 FDA recommended checklist was unwieldy and unlikely to be followed, the Risk Management Committee of the Harvard Medical School Department of Anesthesia[19] devised a very simple, generic preanesthetic apparatus checkout (Box 22-3). This document is of interest because it specifically separates the items to be checked into two categories: those in the "first-use check" that would be done at the beginning of each work day, and those in the "case check" that must be repeated prior to the start of each anesthetic. It was also required that this case check be documented on the individual anesthesia record by the anesthesiologist who performed it. This case check also went beyond just the machine, listing the need to verify the presence of suction, airway and intravenous infusion apparatus, and both routine and resuscitative medications.

All the various versions of the generic preanesthetic checklist have a common theme. Scrupulous attention to the details of this type of checkout procedure should detect the vast majority of defects in the anesthesia delivery system and thus (assuming appropriate corrective measures are taken before the equipment is used) prevent situations that could or would endanger the patient.

Box 22-3. Department of Anaesthesia, Harvard Medical School Standards of Practice—III
Preanesthetic Apparatus Checkout
Adopted January, 1987

These standards apply to all general, regional, or monitored intravenous anesthetics administered in all anesthetizing locations. In emergency circumstances in any location, immediate life support measures of whatever appropriate nature come first with attention turning to the measures described in these standards as soon as possible and practical. These are minimal standards which may be exceeded at any time based on the judgment of the involved anesthesia personnel. These standards encourage high quality patient care but observing them cannot guarantee any specific patient outcome. These standards are subject to revision from time to time, as warranted by the evolution of technology and practice.

Preanesthetic apparatus checkout shall be done as follows:

The "first-use check"

The function of the anesthesia machine shall be tested prior to its first use during any work day. The specific protocol used shall be at the discretion of the responsible anesthesiologist or anesthetist insofar as it is consistent with the policy of the individual hospital department. At minimum, the following shall be determined:

1. There is no external damage that compromises function.
2. Adequate main and reserve oxygen supplies are available.
3. The following components if present have *no visible damage* and *function correctly:*
   a. Flow sensitive fresh gas ratio protection or warning system.
   b. Inspired gas oxygen analyzer and its audible lower-limit alarm.
   c. Breathing system.
   d. Mechanical ventilator and the monitor for breathing system disconnect.
   e. Waste gas scavenging system.
4. There are no clinically significant leaks in the anesthesia machine or the breathing system.

The "case check"

Prior to the start of *each anesthetic* (including the first one of the day), the responsible anesthesiologist or anesthetist shall verify the following and after so doing, note on the anesthetic record that the case check has been performed. The specific protocol used shall be at the discretion of the responsible anesthesiologist or anesthetist insofar as it is consistent with the policy of the individual hospital department. At minimum, the following shall be verified:

1. Function of the breathing system (patency, absence of leaks, venting through the scavenging system).
2. Flow of oxygen through both flow meter and flush valves.
3. Presence of functioning suction.
4. Presence of apparatus for airway maintenance, including tracheal intubation.
5. Presence of apparatus for starting and maintaining an intravenous infusion.
6. Presence of appropriate anesthetic drugs as determined by departmental policy. When a vaporizer is present, the liquid level should be confirmed and the filler cap tightened.
7. Presence of appropriate resuscitative drugs as determined by departmental policy.

From Eichhorn JH, Cooper JB, Cullen DJ, et al: Anesthesia practice standards at Harvard: a review, *J Clin Anesth* 1:55-65, 1988.
NOTE: Each hospital anesthesia department shall adopt written protocols for the day check and case check of anesthesia apparatus.

EQUIPMENT QUALITY ASSURANCE

As opposed to the acute preanesthesia checkout, the chronic component of anesthesia equipment management is a comprehensive quality assurance program involving equipment evaluation, purchasing, installation, initial inspection, periodic safety inspections, preventive maintenance, repair, record-keeping, and retirement. Coupled with the specific attention to pieces of equipment can be a periodic safety inspection of the anesthetizing environment. An excellent review article[20] includes a 49-point safety inspection that is intended to be performed annually and covers anesthetizing areas, individual anesthetizing locations, and equipment. All facilities in which anesthesia is given should have this type of thorough safety inspection at least annually.

Prepurchase evaluation

The QA, or management, program begins well before any anesthesia equipment is purchased. When new equipment is needed or contemplated, designated members of the anesthesia department must take responsibility for writing specifications for what is needed and then evaluating potential products. Anesthesiologists who will actually be using the equipment must be involved; these tasks should not be delegated to support personnel, purchasing agents, or a product evaluation committee of the facility as a whole. A proposed piece of equipment must meet applicable codes and standards. This usually will be the case when major manufacturers are dealt with. However, certain standards may evolve rapidly or slowly but significantly, as is the case with the most recent anesthesia machine standards.[1] Thorough questioning of sales representatives and further investigation if there are any doubts should prevent the purchase of new equipment that does not meet current standards. Additional information can often be obtained from the ECRI (Plymouth Meeting, Pa.) through its monthly publication *Health Devices*. ECRI conducts evaluations and gives ratings of the various brands and models of a specific type of product. The anesthesia literature occasionally may be of help, and when major purchases are contemplated, a computerized literature search for information may reveal relevant publications.

Incoming inspection

When new equipment arrives, it must be inspected and checked for proper function before it is put into service. Any electrical device must be tested for leakage current and compliance with standards, usually in the facility's own maintenance shop or by an outside evaluator who is not associated with the manufacturer. Complex equipment, such as anesthesia machines, ventilators, and physiologic monitoring systems, should be assembled and then tested for correct function by a person from the equipment manufacturer or an associated manufacturer's agent. This leads to certification that the equipment is safe and ready for use. (Note that these certification documents become the start of the unique file of records and information that will stay in the anesthesia department and track the piece of equipment throughout its life.) Allowing relatively untrained or inexperienced personnel to assemble and certify new equipment, even if they do it perfectly, can present serious adverse medicolegal implications. Any untoward development in the future involving such new equipment will prompt review of the records and virtual automatic assumption of malfeasance if the people initially handling the equipment were not fully qualified to do so.

Record-keeping

As noted, a unique record must be kept for each piece of "capital" equipment (anything that has a serial number) that comes into the anesthesia workplace. This record can be a page or, more likely, a section in a master equipment logbook (which must exist in every anesthesia department or environment). In addition to the certifying document, the exact make, model, serial number, and any in-house identification must be recorded. This not only allows immediate identification of any equipment involved in a future recall or product alert but also serves as the permanent repository of the record of every instance of inspection, problem, problem resolution, maintenance, and servicing until that particular piece is discarded. For electrical equipment that will undergo periodic inspection and testing, it is convenient to create stickers with blanks for all the necessary information to be entered and to have these filled out by the technician performing the inspection. These stickers are then affixed in sequence in the master log over the life of that piece of equipment.[20] This log must be kept up to date at all times. There have been rare but frightening examples of potentially lethal problems with anesthesia machines leading to product alert notices requiring immediate identification of certain equipment, its location, and its service status.

Maintenance and servicing

There is a distinction between equipment failure due to progressive deterioration of components over time from continued use and catastrophic, unexpected failure, which usually is not predictable. Preventive maintenance is intended to anticipate what is essentially predictable failure (such as that of O rings, gaskets, and rubber bellows) and to replace the weakened component before it eventually does fail. Manufacturers, particularly because of the potential liability implications of a catastrophic failure, expend a great deal of effort constructing a preventive maintenance schedule. Preventive maintenance should be performed often enough and thoroughly enough to prevent most predictable failures while still maintaining reasonable cost. Users sometimes believe the manufacturers are too cautious and prescribe too much periodic maintenance in order to generate service business. These users are tempted to lengthen the maintenance cycles or to limit the extent of the service. Although this can save money in the short term, the liability implications in the event of a catastrophic anesthesia equipment failure that contributes to patient harm are unacceptable to the user. This functionally obligates users to attempt to adhere to the prescribed maintenance and service regime that comes with the equipment from the manufacturer.

Safety inspections and functional testing are integral components of the concept of preventive maintenance. Fig. 22-14 shows a sample protocol for one comparatively small piece of equipment. It is organized and presented clearly. In facilities with a large number of each type of equipment, use of such protocols should simplify the repetitive tasks for service personnel and help to assure that all the points are covered for each unit. Of course, copies of the completed form should be stored permanently in the departmental master equipment log.

The question of who should maintain and service anesthesia equipment has been widely debated and is very important. Needs and resources differ. The fundamental options are (1) factory service representatives who are directly employed by the manufacturer or the manufacturer's agent to work on the equipment made by that company; (2) independent service contractors who usually work on all brands of equipment and who may or may not have some type of relationship with the various manufacturers but are not employed by them; and (3) personnel within the anesthesia group or department or the maintenance and engineering department of the health care facility (these can be either formal biomedical engineers or less formal technicians). The order of the three options approximately represents decreasing average cost and increasing liability implications for the practitioners using the equipment. These issues should not necessarily drive the decision as to which to choose, but they certainly can be taken into consideration. The fundamental issue is straightforward: the person performing preventive maintenance and service must be qualified.

A Simplified Inspection Protocol for Incoming Equipment and Preventive Maintenance (O₂ Monitors)		

Unit # _____   Date _____
Sensor # _____   Location _____
                                    Inspected by _____

Materials needed:
Batteries, 4.05 volts, mercury
Sensor
Sensor membrane
Paper towels

Bottle of electrolyte (PO₂ gel)
Small screwdriver
Allen wrench
Metal cable clamp, pliers
Cleaner, soap solution

1.0 Visual Inspection/Cleaning	OK/Action Taken	Action Needed/ Comments
1.1 Clean exterior		
1.2 Clean and inspect: a. Controls b. Face of meter c. Rear sensor connector		
1.3 O₂ sensor —inhalation side —snug in T-piece or dome valve adapter T-piece adapter—snug in breathing circuit		
2.0 Operational Tests		
2.1 Unit upright FUNCTION—STBY | adjust METER ZERO to read "0" % O₂		
2.2 FUNCTION— BATT OK | meter in white BATT OK area between 82-86%		
2.3 FUNCTION—ON 100% O₂ flush | adjust CALIBRATE to read 98% O₂		
2.4 Alarms—with 100% O₂ a. "HI" pointer clockwise (model 404) | Alarm sounds Rotate "LO" pointer CW | Lamp illuminates at 96-100% O₂		
b. Model 404 only: "LO" pointer below 75% O₂ | Alarm sounds Rotate "HI" alarm CCW | Lamp illuminates at 96-100% O₂		
2.5 100% O₂ | adjust CALIBRATE to read 100%		
2.6 Room air | meter reading 21% ± 2% within 30 seconds		
3.0 Final inspection		
3.1 Sensor | secure in T-piece/dome valve		
3.2 Monitor | securely mounted tighten nuts		
3.3 Inspection sticker		

Fig. 22-14. Sample protocol for equipment inspection and preventive maintenance. This detailed checklist for an older style of circuit oxygen monitor is an excellent example of equipment quality assurance in action. Used at the time a new model enters the facility and at the appropriate maintenance intervals thereafter, the checklist facilitates an efficient, complete servicing and evaluation while also creating a complete and valuable record that must be permanently kept in the master equipment log. (Copyright 1986 by The Joint Commission on Accreditation of Healthcare Organizations, Oakbrook Terrace, Ill. Reprinted with permission from *Quality Review Bulletin*: Duberman and Wald.[20])

Whether service personnel are qualified may be somewhat difficult to ascertain, but judicious investigation of references and direct questioning of the service personnel regarding their education, training, and experience is appropriate. Direct contact with the supervisor or manager responsible for the work of the service person is strongly advised, because it indicates the importance that the practitioners attach to maintenance and service. Whether a technician who spent a week at a course at an equipment manufacturer's factory can perform the most complex repairs depends on a variety of factors.

Ultimately, the practitioner using the equipment must decide the competence of individual personnel to repair the equipment. Failure to be involved and have some oversight in this process exposes the practitioner to increased liability in the event of an untoward outcome associated with improperly maintained or serviced equipment. It must be stressed that such situations are, fortunately, very rare. However, as with so many things in modern anesthesia practice, the continual background threat is enough to prompt specific plans and actions.

Daily support

In addition to periodic preventive maintenance and servicing, there must be adequate day-to-day clinical maintenance of anesthesia equipment. Because health care budgets are continually under scrutiny, anesthesia technicians seem to be a popular target for cost cutters. It is dangerous false economy to reduce technicians below the number genuinely needed to retrieve, clean, sort, disassemble, sterilize, reassemble, store, and distribute the equipment of daily anesthesia practice. Inadequate service in this area truly creates an accident waiting to happen. Although it is desirable that all anesthesia practitioners be able to change the carbon dioxide absorbent on their anesthesia machines, some might be sufficiently unfamiliar with the procedure to create a hazard in the process. There are many other sources of potential danger from lack of adequate technical support personnel who are intended to execute tasks such as this.

Retirement of equipment

There is a strong sentiment against using the word "obsolete" to refer to older anesthesia equipment.[1] The concept has adverse medicolegal implications and dwells in the past, whereas a safety improvement effort involving new equipment looks to the future. It has been stated, however, that replacement of obsolete anesthesia machines and monitoring equipment is one key element of a risk-modification program.[21] Ten years has been frequently cited as an estimated useful life for an anesthesia machine, but this is simply an opinion and is probably related to depreciation tables used by hospital actuaries. Certainly, unmodified anesthesia machines much more than 10 years old do not even meet the 1979 ANSI Z-79.9 safety standards[1] (requiring such things as a vaporizer lockout) and do not incorporate the new technology of the past decade that is designed to prevent untoward incidents. Also, the accepted anesthesia machine standards were further modified in 1989 (ASTM F 1161-88)[1] to require oxygen analyzers that are enabled when the machine is turned on, to require alarms of different priority categories for different warning conditions, and functionally to prohibit flowmeter-controlled vaporizers (see also Chapter 2). Furthermore, there is every indication that technology will continue to advance at this accelerated rate. Note that some anesthesia equipment manufacturers, anxious to minimize their own potential liability, have refused to support (with parts and service) some of their older pieces of equipment (particularly gas machines) still in use. This is a very strong message to practitioners that such equipment must be replaced as soon as possible.

The American Society of Anesthesiologists[22] took a position in 1988. It was entitled, "Policy for Assessing Obsolescence" and stated: "The age of an anesthesia gas machine has not been demonstrated to be a factor in anesthetic mishaps. An anesthesia gas machine, however, which no longer functions as designed and is not modified to meet acceptable levels of performance and monitoring should not be used." Other entities can also play a role in this debate. In 1989, the New Jersey State Department of Health issued comprehensive safety regulations for anesthesia practice, which included several specifications for anesthesia equipment such as vaporizer lockout and airway pressure alarms. The medicolegal implications of these regulations in that state were significant. It was reported by anesthesia machine manufacturers that a dramatic surge in sales was directly caused by these regulations, indicating that many comparatively older gas machines were still in use. (See also Chapters 16 and 25.) Gray areas persist in this debate. The summary message is that a great many technologic advances have been made in anesthesia equipment, particularly gas machines, specifically intended to increase the safety of the patients anesthetized with that equipment. Exactly how fast these improvements are incorporated into daily use will depend on the circumstances of a given anesthesia practice, published and de facto standards, applicable regulations, and the medicolegal climate.

Equipment crisis management

Finally, should equipment fail, it must be removed from service and replaced if that anesthetizing location will still be used. Groups or departments are obligated to have sufficient back-up equipment to cover any reasonable incidence of failure (predicted on the basis of past experience and the manufacturer's guidelines). The equipment removed from service must be clearly marked with a sign (so that it is not put back into service by well-meaning support personnel or even other practitioners) that includes the date, time, person discovering the fault, and details of the problem. The responsible personnel must be notified so that they can remove the equipment, make an entry in the log, and initiate repair. A piece of equipment either directly or indirectly involved in causing an anesthesia accident must be immediately sequestered and not touched by anybody—particularly not by any equipment service personnel. There may be strong pressure to return a major piece of equipment, such as a gas machine, to service if there is no spare available; this temptation must be resisted. If a severe accident occurred, it may be necessary for the equipment in question to be inspected at an appointed time by a group consisting of qualified representatives of the manufacturer, the service personnel, the plaintiff's attorney, the insurance companies involved, and the practitioner's defense attorney. Also, major equipment problems involving obvious or suspected hazards should be reported immediately to the Medical Device Problem Reporting system of the United States FDA via the Device Experience Network (telephone 800-638-6725).[23] This system accepts voluntary reports from users and requires reports from manufacturers when there is knowledge that a medical device has been involved in a serious incident. This is a logical progression of an equipment quality assurance process.

Implementation of the acute and chronic components of an anesthesia equipment quality assurance program should help to minimize the likelihood of equipment-related untoward events during anesthesia care. Both the preanesthesia checklists and the equipment management programs outlined in this chapter are intended as models. Individual anesthesia practitioners, groups, and departments must adapt these principles to their own particular situations, taking into account the type of equipment, practice environments, and local characteristics. Incorporation of the spirit more than the letter of the recommendations is the key. It is important to recall that human errors of judgment are implicated in the vast majority of adverse outcomes from anesthesia; overt equipment failure or problems are responsible for only a small fraction of these cases. Nonetheless, this fraction is virtually reducible to zero with rigorous application of the principles of checkout and quality assurance.

REFERENCES

1. Lees DE: *Anesthesia machine and equipment standards.* In Eichhorn JH, editor: *Problems in anesthesia, vol 5, Improving anesthesia outcome,* Philadelphia, 1991, Lippincott, pp 205-218.
2. Petty C: *The anesthesia machine,* New York, 1987, Churchill Livingstone.
3. Dorsch JA, Dorsch SE: *Understanding anesthesia equipment: construction, care and complications,* ed. 2, Baltimore, 1984, Williams and Wilkins.
4. Rendell-Baker L: Problems with anesthetic gas machines and their solutions. In *Problems with anesthetic and respiratory therapy equipment,* Boston, 1984, Little Brown, pp 1-82.
5. Spooner RB, Kirby RR: Equipment-related anesthetic incidents. In Pierce EC, Cooper JB editors: *Analysis of anesthetic mishaps.* Boston, 1984, Little Brown, pp 133-147.
6. Cooper JB, Newbower RS, Long CD, et al: Preventable anesthesia mishaps: a study of human factors, *Anesthesiology* 49:399-406, 1978.
7. Cooper JB, Newbower RS, Kitz RJ: An analysis of major errors and equipment failures in anesthesia management: considerations for prevention and detection, *Anesthesiology* 60:34-42, 1984.
8. Heath ML: Accidents associated with equipment, *Anaesthesia* 39:57-60, 1984.
9. Craig J, Wilson ME: A survey of anaesthetic misadventures, *Anaesthesia* 36:933-936, 1981.
10. Eichhorn JH: Prevention of intraoperative anesthesia accidents and related severe injury through safety monitoring, *Anesthesiology* 70:572-577, 1989.
11. Buffington CW, Ramanathan S, Turndorf H: Detection of anesthesia machine faults, *Anesth Analg* 63:79-82, 1984.
12. Paulus DA, Basta JW, Klie H, et al: Preanesthesia checklist, *Anaesth Analg* 64:264, 1985.
13. Cundy J, Baldock GJ: Safety check procedures to eliminate faults in anaesthesia machines, *Anaesthesia* 37:161-169, 1982.
14. Anesthesia apparatus checkout draft recommendations, CRF 51, 60, 10673, March 28, 1986. Final version: Federal Register 52:36-37, 1987.
15. March MG, Crowley JJ: An evaluation of anesthesiologists' present checkout methods and a test of the validity of the FDA checklist for use by anesthesiologists, *Anesthesiology* 73:A-1020, 1990 (abstract).
16. FDA Center for Devices and Radiologic Health: Medical devices bulletin 7: 1-2, 1990.
17. Canadian Anaesthetists' Society: Guidelines to the practice of anaesthesia. Approved June, 1989.
18. Charlton JE: Checklists and patient safety, *Anaesthesia* 45:425-426, 1990 (editorial).
19. Eichhorn JH, Cooper JB, Cullen DJ, et al: Anesthesia practice standards at Harvard: a review, *J Clin Anesth* 1:55-65, 1988.
20. Duberman SM, Wald A: *An integrated quality control program for anesthesia equipment.* In Chapman-Cliburn G, editor: *Risk management and quality assurance: issues and interactions,* Chicago, 1986, Joint Commission on Accreditation of Healthcare Organizations, pp 105-112. (A special publication of the *Quality Review Bulletin.*)
21. Pierce EC: *Risk modification in anesthesiology.* In Chapman-Cliburn G, editor: *Risk management and quality assurance: issues and interactions,* Chicago, 1986, Joint Commission on Accreditation of Healthcare Organizations, pp 20-23. (A special publication of the *Quality Review Bulletin.*)
22. ASA Board of Directors Summary, *ASA Newsletter* 53:4, April 1989.
23. HHS publication (FDA) No. 85-4196. Food and Drug Administration, Center for Devices and Radiologic Health, Rockville, Maryland.

Chapter 23

MAINTENANCE, CLEANING, AND STERILIZATION OF ANESTHESIA EQUIPMENT

Leslie Rendell-Baker, M.D.

MAINTENANCE OF ANESTHESIA EQUIPMENT

The range of anesthesia equipment has developed from the original simple gas machine to incorporate many ancillary devices, such as ventilators, oxygen analyzers, capnographs, pulse oximeters, and multi channel monitors. All of these devices require routine servicing if they are to function satisfactorily. A patient's life may depend on equipment functioning reliably; therefore, it is essential that equipment be serviced in accordance with the manufacturer's recommendations. This is also important from a medicolegal standpoint. Thus, in the event of a mishap, it is critical to be able to prove that the equipment was serviced in accordance with the manufacturer's recommendations. Most manufacturers offer service contracts under which the equipment is serviced every three or four months. As most manufacturers service only their own equipment, a separate service contract is needed for each kind of equipment.

To eliminate the inconvenience of multiple service contracts and service personnel, independent biomedical companies offer to service the complete range of anesthesia and ancillary equipment. This simplifies the process because all servicing can be accomplished in one visit. Many of the major equipment companies offer training courses for the employees of independent servicing companies, where they learn to service that manufacturer's equipment correctly. Before signing any service contract, it is wise to seek competitive bids and to contact hospitals already using these services to determine whether they have proven satisfactory.

Some large medical centers with bioengineering departments find it convenient to have their own bioengineering staff service most of the medical center's equipment. The staff attends training programs sponsored by manufacturers to acquire the necessary servicing skills and to study service manuals. The advantage of in-house maintenance is that skilled technical help is readily available in the event of unexpected problems. A record should be kept of all servicing and repairs carried out on each piece of equipment so that there is documentation of all maintenance should any problems arise. After any piece of equipment has been serviced, it is essential that the user carefully check it for proper function.

The bioengineers become expert in handling most problems that develop with the equipment, and they can provide valuable expert advice, such as evaluating the technical design of any proposed new purchase. As the design of future anesthesia apparatus inevitably moves from the mechanical to the electronic, expert technical advice and assistance will become increasingly valuable (see Chapter 33).

STERILIZATION OF ANESTHESIA EQUIPMENT
Methods available

Several methods are available to clean anesthesia equipment. These include sterilization, disinfection, and antisepsis. All reusable items must first be cleaned and decontaminated. Cleaning involves washing with a detergent or disinfectant to remove all blood, mucus, and foreign material. The items are then rinsed and dried. This renders the items safe to handle (reasonably free of transmitting infection), or in other words, decontaminated. Antiseptics are chemicals that can be used on living tissues to kill germs. Disinfectants are chemicals used to kill germs but are not used on living tissues. Disinfection is divided into three levels: high, intermediate, and low. High-level disinfection kills bacteria, fungi, and viruses; however, large numbers of endospores may not be killed. Most high-level disinfectants can produce sterilization with sufficient contact time. Intermediate-level disinfection kills bacteria, fungi, and most viruses but not bacteria endospores. Intermediate-level disinfection also kills tuberculosis organisms. Low-level disinfection kills most bacteria and some fungi and viruses; it does not kill tuberculosis bacteria or endospores. Sterilization kills all bacteria, including endospores, fungi, and viruses.

Sterilization can be accomplished by either steam or gas autoclaving. Steam autoclaving is the preferred method for equipment that can tolerate the heat and the steam. Items such as metal laryngoscope blades are ideal for steam au-

toclaving. This method provides the quickest turn-around time. Gas autoclaving with ethylene oxide (ETO) is useful for items that cannot tolerate exposure to high temperatures and steam. This includes items made of plastic and rubber as well as fiberoptic endoscopes. A major disadvantage of ethylene oxide sterilization is that it requires at least a 24-hour turn-around time so that items can be aerated to eliminate residual ethylene oxide gas.

Items can be disinfected by being soaked in alkaline glutaraldehyde (e.g., Cidex) solution. These preparations are caustic to the skin as well as being respiratory irritants. Therefore, when these solutions are used, proper precautions should be taken to avoid prolonged skin contact or inhalation of the vapor. Also, careful and thorough rinsing of any item disinfected in the solution is essential. Phenolic solutions (e.g., Wexcide) are commonly used as a hospital germicidal disinfectant. This solution is also caustic and gloves should be worn when it is handled. Sodium hypochlorite solution (chlorine bleach 1:5 to 1:10 dilution) is an excellent disinfectant for destroying the hepatitis virus. Isopropyl alcohol is considered an intermediate-level disinfectant. Although it is effective against the human immunodeficiency virus (HIV) and the hepatitis B virus (HBV), it is not effective against hydrophilic enteroviruses.

A number of antiseptics that are used mainly for hand-washing and surgical skin prepping can also be used for cleaning instruments. These include iodophor (e.g., Betadine), which when combined with liquid soap is known as povidone-iodine surgical scrub. Chlorhexidine gluconate (e.g. Hibiclens) and hexachlorophene are other useful antiseptics. Benzalkonium chloride is not recommended because it is not effective against gram-negative organisms.

Background considerations

The design and construction of much of the equipment used in anesthesia is such that many of the items are not readily cleaned or sterilized. In times past, a perfunctory rinse of the breathing tubing and mask, which merely served to redistribute the bacteria, was the extent of the anesthesiologist's attempt at cleanliness. There was little interest in routine sterilization of anesthesia breathing systems (except in tuberculosis surgical centers) because there had been few reports of cross contamination related to anesthesia equipment.[1] It was not until the late 1960s, when cardiac and other surgeons reported outbreaks of postoperative chest infections arising from sources in the anesthesia ventilator or breathing bag and tubing, that anesthesiologists realized that a real problem might exist.[2] As increasing numbers of patients were ventilated in intensive care units, the prevalence of contaminated humidifiers and ventilator tubing became recognized, stimulating a review of the poor hygienic status of the anesthesia apparatus and its breathing systems.

Absorber assembly

In the past, if the carbon dioxide absorber needed to be sterilized, not only was it difficult to remove it from the machine but also the pressure gauge built into the housing often could not tolerate the raised temperature and pressure. Also, the plastic absorbent containers often could not withstand either gas or steam sterilization. Fortunately, the North American Dräger absorber manufactured today can be autoclaved once the breathing system pressure gauge, positive end-expiratory pressure (PEEP) valve, and valve assemblies have been removed (for further information, refer to the North American Dräger absorber system operator's instruction manual). The Ohmeda absorbers can be sterilized using ethylene oxide once the valve assemblies and plastic carbon dioxide canisters are removed. The valves and canisters can be cleaned with an appropriate liquid sterilization agent. (For further information, refer to the Ohmeda GMS absorber manual.)

Bacterial filters

Although many have advocated the use of bacterial filters to prevent anesthesia breathing systems from becoming contaminated, Pace, et al.[3] and Garibaldi, et al.[4] showed that use of filters in the breathing system had no effect on the incidence of postoperative pulmonary infections. Similar studies by Feeley, et al.[5] also failed to show any benefit from the use of sterile breathing systems on the incidence of postoperative pulmonary infections. Studies[6] have shown that it is quite difficult to transfer bacteria from the patient through the breathing tubes to the absorber or from the absorber to the patient. Also, the soda lime and the anesthesia gases are inhospitable to bacteria. However, the use of bacterial filters on the machine is still controversial. A recent report by Brooks, et al.[7] found that even when filters were used on the inspiratory and expiratory sides of the machine, 25% of the anesthesia circle systems and 44% of the ventilators cultured were positive for bacterial pathogens. The role that these organisms play in surgical infections is currently unclear. Recent attention to universal precautions in order to protect medical personnel from the rising incidence of HIV,* hepatitis, and pulmonary tuberculosis has renewed interest in the problems of cleaning and sterilizing of the anesthesia equipment.

MYCOBACTERIAL CONTAMINATION OF APPARATUS

The rising incidence of drug-resistant pulmonary tuberculosis in HIV-positive intravenous drug abusers, Haitian-Americans, and other non-Caucasian populations is a serious problem.[9-11] As the immune system becomes increasingly impaired, old pulmonary tuberculosis lesions may become reactivated. Open, active pulmonary tubercu-

---

losis may precede the diagnosis of AIDS.[12] Radiologic diagnosis may also be difficult because the lesions may be indistinguishable from those of Pneumocystis carinii.[13] Some respiratory therapists are reported to have developed pulmonary tuberculosis while administering pentamidine inhalations to patients with Pneumocystis carinii.[14,15] This stresses the need for use of the following precautions when patients are handled who are suffering from pulmonary disease that could be due to tuberculosis:

1. The patient should wear a mask.
2. All OR staff should be notified that the patient is potentially infectious.
3. After use, reusable equipment that was in contact with the patient's airway should be disinfected with an appropriate chemical, such as glutaraldehyde. It should then be thoroughly washed, wrapped, labeled, and sterilized, preferably with steam.
4. If possible, a disposable circle absorber system should be used. If one is not available, the absorber system should be processed as in Item 3 above.
5. Intraoral manipulations should be kept to a minimum. After a single use, suction catheters should be discarded into a container that is designated for and labeled as containing hazardous materials.
6. Used gowns, gloves, shoe covers, and face masks should be discarded into marked containers when their users leave the OR.
7. Traffic and equipment in the OR should be kept to a minimum.

Cleaning

Cleaning is the first step in decontamination. Dirt and dried secretions inhibit the action of the disinfectant by preventing its contact with the surface of the article and by neutralizing the disinfectant's action. Cleaning entails a preliminary soaking in cold water to which detergent has been added and should be performed in a sink in the equipment room by personnel wearing gloves. If available, a Pasteurmatic or ultrasonic cleaner helps to reduce contact with the contaminated equipment. The Centers for Disease Control (CDC)[16] and the Association of Operating Room Nurses (AORN)[17] have published recommended practices for the cleaning and processing of anesthesia equipment. These procedures are recognized by the CDC to be sufficient for preventing transmission of infection from patient to patient and from machine to patient.[18]

Choice of sterilization or disinfection method

Spaulding, et al.[19] separated the sterilization or disinfection procedures necessary for medical devices by dividing them into three categories on the basis of risk of infection associated with their clinical use:

1. *Critical items:* Devices that penetrate the skin or are in contact with sterile areas of the body. Thus spinal nee-

---

*Estimated to be 1 in 75 in the United States in males aged between 15 and 49 years.[8]

dles, cardiac catheters, and surgical instruments require sterilization.

2. *Semicritical items:* Devices that are in contact with mucous membranes, such as endoscopes, temperature probes, or tracheal tubes need high-level disinfection or may be sterilized.

3. *Noncritical items:* Devices that are in contact with unbroken skin and body surfaces, such as stethoscopes and blood pressure cuffs, need only intermediate or low-level disinfection.[18]

STERILIZATION
Steam autoclaving

Steam autoclaving is always the first choice for items that can tolerate the heat and steam. It is the fastest and most effective method available. The moist heat is more effective than dry heat in coagulating cellular proteins, thereby killing organisms at lower temperatures. Water at sea level boils at 100° C. However, if it is confined in a closed vessel, such as the autoclave, as the pressure rises, so does the temperature at which the water boils. This change from liquid to vapor requires a considerable amount of heat (580 cal/g of water). The latent heat in the steam is given up as the steam condenses on the cool items in the autoclave, and this shortens the time required to achieve sterility as compared with a hot air oven. The higher the pressure in the autoclave, the higher is the temperature of the steam and therefore, the shorter is the time required for sterilization. Before the sterilization cycle is begun, it is essential to evacuate the air from the autoclave chamber. If this is not done, the quantity of steam entering the autoclave is reduced and, with this, the temperature achieved at any given pressure is also reduced. As the steam enters the chamber, it enters the load to be sterilized and gives up its latent heat as it condenses on the cooler items. Once the intended temperature is reached, the duration of sterilization is set. At the end of this period the steam is exhausted from the autoclave by vacuum to avoid condensation of water on the load when cool air is admitted. Modern autoclaves have automatic controls that ensure that the correct sequence is followed. Commonly used combinations are 15 minutes at 121° C and 15 psig or 5 to 10 minutes at 132° C and 30 psig. Thus, if a steam autoclave is used, processing of equipment, including washing, packaging, autoclaving, and cooling of the item can be accomplished in well under 1 hour.

Packaging. Items that have been sterilized must remain sterile for some time after removal from the autoclave. Therefore, they should be packed in nylon bags or specially made packets that are easily permeable to steam.

Ethylene oxide gas autoclaving

Ethylene oxide gas autoclaving can be used for plastic items and others that cannot tolerate exposure to the higher temperatures and steam in the steam autoclave. In fact, it was the introduction of ethylene oxide sterilization in 1947 and its perfection in 1962 (Fig. 23-1) that made possible the sterile disposable equipment now so widely used in our hospitals.[20,21] Ethylene oxide gas autoclaving was first used to sterilize anesthesia equipment in the Buffalo General Hospital in 1960 and then by Dr. John Snow of Boston in 1962.[22] Very little was known at that time about the rate of elimination of the gas from polyvinylchloride (PVC) plastic tracheal tubes and other items. Neither was it known how much residual ethylene oxide in the items could be tolerated by human tissue. By 1968 there were numerous reports of chemical burns of the trachea, oropharynx, and skin due to failure to eliminate the residual gas from sterilized items. The introduction of heated aeration cabinets, through which warm bacterially filtered air was drawn to hasten the elimination of the gas from the items sterilized, eventually eliminated the problem. These aerators were introduced as a result of research carried out by the Ethylene Oxide Subcommittee* of the former American National Standards Institute Z79 Anesthesia Standards Committee.

Precautions for safe use of ethylene oxide. Ethylene oxide would not be effective as a sterilant if it were not poisonous. In fact, it is a much more serious hazard to the user's health (Fig. 23-2) than is nitrous oxide pollution in the operating room. The Occupational Safety and Health Administration (OSHA) has set a maximum exposure level of 1 ppm per 8 hour time-weighted average with a permissible exposure limit of 5 ppm averaged over a 15 minute sampling period.[23]

To achieve this low level, sterilizers and aerators should not be located in work areas. They should be installed in separate, well-ventilated areas that have dedicated air extraction systems to remove gas residues to the outside atmosphere (Fig. 23-3). The Environmental Protection Agency (EPA)[23] recommendations and guidelines for the modification of work-place design and practice in hospitals, aimed at reducing the exposure of hospital workers to no more than 1 ppm of ethylene oxide, are given in Appendix A of the OSHA document.[23] These recommendations include the use of nonrecirculating or dedicated ventilation systems to remove the ethylene oxide from all areas around the sterilizer and aerator.

The State of California Air Resources Board[24] estimates that 800,000 pounds of ethylene oxide are emitted each year from sterilizers at 650 facilities in California. "Once the ethylene oxide is emitted, it remains in the air without breaking down for long periods of time. People who live near facilities with sterilizers or aerators may therefore be exposed to airborne ethylene oxide from these

---

*Now a part of the Association for Advancement of Medical Instrumentation's Sterilization Committee.

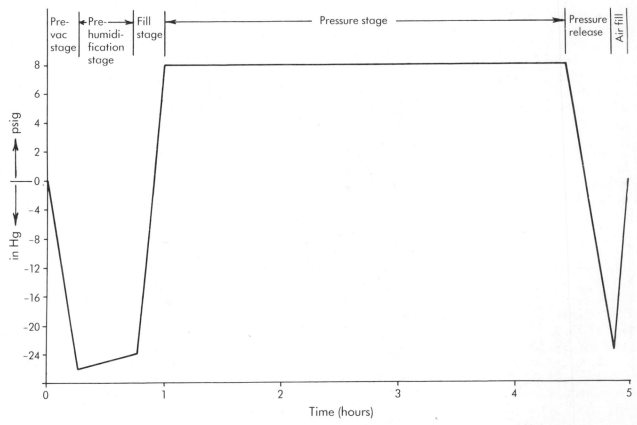

Fig. 23-1. The McDonald ethylene gas sterilization process. The graph indicates the various pressure changes that occur during the cycle. The vertical axis is pressure in units of psig when positive, and in inches of mercury when negative. The horizontal axis is time in hours. (Illustration from McDonald RL: method of sterilizing. US Patent No 3,068, 064; 1962.)

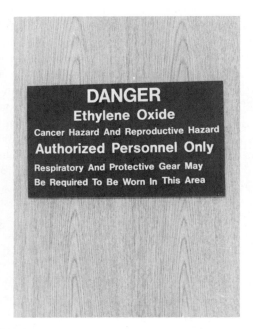

Fig. 23-2. Required warning sign at the entrance to an ethylene oxide cylinder manifold room at the rear of the ethylene oxide sterilizer.

sources. . . . Ethylene oxide has been classified as a probable human carcinogen and its inhalation may lead to an increased risk of contracting leukemia and stomach cancer."[24] The California Department of Health Services has estimated that the release of 800,000 pounds of ethylene oxide into the atmosphere per year translates into 360 to 510 potential excess cancers over a 70-year period. It is for this reason that, starting in August 1993, the Air Resources Board will prohibit the release of ethylene oxide into the atmosphere. Some device will be necessary to convert the ethylene oxide into harmless compounds. Catalytic converters are now available that break down the ethylene oxide into carbon dioxide and water (Fig. 23-4).

Because ethylene oxide gas is highly explosive, in the past large sterilizers used a mixture of 10% ethylene oxide with 90% carbon dioxide or 12% ethylene oxide with 88% fluorocarbon quenching agent, such as Freon 12, which has been implicated in the depletion of the earth's ozone layer. It is anticipated that a new, more environmentally acceptable fluorocarbon mixture called Penngas 2, which contains 90% of a new fluorocarbon with 10% ethylene oxide will be available to permit continued use of an eth-

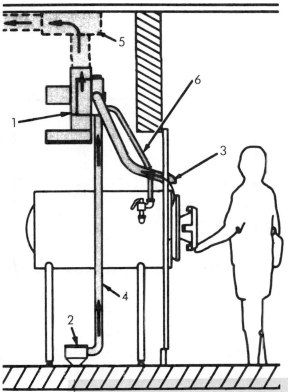

Fig. 23-3. The AMSCO Envirogard system is designed to remove the ethylene oxide gas from the air surrounding the sterilizer. It is operated by an exhaust blower *(1)* mounted above the sterilizer. To this are attached the tubing *(4)* and the gas capture funnel *(2)* mounted on the drain system into which the ethylene oxide gas and water are discharged at the end of the sterilization cycle. The door vent adaptor *(3)* installed above the sterilizer door is designed to remove the gas released when the sterilizer door is opened. Tube *(6)* connects the sterilizer's safety valve to the system. The captured gas is delivered into the hospital's dedicated exhaust system *(5)*, which delivers the gas to the atmosphere outside of the building. Note that this will not be permitted in southern California after December, 1992. (Diagram courtesy of AMSCO/The American Sterilizer Company, Erie, Pa.)

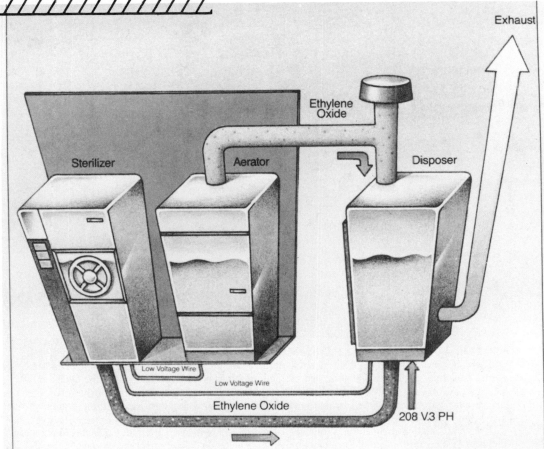

Fig. 23-4. The AMSCO Ethylene Oxide Disposer System takes the ethylene oxide vented from the sterilizer and the aerator and passes it over a manganese dioxide–copper oxide catalyst, which is heated initially to 138° C. Because the reaction between the catalyst and the ethylene oxide is exothermic the temperature commonly rises to 260° C. The ethylene oxide is converted to carbon dioxide and water. This or a similar apparatus will become mandatory in California after December, 1992, for all installations using more than 4 pounds of ethylene oxide per year.[24] (Illustration courtesy of AMSCO, Erie, Pa.)

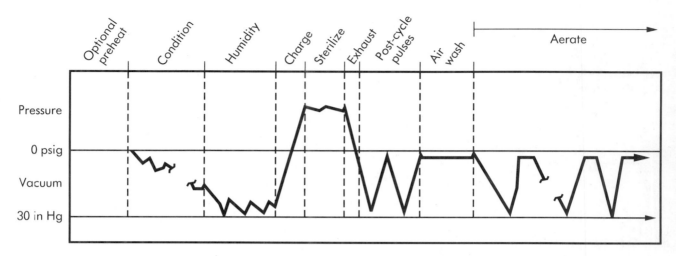

Fig. 23-5. Modern ethylene oxide sterilization and aeration cycle. To the original McDonald process shown in Fig. 23-1 has been added the air wash and repeated vacuum cycles to remove the ethylene oxide from the load. The vertical axis is pressure in units of psig when positive, and in inches of mercury when negative. The horizontal axis is time (no units). (Diagram courtesy of AMSCO, Erie, Pa.)

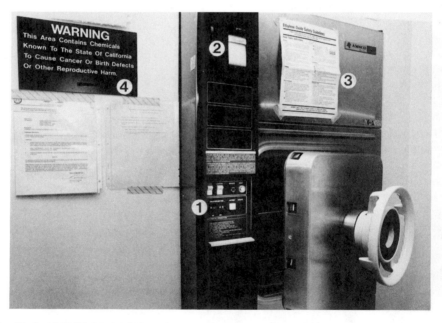

Fig. 23-6. AMSCO Model 2027 Ethylene Oxide Sterilizer and Aerator. The controls (1) permit it to be programmed to carry out the desired sterilization and aeration program. A strip chart recorder (2) prints out the temperature and pressure within the chamber throughout the cycle. In a sample 12% ethylene oxide −88% Freon 12 cycle at 54° C, the humidification of the load after the vacuum had removed the air from the chamber occupied 55 minutes. Sterilization with ethylene oxide at 8.5 psig occupied 1 hour and 46 minutes, and the exhaust purge and aeration cycle took 12 hours and 48 minutes for a total cycle time of 15 hours and 29 minutes. Displayed above the door of the sterilizer are the manufacturer's ethylene oxide safety guidelines (3) and to the left is the warning (4) required by the State of California: "This area contains chemicals known to the State of California to cause cancer or birth defects or other reproductive harm." (Copyright 1991 L. Rendell-Baker, M.D.)

ylene oxide and fluorocarbon mixture.[25-27] Small gas sterilizers often use 100% ethylene oxide.

The ethylene oxide sterilization process. The ethylene oxide sterilization process differs from the steam autoclave cycle in that it has two phases. In the first phase, the gas is forced into the load; and in the second phase, heated, bacterially filtered air at 60° C removes the residues of ethylene oxide from the load in 8 to 12 hours. In the absence of an aerator, elimination of ethylene oxide residues from packages of equipment containing PVC resting on a shelf at an ambient temperature of 21° C takes up to 7 days.

Before items are placed in the ethylene oxide sterilizer, they must be thoroughly cleaned and gross amounts of water must be removed. However, the equipment is not heat-dried because 45% relative humidity is required for ethylene oxide to penetrate the load. Equipment is then packaged in specially designed bags, which are permeable to the ethylene oxide. Nylon cannot be used because it is not permeable to ethylene oxide. The air within the chamber is removed, and steam is added to humidify the load. The humidity allows the ethylene oxide to penetrate the load and kill the bacteria. Items to be sterilized are exposed to ethylene oxide for 2 to 3 hours at a pressure of 8 psig and a temperature of approximately 54° C when the fluorocarbon mixture is used or at 25 psig and 54° C when the carbon dioxide mixture is used (Fig. 23-5). The fluorocarbon facilitates ethylene oxide penetration through the packaging and into the items to be sterilized.

Modern ethylene oxide sterilizers have a purge and aeration cycle. They use alternating cycles of vacuum and filtered air to remove all the gas remaining within the sterilizer (Fig. 23-6). Older sterilizers without this cycle can release a cloud of ethylene oxide gas when the sterilizer door is opened. This necessitates an extraction hood above the sterilizer door with a dedicated exhaust system (Fig. 23-3), and potentially exposes the operator to ethylene oxide gas. When sterilizers without the purge and aeration cycle were used, once the gas had dissipated the load was transferred to an aerator through which bacterially filtered warmed air was passed for 8 to 12 hours. This is the time required to remove ethylene oxide from PVC items. Failure to remove all ethylene oxide by inadequate aeration can easily lead to chemical burns to the patient.

DISINFECTION
Pasteurization

The process of pasteurization is named after Louis Pasteur (1822-1895), the French chemist who discovered bacteria and introduced the process by which milk is heated to 62° C, held at that temperature for 30 minutes, and then rapidly cooled. This method does not destroy spores but does kill Mycobacterium tuberculosis, streptococci, salmonellae, and Brucellae, which were responsible for milk-borne diseases. This method is now widely used to disinfect plastic and rubber anesthesia and respiratory equipment (Fig. 23-7). Blood, secretions, and other contaminants are first removed by a thorough washing process. The equipment is then subjected to hot water at 77° C for 30 minutes. Though this method kills most microorganisms, it does not produce a sterile product; the equipment must be handled when transferred from the washer to the drying cabinet and then again when it is packaged in plastic bags. The interior of the tubing and the face mask will be as clean as the equivalent disposable breathing systems, which are not sterile either.

Most pieces of equipment that the anesthesiologist must clean do not need to be sterile. Sterility is important only for such items as intravenous catheters, epidural and spinal needles, and central venous and pulmonary arterial catheters. In the vast majority of circumstances, these items are disposable and are purchased from the manufacturer already sterilized. It would be unusual for the anesthesiologist to be involved in sterilizing any of these items. However, in the event that an item needs to be sterilized, then steam or ethylene oxide are preferred.

Most items that the anesthesiologist uses are in the semicritical category. These items require a high level of disinfection. They include fiberoptic endoscopes and certain reusable items, such as rubber face masks, anesthesia breathing circuits, tracheal tubes, and temperature probes.[28] These items must first be thoroughly cleaned of all blood and secretions, preferably with a solution such as chlorhexidine gluconate (e.g., Hibiclens), an iodophor (e.g., Betadine), or a detergent soap, and then thoroughly rinsed. Once these items have been cleaned they can then be subjected to high-level disinfection in a 2% solution of alkaline glutaraldehyde (e.g., Cidex). It is important to follow the manufacturer's recommendations for soaking time, but in general a period of at least 20 minutes is required to kill the tuberculosis bacillus and other viruses. It is important to clean the items beforehand because organic matter, such as blood and mucus, may negate the biocidal effects of chemical disinfectants. It should also be remembered that glutaraldehydes are caustic, and contact with the skin, as well as inhalation of the fumes, should be avoided.

If one does not wish to use the glutaraldehyde solutions, items such as metal laryngoscope blades can be washed and then steam or gas autoclaved. Also, after being washed, fiberoptic endoscopes can also be gas autoclaved. It is important to install the venting cap on the endoscope before it is sent for gas autoclaving. This allows the gas that permeates the endoscope to escape without rupturing the outer skin. The cap is then removed before the endoscope is returned to service or immersed in liquids.

Hard surfaces that become contaminated need an intermediate-level disinfection. This is best accomplished with a phenolic (e.g., Wexcide) or sodium hypochlorite (e.g., chlorine bleach 1:5 or 1:10 dilution). Hypochlorite is pre-

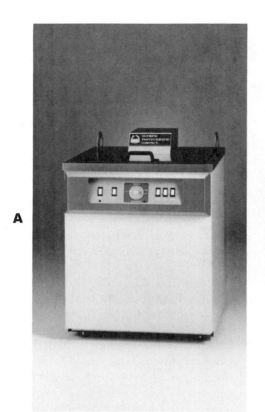
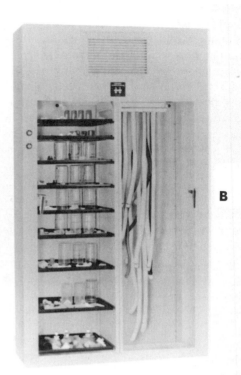

Fig. 23-7. The Olympic Pasteurmatic Compact System. **A,** The rotary washer and pasteurizer can take up to 20 anesthesia breathing system components loaded into its stainless steel basket for a 30-minute wash cycle. As the basket rotates, jets of hot water at 60° C are directed at the contents. The chamber is filled with hot detergent solution, into which the equipment is repeatedly plunged to dislodge contamination. When the 30-minute wash cycle is completed, the pasteurization cycle follows with water at 77° C, in which the equipment is immersed for 30 minutes. **B,** Next, the equipment is transferred to the drying cabinet, where bacteria-free filtered air at 57° C is blown over the equipment to speed up drying. After removal from the dryer, the equipment is sealed in plastic bags, ready for its next use. (Illustration courtesy of Olympic Medical Corp., Seattle, Wash.)

ferred if the area is contaminated with blood. Other instruments, such as stethoscopes, can be cleaned in a detergent and then disinfected with either isopropyl alcohol or hypochlorite solution. It must be remembered that the item must be thoroughly rinsed and dried after any disinfection procedure. A comprehensive review of the guidelines for selection and use of disinfectants can be found in the article by Rutala.[29]

Occasionally, the anesthesiologist is called upon to care for a patient with Creutzfeldt-Jakob disease (i.e., presenile dementia). This is a particularly difficult situation because the Creutzfeldt-Jakob organism is *extremely* resistant to normal decontamination methods and presents a considerable hazard to the medical staff.[31] Indeed, this organism has led to the deaths of a neurosurgeon,[32] a pathologist,[33] and two histopathology technicians.[29,30,34,35] The recommended method for decontamination is steam sterilization for 1 hour at a temperature of 132° C. Also, soaking instruments for 1 hour in 1 N (i.e., 4%) sodium hydroxide (a very caustic solution) has also been reported to be effective. Surfaces and other noncritical items can be disinfected by soaking in full-strength, undiluted bleach for 15

to 30 minutes, thoroughly rinsing, and then repeating.[29] Obviously this is a very difficult situation, and advice from the hospital epidemiologist can be extremely useful in this circumstance.

Although universal precautions are mandatory because any patient is potentially a carrier of an infectious disease, other, special steps are taken when a patient is known to have a highly infectious disease. For instance, if a patient has active pulmonary tuberculosis, it is ideal to use an all-disposable anesthesia circuit. If that is not available, then a system that is easily sterilized, such as a Bain circuit, should be used. This is easier than trying to decontaminate an entire circle breathing system and ventilator. Also, keeping only necessary equipment inside the room and moving nonessential items to a substerile area will also markedly decrease clean-up and turn-around time.

Recommendations for infection control in anesthesia equipment
Anesthesia apparatus and ventilators

1. All machine surfaces including flow control knobs should be cleaned daily with a phenolic solution.

2. The machine's counter top should be covered with a fresh, clean towel for each patient
3. After exposure to an infectious patient (i.e., one with open pulmonary tuberculosis), all surfaces should be cleaned immediately with a phenolic solution.

Disposable equipment to be discarded after each case

1. Syringes and needles should be discarded into a SHARPS container after use.
2. Tracheal tubes of all types and PVC endobronchial tubes should be discarded.
3. Esophageal stethoscopes should be discarded.

Equipment to be sterilized or pasteurized

1. Steam sterilization should be used whenever possible in preference to ethylene oxide sterilization.
2. Pasteurization may be used when clean rather than sterile equipment is acceptable. It applies to:
   a. Rubber breathing systems
   b. Rubber endobronchial tubes
   c. Face masks
   d. Oral airways
   e. Temperature probes
   f. Laryngoscope blades
   g. Ventilator bellows
3. The carbon dioxide absorber assembly should be autoclaved or gas sterilized following use for patients with pulmonary tuberculosis or other pulmonary infection.

PROTECTION OF ANESTHESIA STAFF AGAINST HEPATITIS B AND HUMAN IMMUNODEFICIENCY VIRUSES[15,36,37,38]

Because anesthesiologists daily come into intimate contact with the mucous membranes and saliva of patients, the risk of transmission of hepatitis B (HBV) to the physician is real. The risk of contracting both HBV and human immunodeficiency virus (HIV) is greatest when an infusion is set up, "lines" are inserted, or blood samples are drawn. Between 8% and 20% of personnel receiving needle-stick injuries contaminated with HBV infected blood will develop hepatitis B.[39,40] Hepatitis B is reported to result in 300 deaths of hospital personnel per year.[38,39] Regarding HIV, the Centers for Disease Control report that 0.47% of health care workers receiving needle-stick injuries with HIV infected blood became infected. That is, a little under 1 in 200 needle-stick injuries resulted in HIV infection. However, the average anesthesiologist treats many thousands of patients during his/her working life, so the cumulative risk of occupationally acquired HIV infection may be as high as 1 in 25.[41] "Although the risk of contracting HIV as a result of occupational exposure to a needle-stick may be low compared with HBV, the consequences of in-

fection are far more serious: for whereas only 2% of people infected with HBV die of their infection,[42] 50% of those infected with HIV will develop AIDS within 6 years."[43] There is no protective vaccine against HIV, and prompt treatment with zidovudine after needle-stick injury has so far proved ineffective.[44,45]

Hepatitis B is more highly infectious than HIV. The virus can survive for several days on stainless steel surfaces, needles, or gloves. Because much of the equipment used in anesthesia is a potential route by which this virus can be transmitted and because it is resistant to phenol disinfectants, the use of disposable equipment or steam sterilization is indicated. Vaccine against hepatitis B is now available, all health care personnel at risk should avail themselves of this protection.

Centers for Disease Control recommended universal precautions

The universal precautions recommended by the CDC[38] should be adopted when handling all patients because it is not possible to determine who may be HBV or HIV positive. To protect the practitioner's health, it is essential to prevent exposure of skin or mucous membrane to blood or other body fluids. The CDC recommend the wearing of gloves, goggles, gown, and mask throughout all procedures. The provision of these protective items by hospitals and their use by the staff is now mandated by the OSHA 1990 regulations.[46,47] If hands or other skin surfaces become contaminated with blood or other bodily fluids, they should be washed immediately, because studies suggest that intact skin may transmit HIV infection. The Langerhans cells in the skin and mucous membrane may be the HIV's primary target cells and the route for HIV infection. "The assumption that HIV infection occurs exclusively by entry of the virus through wounds in the skin and mucous membranes into the blood can no longer be considered valid."[48-50]

Needles and other sharp items should be carefully disposed of in a SHARPS container. The CDC recommendation incorporated into the OSHA regulation is that unprotected needles shall not be recapped or removed from disposable syringes.

Impact of HIV positive status on anesthesia staff [51-53]

Although the CDC has not yet published official recommendations on the actions to be taken on the future employment and duties of HIV positive medical staff, it seems likely that such personnel will be excluded from immediate patient contact and performing invasive procedures. The impact, therefore, of this infection on the individual is so severe that many leading centers now provide disability insurance coverage for all their house staff, and no doubt this coverage will eventually be extended to all high-risk personnel.[54,55]

Minimizing the hazards: needle-free anesthesia

Accidental needle-sticks are the most common route whereby hospital workers acquire HIV infection. The elimination, as far as possible, of the use of unprotected needles should help to reduce this hazard. To this end, several items are now available: (1) an intravenous needle cannula set that encloses the needle as the cannula is inserted (Fig. 23-8), (2) intravenous extension sets (Fig. 23-9) with valved Luer injection ports that permit intravenous drugs to be given directly from syringes without the use of needles, (3) minispikes that permit syringes to be filled with drugs from vials without the use of a needle (Fig. 23-10), and (4) shrouded needles (Fig. 23-11) that permit injections into the ports of standard intravenous sets while protecting the user against accidental needle-sticks. The risk of needle-sticks is also eliminated by another system, which uses blunt plastic cannulas combined with special injection caps (Figs. 23-12, 23-13, and 23-14). Intravenous infusion and central venous pressure equipment (Fig. 23-15) designed to limit blood contamination of the user's hands have also been introduced.

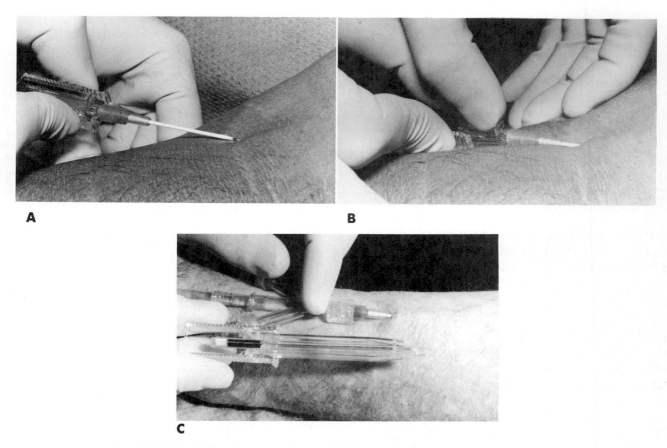

A

B

C

Fig. 23-8. The Critikon Protective System (Critikon Inc., Tampa, Fla.) enables placement of an intravenous catheter without exposing the user to the hazard of a needle stick. **A,** The needle and catheter are inserted into the vein. **B,** The thumb advances the catheter into the vein, and the needle is drawn back into its protective sheath. **C,** The sheath is shown with the needle locked inside. (Copyright 1990, L. Rendell-Baker, M.D.)

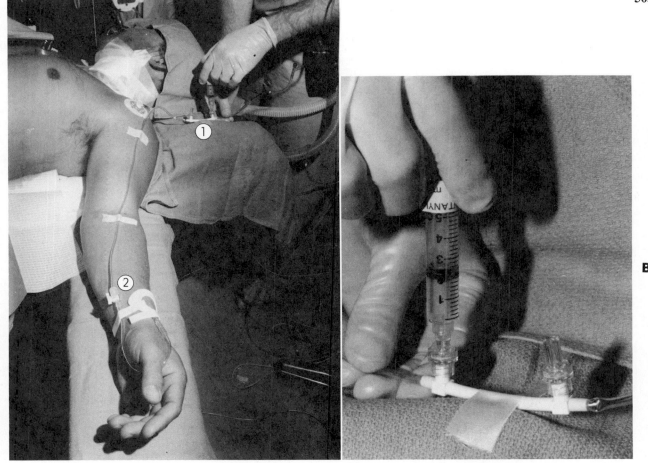

Fig. 23-9. A, The Burron AET-36 Anesthesia Extension Set (Burron Medical Inc., Bethlehem, Pa.) provides two valved injection sites *(1)* close to the anesthesiologist, through which injections can be made without the use of needles. A three-way stopcock *(2)* is also provided. **B,** Close-up of valved injection sites. (Copyright 1991, L. Rendell-Baker, M.D.)

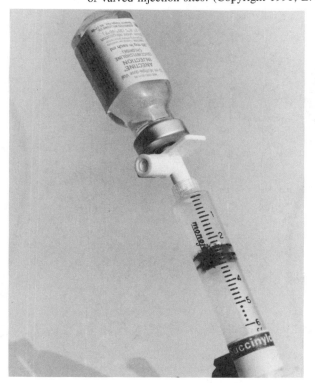

Fig. 23-10. The Burron DP1000 MiniSpike inserted into the vial permits the syringe to be filled with succinylcholine without the use of a needle. (Copyright 1990, L. Rendell-Baker, M.D.)

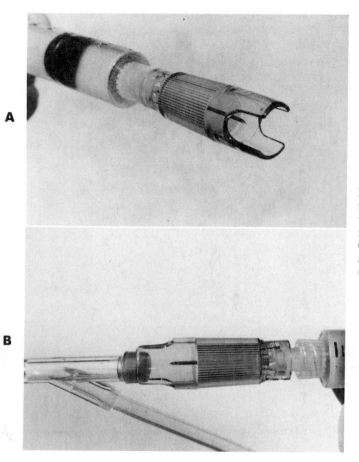

Fig. 23-11. A, The shroud on the IMS 4009 Stick-Gard (International Medication Systems, South El Monte, Calif.) needle prevents accidental needle sticks. **B,** the cutaway on the sides permits injections to be made into the infusion set's injection sites. Combined with a suitable drug vial access cap, this could provide a convenient needleless system using standard infusion sets. (Copyright 1990, L. Rendell-Baker, M.D.)

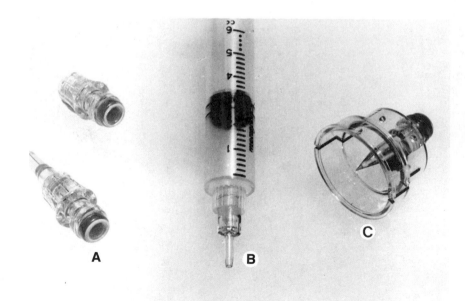

Fig. 23-12. The components of the Baxter Interlink (Baxter Healthcare Corp., Valencia, Calif.) system that eliminate the needle-stick problem. **A,** The injection cap with preformed, normally closed slit, which admits the cannula but prevents leakage. **B,** The blunt plastic cannula replaces needles. **C,** The disposable drug vial access cap. The spike penetrates the cap of the vial. (Copyright 1991, L. Rendell-Baker, M.D.)

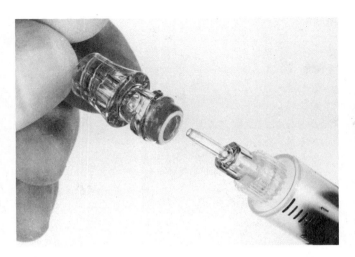

Fig. 23-13. The plastic cannula on the syringe is able to penetrate the special, preformed, normally closed slit in the injection cap without danger of leakage or coring. (Copyright 1991, L. Rendell-Baker, M.D.)

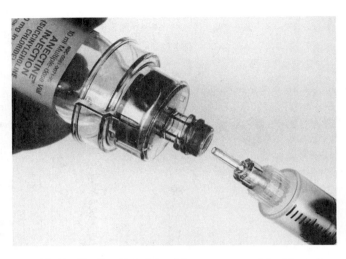

Fig. 23-14. The Interlink drug vial access cap and the blunt plastic cannula eliminate the need for a needle to fill a syringe with drugs from a multidose vial. (Copyright 1991, L. Rendell-Baker, M.D.)

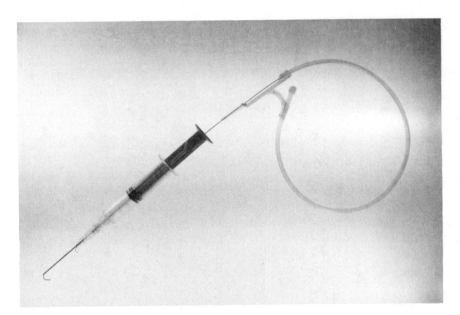

Fig. 23-15. The Arrow Raulerson (Arrow International, Inc., Reading, Pa.) syringe minimizes blood contamination of the user's hands by providing a valved channel for the guide wire through the plunger of the syringe. This eliminates the need to detach the syringe from the introducer needle to insert the guide wire, thus eliminating the opportunity for reflux of a patient's blood and the danger of contaminating the user's fingers. (Copyright 1991, L. Rendell-Baker, M.D.)

DEPARTMENTAL ORGANIZATION FOR CARE OF ANESTHESIA EQUIPMENT

Good communication between the anesthesiologist and nurses in the operating room and the anesthesia ancillary staff is essential. The operating room two-way intercom is conveniently placed for use by the anesthesiologist or the nurses and provides direct contact with essential services. The operating room anesthesia technician call system is placed close to the operating room door so that it can be used as the patient is moved from the operating room to the PACU. The anesthesia technicians in the workroom are alerted (Fig. 23-16) that the room is ready to be cleared of used equipment, cleaned, and restocked with drugs and apparatus.

Adequate receptacles for the disposal of used equipment are essential. Fig. 23-17 shows the result of failure to provide such receptacles. The provision of an anesthesia drug

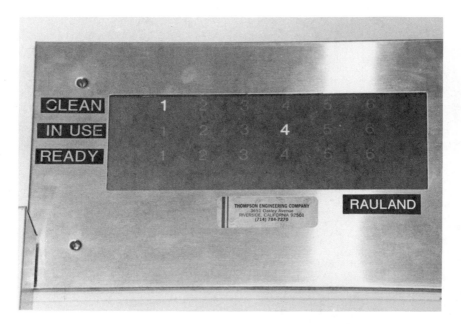

Fig. 23-16. This operating room status monitor in the anesthesia equipment room indicates that operating room 1 is ready to be cleaned and that operating room 4 is in use. (Copyright 1991, L. Rendell-Baker, M.D.)

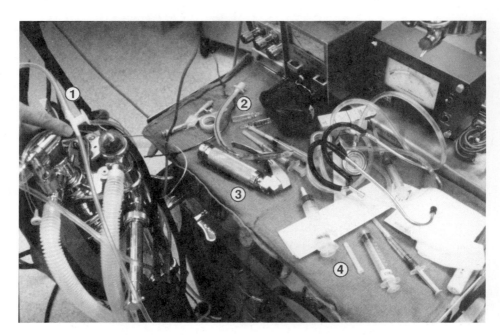

Fig. 23-17. In the absence of an efficient disposal system for used and contaminated items, the anesthesia machine can easily look like this at the end of a busy case. It is difficult to see how this machine could be more contaminated. The suction catheter *(1)* is draped over the absorber, the used tracheal tube *(2)*, and stylette; the laryngoscope *(3)* and innumerable syringes and needles *(4)* are evident on the tabletop. (Copyright 1987, L. Rendell-Baker, M.D.)

and equipment cart (Fig. 23-18) with separate receptacles for contaminated reusables and disposables greatly facilitates the anesthesia technician's work in readying the apparatus for the next case (Fig. 23-19).

When the schedule includes a number of cases to be performed under regional anesthesia, an anesthesia induction area provides a quiet space where blocks can be inserted while the OR is being prepared. This speeds up the turn-around and facilitates the technician's work.

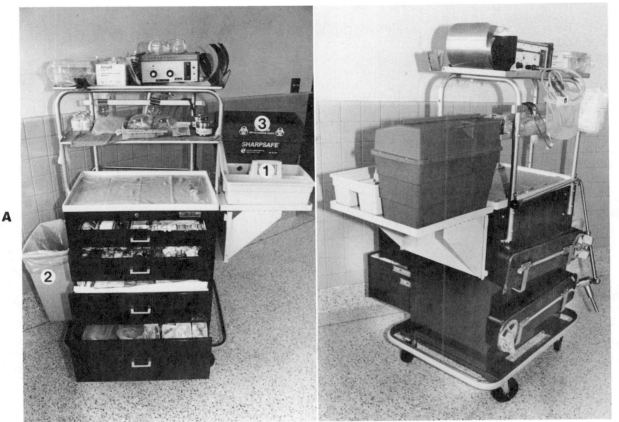

Fig. 23-18. A, This Blue Bell Biomedical (Blue Bell Bio-Medical, Blue Bell, Pa.) anesthesia drug and equipment cart is arranged to separate the used reusable items, such as laryngoscopes, face masks, and airways, that are placed in the plastic basket *(1)* for cleaning and pasteurization, from the disposable items which are placed in the plastic trash bucket *(2)*. All sharp items, such as syringes, needles, and ampules, are placed in the plastic SHARPSAFE *(3)*. **B,** The rear of the cart has hooks that hold the arm boards and the patient screen. (Copyright 1991, L. Rendell-Baker, M.D.)

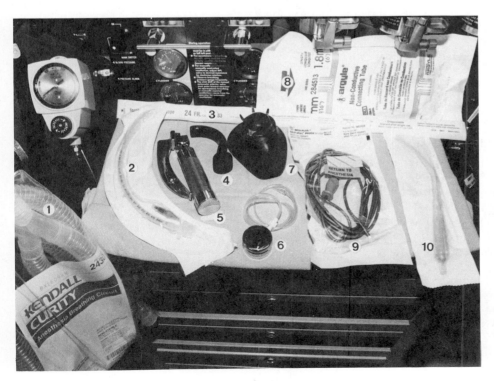

Fig. 23-19. Anesthesia apparatus prepared for use with a clean towel on the tabletop and the following items of equipment: *1,* clear plastic disposable breathing system; *2,* sterile tracheal tube; *3,* esophageal stethoscope; *4,* Guedel oral airway; *5,* laryngoscope with Macintosh blade; *6,* Wenger precordial stethoscope; *7,* face mask; *8,* disposable connecting tubing for suction handle; *9,* telethermometer probe; *10,* Yankauer suction handle. (Copyright 1991, L. Rendell-Baker, M.D.)

Table 23-1. Catheter size colors used in the United States and proposed international standard colors

	Present United States Catheter Colors				
	14 Gauge	**16 Gauge**	**18 Gauge**	**20 Gauge**	**22 Gauge**
Abbocath (Abbot)	Gold/tan	Gray*	Green*	Pink*	Dark blue*
Medicut (Argyle)	Orange/tan*	Gray*	Green*	Dark pink*	Blue*
IV Cath (B-D)	Light gray	Lavender	Light pink	Light yellow	Dark gray
Longdwell (B-D)	Olive	Purple	Pink	Yellow	Black
Angiocath (Deseret)	Pink	Yellow	Tan	Light green	Light blue*
Cathlon (Jelco)	Orange*	Gray*	Dark green*	Pink*	Dark blue*
Quick Cath (Vicra)	Orange*	Gray*	Light green*	Light pink*	Light blue*
Equivalent metric sizes	**2.0 mm**	**1.6 mm**	**1.2 mm**	**0.9 mm**	**0.7 mm**
	ISO/TC84 Proposed International Standard Colors*				
	Orange	Gray	Green	Pink	Blue

*Note these manufacturers already comply with this proposal based on French National Standard.

USE OF STANDARD COLORS HELPS RECOGNITION

The American Society for Testing and Materials (ASTM) standard D4774* for drug syringe labels uses color to identify the group to which a drug belongs. Thus it is easy to distinguish the yellow label on a thiopental induction agent from the blue label of a fentanyl narcotic or the light red label on a muscle relaxant syringe (Fig. 23-20) (see also Chapter 18 and color insert).

Most manufacturers use color-coding by size on the plastic hubs of intravenous cannulas. Unfortunately, there is no accepted standard range of colors to distinguish among the various sizes. Authorities in the European Common Community (ECC) are now exerting pressure on manufacturers to achieve uniform standards by the time the Community becomes effective in 1992. Progress is being made on an intravenous catheter standard incorporating a standard range of colors to identify the size of the cannulas based on the existing French National Standard (see Table 23-1).†

DISPOSABLE BREATHING SYSTEM EQUIPMENT

The first disposable plastic blood and intravenous sets were introduced in 1947, followed by plastic disposable syringes in 1957. However, it was not until 1968 that the first disposable breathing systems were introduced by Thomas J. Mahon, M.D., of New Jersey, with R. Bryan Roberts, M.D., of The Mount Sinai Hospital in New York (Fig. 23-21). Bryan Roberts helped Mahon design the

lightweight breathing system with its plastic swivel-Y mask and tube adapter. This was first shown at the ASA Annual Meeting in Washington, D.C., in October 1968.[56]

One reason for the delay in the appearance of disposable breathing systems was that before the American National Standards Institute Z79 Anesthesia Standards Committee introduced the standard 15-mm and 22-mm breathing system fittings in the early 1960s, each manufacturer had its own size of fitting on the absorber, bag mount, Y piece, and mask.[57,58] The user therefore had to buy masks, bags, and breathing tubes of that size from the original manufacturer. When all manufacturers adopted the standard 15-mm and 22-mm fittings, the user had only to stock one supply of expendable rubber components, and these could be obtained from any supplier.[59] It was the adoption of these standard sizes of fittings that provided a large enough market to make the introduction of disposable equipment economically worthwhile.

Problems with disposable equipment

In the original standard for breathing system fittings the "plug and ring" gauges were designed specifically to test the accuracy of metal components, which, unlike plastic, do not stretch or "flow" when the components are forced together. Also, the gentle 1-in-40 conical taper (1 unit increase in the diameter for each 40 units of length) used for the metal fittings was not satisfactory for plastics, for which a steeper 1-in-20 taper was better. The manufacturers therefore often had difficulty in producing satisfactory fittings that could hold together securely. Much of the problem was due to the widely variable characteristics of the plastics used, which ranged from hard polycarbonate to elastic polyethylene. As a result, accidental disconnection, particularly between the tracheal tube connector and the Y piece, became a chronic problem.[60-63] Fortunately, since

*Contact Margie Lawlor, ASTM, (215) 299-5518 for information on D4774 and other Subcommittee D10-34 standards.
†For information, contact Dawn Helsing, AAMI, (703) 525-4890, Secretary of the US TAG for ISO-TC84, the International Committee working on this project.

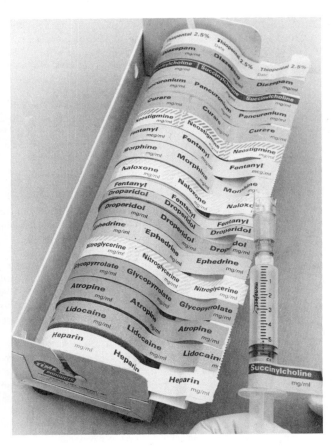

Fig. 23-20. An ASTM D4774 standard colored drug label being applied to a syringe of succinylcholine. In this standard, colors are used to define the group to which a drug belongs. Because the colors used are defined by numbers in the Pantone Matching System (PMS) for printer's ink, any label company should be able to match the standard's colors. For example, labels on induction agents are PMS yellow, those on tranquilizers are PMS 151 orange, those on muscle relaxants are PMS 805 fluorescent red, those on narcotics are PMS 297 blue, those on vasopressors are PMS 256 violet, those on local anesthetics are PMS 401 gray, and those on anticholinergics are PMS 367 green. (Copyright 1991, L. Rendell-Baker, M.D.)

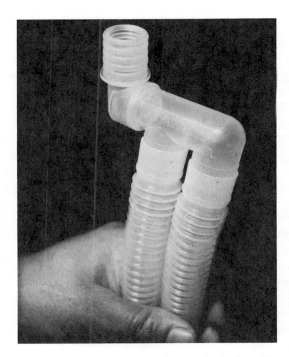

Fig. 23-21. This pioneer disposable anesthesia breathing system with swivel Y was designed by R. Bryan Roberts, M.D., and Thomas J. Mahon, M.D., in 1968. (Copyright 1987, L. Rendell-Baker, M.D.)

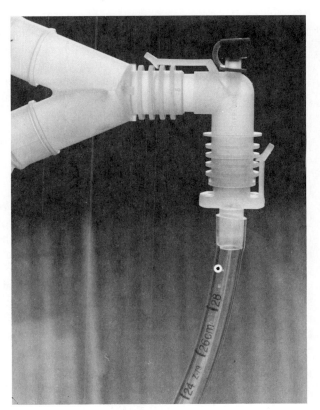

Fig. 23-22. The Kendall Safetrak (Kendall Healthcare Products Co., Mansfield, Mass.) system uses clips on the 15-mm fittings, which engage with the rings on the 22-mm male fittings to prevent accidental disconnection. (Copyright 1990, L. Rendell-Baker, M.D.)

the ASTM F29 Standards Committee* evolved standard gauges and testing procedures specifically designed for plastic† as well as metal components, the problem of accidental disconnection should be considerably reduced. However, to obtain a secure fit, the user must rotate the components into each other while forcing them to engage. Some manufacturers use grooves molded into the 22-mm male fittings as part of an antidisconnect system (Fig. 23-22).

*ASTM F29 took over the functions of ANSI Z76 in 1983.
†Standard F1054-87 Standard Practice for Conical Fittings of 15-mm and 22-mm sizes. For ASTM F29 standards contact Beth Moran, (215) 299-5517.

REUSE OF DISPOSABLE EQUIPMENT

Although many hospitals in the United States are reusing some disposable items[64] such as hemodialysis tubing,[65] cardiovascular catheters, and ventilator breathing systems, according to FDA guidelines[66] the hospital must be able to "demonstrate: (1) that the device can be adequately cleaned and sterilized; (2) that the physical characteristics or quality of the device will not be adversely affected; (3) the device remains safe and effective for its intended use; and (4) they must accept full responsibility for the device's safety and effectiveness." However, Hedley-Whyte[67] has stated that "the reuse of disposable anesthesia devices presents a greater medicolegal hazard than any other type of equipment, commensurate with the relative size of malpractice awards in anesthesiology. Consequently, anesthesia devices intended for single use are not reused in Harvard Medical School's teaching hospitals."

Whether using a disposable or a reusable piece of equipment, the objective is to provide for each patient (1) a sterile tracheal tube; (2) a clean laryngoscope blade; (3) a clean breathing system consisting of breathing bag, breathing tubes, Y piece, mask adapter, and face mask; (4) a clean oral airway; (5) a clean esophageal stethoscope; and (6) a clean telethermometer probe.

Reusables

Clean reusables can be provided by a system such as the Pasteurmatic, which can handle up to 20 breathing systems per load with a technician able to process five loads in an 8-hour shift, making a total of 100 breathing systems per shift. The process has four phases: washing, pasteurization, drying, and packaging, which consumes most of the time. This system will occupy one technician's attention throughout a day to handle the equipment for 20 to 25 operating rooms.

Disposables

Less manual labor is involved with disposables, but extra space in or near the operating room is essential for storing the bulky disposable breathing systems. It may be that the local dealer can arrange to store much of a hospital's requirements if given an annual contract so that deliveries can be made once or twice a month to suit the hospital's storage facilities. If there is doubt as to the best choice, the manufacturers of the Pasteurmatic or similar systems should be asked to produce cost analyses comparing their equipment with use of disposable systems.

REFERENCES

1. Thomas ET: The problem in Practice. *Int Anesthesiol Clin* 10(#2):11-22, 1972.
2. Thomas ET: The sterilization dilemma: where will it end? *Anesth Analg* 47:657, 1968.
3. Pace NL, Webster C, Epstein R, et al: Failure of anesthetic circuit bacterial filters to reduce postoperative pulmonary infections, *Anesthesiology* 51:S362, 1979 (abstract).
4. Garibaldi RA, Britt MR, Webster C, et al: Failure of bacterial filters to reduce the incidence of pneumonia after inhalation anesthesia, *Anesthesiology* 54:364, 1981.
5. Feeley TW, Hamilton WK, Xavier B, et al: Sterile anesthesia breathing circuits do not prevent postoperative pulmonary infection, *Anesthesiology* 54:369, 1981.
6. du Moulin GC, Sauberman AJ: The anesthesia machine and circle system are not likely to be sources of bacterial contamination, *Anesthesiology* 47:353-358, 1977.
7. Brooks JHJ, Gupta B, Baker D: Anesthetic machine contamination, *Anesthesiology* 75:A874, 1991 (abstract).
8. Merson MH: In report of conference on "HIV disease: pathogenesis and therapy" Grenelefe, Florida 13-17 March 1991, *Science* 252:372-373, 1991.
9. Selwyn PA, Hortel D, Lewis VA, et al: A prospective study of the risk of tuberculosis among IV drug users with human immunodeficiency virus infection, *N Engl J Med* 320:545, 1989.
10. Pitchenick AE, Cole C, Russell BW, et al: Tuberculosis, atypical mycobacteriosis and acquired immunodeficiency syndrome among Haitian and non-Haitian patients in South Florida, *Ann Intern Med* 101:641, 1984.
11. Barnes PF, Block AB, Davidson PT, et al: Tuberculosis in patients with human immunodeficiency virus infection, *N Engl J Med* 324:1644, 1991.
12. Chaisson RE, Schecter GF, Theur CP, et al: Tuberculosis in patients with acquired immunodeficiency syndrome, clinical features, response to therapy, *Am Rev Respir Dis* 136:570, 1987.
13. Pitchenick AE, Robinson HA: The radiographic appearances of tuberculosis in patients with acquired immunodeficiency syndrome (AIDS) and pre-AIDS, *Am Rev Respir Dis* 131:393, 1985.
14. Montgomery AB, Corkery KJ, Baunette ER, et al: Occupational exposure to aerosolized pentamidine, *Chest* 98:386-388, 1990.
15. Tuberculosis and acquired immunodeficiency syndrome, MMWR 36, New York City, 1987, Centers for Disease Control, pp 785-795.
16. Garner JS, Favero MS: Guidelines for hand-washing and hospital environmental control, publication no 99-1117, Atlanta, Ga, 1985, Centers for Disease Control.
17. AORN Recommended Practices Subcommittee: Recommended practices: cleaning and processing anesthesia equipment, *AORN J* 41:625-631, 1985.
18. Favero MS: Principles of sterilization and disinfection. In Berry AJ, editor: Infections in anesthesia, *Anesth. Clin. N. America* 7(#4), Philadelphia, 1989, WB Saunders, pp 941-949.
19. Spaulding EH, Cundy KR, Turner FJ: *Chemical disinfection of medical and surgical materials.* In Block SS, editor: *Disinfection, sterilization and preservation,* Philadelphia, 1977, Lea and Febiger, pp 654-684.
20. Phillips CR: The sterilization action of gaseous ethylene oxide. II. Sterilization of contaminated objects and related compounds: time, concentration and temperature relationships, *Am J Hyg* 50:280, 1947.
21. McDonald RL: Method of sterilizing. US Patent No 3,068,064; 1962.
22. Snow JC, Mangiaracine AB, Anderson ML, et al: Sterilization of anesthesia equipment with ethylene oxide, *N Engl J Med* 266:443, 1962.
23. Title 29. Code of Federal Regulations Part 1910, Subpart 1047. June 24, 1984 set 1 ppm exposure limit. Appendix A gave EPA Nonmandatory Recommendations and Guidelines. The 1990 publication set the 5 ppm maximum exposure limit.
24. Proposed ethylene oxide control measures for sterilizer and aerators. Staff Reports, State of California Air Resources Board, March 23, 1990.
25. Pennsylvania Engineering Co, 1107-21 N Howard St, Philadelphia, Pa 10123: Recipient EPA stratospheric ozone protection award for 1991.

26. Talukdar R, Melloulei A. Gierczak T, et al: Atmospheric lifetime of CHF$_2$Br, a proposed substitute for halons, *Science* 252:693-695, 1991.

27. Manzer LE: The CFC-ozone issue: progress in the development of alternatives to CFCs, *Science* 249:31-35, 1990.

28. Drummond DC, Skidmore AG: Sterilization and disinfection in the physician's office, *Can Med Assoc J* 145:937-943, 1991.

29. Rutala WA: APIC guidelines for infection control practice, *Am J Infect Control* 18:99-117, 1990.

30. Brown P, Gibbs CJ, Amyx HL, et al: Chemical disinfection of Creutzfeld-Jakob disease virus, *N Engl J Med* 306:1279-1281, 1982.

31. Brown P, Preese MA, Will RG: "Friendly fire" in medicine: hormones, homografts, and Creutzfeld-Jacob disease, *Lancet* 340:24-27, 1992.

32. Schoene C, Masters CL, Gibbs CT, Jr. et al: Transmissible spongform encephalopathy (Creutzfeld-Jacob disease): atypical clinical and pathological findings, *Arch Neurol* 38:473-477, 1981.

33. Gorman DG, Benson DF, Vogel DG, et al: Creutzfeld-Jacob disease in a pathologist. *Neurology* 42:463, 1992.

34. Miller DC: Creutzfeld-Jacob disease in histopathology technicians, *N Engl J Med* 318:853-854, 1988.

35. Sitwell L, Lack B, Attack E, et al: Creutzfeld-Jacob disease in histopathology technicians, *N Engl J Med* 318:854, 1988.

36. Guidelines for prevention of transmission of HIV and hepatitis B to health care and public safety workers, MMWR 38, June 23, 1989, Centers for Disease Control, p 56.

37. Update: acquired immunodeficiency syndrome and immunodeficiency virus infection among health care workers, MMWR 37, 1988, Centers for Disease Control, p 229.

38. Update: universal precaution for prevention of transmission of HIV, HGV and other blood-borne pathogens in health care settings, MMWR 37, #24, June 26, 1988, Centers for Disease Control.

39. Berry AJ, Isaacson IJ, Kane MA, et al: A multicenter study of the prevalence of hepatitis B viral serology markers in anesthesia personnel, *Anesth Analg* 63:738, 1984.

40. Berry AJ, Isaacson IJ, Hunt D, et al: The prevalence of hepatitis B viral markers in anesthesia personnel, *Anesthesiology* 60:6-9, 1984.

41. Jones ME: A thing about AIDS, *Anaesth Intensive Care* 17:253-263, 1989.

42. Morgan DR: HIV and needle-stick injuries, *Lancet* 335:1280, 1990.

43. Moss AR, Baccetti P, Osmond D, et al: Seropositivity for HIV and the development of AIDS or AIDS related condition: three year follow-up of the San Francisco General Hospital cohort, *Br Med J* 296:745-750, 1988.

44. Occupational infection among anaesthetists, *Lancet* 336:1103, 1990 (editorial).

45. Anon: Zidovudine and needle-stick exposure, *Lancet* 335:1271, 1990.

46. Occupational exposure to blood borne pathogens: OSHA final rules, 29 CFR part 1910:1030, Federal Register Part 2, Department of Labor, OSHA, Dec 6, 1991.

47. Enforcement procedure for occupational exposure to hepatitis B virus (HBV) and human immunodeficiency virus (HIV), OSHA Instruction CPL2-2-44B, Feb 27, 1990.

48. Braathen LR, Romirez G, Kunze RO, et al: Langerhans cells as primary target cells for HIV infection, *Lancet* ii:1094, 1987.

49. Niedecken H, Lutz G, Bauer R, et al: Langerhans cell and primary target and vehicle for transmission of HIV, *Lancet* ii:519, 1987.

50. Kay LA: Immunology of human skin and susceptibility to HIV infection, *Lancet* ii:166, 1987.

51. Angell M: A dual approach to the AIDS epidemic, *N Engl J Med* 324:1498-1500, 1991.

52. Brennan TA: Transmission of the human immunodeficiency virus in the health care setting: time for action, *N Engl J Med* 324:1504-1509, 1991.

53. Bayer R: Sounding board: public health policy and AIDS epidemic—an end to the HIV exceptionalism? *N Engl J Med* 324:1500-1504, 1991.

54. Dunne DW, Keggi JM, Kornick JJ et al: Physicians in training and HIV, *N Engl J Med* 322:1392-1393, 1990.

55. York E: When a house officer gets AIDS, *N Engl J Med* 322:1155, 1990 (letter).

56. Roberts RB: Disposables in anesthesiology and respiratory care. *Int Anesthiol, Clin* 10 (#2): 157-177, 1972.

57. Rendell-Baker L: Standards of anesthetic and ventilatory equipment, *Int Anesthesiol Clin* 20(#3): 171, 1982.

58. Rendell-Baker L: *Standards for anesthesia,* In Brown BR, editor: *The issues in future anesthesia delivery systems.* Philadelphia, 1982, Davis, pp 59-78.

59. *Standard Specification for Conical Fittings of 15-mm and 22-mm sizes,* ASTM Standard F1054-87, 1987, American Society for Testing and Materials, Philadelphia, Pa.

60. Cooper JB, Long CD, Newbower RS, et al: Multihospital study of preventable anesthesia mishaps, *Anesthesiology* 51:S348, 1979 (abstract).

61. Cooper JB, Newbower RS, Long CD, et al: Preventable anesthesia mishaps: a study of human factors, *Anesthesiology* 49:399-406, 1978.

62. Cooper JB, Newbower RS, Kitz RJ, et al: An analysis of major errors and equipment failures in anesthesia: considerations for prevention and detection, *Anesthesiology* 60:34-43, 1984.

63. FDA Contract #225-82-5070 report 86-4205. Accidental Breathing System Disconnection.

64. Greene VW: Reuse of disposable medical devices: historical and current aspects, *Infect Control* 7:508-513, 1986.

65. AAMI Recommended Practices on Reuse of Hemodialyzers, Arlington, Va, 1990, AAMI.

66. Reuse of medical devices, FDA Compliance Policy Guide #7124-16, Washington, DC, 1987, US Government Printing Office.

67. Hedley-Whyte J: *Medicolegal and infection risks of reuses of single use supplies and equipment in anesthesiology.* In *Reuse of disposable medical devices in the 1980s.* Proceedings of an International Conference, March 29-30, 1984, Washington, DC: Institute for Health Policy Analysis. Georgetown Medical Center, 1984, pp 149-155.

Chapter 24

MEDICOLEGAL AND RISK MANAGEMENT ASPECTS OF ANESTHESIA EQUIPMENT

John H. Eichhorn, M.D.
E.S. Siker, M.D.

Medicolegal issues
    Manufacturer's warranty
    Implied warranty
    Express and implied warranty
Risk management principles applied to anesthesia equipment
    Prepurchase evaluation of equipment
    Training and in-service education
    Policy and procedure
    Privileges and responsibilities
    Logs and records
    Maintenance and service
    Back-up equipment
    "Obsolete" equipment and its replacement
    Response to an adverse event involving equipment
    Standardization of equipment within a department

As the workplace of the anesthesiologist becomes ever more complex, users of anesthesia equipment must consider the medicolegal and risk management aspects of the paraphernalia now considered necessary to the conduct of anesthesia care. In all of clinical medicine, anesthesia practice is probably the activity most dependent on devices that range from a simple tongue depressor to complex, computer-driven "smart" gas machines, two-dimensional echocardiograms, and multiplexed mass spectrometry systems. Such equipment has the potential to create annoyance, inconvenience, inefficiency, and, more important,

injury or death. Awareness of the medicolegal considerations coupled with appropriate principles of risk management can minimize adverse outcomes attributable to anesthesia equipment. Such considerations have two basic components: first, efforts to guarantee that the equipment will be free of defects and will not fail and, second, efforts to ensure error-free use of the equipment.

This chapter describes both the medicolegal and risk management perspectives of anesthesia equipment. Viewed in isolation, the perceptions can be distorting. Neither each patient cared for nor every anesthetic administered constitutes a reason for fear that a plaintiff's counsel lurks, waiting for every lapse. Rather, the objective here is to illustrate patterns often overlooked by anesthesia providers that can easily be incorporated into routine practice.

All too often, the structural component of care (i.e., equipment) is taken for granted until there is a catastrophe. The potential for complacency in anesthesia practice exists because equipment is usually so reliable that it is rarely the source of morbidity or mortality. Such complacency significantly increases the risk that unsuspected problems with equipment may endanger patients and create liability exposure for anesthesia providers.

Overt failure of properly maintained anesthesia equipment is a comparatively rare event. The original critical incident study,[1] found that 14% of anesthesia critical incidents involved apparent equipment failure. In a larger follow-up study,[2] only 4% of the incidents "with substantive negative outcomes" involved equipment failure. In the period 1977 to 1984, the Emergency Care Research Institute (ECRI)[3] examined 15 anesthesia incidents involving anesthesia equipment. Analysis of these events revealed that human error was a significant component in most of the cases,[4] as is usually true for critical incidents. "Whereas equipment failure is still a potential component of accidents, it is greatly overshadowed by the potential for human error."[5]

The frequent attempt to implicate anesthesia equipment in malpractice litigation has given the false impression that equipment failure is commonplace. In addition, questions are often raised concerning the inherent safety of equipment design, which may indeed contribute to human error. Medicolegal and risk management issues encompass efforts both to provide perfectly functioning equipment and to promote its proper use.

The original weighted-ball positive end-expiratory pressure (PEEP) valve remains a classic example of the relationship between equipment design and human error. When properly installed, these valves function as intended. The potential for serious error, however, is inherent in the design of the valve. If the valve is placed in the inspiratory limb of the circle system, it can cause a total obstruction of the breathing system with devastating consequences for the patient. However, a comprehensive and continuing risk management program emphasizes the role of anesthesia equipment by those who use it every day. Only such a program genuinely minimizes the rare but possible equipment-related catastrophe.

MEDICOLEGAL ISSUES

Both the manufacturer and the user of anesthesia equipment share the responsibility for that equipment. Issues of cost and profit aside, the two should function as full partners interested only in the safe care of patients. However, the evolution of the medicolegal tort system in the United States in the 1970s and 1980s has imposed additional constraints on this relationship. It has become all too common for the plaintiff's attorney in an anesthesia malpractice case to attempt to involve as an additional defendant the manufacturer of any equipment, however remotely connected to the incident.

The number of product liability cases has increased significantly over the last two decades. A feature common to the large majority of product liability cases is the perception that the manufacturer has a "deep pocket" (excess liability insurance, as well as corporate assets). Consequently, cases that may have little or no merit are occasionally pursued against equipment manufacturers. A company wishing to avoid both the costs and annoyance of litigation may, although faultless, offer to settle for some nominal amount.

This situation occasionally engenders an adversarial relationship between manufacturer and user. Manufacturers have a major financial interest in seeking to avoid blame for injuries to patients. For example, one manufacturer stopped making anesthesia gas machines in the mid-1980s after a rash of serious accidents and subsequent lawsuits that were attributed to a failed vaporizer turret rubber O ring. This allegedly caused the delivery of massive overdoses of volatile anesthetic agents. Equipment manufacturers today are trying to produce items free of both design and manufacturing defects, as well as increasing efforts to assure proper use of the equipment. More detailed and updated operation manuals are now available. Product bulletins are issued that encourage users to report equipment problems. Companies are quick to issue product advisories or recalls when users discover new ways to misuse the equipment that may create a hazard. One effect of this is to help insulate the manufacturer from potential liability when the practitioner is at fault.

Manufacturer's warranty

Recently emphasis on product warranty, which defines the manufacturer's responsibility, has been renewed. The purchaser must be aware of the warranty's contents because it constitutes a *de facto* contract with the manufacturer.

Everyone is familiar with the warranty that accompanies such purchases as radial tires and VCRs. The warranty guarantees that the product has been manufactured to specifications permitting it to function in a defined environment and for described purposes. The warranty also states the circumstances in which the product should not be expected to function (optimally or at all) and specifies abuses of the product that will altogether negate the responsibility of the manufacturer. Most warranties state a time limit after which the company assumes no further responsibility. Furthermore, should the product be defective or fail to function in the prescribed manner, the company may (at its option) replace or repair it and assume the costs for parts and/or labor.

The manufacturer must stand behind the warranty for each product. Where medical devices are concerned, company representatives usually provide maintenance service after the warranty period but do not provide extensions of that warranty in either scope or time.

The United States Food and Drug Administration (FDA) is the federal agency responsible for approving the use of all medical devices. When a defect is found in a medical device, a report to the FDA initiates inquiries to the company. Indeed, the user/purchaser's warranty may be voided if the defect is not reported in a timely fashion to the company. The company, in turn, must notify the FDA with whatever disclaimers it deems appropriate. This may ultimately lead to a certified letter from the manufacturer notifying all registered purchasers of circumstances that may be potentially hazardous, and perhaps even to the recall of the particular model in question.

Implied warranty

It is important to understand the difference between the actual warranty of a product and the concept of implied warranty; it is the concept of implied warranty that lies at the root of product liability lawsuits. Implied warranty goes well beyond what is stated in the written warranty and is based on what the user/purchaser reasonably believes, largely on the basis of experience and industry standards, regarding the product's safety and function. It forms the basis of what should be expected concerning the safety and performance of the product. The legal implications and case law concerning implied warranty are discussed in the next section.

It is on the basis of this doctrine that a patient or purchaser/user who has been injured may seek compensation from the manufacturer of a product, however well the product performed, that was involved in an injury-producing incident. As noted earlier, the perception is that the manufacturer has a "deep pocket," and the plaintiff needs to demonstrate that a standard exists before the manufacturer can be accused of violating it.

Express and implied warranty

Express warranties: by affirmation, promise, description, or sample. This area of the law is under the aegis of the Commercial Code, and express warranties by the seller are set forth in the following[6]:

Any affirmation of fact or promise by the seller to the buyer which relates to the goods and becomes part of the basis of the bargain creates an express warranty that the goods shall conform to the affirmation or promise.

Any description of the goods which is made part of the basis of the bargain creates an express warranty that the goods shall conform to the description.

Any sample or model which is made part of the basis of the bargain creates an express warranty that the whole of the goods shall conform to the sample or model.

Implied warranties. The specifics of implied warranties include what a buyer should reasonably believe about a product that may not be specifically spelled out in the express warranty but rather derives from reasonable reliance on a knowledgeable seller.[7] Implied warranties have become a part of almost every commercial environment, including the selling of medical devices.

In seeking damages on the grounds that the seller failed to satisfy the buyer's belief of implied warranty, the allegations of damage must be based on implied warranty after avoiding exclusions and limitations erected by the seller. The Commercial Code lists four general principles for assessing damage upon review of the case[6]:

1. The court should attempt to place the aggrieved party in the same position as performance would have placed him.
2. The court should require the parties to mitigate damages where possible.

3. The court, where consistent with public and statutory policies, should respect the intentions of the parties.
4. Common sense, commercial practicability, and Code policies should guide the court.

These technical aspects of warranties have become important because of the advent of the potentially adversarial relationship between a medical practitioner using a device at the time of injury to a patient and the manufacturer of that device. The precise wording of the warranty, as well as the other information in the operator's manual, is very important. In the section on response to an adverse event involving anesthesia equipment, specific instructions for action are given that bear on these issues.

RISK MANAGEMENT PRINCIPLES APPLIED TO ANESTHESIA EQUIPMENT
Prepurchase evaluation of equipment

One would expect the users of anesthesia equipment to have an interest in and knowledge about the equipment that they purchase and use. The reality, however, is that some practitioners make decisions regarding equipment purchase solely on the basis of advertising claims and promotions. Although manufacturers' representatives can be extremely valuable sources of pertinent information, it remains the responsibility of the practitioner to evaluate available equipment for purchase. For example, it makes little sense for a practitioner in a small community hospital to do without basic equipment in order to buy a two-dimensional transesophageal echocardiograph.

A common illustration involves the replacement of "obsolete" anesthesia gas machines. Because a variety of models are available with a spectrum of complexity, options, and features, the decision as to which machine to purchase requires careful consideration. First, an evaluation of the practice environment, the personnel involved, and the patient population to be served needs to be conducted. Next, it is important to (1) identify a suitable replacement machine, (2) assess the remaining "useful life" of the current machines, and (3) know how much money is available for the purchase of the machines. Finally, all of these factors are weighed and a decision is made either to phase in expensive top-of-the-line machines over a number of years, or over a short term to purchase modern and functional machines that are neither elaborate nor as expensive. Difficult decisions such as this require sound risk management principles. This involves identifying a problem (old anesthesia machines lacking modern safety features), evaluating it (recognizing the desirability of replacement), and implementing a resolution (purchasing new machines).

Users of anesthesia equipment can make informed prepurchase evaluations of the available brands and models. Does the equipment meet applicable standards for design and manufacture? Standards described as voluntary are usually incorporated as mandatory because industry fears liability implications. Similarly, users may reject equipment that does not meet widely accepted standards for the same reason. Again, focusing on anesthesia machines as the prototypical example, the standards questions were particularly important in the early 1980s. The American National Standards Institute (ANSI) Z-79.9 1979 standard, *Minimum Performance and Safety Requirements for Components and Systems of Continuous-Flow Anesthesia Machines for Human Use,*[8] heralded several important changes. Insistence by users for machines that met these specifications quickly followed. In 1989, the successor, and current standard, the American Society for Testing and Materials (ASTM) F1161-88 *Standard Specification for Minimum Performance and Safety Requirements for Components and Systems of Anesthesia Gas Machines*[9] was implemented. This standard mandates oxygen analyzers, a graded series of three levels of audible and visual alarm signals that cannot be turned off, monitoring of breathing system pressure and either spirometry or capnography on all machines. Purchasers of anesthesia machines in the early 1990s should verify that the model considered meets these standards. Although widely accepted, these standards are required by neither law nor custom. However, the potential liability exposure of using an anesthesia machine that does not meet the standards is quite significant.

Many of the pieces of equipment used in anesthesia are reviewed in *Health Devices,* a publication of ECRI. ECRI also publishes alerts and warnings about specific safety defects either discovered by ECRI or reported to it by users (and subsequently verified). The United States Food and Drug Administration (FDA) has a Problem Reporting System that compiles reports of medical device failures. Although such information could be valuable to the prospective buyer of medical equipment, specific reports are not readily available to individuals.

Once the prospective buyer has learned as much as possible about a particular piece of equipment, it is then desirable to inspect the equipment. The buyer might also wish to obtain from company officials or even the product designers information beyond that available from the local sales representative. Finally, a thorough clinical evaluation in the setting in which the equipment will eventually be used will provide invaluable first-hand experience.

In summary, the prospective purchaser of anesthesia equipment is obligated to evaluate the needs of the practice setting before purchasing appropriate equipment. In addition, efforts must be made to gather the maximum available information about the equipment to facilitate an intelligent purchase. Failure to do either could conceivably set the stage for equipment-related injury to a patient.

Training and in-service education

Once any piece of anesthesia equipment is purchased, a sequence of necessary events follows, leading to the clinical use of the product. These should include on-site training in the use of that equipment for all practitioners who will be eventually be using it. If at all possible, training sessions are best conducted after the arrival of the equipment but before clinical installation. Because this is not always possible, efforts should be made to minimize the time between training and clinical use.

Training sessions on new equipment frequently are conducted by the manufacturer's sales representative. In certain cases, however, especially when there has been a large-scale replacement of equipment, professional trainers are sent to educate the anesthesia personnel. It is critical that all users receive training. Anesthesia providers who are technically facile often believe that they can figure out how to work anything by "playing with it for a few minutes." Although this may be true to a degree, it is no longer good enough. An example demonstrates the complexities involved. At the start of the 1980s, a well-known university anesthesia department decided to order new anesthesia gas machines for newly constructed obstetrical ORs. All the existing anesthesia machines at that time were Harris-Lake Boyle 50s, a relatively older, pneumatically powered design. The model ordered was a state-of-the-art electronically controlled gas machine. Virtually no one in that department had ever worked with an electronic anesthesia machine; therefore, many training sessions were held over an extended period of time. No records were kept to verify that each and every practitioner was trained and checked out on the new machines. One senior attending anesthesiologist, who had seen many anesthesia machines come and go over the years, simply did not attend any of the training sessions. This senior attending anesthesiologist was on obstetric call while all the on-call residents were working in the main OR when there was a call for a stat Cesarean section for profound fetal distress. The attending anesthesiologist found the patient on the table ready for the induction of general anesthesia. The anesthesiologist had never seen the new electronic anesthesia machine and was very surprised to find that turning the oxygen flowmeter knob yielded no flow. Fortunately, there were personnel nearby who knew the machine's main on/off switch had to be turned on before gas would flow to the flowmeters. The machine was correctly activated and the case proceeded without incident. Although this is an unusual example, it illustrates that practitioners expected to use a piece of equipment should know how to do so correctly. The mere *appearance* of lax practice patterns may be enough for the plaintiff's attorney to claim substandard practice.

Another aspect of equipment training involves medical students, anesthesia residents, and other trainees. The beginning resident or student in anesthesiology may feel overwhelmed by the array of monitoring devices and the complexity of today's anesthesia machines. Whereas old hands should have no problem learning to use new equipment, new hands are confronted with the entire spectrum of new devices. Prudent faculty will advise the new residents to pay attention to the patient, leaving the assigned faculty or senior resident to respond to warning bells and whistles until the trainee learns to operate the equipment. With regard to personnel who are novices with the equipment, the anesthesia department support personnel must also receive training in caring for the equipment. It is just as important for workroom technicians to be fully trained for their roles with new equipment as it is for the anesthesia providers.

These principles apply to all supplies and equipment, no matter how trivial the supplies or equipment may seem. Changing the vendor for such routine supplies as epidural catheters or central vascular access kits can cause more problems than can a new anesthesia machine.

In-service education implies demonstration of the equipment in the field. Another forum is the so-called "equipment fair" within a department. This activity, which can be conducted periodically, involves assembling various pieces of equipment—both old and new—used in the department. One person is designated to be available throughout the period (2 hours, for example) to demonstrate the subtleties of the construction and operation of a certain piece of equipment to anyone who wishes to learn or review.

Today's medicolegal realities make it necessary to keep detailed written records of the activities noted in this section. For example, with the introduction of a major new piece of equipment, those who attended the training sessions should be noted on a permanently retained attendance record. This gives the responsible departmental officials the ability to verify that all users have been trained and provides proof after an accident that the user was familiar with that piece of new equipment.

Policy and procedure

Each facility where anesthesia is administered—whether it be a small surgicenter or a large university teaching hospital—must have an anesthesia policy and procedure (P&P) manual. Any practitioner who has had a specific problem and referred to such a manual for some seldom-used but crucial information will appreciate the value of that manual's being both created and updated. Some institutions issue copies of this manual to each anesthesia provider.

All of the policies and plans discussed in the section on maintenance and service, which follows, and in Chapter 22 must be summarized in the P&P manual. This accomplishes several purposes. First, it forces the anesthesia providers to think about what activities are taking place in the department. Second, it provides documentation for inspectors and regulatory agencies. Third, it provides a resource for both old and new department members.

One of the policies deals with departmental meetings, which should include discussions about equipment. Proposals for new equipment, actual purchases, problems with equipment and their resolution, and any related topics should be presented at meetings and recorded in the minutes.

Protocols for equipment not in routine use should be included in the P&P manual. PEEP valves for intraoperative use on anesthesia machines are an excellent topic for inclusion in the P&P manual because of their small yet definite potential for dangerous misapplication. Other examples include the cerebral function monitor and the recording nerve stimulator. Other P&P issues that should be in the manual include all monitoring standards, as well as protocols for the transfer of care during a case because this involves an equipment check.

Privileges and responsibilities

In other medical specialties that are heavily dependent on technology, some of the equipment is so specialized (e.g., lasers) that practitioners must demonstrate specific competence in its operation before being able to use it in their practices. Other examples include laparoscopic procedures in general surgery or new orthopedic prostheses. Are similar processes needed in anesthesia practice today? In the anesthesia community these discussions have centered around the value of *procedure*-specific credentialling—that is, whether a practitioner is qualified and/or able to administer anesthesia for cardiac, obstetric, neonatal, or other specialty cases. It has been suggested that special credentialling be required for use of certain specialized equipment. Whether or not such a practice is in fact warranted, it has certainly not become a national trend. It seems likely that most anesthesia practices will continue to assume that practitioners are qualified to use the equipment available.

It is prudent that identifiable individuals be accountable for the evaluation, purchase, introduction, maintenance, and service of equipment. Often, in medium to large groups, there is at least one anesthesiologist who has an interest in equipment. This person can be assigned the responsibility for departmental equipment. In very large departments, there is usually a committee to deal with equipment-related issues. Another component of responsibility for equipment should include the supervision of anesthesia technicians. Technicians' roles vary in different departments, but they invariably involve the equipment.

Logs and records

Although it has always been good practice to keep detailed records of the history of anesthesia equipment within a department, it is now absolutely mandatory. For all the reasons cited in other sections of this chapter, it is necessary to be able to document the entire history of a piece of major equipment. Other purchases involve supplies, or "consumables." These items do not have serial numbers, but usually they do have a manufacturer's lot number, which allows control of, for example, inventory, quality, and sterility. Any concern related to equipment must be entered into the log. Even minor problems or concerns should be entered in the log. Battery changes for battery-powered or battery-backed-up equipment should also be recorded. A detailed record of all periodic safety checks and scheduled maintenance must be maintained. Strict adherence to this pattern of detailed recording will yield comprehensive "medical histories" on all capital equipment.

The obvious value of such equipment logs is the detailed information they provide in the event that a piece of equipment is implicated in either a critical incident or injury to a patient. There are well-documented cases in which equipment was returned from service in an unsafe condition and subsequently caused injury. One example involved an older vaporizer that was removed and modified with the specific intention of making it safer. It was incorrectly reinstalled on a gas machine, and this apparently led to a cardiac arrest from a massive overdose of potent volatile agent.[13] Accidents like this can be prevented by the requirement that newly serviced equipment be checked for function and safety before clinical use. If there is a possibility that the manner in which the equipment was manufactured or serviced had some role in an anesthesia accident, then these records are vital and may serve to aid in the legal defense of the anesthesia practitioner. If, on the other hand, the records show otherwise, then this should be known at the outset by the anesthesiologist, insurer, and legal counsel.

Maintenance and service

In the same way that commercial airline pilots and passengers depend on aircraft mechanics to insure properly functioning aircraft, anesthesiologists and their patients depend on equipment service personnel to provide fully functional and safe anesthesia equipment. A central question in each practice situation is who will maintain and service the equipment. Maintenance and service can be divided into two areas: (1) routine daily maintenance, such as changing the carbon dioxide absorbent and (2) actual intervention involving assembly and calibration.

Routine daily maintenance can be done either by the anesthesiologist or by qualified support personnel, such as anesthesia technicians trained specifically for this purpose. Departments often have some type of technical support personnel. The technician should have an explicitly and clearly written job description. It is then essential that the technician be trained and able to do the job. Furthermore, because such technical support positions involve restocking of disposables at anesthetizing locations, it is appropriate to expect technicians to understand the potential dangers of failing to provide properly functioning essential apparatus.

Of equal importance is the decision about capital equipment maintenance and repair. In only a few practice settings can this be done by the anesthesia practitioner. As noted earlier, repair or replacement of new capital equipment is part of the purchase agreement for a specified time period (e.g., 1 year). Generally, there are three basic mechanisms for major maintenance and repair service: (1) an in-house bioengineering department, (2) the manufacturer's factory service representatives, and (3) contract service personnel. The choice of one of these depends on the practice setting and its specific needs as well as on the costs, availability, reliability, and other factors of the service. The anesthesia practitioner must ensure that the service personnel responsible for the maintenance and repair of the equipment are both competent and familiar with the particular piece of equipment being serviced. It is important to ascertain that the company providing service has its own adequate liability insurance coverage. In the unlikely circumstance that a service error contributed to or caused injury to a patient, and the servicing entity was found to have inadequate or no liability insurance coverage, then the liability exposure of the involved anesthesia practitioner(s) dramatically increases. Some anesthesiologists choose to contract with the factory service representatives because of the assumption that they are the most knowledgeable and have a vested interest in the product. The trade-off is the potential need to deal with a number of personnel from different companies.

When a decision is made as to who will service the equipment, a service contract will include the parameters of liability. This has additional ramifications because the contract usually mandates adherence to the equipment manufacturer's maintenance and service recommendations, including the schedule for preventive maintenance. Failure to do so can impose adverse liability implications on the practitioner. The maintenance contract is a carefully worded legal document that provides specific details about the following:

1. What maintenance will be undertaken
2. Frequency of routine maintainance
3. What circumstances constitute valid reasons for emergency repairs
4. Whether the maintenance organization will supply a "loaner" if the unit must be removed for off-site repairs
5. The costs of routine annual maintenance and additional charges for emergency repairs
6. The duration of the contract and terms for renewal

Maintenance contracts may require that service personnel be held harmless, or protected by the hospital/department from inclusion as defendants in any liability actions. Whatever the intent, contracts cannot absolve any party of responsibility if negligence is proven, and therefore such clauses serve little purpose.

It is important to emphasize a component of routine maintenance, namely, the calibration of equipment containing continuously variable parameters. The best examples are the gas flowmeters and the output of vaporizers. In several reported cases, gas flowmeters were misassembled or tightened improperly during servicing and were not checked either by the servicing personnel or the anesthesiologist first using the machine after the servicing.[3] Often forgotten are the many routine electronic monitors and devices that need regular calibration. Heart rate counters must be tested to verify their accuracy. The same holds true for such equipment as pressure channels, spirometers, capnographs, and electronic thermometers.

Although not directly associated with the maintenance and service of anesthesia equipment, an additional issue that deserves mention is that of electrical safety in the operating room. This usually is the responsibility of the medical engineering department, but the anesthesia department may be assigned or may assume some responsibility for this area. The points to be covered include the following:

1. Isolation transformers
2. Line isolation monitors
3. Ground fault circuit interrupters
4. Awareness of microshock

Similarly, trace gas testing in the operating room is another issue with regard to risk management. Whether anesthesia waste gas pollution of the operating room environment has any significant deleterious effects has been debated intensely over many years. Various studies have found conflicting results, and the subject remains highly controversial.[11] Accordingly, it seems inherently reasonable that the anesthesia gas machines and breathing systems be maintained so as to be in compliance with accepted federal recommendations from the National Institute of Occupational Safety and Health and regulations of the Occupational Safety and Health Administration.[12] These recommendations state that nitrous oxide levels be limited to less than 25 ppm and that halogenated agents be limited to no more than 2 ppm when administered alone or 0.5 ppm when administered with nitrous oxide. It is necessary for the anesthesia department to ensure that these tests are conducted on at least a quarterly basis. Results must be carefully documented, and these records should be kept indefinitely. Any gas machine that is faulty must be taken out of service immediately, repaired, and then retested. The results must be fully documented in a permanent record before the machine is returned to clinical use.

Personnel policies relating to this issue also have implications for risk management. That anesthesia gas pollution poses a potential hazard is neither proven nor accepted, but a pregnant anesthesia provider's request to be excused from the anesthetizing environment must be carefully evaluated. Advice from risk managers and/or legal counsel who can best evaluate case law of the particular jurisdiction may help to resolve difficult situations. (See also Chapter 5.)

Back-up equipment

A significant problem in risk management can arise if there are exactly the same number of a crucial piece of equipment (i.e., pulse oximeters) as there are operating rooms. If one malfunctions prior to the start of an elective case and there is no substitute, should the case proceed? It is often impractical to postpone the case until later in the evening when a pulse oximeter will become available. Should the anesthesiologist describe the situation in the chart and proceed without a pulse oximeter? The pressure not to cancel is very real, and most anesthesiologists want to maintain the cooperation and goodwill of the surgeon. It would be prudent to anticipate this situation and develop a departmental policy to deal with such circumstances. In the vast majority of cases, no problem will arise, and thus it would seem reasonable to proceed without the equipment. However, major accidents almost always involve a coincidence of circumstances. The absence of a vital piece of equipment, such as a pulse oximeter or an oxygen analyzer, can easily be the first event in a sequence of events that ends in a catastrophe.

Such situations can be avoided by having sufficient back-up equipment. Even in small practices, it is not unreasonable to have a spare anesthesia machine and rapid access to an extra set of monitors. The relative ease of assuring that appropriate back-up equipment is available should eliminate such difficult decisions.

"Obsolete" equipment and its replacement

The prospective useful life of a piece of anesthesia equipment has always been difficult to define. There are undoubtedly well-maintained anesthesia machines that are 20 or 30 years old and that still function properly. Should these gas machines be considered "obsolete" because they do not meet the current voluntary consensus standards for anesthesia gas machines? If so, are they also not safe to use even by someone thoroughly familiar with them? Except for occasional newsletter articles and anecdotes, to date no study has been published that conclusively finds older anesthesia equipment to be a direct cause of catastrophic accidents. The American Society of Anesthesiologists does not have an official policy about equipment replacement, which reflects to a large extent the wide divergence of opinion on the issue. How, then, can the useful life of a device be determined? Taking into consideration practice patterns and the current pace of technical advances, it is possible to generate some estimates for the planned replacement of major equipment. Accordingly, it is reasonable to create a table such as the following:

EQUIPMENT	YEAR PURCHASED	SERIAL NUMBER	PLAN TO REPLACE
X anesthesia machine	1978	A-221-433	1990
Y pulse oximeter	1985	121-00-85	1991
Z capnometer	1987	CN-478	1992

Some manufacturers have decided to retire their oldest models from service. They have implemented this policy *de facto* by refusing to support older gas machines. Analysis of commercial publications dealing with these issues suggests that the companies believe their newer anesthesia machines to be safer. Accordingly, the manufacturers are doing everything possible (such as offering trade-ins) to promote the replacement of older machines with newer, safer models. The question arises as to whether or not there are liability implications for the individual anesthesia practitioner who chooses to continue using a gas machine that has no so-called modern safety devices. There is no clear answer because of the absence of publicized case-law precedents. However, in certain states (e.g. N.J.) recently enacted legislation has made it impossible to continue using many older anesthesia machines (see Chapter 25).

Response to an adverse event involving equipment

Perfect outcomes are not inevitable. Although there may be instances of overt equipment failure, human error is still the most common cause of mishaps. Current statistics suggest that every anesthesiologist will encounter at least one major accident in his or her professional career. Precisely because such events are so rare, the individual anesthesiologist has little or no past experience on which to base a response. Accordingly, it is wise for all anesthesia personnel to consider such issues before a crisis develops and plan for a reasoned and appropriate response.

The moment a major anesthesia complication is recognized, expert help must be summoned. Often, a senior anesthesiologist should assume a supervisory role and identify the source of the problem. All anesthesia equipment and supplies being used when the event occurred must be preserved exactly as they were at the time of the incident. Nothing may be altered, cleaned, reused, or discarded. At least for the moment, the anesthesia machine, monitors, associated equipment, medication, and trash must remain undisturbed. Once the patient has been cared for and moved to another location, the supervisor must: (1) decide whether the equipment may have been in any way responsible for the adverse event; (2) store under lock and key all the equipment that was being used if the equipment may have been responsible (the importance of this cannot be stressed enough!); (3) gather all supplies in use and trash even if there is no suspicion of equipment involvement and (4) return the equipment to clinical service after the decision has been made that none of the major pieces of equipment was involved in the incident. There are countless medicolegal anecdotes of subsequent charges and counter-charges (even up to several years later) concerning the possible role of anesthesia equipment in an adverse event. It is important to know if the equipment was in some way at fault. Likewise, it is important to determine if this was not the case.

Equipment that is implicated in a major accident must be kept locked away and covered with prominent labels. It must not be repaired or, worse, accidentally returned to clinical use until it can be inspected and tested. This may

involve a single meeting attended by all relevant parties during which the equipment is investigated in front of everyone. Although this may sound excessive, it is the best way to guarantee a fair evaluation of the role that the equipment played in the incident. The requirements and recommendations for reporting medical equipment failures are discussed in Chapter 22.

Standardization of equipment within a department

Another issue that is of concern, but lacks scientific studies, involves the training and risk management implications of having different makes and models of equipment in one department. Those responsible for residency training may believe that it is desirable for anesthesia residents to be familiar with several different types of anesthesia gas machines, ventilators, monitors, and other equipment. The argument can be made that because there are many different models of each type of equipment, the resident ultimately will be safer if he or she learns how to adapt to the variations of the different models. From a fiscal point of view, it may not be possible to replace equipment within a time frame that would allow purchase of all the same model of a given piece of equipment.

On the other hand, some might consider it to be inherently dangerous to have several different brands of anesthesia machine in the same operating suite. During a stressful situation this could lead to confusion, and this confusion may be exacerbated with disastrous results. Because adverse events, particularly those related to equipment, are rare, data on this issue do not exist. The premise for this argument is that using the same type of equipment in all the operating rooms will facilitate the ability of the practitioner to rapidly identify and rectify equipment problems. The impending introduction of highly sophisticated anesthesia workstation simulators may, at last, allow genuine research into this question. Until such time, however, the professionals responsible for anesthesia equipment must make purchasing decisions on the basis of the characteristics of their personnel and by using their best judgment.

Legal action resulting from the majority of malpractice suits against anesthesiologists is the result of allegations of inappropriate management. Whenever possible, the plaintiff will involve a manufacturer because of the latter's deep pocket, as explained in this chapter, rather than because of a clear cause-and-effect relationship between an untoward outcome and the equipment involved.

When the equipment has played a role in a mishap, the anesthesia provider should examine the express warranty that accompanied the equipment as well as the expectations for such equipment under the doctrine of implied warranty. Here, the overlap between legal issues and risk management is easier to understand because the latter assumes that the equipment has been maintained in accordance with the manufacturer's recommendations. Each department of anesthesiology should maintain a policy manual, which outlines a precise protocol for familiarizing personnel with new equipment as well as a protocol for the care and maintenance of all equipment.

There is no greater defense than a clear record that documents that the required servicing of equipment has been performed. In addition, the policy manual should delineate physician privileges for highly specialized equipment (e.g., intraoperative echocardiography) and job descriptions for all technical personnel. Sound risk management practices should also inform all members of the department about problem areas, such as electrical hazards, not directly related to anesthesia equipment.

Finally, any approach to risk management must be based upon the special features that characterize every department. No expedient formulas can be prescribed to reduce risk. No simple path avoids legal pitfalls.

REFERENCES

1. Cooper JB, Newbower RS, Long CD, et al: Preventable anesthesia mishaps: a study of human factors, *Anesthesiology* 49:399-406, 1978.
2. Cooper JB, Newbower RS, Kitz RJ: An analysis of major errors and equipment failures in anesthesia management: considerations for prevention and detection, *Anesthesiology* 60:34-42, 1984.
3. Spooner RB, Kirby RR: Equipment-related anesthetic incidents. In Pierce EC, Cooper JB, editors: Analysis of anesthetic mishaps, *Int Anesthesiol Clin* 22(2):133-147, 1984.
4. Gaba DM: Human error in anesthetic mishaps. In Pierce EC, editor: Risk management in anesthesia, *Int Anesthiol Clin* 27:137-147, 1989.
5. Cooper JB, Gaba DM: A strategy for preventing anesthesia accidents. In Pierce EC, editor: Risk management in anesthesia, *Int Anesthiol Clin* 27:148-152, 1989.
6. United States Uniform Commercial Code, 332:313-318.
7. *Cornell Law Review*, 72:1190, 1987.
8. *Standard Specification for minimum Performance and Safety Requirements for Components and Systems of Continuous-Flow Anesthesia Machines for Human Use*. Z79.8-1979, New York, 1979, American National Standards Institute.
9. *Standard Specification for Minimum Performance and Safety Requirements for Components and Systems of Anesthesia Gas Machines*. F1161-88, Philadelphia, 1989, American Society for Testing and Materials.
10. Eichhorn JH: Prevention of intraoperative anesthesia accidents and related severe injury through safety monitoring, *Anesthesiology* 70:572-577, 1989.
11. Shackleton S, Harrington JM: *The pollution controversy*. In Lunn JN, editor: *Epidemiology in anesthesia*, London, 1986, Edward Arnold, pp 93-122.
12. *National Institute for Occupational Safety and Health criteria for a recommended standard for occupational exposure to waste anesthetic gases and vapors*, Publication 77-140, 1977 Department of Health and Human Service (NIOSH).

Chapter 25

STANDARDS AND REGULATORY CONSIDERATIONS

David Eric Lees, M.D.

Until recently, it was possible to practice safe and modern anesthesia without any knowledge of the regulatory and voluntary standards governing anesthesia equipment. This is changing, however, and individual practitioners are now subject to federal and state regulations regarding the use of these devices and may even be strongly influenced by international standards and agreements. The arena of medical device standards and regulations is complex and arcane, and there is much overlap of authority. This chapter reviews the history, present status, and pending developments that will affect the clinician over the next decade. The reader should be left with a good understanding of both the processes and the players in this now international setting of standards and regulations.

REGULATION OF MEDICAL DEVICES
Early federal efforts

Increasing public concern over the safety and effectiveness of medical devices in the late 1960s and early 1970s led to the formation of a study group within the Department of Health, Education, and Welfare, the predecessor of the present Department of Health and Human Services. This study group, chaired by Dr. Theodore Cooper of the National Heart, Lung, and Blood Institute, estimated (as did other studies at the time) that over the last decade more than 10,000 injuries and hundreds of deaths were linked to medical devices currently on the market.[1]

Recommendations from this study group formed the basis of the Medical Device Amendments of 1976. The members of the group felt that performance standards would be more effective than premarket approval in ensuring the safety and effectiveness of new medical devices.

Medical Device Amendments of 1976. In 1976 the Medical Device Amendments (The Amendments, 21 U. S.

C. Secs. 513-521) were promulgated into law. These amendments supplemented the original Federal Food, Drug, and Cosmetic Act of 1938. This authorized the establishment of the Bureau of Medical Devices to regulate and guide medical device manufacturers. It did not give the Food and Drug Administration (FDA) any control over the individual user or practitioner. Section 201(h) of the Federal Food, Drug, and Cosmetic Act defined a device as

an instrument, apparatus, implement, machine, contrivance, implant, in-vitro reagent, or other similar or related article including any component, part or accessory which is (1) recognized in the official National Formulary, or the United States Pharmacopoeia, or any supplement to them, (2) intended for use in the diagnosis of disease or other conditions, or in the cure, mitigation, treatment or prevention of disease, in man or other animals, or (3) intended to affect the structure of the body in man or other animals and which does not achieve any of its principal intended purposes through chemical action within or on the body of man or other animal and which is not dependent upon being metabolized for the achievement of any of its principal intended purposes.

These amendments provided the FDA with the authority to regulate medical devices by establishing a three-tiered system of regulation. Manufacturers were required, at the very least, to notify the FDA of any new low-risk device prior to its being marketed. High-risk devices, on the other hand, required premarket approval. In all cases, however, the FDA was supposed to conduct postmarketing surveillance of the device after its introduction into clinical use.

Classification of devices

According to the 1976 Amendments, the FDA was required to classify all medical devices into one of three categories. These were as follows:

Classification	Requirements
Class I	General controls
Class II	Performance standards
Class III	Premarket approval

Class I. Class I devices were subject only to general controls to ensure safety and effectiveness. These controlling regulations (1) required that devices be registered, (2) prohibited adulteration or mislabeling of items, (3) provided for notification of risks, repair, replacement, or refund, (4) restricted the sale and distribution of certain devices, and (5) required good manufacturing practices as defined by the FDA.

Class II. Devices in Class II had to meet performance standards because general controls were not considered sufficient to guarantee their safety and effectiveness. These devices had to fulfill all requirements of Class I in addition to FDA performance standards. Because this presented such a daunting task, Class II devices were permitted to

comply only with general controls until such time as performance standards could be established.

Recognizing that their own resources were limited, the FDA gave tacit approval to existing national or international standards. In doing so, the FDA was not relieved of the responsibility to formulate mandatory performance standards. However, the FDA had indicated informally that their limited resources would not be employed where voluntary standards were in effect.

The process by which a mandatory performance standard was developed was quite complex. There first had to be an announcement in the Federal Register providing interested parties the opportunity to present to the FDA (in person or writing) requests for reclassification of devices to either Class I or Class III. If the device was not reclassified, then notices were posted inviting interested parties (either individuals or organizations) to participate in the development of the performance standard. Voluntary standards were sought because they represent an excellent starting point.

At this point the FDA could take one of three actions: (1) accept a voluntary standard: (2) accept the offer of a particular party to draft one; or (3) draft one in house. Once a standard was drafted, an announcement was made in the Federal Register and comments sought. Any issues raised concerning the standard were handled by an FDA-appointed standards advisory committee. After the technical issues were resolved, the revised draft was published by the FDA, the final regulation becoming effective in 1 year.

Class III pre-Amendment. Class III devices were those that were considered to be life-sustaining or life-supporting, that were implanted in the body, or that potentially presented considerable risk of illness or injury. Under Section 515 of the Food, Drug, and Cosmetic Act, these devices required premarket approval (PMA) before they could be marketed. It was assumed that general controls and performance standards alone would not assure the safe and effective use of devices in Class III. However, certain allowances were made for devices marketed prior to enactment of the Amendment. For pre-Amendment devices (marketed before May 28, 1976), immediate premarket approval did not have to be obtained until there were final classification regulations for that device. Even Class III devices with significant risk could be marketed on these grounds until the FDA issued a regulation requiring that PMAs be submitted for such devices.

Class III substantial equivalence. A new Class III device that was available commercially after the enactment date could attempt to claim substantial equivalence to an existing pre-Amendment class III device and thus "ride on the coat-tails" of similar, older devices. This was provided for under section 510(k) of the Food, Drug, and Cosmetic Act. If a manufacturer chose the 510(k) route, the FDA needed premarket notification. Should the FDA have decided that substantial equivalence did not apply to the particular device, it had to be classified as a Class III. As such, it required premarket approval and review by the Anesthesiology and Respiratory Devices Review Panel before it could be marketed. The manufacturer's only other option was to re-petition for reclassification of their device to a Class I or Class II. The FDA generally ruled that a device was not substantially equivalent if (1) its intended use was different, (2) it raised new questions about safety or effectiveness, or (3) it did not perform as well as devices already on the market.

Class III transitional devices. A third group of Class III devices were referred to as new or transitional devices. These devices were considered neither Class I nor II and had no substantial equivalents. Premarket approval had to be obtained for such devices, which also had to comply with the Investigational Device Exemption (IDE) regulations during their clinical trials.

Premarket approval

To obtain premarket approval (PMA), the manufacturer or importer had to provide the FDA with the following information:

1. Detailed description of the device
2. Description of manufacturing methods
3. Results of preclinical studies
4. Results of clinical investigations
5. Labeling
6. Summary of safety and effectiveness

Section 520(g) of the Food, Drug, and Cosmetic Act allowed the FDA to grant exemptions for devices that were being investigated to determine their clinical effectiveness and safety. The manufacturer was expected to complete an application for an Investigational Device Exemption (IDE), which was equivalent to an Investigational or New Drug Exemption (IND) for a pharmaceutical. This exemption allowed the device to be shipped commercially and used in clinical trials. As with an IND, the clinical use of the device must be approved by an institutional review board (IRB). This applied only to those devices with which one might logically expect significant risk. If risk was insignificant, an IDE was not required, but IRB approval was necessary wherever the clinical trials were being conducted. This determination was made by the manufacturer of the device. In general, a device with significant risk was one that had the potential to cause serious harm to the safety or health of an individual and was (1) implanted, (2) used to sustain human life, or (3) of substantial importance in diagnosing, curing, or preventing impairment of health.

Custom devices. Provision was made for one other area of device manufacture, that of custom devices. Custom devices were defined as those made for a specific physician for personal use and not made available to any other physician. Although a PMA was not required, a custom device had to meet the Class I general control requirements.

Medical device advisory panels. The Amendments also established 17 medical device advisory panels for the purpose of advising the FDA on device classification and performance standards. These advisory panels were as follows:

1. Anesthesiology and respiratory therapy
2. Circulatory system
3. Clinical chemistry and toxicology
4. Dental
5. Ear, nose, and throat
6. Gastroenterology-urology
7. General hospital and personal use
8. General and plastic surgery
9. Hematology and pathology
10. Immunology
11. Microbiology
12. Neurology
13. Obstetrics and gynecology
14. Ophthalmology
15. Orthopedic and rehabilitation
16. Radiology
17. Device good manufacturing practice advisory committee

Each panel had nine members in addition to an FDA employee, who served as the executive secretary. Seven of the panelists were voting members, and the consumer and industry representatives were nonvoting members. The panel could request consultants when necessary. These panels did the following:

1. Advise the FDA on device classifications
2. Review specific issues or problems with regard to investigational studies and guidance documents
3. Advise the FDA on certain risks associated with the use of specific devices
4. Provide recommendations concerning PMA applications
5. Review device reclassification requests

Congressional investigations. In 1982, hearings were held by the House Subcommittee on Oversight and Investigations of the Committee on Energy and Commerce (John Dingell, Democrat from Michigan, Chairman) to undertake a staff review of the FDA's implementation of the 1976 Medical Device Amendments.[2] In passing the Amendments, the original and explicit intention of Congress was for the FDA to develop mandatory performance standards for all Class II devices. Six years later, however, Congressman Dingell's Subcommittee was concerned that nothing had been done.[3]

In defense of its actions, the Office of Medical Devices (the predecessor of the Center for Devices and Radiological Health) offered that the recent emergence of many voluntary standards and their adoption by industry obviated the need for many mandatory standards. The Office also claimed that the process by which mandatory standards were issued was bureaucratically burdensome and that the FDA's resources were inadequate for this task. Finally, the Office of Medical Devices noted that the general controls that currently applied to all medical devices were satisfactory for Class II devices.

The Subcommittee was not pleased with these responses. It disputed the FDA's claim that there were no problems with Class II devices and that voluntary standards would suffice in the absence of mandatory performance standards. The Subcommittee was also critical of the fact that the FDA was not careful in reviewing the decisions of the Device Classification Advisory Panels, which placed the majority of medical devices into Class II without having adequate resources to accomplish the task. The Agency would have done better in the Subcommittee's estimation if it had concentrated its resources on a few devices in Class II.[3]

CENTER FOR DEVICES AND RADIOLOGICAL HEALTH

In 1982, the FDA established the Center for Devices and Radiological Health (CDRH), which was formed from elements of the old Bureau of Medical Devices and the Bureau of Radiological Health. Within the CDRH, four divisions reported to the Director's office: Compliance, Training, Science and Technology, and Device Evaluation. The Office of Device Evaluation was divided into seven scientific divisions:

1. Anesthesiology, neurology, and radiology
2. Cardiovascular
3. Clinical laboratory
4. Gastroenterology, urology, and general use
5. Obstetrics; gynecology; ear, nose, and throat; and dental
6. Ophthalmics
7. Surgical, rehabilitation, orthopedics

The classification of devices (Classes I, II, and III) was determined by panels of experts, who advised the FDA. Of the initial 1750 devices classified, 40% were Class I, 50% Class II, and 10% Class III. Despite the Congressional mandate to write standards for all Class II devices, this overwhelmed the CDRH, which had inadequate resources. Finally, in response to Congressional pressure, the CDRH determined a priority for the writing of performance standards for the following medical devices:

1. Continuous ventilators
2. Vascular graft prostheses
3. Cardiac monitors
4. Ventilator tubing
5. Breathing frequency monitors
6. Central nervous system fluid shunts
7. Toxoplasmosis serological reagents
8. Rheumatoid factor immunological test systems
9. Calibration equipment for hematocrit/hemoglobin measurement
10. Immunoglobulin test systems

Seven years later, despite Congressional intent and Agency promises, no such performance standards have been issued for Class II devices.

CONGRESSIONAL INVESTIGATION OF FOREGGER INCIDENT

In 1984, the Subcommittee on Oversight and Investigations again took up the issue of FDA oversight of medical devices.[4] This time the hearings were initiated as a direct result of four mishaps with anesthesia machines that had been reported in the national press and on television. Within a year, four patients died as a result of problems with the Foregger Model 705 anesthesia machine. A stuck valve in the gas-control manifold caused marked increases in vaporizer output. In addition, although the problem was identified, 41 units (34 U.S., 7 foreign) could not be located. The Director of the Center for Devices and Radiological Health was criticized for failures in premarket approval and postmarketing surveillance of subsequent malfunctioning medical devices.

The Director in turn accused the company of impeding investigation of the deaths by restricting access to company files. These files contained complaints about the equipment from physician and nurse anesthetist users. The CDRH Director, however, was able to point to the newly developed Medical Device Reporting system (MDR), which required manufacturers, distributors, and importers of medical devices to notify the Agency within 5 days of any deaths or serious injuries related to the use of a medical device. In response to this new medical device reporting system, the agency anticipated receiving 25,000 reports annually. In addition, the Agency's director pointed out that a similar program was recently initiated by the American Society of Anesthesiologists (ASA) and the American Association of Nurse Anesthetists (AANA).

The MDR regulations, issued shortly thereafter, required all manufacturers and distributors of medical devices to report deaths and serious injuries from medical devices to the FDA. In addition, any malfunction that had the potential to cause death or serious injury had to be reported in writing. A report was to be made by telephone within 5 days and a written follow-up report within 15 days. A report had also to be filed for malfunctions that could have resulted from design flaws, manufacturing problems, user error, or poor or absent maintenance. The MDR reports were to include (1) identification of the device, (2) manufacturer or importer, (3) reporting individual, and (4) a description of the clinical problem or malfunction encountered.

GENERAL ACCOUNTING OFFICE STUDY OF MEDICAL DEVICE REPORTING

At about the same time, the General Accounting Office (GAO) conducted a similar study, which pointed out that the FDA was aware of fewer than 1% of the device problems occurring in hospitals.[5] Although hospitals usually took local action to prevent problems from recurring with a particular device, the FDA was rarely ever informed by manufacturers who had been notified. As a result of their findings, the GAO recommended that

. . .the FDA attempt to increase the quantity and quality of information available for monitoring device problems by requiring the distributor of medical devices to report problem information to manufacturers. We also recommend that FDA increase its efforts to inform health care professionals as to how to report problem information. . . . We have since pointed out that to ensure that the postmarket surveillance system achieves its "early warning" goal it would be necessary to include virtually all hospitals in a mandatory problem-reporting program.[5]

The FDA generally agreed with the findings, but asserted that these deficiencies would be addressed by the new MDR reporting system instituted at the end of 1984. The GAO then did another study to verify FDA's assertions concerning the MDR.[6] A number of problems were found with the MDR system. Although the number of reports received by the FDA with regard to device problems did increase considerably (approximately 2000 reports annually before and 18,000 afterward), the degree of compliance could not be determined. The FDA could not distinguish between device manufacturers who were not experiencing problems and thus filing no reports, and those who were encountering device problems but were not filing because of either ignorance or negligence. The FDA suspected that only 25% of the manufacturers were complying fully with the MDR system.

The GAO also determined that the FDA's data processing capabilities were not up to the demands imposed by even partial adherence to MDR regulations. At the time of the GAO study, there were more than 10,000 unprocessed reports of device malfunctions. Where analysis had been completed, there was no indication of the final action taken. At this time the GAO recommended that the MDR regulations be modified to require that each manufacturer file an annual report stating either that no device malfunctions were reported or providing a summary and analysis of reports received. The FDA chose not to incorporate this modification into the MDR system at that time.

Although the information was limited, it did reveal interesting patterns among device problems. The top 10 devices reported to the FDA as most frequently malfunctioning were as follows:

Device	Percent of reports
Ventilator	18
Pacemaker	10
Anesthesia machine	8
Glucose monitor	8
Infusion pump	4
Intravascular administration set	4
Pacemaker electrode	4
Intraaortic balloon	2
Respiratory gas humidifier	2
Peritoneal dialysis administration set	2

When the data are reorganized to indicate the devices most associated with deaths of patients from 1985 to 1987, the ranking is as follows:

Device	Percent of reports
Heart valve	16
Defibrillator	15
Pacemaker	6
Ventilator	6
Pacemaker electrode	4
Anesthesia machine	3
Intravascular diagnostic catheter	3
Infusion pump	3
Tampon	3
Intraaortic balloon	2
Top 10 devices	60
All other devices	40

The report summarizes the data by stating the following:

Cardiovascular device problem reports accounted for 708 death reports, or 46% of all problem reports associated with patient deaths over the three year period . . . . Ventilators and anesthesia gas machines, both of which are used in anesthesiology, accounted for 141 deaths, or 9% of all reports received by the FDA from 1985 through 1987. No other single device or group of related devices accounted for more than 3% of device problems that involved patient death. Over 75% of all reported deaths were related to devices in anesthesiology and cardiovascular medical specialities.[6]

SUBSEQUENT GOVERNMENT REPORTS

This was not the last time, however, that the FDA was investigated by the Subcommittee or the General Accounting Office. Testifying before the Subcommittee on Health and the Environment (Committee on Energy and Commerce) in November of 1989, the Comptroller General of the General Accounting Office stated:

Our work reveals several shortcomings in both the premarket review and postmarket surveillance systems for medical devices and raises serious questions about the ability of these systems and related regulations to protect the American people from unsafe and ineffective medical devices.[7]

In particular, the Comptroller General's study pointed out problems with the substantial equivalence provision of the 1976 Amendments:

We see four principal issues that need to be addressed in the current premarket review system: (1) the fact that the pre-1976 devices to which new ones are found substantially equivalent never themselves have been tested at all; (2) the use of an old and often outdated comparison base (of pre-1976 devices) for determining substantial equivalence; (3) the lack of a definition of substantial equivalence; and (4) FDA's failure both to develop the mandated performance standards for medium-risk devices and to implement premarket approval requirements for pre-1976 high risk devices.

As a result of our review of these issues, we have suggested that if Congress is concerned about the way in which the FDA interprets the term substantial equivalence, it may want to consider providing a statutory definition of that term. In addition we have recommended that the Congress amend the Federal Food, Drug, and Cosmetic Act to shift the comparison base from devices introduced prior to 1976 to currently marketed devices.[7]

The Comptroller General also commented that no premarket approval system could assure that problems would not arise once the device was placed into clinical use. Therefore, a postmarket surveillance system should be instituted to serve as an early-warning system for problems encountered with devices in the field.

The GAO was particularly concerned with the constraints under which the FDA had to operate. Contrary to the opinion of most physicians and laypeople, the FDA had no authority under the 1938 Federal Food, Drug, and Cosmetic Act and the subsequent Amendments to recall a product by a device manufacturer. Only by securing a court order could the agency force a manufacturer to comply. More often than not the FDA could do no more than request that a device be recalled. From 1983 to 1988, 1635 products were recalled entirely on the initiative of the manufacturer. None was recalled on the basis of an FDA request. In addition, in more than 50% of cases, the FDA did not learn of the recall directly from the manufacturer.

In conclusion, the Comptroller General stated:

In sum, the statutes that govern medical devices need some adjustment and the existing FDA system for premarket review and postmarket surveillance both need improvement. The evidence is that the nation does not presently have a fully functioning process for ensuring the safety and effectiveness of medical devices. We are gratified that most of the problems we have pointed out and the recommendations we have made are being addressed in these hearings, as well as in H.R. 3095 as introduced by you, Mr. Chairman, and Mr. John Dingell, Chairman of the House Committee on Energy and Commerce, in the current session of this Congress.[7]

SAFE MEDICAL DEVICES ACT OF 1990

The Safe Medical Devices Act of 1990 was signed into law on November 28, 1990 (Public Law 101-629). Some but not all of the specific elements of the new law are given in this section.[8]

User reports

Whenever a device user facility (i.e., hospital, ambulatory surgical center, outpatient treatment center or nursing home) (physician offices are specifically exempted) receives or otherwise becomes aware of information that reasonably suggests that there is a probability that a device has caused or contributed to the death of a patient of the facility, the facility shall, as soon as practicable, but not later than 10 working days after becoming aware of the information, report the information to the Secretary and if the identity of the manufacturer is known, to the manufacturer of the device. In the case of deaths the Secretary may by regulation prescribe a shorter period for the reporting of such information.[8]

Similar language applies whenever a facility is aware that a device has contributed to serious injury or illness. The legislation defines serious illness and serious injury as

illness or injury, respectively, that

i. is life threatening
ii. results in permanent impairment of a body function or permanent damage to a body structure, or
iii. necessitates immediate medical or surgical intervention to preclude permanent impairment of a body function or permanent damage to a body structure[8]

The name of a facility that files a report will not be disclosed except in certain clearly defined circumstances.

Distributor reports

Every distributor, manufacturer, or importer is required to file a report of all device incidents reported by user facilities. The FDA is supposed to receive duplicate reports of every incident that causes serious injury or illness or death. All manufacturers and distributors are required to file an annual statement with the Secretary indicating whether or not they were notified of problems by users.

Substantial equivalence

Every 510(k) submission is now required to prove that the product is as safe and effective as other devices on the market. The manufacturer making a claim of substantial equivalence must be aware of all the problems that have befallen similar devices. For Class III products, the FDA may require additional support and research data. The new law has made advisory panel review of PMA applications optional, but if it is thought to be in the best interest of the institution or organization, a full panel review may be requested.

Classification and reclassification

Those devices previously classified as Class II and for which performance standards were initially required under the 1976 Amendments are now designated as requiring special controls. Special controls apply only to devices that cannot be safely reclassified as Class I, and for which it is evident that special controls will provide an adequate assurance of safety and effectiveness. These special controls may be voluntary consensus standards, postmarket surveillance, or "other appropriate actions" as determined by the FDA. In addition, the FDA will now be forced to review those Class III devices that have never been reviewed for safety and effectiveness. Under the previous law, all reclassifications were reviewed by the appropriate advisory committee. It is now left to the agency to decide whether or not to consult the advisory panel.

Performance standards

The FDA was relieved of the responsibility of creating regulatory standards for Class II devices. Although this was one of the original intentions of the 1976 Amendments, the FDA CDRH never had sufficient money, resources, or personnel to write mandatory standards for the more than 1200 Class II devices in existence. The CDRH can now issue special controls, however, if needed. Ultimately, there will be greater regulation of Class II devices.

Under the 1976 Amendments all performance standards had to be reviewed by the advisory panels. Under the Safe Medical Devices Act of 1990, performance standards are reviewed by the advisory panel only upon request.

Recall authority

The FDA can now order an immediate halt to the manufacture or distribution of a device. Within 10 days, and following an informal hearing, the FDA is authorized to order a product recall without a court order. In addition, the FDA can now demand that users refrain from using the device until the problem is resolved. In the past, the FDA could not proceed with banning a medical device until after consulting with the advisory committee.

Postmarket surveillance

Manufacturers must now submit a plan for postmarket surveillance of devices, which will enable detection of a pattern of problems. This was specifically aimed at preventing recurrences similar to those with the Foregger anesthesia machine. In addition, manufacturers and distributors must develop a device tracking mechanism. This is particularly important with implants (i.e., heart valves and pacemakers), so that all recipients may be located quickly in the event of a problem with a device.

Humanitarian device exemptions

Similar to the orphan drug law, the humanitarian device exemptions encourage the development of implantable devices and equipment that will benefit only a small segment of the population, and otherwise offer the manufacturer no financial incentive. Such a device must present no unreasonable risk and offer a greater benefit than risk.

Penalties

The new legislation gave the FDA greater powers of enforcement. The agency now has the authority to levy civil penalties of up to $1000 per incident, with a $1 million cap for all violations per regulatory proceeding. In addition, the FDA now has the power to subpoena. If necessary, the FDA may issue stop-shipment orders or device recalls without a public hearing. Under the old legislation, the bureaucracy attached to the seizure of a product and its removal from the market was cumbersome. By comparison, the new process is streamlined, although the FDA hopes that most recalls will be voluntary.

The Safe Medical Devices Act of 1990 took effect November 28, 1991. This was done by Congress because many of the proponents of this legislation believe that the FDA has not responded to Congressional mandates fast enough in the past. The Office of Device Evaluation (ODE) is responsible for writing the implementing regulations for this new legislation. The number of scientific review divisions has been reduced from seven to five, and there has been some shifting of product lines. Some of the advisory panels, among them anesthesiology and respiratory therapy, are now under different division management. During the next year, however, the FDA must do the following:

1. Develop regulations to minimize the administrative burden on device user facilities when reporting injuries or deaths related to medical devices.
2. Promulgate regulations that set forth compliance requirements for a manufacturer's postmarketing surveillance program (this went into effect on January 1, 1991).
3. Determine information that must be included with safety and effectiveness summaries as part of the 510(k) substantial equivalence mechanism.
4. Develop regulations for equipment that has never been reviewed for safety and effectiveness.
5. Develop special controls for Class II devices.
6. Develop humanitarian device exemption regulations.

Despite the Congressional mandate, the FDA Commissioner has claimed that he has neither the funds nor the personnel necessary to carry out the law.[9] In fiscal year 1992, the FDA will receive $770 million, of which only $5.2 million will be directed toward implementing the new and additional requirements of the Safe Medical Devices Act—namely, inspection of manufacturers and follow-up on deaths or injuries related to devices. A large backlog of uninvestigated cases grew under the existing MDR regulations; it remains doubtful whether the CDRH will be able to handle the deluge of paperwork expected to follow implementation of the Safe Medical Devices Act of 1990.

One of the most important features of the new law is that it imposes mandatory requirements on the facilities that use medical devices. The user now shares the onus, which previously had fallen to the manufacturer. Thus the FDA has gained regulatory access and control in the local hospital. With this new law, the emphasis has been moved from premarket approval to postmarket control. Consistent with this change in philosophy, the processes by which devices are classified and approved have been relaxed.[10]

All institutions, from major medical centers to small free-standing ambulatory surgical centers, are now required to report any information on the death or injury of a patient that may have been caused by a medical device. Both the FDA and the manufacturer must be notified within a specified period of time and in a prescribed manner. In addition, institutions are required to produce biannual reports summarizing all individual reports filed over the past 180 days.

The 1990 Safe Medical Device Act makes several important changes in the law compared to the 1976 Medical Device Amendments. These changes are summarized in Table 25-1. As previously discussed, the 1990 law also makes certain changes in the requirements for Class I, II, and III medical devices; these are summarized in Table 25-2.

It is interesting to note that within the medical industry, medical devices are now subject to more stringent regulation than is the pharmaceutical industry. This is the case despite the fact that most of the recent congressional investigations and public scandals have been associated with pharmaceuticals.

STATE REGULATIONS
New York

Until recently, medical devices were governed only by federal law. Now, however, medical devices are subject to state law, through state regulation of health care facilities.[11] Although the general medical and hospital community objected strongly to many of the new regulations, little if any objection was heard from community or from academic anesthesiologists. Indeed, most anesthesiologists supported the anesthesia section of the Code (Section 405.13). This represented the first time a state government mandated which equipment had to be present during the administration of anesthesia and set policies governing the use of these devices. Specifically, Section 405.13 Anesthesia Services requires the following in the state of New York:

Anesthesia service policies shall clearly outline requirements for orientation and continuing education programs . . . that are relevant to care provided but must, at a minimum, include instruction in: safety precautions, equipment usage and inspection . . . (405.13.a.2)

All anesthesia machines shall be numbered and reports of all equipment inspections and routine maintenance shall be included in the anesthesia service records. Policies and procedures shall be developed and implemented regarding notification of equipment disorders/malfunctions to the director, to the manufacturer and . . . to the Department (of Health). (405.13.b.1)

Routine checks shall be conducted by the anesthetist prior to every administration of anesthesia to ensure the readiness, availability, cleanliness, sterility when required, and working condition of all equipment used in the administration of anesthetic agents. (405.13.b.2.ii)

During all anesthetics, the heart sounds and breathing sounds of all patients shall be monitored through the use of a precordial

Table 25-1. Federal Medical Device Regulation

	1976 Amendments	1990 Safe Medical Device Act
Enforcement	Court order needed	Can order manufacturer to cease distribution and notify device users
Civil penalties	Generally not applicable	$15,000/violation; $1 million cap
Postmarket surveillance	Not required	Manufacturer must have formal protocol
User facility reporting	Not required	Mandatory with death or injury
Substantial equivalence claim	Premarket notification	Premarket approval
Tracking mechanism for devices	None	Required for implants

Table 25-2. Changes in Device Classification Requirements

DEVICE	1976 Amendments	1990 Safe Medical Device Act
Class I	General controls	Unchanged
Class II	Mandatory performance standards	Special controls
Class III	Premarket notification to FDA of substantial equivalence	Premarket approval by FDA before marketing

or esophageal stethoscope. Such equipment or superior equipment shall by obtained and utilized by the hospital. (405.13.b.2.iii.c)

During every administration of general anesthesia using an anesthesia machine, the concentration of oxygen in the patient's breathing system shall be measured by an oxygen analyzer with a low oxygen concentration alarm. (405.13.b.iii.d)

For every patient receiving general anesthesia with an endotracheal tube, the quantitative carbon dioxide content of expired gases shall be monitored through the use of end-tidal carbon dioxide analysis or superior technology. In all cases where ventilation is controlled by a mechanical ventilator, there shall be in continuous use an alarm that is capable of detecting disconnection of any components of the breathing circuit. (405.13.b.iii.e)

The patient's circulatory functions shall be continuously monitored during all anesthetics. This monitoring shall include the continuous display of the patient's electrocardiogram. . . . (405.13.b.iii.f)

During every administration of anesthesia, there shall be immediately available a means to continuously measure the patient's temperature. (405.13.b.iii.g)[11]

New Jersey

New Jersey has taken New York's regulations one step further. The New York state regulations are considered performance oriented, which means they seek a minimum level of clinical practice. In contrast, those of New Jersey are more design oriented, in that they specify engineering requirements.[12]

The New Jersey regulations state the following:

Diameter index safety systems or its equivalent shall be used on all larger cylinders of medical gases and ceiling outlets of medical gases. (8:43B-18.5.a)

Pin index safety systems with a single washer shall be used on all small cylinders to prevent interchangeability of medical gas cylinders. (8:43B-18.5.b)

All medical gas hoses and adapters shall be color coded. (8:43B-18.5.c)

An oxygen failure-protection device ("fail-safe" system) shall be used on all anesthesia machines to announce and, at lower levels of oxygen pressure, to discontinue other gases when the pressure of the supply of oxygen is reduced. (8:43B-18.5.d)

A vaporizer exclusion ("interlock") system shall be used to assure that only one vaporizer, and therefore only a single agent, can be actuated on any anesthesia machine at one time. (8:43B-18.5.e)

To prevent delivery of excess anesthesia during an oxygen flush, no vaporizer shall be placed in the circuit downstream of the oxygen flush valve. (8:43b-18.5.f)

All anesthesia vaporizers shall be pressure compensated in order to administer a constant non-pulsatile output. (8:43B-18.5.g)

Accurate flow meters and controllers shall be used to prevent the delivery to a patient of an inadequate concentration of oxygen relative to the amount of nitrous oxide or other medical gas. (8:43B-18.5.h)

Alarm systems shall be in place for high (disconnect), low (subatmospheric), and minimum ventilatory pressures in the breathing circuit for each patient under general anesthesia. (8:43B-18.5.i)

An in-circuit oxygen analyzer shall monitor the oxygen concentration within the breathing circuit, displaying the percent oxygen of the total mixture, for all patients receiving general anesthesia. (8:43B-18.7.a)

A respirometer (volumeter) measuring exhaled tidal volume shall be used whenever the breathing circuit of a patient under general anesthesia allows. (8:43B-18.7.b)

The body temperature of each patient under anesthesia shall be continuously monitored. (8:43B-18.7.c)

Pulse oximetry shall be performed continuously during administration of all anesthesia, including intravenous conscious sedation, at all anesthetizing locations, when technically feasible. . . . (8:43B-18.7.d)

End-tidal carbon dioxide monitoring shall be performed continuously during administration of all general anesthesia, where technically feasible. (8:43B-18.7.e)

A precordial stethoscope or esophageal stethoscope shall be used when indicated on each patient receiving anesthesia. If necessary, the stethoscope may be positioned on the posterior chest wall or tracheal area. (8:43B-18-.7.i)

A peripheral nerve stimulator shall be available within the operating suite to monitor the patient's extent of muscle paralysis from muscle relaxants. (8.43B-18.7.j)[11]

This approach, although its design requirements appear to be exact, is quite flawed in that it fails to account for future, inevitable, changes in the standards. For instance, the New Jersey regulations fail to recognize either the ANSI Z-79.8 or the ASTM F1161-88 standards for anesthesia gas machines. It would have been easier and more effective to require that anesthesia gas machines meet certain voluntary consensus standards, which would enable the state regulations to be updated automatically as new standards were issued. As it now stands, the regulations are subjected to a lengthy period of public comment and review before any changes can be enacted. One disadvantage of such design-specific regulations is that they may prevent the introduction of a technologically superior and safer anesthesia gas machine.

MEDICAL DEVICE VOLUNTARY STANDARDS

Voluntary consensus standards are a relatively new phenomenon in medicine. Commercial standards have existed for well over 100 years. Often, however, they reflect the interests of the manufacturer who was initially dominant in the marketplace. These standards then codify commonly used and long-standing practices. Commercial standards may be developed solely within a company, by a trade group, or by a technical society. Generally in the United States the writing of standards is essentially a bottom-up process that formalizes existing and accepted commercial or industrial processes.

The arena of voluntary consensus standards for medical equipment may not appear as orderly and regimented as that of government regulation. In fact, it can be a source of considerable confusion to the practicing anesthesiologist. This is especially true when an anesthesiologist wants to determine the presiding voluntary consensus standard for a particular piece of equipment. Several different sets of voluntary standards from a number of different organizations often apply to a single medical device. Even the "alphabet soup" used to describe the different organizations—AAMI, ANSI, NFPA, IEEE, ASTM—can be confusing.

Developing standards by the voluntary consensus method is faster and more responsive to the marketplace than it is by either state or federal agencies. Organizations that propose voluntary standards are not subject to the cumbersome bureaucratic and legal intricacies that govern both federal and state governments. This is not to say, however, that voluntary consensus organizations can be cavalier or ignorant with regard to legal requirements. In the interest of fairness and to prevent legal ramifications, all interested parties must be allowed to participate in the process of creating standards in accordance with the individual organization's bylaws.

Compliance with voluntary standards is not mandatory because the parent organization has no legal jurisdiction. Voluntary consensus standards, however, often have an influence even before they are finalized. Responsible manufacturers find both legal protection and sales advantages in claiming that their equipment meets various voluntary standards, such as those of AAMI, ANSI, or ASTM. New voluntary standards cannot require that a manufacturer remove from the marketplace earlier equipment that does not conform to the new standard. Only a municipal, state, or federal jurisdiction can demand compliance or remove an item from the market. Often, voluntary consensus standards, such as those of the National Fire Protection Association (NFPA), are adopted by local agencies that have the authority to turn the standards into law. Voluntary equipment standards can also be adopted by a government agency as part of their procurement or purchasing policies. On occasion, however, a governmental regulation may be adopted before the voluntary standard has been finalized. As part of its newly revised 405 regulations that took effect in January of 1989, New York state required quantitative determination of end-tidal carbon dioxide by capnometry. However, the ASTM voluntary standard for capnometry did not receive final approval until 1991. Before 1991, there were no standards defining the performance and calibration characteristics of a capnometer.

National Fire Protection Association

The anesthesia community has been involved with voluntary standards for almost 40 years. Initially, the ASA participated in the development of standards by the National Fire Protection Association (NFPA). NFPA writes standards for many aspects of fire prevention, detection, and suppression. They also address standards for different types of facilities, such as multiple dwellings, factories,

and hospitals. Initially, when cyclopropane and ether were used in operating rooms, the input of anesthesiologists was important in developing standards for anesthetizing locations. Their input was again needed with the advent of centralized medical-gas distribution systems, such as for oxygen and nitrous oxide. What initially developed as fire safety regulations for all occupants of a facility eventually evolved into patient safety standards. An example of this is the present NFPA standard for nonflammable medical-gas piping systems. Anesthesiology input has remained vital to the NFPA throughout the years, both to provide user input and to ensure that proposals by fire professionals for changes or modifications do not adversely affect the hospital's clinical practice. For instance, a firefighter cannot elect to turn off the hospital's entire oxygen supply because of a fire in one wing of the facility. Obviously, the drafting of such a standard would require compromise on the part of both clinicians and fire professionals.

All standards published by the NFPA that affect hospitals are now published in one document: *NFPA 99: Standard for Health Care Facilities*.[13] This document is generally updated every three years and was most recently updated in 1990. It contains standards governing anesthetizing locations, emergency power supplies, high-frequency electricity, medical-gas pipeline systems, and hyperbaric oxygen facilities.

Although ether and cyclopropane are no longer employed in modern operating rooms, the threat of fire has in no way been eliminated. Each year the amount of electrical equipment in the operating room increases. Many of these devices, such as electrosurgical units and lasers, can ignite the drapes, sponges, and other disposable items in an operating room. In the presence of oxygen and/or nitrous oxide, a spark can become a conflagration. The NFPA is currently holding a series of meetings to address the issue of operating room fires in response to an apparent increase in such events over the past few years. This perception was generated in part by the ASA House of Delegates at their October, 1990, meeting, during which the following resolution was passed:

. . . that the President charge the Committee on Equipment and Facilities with developing a mechanism to obtain information regarding operating room fires, with a report to the August, 1991, Board of Directors meeting.

American National Standards Institute

The anesthesia community has a long history of involvement with the American National Standards Institute (ANSI). ANSI, a private, nonprofit organization, was founded more than 70 years ago in order to coordinate and facilitate the development of standards. In 1956 the American Society of Anesthesiologists assumed the secretariat of ANSI Committee Z-79 for Anesthesia and Respiratory Therapy Equipment, and they maintained this position until 1983. During this time, many standards were produced by the Z-79 Anesthesia and Respiratory Therapy Equipment Committee, including those for humidifiers, reservoir bags, ventilators, tracheal tubes, and anesthesia machines.

Probably the most important and best-known standard created by the Z-79 Committee was the Z-79.9 1979 standard for *Minimum Performance and Safety Requirements for Components and Systems of Continuous-Flow Anesthesia Machines for Human Use.*[14] This was the first attempt by the manufacturers and users of anesthesia equipment to ensure compatibility and performance among the various types of anesthesia machines.

The major accomplishments of this standard include:

1. Legibility and visibility requirements for gauges and dials
2. Pin indexing system on gas-tank yokes
3. Elimination of cross filling between tanks
4. Pipeline pressure gauges
5. Pressure regulators to preferentially seek oxygen from central as opposed to tank supplies
6. Diameter-indexed safety system
7. Fail-safe mechanism
8. Single-purpose oxygen flush valves
9. Single flowmeter knobs for each gas
10. Vaporizer "lock out" for multiple vaporizers
11. 15/22 mm standardized connections on the machine

Although this standard contained flaws, it was the best standard that could be developed at the time through voluntary consensus efforts. The standard was deficient in some major areas. It permitted the use of in-circuit vaporizers and required neither oxygen analyzers nor a method to prevent the administration of a hypoxic mixture. It did, however, serve the anesthesia community well, both manufacturer and user, during the 10 years it functioned as the ruling anesthesia machine standard.

American Society for Testing and Materials

In 1983, the ASA left ANSI and began working with the American Society for Testing and Materials (ASTM). It was felt that ASTM offered more protection to participants because it was incorporated in the state of Pennsylvania. In a 1964 ruling, the U.S. District Court of the Eastern District of Pennsylvania declared that ASTM's due process procedures provided the participants with immunity against antitrust prosecution: Under Pennsylvania law, members of a nonprofit organization were not personally liable for the obligations of and any judgments against the corporation.

In 1982, the Supreme Court ruled that organizations that provide informal interpretations on official stationery must ensure that these are not mistaken as official statements by the general public. A legal analysis of the decision provided to members of the NFPA by their general counsel noted that:

> Reasonable technical decisions based on safety considerations are proper and protected. Essentially the Supreme Court has taken the position that standard-setting organizations are important, and that the organizations must exercise reasonable care in supervising the activities of their volunteers.

A good faith interpretation of a standard reasonably supported by health or safety considerations will not be successfully challenged.[15]

Currently, the ASTM handles most of the activities concerning voluntary standards that affect anesthesia durable equipment. Committee F-29 on Anesthetic and Respiratory Therapy Equipment has over 30 subcommittees that focus on safety and performance standards rather than on design or specific engineering standards. Design and engineering decisions are best left to the individual manufacturer. ASTM views standard-writing activities as a method to achieve an orderly approach to a specific activity or problem. All committee members are volunteers; the formal ASTM staff provides only administrative support. ASTM does not fund any participants, nor does it have its own laboratory facilities; individual members must have their own funding. At present, the Chairman of the ASA Committee on Equipment and Facilities serves as the ASA liaison to the ASTM. Other members of the ASA chosen by the Committee on Equipment and Facilities also serve on the parent F-29 Committee and its many subcommittees. Not all anesthesiologists, however, who serve on ASTM committees are funded or nominated by the ASA.

Any ASTM member may solicit membership on a particular committee provided the member has proven knowledge or qualifications in the committee's area. Under the organization's bylaws, the members of any committee should reflect a balance of users, producers, ultimate consumers, technical representatives, insurers, educators, and those with an interest in the area. The last category can include members of the Food and Drug Administration or of nonprofit health care organizations that deal with medical devices directly or indirectly.

Almost anyone can initiate the creation of a standard within ASTM. The proponent must first submit a written request detailing the various companies, individuals, and organizations who would be participating. The executive staff of ASTM then decides whether or not the proposal has merit. If accepted, the proposal is then referred to a particular committee. The ASTM writes standards for everything from tarmac to towels.

The ASTM F1161-88 standard, *Specifications for Minimum Performance and Safety Requirements for Components and Systems of Anesthesia Gas Machines,* was ratified by ASTM at the end of 1988.[16] Although issued by a different organization (ASTM), this standard effectively superseded the ANSI Z-79.8 standard for anesthesia machines, and in many way it was superior to the earlier one. It now has the following requirements:

1. Preoperational checklist
2. Concentration-calibrated vaporizers
3. Oxygen analyzer
4. Alarms enabled by a master switch
5. Alarm hierarchy
6. Breathing system pressure monitoring
7. Volume monitoring or capnometry

Another decade likely will pass before a revised standard for anesthesia machines is issued. Although there have been no voluntary American standards concerning expected equipment life, it is reasonable to assume that by the time the next anesthesia machine standard is issued, before the year 2000, all the machines of the Z-79 era will have been retired. When the F1161-88 standard was issued, many in the anesthesia and regulatory community hoped that all machines predating the Z-79 standard would be retired. Recent studies have shown this not to be the case, and it is unfortunate that many anesthesia machines more than 30 years old are still being used in obstetrical units, radiology suites, and emergency rooms. Although obsolescence is difficult to define, a machine that has been in operation for more than two decades should be retired. Failure to do so may significantly jeopardize the safety of the patient.

Institute of Electrical and Electronics Engineers

The Institute of Electrical and Electronics Engineers (IEEE) has traditionally written standards that directly concern only engineers. The ultimate consumers, although they enjoyed the increased benefits and safety provided by such standards, were oblivious to their efforts. One project within IEEE of particular interest to the anesthesia community concerns the IEEE Committee P-1073, which is trying to develop the Medical Information Bus (MIB). Work on this was begun in 1987, although the idea originated during the early 1980s. In 1982, the Association for the Advancement of Medical Instrumentation (AAMI) sponsored a roundtable discussion on "Developing Standards for Data Management in Monitoring." Many of those attending the session thought that a standardized method for data communication among monitoring equipment was needed in the operating room. A proposal was subsequently made by the AAMI Standards Board that a technical committee be formed to develop standards for monitoring system data management. However, no further action was taken by AAMI.

The IEEE then became interested in this project. In 1987, it was taken up by Committee P1073 of the IEEE Engineering in Medicine and Biology Society (EMBS), which consisted of device manufacturers, computer experts, clinicians, and biomedical engineers.[17] The Com-

mittee undertook to produce an international standard for local area networks (LANs) that will enable communication between free-standing monitors, infusion and life-support devices, and a host computer system. This will not serve laboratory or pharmacy functions but rather is intended solely to support the clinician in an acute patient care setting, such as the intensive care unit or the operating room.

The standard specifically makes provision for anesthesia machines and ventilators with the purpose of developing an automated anesthesia record using "local intelligence," which can be up-loaded to a large host computer system. The goal is to eliminate the need for individual institutions to write software or design connectors for devices. The standard therefore is vendor-independent.

At present, the MIB Committee has completed draft standards for both the interbed network, (IEEE P1073.1), which deals with the overall architecture of the MIB including the required features and common facilities to which the various applications may communicate, and the Bedside Communications Subnet (IEEE P1073.2), which deals with communication among the individual devices and the bedside terminal. The IEEE affirmation process is now underway. Work has also begun on IEEE P1073.3, which will ultimately deal with connecting the bedside local intelligence with the master host computer.

International standards and regulations

Unlike European and Pacific rim countries, the United States is not represented at international standards organizations by any official governmental representative. The United States does not have a single body that speaks for all standards activities within the country. However, the National Institute for Standards and Technology (NIST), a branch of the federal government, has proposed the creation of a Standards Council of the United States (SCUSA). As envisioned by NIST, SCUSA would coordinate relations between governments with regard to standards. It would also grant accreditation to programs and laboratories as well as to the various voluntary associations that write standards.

On the international level, standards are dichotomized much as they are nationally. There are older multinational standards organizations, such as the International Standards Organization (ISO) and the International Electrotechnical Commission (IEC), which work on the basis of voluntary consensus. Other, newer multinational organizations with official regulatory authority are now emerging.

At present ANSI serves as the coordinator and representative for the United States before the ISO and the IEC. Under the General Agreement on Tariffs and Trade (GATT), to which the United States has been a signatory for over 40 years, there exists a Standards Code that provides ground rules for preparing, ratifying, and implementing international technical standards. ANSI has assumed the role of representative for the United States, but, in contrast to many of its counterparts in Europe, it has no official governmental sanction.

In 1992, the 12 member nations of the European Community (EC) will unite economically. In anticipation of this, the EC has contracted with two private European standards organizations—the Committee for European Standardization (CEN) and the Committee for European Electrotechnical Standardization (CENELEC)—to merge the various national standards of its component members into one encompassing document for approval by the 12 members. It is the intention of CEN and CENELEC to develop standards that closely follow those of the ISO and IEC.

Anesthetic workstations. The CEN is currently working on a project entitled *Anesthetic Workstations and Their Modules: Essential Requirements*.[18] The Anesthetic and Respiratory Devices Committee of the ISO was actively involved in the development of this European draft standard, which establishes the essential requirements for anaesthetic workstations, or anesthetizing locations, as they are known in the United States. The standard outlines the complete requirements for individual modules that together constitute a complete anesthetic workstation (i.e., anesthesia ventilator, breathing system, scavenging system, vaporizers, monitors, and alarm systems). Here, the goal is not to specify a universal world anesthesia machine, but rather to ensure that each component utilized clinically meets minimum, specific, identifiable requirements.

The CEN draft applies the same standards to both the workstation as a whole and the individual modules. These standards concern environmental conditions, electrical shock hazards, mechanical hazards, excessive or unwanted radiation, and excessive temperature. The standard sets requirements for construction as well as for minimum accuracy. Although this draft standard recognizes the practice standards both in the United States and in other countries, it does not produce its own minimum monitoring configurations. Instead, it requires only that certain performance standards be met for those elements that are present.

The draft recognizes, however, the need to better integrate and display information from both patient and equipment monitors in order to improve anesthetic data collection and alarm function. To accomplish this, the draft requests that a medical information bus system be incorporated in the workstation to enable communication between individual monitors and the workstation as a whole.

Both voluntary consensus standards and governmental regulations can coexist harmoniously in the future. Although the clinician, the industry, and the patient undoubtedly benefit from standards, there is no clear evidence that mandatory standards are better at preventing problems than are voluntary standards. A voluntary standard can be developed in a relatively short time by assembly of a group that represents the interested parties. Voluntary standards can be easily modified or amended and therefore can respond more quickly to changing technology. Government regulations have the force of law and can require a minimum performance standard for manufacturers and users. Unlike voluntary standards, government regulations can remove unsafe devices from the market or mandate modifications. However, involved bureaucratic procedures frequently delay the implementation of these standards and can make modifications difficult. Voluntary standards serve to influence the manufacturers of new products. However, only a governmental regulation can mandate that obsolete equipment be removed from service.

REFERENCES

1. *Everything you always wanted to know about the medical device amendments. . . and weren't afraid to ask*, ed 2, HHS Publication FDA 84-4173. U.S. Department of Health and Human Services, Public Health Service, Food and Drug Administration, Center for Devices and Radiological Health, 1984.
2. *Medical device regulation: the FDA's neglected child*, Subcommittee on Oversight and Investigation of the Committee on Energy and commerce, U.S. House of Representatives, May 1983.
3. Munsey RR: House report rebukes FDA on performance standards, *Med Instrum* 17:279-280, 1983.
4. FDA defends investigation of anesthesia machines, *American Medical News*, October 19, 1984.
5. *Medical devices: early warning of problems is hampered by severe underreporting*, GAO/PEMD-87-1, Washington, DC, December 1986.
6. *Medical devices: FDA's implementation of the medical device reporting regulation*, GAO/PEMF-89-10, Washington, DC, February 1989.
7. *Medical devices: the public health at risk*, GAO/T-PEMD-90-2, Washington, DC 1989.
8. *Safe medical devices act of 1990*. 21 C.F.R. Part 821, Federal Register Vol. 57, No. 60, March 1992.
9. *Medicine and health*, Volume 45, No.9, Washington, DC, March 4, 1991, Faulkner and Gray (newsletter).
10. Wechsler J: A full plate for FDA. Washington Report: *Medical Design and Material*. pp 9-11, February 1991 (newsletter).
11. Hospital: minimum standards, Part 405, Article 2, Subchapter A, Chapter V, Title 10, *Official Compilation of Codes, Rules and Regulations of the State of New York 1988*.
12. *Health facilities evaluation and licensing:* Hospital Licensing Standards Anesthesia Care, New Jersey Annotated Code 8:43B-18, 1989.
13. *NFPA 99: Standard for Health Care Facilities*, Batterymarch Park, Mass, 1990, National Fire Protection Association.
14. *Minimum performance and safety requirements for components and systems of continuous-flow anesthesia machines for human use*, ANSI Z-79.8, New York, 1979, American National Standards Institute.
15. Daniel J. Piliero II, General Counsel to the National Fire Protection Association: private communication to Robert W. Grant, President, National Fire Protection Association, May 20, 1982.
16. *Standard specifications for minimum performance and safety requirements for components and systems of anesthesia gas machines*, ASTM F-1161-88, Philadelphia, Pa, 1989, American Society for Testing and Materials.
17. Figler AA, Stead SW: The medical information bus, *Biomed Instrum Technol*, 101-111, 1990.
18. *Anesthetic workstations and their modules: essential requirements*, CEN/TC 215/ WG1 N36 Lubeck, Germany, 1990.

Part VI

SPECIAL SITUATIONS

Chapter 26

PEDIATRIC ANESTHESIA SYSTEMS AND EQUIPMENT

Simon C. Hillier, M.B., Ch.B., F.F.A.R.C.S.
William L. McNiece, M.D.

The ultimate goal of the anesthesiologist during pediatric surgery is to provide the patient with a safe and smooth anesthetic. What is not always obvious is the best method of achieving this end. Which breathing system is appropriate for the pediatric patient? How do the maturational changes in respiratory physiology affect the selection and use of equipment? A ventilator and breathing system that works well for adults may not function ideally for the pediatric patient. Are the routine monitors primarily designed for adults equally applicable to pediatric patients of all sizes? Furthermore, understanding how equipment works and using it correctly can mean the difference between providing safe anesthesia and inviting disaster. This chapter reviews pediatric anesthesia systems, including a description of the equipment, and discusses how to select and use the equipment correctly.

PHYSIOLOGY
The work of breathing under anesthesia

A brief review of some aspects of the respiratory physiology of infants and children during anesthesia will provide the background for the recommendations presented in this chapter. Several factors may increase the work of breathing under anesthesia (Box 26-1). These factors can be broadly divided into two groups. First is the increased work of breathing that may be imposed by the anesthesia breathing system, including inspiratory and expiratory resistance of breathing circuits, circuit dead space, and rebreathing of carbon dioxide. Second are changes in the mechanics and the control of breathing induced by general anesthesia. These include decreased total respiratory compliance, decreased lung volume, airway closure, and partial upper airway obstruction. Thus, during general anesthesia in children many factors may act to increase the demands on the respiratory system while simultaneously decreasing its ability to cope with these demands.

Box 26-1. Perioperative factors increasing the work of breathing*

Anesthetic circuit	*General anesthesia*
Increased resistance	Decreased lung volume
Increased dead space	Decreased compliance
Valvular resistance	Airway obstruction
Rebreathing of carbon dioxide	

*Both the induction of general anesthesia and the anesthesia breathing system may contribute to the increased work of breathing under anesthesia.

Table 26-1. A comparison of some selected normal respiratory variables in infants and adults

Normal value	Infants	Adults
Weight (kg)	3.0	70
Surface area (m²)	0.2	1.8
Surface area/weight (m²/kg)	0.06	0.03
Respiratory frequency (breaths/min)	30-40	10-16
Tidal volume (V_T)	7	7
Dead space (V_D)	2.2	2.2
V_D/V_T ratio	0.3	0.3
Functional residual capacity (ml/kg)	30	30
Lung compliance (ml/cm H_2O)	5	200
Specific compliance (ml/cm H_2O/ml)	0.05	0.05
Airways resistance (cmH_2O/L/sec)	25-30	1.6
Work of breathing (g/cm/L)	2000-4000	2000-7000
Alveolar ventilation (ml/kg/min)	100-150	70
Oxygen consumption (ml/kg/min)	6-8	4

Table 26-1 compares some selected normal respiratory physiologic values between infants and adults. Neonates and infants have less respiratory reserve than adults and may demonstrate an unpredictable response to the added work of breathing through a circuit under general anesthesia. For example, patients breathing spontaneously with the Mapleson D, E, and F circuits may rebreathe some alveolar gas if the fresh gas flow is less than 2.5 to 3 times the predicted minute ventilation.[1] Under normal circumstances the patient is able to increase appropriately his/her minute ventilation in response to rebreathing and thus prevent significant hypercarbia. However, it is known that some anesthetized *adults* are unable to respond to increases in inspired carbon dioxide by hyperventilation, and therefore become hypercarbic.[2] The response of spontaneously breathing anesthetized (nitrous oxide and 1% to 1.5% halothane) *infants* to an increase in inspired carbon dioxide was examined by Olsson and Lindhal.[3] Patients younger than 6 months of age did not increase their minute ventilation in response to the added carbon dioxide, while patients older than 6 months of age increased their minute volume by 16% and 34% in response to inspired carbon dioxide concentrations of 2.22% and 3.71%, respectively. When the halothane concentration was reduced to 0.8% the ventilatory response to carbon dioxide returned in those patients less than 6 months of age. Thus, deep inhalational anesthesia attenuates the ventilatory response to carbon dioxide in small infants. General anesthesia has also been shown to adversely affect the ventilatory response to increased respiratory work in the forms of tubular resistance, dead space, and valvular resistance. Charlton et al.[4] noted that for a given increase in apparatus dead space, the infant must increase minute ventilation to a proportionately greater degree in order to maintain normocarbia when compared with the older child. The neonate may be particularly prone to respiratory compromise in the face of prolonged increases in respiratory work. The newborn's diaphragmatic muscle is immature, having a smaller proportion of fatigue-resistant high-oxidative muscle fibers.[5] In addition to its potential for fatigue, the infant diaphragm is less able to generate a maximal inspiratory force than

the adult diaphragm.[6] Thus, it is not surprising that several authors have recommended that the newborn and infant should not breathe spontaneously for a prolonged period of time under general anesthesia.[7,8]

PEDIATRIC ANESTHESIA EQUIPMENT

Face masks

It is essential that the pediatric face mask be able to provide a good seal to the patient's face. This facilitates effective positive pressure ventilation, avoids entrainment of room air during spontaneous ventilation, and reduces operating room pollution. Other desirable features include low dead space, comfort for the patient, and construction of transparent material to allow observation of the patient's color and the presence of secretions or vomitus. Clear masks may also be considerably less threatening to the patient.[9] The Vital Signs (Vital Signs, Inc., Totowa, NJ) face masks have most of these desirable characteristics (Fig. 26-1). While the ability to ventilate the patient by mask is of the utmost importance, the requirement of a low dead space is also important to avoid retention of carbon dioxide and increased respiratory work. The measured dead space of most face masks is significantly greater than the functional dead space actually encountered in clinical practice.[4] It is postulated that streaming of gas reduces the functional dead space and reduces rebreathing.[10] The Rendell-Baker-Soucek mask (Fig. 26-2) has a very low dead space, but requires practice to obtain an airtight fit consistently. Maintaining an airway can be difficult in the child because the anesthesiologist's fingers holding the face mask can cause external compression of the compliant upper airway. Care should be taken to ensure that fingers do not accidentally stray from the mandible onto the soft tissues surrounding the airway. Mask anesthesia is usually

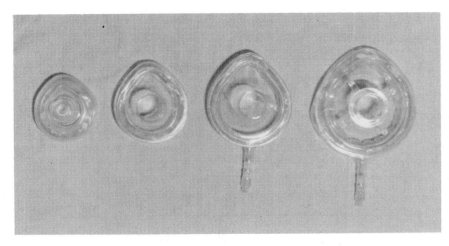

Fig. 26-1. Vital Signs transparent anesthesia face mask with adjustable air cushion.

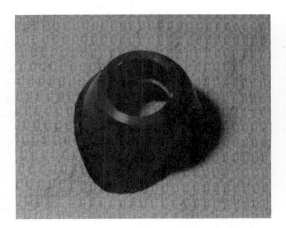

Fig. 26-2. Rendell-Baker-Soucek low dead space pediatric face mask.

given for short procedures and prior to and following tracheal intubation. Mask anesthesia with spontaneous ventilation should not be used for long periods of time in small infants who are unable to tolerate the increased work of breathing and may respond with apnea or hypoventilation. Inhalational induction of anesthesia may often be facilitated by the application of pleasant flavoring to the inside of the face mask to disguise the smell of the potent volatile agents and the unpleasant plastic odor of the mask and breathing circuit (Fig. 26-3).

Tracheal tubes

Selecting the correct tracheal tube type and size, along with its accurate and secure positioning, is vitally important.

Selecting the correct diameter. In children less than 10 years of age, the narrowest part of the upper airway is

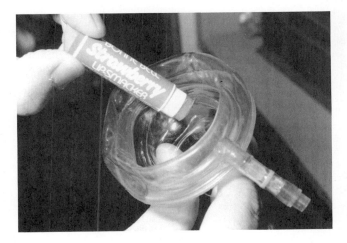

Fig. 26-3. Inhalational induction of anesthesia can be made pleasant for the patient by the application of an odorant to the face mask.

the subglottic region. At this location the cricoid forms a complete ring of cartilage around the airway that is lined with loosely bound pseudostratified epithelium. Trauma to the subglottic area (e.g., intubation with a tube of too large a diameter) results in edema that may decrease the lumen of the airway and increase resistance to gas flow after extubation. At birth, the cross-sectional area of the airway at the cricoid level is 14 mm^2. It should be noted that during laminar flow, resistance is inversely proportional to the fourth power of the radius. A 1-mm ring of edema in the newborn will reduce the cross-sectional area of the airway by 65%, thus significantly increasing airway resistance. A similar ring of edema in the adult would have a minimal effect on airway resistance.

The optimal size of tracheal tube is the largest that will pass easily into the trachea without traumatizing the larynx. To determine the leak pressure after tracheal intubation, the reservoir bag should be slowly inflated and circuit pressure measured while listening with a stethoscope either at the mouth or in the sternal notch for a leak. The optimal leak pressure is not known, but it is known that the incidence of postextubation stridor increases as the leak pressure increases, particularly to greater than 25 cm H_2O. Most patients' lungs can be ventilated adequately at leak pressures of 15 to 20 cm H_2O. If the patient has lung disease, or an intrathoracic or high abdominal procedure is planned, a higher leak pressure, such as 25 to 30 cm H_2O, may be necessary to allow adequate ventilation when pulmonary compliance is reduced. Occasionally an unacceptably large leak is present with one size of tube and no leak is present with a tube 0.5 mm larger in diameter. Under these circumstances a cuffed tube of the smaller size with the cuff deflated may produce an acceptable leak. Using a tube that is too small with a large leak may lead to difficulty in ventilating the lungs, difficulty in obtaining accurate end-tidal carbon dioxide measurements, increased risk of aspiration, and increased incidence of tube obstruction by secretions. Suction catheters appropriate to all tube sizes must be immediately available to remove secretions from tracheal tubes.

Formulas to predict correct tracheal tube size are based on weight and age (Box 26-2) One should have available tubes sized 0.5 mm above and below the predicted requirement, as well as that predicted by the formulas. The use of clear, thin-walled tubes is recommended (Fig. 26-4). All tubes should be Z79 Committee approved and polyvinyl chloride (PVC) implant tested.

The peak incidence of postextubation stridor appears to be between 1 and 4 years of age.[10] Other factors that have been shown to contribute to the incidence of postextubation stridor include a tight-fitting tracheal tube, that is, a leak at greater than 25 cm H_2O; traumatic or multiple intubations; coughing with the tracheal tube in place during emergence from anesthesia; changing the patient's head position while intubated; intubation of greater than 1 hours' duration; and operations in the neck region. Interestingly, although the presence of an upper respiratory tract infection was not found to be a contributing factor in earlier studies, recent data show that respiratory tract infections in patients less than 1 year of age increased the risk of postextubation stridor by 27-fold.[11] Patients with Down syndrome may have a narrow subglottic region and are thus prone to postextubation stridor.

Selecting the correct insertion depth. The newborn trachea is only 4 cm long. Therefore, the margin of error for a tube that is located in the midtrachea is only 2 cm in either direction, resulting in either bronchial intubation or accidental extubation. One approach to determining the correct insertion depth is as follows: While the tube is gently advanced after intubation, the chest is auscultated bilaterally to determine the depth at which bronchial intubation occurs. Then, the tube is carefully withdrawn and secured

---

Box 26-2.   Determination of tracheal tube size and depth of insertion

Size of tracheal tube

Premature infants (1000 g)	2.5 mm I.D.*
Premature infants (1000-2500 g)	3.0 mm I.D.
Children less than 6 years	(age ÷ 3) + 3.75 mm I.D.
Children greater than 6 years	(age ÷ 4) + 4.5 mm I.D.

Alternative formula based on weight	[weight (kg) + 35] ÷ 10 mm I.D.

Tubes 0.5 mm I.D. larger and smaller than calculated from these formulas should be immediately available

Depth of insertion

7 cm for a 1-kg infant; one additional cm per kg body weight up to 4 kg
> 4 kg and up to 1 year of age: 10 cm at the alveolar ridge
After 1 year of age: (age ÷ 2) + 12 cm
*I.D. = internal diameter.

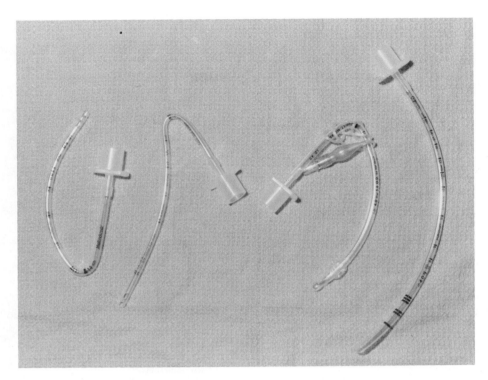

Fig. 26-4. A selection of pediatric tracheal tubes. From left to right: oral RAE tube, nasal RAE tube, cuffed oral RAE tube, standard oral uncuffed tube.

at the appropriate depth. It should be noted that when the tube has a Murphy eye it may be difficult to determine tube position by auscultation because the eye may transmit sufficient gas to produce breath sounds, despite the tube tip being located in a mainstem bronchus. In small infants, particularly those with lung disease, it is not always easy to determine by auscultation alone at what depth the tube should be secured. When accurate tube position is crucial (e.g., for repair of a tracheoesophageal fistula), a small diameter flexible fiberoptic bronchoscope or a chest film may be used to determine the tube location. Use of 1.8-mm (Olympus PF 18M) and 2.2-mm (Olympus LF-P) external diameter flexible fiberoptic bronchoscopes aid in tube positioning. The larger of these bronchoscopes has a directable distal tip. However, neither has a suction channel. Both bronchoscopes can be passed through a 2.5-mm internal diameter tracheal tube. Armored tubes are also available in some pediatric sizes (Fig. 26-5).

Using the oral RAE tracheal tube. The preformed Ring, Adair and Elwyn tube (RAE, Mallinckrodt, Argyle, NY; Fig. 26-4) is often used during pediatric ENT and other head and neck procedures.[12] The tube has many advantages, but there are potential hazards.

The tube was designed for use in cleft lip and palate surgery, at an institution where the surgeon preferred to leave the tube untaped so that it could be moved during the procedure. The designers of the tube intended the distal tip of the tube to lie nearer to the carina than a conventional

tube in order to reduce the likelihood of accidental extubation. Two Murphy eyes, located at the distal end of the tube, are intended to allow continued ventilation should bronchial migration occur. The acute angle in the RAE tube, the part of the tube most likely to kink, is located outside the mouth, and is therefore readily visible.

While these design features are useful, some potential hazards have recently been described in the literature. When using a RAE tube that is positioned with the acute angle at the lower lip, it should not be assumed that the distal tip of the tube is located correctly. A recent study demonstrated that the distal tips of 32% of RAE tubes positioned in this way were located at the carina or down a mainstem bronchus.[13] In addition, the Murphy eyes do not always assure adequate ventilation when the distal end of the tube is located in a mainstem bronchus. However, the Murphy eyes may allow sufficient ventilation to confuse the issue when the chest is auscultated to confirm bilateral breath sounds. The manufacturer suggests tube sizes appropriate to each age, but these recommendations should be interpreted with caution as they advocate a larger internal diameter tube than that predicted by standard formulas for pediatric tracheal tubes. Oral uncuffed RAE tubes have a slightly smaller outside diameter (0.1 mm less) than standard Mallinckrodt tracheal tubes. It is recommended that a left precordial stethoscope be used with a RAE tube to detect bronchial migration. Another potential problem when using a RAE tube is difficulty suctioning the tracheal

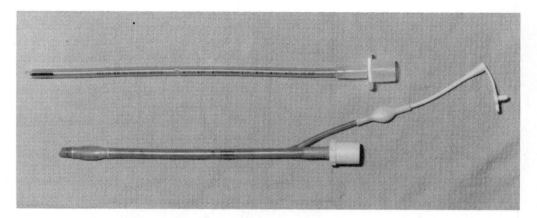

Fig. 26-5. Examples of two pediatric armored tubes. *Top:* anode tube. *Bottom:* cuffed Rusch armored tube.

tube; passing a catheter beyond the acute angle in the tube can be difficult. Despite these potential problems, many anesthesiologists have found the RAE tube to be extremely useful during many surgical procedures of the head and neck.

PEDIATRIC BREATHING SYSTEMS

The anesthesia machine used for pediatric cases is basically similar to that used for adult anesthesia. However, it is very important that the machine have the capability of delivering air. A significant number of pediatric patients presenting for surgery are premature neonates. These patients may be at risk for retinopathy of prematurity (ROP); it is often desirable to avoid the administration of high concentrations of oxygen to such patients. These patients will often require an FIO_2 approaching that of room air. Similarly, many of the newborns presenting for emergency surgery have intraabdominal disease such as necrotizing enterocolitis with pneumatosis intestinalis and bowel obstruction. Both conditions are contraindications to the use of nitrous oxide. In these circumstances air is required to decrease the FIO_2 in the absence of nitrous oxide.

The pediatric breathing system should be of low resistance and dead space, easily adapted to a wide range of patient sizes. It should also be efficient for use with both spontaneous and controlled ventilation and easy to humidify and scavenge (Box 26-3). If the circuit contains valves, they should offer minimal resistance to gas flow and be reliable. In addition, the circuit should have a low compressible volume and be lightweight and compact. Currently, the most commonly used circuits are the Mapleson D, E, and F systems, including the Bain modification of these circuits; the Magill attachment (Mapleson A); and the circle system with absorber.

Mapleson D, E, and F system development

The Mapleson D, E, and F systems are direct descendants of the original T-piece system that was introduced in

Box 26-3. Characteristics of an ideal pediatric anesthesia breathing system

Low dead space
Low resistance
Lightweight and compact
Low compressible volume
Easily humidified
Easily scavenged
Suitable for both controlled and spontaneous ventilation
Economy of fresh gas flow

1937 by Philip Ayre of Newcastle, England.[14] The original Ayre's T-piece has been greatly modified over the years and is rarely used today. The most commonly used configurations are the Mapleson D and F systems (Figs. 26-6 and 26-7). The Mapleson F system is a modification that is generally attributed to Jackson Rees, who added a reservoir bag with an adjustable valve to the expiratory limb.[15] When used with the valve open, the movement of the reservoir bag allows monitoring of spontaneous ventilation. With the valve partially closed, manual compression of the bag allows controlled ventilation. The Mapleson D system has an expiratory valve located at the end of the expiratory limb and functions in a manner similar to the Mapleson F circuit. The volume of the expiratory limb and reservoir bag should exceed the patient's tidal volume. The Mapleson D and F circuits can be used with mechanical ventilation by removing the reservoir bag and connecting a ventilator. These circuits have been described as coming the closest to meeting the requirements of an ideal pediatric anesthesia circuit.[16]

Functional analysis

Before the advent of continuous end-tidal carbon dioxide monitoring, it was difficult in these circuits to predict accurately the fresh gas flow and minute ventilation re-

Ayre's T-piece

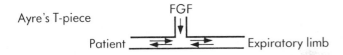

Mapleson D

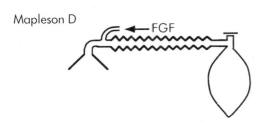

Mapleson E

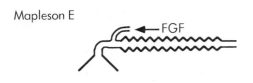

Mapleson F
Jackson-Rees modification

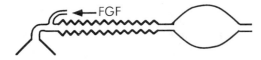

Fig. 26-6. The Ayre's T-piece and its direct descendants, the Mapleson D, E, and F circuits. FGF = fresh gas flow.

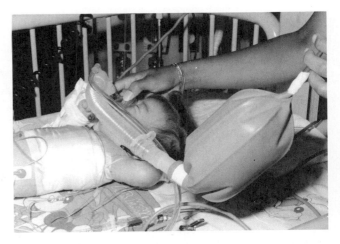

Fig. 26-7. A portable disposable Jackson-Rees circuit (Mapleson F) in use during transport of an infant.

quirements to produce a desired arterial carbon dioxide tension ($PaCO_2$. The published reports about the fresh gas flow and minute ventilation requirements of these circuits were not always consistent. The functional characteristics of these circuits are essentially similar, but differ between spontaneous and controlled ventilation. Many factors affect the performance of these systems with regard to carbon dioxide elimination, including fresh gas flow, minute ventilation, carbon dioxide production, respiratory rate, tidal volume, and expiratory pattern. Not all of these factors are predictable or under the direct influence of the anesthesiologist (see also Chapter 4).

Clinical use

Spontaneous ventilation. During spontaneous ventilation, the expiratory valve of the circuit is open (or partially closed to provide CPAP). At the start of expiration, gas flows along the expiratory limb toward the reservoir bag and expiratory valve. This gas is a mixture of fresh gas, dead space gas, and alveolar gas. In early expiration, fresh gas and dead space gas will predominate. Later in expiration alveolar gas and fresh gas will predominate. As expiration proceeds, the reservoir bag fills and the pressure within the circuit increases. Eventually some of the gas

contained within the reservoir bag is vented through the expiratory valve. The composition of the gas that is vented depends in part upon the degree of longitudinal mixing that occurred in the expiratory limb and reservoir bag. [17] If an end-expiratory pause occurs, fresh gas will continue to accumulate within the expiratory limb of the circuit and will drive the mixture of alveolar, dead space, and fresh gas toward the reservoir bag. During inspiration, the patient will inspire a mixture of fresh gas and gas from the expiratory limb and reservoir bag. The relative proportions of these gases will depend upon the relative proportions of the peak inspiratory flow and the fresh gas flow (Fig. 26-8.). If the fresh gas flow exceeds the peak inspiratory flow, little gas will be entrained from the expiratory limb of the circuit. When the fresh gas flow is less than the peak inspiratory flow, some inspired gas will be entrained from the expiratory limb. Thus it becomes apparent that rebreathing can be avoided completely if the fresh gas flow exceeds the peak inspiratory flow. For most patients this usually requires a fresh gas flow that is in excess of three times the minute ventilation.

However, normocarbia can usually be achieved with fresh gas flows that are less than the peak inspiratory flow. This occurs for two reasons.

1. Even if fresh gas flow does not exceed peak inspiratory flow, some fresh gas will accumulate in the expiratory limb during expiration, during the expiratory pause, and during inspiration when fresh gas flow exceeds inspiratory flow. This fresh gas will then be inhaled during inspiration when inspiratory flow exceeds fresh gas flow (see Fig. 26-8). This requires minimal mixing between fresh gas and alveolar gas in the expiratory limb if the fresh gas flow is to be reduced substantially. The end-expiratory pause is usually nonexistent or very short during spontaneous ventilation with halothane anesthesia;

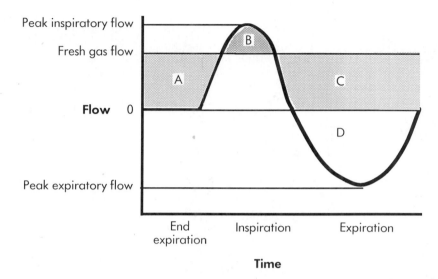

Fig. 26-8. Schematic representation of gas flow patterns with a T-piece circuit with partial rebreathing (i.e., fresh gas flow is less than peak inspiratory flow). During the end-expiratory pause fresh gas (A) flushes alveolar gas down the expiratory limb of the circuit. As inspiration commences inspiratory flow exceeds fresh gas flow. The difference (B) is inhaled from the expiratory limb and reservoir bag. The composition of this gas (B) depends upon the relative proportions and mixing of exhaled gas (D) and fresh gas (C) during expiration. As fresh gas flow exceeds peak inspiratory flow, (B) will no longer exist and no rebreathing will occur.

however, enflurane may produce a longer end-expiratory pause. The fresh gas flow requirements for adults breathing spontaneously are lower when they are anesthetized with enflurane than with halothane.[18]

2. Patients can maintain normocarbia, despite having fresh gas flows that are less than the peak inspiratory flow, even though they may rebreathe a mixture of alveolar, fresh, and dead space gas. In that circumstance, normocarbia can be maintained only by increasing alveolar ventilation.[2] Some degree of rebreathing may be beneficial to the patient, in that warmed and humidified gas is inhaled. However, not all patients are capable of increasing their minute ventilation in this manner. Some patients, termed "poor-responders," simply allow their end-tidal carbon dioxide ($P_E'CO_2$) to increase when rebreathing alveolar gas.[2] Even if the patient does maintain a normal $P_E'CO_2$ by hyperventilating, it is not certain whether small infants and children are able to sustain this increase in ventilation for a prolonged time. The use of capnometry to determine if there is rebreathing ($P_ICO_2 > 0$) allows titration of the fresh gas flow to eliminate rebreathing if desired. Generally speaking, a fresh gas flow of not less than 2.5 and up to 3 times the minute ventilation will usually eliminate rebreathing (Box 26-4).[19] Significant fresh gas flows will be required in larger children and adults to prevent rebreathing, where peak inspiratory flows may exceed 20 L/min. Fresh gas flows of this

magnitude are difficult to humidify, and are expensive. In older children and adults a circle system or Mapleson A (Magill) circuit is more efficient in terms of fresh gas flow requirements during prolonged spontaneous ventilation.

Controlled ventilation. During controlled ventilation the expiratory valve is kept partially closed. As with spontaneous ventilation, during expiration a mixture of alveolar, dead space, and fresh gases enter the expiratory limb and reservoir bag. During the end-expiratory pause this gas mixture is propelled toward the reservoir bag by the continuing fresh gas flow. As inspiration commences, the pressure in the expiratory limb increases and some of the gas mixture in the reservoir bag is vented. The patient will receive a gas mixture that is composed of the ongoing fresh gas flow and the gas that was in the expiratory limb at the end of expiration (a mixture of alveolar, dead space, and fresh gas). In practice, fresh gas flow requirements during controlled ventilation may be less than those during spontaneous ventilation as a certain amount of controlled rebreathing is acceptable. Several recommendations have been made for the fresh gas flow and minute ventilation requirements when using the T-piece derivatives. These are summarized in Box 26-4. When the fresh gas flow is sufficient to flush the alveolar gas from the expiratory limb, no rebreathing will occur. Any increase in fresh gas flow above this point will not affect end-tidal carbon dioxide tension ($P_E'CO_2$) except by augmenting tidal volume (see the section on ventilation). When fresh gas flow is suffi-

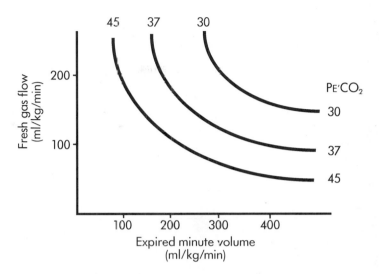

Box 26-4. **Fresh gas flow (FGF) requirements to prevent rebreathing in a T-piece system**

Spontaneous ventilation

Mask anesthesia <30 kg:FGF = 4 × [1000 + (100 × kg body weight)]

>30 kg:FGF = 4 × [2000 + (50 × kg body weight)]

Intubated <30 kg:FGF = 3 × [1000 + (100 × kg body weight)]

>30 kg:FGF = 3 × [2000 + (50 × kg body weight)]

Controlled ventilation

10–30 kg: 1000 ml + 100 ml/kg
>30 kg: 2000 ml + 50 ml/kg

From Rose DK, Byrick RJ, Froese AB: Carbon dioxide elimination during spontaneous ventilation with a modified Mapleson D system: studies in a lung model, *Can Anaesth Soc J* 25:353, 1978.

Fig. 26-9. Fresh gas flow and minute ventilation requirements for three levels (30, 37, and 45 mm Hg) of end-tidal carbon dioxide (PE'CO$_2$) during controlled ventilation with a T-piece. (Redrawn with permission from Conway CM: *Anaesthetic breathing systems.* In Scurr C, Feldman SA, editors: *Scientific foundations of anaesthesia.* St Louis, 1982, Year Book Medical Publishers.)

cient to prevent rebreathing, PE'CO$_2$ is determined primarily by alveolar ventilation. When fresh gas flow is reduced to the point at which rebreathing occurs and minute ventilation is greater than the predicted minute ventilation for the patient, fresh gas flow becomes the primary determinant of PE'CO$_2$ (Fig. 26-9). In practice, a fresh gas flow is selected that allows some controlled rebreathing. This permits the use of relatively generous tidal volumes in an effort to prevent atelectasis and shunting, without an excessive reduction in PE'CO$_2$. Capnography enables frequent and accurate titration of the fresh gas flow to produce the desired PE'CO$_2$.

A commonly applied formula to determine fresh gas flow requirements is that of Rose et al.,[19] who recommend a fresh gas flow twice the minute ventilation (see Box 26-4). Neonates require a fresh gas flow of 3 L/min. Fresh gas flows may need to be increased in the presence of a large tracheal tube leak. When using controlled ventilation, it should be appreciated that increasing the rate of ventilation may not always produce a decrease in end-tidal carbon dioxide tension (PE'CO$_2$) and may in fact *increase* the PE'CO$_2$.[20] This occurs because the duration of expiration and the expiratory pause determine how much alveolar gas is flushed from the expiratory limb by the ongoing fresh gas flow. An increase in respiratory rate will decrease the time available for alveolar gas to be flushed from the expiratory limb. When determining the minute ventilation to be delivered to the pediatric patient, the effects of compressible circuit volume, tracheal tube leaks, inspiratory time, and tidal volume augmentation by fresh gas flow should be taken into account.

The Mapleson D and F circuits are lightweight and have low resistance and dead space. Some means of humidification is necessary because of the high fresh gas flows required by these circuits. Fresh gases entering the circuit can be passed through a heated humidifier, or a heat and moisture exchanger can be placed between the circuit and the tracheal tube. Despite the high fresh gas flows several scavenging systems have been found to be effective.[21] These circuits are effective for both controlled and spontaneous ventilation; however, in larger patients one may prefer to use a Mapleson A or circle system during spontaneous ventilation. Most newborns and small infants will not be breathing spontaneously while anesthetized for prolonged periods. During spontaneous ventilation in infants and children it is probably advisable to avoid rebreathing in view of their unpredictable response to the increased work of breathing. During controlled ventilation a certain amount of rebreathing is acceptable and may even be advantageous. Capnometry allows the monitoring of inspired carbon dioxide to detect rebreathing and has improved the anesthesiologist's ability to accurately adjust fresh gas flows.

The Bain modification of the Mapleson D system. The Bain circuit, described by Bain and Spoerel in 1972, is functionally identical to the Mapleson D system from which it is derived.[22] In the Bain circuit the fresh gas flow is carried within the expiratory limb in a smaller inner hose, and is attached to the machine using a special adapter (Fig. 26-10). The outer expiratory limb is 22 mm in internal diameter and the inner fresh gas tubing is 7 mm in internal diameter. Fresh gas flow requirements for the Bain system are the same as those recommended for the Mapleson D and F systems. The Bain circuit is lightweight and less bulky than traditional T-piece systems, and has

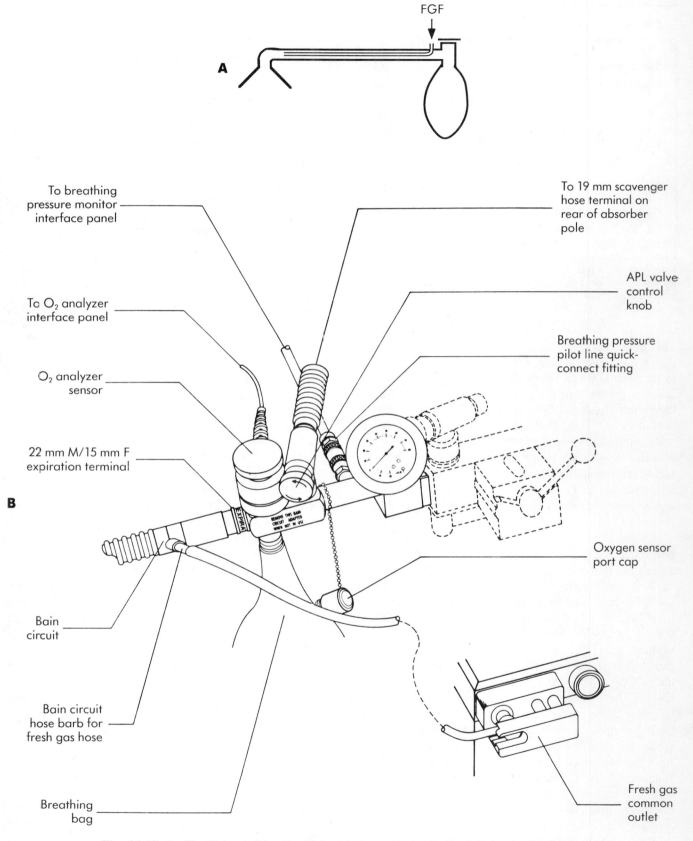

Fig. 26-10. A, The Bain modification of the Mapleson D circuit. **B,** A Bain circuit adapter, which incorporates a bag mount, pressure gauge, adjustable pressure limit (APL) valve, and a 19-mm scavenging connector. (Courtesy North American Dräger, Telford, Pa.)

been used successfully for neurosurgical and head and neck procedures.

Before using the Bain circuit it is important to verify that the fresh gas inner tube is not fractured or disconnected. In this situation fresh gas will enter the expiratory limb near the reservoir bag and a huge dead space will result.[23] "Pethick's maneuver" has been recommended to test the integrity of the circuit.[24] In this maneuver the patient end of the circuit is occluded and the reservoir bag filled. Then the patient end is opened and a high flow of oxygen is passed through the circuit using the oxygen flush. The high flow of oxygen exiting from the patient end of an intact fresh gas hose will cause a reduction in pressure in the expiratory limb via the Venturi effect, which will collapse the reservoir bag. If the inner tube is disrupted, oxygen under pressure will enter the expiratory limb and distend the reservoir bag. This technique has been criticized because small leaks may go undetected and the test itself may cause circuit disruption. Similarly, if the inner tube is intact but does not extend completely to the end of the expiratory limb, significant dead space will exist that may not be detected. A new adapter has recently been described that tests the integrity of the inner and outer tubing separately (Fig. 26-11).[25] Another method of checking the Bain circuit is to set 50 ml/min of gas flow on the oxygen flowmeter and then occlude the distal (patient) end of the inner tube using the plunger of a small syringe. If the inner tube is intact, a decrease in gas flow should result and the flowmeter bobbin will sink.[26]

Mapleson A (Magill) circuit

The Mapleson A (Magill) circuit has the advantage of economy of fresh gas flow when used for the spontaneously breathing patient (Fig. 26-12). When used for controlled ventilation the advantage of economy of fresh gas flow is lost and a Mapleson D or circle is a better choice. The circuit is not as light as the Mapleson D and has a larger dead space, which may reduce its efficiency in smaller children.[27] The Mapleson D system may be more appropriate for use in the infant or small child because these children will usually be breathing spontaneously for only a short period at induction and emergence, requiring controlled ventilation for all but the shortest procedures. Current recommendations during spontaneous ventilation with a Mapleson A circuit are that a fresh gas flow equivalent to the patient's alveolar ventilation (or approximately 70% of the minute ventilation) will prevent rebreathing.[28] However, because of the difficulty in predicting accurately an individual patient's alveolar ventilation, higher fresh gas flows are often used. During controlled ventilation inefficiency of the circuit occurs because the patient will preferentially rebreathe alveolar gas while fresh gas and dead space gas is vented at the expiratory valve. Fresh gas flows of up to 20 L/min have been recommended for controlled ventilation in adults. For anything but the shortest

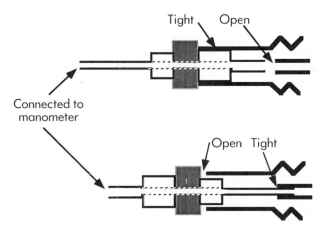

Fig. 26-11. Bain circuit test adapter. One end of the device is connected to a manometer and a sphygmomanometer bulb to allow inflation and pressure measurement. The other end of the device is inserted into the patient end of the Bain circuit. The specific calibers and lengths of the components of this device allow it to be inserted in one of two ways. In the top illustration, by occluding the outer lumen of the Bain circuit, the integrity of the entire circuit is determined. If the device is removed, reversed, and reinserted the inner inspiratory limb can now be isolated from the outer expiratory limb and its integrity determined separately. (Redrawn with permission from Berge JA, Gramstad L, Budd E: Safety testing the Bain circuit—a new test adaptor, *Eur J Anaesthesiol* 8:309, 1991.)

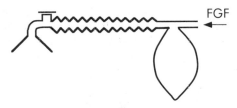

Fig. 26-12. The Mapleson A (Magill) circuit.

duration of controlled ventilation there are much more appropriate alternatives to this system.

Circle systems

The circle system is the most commonly used breathing circuit in the United States today. Its main advantages are those of economy of anesthetic gas use, decreased environmental pollution, and conservation of heat and moisture. The early experiences with the use of adult circle systems to anesthetize pediatric patients resulted in respiratory compromise in spontaneously breathing children less than 2 years of age.[29] This compromise was attributed to the relatively high resistance of the valves, tubing, and soda lime and the relatively large dead space. These factors led to early recommendations that the circle system not be used for children less than 6 years of age.[30] Since that time developments in circuit design have led to the introduction of circle systems with smaller canister and tubing volumes, decreased compliance, and lower resistance valves and connectors.

In contrast to the early experience of using older-design adult circles, recent clinical experience using the circle system in pediatric patients has been favorable. In comparison with the Mapleson D or F circuit, the circle is more economical, conserves heat and moisture better, and is easier to scavenge.[1] The resistance of circle systems has been found to be slightly higher than that of a Mapleson D or F system, but not to the extent that it affects the minute ventilation or blood gas homeostasis of spontaneously breathing infants.

The resistance of the current design of circle system has been compared with that of a Mapleson F system.[31] The resistance to breathing is similar in spontaneously breathing older infants. Both have resistances that are significantly less than that of a size 3 or 3.5 mm tracheal tube. Hence both types of circuits appear to be acceptable for short-term spontaneous ventilation for healthy older infants.

In contrast to resistance, the compliance of circle and Mapleson D circuits differs significantly. The compliance of the Mapleson D circuits of several different manufacturers is lower than that of several different circles. The circle compliances differ widely with different types of tubing. The compliance of the system assumes great importance during the controlled ventilation of small infants. The small tidal volumes of the neonate and young infant are dwarfed by the compression volume of some adult circuit/ tubing combinations. As a result, most of the tidal volume delivered by a mechanical ventilator may be used to distend the circuit tubing rather than to ventilate the patient's lungs. The tidal volumes that are delivered by the ventilator are often much greater than predicted based on the patient's weight because of this compression volume. The difference may be so great that tracheal tube obstruction will be difficult to detect using airway pressure manometry. These factors make consistent ventilation more difficult with the circle system than with the Mapleson D or F system. Hence, if circle systems are to be used during mechanical ventilation of an infant, careful monitoring of respiratory parameters, including airway gas analysis and pressure manometry, is essential.

VENTILATORS AND VENTILATION

Most ventilators that are commonly used in the operating room (e.g., Dräger AV-E, Ohmeda 7000/7800 series, Fig. 26-13) were not designed specifically for pediatric use. These ventilators are pneumatically driven, have a double circuit, and are time-cycled, constant-flow generators (see also Chapter 6). Most relatively healthy children can be ventilated in a satisfactory manner using these devices, provided that the adequacy of ventilation is continuously monitored. When ventilating infants and children it is important to note that measurements of tidal volume from the ventilator bellows, or of expired minute volume from spirometers, will not necessarily reflect delivered patient volumes and should be interpreted with extreme caution. The reasons for these discrepancies will be discussed in the next section.

The requirements for the ideal pediatric operating room ventilator may differ somewhat depending upon the patient population encountered. The pediatric patient with cardiopulmonary disease, changing lung compliance, obstructive airways disease, or extreme prematurity will often require a more sophisticated approach to mechanical ventilation than that required for relatively healthy children. The ideal ventilator should be simple, reliable, affordable, and easy to understand and operate. It should be capable of ventilating patients of all ages and sizes, with and without pulmonary disease, and be easily incorporated into whatever anesthetic breathing system is being used. The ventilator should be able to ventilate the patient in a pressure or volume preset mode and be able to administer PEEP. The anesthesiologist should be able to adjust continuously the respiratory parameters between those of an adult and those of a premature newborn.

Practical aspects of ventilating infants and children

Factors that affect tidal volume delivered to the patient. Several factors can make the patient's delivered tidal volume significantly different from that delivered into the circuit by the ventilator. These include compression volume, tracheal tube leak, and augmentation of tidal volume by fresh gas flow. The volume delivered to the patient may be less than or greater than that expected by the anesthesiologist. The variable and unpredictable nature of these discrepancies is a compelling indication for the use of continuous end-tidal carbon dioxide monitoring in pediatric anesthesia.

Compression volume. When a ventilator bellows delivers a tidal volume into a breathing circuit, a portion of that volume will not enter the patient's lungs. This is wasted ventilation, and is partly due to the compression volume.[32]

The compression volume is that volume lost owing both to the compliance of the circuit and the compression of the gases within the circuit. The loss of gas due to distention of the circuit is determined by the volume of the circuit, the circuit compliance, and the peak inflation pressure. Disposable plastic circuits are more distensible than wire-reinforced circuits, and the nondisposable rubber circle system is more distensible than a nondisposable Mapleson D circuit.[1] Breathing circuits expand both in diameter and length when internally pressurized. The ventilator itself may also contribute to the compression volume. An adult ventilator bellows usually has a significantly larger compression volume than a pediatric bellows (4.5 ml/cm H_2O versus 1 to 2.5 ml/cm H_2O).[33]

Volume loss due to compression of gases is a separate entity from that due to circuit distention and is determined by Boyle's law ($P_1 \times V_1 = P_2 \times V_2$). Volume loss from gas compression is therefore solely dependent upon circuit

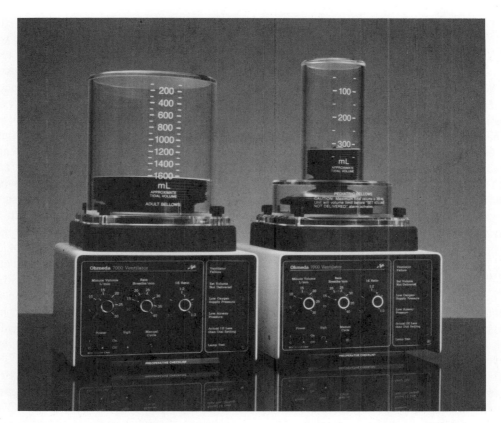

Fig. 26-13. The Ohmeda 7000 anesthesia ventilator. This device is shown with adult *(left)* and pediatric *(right)* bellows attachments.

volume and peak inflation pressure. The total amount of wasted ventilation is determined by the relative compliances and resistances of the circuit and the patient's lungs. A patient with restrictive lung disease and poor pulmonary compliance will receive a smaller tidal volume than a patient with normal lungs for the same inflation pressure. Similarly, for the same inflation pressure, compressible volume becomes increasingly more significant as the desired delivered volume to the patient decreases. This principle is illustrated in the following example.

A ventilator and circuit combination with a compression volume of 5 ml/cm H_2O is adjusted to deliver a tidal volume of 10 ml/kg to the patient at an inflation pressure of 20 cm H_2O. If the patient weighs 20 kg and a 200-ml tidal volume is desired, the total delivered volume must be 300 ml (100 ml compression volume plus 200 ml tidal volume). However, if the patient weighs only 5 kg, and a 50-ml tidal volume is required, at an inflation pressure of 20 cm H_2O, the total delivered volume must be 150 ml (50 ml tidal volume plus 100 ml compression volume). In the latter case, the total volume delivered by the ventilator is three times the patient's actual tidal volume. This example illustrates how tidal volume as indicated on the ventilator bellows may not accurately represent the volume that actually enters the patient's lungs. Furthermore, the disparity between the indicated tidal volume and the delivered tidal

volume becomes greater as patient size decreases. Compressible volume can also be significantly increased by including a humidifier chamber into the circuit. This effect is particularly marked when a heated humidifier chamber is added to a pediatric (compared with an adult) circle system, producing a proportionately larger increase in circuit volume. Compressible volume can be significantly reduced by using circuits that are specifically designed for particular patient sizes. For example, the anesthetic circuits manufactured by Baxter Healthcare Corp. (Deerfield, Ill.) for neonatal, pediatric, and adult use have significantly different compressible volume factors (1.0, 1.2, and 2.5 ml/cm H_2O, respectively). The decreased compliance of the neonatal and pediatric breathing circuits is attributable to the reduced volume of these circuits and the smaller radius of curvature of the tubing which makes them less distensible (Laplace's Law: $P = 2t/r$).

Tracheal tube leaks. The presence of a leak around the tracheal tube results in a portion of the delivered tidal volume being lost during inhalation and exhalation if the airway pressure is greater than the leak pressure of the tracheal tube. *Maintaining constant minute ventilation in the presence of a variable tracheal tube leak can be a particularly difficult problem.* In this situation pressure-preset ventilation has some advantages (see also Chapter 6). An alternative approach is to use a cuffed tube, provided that the leak pressure is carefully adjusted and intermittently monitored.

Tidal volume augmentation by fresh gas flow. Depending on the type of anesthetic breathing system in use, and its fresh gas flow requirements, the tidal volume delivered by a ventilator can be significantly augmented by continuous fresh gas inflow from the anesthesia machine.[34,35] For example, when the fresh gas flow is 5 L/min and the inspiratory time is 0.6 second, the delivered tidal volume will be augmented by 50 ml ([5000/60] × 0.6). The practical implication is that *if the fresh gas flow is altered during the course of anesthesia, a change in minute ventilation is likely to occur that may not be reflected by a change in the ventilator bellows displacement.*[36] (See also Chapter 16, Figs. 16-4, *A* and 16-4, *B*.)

Monitoring ventilation

From the foregoing it can be seen that unpredictable changes in alveolar minute ventilation may occur during anesthesia that may not be detected by monitoring the ventilator bellows excursion. These alterations are likely to have greater physiologic significance in smaller patients. Adequacy of carbon dioxide elimination is the most important end point to monitor during controlled ventilation. Thus, continuously measuring end-tidal carbon dioxide and intermittent arterial blood gas analyses are the most reliable methods of ensuring the adequacy of ventilation of a patient in the operating room.

Exhaled volume measurement. Determining the adequacy of ventilation via the measurement of exhaled volume in small children is difficult. Before the advent of capnometry, adequacy of ventilation was determined by estimating the tidal volume from the ventilator bellows or from expiratory limb spirometry. Measurements of exhaled volume made at the expiratory limb may not accurately reflect the patient's exhaled volume because the spirometer or flow transducer cannot differentiate between gas that returns from expanding the patient's lungs and gas that simply distended the breathing system during positive pressure inspiration. Similarly, gas that is lost from a tracheal tube leak during exhalation will have contributed to the patient's inspiratory volume but will not be measured. Only in the absence of a tracheal tube leak, and if the bellows, circuit, and humidifier compressible volumes are known, is it possible to estimate accurately the patient's delivered volume from expired spirometry.

Ventilation methods used commonly in the operating room

Most operating room ventilators (e.g., Dräger AV-E, Ohmeda 7000/7800 series) are volume preset, flow generators, i.e., stable tidal volume, stable inspiratory flow (see Chapter 6). The combination of inspiratory flow and time then determines the volume that is delivered to the circuit. In effect, the ventilator functions as a constant volume device. Although the device may deliver a constant volume to the patient circuit, the volume delivered to the patient may be somewhat different, and may vary considerably during the course of anesthesia owing to the factors discussed previously. Before the routine use of capnometry, the inability to deliver and measure accurately and consistently a desired patient tidal volume was a significant clinical problem.

Constant flow, time-cycled ventilation without pressure limit. The Narco Air-Shields Ventimeter,[*] Dräger AV-E,[†] and Ohmeda 7000/7800 series[‡] are the most commonly used operating room ventilators (see also Chapter 6). In the Air-Shields Ventimeter the inspiratory time and flow determine the tidal volume (Fig. 26-14). The inspiratory time and the expiratory time are adjusted to determine the respiratory rate and the I:E ratio. Other constant-flow, time-cycled ventilators, such as the Ohmeda 7000/7800 series, differ in the manner in which the I:E ratio and respiratory rate are adjusted, but the principle of operation is similar. A commonly used technique to initiate controlled ventilation of pediatric patients begins with selecting an inspiratory time and rate prior to connecting the patient to the ventilator. The inspiratory flow is set initially at its lowest level and then gradually increased until chest wall movement, inspiratory pressure, and gas entry as determined by auscultation are appropriate. Continuous fine adjustment of minute ventilation is then made according to determinations of end-tidal carbon dioxide. In the past many pediatric anesthesiologists recommended that once an acceptable inspiratory volume was determined, the patient draped, and chest excursion no longer readily visible, it is probably safer to adjust minute ventilation by adjusting the respiratory rate rather than the tidal volume. The presumption was that in the absence of direct observation of chest excursion, adjusting the rate rather than the tidal volume assured that the patient continued to receive an appropriate tidal volume. However, with continuous monitoring of airway pressure, breath sounds, and end-tidal carbon dioxide, and with an understanding of the factors that can affect delivered patient tidal volume, this recommendation may no longer apply.

The use of constant-flow, time-cycled ventilation has the advantage that increases in airway resistance, such as the presence of secretions in the tracheal tube, will be reflected as an increase in airway pressure. Changes in compliance will also produce a change in inflation pressure. In the presence of a variable tracheal tube leak, however, tidal volume will decrease as the leak increases (see Chapter 6).

The use of the pediatric bellows allows easier visualization of smaller excursions, but the tidal volume indicated may still differ significantly from that delivered to the patient. The maximum marked volume on the adult Ohmeda

*Healthdyne, Hatboro, Pa.
†North American Dräger, Inc., Telford, Pa.
‡Ohmeda, Madison, Wis.

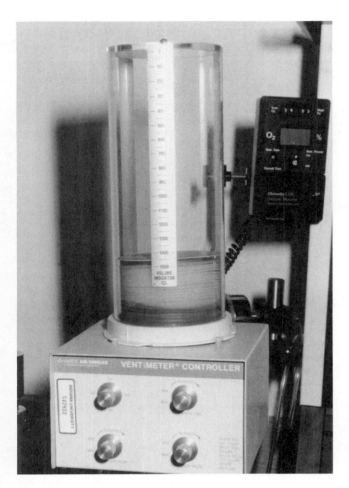

Fig. 26-14. The Narco Air-Shields Ventimeter ventilator. (Courtesy of Healthdyne, Hatboro, Pa.)

bellows is 1600 ml, versus 300 ml on the Ohmeda pediatric bellows (see Fig. 26-13). The discrepancy between indicated and actual delivered tidal volume, due to compression volume, may be less when using a pediatric bellows because of its smaller compression volume compared with that of the adult bellows (e.g., the Ohmeda 7800 adult bellows compliance is 3 ml/cmH$_2$O, versus a pediatric bellows compliance of 1.5 ml/cmH$_2$O).[37] An advantage of using the pediatric bellows with the Dräger AV-E ventilator is that when using the pediatric bellows the driving gas used to compress the bellows is reduced, thus allowing better control of lower inspiratory flow rates.[38]

Constant-flow, time-cycled ventilation with pressure preset (stable inspiratory flow, unstable tidal volume). This method of ventilation allows inspiratory flow to be limited when a preset inspiratory pressure is reached. When this type of ventilation is used the inspiratory flow is usually set at a level that is higher than when a pressure limit is not used. *Thus, the flow to the circuit is limited by the pressure and not by the inspiratory flow set by the operator.* In theory, a wide range of sizes of healthy infants and children can be ventilated by this system with little adjustment to the inspiratory flow. This is because the tidal

volume is determined by pulmonary compliance and resistance and is limited by the preset pressure. By using a preset pressure of between 15 and 20 cm H$_2$O, and providing adequate inspiratory flow, the patient with normal pulmonary compliance and resistance can usually be ventilated safely. Inspiratory time and expiratory time, or I:E ratio and respiratory rate, are adjusted as appropriate for the child. The potential advantages of pressure preset ventilation over constant-flow, time-cycled ventilation without pressure preset include the ability to compensate for a variable degree of leak, and to avoid excessive airway pressure should compliance change abruptly (e.g., the surgeon leaning on the patient's chest). This system will deliver a relatively constant tidal volume in the face of a changing tracheal tube leak, but will deliver a more variable tidal volume in the face of changing pulmonary compliance. A disadvantage of this method of ventilation is that airway pressure will not change in the face of varying lung compliance or tube blockage or leak, all of which are relatively common in pediatric anesthesia practice. However, the volume will change as much or as little as the pressure would in a volume preset machine. Therefore, the tidal volume is now the appropriate variable to monitor. This, however, may be difficult to achieve clinically. Careful attention to the end-tidal carbon dioxide concentration is a satisfactory alternative.

As with volume-controlled ventilation, when using pressure preset ventilation the tidal volume delivered to the patient may be markedly different from that indicated either by the bellows or measured by an expiratory limb spirometer. Adequate ventilation must be assessed by monitoring end-tidal carbon dioxide concentration.

Certain models of the Dräger AV-E standing bellows ventilator can be supplied or retrofitted with a pressure-limiting valve called the Dräger Pressure Limit Control (DPLC). When used in conjunction with the DPLC, the AV-E functions as a time-cycled, pressure preset ventilator. The unit may be used with a pediatric bellows, allowing better visualization of delivered volumes and reducing the compressible volume of the system. With the DPLC, inspiratory pressure is continuously adjustable (Fig. 26-15). The minimum inspiratory pressure possible with this device is 15 cm H$_2$O with a fresh gas flow of 4 L/min. The inspiratory pressure may deviate from that indicated by the DPLC and should always be measured directly. If the pressure limit is reached before the bellows has fully descended, the delivered tidal volume may be significantly less than that indicated by the bellows (see also Chapter 6).

The Ohmeda 7800 is another example of a constant-flow, time-cycled ventilator that may be used in the pressure preset mode. However, there is an important functional difference between the Ohmeda 7800 and the Dräger AV-E when used in the preset pressure mode. When using the Ohmeda 7800, inspiration is terminated when the preset pressure is reached and the ventilator immediately cy-

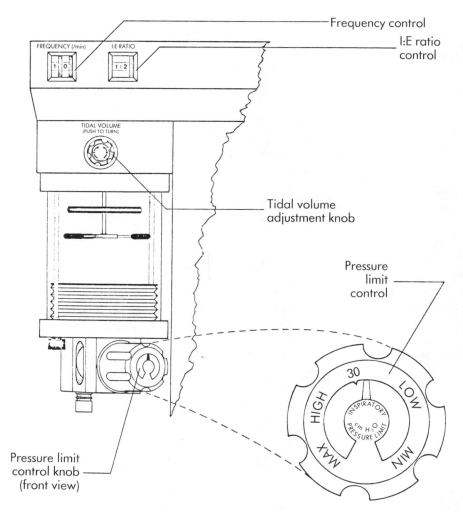

Fig. 26-15. The Dräger Pressure Limit Control. See text for details. (Courtesy of North American Dräger, Telford, Pa.)

cles to expiration. When using the AV-E with the DPLC (i.e., pressure preset), inspiration will continue if the pressure limit is reached before the end of the inspiratory time, because the inspiratory time is determined solely by the ventilator's respiratory rate and I:E ratio settings. In effect, this produces an inspiratory pause at an airway pressure that is determined by the pressure setting on the DPLC. In practical terms, this distinction between these two devices may become important when ventilating newborns and small infants (see below).

Siemens Servo 900C ventilator. The Siemens Servo 900 series of ventilators are pneumatically and electronically controlled time-cycled ventilators. Their flexibility allows constant or nonconstant inspiratory flow patterns and pressure- or volume-controlled ventilation (Fig. 26-16). Primarily designed as an intensive care ventilator, various modes of ventilation are possible and varying amounts of PEEP and CPAP may be applied. Pediatric anesthesiologists working in a tertiary referral center may encounter patients weighing between 500 g and 150 kg, many with significant cardiopulmonary disease. The Sie-

mens system offers several advantages in pediatric anesthetic practice, including the ability to ventilate any size of patient, apply varying degrees of PEEP, deliver very rapid respiratory rates, and operate in either the pressure preset or the volume preset mode. This ventilator is reliable and effective for virtually every patient that the pediatric anesthesiologist is likely to encounter.

However, the Siemens Servo system has a limitation that is very important to the pediatric anesthesiologist. Difficulty may be experienced when this system is used in the manual mode with small patients breathing spontaneously during mask anesthesia. Normally, when using a Mapleson or circle system during mask anesthesia, the anesthesiologist receives tactile and visual feedback from the reservoir bag about the patient's respiratory effort, the degree of leak, and the adequacy of the airway. One is able to see and feel the movement of the reservoir bag during both inspiration and expiration. This is important information, particularly during the induction of anesthesia in patients who are very small or have airway problems. When using the Servo system in the manual mode with an infant

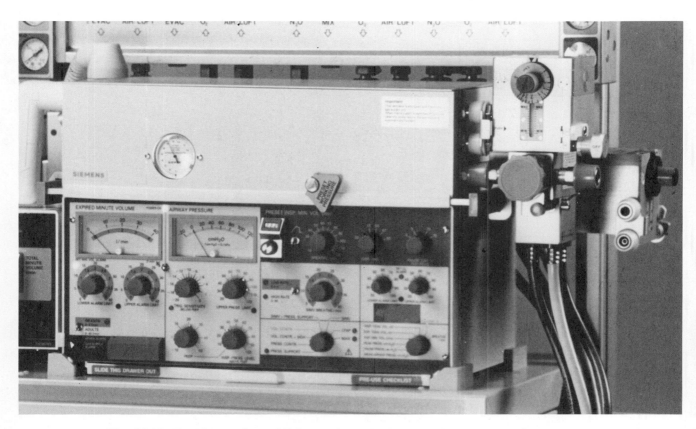

Fig. 26-16. The Siemens Servo 900C control panel. (Courtesy of Siemens-Elema AB, Solna, Sweden.)

breathing spontaneously this information is largely lost. After inspiration the reservoir bag intermittently refills from the gas reservoir bellows. This intermittent filling from the bellows is difficult to distinguish, by touch or visually, from the respiratory effort of the patient, particularly when the patient is very small (<10 kg). The rate of filling depends on the preset minute volume determined by the operator. In addition, during exhalation the expired gas does not return to the reservoir bag but is vented via the exhaust valve. This lack of feedback from the gas delivery system can make an inhalational induction of small infants more difficult. To overcome these problems, at the authors' institution a separate gas supply, blender, and vaporizer supplying a Mapleson D system are used during the induction and emergence phases of anesthesia.

Sechrist Infant Ventilator. Sechrist Infant Ventilator (Sechrist Industries, Anaheim, CA) is an electrically powered, pneumatically operated, continuous-flow, time-cycled ventilator (Fig. 26-17). It is designed specifically for patients weighing less than 10 kg. This device has been described as a "mechanical thumb" and is often used during anesthesia in conjunction with a Mapleson D system. Fresh gas flow is directed from a gas mixing module and humidifier past the patient connection to the exhalation valve (Fig. 26-18). Inflation of the patient's lungs is accomplished by closing the exhalation valve. Exhalation occurs when the exhalation valve is opened. Thus the exha-

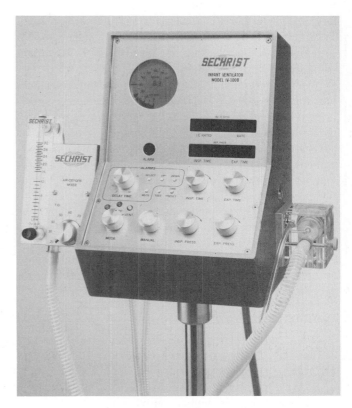

Fig. 26-17. The Sechrist Infant Ventilator. (Courtesy of Sechrist Industries, Inc., Anaheim, Calif.)

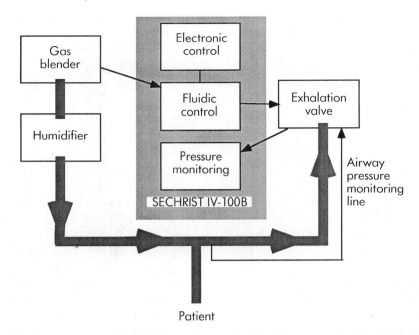

Fig. 26-18. The working principle of the Sechrist Infant Ventilator. Flow is directed from the gas blender via a humidifier to the patient. When the exhalation valve is open the patient's lungs will discharge to the atmosphere via the exhalation valve. Hence the ventilator functions as a "mechanical thumb" or T-piece occluder.

lation valve is the principal active component of this ventilator. The microprocessor controls the inspiratory and expiratory times. Adjustment of the inspiratory and expiratory times determines the respiratory rate and the I:E ratio. Tidal volume is determined by the inspiratory time and inspiratory flow controls, but may also be limited by the inspiratory pressure control.

When the ventilator is used during anesthesia in conjunction with a Mapleson D circuit, tidal volume is augmented by fresh gas flow from the anesthesia machine into the breathing circuit. This ventilator permits delivery of adjustable levels of PEEP and CPAP. This device has several advantages: it has a pressure limit function; it can provide varying amounts of PEEP or CPAP; it provides a continuous display of inspiratory and expiratory time, I:E ratio, respiratory rate, and airway pressure; and rapid respiratory rates may be delivered. However, the total inspiratory flow is limited to the sum of ventilator gas flow and the anesthesia circuit fresh gas flow. The total inspiratory flow available with this device may be insufficient for patients weighing more than 10 kg.

Positive end-expiratory pressure

During general anesthesia several factors may decrease the patient's functional residual capacity (FRC) (Box 26-5). This fall in FRC can lead to airway closure, ventilation/perfusion mismatch, and hypoxemia.[39] It has been demonstrated that the application of 5 cm H_2O PEEP can partially restore FRC and increase oxygenation.[40,41] If

---

> **Box 26-5.   Factors that decrease FRC in infants during the perioperative period**
>
> Decreased intercostal muscle tone
> Loss of diaphragmatic muscle tone
> Abolition of glottic tone/absence of PEEP
> Apnea during intubation

PEEP is applied, airway pressure should be carefully monitored to allow the detection of excessive airway pressure. Ideally, airway pressure should be monitored as close as possible to the tracheal tube. In practice, airway pressure is usually monitored in the expiratory limb of the circuit. It should be noted that the application of PEEP may decrease the tidal volume delivered, depending upon the design of the ventilator.[42] Many anesthesia ventilators (including the Dräger AV-E and Ohmeda 7000/7800 series) with an ascending bellows will continuously apply a minimum of 2 to 3 cm H_2O PEEP. The PEEP is produced by the ventilator relief valve to prevent premature outflow of gas into the scavenging system during exhalation[43] (see also Chapter 6).

Ventilating neonates and very small infants

The healthy newborn has a normal spontaneous respiratory rate of approximately 38 breaths per minute.[44] However, most healthy newborns undergoing anesthesia can be safely ventilated at respiratory rates that are somewhat

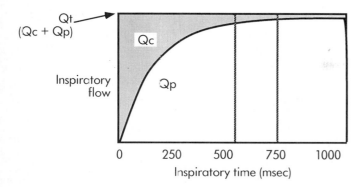

Fig. 26-19. A schematic of the inspiratory flow pattern during constant flow ventilation. The total flow from the ventilator (Q_t) is constant throughout inspiration. The proportion of flow that is spent in distending the anesthesia circuit (Q_c) is large at the start of inspiration and decreases as inspiration continues. Thus, longer inspiratory times may be more effective when the circuit compliance is high compared with that of the patient because the early part of inspiration is spent distending the circuit. (Adapted from Epstein MAF, Epstein RA: Airway flow patterns during mechanical ventilation of infants: A mathematical model, *IEEE Trans Biomed Eng* 26:299-306, 1979.)

lower, such as 20 to 30 breaths per minute.[45,46] Some of the factors determining the adequacy of ventilation of the neonate have been modeled mathematically.[47]

The anesthesia circuit, ventilator bellows, and humidifiers all have significant compliance. During inspiration a portion of the flow delivered by the ventilator (Q_t) is expended in distending the circuit (Q_c), thus the inspiratory flow to the patient (Q_p) will be reduced accordingly ($Q_t = Q_c + Q_p$; Fig. 26-19). This partly explains why very small infants can be ventilated safely with ventilators that have minimum inspiratory flows that exceed those of a spontaneously breathing infant. For example, the Air-Shields Ventimeter has a minimum inspiratory flow of 1.5 L/min, compared with that of 1 L/min for a premature newborn.[9]

The total delivered flow from the ventilator, Q_t, equals the sum of Q_p and Q_c. The disparity between Q_p and Q_t is greatest at the start of inspiration and decreases as inspiration proceeds. During the latter portion of the inspiratory period (e.g., after 360 msec) Q_p approximates Q_t ($Q_p/Q_t = 0.9$) as the circuit is pressurized. Thus, late inspiration is the time when the most effective patient ventilation occurs. However, when the inspiratory time is short, Q_p will be a very small portion of Q_t for a significant proportion of the inspiratory period. However, when the patient is ventilated very rapidly, it should be noted that shorter inspiratory times (e.g., 500 msec) may occasionally be necessary to allow sufficient time for expiration. Therefore, at rapid ventilatory rates with short inspiratory times, significantly higher inspiratory flows and pressures may be required to ventilate the patient effectively. However, when using lower respiratory rates and when inspiratory time is prolonged, a proportionately larger increase in the duration of the later, more effective, period of inspiration occurs. This may explain the apparently paradoxical deterioration in gas exchange that is occasionally observed in small infants when they are ventilated at rapid respiratory rates if the inspiratory time is reduced.

Manual versus mechanical ventilation of neonates and infants. It has been frequently recommended that the neonate or small infant be ventilated by hand rather than mechanically.[48] A potential advantage of manual ventilation is that it would allow the rapid detection of changes in respiratory compliance by the "educated hand" of the pediatric anesthesiologist. In the past, manual ventilation was common owing to the lack of both reliable respiratory monitoring and ventilators suitable for neonates. However, with the advent of pulse oximetry, capnography, routine monitoring of airway pressure, and reliable operating room ventilators, the arguments for manual ventilation are less convincing than they were in the past.

Recent data suggest that even experienced pediatric anesthesiologists are unable to consistently detect large changes in respiratory compliance (e.g., complete occlusion of the tracheal tube) in a test lung ventilated manually using a Mapleson D or pediatric circle system.[49] Smaller changes in compliance than those that went undetected in the study would probably produce clinically significant changes in ventilation and oxygenation in a neonate. It has been postulated that the pressure-volume characteristics of the reservoir bags, and the relatively large compressible volume of many pediatric breathing circuits (compared with the neonate's small tidal volume) made manual detection of compliance changes unpredictable. The study did not address the ability of the "educated hand" to detect leaks from the breathing circuit.

Mechanical ventilation produces more consistent ventilation, and also frees the anesthesiologist's hands to perform other essential tasks. It has been argued that the large compressible volume of the breathing circuit makes mechanical ventilation unpredictable in the neonate, but these arguments also apply to manual ventilation of the neonate.[50,51] When using volume-preset mechanical ventilation the volume delivered to the circuit is constant. Although changes in the patient's compliance may change the tidal volume delivered to the patient, changes in tidal volume will be accompanied by changes in airway pressure, thus enabling the rapid detection of changes in the patient's compliance. Manual ventilation has no advantage over mechanical ventilation for the detection of changes in the patient's compliance, provided that mechanical ventilation is accompanied by continuous measurement of airway pressure, chest excursion, breath sounds, oxygen saturation, and end-tidal carbon dioxide concentration. However, in the case of acute adverse changes in respiratory function it is usual to revert to manual ventilation of the patient to confirm adequate lung inflation and allow breath-to-breath adjustment of ventilation.

Most *healthy* children can be ventilated adequately with ventilators that were primarily designed for adults, provided they are used with appropriate respiratory monitoring. These "adult" devices have the advantage of being familiar to most anesthesiologists, and their operating characteristics are well understood. These devices are safest when the alveolar ventilation is continuously monitored using capnometry, oximetry, airway pressure, exhaled tidal volume, and continuous auscultation of breath sounds. Pressure-limited ventilation and volume-controlled ventilation each have advantages and disadvantages under different circumstances. The operator should be aware that variable tube leaks, tube obstructions, and changes in pulmonary compliance and resistance may have differing presentations and effects depending upon the mode of ventilation.

HUMIDIFICATION

The humidification of inspired gases is of particular importance during anesthesia in infants and children (see also Chapter 7). The safe and precise function of the components of a modern anesthesia machine requires a supply of clean, dry anesthetic gases. The inhalation of dry, cold gases is suboptimal for the patient. Therefore, inhaled gases should be humidified before being delivered to the patient's respiratory tract.

Beneficial effects of humidification

Effective humidification can help to circumvent several problems that are attributed to the breathing of dry gases. Beneficial effects of humidification include the reduction of heat and water loss from the respiratory tract, the prevention of airway damage, and the prevention of inspissation of secretions that could cause tracheal tube obstruction.

Energy and water loss from the respiratory tract. During the course of normal breathing, cold, dry atmospheric air is inhaled, warmed to body temperature, and saturated with water vapor by the time it reaches the distal bronchi. Air fully saturated with water vapor at 37°C contains 44 mg/L of water (absolute humidity 44 mg/L, relative humidity 100%). To humidify inhaled gases, heat and water vapor are transferred from the mucosal lining of the airway. Under normal circumstances, most of the heat and water is returned to the respiratory mucosa as cooling and drying of the patient's gas occurs during expiration. If the upper airway is bypassed by a tracheal tube, significant heat and water loss will occur from the patient if inspired gases are not humidified prior to their administration. Because of the very low specific heat and thermal capacity of dry gas, it is difficult to provide sufficient energy to the patient to prevent intraoperative hypothermia without causing thermal injury to the airway. A 3-kg infant with a minute ventilation of 500 ml/min will expend 0.0035 kCal/min to raise the temperature of cold, dry inspired gases to

body temperature. However, if in addition, another 0.012 Kcal/min are required for the heat of vaporization to saturate the dry inspired gases with water vapor at body temperature,[52] the total amount of energy expended will be ~0.015 kCal/min. This energy expended in warming and humidifying cold anesthetic gases amounts to approximately 10% to 20% of the total energy expenditure of the infant. Similarly, the infant who is not tracheally intubated may also benefit from humidification because minute ventilation, and therefore heat and water loss, is relatively high compared with that of the adult.

Respiratory tract mucociliary dysfunction. The inhalation of dry gases halts mucociliary transport.[53] This is probably secondary to both ciliary paralysis and decreased mucous flow. Decreased humidity causes the viscosity of mucus to increase markedly. Greater than 50% relative humidity is required to allow continued flow of mucus.[54] Providing humidified inspired gases can reduce the incidence of postoperative pulmonary complications in adults.[55] Similar data in pediatric patients are lacking.

Tracheal tube obstruction. Given the small internal diameter of pediatric tracheal tubes, even a small amount of inspissated mucus within the lumen of the tube may produce significant airway obstruction. A small premature infant may require a 2.5-mm internal diameter tracheal tube. These small patients, who desaturate very rapidly and have the smallest tracheal tubes, benefit the most from humidification of inspired gases. No data presently available demonstrates that humidification decreases the incidence of tracheal tube obstruction. Despite this, the clinical impression in the authors' department is that tracheal tube obstruction has become less common since the introduction of routine active humidification of inspired gases.

Methods of providing humidification in pediatric systems

Several methods are available to reduce heat and water loss from the airway during anesthesia. It is interesting to note that the tracheal tube itself may act as a passive heat and moisture exchanger, as the moisture in exhaled gases condenses within the tube and is then added to the inspired gas mixture. However, the humidifying efficiency of the tracheal tube alone is low. Most studies that have measured humidity at the distal end of the tracheal tube during anesthesia demonstrate that, in the absence of either active or passive humidification, the tracheal tube will supply sufficient moisture to produce an inspired relative humidity of 30% at its distal end.[56] This is less than the 50% relative humidity that is reported to be necessary to allow normal mucus flow.

Humidifiers in common use are either *active*, adding exogenous heat and water to the breathing system, or *passive*, conserving and allowing the rebreathing of the patient's endogenous heat and moisture. Alternatively, the use of a circle system with low fresh gas flows and carbon

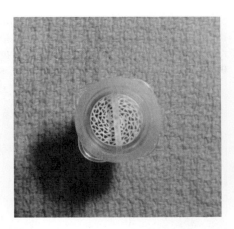 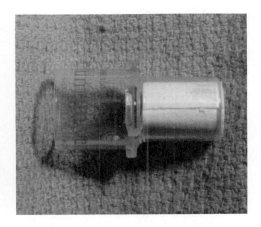

Fig. 26-20. A low-dead-space, high-efficiency pediatric heat and moisture exchanger (Mini Humid-Vent, Gibeck-Dryden Corp, Indianapolis, Ind.)

dioxide absorption will generate heat and humidity that can be inhaled by the patient. Each method of humidification has its specific advantages and disadvantages.

Passive humidification. The simplest method of humidification is passive humidification, using a heat and moisture exchanger (HME). Heat and moisture exchangers do not add heat or water to the inspired gas other than that exhaled by the patient in the preceding breaths. These devices are placed between the tracheal tube and the breathing system. The HME contains an exchange medium with a large surface area. It is simple and has been shown to be effective. Its ability to humidify inspired gas depends upon the ambient conditions. When breathing room air (20°C, 50% relative humidity, 7 mg H_2O/L absolute humidity), HMEs can produce a relative humidity of almost 100% in the inspired gas. When breathing cold, dry anesthetic gases (0 to 20°C, 0% relative humidity) the inspired gas relative humidity may be as low as 60% at 37°C. However, recent improvements in the design of these devices have increased their efficiency. Concerns about the use of these devices in pediatric anesthesia practice relate to the issues of dead space, resistance, and efficiency. Recently, several HMEs have been developed specifically for use in infants. The characteristics of one such device (Mini Humid-Vent, Gibeck-Dryden; Fig. 26-20) have been measured.[57] Although the device has a dead space of 4.2 ml when measured in isolation, when added to the circuit its dead space decreases to 2.7 ml because of the volume occupied by the circuit and tracheal tube connectors. The dead space is likely to be small in relation to the tidal volume (50 ml) of the pediatric patient, for whom this device is recommended. The resistance of the device at gas flows between 2 and 10 L/min approximates that of a 5.0-mm tracheal tube. At a gas flow of 10 L/min the pressure drop across a 3.0 mm tracheal tube was increased from 9.6 cm H_2O to 10.4 cm H_2O by the addition of an HME. The resistance to flow across the HME was increased by 10% to 30% when humidified air was compared with dry air.

In contrast, Rodee et al.[58] determined that the increased work of breathing imposed by HMEs is significant. The Mini Humid-Vent was found to increase the work of breathing by up to 60% when dry, and more when saturated. The authors of that study suggest that the HME be removed from the circuit during spontaneous ventilation. Bissonnette et al.[59] compared the performance of the same HME with that of active humidification in ventilated anesthetized children weighing between 5 kg and 30 kg. These investigators found that while passive humidification was less efficient than active humidification, it was significantly better than no humidification. While the relative humidity of inspired gases with passive humidification was initially only 50%, after 80 minutes of anesthesia the relative humidity of the inspired gases had increased to a level (80%) that was not significantly different from that of active humidification (90%). Passive humidification effectively reduced the mean temperature drop that occurred during surgery from 0.75°C to 0.25°C.

It appears that HMEs are capable of immediately supplying sufficient humidity to prevent airway damage (>50% relative humidity). After 80 minutes of anesthesia their ability to humidify inspired gases is similar to that of an active device. The delay in reaching peak efficiency is related to the time required to saturate the hygroscopic membrane. The manufacturers do not recommend that the membrane be saturated before use.[60] The application of a large amount of water to the HME ("prewetting") may cause a massive rapid release of lithium chloride (the hygroscopic component of some HMEs) into the lung, producing a plasma lithium concentration comparable to that of a therapeutic intravenous injection. Lithium chloride has a very narrow therapeutic range. For the same reason, the manufacturers do not recommend that HMEs be used in combination with active humidification.

Heat and moisture exchangers are effective in reducing heat loss during the perioperative period. Their resistance and dead space appear to be acceptable, especially considering that most infants and children undergoing surgery for an appreciable length of time will be ventilated rather than be allowed to breathe spontaneously. There are at present little data concerning the use of HMEs in patients weighing less than 5 kg, but such devices are undergoing development. The humidification efficiency of HMEs is predicted to be decreased in the presence of a large leak around the tracheal tube because a variable proportion of the exhaled, heat- and moisture-rich gas will bypass the HME.

Active humidification. In many pediatric centers inspired gases are humidified using a heated water humidifier (e.g., Fisher-Paykel, Auckland, New Zealand; Fig. 26-21) for even the shortest procedures in an attempt to prevent energy and water loss from the respiratory tract. The temperature of the inspired gases is continuously monitored to avoid hyperthermia or thermal injury to the respiratory tract. While active humidification may be more efficient than passive humidification, it is more cumbersome and costly. The presence of the humidifier chamber in the breathing system adds significant compressible volume to the circuit. The potential for circuit disconnections is increased because of the additional connections required for both the humidifier chamber and the temperature monitoring equipment. Other potential hazards of humidifiers, particularly with ultrasonic nebulization, include overhydration and increased airway resistance. Ultrasonic nebulization adds small droplets (1 to 10 μm diameter) of unheated water to the airway in the form of an aerosol. Molecular humidification (i.e., heated water bath or HME) simply adds molecular water vapor to the airway (see also Chapters 7 and 16).

Active humidification using the heated water system has the advantages of being applicable to all sizes of patients (including those weighing less than 5 kg), being highly efficient, and avoiding the problems of dead space and resistance encountered with HMEs. Thus, active humidification can be used safely during both controlled and spontaneous ventilation. However, with recent developments in the design of small HMEs many of the advantages of active humidification may soon be less important.

CAPNOGRAPHY AND RESPIRATORY GAS ANALYSIS IN PEDIATRIC PATIENTS

There is no question that capnography has an important role in monitoring the adequacy of alveolar ventilation and fresh gas flow during anesthesia (see also Chapter 8). Capnography is also used to confirm tracheal tube placement and can aid in the diagnosis of several complications occurring during anesthesia, including venous air embolism and malignant hyperthermia. However, there are potential problems in obtaining accurate capnometric data from small children (Table 26-2).

Capnometers can be divided broadly into two groups, mainstream or flow-through devices, and sidestream or aspirating devices (see also Chapter 8). Sidestream devices

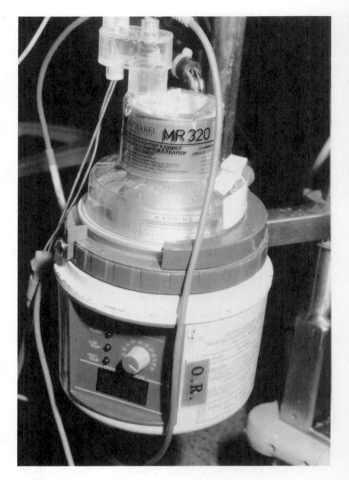

Fig. 26-21. A Fisher-Paykel heated humidifier.

are commonly used in the operating room. Sidestream devices have the advantage of being able to analyze all of the inspired gases, a property that is not presently true of mainstream devices.

The accuracy (defined in this context as the degree to which end-tidal carbon dioxide tensions approximate arterial carbon dioxide tensions) of the sidestream device when used for pediatric patients has been investigated by several groups. Several factors appear to be important. The site of gas sampling from the breathing circuit appears to be important in patients weighing less than 12 kg.[61] When gas is sampled from the distal end of the tracheal tube using a sampling catheter, the accuracy of measurement was improved considerably over measurements made at the tracheal tube circuit connector (proximal sampling). However, distal versus proximal sampling may not affect the accuracy of measurement when a nonrebreathing circuit and ventilator such as a Siemens Servo system is used.[62]

Recently it has been demonstrated that gas need not be sampled from the distal tip of the tracheal tube, but may be sampled with similar accuracy at the point of narrowing of the tracheal tube adapter (Fig. 26-22).[63] When the Mapleson D circuit is used, end-tidal values are often de-

Table 26-2. Techniques to improve accuracy of end-tidal carbon dioxide monitoring in infants and children

Technique	Advantage	Disadvantage
Distal sampling	Decreases dilution by fresh gas flow (FGF)	Requires special sampling port (purchased or made)
Cuffed tube (absence of leak)	Decreases dilution by ambient air in oropharynx	Increases incidence of subglottic stenosis
Sechrist ventilator	Uses low FGF (250 ml/min) and simulates a nonrebreathing system by venturi effect on expiration	Not commonly used in operating rooms
Circle system	Valves isolate FGF to minimize dilution of sample	Valves increase work of breathing in infants who are spontaneously ventilating
Low FGFs	Decreases dilution of expired sample	May increase rebreathing in a Mapleson D or Bain system
Lower sampling rates	Minimizes dilution by FGF	Decreases accuracy by increasing lag time and reducing response time, especially at rapid respiratory rates and low tidal volumes (does not record true carbon dioxide peak)
Long I:E ratios (1:3.5)	Prevents rebreathing	Probably not significant
Controlled ventilation	Increases tidal volume relative to FGF	Prevents weaning from mechanical ventilation
Discontinuation of FGF during sampling	Prevents dilution of sample	Interrupts normal ventilation
Mainstream capnometer	Prevents plugging of the sampling catheter with secretions or humidity; decreases response time; minimally affected by FGFs	Adds dead space and weight; patient must be tracheally intubated

Adapted from Dubose R: *Pediatric equipment and monitoring*. In Bell C, Hughes C, Oh T, editors: *The pediatric anesthesia handbook*, St. Louis, 1991, Mosby–Year Book.

creased when compared with arterial values. The high fresh gas flow required in these circuits dilutes the end-expired carbon dioxide, thereby artifactually lowering the end-tidal carbon dioxide reading. However, when using this anesthesia breathing system the carbon dioxide "dilution" effect may also be reduced when certain ventilators, such as the Sechrist Infant Ventilator, are used.[64] The Sechrist Infant Ventilator aspirates expired gas from the circuit during expiration using a venturi device. The purpose of this device is to reduce unintentional PEEP caused by the high expiratory resistance of the ventilator.

The sampling rate of sidestream capnometers may variably affect their accuracy. High gas sampling rates (>250 ml/min) may exaggerate the end-expiratory dilution effect by entraining fresh gas and diluting expired carbon dioxide. On the other hand, low sampling rates (<100 ml/min) may prolong the response time of the capnometer such that the ability to display a valid waveform at rapid respiratory rates is lost.[65]

Mainstream capnometers have been compared with sidestream analyzers in children. The investigators found them to be as accurate as distally sampling sidestream analyzers and considerably more accurate than proximally sampling sidestream analyzers.[66] Presently available mainstream analyzers measure only carbon dioxide.

In general, the accuracy of sidestream measurements is reduced when used with small infants, in a partial rebreathing system requiring high fresh gas flows, with very high or very low gas sampling rates, and by the presence

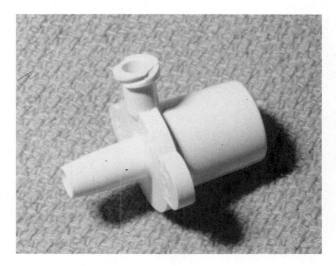

Fig. 26-22. A low dead-space tracheal tube connector with a gas sampling port.

of lung disease (see also Chapter 8). Neonatal lung disease is a situation in which measurements of end-tidal carbon dioxide do not accurately reflect arterial carbon dioxide.[67] Patients with cyanotic heart disease having either reduced pulmonary blood flow or mixing lesions will also tend to have reduced end-tidal carbon dioxide values when compared with arterial measurements.[68] The author of that study emphasizes that in order for capnometry to be useful as a monitor of trend it is important that the arterial-to-end-tidal carbon dioxide difference remains constant. Unfortunately, patients with cyanotic heart disease may have variations in both their shunt fraction and dead-space/tidal volume ratios during anesthesia and surgery. These variations will produce a variable arterial-to-end-tidal carbon dioxide difference, thereby reducing the utility of capnometry, even as a monitor of trend, in these patients.

Despite the fact that expired carbon dioxide measurement may not always accurately reflect arterial carbon dioxide tension in children, it does appear to be very useful as a trend monitor in patients without cyanotic heart disease and has an extremely important part to play in improving the safety of pediatric anesthesia.

BLOOD PRESSURE DETERMINATION

Periodic blood pressure determination is an essential part of monitoring during anesthesia.[69] A variety of techniques and equipment are available[70] (see also Chapter 13). All noninvasive forms of blood pressure determination depend in part on a snugly fitting cuff containing an air-filled bladder that can be inflated to controlled pressures. The American Heart Association has developed recommendations for indirect blood pressure determination, including cuff sizes.[71] The width of the inflatable bladder of the cuff should be 0.4 times the circumference of the extremity. The length of the bladder should be at least twice its width to cover at least 80% of the extremity circumference. Cuffs that are too narrow will result in an overestimation of the blood pressure, while cuffs that are too wide will underestimate the blood pressure.[72,73] Given the same degree of mismatch, cuffs that are somewhat too wide will result in less error than cuffs that are too narrow.[74] As a result, a series of blood pressure cuffs of various sizes must be available for the accurate noninvasive determination of blood pressure in pediatric patients.

Most methods of indirect blood pressure determination depend on the occlusion of blood flow combined with some method of detecting and analyzing the return of the arterial flow. Manual methods of detecting this flow include flush, palpation, and auscultation. Some care must be taken when using auscultation in infants and children, as the pressure of the stethoscope head may result in artifactual Korotkoff-like sounds.[71]

Doppler ultrasound detection of arterial flow is a useful method of determining systolic blood pressure even in small infants.[75] One commonly used unit is battery powered, and has an ultrasonic emitter and detector capable of identifying arterial blood flow and converting that information into an audible sound (Parks Medical Electronics, Inc. Beaverton, Oreg.) The return of arterial flow with the onset of systole is easily recognized and correlates well with both auscultatory assessment and intraarterial pressure measurement.[75,76]

Ultrasonic blood pressure determination has several advantages. It can be utilized even in hypovolemic patients and does not require a regular heart rate. It provides a method of beat-to-beat confirmation of cardiac contraction. A blood pressure determination can be obtained rapidly with minimal effort once the monitor has been positioned and secured. However, it has two primary limitations. It results in some additional room noise, and it requires some operator action to obtain each value.

Using the pulse oximeter in infants to detect the return of arterial flow has also been evaluated.[77] Blood pressures obtained with the pulse oximeter tend to be lower than those obtained by Doppler flow assessment. Moreover, if the arterial flow is occluded for any but a brief period, the pulse oximeter may shift to a search mode and not detect the initial few pulses. Korotkoff sound detection can also be used to determine systolic pressure.

Most automated noninvasive blood pressure determining systems use an oscillometric method.[78] The oscillometric method uses a rapid inflation of the blood pressure cuff until the artery is occluded followed by incremental reductions in cuff pressure. As arterial blood flow resumes, oscillations in the cuff pressure occur, indicating systole. Maximal oscillations appear to correlate with mean arterial pressure, with dampening of the oscillations indicating diastole.

Noninvasive blood pressure devices that use an oscillometric method are available from several manufacturers. The Dinamap unit (Device for Indirect Noninvasive Automated Mean Arterial Pressure, Critikon Inc., Tampa, Fla.) was the first type of this device and has continued to be investigated in a variety of clinical settings.[72,79-84] The Dinamap provides a safe, easy, method of periodic automated blood pressure determination in pediatric patients, including neonates. Individual readings may be inaccurate but most investigations have reported the accuracy to be within 5 mm Hg of the actual value.[78] Accuracy may decrease in severely ill patients. The method does require several heart beats to determine the blood pressure value. As a result, it cannot be applied in situations where beat-to-beat information is needed and may fail when the heart rhythm is irregular.

It is important to recognize that whatever method is used to determine the blood pressure, the value must be compared with the expected values for a patient of that age. Various tables of normal values are available in standard texts and other sources.[85-87]

ELECTROCARDIOGRAPHIC MONITORING

The electrocardiogram (ECG) is an excellent, easily positioned, noninvasive monitor of heart rate and rhythm (see also Chapter 14). Apart from sinus bradycardia and tachycardia, rhythm changes are not common in pediatric patients. Premature atrial and ventricular contractions, junctional rhythms, and respiratory variations are seen on occasion. The rhythm changes generally relate to some aspect of the ventilatory, metabolic, anesthetic, or surgical management rather than to a primary cardiac event. They can generally be identified using standard limb lead electrode positions, although special leads may be helpful in some instances.[88]

While the ECG is a very useful monitor of heart rate and rhythm, it can continue to be normal even in the presence of moderate to severe circulatory or ventilatory abnormalities. Indeed, the ECG can appear normal (at least briefly) without systemic perfusion. As a result, additional monitors must be used to supplement the ECG to assess the adequacy of systemic perfusion.

Pediatric electrocardiographic monitoring requires equipment capable of processing higher frequency signals.[89] At a minimum, the equipment must be able to identify individual heart beats and provide accurate rate analy-

Table 26-3. Common sources of inaccurate saturations (SpO_2) obtained using pulse oximetry (See also Chapter 11)

Type of interference	Cause	Solution
Excessive ambient light	• Operating room light • Bilirubin lights • Bright fluorescent lighting • Infrared heating lamps • Sunlight • Xenon surgical lamps	• Cover sensor with opaque material (e.g., blanket, foil)
Optical shunt	• Too large a sensor allows light to reach the sensor without passing through a pulsatile bed	• Sensor must be completely adherent to skin and be of the appropriate size
Optical cross talk	• Multiple sensors too close to one another	• Cover each sensor with opaque material or separate sensors (one per extremity)
Movement artifact	• Shivering • Active child	• ECG pulse rate must correlate with that displayed by the oximeter before credence can be given to oximeter SpO_2 reading • Move the probe to a more central location (ear vs. finger) • Change the oximeter mode to a longer averaging time
Absorption of light by nonhemoglobin sources	• IV dyes • Nail polish • Bilirubin	• Removal of nail polish • Verify readings with laboratory co-oximetry
Electrical interference	• Usually caused by electrocautery; can be affected by 60-Hz interference	• 60-cycle interference may be improved by changing the plug to another outlet • Some machines have built-in mechanisms to decrease interference by cautery
Low perfusion	• Cold extremities • Decreased cardiac output • Peripheral vasoconstriction	• Warm extremities • Use of inotropic agents or vasodilators • Use of a more central location for probe site (tongue or ear)
Active venous bed	• Right heart failure • Tricuspid regurgitation	• Using an oximeter with visual display of plethysmograph waveform may help interpretation
Altered hemoglobin	Hemoglobin F: • Oximeter remains in the range of acceptable accuracy Hemoglobin S: • Possibly accurate if oxygenated; probably very inaccurate in crisis Methemoglobin: • R = 1.0, S_pO_2 = 85% (see Chapter 11) Carboxyhemoglobin: • Falsely elevated S_pO_2	• Verify readings with laboratory co-oximetry

Adapted from Dubose R: *Pediatric equipment and monitoring*. In Bell C, Hughes C, Oh T, editors: *The pediatric anesthesia handbook*, St Louis, 1991, Mosby–Year Book.

sis. Sampling frequency is particularly important for digitized, diagnostic (12-lead) ECG analysis.[90] Normal values for QRS amplitudes can vary depending on the frequency of sampling in digitized systems, because slower sampling frequencies may miss the peak QRS amplitudes.[90,91]

Electrocardiographic monitoring for ST changes is of limited use during most pediatric anesthesia since cardiac ischemia is unusual in pediatric patients. However, it can occur in some circumstances.[92] Kawasaki disease is an acute exanthematous condition usually seen in infants and children less than 5 years of age.[93] The illness is associated with coronary artery aneurysms in 20% to 25% of patients. These aneurysms generally resolve over time, but the lesions may become stenotic. Cardiac ischemia is well recognized in these patients and appropriate electrocardiographic monitoring is indicated perioperatively.[94] Other pediatric clinical situations in which cardiac ischemia may occur include surgery involving the coronary arteries, congenital coronary artery abnormalities, and systemic air embolism.

PULSE OXIMETRY

Hypoxemia is a major concern during any anesthesia procedure. Its incidence is increased during anesthesia administered to children age 2 years and younger.[95] Pulse oximetry provides a reliable method to detect hypoxemia prior to the time it is detected clinically (see also Chapter 11).[96] While pulse oximetry values may change several seconds after the arterial saturation changes,[97] it is a clinically rapid detector of changes in oxygen saturation.

Pulse oximetry is applicable to all pediatric patients, including neonates.[98,99] It has replaced transcutaneous oxygen tension measurement for most applications. However, pediatric patients present several problems for pulse oximetry measurement. The smaller patients generally require specifically designed probes. The probes must allow the emitter and detector portions of the probe to face each other across some pulsatile bed. Careful attention to probe placement is essential. Oximetry during anesthesia induction and emergence can also be difficult as the probes may move with the patient's movements. The effect of the presence of fetal hemoglobin (HbF) on pulse oximetry has not been fully elucidated but it appears to be minimal.[100] Common sources of inaccurate SpO_2 values are summarized in Table 26-3.

Unlike adult patients, hyperoxia is of concern in neonates with immature retinas because elevations in arterial oxygen tension are associated with the development of retinopathy of prematurity. The upper limit of desirable oxygenation varies from infant to infant depending on a variety of factors, including postconceptual age and the clinical stability of the infant. In infants with a patent ductus arteriosus, the pulse oximetry probe should be located at a site that indicates preductal saturation.[101] Typical upper limits for SpO_2 in the stable preterm infant are 90% to 95%.[102] No matter what number is selected for the upper limit, the value lies in the flat portion of the oxyhemoglobin dissociation curve where large changes in oxygen tension occur with small changes in hemoglobin saturation. While pulse oximetry can be used to detect hyperoxia in this setting, its performance is not optimal.[100,102] Nonetheless, pulse oximetry is a valuable aid to the anesthesiologist caring for any patient, particularly the neonate, infant, and young child.[103]

REFERENCES

1. Rasch DK, Bunegin L, Ledbetter J, et al: Comparison of circle absorber and Jackson-Rees systems for paediatric anaesthesia, *Can J Anaesth* 35:25-30, 1988.
2. Byrick RJ, Respiratory compensation during spontaneous ventilation with the Bain circuit, *Can Anaes Soc J* 27:96-105, 1980.
3. Olsson AK, Lindhal SGE, Pulmonary ventilation, CO_2 response and inspiratory drive in spontaneously breathing young infants during halothane anaesthesia, *Acta Anaesthesiol Scand* 30:431-437, 1986.
4. Charlton AJ, Lindhal SGE, Hatch DJ: Ventilatory responses of children to changes in dead space volume, *Br J Anaesth* 57:562-568, 1985.
5. Keens TG, Bryan AC, Levison H, et al: Developmental patterns of muscle fiber types in human ventilatory muscles, *J Appl Physiol* 44:909-913, 1978.
6. Scott CB, Nickerson BG, Sargent CW, et al: Developmental pattern of maximal transdiaphragmatic pressure in infants during crying, *Pediatr Res* 17:707-709, 1983.
7. Reynolds RN: Acid-base equilibrium during cyclopropane anesthesia and operation in infants, *Anesthesiology* 27:127-131, 1966.
8. Todres ID, Firestone S: *Neonatal emergencies.* In Ryan JF, Todres ID, Coté CJ, editors: *A practice of anesthesia for infants and children,* Orlando, Fla, 1986, Grune & Stratton.
9. Fisher DM: *Anesthesia equipment for pediatrics.* In Gregory GA, editor: *Pediatric anesthesia,* New York, 1990, Churchill Livingstone, p 470.
10. Koka BV, Jeon IS, Andre JM, et al: Post intubation croup in children, *Anesth Analg* 56:501-505, 1977.
11. Cohen MM, Cameron CB: Should you cancel the operation when a child has an upper respiratory tract infection? *Anesth Analg* 72:282-288, 1991.
12. Ring WH, Adair JC, Elwyn RA: A new pediatric endotracheal tube, *Anesth Analg* 54:273-274, 1975.
13. Black AE, Mackersie AM: Accidental bronchial intubation with RAE tubes, *Anaesthesia* 46:42-43, 1991.
14. Ayre P: Anaesthesia for intracranial operation: a new technique, *Lancet* 1:561-563, 1937.
15. Rees GJ: Anaesthesia in the newborn, *Br Med J* 1:1419, 1950.
16. Steward DJ: *Manual of pediatric anesthesia,* New York, 1985, Churchill Livingstone, p 57.
17. Bruce W: *Anesthetic breathing systems.* In Scurr C, Feldman S, Soni N, editors: *Scientific foundations of anesthesia,* Oxford, 1990, Heinemann, p 673.
18. Johnsson LO, Zetterstrom H: Flow pattern and respiratory characteristics during halothane anaesthesia, *Acta Anaesthesiol Scand* 29:309-314, 1985.
19. Rose DK, Byrick RJ, Froese AB: Carbon dioxide elimination during spontaneous ventilation with a modified Mapleson D system: studies in a lung model, *Can Anaesth Soc J* 25:353-365, 1978.
20. Nightingale DA, Richards CC, Glass A: An evaluation of rebreathing in a modified T-piece system during controlled ventilation of anaesthetized children, *Br J Anaesth* 37:762-771, 1965.
21. Hatch DJ, Miles R, Wagstaff M: An anaesthetic scavenging system for paediatric and adult use, *Anaesthesia* 35:496-499, 1980.

22. Bain JA, Spoerel WE: A streamlined anaesthetic system. *Can Anaesth Soc J* 19:426-435, 1972.
23. Hannallah R, Rosales JK: A hazard connected with the use of the Bain circuit: a case report, *Can Anaesth Soc J* 21:511-513, 1974.
24. Pethick SL: *Can Anaesth Soc J* 22:115, 1975 (letter to the editor).
25. Berge JA, Gramstad L, Bodd E: Safety testing the Bain circuit: A new test adaptor, *Eur J Anaesthesiol* 8:309-310, 1991.
26. Seed RF: A test for coaxial circuits, *Anaesthesia* 32:676, 1977 (letter).
27. Voss TJV: Dead space in paediatric anaesthetic apparatus, *Br J Anaesth* 35:454-460, 1963.
28. Norman J, Adams AP, Sykes MK: Rebreathing with the Magill attachment, *Anaesthesia* 23:75-81, 1968.
29. Adriani J, Griggs T: Rebreathing in pediatric anesthesia: recommendations and descriptions of improvements in apparatus, *Anesthesiology* 14:337-347, 1953.
30. Stephen CR, Slater HM: Agents and techniques employed in pediatric anesthesia, *Anesth Analg* 20:254, 1950.
31. Conterato JP, Lindahl SGE, Meyer DM, et al: Assessment of spontaneous ventilation in anesthetized children with use of a pediatric circle or a Jackson-Rees system, *Anesth Analg* 69:484-490, 1989.
32. Coté CJ, Petkau AJ, Ryan JF, et al: Wasted ventilation measured with eight anesthetic circuits with and without inline humidification, *Anesthesiology* 59:442-446, 1983.
33. Binda RE, Cook DR, Fischer CG: Advantages of infant ventilators over adapted adult ventilators in pediatrics, *Anesth Analg* 55:769-772, 1976.
34. Ghani GA: Fresh gas flow affects minute volume during mechanical ventilation, *Anesth Analg* 63:619, 1984 (letter).
35. Scheller MS, Jones BL, Benumof JL: The influence of fresh gas flow and *I:E* ratio on tidal volume and arterial Pco₂ in mechanically ventilated surgical patients, *J Cardiothorac Anesth* 3:564-567, 1989.
36. Aldrete JA, Castillo RA, Bradley EL: Changes in fresh gas flow affect the tidal volume delivered by anesthesia ventilators, *Anesth Analg* 65:S4, 1986 (abstract).
37. Ohmeda 7800 ventilator operation and maintenance manual. Madison, Wis, 1990, Ohmeda, A Division of BOC Health Care, Inc.
38. North American Dräger. Pediatric bellows operator's instruction manual. Telford, Pa, 1988, North American Dräger, Inc.
39. Mansell A, Bryan C, Levison H: Airway closure in children, *J Appl Physiol* 33:711-714, 1972.
40. Katayama M, Motoyama EK: Respiratory mechanics in children under general anesthesia with and without PEEP, *Anesthesiology* 61:A514, 1984 (abstract).
41. Motoyama EK, Brinkmeyer SD, Mutich RL, et al: Reduced FRC in anesthetized children: effects of low PEEP, *Anesthesiology* 57:A418, 1983 (abstract).
42. Mukkada TJ, Khathiwada S, Fernandez J, et al: Effect of positive end expiratory pressure on tidal volume, *Anesthesiology* 69:A269, 1988 (abstract).
43. Eisenkraft JB: *Anesthesia delivery system.* In Rogers MC, Tinker JH, Covino BG, et al: *Principles and practice of anesthesiology,* St. Louis, 1992, Mosby–Year Book.
44. Cook CD, Sutherland JM, Segal S, et al: Studies of respiratory physiology in the newborn infant. III. Measurements of mechanics of respiration, *J Clin Invest* 36:440-448, 1957.
45. Hatch DJ, Sumner E: *Post-operative care.* In Hatch DJ, Sumner E, editors: *Neonatal anesthesia and perioperative care,* London, 1986, Edward Arnold.
46. Smith PC, Schach E, Daily WJR: Mechanical ventilation of newborn infants, *Anesthesiology* 37:498-502, 1972.
47. Epstein MAF, Epstein RA: Airway flow patterns during mechanical ventilation of infants: a mathematical model, *IEEE Trans Biomed Eng* 26:299-306, 1979.
48. Steward DJ: *Pediatric anesthetic techniques and procedures.* In Steward DJ, editor: *Manual of pediatric anesthesia,* ed 2, New York, 1985, Churchill Livingstone, p 59.
49. Spears RS, Yeh A, Fisher DM, et al: The "educated hand:" can anesthesiologists assess changes in neonatal pulmonary compliance manually? *Anesthesiology* 75:693-696, 1991.
50. Picca SM: Mechanical versus manual ventilation of the lungs of infants in the operating room. *Anesthesiology* 76:479, 1992 (reply).
51. Steward DJ: *Anesthesiology* 76:479, 1992 (letter).
52. Ryan JF, Vacanti FX: *Temperature regulation.* In Ryan JF, Todres ID, Coté CJ, editors: *A practice of anesthesia for infants and children,* Orlando, Fla, 1986, Grune & Stratton, pp 19-23.
53. Dalham T: Mucous flow and ciliary activity in the trachea of rats and rats exposed to respiratory irritant gases, *Acta Physiol Scand* 123:36, 1956.
54. Forbes AR: Humidification and mucous flow in the intubated trachea, *Br J Anaesth* 45:118, 1973.
55. Chalon J, Patel C, Ali M, et al: Humidity and the anesthetized patient, *Anesthesiology* 50:195-198, 1979.
56. Bissonnette B, Sessler DI, LaFlamme P: Passive and active inspired gas humidification in infants and children, *Anesthesiology* 71:350-354, 1989.
57. Jones BR, Ozaki GT, Benumof JL, et al: Airway resistance caused by a pediatric heat and moisture exchanger, *Anesthesiology* 69:A786, 1988 (abstract).
58. Rodee WD, Banner MJ, Gravenstein N: Variation in imposed work of breathing with heat and moisture exchangers, *Anesth Analg* 72:S226, 1991 (abstract).
59. Bissonnette B, Sessler DI: Passive or active inspired gas humidification increases thermal steady state temperatures in anesthetized infants, *Anesth Analg* 69:783-787, 1989.
60. Gibeck-Dryden corporation: Personal communication,
61. Badgwell JM, McLeod ME, Lerman J, et al: End-tidal Pco₂ measurements sampled at the distal and proximal ends of the endotracheal tube in children, *Anesth Analg* 66:959-964, 1987.
62. Badgwell JM, Heavner JE, May WS, et al: End-tidal Pco₂ monitoring in infants and children ventilated with either a partial-rebreathing or a non-rebreathing circuit, *Anesthesiology* 66:405-410, 1987.
63. Halpern L, Bissonnette B: A new endotracheal tube connector for sampling end-tidal CO₂ in infants. *Anesthesiology* 75:A930, 1991 (abstract).
64. Hillier SC, Badgwell JM, McLeod ME, et al: Accuracy of end-tidal measurements using a sidestream capnometer in infants and children ventilated with the Sechrist infant ventilator, *Can J Anaesth* 37:318-321, 1990.
65. Gravenstein N: Capnometry in infants should not be done at lower sampling flow rates, *J Clin Monit* 5:63-64, 1989.
66. Hillier SC, Lerman J: Mainstream vs. sidestream capnography in anesthetized infants and children, *Anesthesiology* 71:A357, 1989 (abstract).
67. McEvedy BAB, McLeod ME, Mulera M, et al: End-tidal, transcutaneous, and arterial Pco₂ measurements in critically ill neonates: a comparative study, *Anesthesiology* 69:112-116, 1988.
68. Burrows FA: Physiologic deadspace, venous admixture, and the arterial to end-tidal carbon dioxide difference in infants and children undergoing cardiac surgery, *Anesthesiology* 70:219-225, 1989.
69. American Society of Anesthesiologists: *Standards for basic intraoperative monitoring,* Park Ridge, Ill, 1990, American Society of Anesthesiologists.
70. Sanford TJ Jr, Jones BR, Smith NT: Noninvasive blood pressure measurement, *Anesth Clin North Am* 6:721-741, 1988.
71. Frohlich ED, Grim CP, Labarthe DR, et al: Recommendations for human blood pressure determination by sphygmomanometers: report of a special task force appointed by the steering committee, American Heart Association, *Circulation* 77:502A-514A, 1988 (abstracts).
72. Kimble KJ, Darnall RA Jr, Yelderman M, et al: An automated oscillometric technique for estimating mean arterial pressure in critically ill newborns, *Anesthesiology* 54:423-425, 1981.
73. Okahata S, Kamiya T: Influencing factors on indirect measurement of blood pressure in children, *Jpn Circ J* 51:1400-1403, 1987.
74. Geddes LA, Whistler SJ: The error in indirect blood pressure measurement with the incorrect size of cuff, *Am Heart J* 96:4-8, 1978.

75. Gordon LS, Johnson PR Jr, Penido JR, et al: Systolic and diastolic blood pressure measurements by transcutaneous Doppler ultrasound in premature infants in critical care nurseries and at closed-heart surgery, *Anesth Analg* 53:914-918, 1974.

76. Reder RF, Dimich I, Cohen ML, et al: Evaluating indirect blood pressure measurement techniques: a comparison of three systems in infants and children, *Pediatrics* 62:326-330, 1978.

77. Wallace CT, Baker JD III, Alpert CC, et al: Comparison of blood pressure measurement by Doppler and by pulse oximetry techniques, *Anesth Analg* 66:1018-1019, 1987.

78. Ramsey M: Blood pressure monitoring: automated oscillometric devices, *J Clin Monit* 7:56-67, 1991.

79. Cullen PM, Dye J, Hughes DG: Clinical assessment of the neonatal Dinamap 847 during anesthesia in neonates and infants, *J Clin Monit* 3:229-234, 1987.

80. Dellagrammaticas HD, Wilson AJ: Clinical evaluation of the Dinamap non-invasive blood pressure monitor in pre-term neonates, *Clin Phys Physiol Meas* 2:271-276, 1979.

81. Friesen RH, Lichtor JL: Indirect measurement of blood pressure in neonates and infants utilizing an automatic noninvasive oscillometric monitor, *Anesth Analg* 60:742-745, 1981.

82. Park MK, Menard SM: Normative oscillometric blood pressure values in the first 5 years in an office setting, *Am J Dis Child* 143:860-864, 1989.

83. Ramsey M: Noninvasive automatic determination of mean arterial pressure, *Med Biol Eng Comput* 17:11-18, 1979.

84. Wareham JA, Haugh LD, Yeager SB, et al: Prediction of arterial blood pressure in the premature neonate using the oscillometric method, *Am J Dis Child* 141:1108-1110, 1987.

85. Burke GL, Voors AW, Shear CL, et al: Blood pressure, *Pediatrics* 80(suppl):784-788, 1987.

86. De Sweit M, Fayers P, Shinebourne EA: Systolic blood pressure in a population of infants in the first year of life: the Brompton study, *Pediatrics* 65:1028-1035, 1980.

87. Nielsen PE, Clausen LR, Olsen CA, et al: Blood pressure measurement in childhood and adolescence: international recommendations and normal limits of blood pressure, *Scand J Clin Lab Invest Suppl* 192:7-12, 1989.

88. Greeley WP, Kates RA, Bushman GA, et al: Intraoperative esophageal electrocardiography for dysrhythmia analysis and therapy in pediatric cardiac surgical patients, *Anesthesiology* 65:669-672, 1986.

89. Weinfurt PT: Electrocardiographic monitoring: an overview, *J Clin Monit* 6:132-138, 1990.

90. Garson A Jr: Clinically significant differences between the "old" analog and the "new" digital electrocardiograms, *Am Heart J* 114:194-197, 1987.

91. Macfarlane PA, Coleman EN, Pomphrey EO, et al: Normal limits of the high-fidelity pediatric ECG, *J Electrocardiol* 22(suppl):162-168, 1989.

92. Bell C, Rimar S, Barash P: Intraoperative ST-segment changes consistent with myocardial ischemia in the neonate: a report of three cases, *Anesthesiology* 71:601-604, 1989.

93. Committee on Infectious Diseases, American Academy of Pediatrics: *Report of the Committee on Infectious Diseases, 1991*, Elk Grove Village, Ill, 1991, American Academy of Pediatrics, pp 282-286.

94. McNiece WL, Krishna G: Kawasaki disease: a disease with anesthetic implications, *Anesthesiology* 58:269-271, 1983.

95. Coté CJ, Goldstein EA, Coté MA, et al: A single-blind study of pulse oximetry in children, *Anesthesiology* 68:184-188, 1988.

96. Coté CJ, Rolf N, Liu LMP, et al: A single-blind study of combined pulse oximetry and capnography in children, *Anesthesiology* 74:980-987, 1991.

97. Severinghaus JW, Naifeh KH: Accuracy of response of six pulse oximeters to profound hypoxia, *Anesthesiology* 67:551-558, 1987.

98. Deckardt R, Steward DJ: Noninvasive arterial hemoglobin oxygen saturation versus transcutaneous oxygen tension monitoring in the preterm infant, *Crit Care Med* 12:935-939, 1984.

99. Hay WW Jr, Brockway JM, Eyzaguirre M: Neonatal pulse oximetry: accuracy and reliability, *Pediatrics* 83:717-722, 1989.

100. Bucher H-U, Fanconi S, Baeckert P, et al: Hyperoxemia in newborn infants: detection by pulse oximetry, *Pediatrics* 84:226-230, 1989.

101. Dimich I, Singh PP, Adell A, et al: Evaluation of oxygen saturation monitoring by pulse oximetry in neonates, *Can J Anaesth* 38:985-988, 1991.

102. Kelleher JF: Pulse oximetry, *J Clin Monit* 5:37-62, 1989.

103. Cohen DE, Downes JJ, Raphaely RC: What difference does pulse oximetry make? *Anesthesiology* 68:181-183, 1988 (editorial).

Chapter 27

ANESTHESIA EQUIPMENT IN REMOTE HOSPITAL LOCATIONS

Cindy W. Hughes, M.D.
Charlotte Bell, M.D.

REMOTE MONITORING

Familiarity with anesthesia equipment, as well as with basic monitoring principles, is vital to the successful administration of anesthesia outside the operating room (OR). It should be determined well in advance what equipment is essential for the safe conduct of anesthesia in parts of the hospital remote from the OR suite. Thought must also be given to back-up systems and the minimum essential equipment that will suffice should all else fail. An appreciation of the technical problems related to anesthesia is only half the battle. Monitoring in certain extreme environments (i.e., magnetic resonance imaging [MRI] and extracorporeal shockwave lithotripsy [ESWL] requires an understanding of the underlying principles of the techniques in order to select appropriate equipment and safely monitor the patient.

The number of procedures performed outside the operating room has risen sharply over the past decade. This is mainly due to major technical advances in diagnostic imaging (computerized tomography [CT], MRI and the aggressive pursuit of less invasive therapeutic techniques, such as lithotripsy, angioplasty, embolization, and umbrella closure of congenital cardiac defects (Table 27-1). Among the patients who routinely require the services of an anesthesiologist for these procedures are young children, the mentally retarded, and the critically ill. An anesthesiologist may be necessary for a number of reasons, including airway management, sedation, analgesia, the patient's inability to cooperate, and the need for close hemodynamic monitoring.

The American Society of Anesthesiologists (ASA) standards for basic intraoperative monitoring[1] (originally approved October 1986 and periodically updated since then) should be incorporated into the anesthetic plan (Box 27-1). Many of the seemingly overwhelming problems encountered when monitoring was first performed in extreme environments, particularly because of the powerful magnetic field of MRI and immersion of the patient in a water bath

---

Box 27-1. ASA standards for basic intraoperative monitoring (approved October 21, 1986 and last amended on October 23, 1990 to become effective by January 1, 1991)

STANDARD I

QUALIFIED ANESTHESIA PERSONNEL

Qualified anesthesia personnel shall be present in the room throughout the conduct of all general anesthetics, regional and monitored anesthesia care.

STANDARD II

OXYGENATION, VENTILATION, CIRCULATION, AND TEMPERATURE SHALL BE CONTINUALLY EVALUATED.

Oxygenation	a)	oxygen analyzer for inspired gases
	b)	observation of patient
	c)	pulse oximetry
Ventilation	a)	auscultation
	b)	observation of patient
	c)	observation of reservoir bag
	d)	end-tidal carbon dioxide analysis
Circulation	a)	continuous display ECG
	b)	heart rate and blood pressure recorded every five minutes
	c)	evaluation of circulation:
		auscultation of heart sounds
		palpation of pulse
		pulse plethysmography
		pulse oximetry
		intraarterial pressure tracing
Temperature	a)	core temperature:
		thermistors, thermocouple, thermometer
	b)	skin temperature:
		thermistor, liquid crystal thermometer

Table 27-1. Locations and procedures outside the OR

Location	Procedure
Computerized tomography (CT scan)	Diagnostic imaging
Magnetic resonance imaging (MRI)	Diagnostic imaging
Lithotriptor	Extracorporeal shock wave lithotripsy
Fluoroscopy suite	Myelograms
	Arthrograms
	Percutaneous biopsy
	Endoscopic retrograde cholangiopancreatography (ERCP)
Angiography suite	Angiograms
	Angioplasty
	Embolization
	Greenfield filter placement
	Percutaneous nephrostomy
	Percutaneous biliary drainage
Cardiac catheterization laboratory	Cardiac catheterization
	Valvuloplasty
	Angioplasty
	Umbrella closures (ASD,* PDA,† VSD‡)
Radiation therapy	Radiation therapy (RT)
Clinics	Percutaneous biopsy
	Bone marrow biopsy
	Endoscopy

*ASD: atrial septal defect
†PDA: patent ductus arteriosus
‡VSD: ventricular septal defect

for ESWL, have been greatly reduced if not eliminated altogether. Equipment is now available for use in the proximity of MRI, and newer ESWL machines no longer require that the patient be immersed in water. Although it may not be possible to follow the same standards in all environments, some standards, tailored to fit the particular environment, should always exist. The following discussion concerns some of the general problems encountered with equipment and monitoring in sites outside the operating room and gives specific recommendations for such extreme environments as MRI and ESWL. Table 27-2 summarizes the equipment available for use in the seven most common remote locations.

BASIC PROBLEMS OUTSIDE THE OPERATING ROOM

Remote locations where radiation is used (i.e., CT scanner, angiography, cardiac catheterization laboratory) do not impose physical limitations on the type of anesthesia equipment that can be used. (This is not the case for extreme environments, such as MRI). All commonly used monitors and machines can be safely used in any radiology suite. The major problems encountered have more to do with the actual logistics of utilizing this equipment in foreign environments. Problems and solutions for each aspect of patient monitoring and care are discussed in the following subsections.

Table 27-2. Remote location and equipment for monitoring

		ASA standard			
	Presence of qualified personnel	**Oxygenation**	**Ventilation**	**Circulation**	**Temperature**
MRI	Minimal biologic hazards	O₂ analyzer • Ohmeda 5125 (MRI compatible) • Oxycheck 2000 (Critikon, Tampa, FL) Pulse oximeter • Biochem Microspare 1040 (Waukesha, WI) • Invivo (fiberoptic) Winter Park, FL • Ohmeda Biox 3700 (Englewood, CO) • Nonin 8604 (Plymouth, MN) • Criticare 503 (Milwaukee, WI) • Nellcor N-100 (Hayward, CA) Observation	Capnometry • Biochem 515 (Waukesha, WI) • Ohmeda 5200 (Englewood, CO) Auscultation • Plastic precordial stethoscope Observation	ECG MRI compatible systems for cardiac gating are available with General Electric or Siemens magnets • Omni-Trak 3100 (Invivo, Winter Park, FL) • Sirecust 400 (Siemens) • Hewlett-Packard HP78352C Noninvasive blood pressure • Dinamap 1846 XT or SX-P (Critikon, Tampa, FL) • Omni Trak 3100 (Winter Park, FL) • Omega 1400 (Winter Park, FL) • Sirecust 404 (Siemens, Needham Heights, MA) Auscultation Plethysmograph Available with cardiac gating feature on General Electric or Siemens magnets	Liquid crystal thermometer and thermistor
Cardiac catheterization lab	Radiation hazard	O₂ analyzer Pulse oximetry Observation	Capnography/capnometry Auscultation • Precordial stethoscope • FM transmitter • Infrared transmitter	ECG Noninvasive blood pressure (automated oscillometry) or arterial pressure transduction Auscultation (as for ventilation) Palpation of pulse Pulse oximetry	Thermistor
Fluoroscopy	Radiation hazard	O₂ analyzer Pulse oximetry Observation	Capnography/capnometry Auscultation • Precordial stethoscope • FM transmitter • Infrared transmitter	ECG Noninvasive blood pressure (automated oscillometry) Auscultation (as for ventilation) Palpation of pulse Pulse oximetry	Thermistor

Continued.

Table 27-2. Remote location and equipment for monitoring—cont'd

	Presence of qualified personnel	ASA standard			
		Oxygenation	Ventilation	Circulation	Temperature
Lithotriptor	Radiation hazard	O_2 analyzer Pulse oximetry Observation	Capnography/capnometry Auscultation • Precordial stethoscope • FM transmitter • Infrared transmitter	ECG Noninvasive blood pressure (automated oscillometry) or arterial pressure transduction Auscultation (as for ventilation) Palpation of pulse Pulse oximetry Central venous or pulmonary artery transduction	Thermistor Liquid crystal
CT scanner	*Must be waived* Windows for observation	Remote monitors: O_2 analyzer Pulse oximeter Observation of patient through window	Remote monitors: Capnometry/capnography Auscultation • FM transmitter • can be waived Remote observation	ECG Noninvasive blood pressure (automatic oscillometry) Auscultation (as for ventilation) Palpation of pulse not possible Pulse oximetry	Thermistor
RT (radiation therapy)	*Must be waived* Television monitors	Remote monitors: O_2 analyzer Pulse oximeter Observation of patient on TV screen	Remote monitors: Capnometry/capnography Auscultation • FM transmitter • can be waived Remove observation	ECG Noninvasive blood pressure (automatic oscillometry) Auscultation (as for ventilation) Palpation of pulse not possible Pulse oximetry	Thermistor
Angiography	*Radiation hazard* • Leaded shields • Leaded glasses • Lead screens	O_2 analyzer Pulse oximetry Observation	Capnography/capnography Auscultation • Precordial stethoscope • FM transmitter • Infrared transmitter Observation	ECG Noninvasive blood pressure (automatic oscillometry) or arterial pressure transduction Auscultation (as for ventilation) Palpation of pulse Pulse oximetry	Thermistor

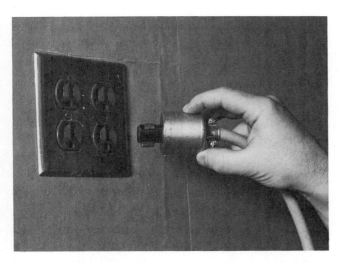

Fig. 27-1. OR equipment is frequently fitted with twist-lock (Hubble) plugs. In remote locations, compatible electrical receptacles may not be available and "cheater" arrangements may be required.

Electrical plugs and receptacles

Electrical outlets may not accommodate the plugs of standard operating room equipment, or they may not be in sufficient supply (Fig. 27-1). Historically, the use of flammable agents made it necessary to supply anesthesia machines and monitoring equipment with explosion-proof plugs.[2] These plugs are large, round, slotted discs that fit only into explosion-proof outlets. When the disc is rotated clockwise in the outlet, the contacts in the receptacles are engaged, preventing the plug from being pulled out of the outlet. This also seals the system from any flammable vapors to prevent the escape of sparks (even static sparks) that might cause an explosion.[3] Operating room equipment is commonly fitted with these explosion-proof plugs. The solution to this problem is simply to take an adaptor and extension cords ("cheater" plugs) to the remote location when necessary (Fig. 27-2).

Suction

Central wall suction is a basic necessity for any anesthetizing location. Although the radiology suites and clinics in newer hospitals are usually equipped with wall suction, this is not so in many older facilities. If central wall suction is not available, arrangements must be made to obtain a portable suction machine.

A related problem is the need for gas scavenging when inhaled agents are to be used. If a gas evacuation system is not available, central wall suction can be used to scavenge gases. Then, a portable suction machine can be used to aspirate oral and gastric secretions. Alternatively, an adaptor can be used to provide simultaneous connections when only one suction outlet is available. If adequate scavenging is not possible, inhaled agents should not be used; an intravenous technique should be selected instead.

Oxygen

Central wall oxygen is available in most remote anesthetizing locations, even in many MRI centers. However, it is advisable in all situations, with or without central wall oxygen, to have on hand a full tank of oxygen and portable ventilating system (Ambu bag or modified Mapleson D circuit). Nonferromagnetic aluminum tanks are available for use in the proximity of an MRI scanner. A back-up ventilation system is an absolute necessity. Such a system is also needed when a patient is transported from a remote anesthetizing location to the postanesthesia care unit.

Monitoring

Electrocardiography. Electrocardiography (ECG) is a de facto standard for patient monitoring during anesthesia. Its value has been well established since the 1960s.[4,5] Although heart rate can be measured by a pulse oximeter, the ECG is a first-line monitor for arrhythmia detection. Many radiologic procedures rely on the use of dyes or wires to manipulate catheters. The incidence of life-threatening reactions associated with angiography or other studies utiliz-

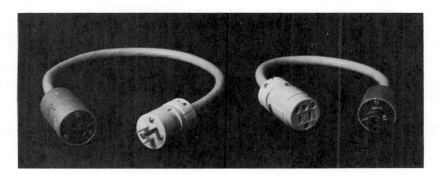

Fig. 27-2. Electrical power cord pigtails can be made so that OR equipment can be used in remote locations that do not possess OR receptacles. Shown on the *left* is an adaptor that converts a twist-lock plug for use in a three-prong receptacle. Shown on the *right* is an adapter that allows a three-prong plug to be connected to a twist-lock receptacle. Appropriate adaptors should always be taken to remote locations.

ing dye is approximately 1:1000.[6,7,8] Arrhythmias are frequently the harbinger of an untoward reaction, making the ECG of paramount importance in remote locations. When the ECG electrodes are placed, care must be taken to avoid interfering with radiologic imaging. Care must also be taken to ensure that the anatomic areas being examined are not obscured by electrodes or wires. The skin should be well prepared and the leads placed on the arms and legs, especially during angiography or CT scans of the thorax and abdomen. Advance consultation with the radiologist to confirm exactly which areas are to be imaged can avoid any problems.

Automated oscillometry is an accurate and efficacious method for measuring blood pressure indirectly.[9,10] An automated system is advisable because it allows personnel to be removed from the patient during periods either of exposure to extremely high radiation (CT, RT) or of prolonged exposure to radiation (cinematography during an angiogram or cardiac catheterization). An automated system provides intermittent blood pressure monitoring, and its display can be viewed through a leaded window or on a video monitor. An automated system also allows the anesthesiologist greater freedom to attend to the patient.

Pulse oximetry. Pulse oximetry has been one of the most significant developments in the past decade, and its utility is widely recognized by almost every medical discipline.[11,12] More information can be obtained from the pulse oximeter than just arterial oxygen saturation (SpO_2). All models feature a tachometer, and many include a visual plethysmographic display as well. Several reports in the literature[13-15] have attested to the expanding role of oximetry in assessing heart rate, perfusion, and intravascular volume status. However, the oximeter should never be the sole monitor used by the anesthesiologist in remote locations, even for the patient who is only minimally sedated. When access to the patient is limited, complete reliance on one monitoring device may be hazardous despite its recognized value.

Temperature. The value of temperature monitoring, well recognized in anesthesiology, is of particular significance in several remote locations. Radiology suites are maintained at colder temperatures to accommodate the computer systems that reconstruct images in CT, angiography, and MRI. These systems are extremely sensitive to atmospheric temperature and can easily overheat. In addition, warming techniques commonly used in the OR are limited. For instance, radiant heat lamps or warming blankets may interfere with imaging. Finally, cold fluids that come into contact with the patient's skin further contribute to evaporative heat loss. For these reasons, use of a standard thermistor is strongly advised to enable prompt recognition and treatment of hypothermia or hyperthermia. Liquid crystal thermometers are not as accurate and may be difficult to read in these settings.[16]

Auscultation. Auscultation of heart and breath sounds has long been the mainstay of monitoring during anesthesia. However, auscultation in remote locations is complicated by the distance between the patient and the anesthesiologist. The recently developed FM wireless transmitter is better suited for the remote monitoring of heart and breath sounds.[17] However, this system does not work in the vicinity of the MRI, due to interference from the radio frequency (RF) waves. The FM signal is not transmitted well through shielded walls but is transmitted through glass.

An infrared remote auscultation unit can be used if the anesthesiologist remains in the procedure room.[18] Such a unit is ideal if the anesthesiologist needs freedom of movement or wishes to avoid an excessive length of extension tubing. Infrared signals are not transmitted through walls (they rely on a beam of light) and therefore cannot be used when the anesthesiologist must remain outside the patient's room. This system is well suited for monitoring during angiography, fluoroscopy, and cardiac catheterization; in the MRI suite, however, interference may be caused by magnetic saturation of the transmitting system.

End-tidal carbon dioxide. Monitoring of end-tidal carbon dioxide is a simple and efficacious method of assuring that ventilation is adequate.[19] Several anesthesia machines (e.g., Dräger Narkomed 3 and 4* and Ohmeda Modulus II†) are available with built-in capnometers. Similarly, a number of currently available free-standing modules are useful in the radiology suite (other than MRI). End-tidal carbon dioxide monitoring is also possible in the sedated, spontaneously ventilating patient who has not undergone intubation. Respiratory gas analyzer sampling/aspirating systems can be attached to a shortened IV catheter and placed inside nasal oxygen prongs (Fig. 27-3). An oxygen nasal cannula is available with an integral port for a sidestream anesthesia gas analyzer (Salter Labs, Arvin, Calif.) (Fig. 27-4). These cannulas are commercially available in small sizes for use in pediatric cases.

Compact monitoring systems. Many of the compact monitoring systems now available are ideal for use in remote locations, because it is usually necessary to transport all anesthesia equipment to these remote locations. This entails the stacking of monitoring equipment, which risks serious damage to expensive equipment (Fig. 27-5). Many of these new transport monitors weigh less than 10 pounds and may contain in one small box an ECG; two invasive pressure channels; and monitoring for noninvasive blood pressure, oximetry, apnea, and temperature. Some of the compact models currently available are PC Express,‡ Es-

---

*North American Dräger, Inc., Telford, Pa.
†Ohmeda, Madison, Wis.
‡Space Labs, Redmond, Wash.

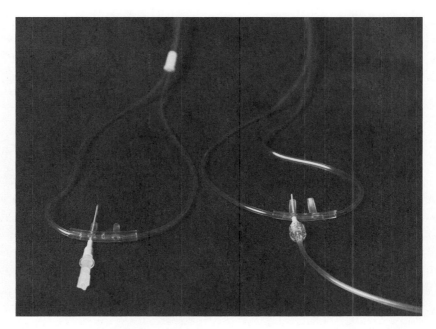

Fig. 27-3. A standard oxygen nasal cannula can be adapted to monitor end-tidal carbon dioxide in a spontaneously breathing patient. An IV catheter is inserted into one of the nasal prongs. The metal needle is then removed, the catheter trimmed, and the gas aspirating tubing attached to the IV catheter. It should be noted that this system works only with the aspirating or sidestream type of gas analyzers.

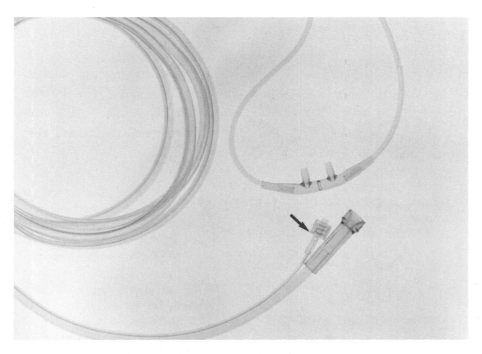

Fig. 27-4. A nasal oxygen cannula with an integral port for end-tidal gas sampling. The *arrow* points to the connector for the gas sampling tubing. One of the nasal prongs delivers oxygen; the other is used for sampling gas.

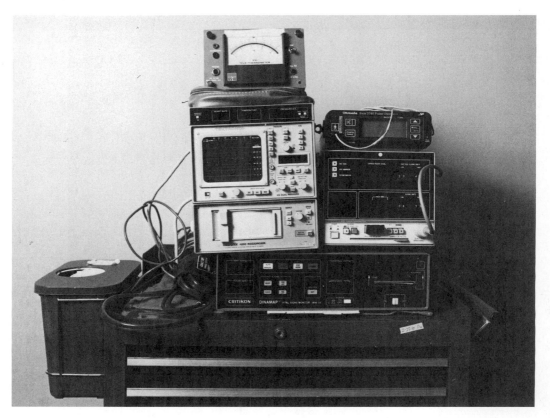

Fig. 27-5. Equipment used to monitor patients in remote locations often consists of many individual pieces. These individual pieces of equipment are frequently stacked precariously on top of one another. This equipment must be carefully secured to a cart; otherwise, damage is inevitable.

cort 300,* Propaq 106,† Tram 7200,‡ and Cardiac Plus§ (still in development).

MAGNETIC RESONANCE IMAGING

Magnetic resonance imaging (MRI) was first described by Rabi in 1939 and is one of the most significant developments in medical diagnosis. It was utilized for biological purposes in 1946 by Block and Purcell, but several decades passed before it was refined sufficiently for clinical use. The simultaneous explosion in computer and superconductor technology served to make MRI a practical reality. It was not until 1977 that Damadian was able to produce the first human images with this technology.[20] Administering anesthesia for MRI has presented a similar challenge.

The difficulties associated with using standard monitors in the presence of a powerful magnetic field have required considerable ingenuity and flexibility. The principles of MRI must be understood, as well as its physiologic and

electronic effects on both patient and equipment, so that new equipment can be designed to maintain the same monitoring standards currently used in other locations. This understanding of magnetic fields also helps the clinician to adapt currently available monitors for adequate patient care.

Magnetic resonance imaging process

The creation of an image involves six sequential steps:[20]

1. *Magnetic field.* First, a powerful uniform magnetic field which aligns all randomly oriented nuclei is created. The field strengths used for medical imaging are 0.5 to 1.5 Tesla (T), where 1 T is equal to 10,000 gauss (G). The earth's magnetic field is just under 1 G. Fields of 1.5 T produce the best resolution.
2. *Radiofrequency pulses.* Next, radiofrequency (RF) pulses are directed at the patient. In the presence of an external magnetic field, cell nuclei absorb more energy. The so-called magnetic resonance is created when these cells are super-energized by RF waves in a magnetic field.
3. *Recovery of alignment.* After nuclei have been super-energized with RF, they recover their original alignment within the magnetic field. Each tissue emits an

*Medical Data Electronics, Arleta, Calif.
†Protocol Systems, Beaverton, Ore.
‡Marquette Electronics, Milwaukee, Wis.
§Ohmeda, Boulder, Colo.

RF signal proportional to the difference between the energized magnetic resonance state and the original alignment. Tissue contrast develops as a result of the different rates of realignment.

4. *Time-varied magnetic fields.* Time-varied magnetic fields (TVMF), the contribution of Lauterbur in 1972, finally made MRI a practical imaging modality. Magnetic field gradients are briefly applied to encode spatially the RF signals emitted from the patient. Before this development, two-dimensional and three-dimensional images were not possible.

5. *Signal readout.* Signal readout times must be determined for each patient before the exam for the recording of RF signal after initial excitation. This process is done before the actual MRI procedure.

6. *Fourier transformation.* The signal from the patient is collected by the RF coil, which surrounds the patient, and is then transformed by computer into a two-dimensional or three-dimensional image.

The difficulties encountered during monitoring in the MRI environment are related to three of the above processes. They are the powerful magnetic field, the RF pulses, and the TVMF. The implications of each are discussed separately in the following subsections.

Magnetic interference. The most obvious hazard of the high static magnetic field created by MRI (usually 1.5 T) is that it attracts ferromagnetic objects into the magnet, and many MRI centers have experienced a projectile-related accident. Even a ballpoint pen or metal jewelry can present a hazard. Before an installation site is selected for an MRI center, all potential sites must be thoroughly surveyed, because all environmental iron is magnetized. It may be necessary to reroute pipes and electrical wiring and remove all stationary environmental iron (i.e., structural steel, floor decking, and concrete reinforcing rods). In spite of such precautions, it is still not possible to isolate the field completely. There is always some magnetization of the environment immediately surrounding the magnet. This effect is readily apparent to anyone who has ever transported anesthesia equipment through the hallways to the MRI center. Thus safety precautions should apply not only within the imaging room but also outside.

As previously stated, considerable creativity and flexibility has been necessary to adapt anesthesia equipment for use in the MRI environment. In general, replacing the machine's ferrous material with stainless steel, brass, or aluminum enables its placement in the imaging room. However, even with the reduced ferrous load, much of the equipment's smaller, more delicate instrumentation is still ferromagnetic and subject to constant torque, which is the alignment of ferromagnetic material within a magnetic field. Constant torque can cause serious damage to sophisticated precision electronic equipment. Therefore, all equipment should be removed from the site when not being used.

Another hazard of working in the magnetic field is the erasure of all magnetic media, such as credit cards, pass keys, floppy discs, and videotapes. Most centers provide lockers outside the most damaging magnetic field for storage of such items and all potential projectiles.

Magnetic interference affects the functioning and accuracy of all equipment within its immediate vicinity. Computer or oscillometric images are distorted by the bending of electronic beams into circular arcs. MRI-compatible equipment is designed to compensate for these distortions.

MRI interference also causes transformers to be saturated. Any piece of equipment powered by alternating current can be damaged in a high magnetic field.[21] Saturation of the transformer prevents the production of inductive voltage, and excessive currents can burn out the power transformer.

Quartz-driven analog watches stop running in a magnetic field but resume function outside the field. Digital clocks are not affected, and most MRI units include one in the control panel. This is helpful for anesthetic record-keeping.

Radiofrequency interference. The two large RF coils that surround the patient present some significant challenges to monitoring in the MRI suite. The outer coil transmits the RF; the inner one receives the RF emitted from the patient. The scanning room must be shielded from outside RF interference, such as television transmitters, beeper paging systems, two-way radios, and commercial radio stations, which may affect RF transmission and reception. In addition, any cables or leads can behave as antennas for the RF. The MRI suite can be RF-shielded if the walls and windows are lined with thin continuous sheets of copper and if wave guides are used in the walls (see the section on wave guides).

Radiofrequency pulses are also capable of inducing electrical eddy currents and short circuiting electrical equipment. It is therefore necessary to shield monitors and cables from the RF. For passive shielding, cables can be wrapped with a thin layer of aluminum foil, and small copper boxes can be used to house electrical equipment. The best location for both the electrical power source and the ground is outside the room. The ground absorbs the RF and thereby actively shields the monitor.[22] Electrical cords should be routed through low-pass wave guides in the wall. The development of more sophisticated MRI equipment will eliminate the need to shield conventional monitors from RF.

Time-varied magnetic field. With the introduction of TVMF (magnetic field gradients), MRI became clinically useful. TVMF enables the computer to encode spatially the RF emitted from the patient to construct two-dimensional or three-dimensional images. Of purely theoretical concern is that TVMF can induce electrical eddy currents in both biologic tissue and electrical wiring. Although the biologic effects are usually minimal, a very large TVMF (> 10,000 T/sec) has the potential to interfere with nerve conduction, to induce seizures, or to cause ventricular fibrillation. For this reason, coils in any cables or leads should be avoided. However, this current is beyond present clinical capabilities, because the TVMF for presently available units is well within the range of biologic current densities (1 to 10 mA/m^2).[23]

An innocuous, albeit annoying, effect of TVMF on personnel is the presence of flickering illuminations known as magnetophosphenes. These are caused by the torque from the magnetic field gradients on the retinal cones. This effect has been completely reversible thus far, and no long-term effects have been reported.[24]

Monitoring in the magnetic resonance imaging suite

Basic set-up. Systems for central wall suction and oxygen are now commercially available for MRI centers. It is advisable to have these installed during construction of the MRI suite after consulting with biomedical engineers and architects. Wave guides (see the next section) are specially designed passages through which cables or tubes can be passed without compromising the integrity of the RF-shielded room.

Electrical power sources for monitoring systems are usually available in the magnet room itself. These consist of isolated duplex power circuits with filtered 120 V (alternating current) to prevent electrical noise artifacts from interfering with the images.[25] Any monitors that are plugged into these outlets should be located as far from the core of the magnet as possible. In addition, they should have little or no ferromagnetic material and be RF-shielded (either encased in a copper box or wrapped in aluminum foil). If possible, monitors should be kept outside the magnet room, and an external power source should be used. When monitors are thus located, only the cables should be passed through wave guides in the wall in order to limit the effects of magnetization, RF, and TVMF on the equipment. It is beneficial to locate the equipment outside the magnet area because the RF will be absorbed by the ground, torque on sophisticated instrumentation will be limited, and the monitor will not become a projectile.[22]

WAVE GUIDES

Wave guides are necessary for all pipes, cables, ducts, and electrical wires entering an RF-shielded room. Wave guides prevent both leakage of RF pulses from the magnet room and interference from outside RF (beepers, radio, or TV signals). In addition, electrical wiring and cables for monitoring equipment can act as antennas for RF, causing interference.

Several different types of wave guide are available, depending on its intended use. A low-pass filter is necessary for passing electrical signals through an RF-shielded wall, including electrical lighting and outlets. These filters were originally placed low in the wall, at the position furthest from the magnetic field and RF coils. The filter consists of

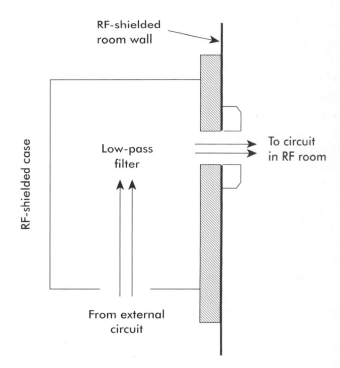

Fig. 27-6. Low-pass filter for passing electrical signals through the wall of an RF-shielded room. (Redrawn from Koskinen MF: *Site planning.* In Edelman R, Hesselink J, editors: *Clinical magnetic resonance imaging,* Philadelphia, 1990, Saunders, pp 341-354.)

an RF-shielded copper box covering the external passage into the room. Cables or wiring pass through this box and then zigzag into the wave guide[21] (Fig. 27-6). Again, if possible, wave guides for monitoring systems should be included during construction of the MRI suite. Newer magnets are now installed with wave guides available in the control panels so that monitoring systems can be added conveniently after construction.

Specific monitoring concerns

Electrocardiogram. An ECG is installed with most MRI units as a requirement for cardiac gating studies (GE and Siemens). The ECG complex is always distorted in an MRI unit because the flow of an electrical conductor (blood) within a magnetic field creates small eddy currents that change the ECG vector.[26] Therefore, the ECG cannot be used for the diagnosis of acute pathological disorders such as ischemia or arrhythmias while the patient is in the magnet.

Besides distorting the ECG, eddy currents can produce electrical fields that can oppose blood flow, thereby reducing cardiac output. This is of greater theoretical than practical concern, however, because only a 1% reduction of output is seen with a 1.0 T field.

Several MRI-compatible ECG systems are currently available, for which the ECG electrodes used are made of carbon graphite to lower resistance, eliminate ferromagnetism, and minimize RF interference. In order to optimize the ECG signal, the skin must be adequately prepared (dried or abraded).

Some controversy surrounds the use of ECG telemetry in the MRI suite. Telemetry may sound appealing because it reduces the amount of wiring and cables needed through the walls of the suite. However, because very high frequency (VHF) telemetry units transmit via RF waves, it should be anticipated that their use will interfere with the RF used for imaging. However, this interference is not seen with ultrahigh frequency (UHF) units, such as the one made by Hewlett-Packard for use with the GE Signa (1.5 T),[27] which transmits in a frequency band well outside the range of the RF used for imaging. However, UHF telemetry units are limited to QRS complex detection for gating studies and cannot be used for diagnostic purposes.

Many authors have reported with enthusiasm on the value of telemetry units. Current reports in the literature[28,29] on the value of telemetry are limited to MRI scanners with weaker magnetic fields (0.6 T). ECG monitoring is improved when telemetry is not used but rather RF-shielded cables carry the signal to an oscilloscope outside the room (Omni-Trak 3100* or Sirecust 404†). Hewlett-Packard also manufactures an MRI-compatible system (HP78352C) which utilizes cables that are RF-shielded and that are installed during the construction of the magnet room.[27]

Blood pressure. Automated oscillometric blood pressure monitoring eliminates the problems of electromagnetic interference because it is based on pneumatic principles. The Sirecust 404 and Omni-Trak 3100 both have automated oscillometry units for MRI, that are being used successfully.[30] Conventional oscillometric units that are not MRI-specific, such as the Dinamap 1846 series,‡ are also being used.[31] These units should be placed well away from the magnet's core, and the tubing should be extended to accommodate this distance. A conventional noninvasive blood pressure unit is not shielded from either RF or the magnetic field and requires a 120-V electrical outlet. Consequently, there is usually some interference with RF during scanning, and if the patient is stable, blood pressures may be recorded using the manual mode between RF pulses. Manual mercury sphygmomanometers have been adapted in a similar manner for use during MRI by replacement of all ferromagnetic hardware with brass or aluminum pieces.[25] This enables more frequent measurement of systolic blood pressure by the "bounce" methods as well as permitting closer proximity of the blood pressure monitoring units to the magnet.

Invasive blood pressure monitoring in the MRI suite has certain practical limitations. It has been necessary to make extensive adaptations to conventional intraarterial catheters and pressure transducers for use in the MRI suite. A case

has been described[28] in which it was necessary to fill 16 feet of pressure tubing with heparinized saline to reach the monitoring unit placed outside the magnet room. Fiberoptic transmission may be the solution to invasive blood pressure monitoring as well as to monitoring problems caused by RF, TVMF, and the magnetic field. The fiberoptic signal can be converted to an electrical signal outside the room.[32]

Ventilation. Capnography has been used successfully in the magnet room.[30,31] Carbon dioxide monitoring is very helpful because breath sounds auscultated through a plastic precordial stethoscope are obscured during RF pulsing. The Biochem 515,* a battery-powered aspirating system, uses cannulas that come in a range of sizes from infant to adult. It is a qualitative rather than a quantitative system and therefore is best used as an apnea monitor. Other conventional carbon dioxide monitors have been used in the magnet room itself.[30] Aspirating systems allow for remote monitoring and cause less image interference than flow-through infrared systems. The flow-through infrared capnograph can be used only for patients who have undergone intubation, and the sensor requires shielding from RF by aluminum foil.

Oxygenation. Most commercially available pulse oximeters will work in the magnet room (Table 27-2).[31] The monitor should be shielded and placed as far from the magnet as possible. At some centers, all monitoring equipment in the magnet room is enclosed in small copper or aluminum boxes for the purpose of RF shielding. The probe of an oximeter should be placed on the extremity that is furthest from the RF coils. Probes can overheat, particularly if the cable connecting the patient to the monitor is coiled. Super electromagnetic fields are created within these coils. Burns can be avoided if the wire is kept free of coils and the digits are protected with clear plastic covering.[33] The most recent advances in pulse oximetry for MRI have been made by the Invivo Research Laboratories of Winter Park, Fla. The oximeter included with the Omni-Trak system utilizes fiberoptic cables. These minimize both RF and TVMF interference and improve the quality of monitoring during RF pulsing and image reconstruction.

Anesthesia equipment. Until recently, existing anesthesia machines required modification before they could be used in a magnetic field.[25] When the machine's ferromagnetic components are replaced with brass, aluminum, and plastic, the ferromagnetic content can be reduced to less than 2% of the total weight. The back bars and vertical supports are among the largest components that should be replaced. Ohmeda now manufactures an MRI-compatible machine, the Excel-210 MRI,† which is 99.8% stainless steel, brass, aluminum, and plastic. Anesthesia machines should be kept 30 to 40 feet away from the core of the

*Invivo, Winter Park, Fla.
†Siemens, Needham Heights, Mass.
‡Critikon, Tampa, Fla.

*Biochem, Waukesha, Wis.
†Ohmeda, Madison, Wis.

magnet because the magnetic field decreases significantly with increasing distance from the core. Medical gas cylinders constructed from aluminum should be used on an anesthesia machine in the MRI suite. Vaporizers, however, are affected little by the powerful magnetic field and function accurately in this environment.

For tracheal intubation, plastic, battery-operated laryngoscopes can be used. One such laryngoscope is manufactured by North American Medical Products of Londonville, New York. Batteries will last longer if shielded with a paper casing or if plastic coated. If MRI-compatible laryngoscopes are not available, the airway can be secured outside the magnet room with conventional ferromagnetic laryngoscopes before the patient is moved into the scanner.

Both circle and nonbreathing anesthesia systems can be used for ventilation in the MRI suite. A Bain circuit or other type of Mapleson D circuit with long extension tubing has been used for both assisted and controlled ventilation.[29] Circle systems have also been used but require long extension tubing, especially if an anesthesia machine remote from the magnet is used. Mechanical ventilation can be accomplished with MRI-compatible equipment, such as the Monaghan 225 SIMV Volume Ventilator.*[34] This particular ventilator is made entirely of plastic and is powered by compressed oxygen at 50 psig. Another nonmagnetic ventilator is the Omni-vent.† This is a time-cycled, volume-preset ventilator also powered by compressed gas at 40 to 140 psig. Many other centers have used standard ventilators on anesthesia machines that have been modified by reduction of the ferromagnetic content. A standard Air Shields Ventimeter Controller II‡ has been used successfully at a distance of 12 feet from the core of the magnet at the 70-G line.[25]

Temperature. Temperature monitoring is necessary during MRI because RF raises body temperature. While no biologic damage has been documented to date, tissues that dissipate heat poorly are at risk (i.e., the lens and the scrotum). Thermistors and liquid crystal thermometers are employed routinely.

Monitoring in the MRI suite provides a number of unique challenges. An understanding of how the monitors are affected by the magnetic field, RF, and TVMF used to construct images is essential. The administration of anesthesia in the MRI suite is now common.[35] With further advances in engineering, magnetically shielded transformers, RF-isolated cables, and fiberoptic transmission will be more readily available for application in anesthesia equipment.

LITHOTRIPSY

Since the early 1980s, the use of lithotripsy to fragment renal stones has become commonplace. This noninvasive

*Monaghan, Plattsburgh, N.Y.
†CMS Medical, Topeka, Kan.
‡Air Shields, Hatboro, Pa.

technique is now the treatment of choice for this procedure because it removes most renal stones safely and effectively without the morbidity and prolonged recovery usually associated with open operative procedures. Unfortunately, this technique has not been as successful in the removal of biliary stones because (1) the gall stones tend to recur; (2) candidacy depends on the number and composition of the stones; and (3) this, along with other treatment modalities, has been replaced by laparoscopic cholecystectomy, which is more successful and carries minimal morbidity. The following discussion therefore considers only urologic lithotripsy.

Despite the continued development of lithotriptors that offer greater convenience and are less painful than the original prototypes, the role of the anesthesiologist on the lithotripsy team appears to be well established. In addition to the hazards associated with anesthetic management in remote locations, the anesthesiologist must be thoroughly familiar with the type and model of lithotriptor being used in order to anticipate patient needs and design appropriate monitoring. This section includes a discussion on the different types of lithotriptors currently available, specific monitoring needs and modifications, and environmental hazards.

The lithotriptor

The original lithotriptor was marketed for patient use by Dornier Systems, an aerospace company, which discovered that jets traveling at speeds greater than Mach 1 sustained fuselage damage from the shock waves of rain drops.[36] The subsequent application of shock waves for bursting calculi was based on the following principles: (1) The mechanical stress from the shock waves is greater than the strength of the renal calculus; (2) shock waves can be transmitted through water (and therefore body tissue) without losing energy until they encounter a nontissue substance (air or stone); (3) shock waves can be focused by reflectors to direct the point of impact; and (4) shock waves can be reproduced reliably.[37]

The Dornier HM-3, the original model and prototype lithotriptor, was designed on the basis of these principles of shock waves and is still being used today in many facilities. In this spark-gap type of lithotriptor, an electric spark is generated under water and the resultant shock wave is focused with the help of an ellipsoid.[36,38,39] The shock wave is propagated approximately three times more effectively in water than in air. Water also provides the same acoustic impedance (density) as body tissue. Consequently, no energy is lost by the shock wave until it reaches a nontissue (nonwater) interface (water-stone or water-air). Upon impact with the particular focal point, a burst of short-term high energy is released, which is greater than the tensile strength of the calculus. Repeated shock waves pulverize or disintegrate the stone into smaller particles, which subsequently can be eliminated through the ureter.

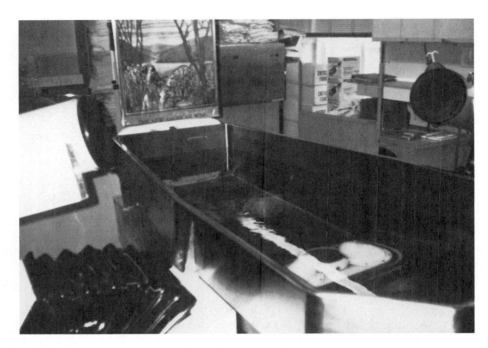

Fig. 27-7. The water bath for the HM-3 lithotriptor. The fluoroscopy tubes can be seen at the sides of the water bath. After being anesthetized, the patient is placed in a gantry (not shown) and then lowered into the water bath.

The force of the shock wave varies from 18 to 24 kV and is determined by the voltage across the electrode.[36,40] Depending on this voltage, as much as 15,000 psig of pressure may be generated by the shock wave.[41] The federal Food and Drug Administration (FDA) has placed a limit on the maximum number of shocks (2000) within the range of 18 to 24 kV permissible for each treatment episode on the HM-3.[42] The patient is immersed in a water bath through which the impulse is propagated (Fig. 27-7). Degasified and demineralized water is used to prevent the dissipation of energy prior to stone impact at a nonwater interface.

Although ultrasound and shock waves obey the same laws of acoustics, ultrasound is not effective for fracturing calculi. Ultrasound creates a sinusoidal wave form, whereas shock waves present as a pressure front of multiple frequencies. As a result, it is not possible to focus ultrasound with precision over long distances.[37,43] Conversely, shock waves can be focused by reflection from the walls of the semiellipsoid from which the initial spark is generated.[37] The stone is positioned in the area of maximal energy density by way of biplanar three-dimensional fluoroscopy. Although focusing by ultrasound eliminates radiation exposure to patient and personnel, it is not precise enough for use with the Dornier HM-3.

The original Dornier HM-3 requires that the patient be immersed to the level of the clavicles in order to keep both the entrance and exit of the shock waves below water. Either general or regional anesthesia is necessary with this method because pain is caused when the waves enter and exit the skin.

Several improvements have been made in the newer generations of spark-gap type lithotriptors. With the Dornier HM-4 (Fig. 27-8) and Med Stone 1000,* the water bath has been replaced by a water cushion, although fluoroscopy is still necessary for focusing.[37,42] The lower pressure released by the shock waves reduces the pain of the procedure and therefore the anesthetic requirement. The MPL 9000[†] and Sonolith 2000[‡] are two newer spark-gap type lithotriptors, which use a water cushion or water basin and are associated with decreased anesthetic requirements. These two machines also use ultrasound instead of fluoroscopy for focusing.[42,44,45] The debate regarding the use of fluoroscopy versus ultrasound for stone localization goes beyond the obvious desire to reduce radiation exposure. One study found that ultrasound was unable to localize 58% of ureteral calculi because of overlay by either pelvic or intestinal gas. Conversely, fluoroscopy failed to localize the majority of slightly opaque or nonopaque calculi.[46]

In 1986, Siemens[§] introduced its second generation Lithostar,[47] which used an electromagnetic shock wave source, allowing the shock wave head to be coupled to the patient without the use of a water bath. In this machine, a high-voltage pulse from a capacitor is passed through an electromagnetic coil discharging 15 to 20 kV. The energy pulse passes through a thin, isolating layer to a metal

*Medstone, Irvine, Calif.
[†]Dornier Medical Systems, Kennesaw, Ga.
[‡]Technomed, Danvers, Mass.
[§]Siemens-Lithostar, Erlanger, Germany.

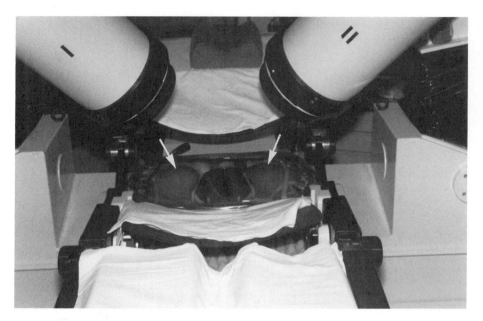

Fig. 27-8. The treatment table for the HM-4 lithotriptor. The water bath is replaced by a water cushion *(arrows)*, which greatly facilitates access to the patient. The fluoroscopy tubes (I and II) are shown in the treatment position.

membrane, which actually generates the shock wave. The shock waves move at the speed of sound through water to an acoustical lens system, which focuses the waves. The shock wave is coupled to the patient through the use of a soft silicone coupling head that abuts the patient's flank. The stone is localized with biplanar fluoroscopy units.[47,48] The relatively low shock-wave pressure and large coupling area between the shock head and the skin produce very little pain for the patient.[49]

The Piezolith 2200* and the EDAP LT-01[†] use a piezoelectric energy source. A concave disc approximately 50 cm in diameter is mounted with mosaic-like piezoceramic crystals. Charged with a high-voltage signal, each crystal emits a brief (<1 μsec) unipolar, high-energy impulse.[50] The shock wave generated is automatically focused by the spherical shape of the concave disc.[50,51] The cavity is filled with water and covered with a soft rubber membrane over which a gel is placed to achieve good contact with the skin.[51] An ultrasound probe is located in the center of the disc permitting continuous real-time imaging throughout the procedure.[51,52] This type of lithotriptor can generate multiple impacts per second, and because the shock wave enters the skin at a lower pressure, there is almost no pain.[53,54]

The piezoelectric lithotriptor requires no special water tub or patient positioning devices. It can be placed easily in a mobile unit with no special room adaptations, and standard power and water sources can be used.[50] How-

ever, the lower pressure of the shock wave may also necessitate the use of more shock waves, or even repeat procedures, to disrupt the stones.

Anesthesia equipment

No special anesthesia machine or circuit is required for anesthetizing a patient in the lithotriptor. However, if a patient being treated in the water bath lithotriptor requires general anesthesia, then the anesthesia hoses will need to be approximately 12 feet long. This will increase the compression volume in the circuit, and the ventilator will have to be adjusted accordingly. A volume monitor can help in setting the ventilator correctly. Finally, the extra length of hose in the circuit creates additional sources of potential leaks and disconnects.

PATIENT MONITORING
Monitors of cardiovascular function

The first-generation lithotriptors (Dornier HM-3) require that the patient be immersed in warm water up to the level of the clavicles while seated semiupright in a hydraulic chair (gantry). Before appropriate monitors of cardiovascular function are selected for use during lithotripsy, it is vital to have a basic understanding of the physiologic changes that occur during immersion and shock wave therapy. Physiologic changes with immersion are compounded by the use of anesthesia and by having the patient seated in an upright position. Vasodilation causing peripheral venous pooling and hypotension is even more pronounced with regional anesthesia than with general because of the resultant sympathetic blockade.[55,56,57]

---

*Wolf, Kniltlingan, Germany.
[†]EDAP International Co., Croissy, Beaubourg, France.

During immersion, increased hydrostatic pressure on the legs and abdomen compresses the peripheral capacitance vessels, causing the intravascular volume to shift to the intrathoracic compartment.[36,41,55,56] The increased intrathoracic pressure manifests as an increase in central venous pressure, right atrial pressure, mean pulmonary capillary wedge pressure, and peak airway pressure during positive-pressure ventilation.[41,55,56,57] Acute changes in right atrial and right ventricular wall tension caused by a rapid increase or decrease in preload may lead to arrhythmias.[58,59] The warm temperature of the bath may increase peripheral vasodilation and increase the difficulty of maintaining hemodynamic stability.[56] Metabolic changes produced by immersion include kaliuresis, natriuresis, diuresis secondary to decreased antidiuretic hormone (ADH), and renin production.[41]

Anesthesia may inhibit the patient's usual ability to compensate for these changes by blocking normal physiologic reflexes. Although such changes are generally well tolerated by young, healthy patients, they may not be tolerated by patients with coronary artery disease, congestive heart failure, or significant valvular disease. Some of the cardiovascular changes caused by immersion can be tempered by immersing the patient slowly and for a brief period, with slow emersion as well.[58,60]

It is not always possible to predict the magnitude to which the cardiovascular system will be altered by immersion. In addition, it may be necessary to increase intravascular volume as well as to administer diuretics in order to eliminate all stone fragments. Therefore, a pulmonary arterial catheter may be required for patients with cardiac disease to detect and treat acute changes in ventricular wall tension caused by rapid changes in intravascular fluid volume.[42] Because patients are immersed to the level of the clavicle, it is important that the catheter insertion site be covered and protected adequately with a sterile plastic adhesive dressing to decrease the risk of infection. The presence of any catheter within the heart also increases the risk of microshock; consequently, all equipment that may come in contact with either the patient or the intracardiac catheter should be carefully checked for leakage of current.

The shock wave generated by lithotripsy may affect cardiac conduction. When lithotriptors were first being used, arrhythmias were frequently seen if the shock waves were delivered during the cardiac repolarization phase.[37,61] Consequently, cardiac gating was added to the original machine, and this enabled recognition of the QRS complex so that the shock could be delivered approximately 20 msec later.[61] Cardiac gating has greatly reduced the incidence of serious arrhythmias, particularly ventricular tachycardia. A normal sinus rhythm at a rate of 100 to 120 beats per minute or less is necessary for the gating to function properly, because the capacitor does not have time to recharge fully before the next triggered discharge if the R-R interval is less than 0.55 seconds.[57]

It is important that the ECG lead system be free from interference that might trigger the shock wave and inhibit recognition of the actual QRS complex. Amplitude and slope criteria are used to assess the QRS and prevent erroneous recognition of noise.[62] Materials and objects capable of emitting a significant electrical charge should be kept away from the ECG to prevent random shock waves. Interference has been reported from pacemakers, shivering, peripheral nerve stimulators, electrode movement, defective wires, and signals from other equipment.[61] Static electrical charges caused by a technician accidentally hitting styrofoam reportedly produced high-amplitude energy spikes that interfered with cardiac gating.[62]

It is important that the ECG leads be attached to dry skin for good contact and to maintain an accurate signal. The electrode leads must be appropriately covered with a dry adhesive dressing to maintain good contact throughout the procedure. Maintaining a five-lead system for ischemia detection may be technically difficult. The Prince Henry ECG montage[63] has been used in Australia and reportedly has a reasonable sensitivity and specificity with a three-lead system during immersion procedures. In this system, the right arm electrode is placed at the manubrium, the left arm electrode at the xiphoid, and the left leg electrode in the V_5 position. This system gives larger P and R waves than usually seen in the lead II position and decreased muscle and respiratory artifact. When the ECG lead selector is turned to lead I, the P wave appears almost as big as when an esophageal electrode is used.

The safety of extracorporeal shock wave lithotripsy for patients who are dependent on pacemakers remains controversial. Currently in the United States, lithotripsy is not approved for patients with pacemakers.[64] The pacemaker spike may be erroneously perceived as a QRS complex by the lithotriptor. If this occurs, the shock might not be generated during the quiescent period of the heart, causing ventricular arrhythmias. Conversely, the pacemaker may malfunction if the shock wave is recognized as a QRS complex. Some authors feel that contemporary pacemakers sufficiently filter extraneous electrical energy so that shock waves have little effect on pacemaker function.[36] Nevertheless, it has been suggested that before treatment is begun, the lithotripsy team should ensure that the pacer is at least 10 cm from the "blast path" to avoid possible damage to timing crystals. As in all situations involving patients dependent on pacemakers and possible interference, the anesthesiologist should have access to back-up assistance, including an appropriate magnet, programmer, cardiologist, or noninvasive temporary pacemaker (see Chapter 31).[64]

Blood pressure monitoring, standard during anesthesia care, must be accurate and reliable during ESWL because of the anticipated hemodynamic changes brought on by immersion. Furthermore, significant postoperative hypertension has been documented in approximately 4% of patients as a result of perirenal hematoma or renal vascular damage.[65] This hypertension is usually seen during the postanesthesia recovery phase but may occur much later, necessitating prolonged accurate blood pressure monitoring.

An automated (oscillometric) blood pressure device is recommended because of the patient's distance from the anesthesiologist.[57] Elevation of the arms may change oscillometric blood pressure readings by as much as 15 mm Hg.[58] This inaccuracy may be a problem with older gantry devices, in which the arms were suspended above the patient's head out of the water bath. More recently, most institutions have elected to float the patient's arms loosely in the water in order to avoid peripheral neuropathy. Although the ulnar nerves may be spared with this procedure, the problem is now that of a wet blood pressure cuff. Transducers or microphones in some automatic blood pressure cuffs do not function when wet.[57] Blood pressure cuffs with Velcro may lose their adhesive ability when immersed for extended periods.[42] A blood pressure cuff with a metal band and clip is more likely to remain correctly positioned on the patient's arm.[42]

An intraarterial catheter with continuous waveform monitoring is recommended for patients in whom blood pressure lability is anticipated, for those whose hemodynamic status requires continuous monitoring, and for those who may require frequent blood sampling. The catheter insertion site can be covered with a sterile plastic adhesive dressing to prevent possible contamination or infection.

Respiratory monitoring

Immersing the patient to the level of the clavicles results in a decrease in both functional residual capacity and vital capacity because of increased hydrostatic pressure.[36,41,42,66] Perfusion shifts to the upper lobe of the lung, causing a mismatch in the ventilation/perfusion ratio. Intrapulmonary shunt is also increased because closing capacity exceeds tidal ventilation, which in turn increases the work of breathing.[41,66] Finally, many consider the danger of airway obstruction to be greater with the lithotripsy patient simply because the patient is remote from the anesthesiologist during general anesthesia or sedation.[41] As a result of this respiratory compromise, Vegfors and his colleagues[66] noted a 2% decrease in oxygen saturation (measured by oximetry) in ASA 1 and 2 patients undergoing lithotripsy. A decrease of up to 4% was noted in patients classified as ASA 3. They also found that premature ventricular contractions occurred more frequently in patients whose oxygen saturations decreased to 92% and that ectopy was resolved by administration of higher concentrations of oxygen. There is apparently little difference in lung function regardless of whether regional or general anesthesia is used for the immersion procedures.[67]

The compromised respiratory physiology and technical difficulties of patient management make it particularly im-

portant that adequate systems be available for ventilation as well as for respiratory monitoring. The precordial stethoscope is useless during lithotripsy because the loud shock wave occurs at the same time as the QRS complex, which obscures the heart tones. Furthermore, with immersion type lithotriptors, it is difficult to secure the precordial stethoscope to the chest wall. Although the esophageal stethoscope can be placed with general anesthesia, the heart sounds cannot necessarily be auscultated over the shock waves.[36,42] Radio telemetry overcomes the problem of remoteness by eliminating the need to extend the stethoscope with additional tubing but does not provide improved acoustics when the shock waves are firing.

Pulse oximetry and capnography are particularly important in remote and hostile environments, where resuscitation is difficult and early information about respiratory malfunction is critical. Ohmeda produces a fully immersible oximeter probe, Softprobe,* which offers a very bright LED, can be molded to fit almost any size of patient, and is electrically safe in the water bath. Furthermore, the probe can be adapted to fit on the ear, nasal septum, or tongue; and thus it is accessible outside the water bath (Fig. 27-9). Placing the oximeter probe on the ear offers the additional advantage of decreased lag time during desaturation or resaturation.[68]

Infrared capnography systems are available in efficient portable units and can be adapted easily to a remote environment or even a mobile van. A nasal oxygen cannula can be adapted for carbon dioxide monitoring in the spontaneously breathing patient (Figs. 27-3 and 27-4). In patients who are undergoing lithotripsy without immersion, apnea monitoring by impedance enables remote monitoring of respiratory rate. The 556 Physiologic Monitor by Corometrics† is a small, easily portable unit, which contains impedance apnea monitoring as well as ECG, pressure transduction, noninvasive blood pressure monitoring, oximetry, transcutaneous oxygen and carbon dioxide monitoring, and temperature monitoring. The screen can be moved approximately 10 feet from the monitor, allowing the anesthesiologist to continue effective monitoring from behind a radiation shield. Impedance apnea monitoring indicates, however, neither that ventilation is adequate nor that it is actually occurring, because it detects only chest movement and does not monitor exhalation of carbon dioxide.

The goal of mechanical ventilation during lithotripsy is to minimize stone movement while maximizing respiratory function. Deep "sigh" breaths may decrease intrapulmonary shunting, but they also increase movement of the diaphragm and therefore the kidney.[58] This may expose parts of the lung field to shock waves, resulting in pulmonary parenchymal injury and hemoptysis. More com-

---

*Ohmeda, Boulder, Colo.
†Corometrics, Wallingford, Conn.

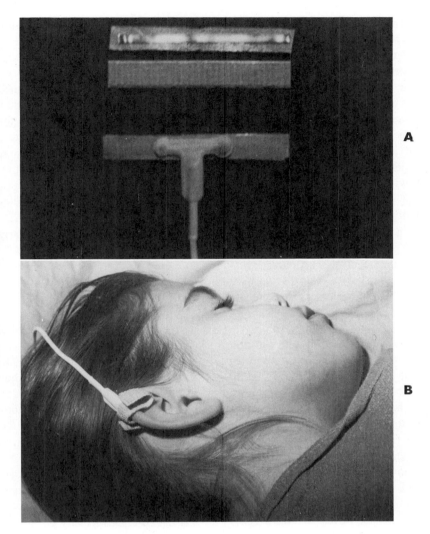

Fig. 27-9. A pulse oximetry probe (Ohmeda) can be adapted for use in different locations. **A,** A piece of aluminum removed from the nose of a surgical mask is placed between two pieces of adhesive dressing. The pulse oximetry probe is then attached to the dressing with double-sided adhesive tape. **B,** The probe can now be molded to fit a number of different locations without the use of any additional tape. In this case, the probe is attached to the helix of the ear. (Stenger MN: *Anesthetic management of pediatric and neonatal emergencies.* In Bell C, Hughes CW, Oh TH, editors: *The pediatric anesthesia handbook,* St. Louis, 1991, Mosby–Year Book.)

monly, increased movement of the kidney causes shock waves to be fired with decreased precision of focus, impeding the accuracy of the shock waves. This results in longer procedures and possibly incomplete stone destruction because less energy is delivered to the stone.[69] The stone must be within one cubic centimeter of the shock wave to be completely disintegrated.[61] Also, more energy reaches nonstone tissue or surrounding perirenal parenchyma.[69]

Because of these problems with conventional mechanical ventilation, many centers use high-frequency jet ventilation to decrease stone movement. Carlson, et al.[61] showed that stones may move as much as 15 to 68 mm with conventional positive-pressure ventilation or spontaneous ventilation. Several studies[61,70,71] have shown that mean

stone movement can be decreased by as much as 90% with high-frequency jet ventilation. Either high-frequency jet ventilation or high-frequency positive-pressure ventilation with a conventional ventilator will minimize the stone movement.[71] This provides for better disintegration with fewer shock waves, shorter fluoroscopy time, less trauma to surrounding tissue, shorter immersion time, and the need to use fewer spark plugs.[41,71] However, some investigators[72] reportedly found no statistically significant difference in the number of shock treatments with either conventional mechanical ventilation or high-frequency jet ventilation.

The use of high-frequency jet ventilation is accompanied by its own set of problems. Special equipment is required, which may or may not be available at a given institution, along with personnel specially trained and comfortable in the use of that equipment. System alarms become more important when unconventional equipment is being used in areas remote from the anesthesiologist and from other back-up support personnel.[57] The system must be specially modified for use with anesthetic agents, to scavenge gases, or to successfully monitor end-tidal carbon dioxide.[71,73] However, during jet ventilation, end-tidal carbon dioxide can be measured intermittently by periodically shutting off the jet and giving manual deep sigh breaths.[71,74] Finally, the jet ventilator may fail to ventilate adequately in patients with bronchospasm, because increased airway resistance will necessitate higher inflation pressures, which eventually stalls the jet, halting gas flow. This may compromise ventilation markedly and may necessitate a change to conventional ventilatory techniques.[73,74] Regardless of the benefit to risk ratio of using high-frequency ventilation, the use of general anesthesia cannot be justified simply to minimize stone movement if the regional technique would be more appropriate for a given patient and procedure.[71]

Another technique that has been used to decrease stone movement is ECG-synchronized ventilation.[69] With this technique, the mechanical breath, and therefore stone displacement, occurs at a fixed interval after the shock wave. Because the shock wave hits the stone during end-expiration only, the stone is totally motionless and does not leave the area of primary focus.[75] Furthermore, this type of ventilation eliminates shock waves during aortic pulsation, which may cause movement of stones located on the left side.[69] QRS-activated ventilation requires the ECG to be connected to a heart rate meter and a trigger delay unit.[75] Besides ventilation, shock waves are still triggered by the QRS to prevent arrhythmias. Therefore, a low tidal volume mechanical breath (3 ml/kg) starts 50 to 100 msec after the shock wave is fired and ends 20 to 50 msec before the next QRS complex begins.[76]

It has been argued[77] that there is less stone movement with ECG-synchronized ventilation simply because the tidal volume is lower. In either case, the higher ventilatory frequency increases dead space, raising the gradient between end-tidal and arterial carbon dioxide. Consequently, monitoring arterial blood gases may be more effective than monitoring end-tidal carbon dioxide. Alternatively, the high-frequency ventilation can be interrupted with a period of conventional ventilation, after which intermittent end-tidal carbon dioxide readings can be obtained. Patients with pulmonary disease may be especially susceptible to greater arterial to end-tidal gradients. With these patients, higher concentrations of inspired oxygen and larger ventilatory volumes should be considered.

Temperature monitoring

Even though it is assumed that the temperature of the water bath is reliably constant, aberrations of core temperature are not uncommon. Therefore, precise temperature monitoring of both the patient and the water bath are im-

perative. Significant hyperthermia may be manifested as increased sweating, increased minute ventilation, decreased urine output, and increased heart rate and and cardiac output.[78] If hyperthermia is left untreated, multiple organ system failure can occur. Conversely, immersion may cause hypothermia even when the water bath is maintained at 36° C.[57] In addition to the common complications of hypothermia, including decreased peripheral perfusion and cardiac ectopy, shivering may also be a problem because it affects stone movement and shock wave accuracy. Shivering from hypothermia appears to be worse with epidural anesthesia but usually stops when the patient is placed in the heated water bath.[40]

Liquid crystal temperature strips can be placed on the forehead of the immersed patient. However, this technique is more accurate for trending than for precise monitoring and also requires that the anesthesiologist be close enough to the patient to be able to read the temperature strip. Esophageal, nasopharyngeal, or tympanic membrane probes can be used with general anesthesia. Care must be taken to avoid submerging the connection of the temperature probe to the main cable, which often causes malfunction. A skin disc can be used above the level of the clavicle with regional anesthesia. Conversely, a rectal probe can be used as long as connections are either covered with waterproof wrap or kept out of the water bath.

Mobile lithotripsy units

In an effort to contain costs and make expensive lithotripsy units more accessible, mobile trailers or vans with self-contained units are being used in many areas (Fig. 27-10). These vans usually become modular extensions of the hospital interior for convenient transport of patients and personnel. Mobile units are subject to the same standards as any operating room with regard to oxygen, suction, and scavenging of anesthetic gases. Some even have separate hookups connecting the van to the hospital's central supply for nitrous oxide and air. To avoid having multiple gas hoses along the floor, which might constitute an environmental hazard, hoses are supported by rings or hooks along the ceiling (Fig. 27-11).

Full electrical capabilities, as in a regular operating room or radiology suite, should be present, along with access to the hospital's back-up generator. An isolated electrical power supply with a line isolation monitor should be considered, particularly for water bath units. The specific details of electrical, architectural, pneumatic, and electronic interfacing with the main hospital from the mobile unit are beyond the scope of most clinicians and demand the expertise of biomedical engineers. However, an anesthesiologist should be part of the planning and design committee to ensure that all safety and risk management principles are observed.

Having a separate monitoring system located in the mobile van along with a fully stocked anesthesia cart is not only convenient but also decreases the wear and tear that

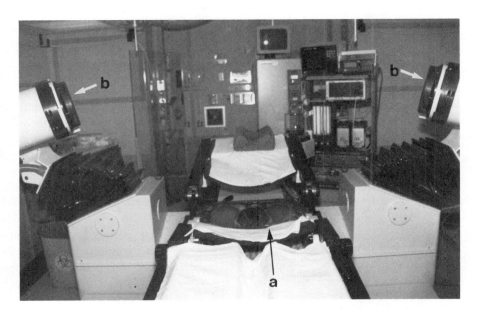

Fig. 27-10. The HM-4 lithotriptor has been installed in a mobile van. The figure shows the patient bed in the treatment position with the water cushion *(a)* and the fluoroscopy tubes *(b)*. In the background are the anesthesia machine and monitors.

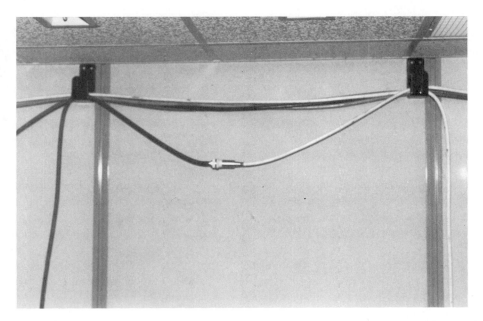

Fig. 27-11. Oxygen, nitrous oxide, air, and vacuum sources are supplied to the mobile van via connections with the hospital's central supply. The gas hoses are then strung around the van to the desired location. L-shaped hooks hold the gas hoses in place. These hooks greatly facilitate setting up and removal of the hoses on a weekly basis. The eyelet type of hook is less desirable because installation and removal of the hoses takes longer and, with repeated set-ups, may actually damage the gas supply hoses.

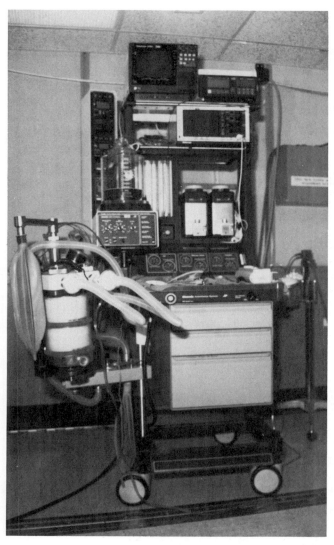

Fig. 27-12. Because space is at a premium in a mobile van, the anesthesia machine (Ohmeda Excel) and the patient monitors have been chosen to provide full monitoring capabilities while occupying a minimal amount of floor space.

occurs when equipment is transported to the van on a daily basis. Many companies now manufacture small, efficient multifunctional monitoring units that can be mounted easily on an anesthesia machine, even in areas with limited space. These units should be selected on the basis of a number of factors, including financial constraints and the company's previous service record with the hospital or department. Any system selected should include basic monitoring capabilities, including ECG, invasive pressure transduction, noninvasive blood pressure monitoring, oximetry, and temperature monitoring. Although also important, end-tidal carbon dioxide and apnea monitoring are not always present in the smaller, self-enclosed units. An acceptable alternative is a separate infrared end-tidal gas analyzer with the capability of measuring halogenated agents (Fig. 27-12).

The patient is usually at a distance from the anesthesiologist because of either the size and shape of the lithotripsy unit or the need to protect the anesthesiologist from radiation exposure. For this reason, the monitoring unit may be near the anesthesiologist and distant from the patient, which will require some modification of connections or extension tubing. On the other hand, the monitoring equipment can be placed near the patient and away from the anesthesiologist. In this scenario, the monitor screen should be easy to read from a distance of 6 feet, and it may have a keyed function pad that can be used separately. The previously mentioned monitor unit (Corometrics 556 Physiologic Monitor*), which has a removable screen that can be located approximately 10 feet away from the basic monitoring system, may be very useful in this situation. This monitor has a 4-hour battery pack that is useful for transporting patients from the van to recovery areas or if further procedures are necessary (i.e., stent placement).[42]

Environmental hazards in the lithotripsy unit

Much of what is required for successful stone pulverization is also the source of potential hazard for both patients and personnel. The room itself may have less direct lighting than the usual operating room suite, making it difficult to see the patient, monitors, and chart. The light is often dimmed during fluoroscopy to enhance imaging, further reducing visibility.[40]

Noise pollution is of the high-impact type, which, though irritating, is not likely to cause permanent damage to hearing.[42] Because the HM-3 lithotriptor is louder than newer models, ear plugs can be useful for the anesthesiologist. Providing the patient with earphones can reduce noise pollution as well as improve the effectiveness of sedation or analgesia. Earphones that provide a musical background may be a worthwhile addition, but they may pose an electrical hazard if the patient is seated in a water bath. Commercially available earphones that use batteries are less hazardous than those that require electrical wiring, but both types should be checked and approved by the biomedical engineers before they are used with the immersion type of lithotriptors. Noise pollution also interferes with monitoring by making it more difficult to perceive breath sounds, heart tones, monitoring pitches on oximetry and ECG units, and alarms.

Electrical safety for both patients and medical personnel is of particular concern with the immersion type of lithotripsy unit. The tank and all monitors must be carefully grounded and the entire suite electrically isolated whether in a mobile unit or not.[62] Hepp[79] used a model to show that electrical hazards are minimal as long as the patient does not touch the ellipsoid rim of the water bath while simultaneously grounded.

When defibrillation is necessary, a potential hazard arises if the person delivering the countershock has wet

*Corometrics, Wallingford, Conn.

hands and is also standing on the wet floor.[61] In this situation, the internal safety devices of the defibrillator must be relied on for protection. When the skin is wet, the delivered countershock follows the path of least resistance along the skin, and the amount of energy that actually reaches the heart may be inadequate.[61]

It is difficult to position the patient in the water bath and avoid nerve injuries.[59] During the procedure, the patient must be suspended in a hydraulic chair (gantry), which presents the two-fold problem of possibly unrecognized pressure and the difficulty of removing the patient quickly should resuscitation be required.[40] Malhotra[39] has described an adaptation of the Surgilift Stretcher Lifter* that assists in the placement of anesthetized patients in the gantry as well as in their prompt removal. This system prevents the patient's monitors or catheters from being dislodged, reduces the risk of back injuries to personnel, and minimizes exposure of personnel to water, with its attendant electrical hazards. Pressure injuries can also be minimized by floating the patient's arms in the water bath rather than securing them either laterally or above the head.

The use of biplanar fluoroscopy to localize stones adds radiation exposure to the list of potential hazards.[38] In addition, spot films, which require more radiation exposure, are necessary to monitor the location and disintegration of the stone. Jocham, et al.[37] reported that radiation exposure during shock wave lithotripsy is approximately half that of percutaneous nephrolithotomy and approximately double that received during intravenous pyelography. The actual amount of radiation to which the patient is exposed depends on a number of factors, including the imaging technique used (fluoroscopy versus spot pictures), the x-ray tube output (voltage and amperage), total exposure time, patient weight and body surface area, and stone size and position.[38] Tube collimators are used to reduce the field size and therefore the amount of exposure.[38] The type of anesthesia administered, whether general or regional, does not seem to affect the amount of radiation exposure.[38]

It is almost impossible to shield patients successfully within the water bath. However, the genitalia, thyroid, and eyes can be shielded with other types of lithotriptors. Exposure of medical personnel to radiation appears to be negligible at a distance of approximately three feet from the lithotriptor.[42] However, all personnel should be appropriately protected with lead shielding or stand behind leaded glass, and those exposed on a routine basis should wear dosimeters.[38]

Equipment modification for pediatric lithotripsy

The original Dornier HM-3 lithotriptor was not built for patients under 30 kg in weight or 135 cm in height. Because approximately 3% of all patients treated for renal calculi are children, many institutions have found it necessary to modify present equipment and monitoring techniques for the safe treatment of children.[80]

Children are at higher risk than adults for complications from lithotripsy. By virtue of their small size, a relatively larger portion of the kidney and surrounding structures are exposed to the focal zone. Shock waves and radiation exposure may be detrimental to growing organs. Finally, the child's relatively small ureter makes it necessary for stone fragments to be smaller in order to pass into the bladder.[81] Even so, shock wave lithotripsy has been approved by the FDA for use in children.[82]

The use of piezoelectric or electromagnetic types of lithotriptors avoids many of the problems encountered when the water bath is used for pediatric patients. The patient can be supine or somewhat lateral, permitting ready access to the airway.[83] These machines are associated with a decreased anesthetic requirement by the patient, making possible the use of a dissociative anesthetic (ketamine), and thereby decreasing the need for special pediatric ventilators.[84] In particular, the piezoelectric technique uses ultrasound instead of fluoroscopy for stone localization, thus eliminating the hazards of radiation exposure.[81] Abdominal counterpressure has been used to ensure that the water-fitted bellows with electromagnetic lithotriptors fit snugly against the patient's flank.[84]

If the original water bath lithotriptor is used for a pediatric patient, the gantry must be adjusted to the patient's size. This helps to protect the lungs, which are susceptible to damage because of the air-tissue interface, as well as to maintain the water level so that it entirely covers shock wave sites but leaves the head completely exposed.[82] If the water level is not high enough to cover abdominal exit sites while leaving the head exposed, intravenous fluid bags can be used at the exit site to maintain the tissue-water interface.[82]

Hemoptysis has been reported in children after as little as three minutes of shock wave exposure.[85] To prevent hemoptysis, the lungs can be protected with polystyrene foam. A 4-cm styrofoam board found in the Dornier electrode packing box can be used to both protect the lungs and extend the back of the gantry chair to support the smaller patient.[85] Although bags of styrofoam pastilles work well for positioning and for minimizing pressure injury, they have been found to float out of position in the water bath, increasing susceptibility to lung damage.[85] For very small infants, an infant seat with a hole cut in the back has been used and secured to the gantry, with a styrofoam board protecting the lung bases.[80] Soft foam with adhesive backing (Reston, 3M) applied directly to the patient also may provide slightly better protection of the lung bases.[86] Regardless of the type of styrofoam protection used, a small radio-opaque wire placed around the edges of the foam allows for visualization on fluoroscopy to ensure that the bases of the lung remain out of the shock wave's pathway.[82,39]

*Trans-D Corporation, Carson, Calif.

Jansson, et al.[69] have reported that heart-synchronized ventilation is especially useful in children to minimize diaphragmatic movement and therefore possible lung damage. An apneic technique in which ventilation occurs only between episodes of shock waves has also been found to minimize the potential for lung injury.[86] With this technique, shock wave episodes are not begun until the patient has been adequately ventilated to lower the end-tidal carbon dioxide to less than 30 mm Hg. A brief period of apneic oxygenation is then alternated with periods of ventilation.

REFERENCES

1. ASA Newsletter, ASA, Park Ridge, Ill, October 21, 1986.
2. National Electrical Code, NFPA no 70-1987, by exception to article 517-101 (b)(2). Articles 517-101 (b)(5) and (c)(2) require connectors "listed for hospital use."
3. Bruner JMR, Leonard PF: *Controversies and confusions. In Electricity, safety and the patient,* Chicago, 1989, Mosby–Year Book, pp 300-319.
4. Eichhorn JH, Cooper JB, Cullen DJ, et al; Standards for patient monitoring during anesthesia at Harvard Medical School, *JAMA* 256:1017-1020, 1986.
5. Cannard TH, Dripps RD, Helwig J, et al: The ECG during anesthesia and surgery, *Anesthesiology* 21:194-202, 1960.
6. Ansell G, Tweedie MCK, West CR, et al: The current status of reactions to intravenous contrast media, *Invest Radiol* 15:S32-39, 1980.
7. Shehadi WH, Toniolo G: Adverse reactions to contrast media: a report from the Committee on Safety of Contrast Media of the International Society of Radiology, *Radiology* 137:299-302, 1982.
8. Hartman GW, Hattery RR, Witten DM, et al: Mortality during excretory urography: Mayo Clinic experience, *Am J Radiol* 139:919-922, 1982.
9. Yelderman M, Ream AK: Indirect measurement of mean blood pressure in the anesthetized patient, *Anesthesiology* 50:253-256, 1979.
10. Bruner JMR, Krenis LF, Kunsman JM, et al: Comparison of direct and indirect methods of measuring arterial blood pressure. III. *Med Instrum* 5:182-198, 1981.
11. Yelderman M, New W: Evaluation of pulse oximetry, *Anesthesiology* 59:349-352, 1983.
12. Kelleher JF: Pulse oximetry: a review, *J Clin Monit* 5:37-62, 1989.
13. Wong DH, Tremper K, Davidson J, et al: Pulse oximetry is accurate in patients with dysrhythmias and a pulse deficit, *Anesthesiology* 70:1024-1025, 1989.
14. Graham B, Paulus D, Caffee H: Pulse oximetry for vascular monitoring in upper extremity replantation surgery, *J Hand Surg* 11A:687-692, 1986.
15. Partridge BL: Use of pulse oximetry as a noninvasive indicator of intravascular volume status, *J Clin Monit* 3:263-268, 1987.
16. Lees D, Schutter N, Bull J, et al: An evaluation of liquid crystal thermometry as a screening device for intraoperative hypothermia, *Anesth Analg* 57:669-674, 1978.
17. Mitzutani A, Ozaki G, Benumof J: A low-cost high-fidelity FM wireless precordial radiostethoscope for continuous monitoring of heart and breath sounds, *J Clin Monit* 6:61-64, 1990.
18. Moretti E, Monti R, Zeig N: A cordless infrared headphone system for monitoring heart and breath sounds, *Anesth Analg* 71:309, 1990.
19. Murray IP, Modell J: Early detection of endotracheal tube accidents by monitoring carbon dioxide concentration in respiratory gas, *Anesthesiology* 59:344-346, 1983.
20. Edelman R, Kleefield J, Wentz K, et al: *Basic principles of magnetic resonance imaging.* In Edelman R, Hesselink J, editors: *Clinical magnetic resonance imaging,* Philadelphia, 1990, Saunders.
21. Koskinen MF: *Site planning.* In Edelman R, Hesselink J, editors: *Clinical magnetic resonance imaging,* Philadelphia, 1990, Saunders.
22. O'Connor J, Engineering Division of Invivo Labs (Winter Park, Fla.): Personal communication, 1991.
23. Pavlicek W: *Safety considerations.* In Stark D, Bradley W, editors: *Magnetic resonance imaging,* St Louis, 1988, Mosby–Year Book.
24. Budinger TF: Thresholds for physiologic effects due to RF and magnetic fields used in NMR imaging, *Trans Nucl Sci* 26:2821-2825, 1979.
25. Karlik SJ, Heatherley T, Pavan F, et al: Patient anesthesia and monitoring at a 1.5T MRI installation, *Magnetic Resonance in Medicine* 7:210-221, 1988.
26. Budinger TF: Nuclear magnetic resonance (NMR): In vivo studies—known thresholds for health effects, *J Comput Assist Tomogr* 5:800-811, 1981.
27. Fletcher D, Hewlett-Packard MRI Equipment Division, Madison Wis: Personal communication, 1991.
28. Barnett GH, Ropper AH, Johnson KA: Physiologic support and monitoring of critically ill patients during magnetic resonance imaging, *J Neurosurg* 68:246-250, 1988.
29. McArdle CB, Nicholas DB, Richardson CJ, et al: Monitoring of the neonate undergoing MR imaging: technical considerations, *Radiology* 159:223-226, 1986.
30. Davis PJ, Gillen C, Kretchman E, et al: Experience with anesthesia for children requiring nuclear magnetic resonance imaging, *Anesth Review* 17:35-40, 1990.
31. Burk NS: Anesthesia for magnetic imaging, *Anesth Clin N Amer* 7:707-721, 1989.
32. Roos CF, Canole FE: Fiberoptic pressure transducer for use near MR magnetic fields, *Radiology* 156:157, 1985.
33. Hughes CW: Anesthesia outside of the operating room, *Semin Anesth* 9:190-196, 1990.
34. Dunn V, Coffman CE, McGowan JE, et al: Mechanical ventilation during magnetic resonance imaging, *Magn Reson Imaging* 3:169-172, 1985.
35. Patteson SK, Chesney JT: Anesthetic management for magnetic resonance imaging: problems and solutions, *Anesth Analg* 74:121-128, 1992.
36. Moyer MK, O'Gara JP, Burrus LE: General anesthesia for ESWL, *AANA J* 56:121-127, 1988.
37. Jocham D, Liedl B, Schuster C, et al: Pain-free ESWL with the tub-free Dornier HM-4 lithotriptor: longterm results, *J Urol* 139:227A, 1988 (abstract).
38. Carter HB, Naslund EB, Riehle RA Jr: Variables influencing radiation exposure during ESWL, *Urology* 30:546-550, 1987.
39. Malhotra V: A modified stretcher-lifter device for transfer of patients during ESWL, *Anesth Analg* 68:699, 1989.
40. Silbert BS, Kluger R, Dixon GCE, et al: Anaesthesia for ESWL at the Victorian Lithotripsy Service: the first 300 patients, *Anaesth Intensive Care* 16:310-317, 1988.
41. London RA, Kudlak T, Riehle RA: Immersion anesthesia for ESWL, *Urology* 28:86-94, 1986.
42. Mulroy, MF: Anesthesia for extracorporeal shock wave lithotripsy, *ASA Refresher Courses* 17:201-213, 1989.
43. Heine G: *Physical aspects of shock-wave treatment.* In Gravenstein JS, Peter K, editors: *Extracorporeal shock-wave lithotripsy for renal stone disease,* Boston, 1986, Butterworths.
44. Tomera KM, Benson C, Segura JW: Initial results of ultrasound-guided second generation lithotriptor, *J Urol* 139:228A, 1988 (abstract).
45. Schmidt A, Kohl H, Eisenberger F: Advanced technology in ESWL: the Dornier multi-purpose lithotriptor MPL9000 vs upgraded Dornier HM3, *J Urol* 139:227A, 1988 (abstract).
46. Rassweiler J, Kohl H: Wolf Piezolith 2200 vs modified Dornier HM3: range of indications, anesthesia and efficacy, *J Urol* 139:228A, 1988 (abstract).

47. Grace PA, Gillen P, Smith JM, et al: ESWL with the Lithostar lithotriptor, *Br J Urol* 64:117-121, 1989.
48. Staritz M, Rambow P, Mildenberger P, et al: Electromagnetically generated extracorporeal shock waves for gallstone lithotripsy: *in vitro* experiments and clinical relevance, *Eur J Clin Invest* 19:142-145, 1989.
49. Jenkins AD, Gillenwater JY: Initial experience with the Siemen's Lithostar, *J Urol* 139:227A, 1988 (abstract).
50. Marberger M, Turk C, Steinkogler I: Painless piezoelectric lithotripsy, *J Urol* 139:695-699, 1988.
51. Kim SC, Moon YT, Kim KD: ESWL monotherapy: experience with piezoelectric second generation lithotriptor in 642 patients, *J Urol* 142:674-678, 1989.
52. Neisius D, Zwergel T, Sarafidis P, et al: Extracorporeal lithotripsy with the Wolf Piezolith lithotriptor: initial clinical experience, *J Urol* 139:227A, 1988 (abstract).
53. Vallancien G, Aviles J, Munoz R, et al: Piezoelectric extracorporeal lithotripsy by ultrashort waves with the EDAP LT 01 device, *J Urol* 139:689-694, 1988.
54. Segura JW, Patterson DE, LeRoy AJ: Piezo-electric lithotripsy in the treatment of renal calculi, *J Urol* 139:263A, 1988 (abstract).
55. Frank M, McAtees EJ, Cohen DG, et al: One hundred cases of anaesthesia for extracorporeal shock wave lithotripsy, *Ann R Coll Surg Engl* 67:341-343, 1985.
56. Weber W, Madler C, Keil B, et al: *Cardiovascular effects of ESWL*. In Gravenstein JS, Peter K, editors: *Extracorporeal shock-wave lithotripsy for renal stone disease*, Boston, 1986, Butterworths.
57. Abbott MA, Samuel JR, Webb DR: Anaesthesia for ESWL, *Anaesthesia* 40:1065-1072, 1985.
58. Lehmann P, Weber W, Madler C, et al: *Anesthesia and ESWL: five years of experience*. In Gravenstein JS, Peter K, editors: *Extracorporeal shock-wave lithotripsy for renal stone disease*, Boston, 1986, Butterworths.
59. Roth RA, Beckmann CF: Complications of ESWL and percutaneous nephrolithotomy, *Urol Clin North Am* 15:155-166, 1988.
60. Behnia R, Shanks CA, Ovassapian A, et al: Hemodynamic responses associated with lithotripsy, *Anesth Analg* 66:354-356, 1987.
61. Carlson CA, Gravenstein JS, Gravenstein N: *Ventricular tachycardia during ESWL: etiology, treatment and prevention*. In Gravenstein JS, Peter K, editors: *Extracorporeal shock-wave lithotripsy for renal stone disease: technical and clinical aspects*, Boston, 1986, Butterworth.
62. Schiller EC, Heerdt P, Roberts J: Life-threatening ECG artifact during ESWL, *Anesthesiology* 68:477-478, 1988.
63. Wicks M, Hunt J, Walker R, et al: An electrode montage for electrocardiographic monitoring, *Anaesth Intensive Care* 17:74-77, 1989.
64. Walts LF, Gravenstein N: The first international symposium on anesthesia and ESWL, *Anesthesiology* 66:109-110, 1987.
65. Peterson JC, Finlayson B: *Effects of ESWL on blood pressure*. In Gravenstein JS, Peter K, editors: *Extracorporeal shock-wave lithotripsy for renal stone disease*, Boston, 1986, Butterworths.
66. Vegfors M, Gustafson M, Sjoberg F, et al: Pulse oximetry during extradural analgesia for ESWL, *Br J Anaesth* 61:771-772, 1988.
67. Kelly RE, Binion M, Malhotra V, et al: Pulmonary function after ESWL: a comparison of general and regional anaesthesia, *Can J Anaesth* 36:137-140, 1989.

68. Tremper KK, Barker SS: Pulse oximetry, *Anesthesiology* 70:98-108, 1989.
69. Jansson L, Bengtsson M, Carlsson C: Heart synchronized ventilation during general anesthesia for ESWL, *Anesth Analg* 67:706-709, 1988.
70. Warner MA, Warner ME, Buck CF, et al: Clinical efficacy of high frequency jet ventilation during ESWL of renal and ureteral calculi: a comparison with conventional mechanical ventilation, *J Urol* 139:486-487, 1988.
71. Perel A, Hoffman B, Podeh D, et al: High frequency positive pressure ventilation during general anesthesia for ESWL, *Anesth Analg* 65:1231-1234, 1986.
72. Finlayson B, Newman RC, Hunter PT II, et al: *Efficacy of ESWL for stone fracture*. In Gravenstein JS, Peter K, editors: *Extracorporeal shock-wave lithotripsy for renal stone disease*, Boston, 1986, Butterworths.
73. Boysen PG, Carlson CA, Banner MJ, et al: *Ventilation during anesthesia for ESWL*. In Gravenstein JS, Peter K, editors: *Extracorporeal shock-wave lithotripsy for renal stone disease*, Boston, 1986, Butterworths.
74. Berger JJ, Boysen PG, Gravenstein JS, et al: Failure of high frequency jet ventilation to ventilate patients adequately during ESWL, *Anesth Analg* 6 262-263, 1987.
75. Perel A, Segal E, Pizov R, et al: QRS-activated ventilation during general anesthesia for ESWL, *J Clin Anesth* 1:268-271, 1989.
76. Segal E, Perel A: Heart synchronized ventilation during ESWL, *Anesth Analg* 69:139, 1989.
77. Pond WW, Lindsey RL, Weaver GA: Value of heart-synchronized ventilation during ESWL remains unproven, *Anesth Analg* 68:823, 1989.
78. Higgins TL, Miller EV, Roberts J: Accidental hyperthermia as a complication of extracorporeal shock wave lithotripsy under general anesthesia, *Anesthesiology* 66:389-391, 1987.
79. Hepp W: *Electrical safety of the Dornier lithotriptor*. In Gravenstein JS, Peter K, editors: *Extracorporeal shock-wave lithotripsy for renal stone disease*, Boston, 1986, Butterworths.
80. Caldwell C, Butcher B: ESWL in infants and small children: gantry modification, *Anesthesiology* 68:658-659, 1988.
81. Marberger M, Turk C, Steinkogler I: Piezoelectric extracorporeal shock wave lithotripsy in children, *J Urol* 142:349-352, 1989.
82. Kramolowsky EV, Willoughby BL, Loening SA: ESWL in children, *J Urol* 137:939-941, 1987.
83. Wilbert DM, Schofer O, Reidmiller H: Treatment of paediatric urolithiasis by extracorporeal shock wave lithotripsy, *Eur J Pediatr* 147:579-581, 1988.
84. Abara E, Merguerian PA, Mchorie GA, et al: Lithostar extracorporeal shock wave lithotripsy in children, *J Urol* 144:489-491, 1990.
85. Malhotra V, Gomillion MC, Artusio JF: Hemoptysis in a child during extracorporeal shock wave lithotripsy, *Anesth Analg* 69:526-528, 1989.
86. Tredrea CR, Pathak D, From RP, et al: Lung protection in children during ESWL, *Anesth Analg* 66:S178, 1987 (abstract).

Chapter 28

ANESTHESIA AT DIFFERENT ENVIRONMENTAL PRESSURES

Enrico M. Camporesi, M.D.

In the course of common anesthetic practice, it is unusual, to worry about alteration in total environmental pressure because the largest number of anesthetic procedures are conducted normally within a limited range of pressure. Most organized hospital settings, in fact, have developed in a narrow span of altitudes not far from sea level, although a significant portion of the world's population continues to live at high altitude. In recent years, traditional surgical and anesthetic techniques have been expanded to countries in development, such as Nepal in Asia, the Andean Highlands of South America, and elevated African regions such as Zimbabwe. Utilization of gas-based anesthesia has increased at altitudes where total barometric pressure is reduced.

In contrast, the historical record is more complex for provision of anesthesia at increased barometric pressure, as it was first described by Paul Bert in 1879. His aim was to use nitrous oxide in anesthetic doses and to be able simultaneously to provide adequate oxygenation. An account of this idea was more recently given by Smith, et al.[1] During the late 1940s, interest in the surgical treatment of congenital heart malformations grew rapidly after Blalock performed the first successful procedure for tetralogy of Fallot in 1944. When surgical correction of the septal and valvular abnormalities was attempted, deep hypothermia and cardiopulmonary arrest were used to provide a motionless heart. Limitations of the technique were primarily the short times of total circulatory arrest (less than 10 minutes) without significant ischemic central nervous system (CNS) sequelae. General anesthesia under hyperbaric oxygenation (HBO) provided an added degree of protection and increased the time of safe cardiac arrest to 30 minutes. Several groups reported their experiences with anesthesia under hyperbaric conditions, including Smith[2] at the Massachusetts General Hospital, Boerema[3] in Holland, and McDowall[4] at the Royal Infirmary in Glasgow. Anesthesia was usually achieved and maintained through the use of nitrous oxide, halothane, or methoxyflurane. In

1953 the extracorporeal circulatory system developed by Gibbon was successfully utilized for correction of an atrial septal defect. It was not until the mid-1960s, however, that a practical cardiopulmonary bypass machine was perfected for wider use. With the introduction of safe cardiopulmonary bypass pumps, cardiac surgery no longer needed to be performed in the hyperbaric chamber. Carotid endarterectomies had also been performed under hyperbaric conditions in order to extend ischemia time and provide cerebral protection, but the practice was never firmly demonstrated to be beneficial.

In 1965 a landmark report appeared by Severinghaus,[5] in which the practice of anesthesia under hyperbaric conditions was reviewed. No recommendations on choice of anesthetic were made in this report; rather, the advantages and disadvantages of commonly used techniques were presented. However, it was stated that intravenous techniques could prove especially useful in the hyperbaric setting. A recent renewal of interest in the field of hyperbaric anesthesia has been caused by explorations of undersea regions (deep-sea drilling for oil), which exposes workers in the diving industry to prolonged stays at significantly increased environmental pressure inside staged hyperbaric chambers. Plans to provide emergency surgery inside these high-pressure vessels have dictated a revision of anesthetic techniques that could be useful in emergencies.

It is interesting to explore both environments—low barometric pressure at high altitudes and high barometric pressures in the undersea world—with attention to the physiological changes commonly associated with anesthesia. The results provide principles and insights applicable to daily practice at "normal" environmental pressure. The first part of the chapter provides a description of the principal physiological challenges introduced by low-pressure and high-pressure environments; the second part summarizes the anesthetic considerations at the different barometric pressures.

THE GASES AROUND THE BODY

The pressure exerted by gas molecules upon all surfaces of the body constitutes the environmental pressure. This pressure is the result of both the atmospheric column of gases prevailing at any one site and the composition of the gases in the column of air above the location. Total environmental pressure at sea level amounts to 760 mm Hg. This value undergoes frequent, often daily, changes, at most ranging up and down by 10 to 15 mm Hg as a consequence of weather fluctuations. The composition of atmospheric air, on the other hand, is singularly constant in its original constituents, and is summarized in Table 28-1.

Only water vapor content varies significantly as a function of total humidity, and the partial pressure of the water molecules may contribute various amounts to the total pressure. Water vapor pressure (P_{H_2O}) is dependent on available water molecules in the atmosphere at a certain

Table 28-1. Composition of atmospheric gas (dry, sea level)

Gas	mm Hg	% of Total
Nitrogen	594	78.09
Oxygen	159	20.95
Carbon dioxide	0.2	0.03
Other inert gases	7	0.93
Water vapor	0	0.00
TOTAL	760.2	100.00

Table 28-2. Approximate composition of inspired gases at atmospheric pressure at sea level

Gas	Dry Air (mm Hg)	Moist Tracheal Air (mm Hg)	Alveolar Gas (mm Hg)
Nitrogen	601	564	568
Oxygen	159	149	105
Carbon dioxide	0.2	0.2	40
Water vapor	0	47	47
TOTAL	760	760	760

temperature. At 0° C, air that is fully saturated has a water vapor pressure of approximately 5 mm Hg, whereas at body temperature (37° C) the water vapor pressure is increased to 47 mm Hg. Whatever humidity and temperature prevail in the gas outside the body, as soon as air is inspired and equilibrated with moist tracheal gas, it is rapidly fully saturated and is heated (or cooled) to body temperature. Water vapor is added to gases in the respiratory airways by the moist linings of the respiratory tract (see also Chapter 7).

The addition of water vapor to atmospheric gases and the usual heating of the inspired gas to body temperature both induce substantial changes in the partial pressure of all gases, and in particular to the partial pressure of oxygen. Table 28-2 summarizes the composition of respired gases. Nitrogen and oxygen are the only gases present in substantial concentration in dry air. Moist, warm tracheal air contains significant amounts of water vapor.

Because the total barometric pressure is unchanged in the trachea, water vapor displaces each of the other gases, thereby decreasing their partial pressures. Alveolar gas contains approximately 100 to 105 mm Hg of oxygen. Commonly, oxygen is taken up by the blood in the lungs and carbon dioxide is released into the alveoli. During the respiratory acts, the gases are primarily moved by convection from the atmosphere to the alveolar space and back to the expired gas outside the body. In the alveolar compartment, diffusion is the primary mechanism for oxygen and carbon dioxide exchange. Therefore, changes in oxygen partial pressure in the inspired gas lead to proportional changes in alveolar PO_2.

High-altitude environments are characterized by a decreased barometric pressure and a reduced partial pressure of inspired oxygen when compared with sea-level values. Conversely, when total atmospheric pressure is increased, for example, inside a diving bell immersed in an underwater environment, all inspired gas partial pressures increase. The range of total atmospheric pressure changes that is still compatible with adequate gas exchange while breathing air is large, from pressures on the highest mountains (about 300 mm Hg total pressure) to those at several hundred feet underwater (about 6 to 7 times 760 mm Hg). The limits can be extended, especially at altitude, by slow adaptive phenomena that require several days to weeks to unfold fully; these phenomena are in part under hereditary control. Much less is known of adaptive phenomena at increased pressure because habitats that expose people to high pressure do not usually allow for safe exposures lasting much more than a few days. Exposure to even higher pressures has been achieved by complex modification of respiratory gases, up to the present maximum of 69 atmospheres.[6]

REDUCED ENVIRONMENTAL PRESSURE

Acute awareness of the adverse effects of the low barometric pressure of high altitude is recorded in literature regarding the Spanish invasion of South America; and these effects were commonly attributed to the "thinness of the air." Acute mountain sickness, at an elevation of about 10,000 feet, was first described in 1671 by the physiologist Borelli. A whole spectrum of disturbances and diseases was described for sojourners and exercisers into altitude, ranging from mild alterations in judgment at low altitude to severe, often deadly, pulmonary edema, often exacerbated by exercise, at high altitude. The decrease in total barometric pressure with altitude, and the attending reduction in inspired PO_2, are shown in Fig. 28-1. Figure 28-2 illustrates the approximate values for PO_2 in inspired air, moist tracheal air, alveolar gas, and arterial and mixed venous blood.

Acute exposure to altitude

Acute exposure to altitude can be achieved in a decompression chamber, by rapid ascent in an airplane, or by a brisk climb on a mountain. In general, the effects of a sudden ascent are comparable to exposure to low oxygen partial pressure. In the range of altitude from 10,000 to 15,000 feet, the increase in altitude causes an increase in ventilation proportional to the decrease in density of the air. Thus the increase in ventilation approximates the amount required to produce equivalent delivery of oxygen to the alveolar spaces. This is primarily achieved by an increase in tidal volume. This increase in ventilation is generally sustained for several days, and it may not reach a plateau until several days at altitude. The arterial hypoxia results in stimulation of peripheral chemoreceptors, which causes an increase in alveolar ventilation. Carbon dioxide

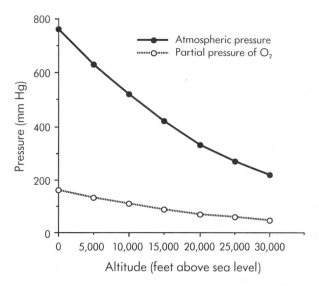

Fig. 28-1. Effect of altitude on total barometric pressure and partial pressure of oxygen (PO_2). Note that PO_2 is a fixed proportion (20.95%) of total barometric pressure. At sea level, PO_2 is 159 mm Hg, and this value is approximately halved at 18,000 feet.

is washed out of the alveoli at an increased rate, and the arterial PCO_2 is decreased. The reduction of $PaCO_2$ leads to a respiratory alkalosis, with an associated increase of arterial pH. These changes stimulate the excretion of bicarbonate from the blood and the kidneys. As a consequence, during the following days the blood bicarbonate is reduced, and a new level appropriate for the level of hyperventilation is established, with a near-normal pH. Thus the respiratory alkalosis is compensated.

The respiratory adaptations and the bicarbonate excretion affect the electrolyte status of spinal fluid and alter subsequent ventilatory responses. As the bicarbonate is excreted from the blood, bicarbonate is also lost from cerebrospinal fluid (CSF). In view of this decreased buffer capacity, changes in carbon dioxide in the CSF result in faster changes in hydrogen ion concentration and lead to an increased sensitivity to carbon dioxide. At this point in adaptation, ventilatory sensitivitiy to carbon dioxide is enhanced. The ventilatory response to hypoxia remains unchanged during the sojourn at high altitude. At extreme altitude, resulting in an arterial PO_2 in the range of 20 mm Hg, a profound depression of the central nervous system is unmasked, with depressed ventilatory drive.

Additional effects on lung function have been demonstrated with exposure to altitude, including an increase in carbon monoxide diffusing capacity, an increase in pulmonary blood flow to the apical lung regions, and an increase in pulmonary vascular pressures. As a result, increases in right-ventricular pressure for extended periods of time induce right-ventricular hypertrophy, with predictable electrocardiographic changes of right-axis deviation and right-ventricular strain.

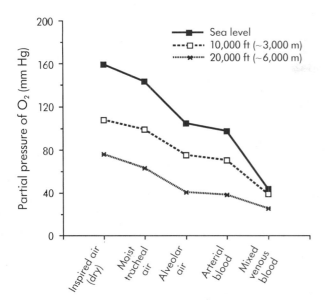

Fig. 28-2. Effect of altitude on partial pressures of oxygen in the respiratory and blood compartments. Average values are shown at sea level, at 10,000 feet, and at 20,000 feet. Although the changes in the gas phase and in arterial blood are reduced in physical proportion, mixed venous PO_2 changes with altitude are reduced by adaptive responses (mainly an increase in cardiac output). Thus mixed venous blood and tissue values reflect much smaller changes in partial pressure of oxygen than does arterial blood.

Oxygen transport at altitude

Hemoglobin concentration increases rapidly at altitude, within hours, due to rapidly rising hemoconcentration. Eventually, however, a real increase in erythropoiesis and a true increase in red cell mass ensues, which is not fully realized for several weeks. As the red cell mass and hemoglobin concentration rise, the erythropoietin level decreases. Soon after development of the hypoxic state, there is an increase in production of 2, 3 diphosphoglycerate (2, 3 DPG). This increase in 2,3 DPG causes a rightward shift of the oxyhemoglobin dissociation curve. The practical significance of this shift has yet to be established.

Cardiac output is characteristically increased in response to hypoxia, but this response adapts during continuing exposure. Despite these adaptive responses to altitude, there is no significant change in either resting oxygen consumption or the ability to perform high levels of exercise at moderate altitude. At altitude levels exceeding 10,000 feet, exercise tolerance is limited with acute exposure, and other symptoms of acute hypoxia manifest themselves by interference with several organ systems. Central nervous system manifestations may present a spectrum of symptoms, including impaired judgment, loss of memory, hallucinations, coma, and death. Cardiovascular manifestations may include severe hypertension, arrhythmias, and right-ventricular and sometimes also left-ventricular failure.

High-altitude pulmonary edema

High-altitude pulmonary edema (HAPE), an extreme manifestation of high-altitude exposure, is often unpredictably seen in lowland dwellers ascending to high altitude. It can also affect natives of high-altitude areas, returning after several weeks at sea level. Its major symptomatology may be limited to nocturnal dyspnea, or "nocturnal asthma," with an increase in fluids in the lungs. It may also occur unexpectedly in individuals who have been many times before to high altitudes without side effects. Infection, exertion, age, sex, or physical exercise do not appear to be predisposing factors. Clinical manifestations consist of tachypnea and nausea, progressing gradually to overt pulmonary edema with copious secretions and cough. Pulmonary arterial pressures are severely elevated, whereas pulmonary venous pressures are normal. Conventional therapy for pulmonary edema is ineffective, and only oxygen administration and return to lower altitudes has proven effective in treatment. Because it may progress to death, this disturbance requires immediate medical attention.

ENVIRONMENTS WITH INCREASED PRESSURE

The only natural exposure to increased barometric pressure is produced underwater, where the pressure increases approximately 1 atmosphere with each 33 feet of descent. During diving, significant physiologic changes are induced by body immersion in water, in addition to the respiratory exposure to elevated total pressure of the inhaled gases. A dry environment can be experienced with increased total pressure around the body, without the effects of water immersion, inside caissons, locks, diving bells, or underwater habitats. Construction of underwater spaces frequently leads to the need for compressed air to ventilate construction works in tunnels and caissons. Conventional submarines, like high-flying airplanes, are pressurized at levels very close to atmospheric, and the occupants are not exposed to changes in pressure.

The dangers of high-pressure environments are similar in part to those produced by small closed environments, and the usual difficulties are often caused by inappropriate carbon dioxide removal. Inspired gas, usually air, contains only small traces of carbon dioxide, therefore, adequate alveolar ventilation removes carbon dioxide from alveolar gas while providing for adequate oxygenation. Within an enclosed environment at increased gas pressure, increased levels of oxygen (increased partial pressure of oxygen inspired gas, or PIO_2) may increase the availability of oxygen supply to alveolar gas, but carbon dioxide may accumulate if the removal is not sufficient. An accumulation of even small amounts of carbon dioxide for example, 0.3% at 3 atmospheres (atm), may increase $PICO_2$ to significant levels (e.g., $PICO_2 = 7$ mm Hg), with an appropriate increase in ventilation, which should be sustained to avoid alveolar and arterial carbon dioxide accumulation. This increased level of ventilation often abates within a short time, producing an increased level of $PaCO_2$, with concomitant disturbances. Other limitations are typical of increased environmental pressure: namely, high oxygen partial pressures resulting in oxygen toxicity at pressures exceeding 3 to 4 atm with compressed air; inert gas (nitrogen) narcosis at pressures exceeding 4 to 7 atm; and decompression sickness, if decompression is carried out rapidly from pressures exceeding 2 to 2.5 atm.

Oxygen toxicity

At pressures up to 3 atm the inspired oxygen partial pressure in air is raised to levels exceeding 450 mm Hg. This appears safe, even for prolonged periods. At higher pressures, however, manifestations of oxygen toxicity appear; and these manifestations affect various organs with variable latencies. High levels of oxygen lead to rapid onset of central nervous system excitatory symptoms, with motor twitching and even seizures. Breathing pure oxygen at 3 atm results in a predictable incidence of grand mal seizures in 7% to 10% of individuals exposed for 1 hour.[7] Numerous other manifestations of organ toxicity have been described, such as endothelial cell damage, interstitial pulmonary edema, and alterations in epithelial cells at the alveolar level. Other symptoms may be caused by acute hemolysis.

Nitrogen narcosis

Inspired nitrogen in compressed air does exert pharmacologic effects at pressures exceeding 4 or 5 atm. Its effects on performance and subjective sensations are similar to those of alcohol ingestion or the inhalation of subanesthetic concentrations of nitrous oxide. Marked variability has been reported among individuals. At pressures exceeding 8 to 10 atm the impairment from nitrogen makes performance of even minimal tasks impossible. Other inert gases, when substituted for nitrogen, have a variable effect. Helium is devoid of narcotic effects and has been used with great success to create a gas environment for prolonged survival at pressures up to 40 to 50 atm. Excitatory effects from breathing helium at elevated pressures ("helium tremors") become significant with other difficulties, such as nausea. Because of this, gas mixtures of helium and nitrogen have been used with success (Atlantis Dives) to expose people in hyperbaric chamber simulators to pressures of up to 69 atm.[6]

A prolonged stay at elevated pressure induces equilibration of all body compartments with the increased gas pressures. A subsequent reduction of pressure causes a decrease of partial pressure of all inspired gases to a lower pressure and induces evolution of the excess gas to the alveoli but often results in supersaturation of certain body compartments. If the decompression is too rapid, gas bubbles may form in the blood and tissues that were previously saturated. This produces a variety of symptoms, as a function of the location of the blockage of tissue blood-

flow and the mechanical tissue disruption. Symptoms may include pain, neural distribution of symptoms with spinal cord or cerebral involvement, loss of sphincteric function of the bladder and rectum, neuroplegia, and all symptoms deriving from localized cerebral edema (these symptoms constitute decompression sickness).

ANESTHETIC PROBLEMS AT MODERATE ALTITUDE

Two main problems can be identified in the administration of anesthetics at altitude: the relative hypoxic background of air at lower ambient pressure, especially before and after anesthetic administration; and the prevailing technical problems associated with delivery of anesthetic vapors from vaporizers when the total ambient pressure is reduced. Significant alterations in the effectiveness of intravenous agents and of regional anesthetic techniques have not been reported, and these agents and techniques may still be used with the same precautions as at sea-level.

At an altitude approximating 5000 feet, the partial pressure of oxygen in air is reduced from the sea-level value of approximately 160 mm Hg to about 125 mm Hg. While room air is breathed at altitude, arterial PO_2 is consequently lowered to approximately 80 mm Hg in normal individuals. Powell and Gingrich[8] recommended administering a gas mixture containing no less than 40% oxygen during anesthesia at an altitude of 1 mile (approximately 5000 feet) in order to compensate for the reduced arterial PO_2 commonly observed during anesthesia. When this altitude is doubled to about 10,000 feet, the inspired PO_2 is reduced to 110 mm Hg and PaO_2 to 65 mm Hg in air. At this hypoxic level, alveolar ventilation increases and $PaCO_2$ is steadily reduced (34 mm Hg at rest).

The effective anesthetic power of nitrous oxide is also reduced as total barometric pressure decreases. It has been shown that analgesia induced by 50% nitrous oxide is reduced by nearly 50% at 5000 feet and it becomes insignificant at 10,000 feet.[9] Therefore, nitrous oxide is not a useful anesthetic gas at altitude. Safar and Tenicela[10] and James and White[11] condemn the use of nitrous oxide for anesthesia at altitude.

Vapors and vaporizers at altitude

The saturated vapor pressure of a volatile anesthetic agent depends only on temperature[12] and is practically independent of total environmental pressure. Consequently, for a given vaporizer temperature, the concentration of a given mass of vapor increases as the barometric pressure is reduced, because the same mass of volatile agent is vaporized in less and less dense carrier gas. However, the partial pressure (expressed in mm Hg) of the agent remains unchanged, and so does its biological effect on the neural tissue where the anesthetic effect is produced (see also Chapter 3). Table 28-3 reports the result of vaporizing halothane at different altitudes. This results in a constant par-

Table 28-3. Concentration and partial pressure of halothane vaporized at different environmental pressures

Barometric Pressure (mm Hg)	Actual Halothane Concentration (%)	Vaporizer Scale Reading (%)	Halothane Partial Pressure (mm Hg)
760	1.16	1.05	8.8
624	1.36	1.00	8.5
518	1.66	1.10	8.6

Modified from James MFM, White JF: Anesthetic considerations at moderate altitudes, *Anesth Analg* 63:1097-1105, 1984.

tial pressure of the agent and a constant scale reading from a vapor analyzer whose principle of operation is based upon measuring the number of molecules present (e.g., infrared, Raman, piezoelectric crystal, but *not* mass spectrometry—see Chapter 8), but produces an increased total halothane concentration in the dilutional gas.

With modern vaporizers, the partial pressure of the vapor should remain unaltered by barometric pressure changes. In fact, McDowell[4] showed that the output of the Fluotec Mk II vaporizer was modified by only a small amount from the theoretical prediction, and those changes could be attributed to the slight change in the density of the carrier gas. However, Safar and Tenicela[10] studied the Foregger vaporizer at 10,000 feet and showed (contrary to the theory) that a higher partial pressure of gas was produced at increased altitude. However, James and White,[11] with a more precise analytical technique (Engström EMMA vapor analyzer, whose principle of operation is a vibrating, lipophilic-coated, piezoelectric crystal), studied the accuracies of a Fluotec Mk II vaporizer and a Dräger Vapor halothane vaporizer inside a pressure chamber simulating altitude. They were unable to show differences in halothane partial pressure with decreased environmental pressure. These authors concluded that because the reading of the vapor analyzer remained constant, the last two types of vaporizers produced a relatively constant partial pressure of halothane even at reduced environmental pressure (see also Chapter 3).

Gas analyzers at altitude

Most of the gas analyzers used by anesthesiologists are based on one of the various physical properties of the agent being measured. Most analyzers respond to the number and activity of molecules of that agent present, independently of the presence of additional gas molecules. Such instruments, therefore, measure partial pressure, not concentration of agents. Most often, however, such devices are traditionally calibrated in percentages. This calibration scale might introduce important errors, which must be prevented when specialized equipment is to be used at increased altitude (see Chapter 8).

Oxygen analyzers

All presently utilized oxygen analyzers (paramagnetic, fuel cell, oxygen electrode devices) respond to partial pressure of oxygen alone and produce alterations of the total measurement output as barometric pressure changes. An oxygen analyzer calibrated at sea level to measure 21% oxygen in air gives a reading of 17.4% oxygen when reading air at 5000 feet. Of course, the analyzer must be recalibrated at altitude to read 21% when air is injected. If the oxygen activity were to be presented as partial pressure (e.g., mm Hg of oxygen), then the device would indeed reflect oxygen availability to the patient's lungs and blood at any pressure. As noted above, the key issue is that air at an altitude above 5000 feet is relatively hypoxic, and it approaches a clinically significant hypoxic level at 10,000 feet. The same principle applies in hyperbaric conditions: compressed air at 5 atm contains 21% oxygen, but total oxygen exerts a partial pressure of approximately 800 mm Hg (21% × 5 × 760 = 798 mm Hg).

Carbon dioxide analyzers

Carbon dioxide analyzers most frequently operate on the principle of infrared absorption. As indicated above, most analyzers have scales that read in percentages, although the sensitive element is responding to the increasing partial pressure of carbon dioxide. By the use of precise gas mixtures, it is possible to calibrate these analyzers to read exact percentages at a fixed altitude. If, however, the analyzer is calibrated at sea level and the same gas containing a fixed percentage of carbon dioxide is injected into the analyzer at a different altitude, then the reading of the analyzer decreases in the percentage scale in proportion to the total barometric pressure.

Gas density and flow

Alteration of total barometric pressure induces a proportional change in gas density. In fact, density reflects closely the number of molecules per unit volume. Gas flowmeters and variable-flow resistors used to produce oxygen-enriched mixtures represent critical devices that use indicators which depend upon gas density.

Flowmeters

The principle of action of most flowmeters is the decrease in pressure that occurs when a gas passes through a fixed resistance, as an indication of total gas flow. If this fixed resistance is represented by an orifice, then resistance depends primarily on gas density. If, however, the fixed resistance is of a laminar nature, then viscosity becomes the prime determinant of the magnitude of the pressure reduction provided by the flow. Most flowmeters currently in use utilize a floating bobbin supported by the stream of gas inside a tube with a tapered diameter.

The density of a gas changes in proportion to the change in total barometric pressure, but viscosity changes relatively little or not at all because viscosity depends mostly on temperature. In a tapered tube, at low levels of flow, the movement of the bobbin primarily depends on laminar flow. As the float moves up the tube, the resistance behaves progressively more like an orifice. In practice, only minor errors, usually 1% per every 1000 feet of altitude, have been reported for most gas flowmeters, such that minor corrections to the total flow can be easily applied.[13] However, if total environmental pressure changes by more than one atmosphere, Halsey and White[14] recommended a complete recalibration, because a single correction factor will be significantly in error. The following equation can be used to derive an approximate correction factor, both at altitude and at increased pressure:

$$F_1 = F_0 \times \sqrt{\frac{d_0}{d_1}}$$

where:

F_1 = Flow at the present ambient pressure
F_0 = Indicated flow on the scale calibrated at sea level
d_0 = Density of gas at sea level
d_1 = Density of gas at the present pressure.

The correction factor may be significant at increased pressure but seldom exceeds 10% at altitudes up to 5000 feet.

James and White[11] tested oxygen and nitrous oxide flow indicators (despite the warning not to use nitrous oxide at altitude) and measured the percentage error at flowmeter settings ranging from 1 to 8 L/min. They demonstrated that errors were larger at higher flow settings, and ranged from 3% to 8% at 5000 feet but from 5% to 20% at 10,000 feet.

High-flow oxygen-enrichment devices

Fixed-orifice Venturi devices are commonly used to provide an enriched gas mixture with elevated oxygen content. Fixed settings (usually 28%, 35%, or 40%) are produced by variable orifices, which produce different amounts of entrainment of air into an oxygen stream. Most of these devices "run rich" at altitude because the total gas density decreases.[11] Therefore, the Venturi type of mask might be used safely at altitude, provided the flowmeter used to quantitate total oxygen flow is properly calibrated for the altitude at which it is being used.

RECOMMENDATIONS FOR ANESTHESIA AT ALTITUDE

The major risk of anesthesia at high altitude is that anesthetized patients can become hypoxic despite the fact that adequate oxygen concentrations are being administered. The effectiveness of nitrous oxide is so reduced by the decrease in partial pressure at altitude that no significant contribution by nitrous oxide to the anesthetic mixture is of clinical use. In addition, it is important to maintain a higher concentration of oxygen both during and after administration of the anesthetic to support adequate oxygenation. It is suggested that 30% oxygen be the minimum at 5000 feet and that 40% oxygen be the minimum at 10,000 feet, for both intraoperative anesthetic management and postoperative recovery.

The problem may be compounded by inaccuracies in flow measurement, because the only way to obtain accurate flow rates at fixed altitude is to utilize flowmeters appropriately calibrated at altitude. Surface calibrated equipment may produce small errors at 5000 feet, but it certainly will deviate significantly, up to 20% at 10,000 feet. Finally, it is important to think of oxygenation and anesthetic vapor activity in terms of partial pressures of oxygen and partial pressures of anesthetic agent, rather than as volumetric percentages (see also Chapter 8).

PHYSIOLOGICAL CONSIDERATIONS AT INCREASED PRESSURE

The major alterations of hyperbaric pressures are reflected in the respiratory system, the heart, and the central nervous system. Exposures of as little as 24 hours to high levels of oxygen (90% to 100%) at 1 to 2 atm can rapidly damage the mucosa of the tracheobronchial tree, manifested by mucosal hyperemia, increased secretions, and atelectasis. This might be of special importance to the patient with reactive airways disease or chronic obstructive pulmonary disease. Airway irritation could complicate tracheal intubation because of the patient's increased tendency to laryngospasm.

In the presence of chronic obstructive pulmonary disease, and any other pulmonary process that narrows the caliber of the airways, increased secretions and increased work of breathing at increased ambient pressure may lead to severe ventilatory difficulties. In addition, pulmonary bullae and other slow exchange zones, as well as mucous plugging, may cause a disastrous problem during decompression because they can lead to parenchymal rupture, pneumothorax, or air embolism secondary to barotrauma.

A reduction in vital capacity has been measured as an index of atelectasis, which correlates with the length and pressure of oxygen exposure and is predicted by empirical units known as units of pulmonary toxicity dose (UPTD).[7] Reductions of vital capacity reverse within hours after termination of oxygen exposure.[15,16]

Loss of pulmonary surfactant has been described after exposure to hyperbaric oxygen. It is not clear whether peroxidation of surfactant plays a significant role in its destruction, but it is clearly demonstrated that surfactant production is inhibited. There is evidence, especially in practice, that adequate humidification of inspired gases protects against some of these pulmonary problems, especially airway irritation.[17] The work of breathing is increased at increased ambient pressures. This is a result of increased turbulent flow due to increased gas density. These pressure-induced changes can be minimized by use of tracheal tubes with the largest possible internal diameter.

Cardiovascular effects

It has been demonstrated that significant peripheral vasoconstriction occurs with the exposure to high blood oxygen tensions. Barratt-Boyes and Wood[18] showed in humans that whereas peripheral vasoconstriction does occur, the pulmonary vascular resistance was decreased. Because of the peripheral vasoconstriction medications should not be given via intramuscular or subcutaneous routes.

Vasoconstriction can also occur in coronary vessels. Studies have demonstrated that coronary blood flow is significantly decreased during exposure to hyperbaric oxygen. Krishnamurti, et al.[19] reported two patients who suffered myocardial infarctions (one of whom sustained sudden death) while being treated with hyperbaric oxygen. Patients with significant obstructive coronary disease should be approached cautiously, especially in the delivery of a general anesthetic under hyperbaric oxygen conditions.

Some studies have demonstrated that cardiac output can be reduced by as much as 12% during hyperbaric hyperoxia, probably as a result of increased afterload. No significant changes in contractility have been demonstrated in a sophisticated dog model exposed to 3 atm of oxygen.[20]

Central nervous system

Oxygen is also a potent cerebral vasoconstrictor that affects pial as well as cerebral arterioles. This principle becomes important when patients with closed head injuries are treated, because one would expect a protective effect of oxygen on neural structures in patients with closed head injuries or intracranial masses. Although few data on this subject are available, practice suggests that seizure threshold may be reduced during general anesthesia in patients who are already at higher risk for seizures. The risk of seizures induced by high oxygen tensions warrants the administration of prophylactic anticonvulsant medications to patients who will have significant exposures to hyperbaric oxygen (e.g., patients treated for gas gangrene at 3 atm in oxygen).

The ability of the attending personnel in the chamber to make sound clinical decisions may be impaired while they are exposed to breathing air at high pressure. Inert gas narcosis is a well described phenomenon in humans breathing air at increased atmospheric pressure. Although not always a significant problem, inert gas narcosis can be observed at pressures of 2 atm and greater. Nitrogen narcosis is not unpleasant; it has been compared to alcohol intoxication. The affected individual may also experience drowsiness and euphoria, and judgment can be negatively affected. The severity of nitrogen narcosis is directly proportional to the pressure exposure. Patients are usually not at risk because they are breathing high oxygen concentrations.

ANESTHETIC GASES UTILIZED UNDER INCREASED PRESSURE

Measured flow vaporizers (e.g., Copper Kettle, Verni-Trol) work by forcing a gas, usually oxygen, at a known flow rate through a sintered bronze disk at the bottom of a pool of liquid anesthetic. The amount of anesthetic agent delivered to the patient depends on four factors: (1) the particular vapor pressure of the agent (a function of van der Waals forces), (2) the temperature of the liquid agent in the vaporizer, (3) the flow of gas through the liquid, and (4) the dilution of the anesthetic vapor with by-pass flow to constitute the desired concentration for delivery.

The key point in calculating the required flows at various ambient pressures is that the vapor pressure of a liquid remains constant with variations in ambient pressure.[12] For example, the vapor pressure of halothane at 20° C is 243 mm Hg. According to Dalton's law of partial pressures, saturated halothane vapor at 1 atm (760 mm Hg) contains 32% halothane (243/760), and at 4 atm (3040 mm Hg) the same halothane partial pressure produces a concentration of 8% (243/3040) by volume. The amount of carrier gas required to dilute the saturated vapor to the desired inspired concentration (0.5% to 1%, as a clinically useful dose) remains constant with changing ambient pressure. If the desired inspired partial pressure is 7.6 mm Hg (1% halothane at 1 atm), then each volume of saturated vapor must be diluted with 32 volumes of carrier gas at 1 atm, or with 8 volumes at 4 atm (which represents the same number of molecules) (see also Chapter 3).

Empirical observations in this area are few; McDowall[4] used a concentration-calibrated variable bypass (Fluotec) vaporizer at pressure and measured actual concentrations of gas delivered at different dial settings. The Fluotec vaporizer works by directing a stream of gas over a surface of liquid anesthetic and diluting the total gas output. McDowall found that the particular vaporizer tested (Fluotec) deviated at low settings (0.5% to 1%) by delivering nearly twice the anesthetic gas concentration while at 2 atm. Gas concentrations did not vary significantly from 1 atm at higher concentration dial settings (from 2% to 4%) (see also Chapter 3).

PHARMACOKINETICS OF INTRAVENOUS AGENTS AT PRESSURE

In 1976, Winter, et al.[21] described the phenomenon of pressure reversal of barbiturate anesthesia in mammals. They observed the reversal of barbiturate anesthesia in rats at pressures of 103 atm. However, the clinical relevance of these findings is of limited value, because therapeutic pressures of clinical relevance are most often restricted to a few atmospheres. A comprehensive review of this argument was published by Kendig and Cohen in 1977.[22] Few data are published concerning the pharmacokinetics of intravenous anesthetics in the literature. A few studies have been performed with specific agents using animal models. Drugs studied include meperidine and pentobarbital. No significant differences were observed in either the half-life, volume of distribution or the plasma clearance of the drugs when pentobarbital and meperidine were measured at 2.8 or 6 atm. Despite the fact that absolute pharmacokinetic values for the dog differ considerably from those for humans, these observations support the concept that intravenous anesthetic agents commonly used at 1 atm can be judiciously administered at pressures of 2 to 6 atm. Pressure reversal was addressed by Kramer, et al.[23-25] who showed no significant differences in the pharmacokinetics of pentobarbital when given at 1, 2.8, and 6 atm. Pressure reversal can still play a role if anesthesia is delivered at much greater depths (e.g., >50 atm) (See Table 28-4).

Ross, et al.[26] were among the first groups to advocate intravenous anesthesia for use in the hyperbaric chamber. This was a result of considering the problem of anesthetic gas pollution inside an enclosed pressure vessel while delivering gaseous anesthetics at pressures of up to 35 atm. Wen-ren, et al.[27] reported the successful use of ketamine anesthesia in 48 patients undergoing open heart surgery while having oxygen administered at 3 atm. Camporesi and Moon[28] reported on the use of ketamine and benzodiazepines along with muscle relaxants in the delivery of anesthesia to patients undergoing therapeutic lung lavages. Approximately 20 patients have been treated with this anesthetic regimen without complications.

Practical considerations for anesthesia in a pressure chamber

During decompression and compression, the air entering or escaping from the chamber generates significant noise, which can interfere with auscultation or the ability to hear equipment alarms. These "traveling" periods are precisely when the anesthesiologist must be especially alert to the condition of the patient. Most complications in anesthetic management happen during changes in chamber pressure (Fig. 28-3).

A laryngoscope is not greatly affected by increased pressure as long as the battery handle is vented and can exchange gas at pressure. Sealed batteries have been shown to function adequately up to 35 atm. Tracheal tubes should be the largest appropriate for the patient. When the pressure is increased, turbulent flow increases and causes an increase in airway resistance and an increase in ventilatory work. Tracheal tube cuffs should be filled with saline rather than air, because water is incompressible and thus the danger of volume variations in the cuff with changing ambient pressure is avoided.

It is imperative to minimize the amount of electrical equipment in the hyperbaric chamber because oxygen par-

Table 28-4. Pharmacokinetic parameters for meperidine (M) and pentobarbital (P) under normal and hyperbaric conditions

Parameter/Drug	1 atm	6 atm	2.8 atm
$t\frac{1}{2}$* (min)/M	60.4±43.6	55.7±17.5	44.9±22.7
$t\frac{1}{2}$(h)/P	4.49±1.11	6.08±2.29	4.88±1.89
CL_T† (ml/[min/kg])/M	75.2±49.8	75.4±40.0	84.4±37.4
CL_T (ml/[min/kg])/P	2.82±0.32	2.67±0.85	3.69±1.23
V‡ (L/kg)/M	4.56±2.06	5.54±1.63	5.18±2.77
V (L/kg)/P	1.11±0.37	1.29±0.24	1.44±0.42

Modified from Kramer WG, Gross DR, Moreau PM, et al: Drug disposition under hyperbaric and hyperbaric hyperoxic conditions: meperidine in the dog, *Aviat Space Environ Med* 54:410-419, 1979; and Kramer WG, Welch DW, Fife WP, et al: Pharmacokinetics of pentobarbital under hyperbaric and hyperbaric hyperoxic conditions in the dog, *Aviat Space Environ Med* 54:1005-1008, 1983.
*$t\frac{1}{2}$ = half life.
†CL_T = clearance.
‡V = volume of distribution.

tial pressure is high and thus the dangers of fire and explosion are increased. Ventilators that are driven by compressed air are preferable. These ventilators work through a pressure differential of about 50 psig. Therefore, as long as the driving gas (oxygen) supply line is adjusted to maintain this differential gradient above ambient pressure, the ventilators should work well at increased pressure, although their peak flow rates will be somewhat lower.

Another safety consideration is the rate of oxygen leaking from the ventilator. This must be kept to a minimum, because standard operating procedure for multiplace hyperbaric units dictates that ambient oxygen concentration should not exceed 23%. This usually can be achieved by scavenging and venting to the outside the excess chamber oxygen overflow from the ventilator. Oil lubrication presents a high risk of fire. Lubrication used for the ventilator must be compatible with high oxygen tensions (e.g., tetrafluorethylene polymer–based lubricants). Moon, et al.[29] reported on the use of the Monaghan 225 ventilator under hyperbaric conditions. He found that this ventilator, after minor modifications, provided adequate ventilatory support at pressures of up to 6 atm.

Monitoring

Monitoring should include the usual monitors for vital signs, which are prudently used at any ambient pressure. The need for accurate blood pressure readings and access for arterial blood sampling suggests that an arterial line should be in place prior to any procedure that will require prolonged anesthesia under hyperbaric conditions.

Arterial oxygen measurements present a problem in the hyperbaric chamber. When a blood sample is drawn and passed through a lock to the surface, gas bubbling may oc-

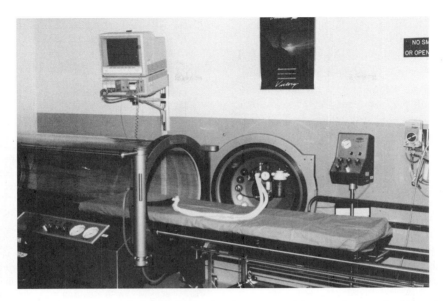

Fig. 28-3. A modern monoplace hyperbaric chamber can provide extensive monitoring and controlled ventilation capabilities. A pressure-preset ventilator is connected through the hatch of this unit and has been used at pressures of up to 3 atmospheres.

cur during decompression of the sample, and the time that the sample remains in transit is also critical. Most blood gas analyzers used in clinical practice are not calibrated to measure oxygen tensions as high as those observed during hyperbaric therapy; therefore oxygen content is only an approximation when it is measured outside the chamber. A direct solution to the problem is to maintain blood gas measuring equipment inside the chamber. The disadvantage of this approach is that although accurate blood gas measurements can be performed at pressure, trained personnel must remain available in the chamber to carry out the measurements.

Pulse oximetry can also be used by splicing cables through chamber walls. Its use has been of value when patients with high pulmonary shunts are treated, in order to increase the ambient partial pressure of oxygen until high saturation (S_pO_2) levels are achieved. A respiratory mass spectrometer can be set up outside the chamber with a sampling line that exits through the wall of the chamber, in order to continuously monitor actual concentrations of oxygen, carbon dioxide, nitrogen, nitrous oxide, and inhalation agent. Appropriate calibrations and constant sampling flow-rates render this extensive measurement system complicated and specialized.

Convulsions are often the first signs of CNS toxicity, and the EEG may represent the only way to detect a seizure in an adequately paralyzed patient. Electrical activity from the ECG must be monitored as usual, but the monitor itself will usually remain outside the chamber because it most often utilizes a CRT-based display. The monitor must remain visible to the attendants inside the chamber through a porthole window. The leads can be passed through a pressure-tight access to the outside of the chamber. More recently, a variety of flat-screen display monitors have been introduced that can be used to record digital and analog signals directly at pressure.

Defibrillation is possible while at pressure in the hyperbaric chamber. Martindale, et al.[30] reported on the use of an R2 defibrillator adaptor on a Life Pak unit. Self-adhering pads were used in order to reduce the danger of fire caused by arcing between defibrillator paddles. As with ECG monitors, the defibrillator unit must be kept outside the chamber, and its wires must be passed through the chamber wall and attached to the patient. Standard defibrillator paddles can be used if care is taken to make good contact between paddle and skin through the use of a low-resistance gel and if the paddles are positioned far enough away from each other to prevent electric arcs. Neuromuscular transmission can be monitored in the chamber without fear of fire or explosion because the amperage delivered is quite low. Any electrical equipment to be used inside the hyperbaric chamber must be flushed with nitrogen in order to provide an inert gas atmosphere in case of spark generation.

PRESENT INDICATIONS FOR ANESTHESIA AT HIGH PRESSURE

Today, anesthesia care may be required at increased pressure for the treatment of conditions that produce transient, reversible hypoxemia. These include whole-lung lavage (usually performed at 2 to 4 atm), and delivery of anesthesia as a result of emergent surgical procedures required on a patient involved in a diving accident, which might occur at pressures of up to 35 atm (depth of saturation in deepest practical commercial diving). In the first setting, anesthesia is likely to require elevated FIO_2 levels, probably up to 2 atm, intravenous maintenance, topical anesthesia of the trachea for intubation, and, possibly, muscle relaxants. In the second setting (i.e., trauma or emergency surgery at very high pressure), preference should be given to regional anesthesia and spontaneous ventilation with oxygen-enriched gas mixtures. This allows for simplicity of patient management in the limited quarters of a confined pressure chamber. Intravenous anesthesia and sedation probably have the flexibility to provide an adequate surgical field in any region of the body in these settings, but this flexibility comes at the price of requiring controlled ventilation, a difficult task at very elevated pressure. In all cases, the plan to decompress as promptly as possible to 1 atm will be implemented in order to provide a safe and speedy egress from the high-pressure environment.

REFERENCES

1. Smith WDA, Mapleson WW, Siebold K, et al: Nitrous oxide anaesthesia induced at atmospheric and hyperbaric pressures. I and II, *Br J Anaesth* 46:3-28, 1974.
2. Smith RM: Anesthesia during hyperbaric oxygenation, *Ann NY Acad Sci* 117:768-773, 1965.
3. Boerema I: An operating room with high atmospheric pressure, *Surgery* 49:291-298, 1961.
4. McDowall DG: Anaesthesia in a pressure chamber, *Anaesthesia* 19:321-336, 1964.
5. Severinghaus J: Hyperbaric oxygenation: anesthesia and drug effects—a committee report, *Anesthesiology* 26:812-824, 1965.
6. Salzano JV, Camporesi EM, Stolp BW, et al: Physiological responses to exercise at 47 and 66 ATA, *J Appl Physiol* 57:1055-1068, 1984.
7. Clark JM: Oxygen toxicity. In Bennett PB, Elliott DH, editors: *The physiology and medicine of diving*, ed 3, London, 1982, Baillière, Tindall & Cox, pp 200-238.
8. Powell JN, Gingrich TF: Some aspects of nitrous oxide anesthesia at an altitude of one mile, *Anesth Analg* 48:680-685, 1969.
9. James MFM, Manson EDM, Dennett JE: Nitrous oxide analgesia and altitude, *Anaesthesia* 37:285-288, 1982.
10. Safar P, Tenicela R: High altitude physiology in relation to anesthesia and inhalation therapy, *Anesthesiology* 25:515-531, 1964.
11. James MFM, White JF: Anesthetic considerations at moderate altitude, *Anesth Analg* 63:1097-1105, 1984.
12. Hill DW: *Physics applied to anesthesia*, ed 4, Boston, 1980, Butterworths, pp 336-337.
13. Friedman MD, Lightstone PJ: The effect of high altitude on flowmeter performance, *Anesthesiology* 55:A117, 1981 (abstract).
14. Halsey MJ, White DC: *Gas and vapour supply*. In Gray TC, Nunn JF, Utting JE, editors: *General Anaesthesia*, ed 4, London, 1980, Butterworths, pp 953-961.
15. Don HF, Wahba M, Cuadrado L, et al: The effects of anesthesia and 100 percent oxygen on the functional residual capacity of the lungs, *Anesthesiology* 32:521-529, 1970.
16. Hickey RF, Visick HD, Fairley HB, et al: Effects of halothane anesthesia on functional residual capacity and alveolar arterial oxygen tension difference, *Anesthesiology* 38:20-24, 1973.
17. Miller JN, Camporesi EM, McLeod M, et al: Studies of early pulmonary oxygen toxicity in man, *Anesthesiology* 55:A369, 1981 (abstract).
18. Barratt-Boyes BG, Wood EH: Cardiac output and related measurements and pressure values in the right heart and associated vessels, together with an analysis of the hemodynamic responses to inhalation of high oxygen mixtures in healthy subjects, *J Lab Clin Med* 51:72-90, 1958.
19. Krishnamurti S, Akhtar M, Krishnan NR: Myocardial infarction in patients undergoing hyperbaric oxygen therapy, *Indian Heart J* 25:107-110, 1971.
20. Savitt MA, Elbeery JR, Owen CH, et al: Mechanism of decreased coronary and systemic blood flow during hyperbaric oxygenation. *Undersea Biomed Res* 16(suppl):77, 1989.
21. Winter PM, Smith RA, Smith M, et al: Pressure antagonism of barbiturate anesthesia, *Anesthesiology* 44:416-419, 1976.
22. Kendig JJ, Cohen EN: Pressure antagonism to nerve conduction block by anesthetic agents, *Anesthesiology* 47:6-10, 1977.
23. Kramer WG, Gross DR, Moreau PM, et al: Drug disposition under hyperbaric and hyperbaric hyperoxic conditions: meperidine in the dog, *Aviat Space Environ Med* 54:410-412, 1983.
24. Kramer WG, Welch DW, Fife WP, et al: Pharmacokinetics of pentobarbital under hyperbaric and hyperbaric hyperoxic conditions in the dog, *Aviat Space Environ Med* 54:1005-1008, 1983.
25. Kramer WG, Welch DW, Fife WP, et al: Salicylate pharmacokinetics in the dog at 6 ATA in air and at 2.8 ATA in 100% oxygen, *Aviat Space Environ Med* 54:682-684, 1983.
26. Ross JAS, Manson HJ, Shearer A, et al: *Some aspects of anaesthesia in high pressure environments*. In *Proceedings of the sixth international congress on hyperbaric medicine*, Aberdeen, 1977, Aberdeen University Press, pp 449-452.
27. Wen-ren L, Zhen-zhi Z, Chong-xian L et al: *Open heart surgery with extra-corporeal circulation under hyperbaric oxygenation at 3 ATA*. In Kindwall ER, editor: *Proceedings of the eighth international congress on hyperbaric medicine*, San Pedro, 1987, Best, pp 177-180.
28. Camporesi EM, Moon RE: *Hyperbaric oxygen as an adjunct to therapeutic lung lavage in pulmonary alveolar proteinosis*. In Bove AA, Bachrach AJ, Greenbaum LJ, editors, *Ninth international symposium on underwater and hyperbaric physiology*. Bethesda, Md, 1987, Underwater Hyperbaric Medical Society, pp 449-452.
29. Moon RE, Bergquist LV, Conklin B, et al: Monaghan 225 ventilator use under hyperbaric conditions, *Chest* 89:846-851, 1986.
30. Martindale LG, Milligan M, Fries P: Test of an R-2 defibrillation adapter in a hyperbaric chamber, *J Hyperbaric Med* 2:15-25, 1987.

Chapter 29

EQUIPMENT FOR ANESTHESIA IN DIFFICULT AND ISOLATED ENVIRONMENTS

Hansel de Sousa, M.D.

Inhalational anesthesia
    Using conventional continuous gas flow
    Using the draw-over method with air
    Using the to-and-fro system
Total intravenous anesthesia
Regional and local anesthesia
Some useful accessories
    The oxygen concentrator
    The laryngeal mask and the binasal pharyngeal airways
    The emergency aspirator

Good training and specialization imply adaptability.[1] Yet an anesthesiologist trained within the last 15 years may be unable to provide safe surgical anesthesia without the security of equipment, drugs, and compressed gases that are now considered to be essential for modern anesthesia.

The importance of being able to adapt to adverse situations, where such extensive technical support may not be available, is no longer obvious. There have been no overwhelming military or natural catastrophes in the United States in recent years. Emergency medical crews are able to extricate victims from practically any accident without requiring limb amputation, and patients in remote areas who require surgery can usually be transported to facilities that are equipped with standard anesthesia apparatus. This chapter provides information on how to administer safe clinical anesthesia in a simple and satisfying manner.[2] It provides an overview of modern anesthesia equipment and principles for use in the field, or perhaps in the reader's hospital in the event of a catastrophe.

Several factors have contributed to a dependency on inflexible, albeit safe, anesthesia. These include mishaps from the improper use of simpler apparatus, misapplication of published standards for anesthesia equipment and practice, and perceived socioeconomic pressures rather than real professional requirements.

A common theme of authors on this subject is that familiarity with equipment is of vital importance. Clinical experience can be difficult to obtain for the same reasons that have led to the increasing complexity of modern equipment. Most contemporary anesthesiologists who have acquired experience with field techniques have done so in countries where educational facilities are often only rudimentary. Nevertheless, when a practitioner visits a less privileged region, the reward in terms of experience gained often more than compensates for any services provided.

This chapter reviews some of the equipment that can be used for anesthesia under mobile disaster circumstances rather than in static but isolated and economically deprived conditions. Techniques for providing anesthesia are not described in detail. Apparatus must be compact, portable, and robust. Surgery can be performed in a hazardous location but must be rapid and essential. Evacuation, even of mass casualties, should be prompt. Cost is not a limiting factor, and anesthesia is normally administered by an expert specialist anesthesiologist, using intravenous induc-

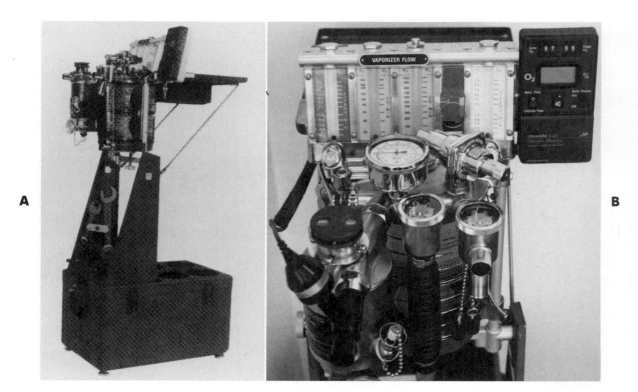

Fig. 29-1. A, The United States military's standard field machine, the Ohmeda Model 885A and carrying case. **B,** Close-up of 885A anesthesia machine components. (From Ohmeda, a Division of BOC Health Care Inc., Madison, Wis.)

tions followed by nonflammable inhaled agents, if indicated.[1] Regional anesthesia for surgery in conscious patients may not be as useful under these conditions as when it is used as an analgesic supplement or in more controlled conditions.

Apparatus that is no longer manufactured is not discussed in detail. Nevertheless, obsolescence in anesthesia is only a relative term, and knowledge of the development of anesthetic apparatus is a useful tool for learning adaptability, provided that the working principles are understood. Anesthesia apparatus suitable for field use is described as standard equipment in books on the historical aspects of anesthesia.[3] Until relatively recently, anesthesia texts written by clinicians often included descriptions of novel and portable apparatus for regional or general anesthesia.[4] Necessity is the mother of invention: a precordial stethoscope can be fashioned from largely scrap material,[5] and vaporizing ether in a can allows performance of complex facial surgery.[6]

Several excellent books describe anesthesia for less technically sophisticated countries,[7-9] and numerous articles have been published about emergency anesthesia in the field.[10-13] These texts and articles should be consulted by anyone who is planning to practice without the re-

sources found within modern, well equipped hospitals in the United States.*

Appropriate portable electronic equipment capable of pulse oximetry or capnometry, measuring noninvasive blood pressure, and displaying the electrocardiogram is continually being improved for use in transporting critically ill patients. Some anesthesiologists believe that if only one monitor were available in the field, the pulse oximeter would be their choice. Because it can also be used as an indicator of perfusion, the pulse oximeter has also been used as the sole monitor in the air evacuation of critically wounded patients.[14]

INHALATIONAL ANESTHESIA

Using conventional continuous gas flow

The Ohmeda Model 885A Anesthesia Apparatus (Fig. 29-1) is the United States military's standard field anesthesia machine.[15] This is presumably because of its similarities to what was at one time a conventional anesthesia ma-

*One week residential courses on anesthesia for developing countries and difficult locations are offered through the Department of Anaesthetics at the University of Oxford and the Frenchay Hospital, Bristol, U.K. The University of Arizona, in conjunction with Health Volunteers Overseas, offers a condensed version in Tucson, Ariz.

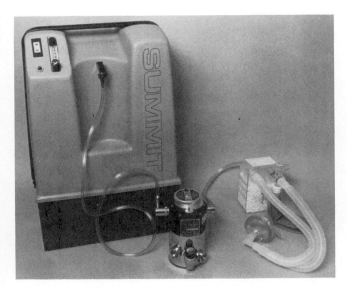

Fig. 29-2. An oxygen concentrator as an alternative source of oxygen for an otherwise familiar anesthesia delivery system. Note the free-standing vaporizer.

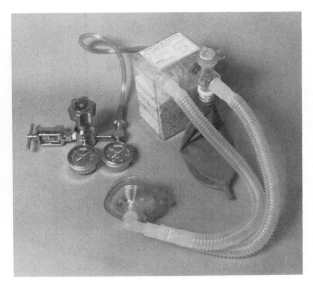

Fig. 29-3. An oxygen cylinder yoke and reducing valve connected to a disposable circle system.

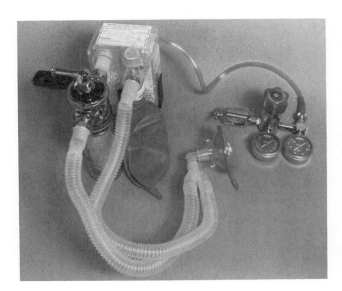

Fig. 29-4. An Ohio #8 vaporizer within a disposable anesthesia circuit. This is a very practical system for those accustomed to it but can be lethal in unfamiliar hands.

chine and breathing circuit. Vaporization is through a Verni-Trol, which, although suitable for most volatile agents, requires familiarity with the system and knowledge of the liquid anesthetic's vapor pressure (see Chapter 3). The Ohmeda 885A machine is bulky, heavy (weighs 52 kg without the necessary gas cylinders), collapsible into a case, and can hardly be considered readily portable. The 885A can be used effectively in a static field hospital, but it requires a ready supply of compressed gases, which may not always be available.

Portable inhalational anesthesia can easily be improvised with familiar equipment and breathing systems consisting of an oxygen source, a standard plenum (Tec-type) vaporizer, and a breathing circuit (Figs. 29-2, 29-3, and 29-4). The breathing circuits illustrated include an inexpensive disposable carbon dioxide absorber unit made by Gibeck-Dryden Corporation (Indianapolis, Ind). It is constructed of K-resin and polystyrene, weighs 1 kg, and contains 650 g of soda lime impregnated with a color indicator. The manufacturer claims the soda lime is good for at least 6 to 8 hours of anesthesia in adults. This is a conservative estimate, based on the absorber's use for in-hospital transportation[16] and in aircraft.[17] Oxygen supplies can be conserved by use of a closed circuit, the average adult requiring no more than 250 ml of oxygen per minute. Insufficient fresh oxygen flows simply cause the reservoir bag to slowly deflate while a high oxygen concentration is maintained. This is the most practical way of providing inhalational anesthesia in a confined space where waste gas scavenging may not be available, such as in an underground entrapment situation or in a dentist's office with minimal ventilation. An oxygen concentrator (see the sec-

tion on oxygen concentrators) can also be used as the gas source for the same system, but a minimum fresh-gas flow of 0.5 L/min must be used to avoid accumulation of condensed atmospheric argon.[18] If a closed circuit is being used and the inhalational anesthesia needs to be deepened quickly, then sufficient agent can be delivered through a plenum vaporizer only if fresh-gas flow rates can be adequately augmented. If this is not practical, or if gas or agent needs to be conserved, additional anesthetic agent can be delivered by direct injection from a syringe into the circuit,[19] into the oxygen supply tubing,[20] or by using a

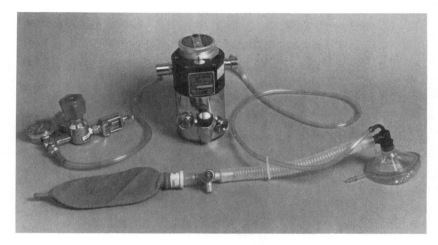

Fig. 29-5. A simple and familiar Mapleson D system for portable inhalational anesthesia. Note the free-standing vaporizer. Care must be taken to ensure that the vaporizer is not tipped.

low-resistance vaporizer within the circle,[21] such as an Ohio #8 vaporizer (Fig. 29-4). This has the added advantage of a built-in servo-control during spontaneous ventilation.[21] It cannot be overemphasized that in order to avoid repeating fatal mistakes, experience with these techniques needs to be acquired before their use in an emergency. At a minimum, the practitioner should understand clearly the way in which alveolar concentration, and hence depth of anesthesia, depends on the factors of ventilation, fresh-gas flow, and vaporizer characteristics.[21] Even during elective surgery, several patients were overdosed with halothane when, in the 1950s, ether was replaced with the much more depressant halothane in draw-over vaporizers placed within the circle.[22]

The Ohio #8 vaporizer is far more difficult to use and more dangerous than modern draw-over vaporizers, such as the one included in the Ohmeda Portable Anesthesia Complete (PAC) unit (see next section). It is mentioned here because, although no longer available from the manufacturer, until the 1970s and early 1980s, it was mounted onto the breathing circuits of many anesthesia machines in obstetric suites for use with ether and then methoxyflurane, and it may still be found in anesthesia workrooms. The PAC unit contains the only low-resistance vaporizer approved for sale by the Food and Drug Administration (FDA) and the only vaporizer that can be used safely during transportation because it will not spill liquid agent when tipped. The irony is that in the United States, the PAC vaporizer is available only to the military, who are forbidden to use it in their hospitals.

The arrangement shown in Fig. 29-5 uses a modified T-piece system, with a Norman mask elbow for the breathing system. Classified as one of a number of configurations of the Mapleson D, these systems are lightweight, require little maintenance, and are used by surgical teams, such as Interplast, when supplies of volatile anesthetic agent and oxygen or air are readily available. Relatively high fresh-

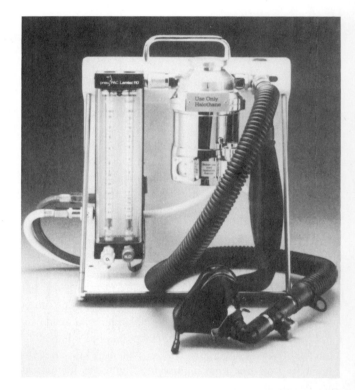

Fig. 29-6. The Lamtec 110 Anaesthetic Unit, manufactured by pneuPAC, Luton, U.K.

gas flows must be used to avoid rebreathing, and the utmost care must be taken to avoid tipping the vaporizer, which would cause liquid anesthetic to enter the breathing system (see Chapter 3).

The Lamtec 110 Anaesthetic Unit* (Fig. 29-6) is a hand-transportable unit, weighs 4 kg, and has standard fittings that can be used with any continuous flow breathing system. The basic unit accepts one of four vaporizers; an

*PneuPAC Ltd. Luton, Bedfordshire, U.K.

extended version accepts two vaporizers. The apparatus requires a source of compressed oxygen.

Using the draw-over method with air

The oldest method of providing inhalational anesthesia involves breathing air, perhaps enriched with oxygen, drawn over a volatile anesthetic agent. This principle was employed when a handkerchief containing anesthetic was held to the face, with various Schimmelbusch types of masks, with the Flagg can, and with numerous hand-held or table-top inhalers. Few vaporizers were calibrated to deliver a known concentration of anesthetic agent. This knowledge was not considered essential for anesthesia, because more reliance was placed on clinical signs than on achieving minimum alveolar concentrations (MAC) in the end-tidal gas.

Two pieces of equipment are commonly used to provide draw-over anesthesia: a vaporizer (Figs. 29-7 and 29-8) and a bellows or self-inflating bag (e.g., Ambu-bag) to inflate the patient's lungs. These are linked together and to the patient by incorporation of one or more one-way valves to isolate the vaporizer and to prevent the rebreathing of exhaled gas, which may have a low concentration of oxygen (Fig. 29-9). The inlet of the apparatus must be open to the atmosphere to enable air to be drawn in, either by the patient's inspiratory effort or by the recoil of the

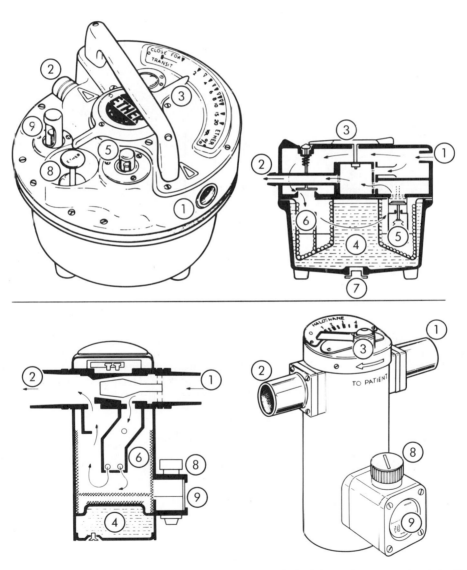

Fig. 29-7. Schematics of the EMO (Epstein, Macintosh, Oxford) Vaporizer *(upper)* and the Oxford Miniature Vaporizer *(lower)*. *1,* inlet port; *2,* outlet port; *3,* concentration control; *4,* water jacket; *5,* thermocompensator valve; *6,* vaporizing chamber; *7,* filling port for water; *8,* filling port for anesthetic; *9,* anesthetic level indicator. (From Dobson MB, *Anaesthesia at the district hospital,* Geneva, 1988, World Health Organization. Reproduced by permission.)

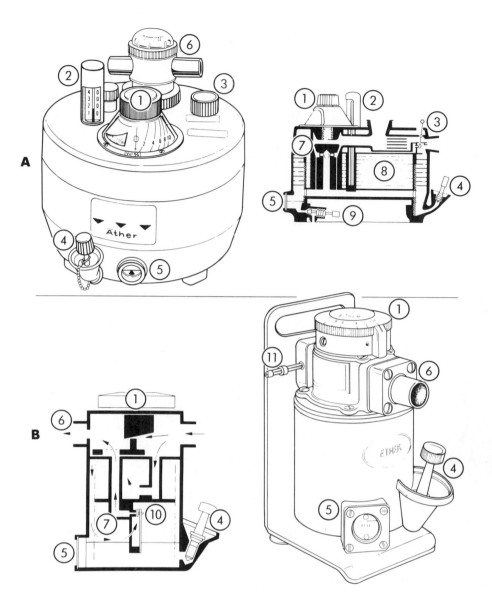

Fig. 29-8. A, AFYA vaporizer (Dräger). **B,** PAC vaporizer (Ohmeda). Both are draw-over vaporizers. *1,* concentration control; *2,* thermometer; *3,* on/off control; *4,* filling port for ether; *5,* ether level gauge; *6,* outlet and one-way valve; *7,* vaporizing chamber; *8,* water-filled heat reservoir; *9, drainage port for ether; 10, thermocompensator valve; 11,* port for oxygen enrichment. (Reproduced by permission of the World Health Organization.)

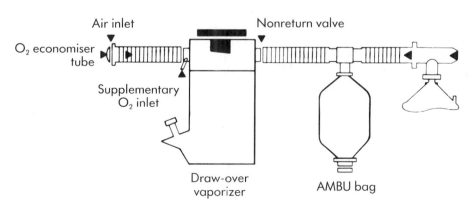

Fig. 29-9. Principle of modern draw-over anesthesia (From Dobson MB, *Anaesthesia at the district hospital,* Geneva, 1988, World Heath Organization. Reproduced by permission.)

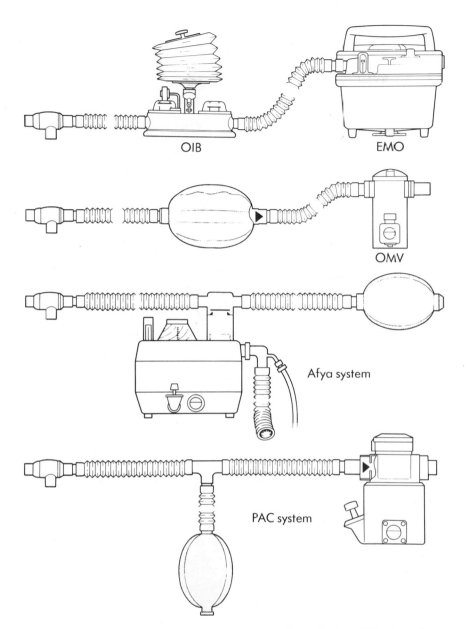

Fig. 29-10. Several arrangements of draw-over systems. (From Dobson MB: *Anaesthesia at the district hospital,* Geneva, 1988, World Health Organization. Reproduced by permission.)

self-inflating bag (Fig. 29-9). Figure 29-10 shows several arrangements of draw-over apparatus. The Oxford Inflating Bellows (OIB) is usually supplied with the Epstein, Macintosh, Oxford (EMO) system. If oxygen enrichment of inspired air is required, a flow rate of 1 L/min of oxygen into the system produces an average oxygen concentration of over 30% when ventilation is 6 L/min. Introducing supplemental oxygen between the vaporizer and the patient dilutes the anesthetic vapor but obviates the need for a reservoir at the vaporizer inlet. If high gas flows are required, such as when a collapsible reservoir bag is being used in an Ayre's T-piece or Magill breathing system, sup-

plies of compressed oxygen can be conserved by entraining ambient air using a Farman type of entrainer or by using compressed oxygen flowing into a venturi tube. The venturi tube entrains air at a rate of at least 1.5 times the oxygen flow into the breathing system.[9]

The EMO vaporizer was produced in 1956 by Epstein and Macintosh as an improved version of the Oxford Ether Vaporizer, which was itself inspired by the Flagg can.[6] It incorporates many ingenious features, requires routine maintenance only every 5 years, and is ubiquitous in developing countries. It is still in production and in common use but is not discussed here in detail because it can be

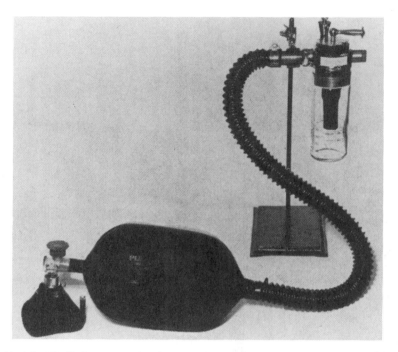

Fig. 29-11. The "Puffa," an example of a portable anesthesia system that could easily be assembled from apparatus in daily use. (From Papantony M, Landmesser CM: Portable unit for fluothane-air anesthesia ("PUFFA"), *Anesthesiology* 21:768-773, 1960. Reproduced by permission.)

used only with ether or methoxyflurane (at 1/10th calibration scale), neither of which is commonly used to provide clinical anesthesia in the United States.

During the Soviet invasion of Hungary in 1956, oxygen supplies in Budapest were depleted within three days. The Civil Defense Department of New York State then purchased 400 EMOs in preparation for a possible catastrophe in the United States. Anesthesia residents were, at the time, taught to provide anesthesia without using supplies of compressed gases.[23] Existing anesthetic apparatus was also easily adapted for use in the field (Fig. 29-11).[24]

In the early 1960s, as ether lost much of its popularity, the Haloxair and Fluoxair,* apparatus were developed (Fig. 29-12) and were evaluated at naval hospitals in Philadelphia and Bethesda.[25-27] The apparatus subsequently was in routine clinical use in the naval hospitals in the continental United States and was stocked by the civil defense in their hospital units. The essential features of the Haloxair include a temperature-compensated vaporizer for halothane, a means for accurately and economically supplementing the inspired air with oxygen, and an automatic valve system that allows for both spontaneous and intermittent positive pressure ventilation.[28]

Another prominent vaporizer, the Oxford Miniature Vaporizer (Fig. 29-7), was developed in the United Kingdom in the early 1960s by the Nuffield Department of Anaes-

*Cyprane Ltd., Yorkshire, U.K.

thetics in Oxford, in conjunction with the Longworth Scientific Instrument Company. This vaporizer is currently manufactured by Penlon Limited, Abingdon, U.K.; their agents in the United States are Eastern Anesthesia Incorporated, of Newton, Pa. The Oxford Miniature Vaporizer was originally conceived as a simple, portable, and robust accessory to the EMO for the induction of halothane anesthesia to be followed by maintenance with ether. Size and weight were kept to a minimum, and new materials were incorporated, such as woven stainless steel wicks. This apparatus has been shown to have a considerably greater versatility than originally intended.[29] With an interchangeable scale, it can accurately deliver known amounts of any of the commonly used volatile anesthetics. It weighs 1.4 kg and has a capacity of 50 ml of anesthetic liquid, which, according to the manufacturers, can provide 1.5% halothane at 20° C for 3 hours.[30] The absence of a built-in back check valve requires that one be included elsewhere in the breathing system.

The Oxford Miniature Vaporizer, incorporated into the Tri-Service apparatus (Fig. 29-13), is popular with the British military. Variations of this vaporizer are still in regular daily use in many parts of Africa and Asia, where it is employed for simple as well as complex cases, such as major trauma and repair of tracheoesophageal fistulas in neonates.[11] In the 1982 Falklands war, this vaporizer, in the form of the Tri-Service apparatus, was used in over half the cases.[31]

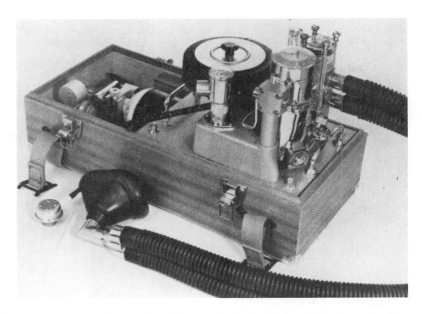

Fig. 29-12. The Haloxaire apparatus. (Cyprane Ltd., Yorkshire, U.K. Reproduced by permission.)

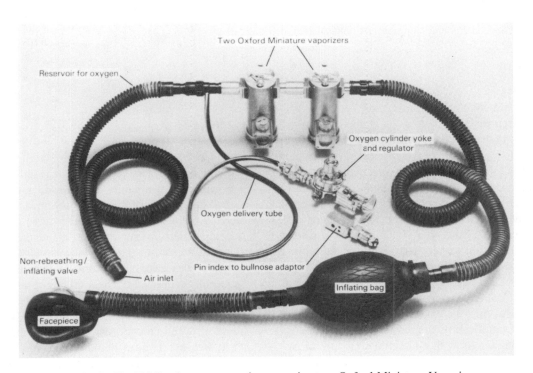

Fig. 29-13. The Tri-Service apparatus, incorporating two Oxford Miniature Vaporizers.

The Oxford Miniature Vaporizer has some disadvantages. Accidental tipping can spill liquid volatile agent into the breathing circuit, and the thermostability of its ethylene glycol jacket was not designed for prolonged use at high gas flows. Thus vapor output decreases as the temperature falls, but some may consider this a safety feature. Although somewhat bulkier and more expensive, the Ohmeda Portable Anesthesia Complete (PAC) system (Fig. 29-14), which incorporates the vaporizer of the Haloxair (Fig. 29-15), does not have these particular drawbacks. The United States military finds the PAC unit more popular than the Oxford Miniature Vaporizer, and both systems were used in United States field hospitals during the 1991 Persian Gulf war when supplies of compressed

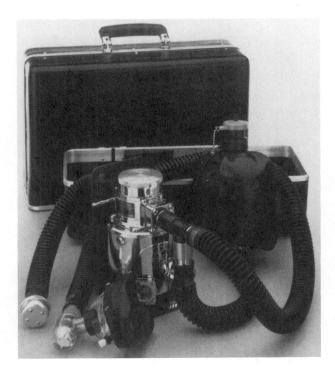

Fig. 29-14. The Ohmeda Portable Anesthesia Complete (PAC) system.

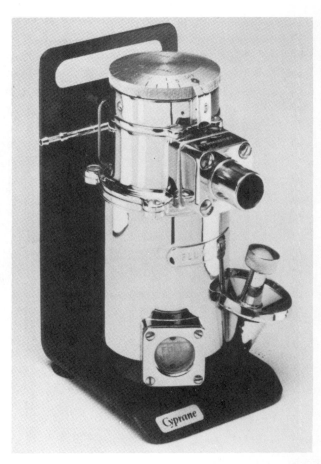

Fig. 29-15. The Ohmeda Portable Anesthesia Complete (PAC) vaporizer.

oxygen for the Ohmeda 885A were in short supply.[32]

Although not currently marketed for civilian use in the United States, the PAC unit is distributed by Ohmeda (Madison, Wis.). The vaporizer weighs 2.3 kg, resembles the familiar "Tec" units, and is agent-specific. The vaporizer can be purchased with either a funnel or key safety filler system. The military version, called the Universal PAC, is calibrated for use with isoflurane, halothane, enflurane, or ether.[33] Because the drain plug is used for changing the calibration scale, the possibility of mixing agents in the vaporizer is minimized. Vapor output concentration for any agent at any dial setting can also be read from an attached scale. A temperature-sensitive valve regulates gas flow leaving the vaporizing chamber, and its function is not significantly altered over a temperature range of 12 to 35° C. As with any calibrated variable bypass vaporizer, the vapor pressure, but not the concentration of anesthetic agent delivered, remains independent of barometric pressure. If the unit is inverted, the force of gravity prevents liquid from entering the breathing system because the inlet to and outlet from the vaporizing chamber are positioned above the maximum liquid level no matter what the position of the vaporizer. Tilting and vibration do not significantly affect performance.[34] This is a major advantage over other vaporizers in certain field conditions, especially for transporting anesthetized patients. Resistance to inhalation is small, being 1 cm of water at a flow of 30 L/min. A nipple at the inlet allows administration of supplemental oxygen, and a back check valve within the gas outlet enables incorporation of a self-inflating bag either within the breathing hose leading to the patient or "teed" in, as the arrangement supplied by the manufacturer. A nonrebreathing expiratory valve with a 15-mm inside diameter/22-mm outside diameter patient port is placed at the end of the breathing hose; this enables the attachment of a face mask or any device with a 15-mm male connector, such as a tracheal tube or a laryngeal mask.

The PAC vaporizer, designed to hold more anesthetic than the Oxford Miniature Vaporizer, requires 85 ml of liquid for a full charge, of which 13 ml are retained by the wick. Because 1 ml of liquid anesthetic produces approximately 200 ml of vapor, an output of 2% vapor at 6 L/hr can be sustained for at least 100 minutes.[33] If the vaporizer is used within a closed circuit, many hours of anesthesia can be provided with a single charge. However, this arrangement is precluded in most emergency situations because the inhaled agent concentration will be unknown, moisture will accumulate within the vaporizer, and unintentional overdosage is easy during controlled ventilation.

In general, plenum vaporizers have an internal resistance some 30 to 50 times that of a draw-over vaporizer, requiring the use of compressed gases for sustained gas flows. However, the Fluotec Mark II vaporizer has been successfully used with a self-inflating bag for draw-over

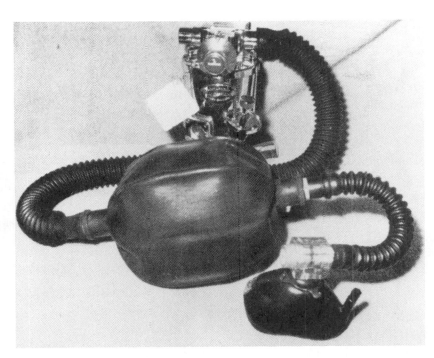

Fig. 29-16. When a Fluotec Mark II is used as a draw-over vaporizer ventilation must be assisted or controlled. (From Counts HK, Jr, Carden WD, Petty WC: Use of the Fluotec Mark II for halothane-air anesthesia, *Anesth Analg* 52:181-187, 1973. Reproduced by permission of the International Anesthesia Research Society.)

anesthesia. However, patients found this device difficult to breathe through, and ventilation had to be assisted or controlled to avoid hypercarbia (Fig. 29-16).[35]

Numerous other arrangements of apparatus, usually assembled from readily available equipment, have been described for draw-over anesthesia.[13] Today, it is difficult to "cannibalize" contemporary apparatus to achieve the same purpose. Even though, in the absence of an antiquated low-resistance vaporizer, a coffee jar would suffice,[6,10] finding a self-inflating bag with an appropriate nonrebreathing valve and a suitable 22-mm male inflow connection is difficult. Some self-inflating bags have a nonrebreathing valve that allows the patient to spontaneously inspire air from downstream, which is of no use for anesthesia. An universal breathing valve must be used at the patient end of the system to ensure that, during spontaneous or controlled ventilation, gas always reaches the patient from the vaporizer (Fig. 29-17).[7]

Using the to-and-fro system

The to-and-fro technique is almost as old as inhalational anesthesia itself. In fact, Morton's first public demonstration of ether anesthesia used a valveless wooden spigot connected to his glass flask. By the very next day, inspiratory and expiratory valves had been incorporated into the mouthpiece, changing the to-and-fro system into a draw-over system.[3] This principle is mentioned here for its simplicity and effectiveness. Rebreathing directly into a 3-L

anesthesia reservoir bag full of oxygen in which 1 to 2 ml of halothane or other similar liquid has been placed rapidly produces anesthesia for a very short surgical procedure. Details of similar techniques are described by Boulton.[10] In Hingson's ingenious portable anesthesia machine,[36] tiny prefilled cylinders of anesthetic and oxygen were discharged into a system incorporating a Waters soda lime canister, and anesthesia of virtually any duration could be provided (Figs. 29-18 and 29-19). This apparatus has been adapted for use with liquid volatile anesthetic by addition of an injection site between the reservoir bag and the soda lime canister.

TOTAL INTRAVENOUS ANESTHESIA

Apparatus required for total intravenous anesthesia (TIVA) is lightweight, familiar, and portable. It consists of sterile syringes, needles, infusion apparatus, and drugs. This is the most common method of producing anesthesia in the field for short surgical procedures such as the amputation of a trapped, unsalvageable limb. Ketamine is usually the primary intravenous anesthetic, and it is also effective when given intramuscularly.[11] Administered by competent personnel, TIVA has proven very satisfactory over a large number of cases, both in emergencies and for elective surgery.[12,37,38]

The concept of total anesthesia in a syringe is so alluring that patients often believe anesthesia for routine surgery consists only of an intravenous injection of thiopental

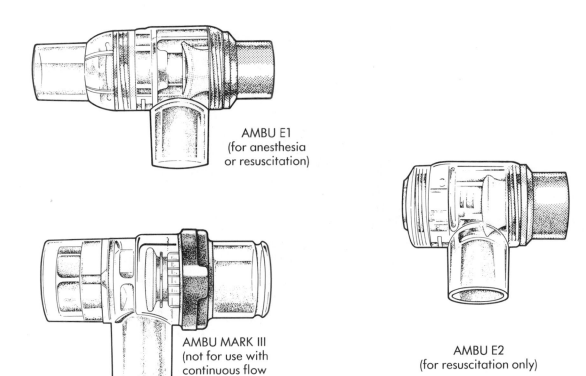

AMBU E1
(for anesthesia
or resuscitation)

AMBU MARK III
(not for use with
continuous flow
anesthesia machine)

AMBU E2
(for resuscitation only)

Fig. 29-17. Three different kinds of nonrebreathing valve. (From Dobson MB: *Anaesthesia at the district hospital,* Geneva, 1988, World Health Organization. Reproduced by permission.)

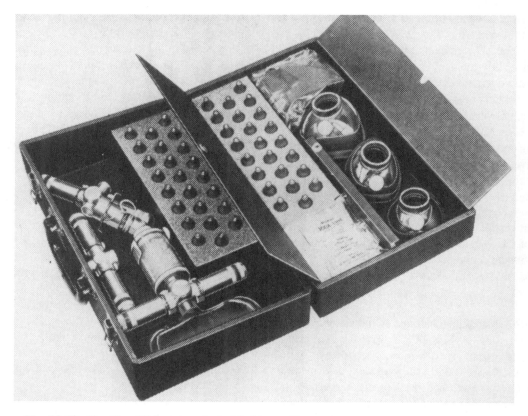

Fig. 29-18. The Case Midget Anesthetic Machine, with supplies for 24 short anesthetics. (Courtesy of RA Hingson, M.D.)

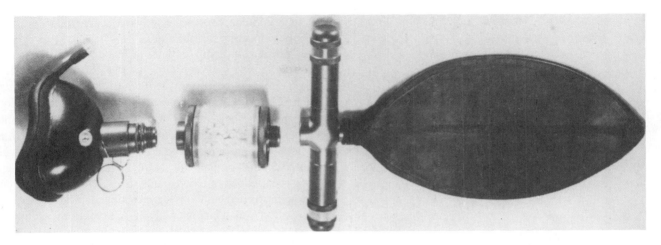

Fig. 29-19. The working components of the Case Midget Anesthetic Machine. (Courtesy of RA Hingson, M.D.)

(Pentothal). Actually, 50 years ago, field experience with TIVA for mass casualties was with thiopental as the sole agent, and results were disastrous.[39] At the present time, TIVA can be provided with many combinations of drugs to achieve hypnosis, analgesia, and muscle relaxation without undue cardiovascular depression. The ablation of the autonomic reflex to surgery, which is necessary when the viscera are stimulated, can be achieved with a sympatholytic drug such as labetalol. The next major development in this field will be the introduction of a drug capable of producing surgical depths of anesthesia without significant respiratory depression or unwanted psychogenic effects. Ketamine was originally marketed as such, as was thiopental, and as is propofol. Stereospecific isomers of ketamine show more promise than receptor-specific opioids.

Total intravenous anesthesia has a major advantage over inhalational anesthesia when contamination of the ambient atmosphere is a problem. In addition, if high inspired oxygen concentrations are needed, (i.e., in the presence of major thoracic trauma or smoke inhalation) and oxygen supplies are limited, a closed circle system utilizing minimal quantities of oxygen can most easily be used in conjunction with intravenous anesthesia. One E cylinder of oxygen (containing 660 L when filled to a pressure of 1900 psig) will last for approximately 40 hours (at a flow rate of 250 ml/min) or one average week of anesthesia use.[37] With the advent of short-acting intravenous drugs; portable, robust, and dependable infusion pumps; and drugs that reverse residual anesthesia, it is surprising that TIVA is not more popular either for elective or field surgery. Despite its attractive simplicity, the technique requires practice and familiarity to achieve sufficient expertise. The requisite of multiple essential drugs, all of which need to be kept sterile, is also a disadvantage in field use. For mass casualties, especially in primitive surroundings where patients must recover without expert supervision,

inhalational and perhaps regional anesthesia are still more popular than TIVA.

REGIONAL AND LOCAL ANESTHESIA

As with TIVA, equipment to provide regional and local anesthesia is compact and portable, and needs to be kept sterile. Disposable syringes, needles, and microcatheters of practically every configuration are readily available, as are a wide variety of local anesthetic preparations. However, major regional anesthesia requires careful planning and constant practice, which will often preclude its use in field situations for anything other than the provision of analgesia for musculoskeletal injuries.[40] Nevertheless, in more static situations, especially for mass casualties when facilities and personnel for general anesthesia are scarce, regional anesthesia may be preferred. In one field hospital dispatched to Armenia immediately after the earthquake of December 7, 1988, regional anesthesia was used for 14 of 26 surgical procedures carried out under difficult circumstances. These 14 anesthetics consisted of 4 epidurals, 6 intravenous regional, and 4 local infiltrations.[14] Apparatus for regional anesthesia in the field does not differ from hospital equipment. If improvisation is necessary, the skill of honing dull needles must be relearned, as must be the knowledge to clean and resterilize needles in order to avoid repeating the disasters of adhesive arachnoiditis caused by detergent residues half a generation ago.[41] Many articles describe techniques for regional anesthesia in difficult situations.[40,42]

SOME USEFUL ACCESSORIES

The oxygen concentrator

Oxygen concentrators, comparable in size to a large portable sewing machine and weighing around 25 kg, have been developed in the past 10 years for medical use as an alternative to compressed or liquid oxygen cylinders (Figs. 29-20, and 29-21). Although commonly used as an oxygen

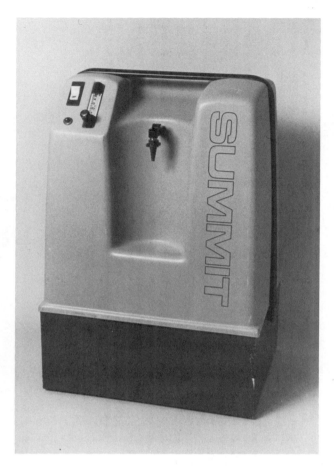

Fig. 29-20. One of many models of portable oxygen concentrator.

source in home health care, oxygen concentrators are routinely employed for anesthesia only when the supply of compressed or liquid oxygen is not dependable. A high concentration of oxygen (85% to 95%) at clinically useful flow rates (up to 5 L/min) is produced by physical separation of oxygen from ambient air. Air from a compressor, which can be powered by electricity or petroleum (portable generators have made electricity practically ubiquitous), is passed through a zeolite column (aluminum silicate with ion-exchange properties). Nitrogen and water vapor are adsorbed, allowing oxygen and rare gases to pass. In order to maintain a continuous oxygen output, a switching device diverts the compressed air stream to an alternative column once the original zeolite column becomes saturated. The first column is then purged of nitrogen so as to be ready for further use. A properly maintained oxygen concentrator can reliably produce a continuous supply of oxygen suitable for draw-over or continuous-flow anesthesia[18,43-46] or, in conjunction with another compressor, can supply standard anesthesia machines.[47] PneuPac Ltd. of Luton, Bedfordshire, U.K., sells an oxygen concentrator combined with an anesthesia machine as a single unit. Some hospitals in the United Kingdom use large oxygen concentrators as a source of pipeline oxygen.

The Mempro Company (Troy, N.Y.) manufactures ultra-thin polymeric membranes that produce from ambient air a product enriched with water vapor and oxygen by using the membranes as a molecular sieve. Gulfstream Medical (Bedminster, N.J.) assembles and markets the device, named the OE Plus, which is used in home applications.

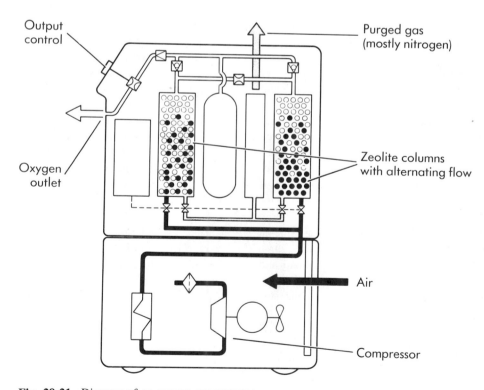

Fig. 29-21. Diagram of an oxygen concentrator.

where humidification as well as oxygenation is important. The 31-kg machine can produce up to 40% oxygen at high or ambient humidity at a rate of up to 8 L/min. It requires an electric power source of 400 watts to power a compressor and two fans. The output pressure of 6 psig is sufficient for use as a gas source for plenum or draw-over vaporizers, as well as for use as an oxygen source for postanesthesia care. The technology of oxygen separation is rapidly improving, and eventually less reliance will be placed on the manufacture, transportation, and storage of liquid oxygen.

The laryngeal mask and the binasal pharyngeal airways

The laryngeal mask (Fig. 29-22) was invented in 1981 in London. Unlike other cuffed pharyngeal airways, it is designed to form a direct connection from the breathing system to the patient's airway by sealing around the laryngeal perimeter rather than the pharyngeal perimeter (Fig. 29-23).[48] Only recently approved for sale in the United States, the laryngeal mask has been available in the United Kingdom since 1988. In the United Kingdom it gained popularity more quickly than either the pulse oximeter or the Dinamap in the United States. Medical trainees can learn to gain control of the airway in unconscious subjects with the laryngeal mask more easily than they can with laryngoscopy and tracheal intubation. The overall success rate was 94% in 20 seconds average time with the laryngeal mask versus 51% in 34 seconds average time with tracheal intubation.[49] Speed and simplicity are of obvious value. Neither a laryngoscope nor muscle relaxants are required. The device is too large to enter the esophagus or trachea, and the dangers of esophageal or bronchial intubation are therefore avoided.[48] An obvious advantage of the laryngeal mask over a face mask and bag ventilation, which requires two operators for optimal ventilation, is that it leaves the hands free.[49] The device has also been life-saving in cases of failed tracheal intubation when ventilation was impossible.[48] Blind intubation through a properly positioned laryngeal mask is successful about 90% of the time.[48]

In general there appears to be an inverse relationship between ease of insertion of the laryngeal mask and ease of laryngoscopy, an anterior larynx apparently being an advantage.[48] The device should always be available for field anesthesia because conditions for laryngoscopy may not be adequate, and attempts at insertion of a laryngeal mask are more likely to be successful than tracheal intubation. Although a properly placed cuffed tracheal tube provides better protection against pulmonary aspiration, the laryngeal mask has been advocated for use in the field for short cases, where the absence of a tube in the trachea allows a reduced depth of anesthesia and more rapid recovery.[11] The device is expensive but reusable and is designed to be sterilized by autoclaving, being made almost entirely of silicone.

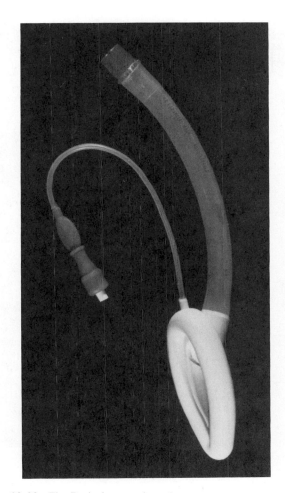

Fig. 29-22. The Brain laryngeal mask.

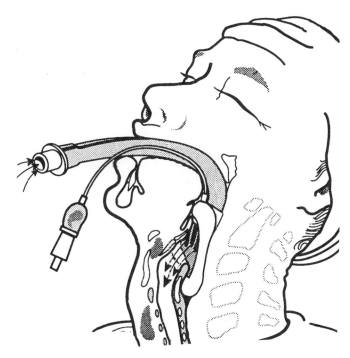

Fig. 29-23. A properly positioned laryngeal mask airway.

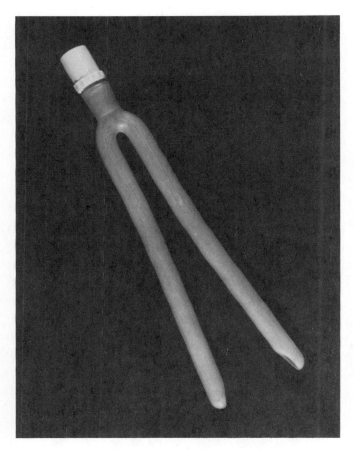

Fig. 29-24. A binasal pharyngeal airway.

The binasal pharyngeal airway (Fig. 29-24) was described in 1969 for airway management during anesthesia and for resuscitation.[50,51] Its applications and advantages are virtually identical to those of the laryngeal mask. A pair of nasopharyngeal tubes, long enough to pass beyond the base of the tongue, are coupled together and connected to a conventional breathing system through a standard 15-mm diameter male connector (Fig. 29-25).[50,51] In a series of over 1000 elective surgical cases and 27 resuscitations, in which muscle relaxants were used as necessary for surgery, there were no problems other than one case of nasal bleeding that stopped spontaneously when tamponaded by the airway. Neither gastric dilatation nor pulmonary aspiration occurred. Securing the airway is quicker than with the laryngeal mask, and the binasal pharyngeal airway is easily used in patients who are unable to open their mouth or extend their atlanto-occipital joint, which may present problems with the laryngeal mask. If unavailable commercially, a binasal pharyngeal airway can be assembled from two long nasopharyngeal airways and a connector similar to those used with conventional double-lumen tracheal/endobronchial tubes.

The emergency aspirator

The emergency aspirator, a portable mechanical aspirator, can be operated with one hand, producing suction up to 450 mm Hg through a large-bore (9-mm) catheter (Fig. 29-26). Excess aspirate is ejected through the rear of the device, allowing continual aspiration. An efficient suction apparatus is essential in the field, where most patients do not have empty stomachs and the incidence of gastric re-

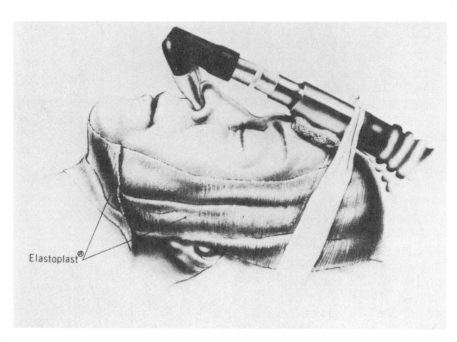

Fig. 29-25. The original form of the binasal pharyngeal airway in use. (From Elam JO, Titel JH, Fenigold A, et al: Simplified airway management during anesthesia or resuscitation: a binasal pharyngeal system, *Anesth Analg* 48:307-316, 1969.)

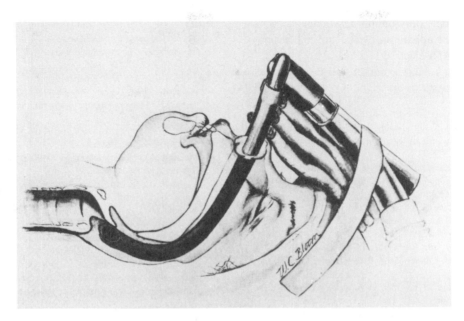

Fig. 29-25, cont'd. For legend see opposite page.

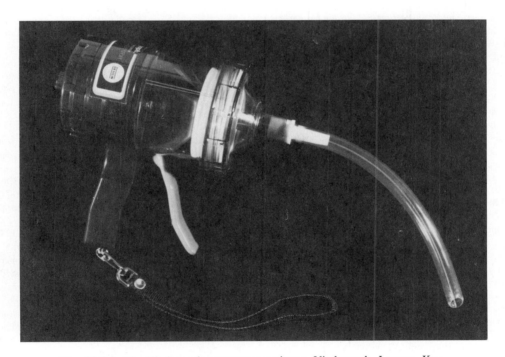

Fig. 29-26. The Vitalograph emergency aspirator, Vitalograph, Lenexa, Kan.

gurgitation may be increased if hypoxemia, respiratory obstruction, or arterial hypotension is also present.[52] The device illustrated is distributed by Vitalograph of Lenexa, Kansas.

It may be argued that the complacent attitude of most anesthesiologists toward field anesthesia can be justified because the rare case requiring field surgery can usually be managed with intramuscular or intravenous ketamine. Nevertheless, the following points are indisputable:

1. On a global level, organized anesthesia in the field during the past decade has depended on draw-over apparatus because compressed gases have invariably been in short supply (for example, in Oman, 1981;[53] Falklands, 1982;[31] Armenia, 1988;[14] Philippines, 1988;[54] Persian Gulf, 1991[32]).

2. Modern draw-over vaporizers are safer and hence easier to use now than ever before. Familiarity with equipment before emergency use is still essential.

3. In the United States, only the military have access to modern draw-over apparatus, which are not permitted to be used in an elective setting.

4. It is still true today that victims of extinction are less well adapted than survivors.[55]

REFERENCES

1. Dobson MB, Boulton TB: Introductory lectures in anaesthesia for developing countries and difficult locations, St. Catherine's College, Oxford, UK, July 8-13, 1990.
2. Macintosh RR: A plea for simplicity, Br Med J ii:1054, 1955.
3. Thomas KB: The development of anaesthetic apparatus, Oxford, UK, 1975, Blackwell Scientific.
4. Flagg P: The art of anesthesia, ed 7, Philadelphia, 1954, Lippincott.
5. Inman MT: A monaural paediatric chest stethoscope for threepence three-farthings, Anaesthesia 21:572-573, 1966.
6. Macintosh RR: Saved by the Flagg 2.1. In Atkinson RS, Boulton TB, editors: The history of anaesthesia, Park Ridge, NJ, 1989, Parthenon Publishing Group.
7. Dobson MB: Anaesthesia at the district hospital, Geneva, 1988, World Health Organization.
8. King MH, editor: Primary anaesthesia, New York, 1986, Oxford University Press.
9. Farman JV: Anaesthesia and the E.M.O. system, London, 1973, English Universities Press.
10. Boulton TB: Anaesthesia and resuscitation in difficult environments. In Hewer CL, editor: Recent advances in anaesthesia and analgesia, ed 11, London, 1972, Churchill-Livingstone.
11. Baskett PJ: The trauma anesthesia/critical care specialist in the field. Critical Care Clinics 6:13-24, 1990.
12. Restall J, Knight RJ: Analgesia and anaesthesia in the field. In Baskett P, Weller R, editors: Medicine for disasters, London, 1988, Butterworth.
13. Olson KW, Kingsley CP: Drawover anesthesia: a review of equipment, capabilities, and utility under austere conditions, Anesth Rev 17:19-29, 1990.
14. Donchin Y, Wiener M, Grande CM, et al: Military medicine: trauma anesthesia and critical care on the battlefield, Critical Care Clinics 6:185-202, 1990.
15. Ohmeda Model 885A instruction and service manual, Revised 12/89, Madison, Wis, Ohmeda.
16. Viegas OJ, Cummins DF, Shumacker CA: Portable ventilation system for transport of critically ill patients, Anesth Analg 60:760-761, 1981.
17. Lanier WL, Weeks DB: Portable semiclosed circuit for prolonged oxygen administration in aircraft, Anesthesiology 63:116-118, 1985.
18. Parker CJ, Snowdon SL: Predicted and measured oxygen concentrations in the circle system using low fresh gas flows with oxygen supplied by an oxygen concentrator, Br J Anaesth 61:397-402, 1988.
19. Lowe JH, Ernst E: The quantitative practice of anesthesia: use of the closed circuit, Baltimore, 1981, Williams & Wilkins.
20. Wolfson B: Closed circuit anaesthesia by intermittent injections of halothane, Br J Anaesth 34:733-737, 1962.
21. Mushin WW, Galloon S: The concentration of anaesthetics in closed circuits with special reference to halothane, Br J Anaesth 32:324-333, 1960.
22. Chang J, Macartney JJ, Graves HB: Clinical experience with Fluothane, a new non-explosive anaesthetic agent, Can Anaesth Soc J 4:187-206, 1957.
23. Harmel M: Personal communication, 1991.
24. Papantony M, Landmesser CM: Portable unit for Fluothane-air anesthesia ("PUFFA"), Anesthesiology 21:768-773, 1960.
25. Coursey JW, Wilson RD: A new draw-over halothane vaporizer, Anesth Analg 44:147-157, 1965.
26. Merrifield AJ, Hill DW, Smith K: Performance of the Portablease and the Fluoxair portable anaesthetic equipment: with reference to use under adverse conditions, Br J Anaesth 39:50-70, 1967.
27. Joyce TH, Vacanti CJ, Van Houten RJ, et al: A draw-over anesthetic system for peace or war, Anesth Analg 48:121-128, 1969.
28. Stephens KF: Transportable apparatus for halothane anaesthesia, Br J Anaesth 37:67-72, 1965.
29. Parkhouse MA: Clinical performance of the OMV inhaler, Anaesthesia 21:498-503, 1966.
30. The OMV Fifty vaporizer (brochure), Abingdon, UK, 1974, Penlon Ltd.
31. Jowitt MD: Anaesthesia ashore in the Falklands, Ann R Coll Surg Engl 66:197-200, 1984.
32. Meeting of Operation Desert Storm Veterans, ASA Annual Meeting, San Francisco, October 28, 1991.
33. Ohmeda Universal PAC: operation and maintenance manual, Ohmeda, BOC Health Care Company, December 1990.
34. Borland CW, Pereira HP, Thornton JA, et al: Evaluation of a new range of draw-over vaporizers: the PAC series laboratory and field studies, Anaesthesia 38:852-861, 1983.
35. Counts HK Jr, Carden WD, Petty WC: Use of the Fluotec Mark II for halothane-air anesthesia, Anesth Analg 52:181-187, 1973.
36. Hingson RA, Brown CA, Gregg E, et al: Noninflammable cyclopropane-helium and oxygen mixtures for use in the Reserve Midget Anesthesia Machine, J Int Coll Surg 30:12-24, 1958.
37. de Sousa H, Snyder G: General anesthesia in the field: total intravenous anesthesia with minimal quantities of oxygen, Anesthesiology 71:A452, 1989 (abstract).
38. Restall J, Tully AM, Ward PJ, et al: Total intravenous anaesthesia for military surgery: a technique using ketamine, midazolam and vecuronium, Anaesthesia 43:46-49, 1988.
39. Halford FJ: A critique of intravenous anesthesia in war surgery, Anesthesiology 4:67-69, 1943.
40. Austin TR: Regional anesthesia in the pre-hospital phase. In Monographs on immediate care, no 2, pain relief, Ipswich, UK, January 1985, The British Association for Immediate Care.
41. Case history of adhesive arachnoiditis produced by spinal anesthesia, Anesth Analg 36:87-92, 1957.
42. Boulton TB: Local anaesthesia in difficult environments. In Lofstrom JB, Sjostrand U, editors: Local anaesthesia and regional blockade, Amsterdam 1988, Elsevier.
43. de Sousa H: Use of an oxygen concentrator as the gas source for general anesthesia, Anesth Analg 70:S82, 1990 (abstract).
44. Carter JA, Baskett PJ, Simpson PJ: The "Permox" oxygen concentrator, Anaesthesia 40:560-565, 1985.
45. Harris CE, Simpson PJ: The "Mini O2" and "Healthdyne" oxygen concentrators, Anaesthesia 40:1206-1209, 1985.
46. Jarvis DA, Brock-Utne JG: Use of an oxygen concentrator linked to a draw-over vaporizer, Anesth Analg 72:805-810, 1991.
47. Easy WR, Douglas GA, Merrifield AJ: A combined oxygen concentrator and compressed air unit, Anaesthesia 43:37-41, 1988.
48. Brain AJ: The Intavent laryngeal mask, instruction manual, ed 2, Henley-on-Thames, Oxford, UK, 1991, Intavent.
49. Davies PR, Tighe SQ, Greenslade GL, et al: Laryngeal mask airway and tracheal tube insertion by unskilled personnel, Lancet 336:977-979, 1990.
50. Elam JO, Titel JH, Fenigold A, et al: Simplified airway management during anesthesia or resuscitation: a binasal pharyngeal system, Anesth Analg 48:307-316, 1969.
51. Weisman H, Weis, TW, Elam JO, et al: Use of double nasopharyngeal airways in anesthesia, Anesth Analg 48:356-360, 1969.
52. O'Mullane EJ: Vomiting and regurgitation during anaesthesia, Lancet I, 1209-1212, 1954.
53. Knight RJ, Houghton IT: Field experience with the Tri-Service anaesthetic apparatus in Oman and Northern Ireland, Anaesthesia 36:1122-1127, 1981.
54. Whitten CE: Experiences in third world anesthesia: peacetime training for operational deployment, Milit Med 153:629-632, 1988.
55. Raup D: Extinction: bad genes or bad luck? New Scientist 131:46-49, 1991.

Chapter 30

CLOSED CIRCUIT ANESTHESIA

James H. Philip, M.E.(E.), M.D.

PRINCIPLES

The basic principle of closed circuit anesthesia is maintenance of a constant anesthetic state by addition of gases and vapors to the breathing circuit at the same rate that the patient's body redistributes (stores) or eliminates them. Often, the desired anesthetic state is first established using a high fresh-gas flow composed of gases (oxygen, nitrous oxide) and vapors (e.g., isoflurane), and the inspired and expired gas tensions are noted. Once these levels are established, maintenance of a steady state (constant gas tensions) is achieved by addition of oxygen, nitrous oxide, and agent vapor to the breathing circuit. The amount of gas and vapor is determined empirically by titration. Several different titration end points can be used. Choices include maintenance of inspired tension, maintenance of expired tension, and maintenance of anesthetic depth judged in some manner. When titrating against the predetermined end point, drugs can be added in a measured or quantified manner or, alternatively, they can be added totally empirically without regard to the total amount administered. In closed circuit anesthesia techniques, gases and vapors are added to the patient's exhaled gas to produce new inhaled gas. One advantage of this technique is that all gases exhaled are already warmed and humidified by the patient and are well-suited for rebreathing.[1]

Thus inhaled gas is formed from two sources. First, the exhaled gas forms most of what the patient will breathe. In addition to exhaled gas, fresh gas is added in the correct quantity and concentration to achieve the inspired gas tensions desired. The same inspired and expired gas tensions are established with a closed circuit as with a semiclosed or open (nonrebreathing) circuit. In this chapter the terms open circuit and nonrebreathing circuit are used interchangeably. Only the method for achieving these levels is altered.

Closed circuit anesthesia can be viewed in several different ways. From one perspective, it is an anesthetic technique unlike all others. The classical closed circuit literature describes theory and practice different from other techniques. In the classical closed circuit approach, once a stable level of anesthesia is established with high-flow oxygen, nitrous oxide, and volatile agent, fresh-gas flow is reduced to the patient's predicted oxygen consumption (243 ml/min for a 70-kg adult), predicted nitrous oxide uptake rate (approximately 100 ml/min after the first 30 minutes), and predicted inhaled agent uptake. Nitrous oxide and agent uptake rates are calculated according to a mathematical formula based on body weight.

The traditional closed circuit anesthesia literature utilizes liquid injection or infusion according to a prescribed time regimen.[2-5] Specifically, the drug administration rate is inversely proportional to the square root of time:

$$\text{Administration rate} = \text{Uptake} = Kt^{-1/2}$$

This empirical relationship was first noted by Severinghaus[6] for nitrous oxide in 1954 and popularized by Lowe[5] beginning in 1972. Severinghaus' original data demonstrated that nitrous oxide uptake followed this power-function relationship fairly closely in the subjects he studied.

There is a scientific explanation for the curious and unexpected mathematical relationship, Uptake $= Kt^{-1/2} = K/\sqrt{(t)}$. It has long been known that body tissues perfused with blood of constant drug concentration or vapor tension have an uptake rate that decreases with time. Specifically, theory and research[7] has demonstrated that uptake into each tissue takes the form of an exponential:

$$\text{Uptake} = Ke^{-t/\tau}$$

where:

t = Time

τ = Time constant (time required to achieve 63% equilibration)

e = Base of natural logarithms (2.7183...)

K = Predictable constant.

Total body uptake is the sum of the individual uptakes by each tissue. In this case, uptake is the sum of a group of exponentials of different amplitudes (K_{tissue}) and time constants (τ_{tissue}). The sum of these exponentials is approximately equal to the power function, $Kt^{-1/2}$. It must be emphasized that, unlike the exponential relationship for a single tissue, the power-function is an empiric relationship and has no underlying mathematical, physical, or theoretical origin, to the best of our current knowledge.

In this classic (Lowe) technique for closed circuit anesthesia, a loading dose is administered to the breathing circuit to bring circuit tension to that desired in the patient's alveoli. A unit dose (for induction and maintenance) is then selected according to the patient's body weight. The relationship with weight follows the relationship first shown by Kleiber[8] and further described by Brody.[9] Kleiber's law states that metabolic processes are proportional to body mass raised to the ¾ power (kg$^{3/4}$). In classical closed circuit anesthesia, unit doses are administered at specific times that have been determined based on the $Kt^{-1/2}$ relationship. It is argued that if uptake can be approximated as $Kt^{-1/2}$, then this is the requisite administration rate to maintain constant alveolar tension. The empiric result is that injections are made at 0, 1, 4, 9, 16, ... minutes. Each administration time is the square of an integer. Lowe points out that the time between injections is 1, 3, 5, 7, ... minutes (i.e., the sequence of odd integers). Even closed circuit enthusiasts, however, advise care and careful observation of the patient and suggest modifying the empiric technique as needed.

It must be noted that this cookbook for drug administration was written in a previous era of more primitive measurement and analysis. In 1972, the digital pocket calculator had not yet replaced the analog slide rule. Anesthetic agent analysis was uncommon; the only clinically available device was the Narkotest,* which consisted of a

*Dräger, Lubeck, Germany.

slowly responding silicone rubber band in a box connected to a mechanical indicator.[10]

With each administration technique—open circuit, semiclosed with high flow, and closed circuit with liquid injection—each patient's inspired, end-expired, and alveolar anesthetic tensions are the same and independent of administration technique. Thus, from the patient's viewpoint, all anesthetic techniques are equivalent.

Although the conventional closed circuit literature used preconceived models, this chapter does not rely on these. Rather, it is assumed that an anesthetic agent monitor is available and in use. The dosage administration scheme therefore is adjusted on the basis of a patient's measured need. Furthermore, if the monitor is a stand-alone unit used by only one operating room, analyzed gases can be returned to the breathing circuit. This simplifies calculations and allows patient uptake to be quantified.

In 1963, Eger[11] introduced the concept of anesthesia at constant alveolar concentration and defined the term minimum alveolar concentration (MAC). As a foundation, he used the pharmacokinetic theory explained by Seymour Kety[12,13]. in 1950. Eger showed that constant alveolar concentration or tension can be produced and maintained when inspired anesthetic concentration is adjusted properly. To compute the proper adjustment sequence (or continuum), he calculated anesthetic uptake into each organ group, adjusting inspired concentration to maintain alveolar concentration constant. Figure 30-1 shows the inspired concentration required to maintain 0.8% alveolar halothane.[11] Inspired halothane concentration (equivalent to partial pressure or tension for a gas or vapor) is begun at 3.3% and is slowly and continuously reduced to 2% at 5 minutes, 1.5% at 20 minutes, and 1% at 3 hours.

In Eger's idealized example, the model patient is perfectly anesthetized when the vessel-rich group reaches 1 MAC as it equilibrates and equalizes with alveolar gas. From the standpoint of achieving constant alveolar tension, the anesthetic is an optimal anesthetic. The target, a step in alveolar tension, is achieved perfectly.

A more realistic clinical end point is a constant anesthetic tension in the brain. That is, the goal of anesthesia is to "anesthetize" the patient's brain. Producing a step change in brain anesthetic tension from its current level to any desired level is a useful clinical target. This is equally true for high-flow anesthesia.

To the clinician, Eger's calculated time course of halothane administration is quite reasonable. It mimics what is administered to many patients. Of course, in today's clinical practice, the vaporizer is not adjusted according to the clock. Rather, the patient's depth of anesthesia is assessed by mental integration of many signs. The pupils are observed for dilation or constriction; and blood pressure, heart rate, and other variables are measured and evaluated. With the convenient availability of anesthetic agent monitors, many clinicians today routinely monitor expired anesthetic concentration (tension) as an important additional

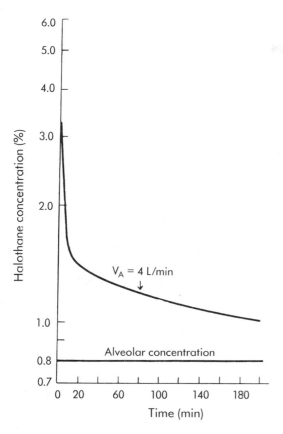

Fig. 30-1. Inspired concentration required to maintain 0.8% alveolar halothane. Halothane inspired concentration begins at 3.3% and is slowly and continuously reduced to 2% at 5 minutes, 1.5% at 20 minutes, and 1% at 3 hours. (From Eger EI II, Guadagni NP: Halothane uptake in man at constant alveolar concentration, *Anesthesiology* 24:299-304, 1963.)

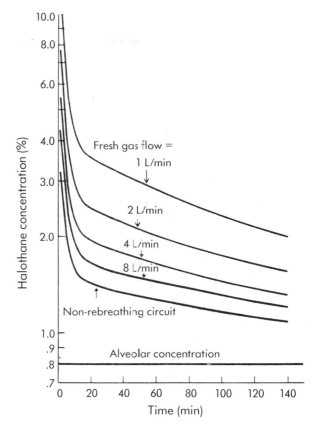

Fig. 30-2. Semiclosed circuit vaporizer settings required for constant alveolar tension of 0.8% halothane at various fresh-gas flows as calculated by Eger. (From Eger EI II, Guadagni NP: Halothane uptake in man at constant alveolar concentration, *Anesthesiology* 24:299-304, 1963.)

sign. To achieve the "ideal" anesthetic, vaporizer setting and fresh-gas flow are adjusted to maintain constant brain anesthetic tension. This is done by allowing a reasonable amount of alveolar overpressure during the period when anesthesia is being deepened. This is described later.

Eger's example (Fig. 30-1) demonstrates anesthesia administration with a perfect nonrebreathing circuit (open circuit). In that system, inspired concentration is perfectly controlled. In contrast, a *semiclosed* breathing circuit with carbon dioxide absorber is the one most commonly used in the United States. With this circuit, inspired concentration or tension is dependent primarily on vaporizer setting but is affected by fresh-gas flow to the breathing circuit and the patient's own exhaled anesthetic tension.

Figure 30-2 shows the semiclosed circuit vaporizer settings required for constant alveolar tension of 0.8% halothane at various fresh-gas flows as calculated by Eger.[11] As flow is progressively decreased from 8 L/min to 1 L/min, vaporizer setting and hence tension delivered to the breathing circuit must be increased. This, again, is because inspired gas is a mixture of fresh gas from the anesthesia machine and gas previously exhaled by the patient.

As fresh-gas flow is decreased, a relatively higher fraction of exhaled gas is rebreathed. Because exhaled gas usually has a lower anesthetic tension than inspired gas, higher vaporizer settings are required to achieve the same inspired concentration.

Note that the initial vaporizer setting at 1 L/min of fresh-gas flow is more than 10% halothane. This is difficult if not impossible to achieve with most modern anesthesia delivery systems. It must be emphasized that the high concentration of anesthetic is delivered *to the breathing circuit,* where it mixes with the 0.8% in the patient's exhaled gas to produce an inspired concentration that must be the same 3.3% as was required in an open circuit. In the two cases, the time course of anesthesia induction is identical because inspired anesthetic concentration is the same. The patient is not aware of how the anesthesiologist created the gas mixture breathed; the patient's body is affected only by the substances present in inspired gas and their concentrations.

Figure 30-3 shows vaporizer settings required to maintain constant alveolar tension for a nonrebreathing circuit (open circuit) and a completely closed circuit with a fresh-

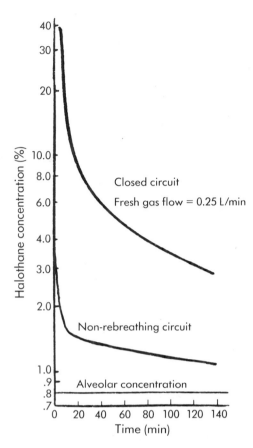

Fig. 30-3. Vaporizer settings required to maintain constant alveolar tension of halothane for a nonrebreathing circuit (open circuit) and a completely closed circuit with a fresh-gas flow of 0.25 L/min.

gas flow of 0.25 L/min. With the closed circuit, the initial vaporizer setting is 40% halothane. In practice, this is impossible for several reasons. First, modern concentration-calibrated vaporizers can be set to administer no more than 5% halothane. Second, the vapor pressure of halothane at room temperature is only 0.33 atm. (33%, or 243 mm Hg) and thus 40% halothane cannot exist under these conditions. Nonetheless, 40% is the theoretical concentration required. This high concentration at the low fresh-gas flow of 250 ml/min into a closed circuit produces the same 3.3% inspired concentration that will achieve the same 1 MAC (0.8% end-expired) anesthetic.

MODEL-ASSISTED UNDERSTANDING OF CLOSED CIRCUIT

Gas Man is an educational computer program[14] designed to teach the pharmacokinetics of inhalation anesthetics. It has been shown to be an effective educational tool, even in centers other than where it was written[15] and when compared to lecture presentation.[16] It provides a strong foundation for teaching uptake and distribution. Various models have been previously described to explain

uptake and distribution[17-19] and other programs (e.g., GUS, Ansim, and others) are also available.[20]

Throughout this chapter, as in Gas Man, the words *tension* and *partial pressure* are used interchangeably. This physical variable represents the effective pressure exerted by a gas, whether it is in the gas phase alone or in combination with another gas, or dissolved in blood or tissue.

Partial pressure is expressed in *percent of 1 atmosphere* (1 atm = 760 mm Hg). Expressing partial pressure this way serves several purposes. When partial pressure is expressed as percent of 1 atm, partial pressure and concentration have the same numeric value for gases. For example, 1 volume percent isoflurane has an isoflurane tension of 1% of 1 atm often shortened verbally to 1%. For blood and tissues, partial pressure is expressed in percent as well. By this definition, a tissue anesthetic measure of 1% does not represent 1% concentration; rather, it represents a partial pressure of 1% of 1 atm (or 1% × 760 mm Hg, or 7.6 mm Hg in terms of absolute pressure).

Next, when partial pressure is expressed as percent of one *standard* atmosphere (i.e., 760 mm Hg), the numbers and concepts work equally well at any atmospheric pressure. Because the physiologic effects of inhaled anesthetics are the results of partial pressure and not concentration,[12,13] anesthetic tensions in the apparatus and patient are the variables shown in the Gas Man windows. The Gas Man Picture represents the model in schematic form and provides a static snapshot of the anesthetic tensions in body tissues (compartments). The Gas Man Graph shows the time course of anesthetic tension in each compartment.

Figure 30-4 shows an annotated Gas Man Picture (top panel) and Gas Man Graph (bottom panel) which represent the time course and current state of the patient and breathing circuit after 15 minutes of 5% isoflurane anesthesia. The picture (Fig. 30-4, *top*) shows anesthetic tension in various locations of interest in the upper half, and it shows flows that conduct drugs from compartment to compartment in the lower half. Compartments are filled to heights representing their respective partial pressures. In the equilibrium state, all compartments are filled to the same height because their partial pressures are equal.

In the Gas Man Graph (Fig. 30-4, *bottom*) it is apparent that tissues in the vessel-rich group (VRG, R) rapidly equilibrate with and almost equal arterial anesthetic tension. Muscle (MUS, M) and fat (FAT, F) equilibrate more slowly. The anesthetic tension in venous blood returning to the heart (VEN) is dominated by blood coming from the vessel-rich group, which receives and returns 75% of the cardiac output. Muscle contributes 20%, and fat contributes 5%. Anesthetic returning to the patient's alveoli is then either exhaled or recirculated to arterial blood according to the relationship between alveolar ventilation and cardiac output. Although this description oversimplifies the situation somewhat, it is sufficient to explain both qualitative and quantitative aspects of inhalation anesthesia.

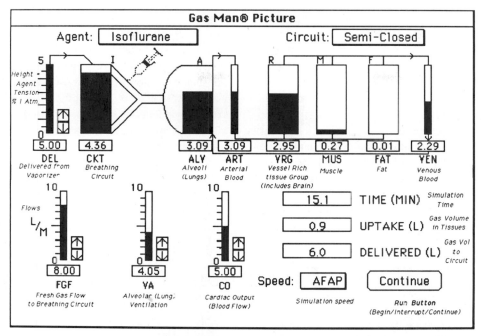

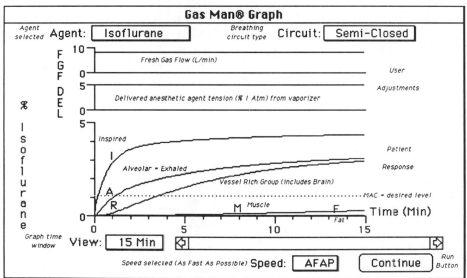

Fig. 30-4. Annotated Gas Man Picture and Gas Man Graph. The Picture shows the current state; compartments are filled to heights representing their respective partial pressures. The Graph shows the 20-minute time course of anesthesia.

In addition to displaying the flow between compartments, the lower half of the Gas Man Picture (Fig. 30-4, *top*) provides additional information about simulation time, patient uptake of anesthetic, and quantity of anesthetic delivered to the breathing circuit. At the end of 15 simulated minutes, anesthetic uptake is 0.9 L isoflurane vapor and volume delivered to the breathing circuit is 6.0 L. The difference between these two values, 5.1 L, is the volume discarded from the breathing circuit through the adjustable pressure-limiting valve during the 15 minutes of anesthetic administration. Efficiency is defined as the ratio of uptake to delivered quantities, expressed as percent.

Here, efficiency = 0.9 L uptake / 6.0 L delivered = 0.15 = 15%. It should be noted that 5.1 L (85%) of the nitrous oxide–oxygen–isoflurane mixture is discarded. This gas is collected by the waste gas scavenging system in the OR, conducted to the hospital chimney, and released to the atmosphere, where it may or may not contribute to ozone layer depletion in the upper atmosphere.

The above example shows how the Gas Man screens can be interpreted. Furthermore, it shows the breathing-circuit response to a constant vaporizer setting and a high fresh-gas flow. This administration technique mimics what is clinically achieved when an attempt is made to provide constant inspired tension using a semiclosed circle system at high fresh-gas flows, except that the resulting clinical concentrations are lower. Anesthesia, however, is not normally administered with a constant vaporizer setting or constant inspired tension. Rather, the trained clinician attempts to maintain anesthesia depth appropriate for surgical conditions by adjusting the vaporizer setting. This is done by observing the response of the patient's clinical signs, as well as by interpreting whatever quantitative measurements are available. Although blood pressure, EEG, and the like may be useful, there is at present no reliable quantified measure of anesthesia depth.

In an attempt to maintain constant anesthesia depth, constant anesthetic tension in the alveoli is a reasonable objective, and end-expired anesthetic tension or concentration is a good measure of alveolar tension.[11,21] The specific measurable objective in administering anesthesia with constant depth, then, is to maintain a constant end-expired anesthetic tension. This is now a quantifiable and achievable objective. It is accomplished by adjusting the vaporizer in whatever manner is required while observing the anesthetic agent monitor that displays inspired and end-expired anesthetic tensions.

The continuum from high-flow to low-flow anesthesia

The continuum from high-flow to low-flow anesthesia can also be well explained by the Gas Man model and simulation. Figure 30-5 shows the picture and graph repre-

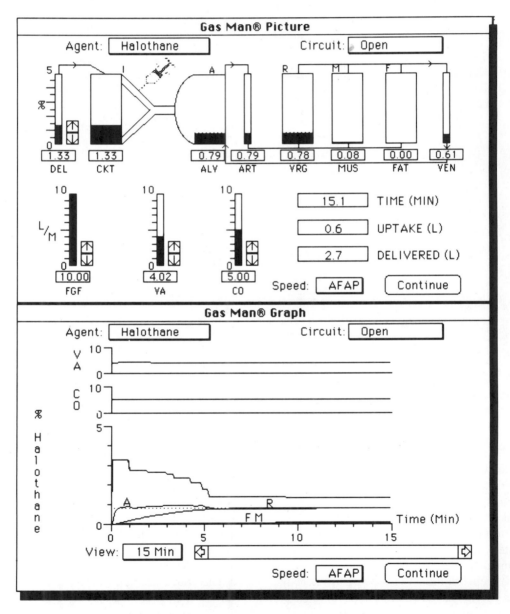

Fig. 30-5. Open circuit constant-alveolar halothane anesthetic. The Gas Man Picture and Graph show constant alveolar tension achieved and maintained with an open (nonrebreathing) circuit and careful adjustment of the vaporizer setting.

senting constant alveolar tension for halothane administered with an open (nonrebreathing) circuit for 15 minutes. The inspired (equal to delivered for the open circuit) halothane tension is initially adjusted to 3.3% and then gradually reduced to produce a flat alveolar tension curve. When this is done carefully, the time course of vaporizer setting and expired anesthetic tension or concentration is indistinguishable from that seen in Eger's example (Fig. 30-1).

Notice that, in the Gas Man Picture, after 15 minutes of anesthesia, the cumulative patient uptake of anesthetic is 0.6 L of halothane vapor. The volume of halothane delivered to the breathing circuit is 2.7 L, computed as if the fresh-gas flow were 10 L/min. Also, the upper half of the Gas Man Graph shows alveolar ventilation and cardiac output; delivered tension and fresh-gas flow are not relevant to an open circuit. Delivered tension and fresh-gas flow are displayed in this location when a semiclosed or closed system technique is simulated.

Figure 30-6 shows the Gas Man Picture and Gas Man Graph of isoflurane administered at constant alveolar isoflurane tension (1 MAC = 1.1%) achieved and maintained by appropriate vaporizer adjustment in a nonrebreathing (open) circuit. Initial inspired isoflurane tension is 2.9%, tapered to 1.5% after 15 minutes.[22]

It was noted earlier that alveolar overpressure (alveolar tension transiently above 1.0 MAC) is sometimes used to produce a more rapid increase in anesthetic tension in the target organ, the patient's brain. Only a brief period of

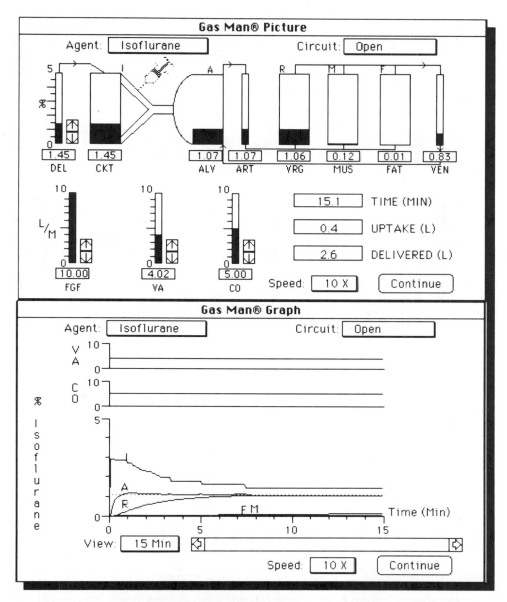

Fig. 30-6. Isoflurane: open circuit constant-alveolar anesthetic tension. The Gas Man Picture and Graph show constant alveolar isoflurane tension achieved and maintained with an open (nonrebreathing) circuit and careful vaporizer adjustment. Note the relative similarity to the halothane open circuit curve in Fig. 30-5.

overpressure is required because brain tension rapidly equalizes with arterial tension, which should by this time have fallen to the desired level. A common target for anesthesia is 1 MAC in the brain; another is 1.3 MAC.

Figure 30-7 shows the picture and graph of isoflurane administered at constant brain isoflurane tension (1 MAC = 1.1%) achieved and maintained by appropriate vaporizer adjustment in a nonrebreathing (open) circuit. Initial inspired isoflurane tension is 5.0%, tapered to 1.5% after 15 minutes. Alveolar tension rises to about 2 MAC for about 2 minutes.

Figure 30-8 shows the Gas Man Picture and Graph depicting constant brain isoflurane tension (1 MAC = 1.1%) achieved in a semiclosed circuit with a fresh gas flow

(FGF) of 10 L/min. The anesthetic tension delivered to the breathing circuit (DEL) begins at 5% isoflurane and is reduced to achieve and maintain a constant brain tension of 1.1%. Just as with the open circuit, it is observed that inspired tension (I) begins at 2.9% and is reduced to approximately 1.5% at the end of 15 minutes. Alveolar tension rises to about 1.6% for about 3 minutes. Constant brain tension is achieved with 3.3 L of vapor delivered to the breathing circuit; the patient's tissue uptake is 0.4 L of vapor. The efficiency is thus about 12% (efficiency = 0.4 L uptake/3.3 L delivered = 12.1%) Hence, in the common high-flow clinical situation, over 80% of the anesthetic agent delivered to the breathing circuit is wasted.

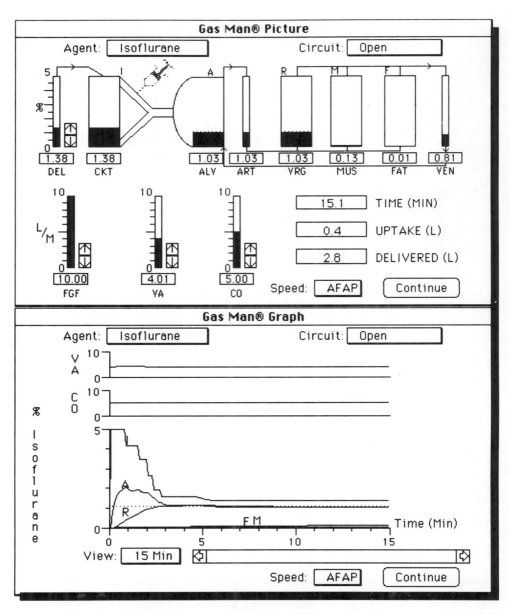

Fig. 30-7. Constant brain anesthetic tension achieved with an open circuit administering isoflurane. The Gas Man Picture and Graph show constant brain tension achieved and maintained with an open (nonrebreathing) circuit and careful vaporizer adjustment.

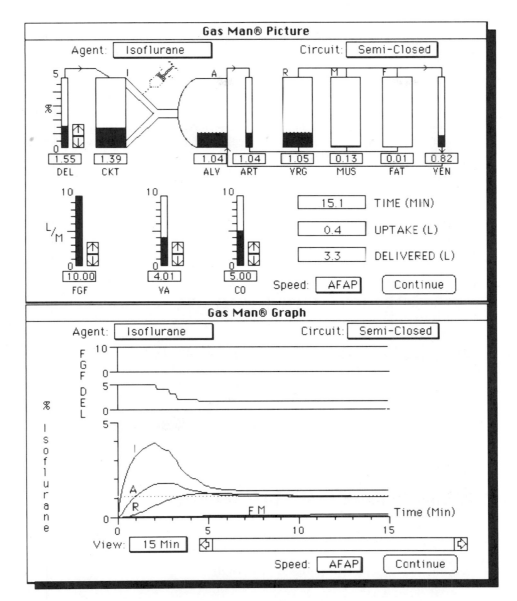

Fig. 30-8. High-flow semiclosed circuit. Gas Man Picture and Graph of constant alveolar isoflurane tension achieved and maintained with a high-flow semiclosed circuit with FGF = 8 L/min.

Figure 30-9 shows a trend of airway anesthetic tension obtained during a high-flow induction with isoflurane, measured with an infrared agent analyzer. Inspired and end-tidal isoflurane tensions are represented by the upper and lower edges of the trend. The isoflurane vaporizer is set to 3%, 2.5%, and 2.2% at 0 minutes, 1 minute and 2 minutes, respectively. Note that constant alveolar anesthetic tension is achieved and maintained after the 1-minute "wash-in" of the patient's lungs.

Use of the breathing circuit can be carried one step further. Instead of decreasing the vaporizer setting, FGF can be reduced to achieve the same decreasing inspired tension. Figure 30-10 shows this. FGF begins at 8 L/min while the vaporizer is set to 5% isoflurane (DEL). At the

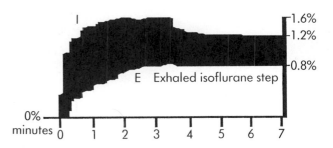

Fig. 30-9. Constant expired anesthetic tension shown on trend from multigas monitor. The graph shows the time course of airway anesthetic tension with the upper and lower edges representing inspired (*I*) and end-expired (*E*) isoflurane tensions, respectively.

end of 2 minutes, rather than decreasing the vaporizer setting, FGF is decreased to 2 L/min. Then, several minutes later, the vaporizer setting (DEL) is decreased as needed. All adjustments are made while the alveolar anesthetic tension (A) is observed and FGF or vaporizer setting is adjusted to achieve 1.1% (1 MAC) expired isoflurane. At the end of 15 minutes with this low-flow anesthetic technique, 1.2 L have been delivered to the breathing circuit, and uptake by the patient's tissues is 0.4 L. This anesthetic administration is then 33% efficient in terms of use of isoflurane vapor (i.e., 0.4/1.2 = 0.333). In other words, with the low-flow technique, the concentration inspired by the patient is identical to that inspired with the high-flow technique; patient response (end-expired anesthetic tension, al-

veolar tension, and anesthesia depth) are also unaffected. The only difference between the two techniques is the manner in which the appropriate gas mixture is created.

Finally, FGF can be reduced to its minimum, thus achieving a completely closed circuit. Figure 30-11 illustrates this in schematic form. In the closed circuit anesthesia technique, FGF is set equal to the patient's uptake of each and every gas employed, including oxygen. When this is achieved, total volume is constant and the concentration or tension of each substance is constant.

Oxygen uptake (usually referred to as oxygen consumption) is a particularly interesting result obtained using a closed circuit. The patient's oxygen consumption is equal to the flow of oxygen to the closed circuit.

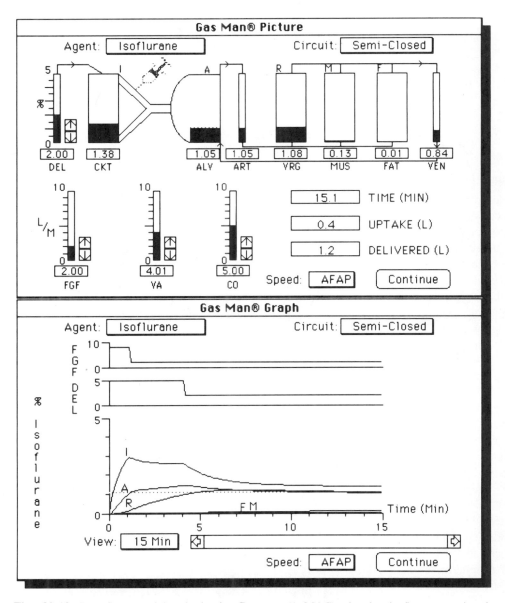

Fig. 30-10. Low-flow semiclosed circuit. Constant (1 MAC) alveolar isoflurane tension is achieved and maintained with a semiclosed circuit. First, high fresh gas flow (FGF = 8 L/min) is used for 2 minutes. FGF is then reduced to 2 L/min (moderately low flow) and the vaporizer setting is reduced as needed to maintain a constant end-expired tension.

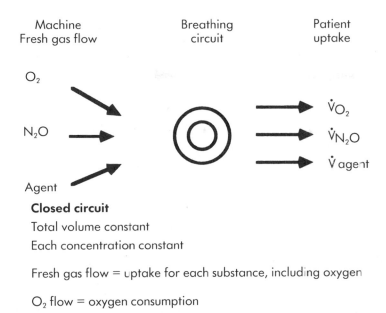

Fresh gas flow = uptake for each substance, including oxygen

O_2 flow = oxygen consumption

Fig. 30-11. The fundamental principle of closed circuit anesthesia is that FGF to the breathing circuit is equal to the patient's uptake for each and every gas and vapor. As a result, the total volume is constant and the concentration and tension (partial pressure) of each gas are constant. The patient's oxygen consumption can be estimated from the oxygen flow to the closed circuit.

Closed circuit anesthesia

To achieve closed circuit anesthesia beginning with induction or to accomplish rapid deepening during anesthesia, a modern concentration-calibrated vaporizer will not suffice. This is because its output at low FGF is insufficient to produce large or rapid changes in inspired tension. For this reason, *liquid* anesthetic agent is injected directly into the breathing circuit by many practitioners of the closed circuit technique. The Gas Man model allows liquid injection to be simulated while the student observes the resulting anesthetic tensions in the circuit and in the patient.

Figure 30-12 shows a Gas Man representation of closed circuit anesthesia administered with 0.5 ml liquid isoflurane injections timed to achieve and maintain 1.1% expired anesthetic partial pressure. Note that 0.5 ml of liquid isoflurane generates approximately 100 ml of vapor at room temperature (see Chapter 3). Liquid isoflurane is injected at empirical times with the objective of maintaining 1.1% alveolar partial pressure. Note that although inspired tension changes dramatically and expired tension varies somewhat, brain tension (VRG, R) is quite stable over time. Alveolar tension can be smoothed by decreasing the liquid bolus volume or, in practice, by converting to a continuous infusion into the circuit.

At the end of 15 minutes of empirical intermittent liquid injection, the Gas Man Graph in Fig. 30-12 shows that patient uptake is again 0.4 L of isoflurane vapor. To achieve this, 0.6 L of vapor were delivered to the breathing circuit as six individual 0.5-ml liquid injections. The discrepancy between the 0.6 L delivered and the 0.4 L uptake is anes-

thetic vapor that remains in the breathing circuit (CKT, 6 L) and the patient's lungs (ALV, 2 L). This same 0.2 L volume of anesthetic vapor was neglected in the previous descriptions for the sake of simplicity. Other than storage in the circuit and lung, the efficiency of agent use is 100% when a closed circuit technique is used as described.

Figure 30-13 shows a Gas Man representation of closed circuit anesthesia administered with injections of liquid isoflurane according to the relationship $t^{-1/2}$. Observe the 1.1% brain isoflurane tension that results. The first injection (0.5 ml) is made at time zero (first DEL spike). Subsequent (0.7 ml) injections are made at 1 minute, 4 minutes, and 9 minutes. Note that almost constant alveolar anesthetic tension (A) is achieved.

At the end of 15 minutes of empirical intermittent liquid injection, Fig. 30-13 shows that patient uptake is again 0.4 L of isoflurane vapor. To achieve this, 0.5 L of vapor were delivered to the breathing circuit as three individual 0.7 ml liquid injections following a loading dose of 0.5 ml. The discrepancy between the 0.5 L delivered and the 0.4 L uptake is anesthetic vapor that remains in the breathing circuit (CKT, 6 L) and the patient's lungs (ALV, 2 L). This same 0.1-L anesthetic volume was neglected in the previous descriptions for the sake of simplicity. Other than this, the efficiency of agent use is 100%.

The initial (average) inspired concentration necessary to achieve 1.1% alveolar tension was approximately 2.9%, as in the previous examples. Average inspired tension was allowed to fall to 1.5% at the end of 15 minutes, as before, this time by lengthening the time between liquid injec-

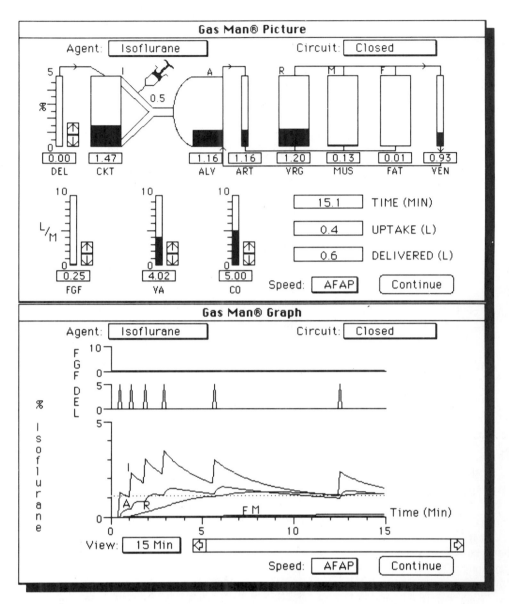

Fig. 30-12. Closed circuit with 0.5 ml injections of liquid isoflurane timed empirically from Gas Man–predicted alveolar tension. 0.5 ml injections are administered to produce and maintain 1.1% alveolar isoflurane on average.

tions. Inspired tension varied considerably between injections, but on the average inspired tension was similar to that for higher flow systems.

PRACTICAL ASPECTS OF CLOSED CIRCUIT ANESTHESIA

The practical aspects of administration of closed circuit anesthesia must be known and understood for this technique to be used effectively. Most contemporary anesthesia machines were not designed to facilitate closed circuit techniques and thus need modification before or during use. The anesthetic record, likewise, must be adapted for the closed circuit technique.

When low-flow or closed circuit anesthesia is administered, certain additional variables should be recorded on the anesthetic record. First, the flows of nitrous oxide and oxygen must, of course, be recorded. Expired tidal volume measured should be carefully observed and recorded because patient ventilation is dependent on both ventilator volume setting and concurrent FGF. Next, the vaporizer setting should be recorded in the conventional manner. Because inspired anesthetic tension is quite different from that delivered from the vaporizer, inspired tension should be measured and recorded to demonstrate that it was known and well controlled. Further, expired anesthetic tension should be recorded to assist in patient manage-

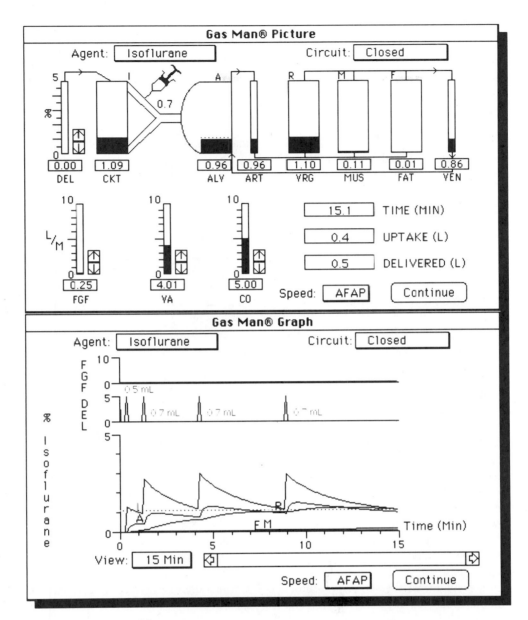

Fig. 30-13. Classic $t^{-1/2}$ closed circuit liquid injection technique. Liquid boluses of 0.5 ml loading dose and 0.7-ml maintenance dose are injected at 0, 1, 4, and 9 minutes. Note that the alveolar isoflurane tension remains near 1 MAC (1.1%) with injections made "by the clock."

ment. The need to monitor and record expired agent tension applies irrespective of FGF; it is equally applicable to high-flow techniques. When all three of these variables (vaporizer setting, inspired tension, and expired tension) are recorded, the anesthetic record documents the patient's receipt of a safe and effective anesthetic. All closed circuit concentrations and flows should be recorded without reservation. Closed circuit anesthesia has been shown to be as safe as a high-flow technique.[23]

Practical administration of closed circuit anesthesia follows the basic principle of the technique: deliver gases and vapors at a rate equal to tissue uptake while maintaining alveolar tension at the desired level. For most adult pa-

tients, the following regimen works as a first approximation. Changes are made to adapt delivery to each patient, as with any clinical technique.

Inhalation anesthesia with isoflurane is induced with high flows and maintained for approximately 20 minutes. During this time, alveolar anesthetic tension is established at the desired level. Mechanical ventilation is usually used. Before flows are reduced, exhaled tidal volume, inspired and expired agent tensions, and inspired oxygen concentration are carefully measured and recorded on the anesthetic record. Flows are then reduced as described below.

With somewhat greater difficulty, the closed circuit technique can be used from the outset, especially when nitrous oxide is omitted. This author prefers sequential 0.5 ml isoflurane injections into the breathing circuit while observing inspired and expired tension on a breath-by-breath basis. Liquid is injected whenever inspired or expired tension falls below that desired. The location of the liquid injection is described below.

When a high-flow technique is used first, FGF is reduced to provide a completely closed circuit. Oxygen flow is reduced to 200 ml/min and nitrous oxide to 100 ml/min. This approximates patient uptake for these gases. To provide the approximately 10 ml/min anesthetic vapor required, the vaporizer is set to 3%. The adjustable pressure limiting (APL, or pop-off) valve is closed to preclude gas from leaving the circuit if the reservoir bag should be used later. The tidal volume setting on the ventilator is increased to provide an undiminished exhaled tidal volume, which is monitored carefully.

The ventilator is then adjusted so that no gas leaves the breathing circuit at the end of exhalation; the exact technique, which depends on the ventilator used, is described below. Typically, the ascending (standing) bellows is adjusted to prevent it from rising to the mechanical stop, which initiates discharge of excess gas. A mark is placed on the bellows housing to signify the correct end-expired bellows position. Deviation of the bellows from this mark signifies inequality between total volume delivered to the circuit and that taken up by the patient and suggests that total FGF should be modified. A change in measured FiO_2 suggests that a change be made in the flow ratio of nitrous oxide to oxygen flow. A rise (or fall) in inspired agent tension requires delay (or repeat) of liquid injection or adjustment of the vaporizer dial setting.

The quantification of these adjustments is not immediately obvious. When the volume of the ventilator bellows changes, flows of nitrous oxide and oxygen are adjusted in proportion to their concentrations in the breathing circuit, *not* according to their proportion in fresh gas. For example, if the respiratory gas monitor indicates an inspired concentration of 66% nitrous oxide and 33% oxygen, then it is in this ratio that additional gas must be added. Therefore, the adjustments in oxygen flow are accompanied by adjustments in nitrous oxide that are twice as large. That is, when oxygen flow is increased by 100 ml/min, nitrous oxide flow is increased by 200 ml/min.

When a change in FiO_2 is noted in the absence of a change in circuit volume, oxygen flow is increased and nitrous oxide flow is decreased, this time by equal amounts. Simultaneous changes in FiO_2 and circuit volume require mixed compensation, which is a combination of the two techniques described.

Finally, when inspired or expired agent tension requires increase, the vaporizer setting is increased or additional liquid is injected into the breathing circuit. To lighten anesthesia, the vaporizer is turned off or a liquid-injection dose is withheld or delayed. An activated charcoal filter may be used to adsorb volatile agent.[24-27] Charcoal functions best when placed in the inspiratory limb of the circle.[28] Anesthesia may also be lightened by flushing the breathing circuit briefly with oxygen or a mixture of oxygen and nitrous oxide and observing the resulting change in inhaled tensions. Avoiding the use of nitrous oxide makes this far simpler then when nitrous oxide is used.

During the administration of any anesthetic, switching between mechanical and manual (controlled or spontaneous) ventilation is often desired. Closed circuit anesthesia offers an additional benefit. Changes in the location of the ventilator bellows can be corrected when alternating between bag and ventilator. To do this, the anesthesiologist maintains a partially filled reservoir bag throughout the case. Meanwhile, the patient is ventilated mechanically. Whenever it becomes necessary to compensate for accumulated circuit volume change, gas is transferred between bellows and bag. This is done by transferring gas via the patient's lungs during exhalation. Deft adjustment of the bag/bellows selector lever is required.

RESPIRATORY GAS SAMPLING

Respiratory gas sampling for analysis complicates low-flow and closed circuit administration unless the sampled gas is returned to the breathing circuit. Although a truly closed circuit cannot be achieved without gas return, circuit loss to sampling can be compensated by the addition of fresh gas to offset the loss. An excessive gas sampling rate can produce negative pressure in the breathing circuit and deplete the volume necessary for patient ventilation.[29,30] To do so, the anesthesiologist increases nitrous oxide, oxygen, and agent flows by an amount equal to the rate of removal by the sidestream, nonreturn gas system. Sample-gas composition equals circuit composition, which is a mixture of inspired and expired gas, weighted according to the inspiratory and expiratory times. Throughout most of the duration of the anesthesia, inspired and expired values do not differ by an amount that affects this minor correction. Because all of the exhaled gas is rebreathed (with carbon dioxide removed) circuit composition is dominated by exhaled gas, with slight alteration by fresh gas. Typical breathing circuit composition is 66% nitrous oxide, 33% oxygen, and 1% isoflurane. Gas sampled from the breathing circuit will approximate this composition. Thus if the sampling rate is 250 ml/min, an additional 165 ml/min (250 × 0.66) nitrous oxide, 82 ml/min oxygen, and 3 ml/min isoflurane must be added to compensate for loss of sampled gas (see Table 30-1). The total resulting flows and concentrations are 265 ml/min nitrous oxide, 282 ml/min oxygen, and 18 ml/min isoflurane or 3% of FGF. Rounding off for convenience, we find that with nonreturn airway gas sampling, FGF is adjusted to 300 ml/min oxygen, and 300 ml/min nitrous oxide, and that the vaporizer is set to 3% (halothane or isoflurane) as a reasonable starting point.

Table 30-1. Flows and concentrations for closed circuit anesthesia with nonreturn airway gas sampling

	N₂O	O₂	Isoflurane	Total
Circuit composition (%)	66	33	1	100
Patient uptake (ml/min)	100	200	15	315
Sample flow (ml/min)	+165	+ 82	+ 3	+250
Total flow required (ml/min)	265	282	18	565
FGF composition required (%)	49	48	3	100
Nominal settings (ml/min)	300	300	18	618
Vaporizer setting	—	—	3%	—

Whenever nitrous oxide is administered to a closed circuit, concentration or tension of oxygen in the breathing circuit must be monitored even more carefully than usual. This is because in a closed circuit, inspired oxygen concentration depends on both gas delivered from the anesthesia machine (FGF) and that exhaled by the patient. Inspired oxygen tension or concentration must be monitored to ensure the safety of gases delivered to the patient. When low flows are used, oxygen concentration alarms should be set tightly above and below the desired FiO₂. Expired as well as inspired tension monitoring is advisable when possible. Arterial oxygen saturation should always be monitored, as for any other anesthetic.

In contrast to high-flow systems, where FGF to the circuit replaces carbon dioxide laden exhaled gas, closed circuit anesthesia requires effective carbon dioxide absorption. Thus, carbon dioxide monitoring (capnography) is even more important with low flows than with high. A functioning carbon dioxide absorber must always be assured.

In a closed circuit system volatile anesthetic agent can be administered either with a concentration-calibrated vaporizer or by direct injection of liquid agent into the breathing circuit. With administration of liquid, most clinicians advocate injection into the expiratory limb of the circuit. Careful monitoring of airway anesthetic tension allows liquid-injection closed circuit anesthesia to be performed quite simply and safely. Figure 30-14 shows the time course of airway anesthetic tension in response to a 1.0 ml injection of liquid isoflurane into the expiratory limb of the breathing circuit connected to a 70-kg patient undergoing surgery. With this agent monitor, concentration is seen to rise with each inspiration and fall with each expiration. Thus the peaks and troughs represent inspired and alveolar anesthetic tensions, respectively. Separate curves connecting all the peaks and all the troughs would follow the I and A curves of the isoflurane analog of the Gas Man figures. Note that inspired tension does not rise for 1 minute. An additional 1½ min are required until peak inspired tension is achieved. At the peak, inspired tension rises by 1.5% to 2.0% from its baseline of 0.5%. Meanwhile, expired tension rises by 0.7% from 0.5% to 1.2%.

Injection of liquid agent into the inspiratory limb is also possible, but greater care is required. Figure 30-15 shows an example of a 1.0 ml liquid isoflurane injection into the inspiratory limb of the circuit. Inspired tension peaks 4%

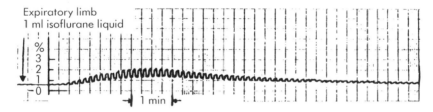

Fig. 30-14. Expiratory limb injection. Time course of airway anesthetic tension after injection of 1.0 ml liquid isoflurane into the expiratory limb of the breathing circuit. Inspired tension begins to rise 1 minute after injection. Inspired and expired tensions begin to rise 2½ minutes after injection.

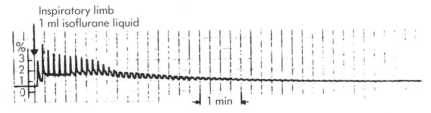

Fig. 30-15. Inspiratory limb injection. Time course of airway anesthetic tension after injection of 1.0 ml liquid isoflurane into the inspiratory limb of the breathing circuit. Inspired tension rises to 4.5% two breaths after injection. Expired tension peaks after two breaths at 1.7% (1.2% above its value two breaths earlier) and remains at this level for several minutes.

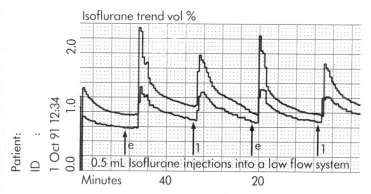

Fig. 30-16. Alternate injections into the inspiratory and expiratory circuit limbs. In each case, inspiratory limb injection *(i)* resulted in an inspired peak within two breaths, and expiratory limb injection *(e)* resulted in a peak approximately 90 seconds after injection. The upper tracing represents inspiratory isoflurane tension and the lower tracing represents expiratory isoflurane tension.

above baseline after two breaths (15 seconds). Expired tension rises by 1.2% within two breaths and remains constant for about 2 minutes. Three minutes after injection the two tracings depicting injection in the two circuit locations become quite similar. A note of caution is in order here. When injected into either the inspired or the expired limb, *liquid anesthetic must never be allowed to reach the patient.* Conventional breathing circuits with a dependent section between the carbon dioxide absorber and the patient easily achieve this. Continuous, breath-by-breath gas monitoring helps assure that inspired and expired tensions are as desired and expected. Figure 30-16 shows alternate injections of 0.5 ml of liquid isoflurane into the inspiratory and expiratory limbs of the circle. In each case, injection into the inspiratory limb resulted in an inspired peak within two breaths, while injection into the expiratory limb resulted in an inspired peak approximately 90 seconds after injection. Injection into the inspiratory limb appears to provide superior control of inspired and expired anesthetic tension.

Many anesthesiologists use a concentration-calibrated vaporizer for closed circuit anesthesia. Some adjust the vaporizer by intermittently selecting between full-on and full-off. With low flow through a concentration-calibrated vaporizer, the time constant, τ, for circuit tension change is long. This is because the circuit time constant is equal to circuit volume divided by circuit flow (τ = Volume/Flow). With a volume of 8 L and a flow of 0.25 to 0.5 L/min, τ is between 32 and 16 minutes. Because of this, even a drastic change in vaporizer setting and fresh gas composition produces a very slow change in the composition of inspired gas.

Closed circuit anesthesia can also be administered via Verni-Trol or Copper Kettle measured-flow vaporizers. However, because of the frequency and potential for error in the calculations required,[31] use of these vaporizing systems is discouraged by this author. (See also Chapter 3.)

BUILD-UP OF TOXIC SUBSTANCES

When high flows are used during anesthesia, gases in the breathing circuit are replaced frequently. Thus, when FGF is high, circuit and exhaled gases are exchanged frequently. Thus any gases that might accumulate in the breathing circuit are removed and replaced with fresh gas. In a closed circuit, all substances entering the breathing circuit remain there unless taken up by the patient, the carbon dioxide absorbent, or circuit materials.

Circuit contaminants can arise from several sources.[32] Anesthetics by themselves or in reaction with soda lime can produce unintended substances. Specifically, halothane produces two metabolites, 2-chloro-1,1,1-trifluoroethane (CF_3CH_2Cl) and 2-chloro-1,1-difluoroethylene (CF_2CHCl), and a metabolite decomposition product, 2-bromo-2-chloro-1,1-difluoroethylene (CF_2CBrCl).[33] Concentrations in a closed circuit are no higher than in a semiclosed circuit. The latter decomposition product is not present in an absorbent-free Bain circuit. These substances are not believed to be a hazard.[34] Enflurane,[35] isoflurane,[36] and desflurane[37] are stable enough to warrant no special concern during closed circuit anesthesia. Sevoflurane[38] has been shown to produce three breakdown products in soda lime. The first is fluoromethyl 2,2-difluoro-1-(trifluoromethyl)-vinyl ether, alternatively called 1,1,1,3,3-pentafluoroisopropenyl fluoromethyl ether (PIFE) [$F_2C=C(CF_3)OCH_2F$]. The second is fluoromethyl 2-methoxy-2,2 difluoro-1-(trifluoromethyl)-ethyl ether, alternatively called 1,1,1,3,3-pentafluoro-3-methoxy-isoproply fluoromethyl ether (PMFE) [$H_3COCF_2CH(CF_3)OCH_2F$]. The third is hexafluoroisopropanol (HFIP). In a closed circuit, PIFE and HFIP concentrations remain low. The safety of PMFE in a closed circuit system is still under investigation.

Patients can produce substances that are better removed from the breathing circuit than rebreathed. One such product is carbon monoxide.[39] In addition, tissue nitrogen continues to be released into the breathing circuit[40] at a rate of approximately 10 ml/min and accounts for a slow exponential rise in circuit nitrogen toward 10%[41] without exceeding this value.[42] Acetone, methane, and other inert gases also build up.[43] It is therefore suggested that the breathing circuit be flushed periodically with a high FGF.

Substances can enter the breathing circuit from other sources. Acrylic monomer is exhaled when joint prostheses are surgically cemented. During this period, the closed circuit should be vented to prevent rebreathing of this chemical.

Some gas monitors sample room air or calibration gases intermittently. The Ohmeda Rascal self-zeros with argon and room air periodically. Argon buildup is insignificant, as is nitrogen accumulation.[41,44] The electronic paramagnetic oxygen monitor used in some multigas monitors (e.g., Datex Capnomac Ultima, Brüel and Kjäer, and Hewlett-Packard Anesthesia Gas Monitors) entrains room air for continuous calibration. If the instrument combines sampled gas with calibration gas, gas returned from the instrument contains room air, and thus nitrogen accumulation in the closed circuit is noticeable and significant.

MACHINE REQUIREMENTS

For an anesthesia machine to facilitate administration of closed circuit anesthesia, several specifications must be met. They are listed in Box 30-1.

USING TODAY'S TECHNOLOGY
Practicalities

Contemporary anesthesia machines generally do not meet the required or desired specifications listed in Box 30-1. Specifically, absence of leaks in gas delivery system, breathing circuit, and ventilator is difficult to achieve. Meticulous maintenance is definitely required. Some machines have low flow capability, while others do not; precise flow control is not available. Some machines provide constant tidal volume independent of circuit volume; others do not.

Quantitative delivery of volatile agent is not offered in any North American machine. Tidal volume varies with FGF with all current anesthesia ventilators. Gas and vapor uptake can be computed only by titration and careful monitoring of concentrations and volumes by the experienced anesthesiologist. Inspired agent tension is dramatically affected by FGF.

To provide liquid injection, adapters are typically purchased specially or fabricated by the user. Many configurations are used.[45] A good example is a straight breathing circuit sampling adapter, 1 inch of disposable breathing circuit, a 15-mm/22-mm straight connector, a rubber-capped injection port, a 22-gauge spinal needle, and a 3-ml Becton-Dickinson syringe (Fig. 30-17). Components are selected to reduce the likelihood of unintentional injection or overdose. The plastic syringe provides the static friction that glass lacks; the 22-gauge spinal needle provides resistance to liquid flow; and the bends in the needle invert the syringe to offset the effect of gravity on the plunger. Some plastics (e.g., polycarbonate) are easily dis-

---

Box 30-1. Specifications for a closed circuit anesthesia delivery system

Required attributes	*Desired attributes*
Leak-free gas delivery system	Quantitative volatile agent delivery
Leak-free breathing circuit	Tidal volume independent of FGF
Nonleaking ventilator	Computation of gas and vapor uptake
Low gas flow capability	High flow and closed circuit
Precise gas flow control	Inspired agent tension independent of FGF
Accurate calibration at low flow	
Delivered tidal volume independent of circuit volume	

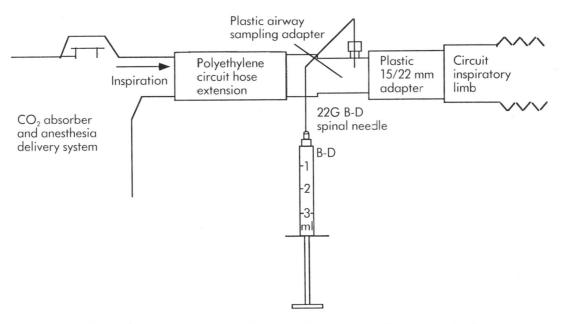

Fig. 30-17. Liquid anesthetic agent injection system that can be used in a closed circuit system.

solved by liquid anesthetics, and so caution is required in the selection of the injection components.

Idiosyncrasies of contemporary anesthesia machines

Some contemporary anesthesia machines make the administration of closed circuit anesthesia difficult. The North American Dräger Narkomed series presents several unique impediments. FGF below 300 ml/min is difficult to produce, and nitrous oxide cannot be administered without annunciation of an alarm when oxygen flow is below 1 L/min. There is also a vent hole in the bag/ventilator selector valve, which must be occluded to prevent loss of reservoir-bag gas to the room during mechanical ventilation. On this machine, end-expiratory bellows height determines delivered tidal volume. Specifically, inspiration is accomplished by bellows descent from its starting volume downward to zero volume. Thus, as circuit volume changes, end-expiratory bellows height changes and tidal volume changes follow.

The Ohmeda Modulus II machine facilitates closed circuit administration in several ways. An optional factory or field modification provides calibrated oxygen flow as low as 50 ml/min. Calibration resolution is no better than 50 ml/min, however. Up to 75% nitrous oxide can be delivered at any oxygen flow; concentrations above this are prevented by a chain linking the oxygen and nitrous oxide flow-control needle valves (see Chapter 2). The 75% limitation still precludes closed circuit nitrous oxide induction, which requires 2 L/min nitrous oxide for a brief period while oxygen consumption is only 250 ml/min. The Ohmeda system has no intentional circuit leaks, and incorrect bellows position (within limits) does not affect tidal volume during mechanical ventilation. This is accomplished by a fixed volume of driving gas compressing the bellows, which delivers the actual inspired tidal volume. Inspired tidal volume diminishes only if there is insufficient volume in the bellows.

THE FUTURE

The future of closed circuit anesthesia is uncertain. Although closed circuit anesthesia has been practiced and advocated for many years, it is currently used in few centers and by few individuals in the United States. Obstacles to its practice fall into two categories: technological and philosophical.

The technological encumbrances to closed circuit are described earlier in this chapter. They make closed circuit administration inconvenient. Philosophical encumbrances usually center on issues of safety. Even though this issue has been addressed amply,[23,46,47] lack of an obvious relationship between control settings and inspired gas is disconcerting to many practitioners. Monitoring of inspired and expired gas tensions and exhaled volume becomes more critical. Finally, a greater understanding of drug kinetics is required for a full understanding of the technique.

In Europe, closed circuit anesthesia has been readdressed in recent years.[48] The PhysioFlex[49,50] anesthesia machine seems to provide most of the needs of closed circuit anesthesia. Because it is not currently available in the United States, it is not described in this chapter. A brief description of this machine is to be found in Chapters 6 and 33. Researchers in Ulm, Germany, have found that isoflurane and enflurane can be safely removed from a charcoal adsorber by heating to 220°C.[51]

Closed circuit anesthesia is a technique that maintains a constant anesthetic state by adding gases and vapors to the breathing circuit at the same rate that the patient's body redistributes (stores) or eliminates them. Some practitioners use liquid anesthetic injection at prescribed time intervals using Lowe's empirical square-root-of-time model; others monitor and maintain inspired or expired anesthetic tensions using a gas monitor that returns analyzed gas to the breathing circuit. A commercial closed circuit anesthesia machine is available in Europe.

REFERENCES

1. Bengston JP, Bengston A, Stenqvist O: The circle system as a humidifier, *Br J Anaesth* 63:453-457, 1989.
2. Lowe HJ: *Dose regulated Penthrane (methoxyflurane) anesthesia,* Chicago, 1972, Abbott Laboratories.
3. Lowe HJ, Mackrell TN, Mostert JW, et al: Quantitative closed circuit anesthesia, *Anesthesiology Review* 12:16-19, 1974.
4. Aldrete JA, Lowe HJ, Virtue RW, editors: *Low flow and closed system anesthesia,* New York, 1979, Grune and Stratton.
5. Lowe HJ, Ernst EA: *The quantitative practice of anesthesia: use of closed circuit,* Baltimore, 1981, Williams & Wilkins.
6. Severinghaus JW: The rate of uptake of nitrous oxide in man. *J Clin Invest* 33:1183-1189, 1954.
7. Zuntz N: Zu pathogenese und therapie der durch rasche luft druck anderungen erzeliegten krankheiten, *Fortschr Med* 15:632, 1897.
8. Kleiber M: Body size and metabolism. *Hilgardia* 6:315-353, 1932.
9. Brody S: *Bioenergetics and growth,* New York, 1945, Reinhold.
10. Lowe HJ, Hagler K: Clinical and laboratory evaluation of an expired anesthetic gas monitor (Narko-test), *Anesthesiology* 34:378-382, 1971.
11. Eger EI II, Guadagni NP: Halothane uptake in man at constant alveolar concentration, *Anesthesiology* 24:299-304, 1963.
12. Kety SS: The physiological and physical factors governing the uptake of anesthetic gases by the body, *Anesthesiology* 11:517-526, 1950.
13. Kety SS: The theory and application of the exchange of inert gas at the lungs and tissues, *Pharmacol Rev* 3: 1-41, 1951.
14. Philip JH: GAS MAN: an example of goal oriented computer-assisted teaching which results in learning, *Int J Clin Mon* 3:165-173, 1986.
15. Garfield JM, Paskin S, Philip JH: An evaluation of the effectiveness of a computer simulation of anesthetic uptake and distribution as a teaching tool, *Med Educ* 23:457-462, 1989.
16. Philip JH, Lema MJ, Raemer DB, et al: Is computer simulation as effective as lecture for teaching residents anesthetic uptake and distribution? *Anesthesiology* 63:3A, A503, 1985 (abstract).
17. Eger EI II: *Anesthetic uptake and action,* Baltimore, 1974, Williams & Wilkins.
18. Mapleson WW: An electrical analogue for the uptake and exchange of inert gases and other agents, *J Appl Physiol* 18:197-204, 1963.
19. MacKrell TN: *An electrical teaching model.* In Papper EM, Kitz RJ, editors: *Uptake and distribution of anesthetic agents,* New York, 1963, McGraw-Hill, pp 215-223.

20. Gravenstein JS: Training devices and simulators, *Anesthesiology* 69:295-297, 1988.

21. Eger EI, Bahlman SH: Is the end-tidal anesthetic partial pressure an accurate measure of the arterial anesthetic partial pressure? *Anesthesiology* 35:301-303, 1971.

22. Philip JH: Gas Man simulation of overpressure is verified by correct alveolar plateaus, *Anesthesiology* 73:3A, A1025, 1990 (abstract).

23. Ernst EA, MacKrell TN, Pearson JD, et al: Patient safety: a comparison of open and closed anesthesia circuits, *Anesthesiology,* 67:3A, A474, 1987 (abstract).

24. Epstein HG: Removal of ether vapour during anaesthesia. *Lancet* 114-116, 1944.

25. Hawes DW, Ross JAS, White WC, et al: Servo-control of closed circuit anaesthesia, *Br J Anaesth* 54:229-230, 1982.

26. Ernst EA: Use of charcoal to rapidly decrease depth of anesthesia while maintaining a closed circuit, *Anesthesiology* 57:343, 1982.

27. Baumgarten RK: Simple charcoal filter for closed circuit anesthesia, *Anesthesiology* 63:125, 1985 (letter).

28. Jantzen JP: More on black and white granules in the closed circuit, *Anesthesiology* 69:437-438, 1988 (letter).

29. Huffman LM, Riddle RT: Mass spectrometer and/or capnograph use during low-flow, closed circuit anesthesia administration, *Anesthesiology* 66:439-440, 1987 (letter).

30. Mushlin PS, Mark JB, Elliott WR, et al: Inadvertent development of subatmospheric airway pressure during cardiopulmonary bypass, *Anesthesiology* 71:459-462, 1989.

31. Keenan RL, Boynan CP: Cardiac arrest due to anesthesia: a study of arrest incidents and causes, *JAMA* 253:2373, 1985.

32. Morita S: Inspired gas contamination by non-anesthetic gases during closed-circuit anesthesia, *The Circular* 2:24-25, 1985.

33. Sharp JH, Trudell JR, Cohen EN: Volatile metabolites and decomposition products in man, *Anesthesiology* 50:2, 1979.

34. Eger EI, II: Dragons and other scientific hazards, *Anesthesiology* 50:1, 1979 (editorial).

35. Eger EI II: *Enflurane: a compendium and reference,* ed 3, Madison, Wis, 1985, Anaquest.

36. Eger EI II: *Isoflurane: a compendium and reference,* ed 2, Madison, Wis, 1985, Anaquest.

37. Eger EI II: Stability of I-653 in soda lime, *Anesth Analg* 66:983-985, 1987.

38. Hanaki C, Fujii K, Morio M, et al: Decomposition of sevoflurane by soda lime, *Hiroshima J Med Sci* 36:61-67, 1987.

39. Speiss W: To what degree should we be concerned about carbon monoxide accumulation in closed circuit anesthesia? *The Circular* 1:8, 1984.

40. Barton FL, Nunn JF: Use of refractometry to determine nitrogen accumulation in closed circuits, *Br J Anaesth* 47:346-349, 1975.

41. Philip JH: Nitrogen buildup in a closed circuit, *Anesthesiology* 73:A465, 1990, (abstract).

42. Bengston JP, Sonander H, Stenqvist O: Denitrogenation and low flow anesthesia, *The Circular* 5:8-9, 1988.

43. Morita S, Latta W, Hambro K, et al: Accumulation of methane, acetone and nitrogen in the inspired gas during closed-circuit anesthesia, *Anesth Analg* 64:343-347, 1985.

44. Coleman, D: Personal communication,

45. Aldrete JA: Vaporizing-adaptors as injection ports for closed anesthesia system, *The Circular* 2:26-28, 1985.

46. Petrella WK: Enhanced discovery of anesthesia related events: an analysis of 400 consecutive low flow and closed circuit cases, *The Circular* 6:14-15, 1989.

47. Hylani MA: Closed circuit anesthesia, *Middle East J Anesthesiol* 8:505-510, 1986.

48. Droh R, Spintge R: *Closed-circuit system and other innovations in anaesthesia,* Berlin, 1986, Springer-Verlag.

49. Rolly G, Versichelen L, Verkaaik, et al: Mass spectrometry analysis of a new closed circuit anesthesia apparatus (Physioflex), *The Circular* 6:5-6, 1989.

50. Verkaail AP, Erdmann W: Respiratory diagnostic possibilities during closed circuit anaesthesia, *Acta Anaesthesiol Belg* 41:177-188, 1990.

51. Groß-Alltag F, Marx T, Friesdorf W: An experimental approach to recycling volatile anesthetics. Proceedings of the second annual meeting of the Society for Technology in Anesthesia, San Diego Calif, 1992.

Chapter 31

NONINVASIVE TEMPORARY PACEMAKERS AND DEFIBRILLATORS

Ross H. Zoll, Ph.D., M.D.

Noninvasive temporary pacemakers* (NTP) and defibrillators are useful devices for treating arrhythmias that may arise during surgery and anesthesia as well as in intensive care or resuscitation settings. Although these are not specifically anesthesia devices, it is important for the anesthesiologist to understand the principles of their function and use.

NONINVASIVE PACING

History

Clinical pacing, first introduced by Paul M. Zoll[2] in 1952, used a device very similar to modern noninvasive pacers. However, it was not well accepted because it was a radical innovation in therapy in that it anticipated subsequent developments in monitoring, medical electronics, and intensive care. Although safe and effective,[3] the technique had problems, such as interference with the electrocardiogram (ECG) signal, which made it difficult to determine effectiveness. In addition, the pacing stimulus produced severe pain. Although useful for resuscitation, noninvasive pacing was not satisfactory for long-term pacing therapy.

Implantable pacemakers followed the development of transistors and tissue-compatible stimulating electrodes.[4] Problems of wire breakage, battery life, and circuit reliability were resolved by about 1980. Following the introduction of transvenous pacing,[5] temporary transvenous pacing became popular for resuscitation, prophylaxis, and short-term pacing. However, in certain situations, the transvenous approach has serious disadvantages. Most important, it is not available rapidly enough for resuscitation of an unexpected cardiac arrest, and in such a situation it

---

*This chapter focuses primarily on the NTP and PD models of noninvasive temporary pacemakers from ZMI, Inc., of which the author was a principal developer. For the record, the author does retain some financial interest. Nevertheless, the author believes these are the only versions that may be satisfactorily used in conscious patients, and there exists objective evidence of their superior effectiveness.[1]

is cumbersome and highly unreliable. As an invasive technique, transvenous pacing carries such risks as hemorrhage, infection, tamponade, embolization, and arrhythmias. For prophylaxis, the need for pacing must be weighed against both the expense of the procedure and the risk of complications.

Electrophysiology

As with all excitable tissue, electrical stimulation of cardiac muscle requires forcing decreases in transmembrane potential to activate voltage-dependent ion channels. Subthreshold stimuli have only very transient and local effects. Suprathreshold stimuli result in action potentials that propagate throughout the cell membrane and, in the case of cardiac muscle, throughout the contiguous muscle mass. If atrioventricular (AV) conduction is intact, propagation is throughout the heart. Stimuli may be introduced either with transmembrane microelectrodes or by current fields from macroscopic electrodes, such as transvenous or epicardial pacing electrodes or external electrodes on the chest wall. Pacing electrodes that are in direct contact with tissue (with surface areas of a fraction of a square millimeter) require only 0.1 to 1.0 mA of current for effectiveness. With long-term electrodes, the development of a millimeter thickness or more of scar tissue increases their effective size and may require several milliamperes of current for stimulation. Electrodes on the chest wall are several centimeters distant from the myocardium and typically require a hundred times as much threshold current. With an external device, unlimited power is available to assure effectiveness. However, large currents passing through the skin, subcutaneous tissue, and muscle may cause considerable discomfort and even burns. The hemodynamic effects are similar to epicardial or endocardial ventricular pacing.[6,7]

Technology

Improvements in the comfort of noninvasive temporary pacing have contributed greatly to the renewed interest in this technique.[8] The original device of 1952 usually caused unacceptable pain in conscious patients, even following sedation and analgesia. Compared with a typical pacing threshold of 150 mA, a sharp stinging pain was produced at 17 mA. With this new device, the pacing threshold has been reduced relative to the threshold for discomfort by modifications to the electrodes and stimulus waveforms (Fig. 31-1). Pacing is usually well tolerated for at least a few minutes at currents of 80 mA or more, even without sedation or analgesia.[9] Pacing thresholds vary from 31 mA to more than 100 mA and average about 55 mA. Sedation or analgesia usually improves acceptance by the patient, especially when pacing is required for several minutes.

The new noninvasive temporary pacemaker (NTP) system consists of a pacemaker pulse generator incorporated into a portable ECG monitor (most models include a por-

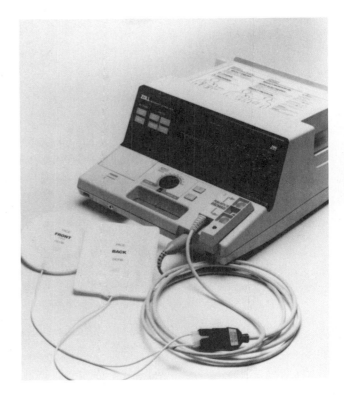

Fig. 31-1. The noninvasive pacemaker and defibrillator combined in a single instrument. (The model illustrated is the PD 1200 from ZMI, Inc., Woburn, Mass.)

table defibrillator as well) and disposable self-adherent electrodes for the anterior and posterior chest wall (Fig. 31-1). A three-lead ECG monitors effective ventricular capture and is required for the VVI (demand ventricular) pacing mode. The pacemaker has three main controls: the on/off switch, the rate selector, and the current amplitude selector. For operation, the electrodes are applied as in Fig. 31-2. A pacing rate (escape rate in VVI mode) is selected according to clinical criteria, and the pacing current's amplitude is gradually increased until ventricular capture occurs.

Theoretically, there should be an optimum size of electrode. At one extreme, the current field of a point source falls off as the inverse square of the distance from that point. Accordingly, a very small electrode on the chest wall would behave like a point source at a distance from the heart. At the other extreme, a very large electrode will have a uniform current field and will stimulate every muscle in the body, including the heart. A range of sizes and positions for electrodes was tested in a variety of patients in order to find the optimal size that would be accepted by most patients and for which precise placement was unnecessary (Fig. 31-2). For the anterior electrode, a diameter of 10 cm was found to be ideal. The posterior electrode is larger and serves as a return path for the current. The negative polarity of the stimulus is applied to the anterior electrode for the lowest threshold.

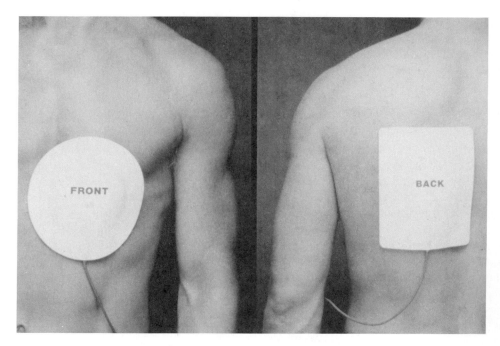

Fig. 31-2. Nominal positions of electrodes for noninvasive pacing.

An additional step was taken to explore the premise that most of the discomfort from noninvasive pacing was related to current density in the skin and subcutaneous tissues. This component of pain, felt subjectively as a sharp or stinging sensation, is different from pain associated with strong muscle contraction, which may also be uncomfortable. Figure 31-3 shows that the threshold current for skin pain (x's), expressed as current density at the skin, is independent of electrode area, except for the smallest electrode, where edge effects or coarseness of sensory organs are important. The cardiac stimulation threshold (circles) is shown for comparison.

To reduce pain, therefore, current density at the skin should be reduced. This can be accomplished by ensuring that the current distribution across the electrode is uniform. Electrodes of relatively high impedance that matches skin impedance help reduce edge effects and avoid hot spots if the skin itself is nonuniform.[10] If practical, perspiration or ECG paste should be cleaned from the skin to achieve the most comfortable stimulation. The skin should not be shaved before the electrodes are applied. Because of the high impedance, up to half the energy supplied by the NTP may be dissipated in the electrodes. The device is designed to supply selected current independent of impedance up to 2000 ohms. However, if the same electrode is to be used for monitoring or defibrillation, a low-impedance medium is necessary.

Electrodes are placed so as to avoid large muscles yet maintain proximity to the myocardium. The optimum location for the anterior electrode can vary considerably among individuals, and some experimentation may be necessary

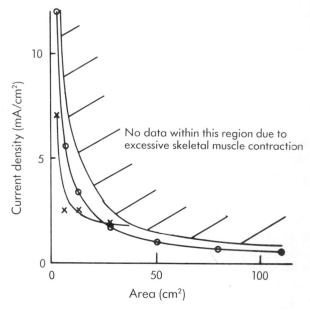

Fig. 31-3. Relationship of current density at threshold to electrode size for cardiac stimulation *(open circles)* and for pain *(x's)*.

to achieve greater comfort. Otherwise, the electrode should be placed just to the left of the sternum and mostly below the pectoral muscle. Stimulation directly over the sternum is usually uncomfortable. Precise positioning of the posterior electrode is not necessary.

The noninvasive pacemaker utilizes the fact that cardiac muscle responds to stimulation somewhat differently than either nerve or skeletal muscle. Nerves and skeletal muscles respond to stimuli of much shorter duration. Stimuli

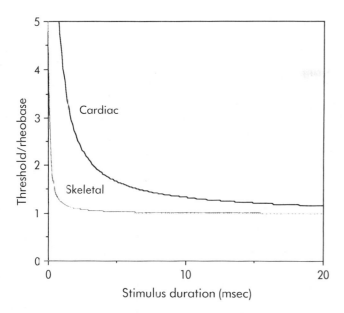

Fig. 31-4. Strength-duration curves for stimulation of skeletal and cardiac muscle.

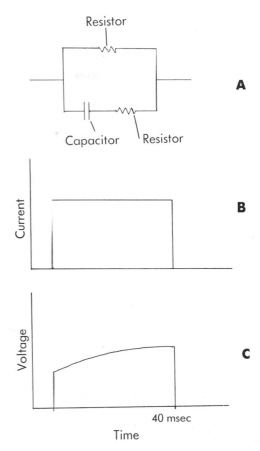

Fig. 31-5. A, Simplified equivalent circuit of tissue and interface. **B,** Controlled current source waveform and, **C,** resulting voltage waveform.

that are long and uniform in time can reliably pace with less discomfort. Figure 31-4 shows normalized threshold curves for muscle stimulation and for pacing as a function of stimulus duration. Increasing the stimulus duration from 0.5 or 2.0 ms to 40 ms greatly reduces the cardiac stimulation threshold. At 40 ms, threshold amplitude is 5% less than at 20 ms and discomfort is subjectively halved. Although the stimuli of long duration feel different, they are no more intense. Again, the controlled current source design of the stimulator produces a long, constant-amplitude current pulse in spite of the complex impedance of the tissue and electrodes (Fig. 31-5). The new stimulus does have the disadvantage of increased interference with ECG monitors, and questions of safety have been raised.

Safety

The most serious potential complication of pacing is that of precipitating arrhythmias. Early electrophysiologic studies implicated stimuli of long duration in the production of arrhythmias.[11] However, the original noninvasive pacer used a waveform of 2 to 3 ms and probably never precipitated arrhythmias. By comparison, various permanent and temporary pacers have produced constant voltage or constant current waveforms from 0.2 to 4.5 ms in duration. Demand modes are often used in pacemakers in part for their hemodynamic benefits but also because of concern about stimulating during the relative refractory, or "vulnerable," period, when the myocardium is partially repolarized and a large, suprathreshold stimulus might precipitate ventricular tachycardia or fibrillation. Indeed, when permanent pacing electrodes with small surface areas were introduced to reduce threshold and extend battery

life, sudden death occasionally resulted when they were used with older pulse generators that produced higher outputs. Especially when there is ischemia or myocardial damage from a recently placed electrode and consequent electrophysiologic inhomogeneity, very large stimuli during the relative refractory period should be avoided. On the other hand, operation of the noninvasive temporary pacer near threshold in the relative refractory period does not produce arrhythmias and is simply ineffective. The maximum output, only four times threshold in the most sensitive patients, is not likely to cause arrhythmias unless the patient's myocardium is so unstable that any extrasystole could degenerate to arrhythmia. Because the purpose of the device is to produce extrasystole, this risk is unavoidable. Mechanical stimulation from temporary pacing wires occasionally triggers arrhythmias, and this cause is avoided as well. Certain patients, who have fibrillated when a temporary wire was passed in the setting of acute myocardial infarction, have done well with noninvasive temporary pacing.

The effect of the long stimulus on safety has been studied in dogs.[12,13] A safety factor (i.e., a therapeutic ratio) was defined as the fibrillation threshold divided by the pacing threshold and measured at various stimulus durations.

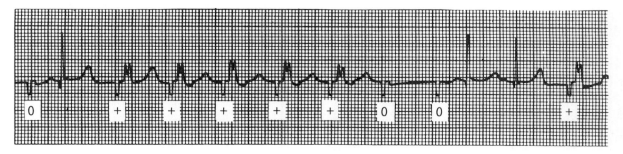

Fig. 31-6. Example of ECG tracing showing effective (+) and ineffective (o, subthreshold) stimulation.

In order to obtain the worst-case result, the stimulus was intentionally applied during the relative refractory period for fibrillation measurements. Episodes of fibrillation occurred at 5 to 10 times the pacing threshold or higher. There appeared to be no change in the safety factor at 40 ms compared with 2 ms.

One significant disadvantage of the long stimulus duration is its interference with ECG monitors. The stimulus artifact is much larger than ECG voltages (1000 times or more) and is within the normal ECG bandwidth. This artifact overloads most monitors, obscuring any real signal. Some monitors include overload recovery circuits and will function normally in this situation. However, the noninvasive temporary pacer is supplied with a rhythm monitor that has preamplifier circuits designed to accommodate the pacing stimulus. The pacemaker circuit inserts a marker on the ECG display to indicate at which point in the cardiac cycle the stimulus occurs. This marker consists of a 40-ms square wave followed by a 40-ms isoelectric period. Following these, the real ECG signal resumes. Usually, part of the QRS response is visible as well as the T wave (Fig. 31-6). Occasionally, it is necessary to switch leads to obtain a clear tracing. The ECG monitor and pacing output are electrically isolated in accordance with Association for the Advancement of Medical Instrumentation (AAMI) standards.

Recent experience

The role of noninvasive external pacing in cardiac arrest situations is currently under investigation. Fibrillation as a mechanism of arrest is probably more common than asystole, although asystole may follow successful defibrillation. Asystole carries a worse prognosis, in part because it often occurs at a late stage in prolonged arrest. Certainly, however, some patients are still viable and can be saved with pacing. Some early studies examining the effectiveness of pacing in arrest situations found that pacing held no advantage except in bradycardia. These studies were probably not sufficiently sensitive to discriminate between the situations in which pacing could be effective and those in which the patient was beyond salvage. More recent studies have found pacing to be of benefit in prehospital arrest situations.[14]

Similar to transvenous pacing, the NTP can be used to interrupt and terminate most supraventricular and ventricular tachycardias using single stimuli, bursts, or overdrive pacing.[15] For tachycardias over 180 per minute, a special rate generator is needed and is easily added. Often all that is required to interrupt the circus movement in a segment of its AV junctional or ventricular path is a single ectopic ventricular beat.

Another potential application of the NTP is stress testing. As with transvenous pacing, noninvasive temporary pacing at rapid rates simulates exercise stress. This technique does not involve the risks accompanying the insertion of a temporary wire. Stress is alleviated immediately upon cessation of pacing, enhancing the safety of the procedure. The pacing is interrupted briefly to look for ischemic changes on the ECG. Although rapid noninvasive pacing may be less comfortable than pacing at normal rates, it usually can be performed with analgesia. The effectiveness of the NTP for stress testing has been confirmed,[16] but extensive experience, and especially correlation to standard protocols, is lacking.

For pediatric use, small electrodes are used for infants and children under 15 kg. Although pacing thresholds are the same for both children and adults,[17] pediatric pacing rates are likely to be two to three times higher than those for adults. For sick or premature neonates, prolonged use may cause burns if the skin is immature and poorly perfused. However, brief use while securing other means of pacing is safe.

In the operating room

Currently, most patients who have significant conduction or sinus node dysfunction have permanent pacers. Although bradycardia or asystole unresponsive to atropine or other chronotropic agents is unusual, it has been reported.[18] Temporary pacing is frequently used during the placement of a pulmonary arterial catheter when the patient has preexisting left bundle branch block. Although complete heart block during catheter placement probably occurs in fewer than 1% of cases, it can be disastrous.[19] The NTP is ideal for this situation.[20] A temporary transvenous pacemaker requires another site of central access and is not without risk.

The NTP is useful for any procedure involving permanent pacer systems. It can assure uninterrupted rhythm during initial implantation of a pacemaker or during revisions or changes of a pulse generator, when mechanical problems occasionally lead to interruption of pacing. The electrodes for the NTP are nearly transparent to x-rays and do not interfere with fluoroscopy.

For patients with permanent pacers, the NTP guarantees pacing capability during surgery should the system be damaged or reprogrammed by electrocautery. Although uncommon, intraoperative failure of a pacing system is occasionally reported. During surgery, electrocautery usually interferes with the sensing function of the NTP, just as it does with permanent pacing systems.

In the event of unexpected arrest, the NTP can be applied within seconds. When applied promptly, it is usually effective in producing an electrophysiologic response even if contractility is inadequate. The presence of an electrophysiologic response to pacing stimuli is the appropriate measure of effectiveness, and other pacing modalities produce no additional hemodynamic benefit.

DEFIBRILLATION
History

Defibrillation, introduced into clinical practice by Beck, et al.[21] in 1947, used electrodes applied directly to the heart. Thoracotomy was advocated as the standard protocol for cardiac arrest. In 1956, Zoll, et al.[22] introduced closed-chest defibrillation with an alternating current (AC) waveform. Lown[23] and Edmark[24] introduced the modern direct current (DC) defibrillator in the early 1960s.

Technology

The basic principle of defibrillation is to interrupt random and chaotic electrical activity in the heart using a large stimulus that excites a large and sufficient fraction of the muscle mass at once.[25] However, the detailed mechanism remains extremely controversial. A number of theories and observations have been proposed. One elegant study in dogs[26] found that one small area of fibrillating tissue (approximately 25%) may remain without the fibrilla-

tion becoming generalized again; however, two such areas usually lead to clinical failure to defibrillate. It has been observed[27] that the defibrillation threshold may be related to the upper limit of vulnerability for producing fibrillation, although the significance of this is unclear. Much of the myocardium is in the refractory state during fibrillation. Therefore, a prolongation of recovery may be involved in the defibrillation mechanism.[28] Unlike pacing, which requires excitement of only a single cell, a defibrillation shock must excite a considerable portion of the myocardium even though part of it may be in a relative refractory state, and 1000 times as much current may be required. Cardioversion of atrial or ventricular tachycardia may require much less current, and a pacing stimulus that produces a single extrasystole will occasionally suffice.

On the other hand, too much current can produce damage to the myocardium that may not be thermal in nature. Damage to the cell membrane and contractile structure may lead to depressed function, necrosis, persistent arrest, or single-cell fibrillation.[29] Therefore, overdose of current may result in failure to defibrillate; but clearly, there exists a therapeutic window for effective defibrillation. A uniform distribution of current throughout the heart assures that no part of the heart is overdosed or underdosed, and this contributes to the success of defibrillation.

Another factor contributing to success is the defibrillator waveform. The capacitor discharge waveform, and to a lesser extent the AC waveform, are less effective than the truncated exponential (trapezoid) or the underdamped harmonic oscillator. Research related to implanted defibrillators has demonstrated new waveforms capable of greater effectiveness with less energy, but these are probably neither practical nor useful for external defibrillation. The large voltages and currents necessary for external defibrillation make engineering considerations of equipment size, weight, and cost significant for complicated waveforms.

The modern defibrillator works by temporarily storing defibrillation energy in a capacitor. A typical circuit for the underdamped harmonic oscillator waveform is shown in Fig. 31-7. The large capacitor is charged to the energy selected by the clinician and then discharged through the

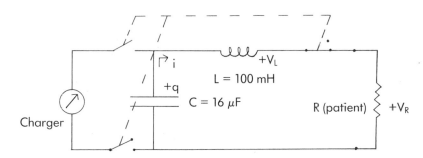

Fig. 31-7. Typical defibrillator circuit (simplified). *C,* Capacitor with a charge of *q,* where capacitance is expressed in microfarads (μF); *L,* inductor with inductance expressed in millihenrys (mH); *R,* patient resistance (impedance); *i* , current in circuit.

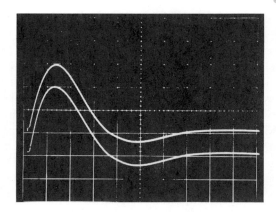

Fig. 31-8. Actual defibrillator waveform at a setting of 400 joules into a 50 ohm impedance. *Upper,* Voltage at 1 kV/division; *lower,* current at 20 amperes/division. The zero current axis is displaced one division lower to separate the traces. Horizontal scale is 1 ms/division.

paddles. The standard formula for the energy (*E*) stored by a capacitor (*C*) at a voltage (*V*) is as follows:

$$E = \tfrac{1}{2}CV^2$$

Most of the energy is delivered to the patient, but some is dissipated by parasitic resistance in the inductor. Therefore, by convention, the defibrillator is calibrated in terms of energy delivered into 50 ohms, roughly the average patient's impedance.

The typical underdamped waveform produced is shown in Fig. 31-8. For example, a typical defibrillator (Electrodyne DS95-M) at a setting of 400 joules has a capacitor voltage of 7.6 kV corresponding to 450 joules stored. At that setting, delivered current into 50 ohms is 66 amperes and delivered peak voltage is 3.3 kV. Depending on patient impedance, however, the underdamped negative component may be absent. Some evidence suggests that a small negative component reduces defibrillation threshold and increases the therapeutic ratio, perhaps by helping to repolarize damaged membranes. The mathematical solution for the output of the circuit shown is demonstrated briefly in the appendix to this chapter.

Factors affecting success

The primary determinants of success for defibrillation are duration of ventricular fibrillation, hypoxemia, and acidosis. These factors are related to the patient's condition, not to the equipment, and they will not be discussed further except to the extent that they influence defibrillation studies. Because metabolic state can vary so widely in ventricular fibrillation, the effects on success rates of changes in technique cannot be discerned. Factors such as weight or paddle location do not seem to affect success rate for ventricular defibrillation in humans. However, these are significant in animal studies of defibrillation and in cardioversion of atrial fibrillation in humans, where metabolic factors are more consistent.

Fibrillation is a random and chaotic, re-entrant arrhythmia. A defibrillation shock at a particular moment finds the myocardium in a unique, unreproducible electrophysiological state, which is part activated, part refractory, part relative refractory, and perhaps part resting. It is not surprising that the threshold for defibrillation fluctuates with each attempt even in the same individual. A sigmoid relationship between dose and response exists in the therapeutic range, as shown in Fig. 31-9. Thresholds vary among individuals for a number of reasons, such as differences in electrophysiologic conditions, geometry, and varying electrical conductivity of the heart and surrounding tissues.

In addition, a number of controllable factors influence the defibrillation threshold, mainly by affecting impedance. Patient impedance can vary widely irrespective of any error in technique. Success in defibrillation correlates better with delivered current than with stored or delivered energy. As with pacemakers, it is the current flow in the myocardium that produces the transmembrane potentials that cause depolarization. Impedance of tissue surrounding the heart and of the electrode interface can vary widely and may absorb a substantial fraction of the delivered energy. Current flow in the myocardium depends almost entirely on delivered current and geometric factors. Peak current can be used as an index of shock strength. Unfortunately, this is practical only for purposes of discussion or research because most defibrillators do not indicate the delivered dose of current. There is some variation in shock duration with impedance, but it is not significant for the underdamped oscillator waveform.

For the defibrillator circuit shown in Fig. 31-7, most of the stored energy is delivered to the patient irrespective of the patient impedance. However, delivered energy is the product of current and voltage, summed over time. Variations in patient impedance cause the delivered dose of current to vary widely. For example, at 100 joules of stored energy, Fig. 31-10 shows the peak current as a function of impedance. Current dose varies by at least a factor of 2 over the domain of common patient impedances. This result is predicted from circuit analysis in the appendix to this chapter.

It has been shown for a wide range of body weights that dose varies with weight (Fig. 31-11).[30] Nonetheless, there has been some controversy about the dose required for defibrillation of very large, obese humans. No dependence of defibrillation threshold on weight has been demonstrated for adults found in ventricular fibrillation.[31] This lack of correlation probably reflects the preponderance of other factors and the relatively narrow range of weights studied.

Shock strength is affected by patient impedance, which in turn is influenced by numerous factors. Even within the same individual, variations in impedance affect clinical outcome and complicate studies of defibrillation threshold. In general, the body presents a complex (i.e., frequency-

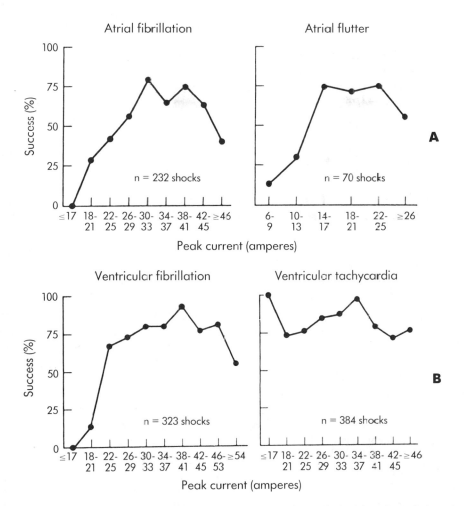

Fig. 31-9. Dose versus response curves for fibrillation and tachycardia in a large population. **A,** Atrial fibrillation and flutter. **B,** Ventricular fibrillation and tachycardia. (From Kerber RE, Martins JB, Kienzle MG, et al: *Circulation* 77:1038, 1988, by permission of the American Heart Association, Inc.)

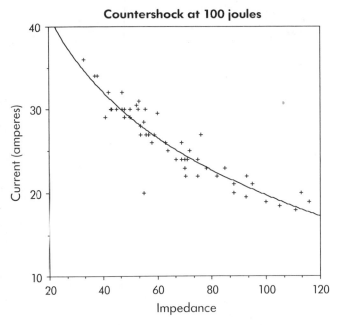

Fig. 31-10. Range of patient impedance at 100 joules and the resulting variation in peak dose of current.

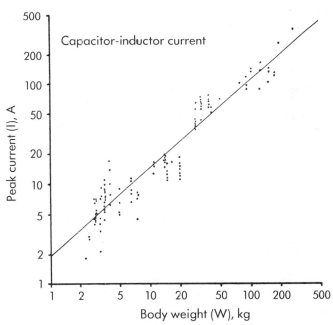

Fig. 31-11. Threshold for defibrillation as a function of weight. (From Geddes LA, Tacker WA, Rosborough JP, et al: Electrical dose for ventricular defibrillation of large and small animals using precordial electrodes, *J Clin Invest* 53:310, 1974, by permission of the American Society of Clinical Investigation.)

dependent) and nonlinear impedance. However, for the large currents involved in defibrillation, the frequency dependence is negligible. The nonlinearity is manifest as a much lower resistance at defibrillation currents than at pacing currents and as a continued decrease as shock strength increases. Resistance probably drops 20% to 30% between 50 and 400 joules. In addition, a history of previous shocks reduces impedance, perhaps through injury or reflex circulatory changes in the skin and other tissues. Burns are unusual, but erythema under the electrodes is normal and usually fades in a few minutes.

Other factors are important in impedance. The interface material usually contributes insignificantly; however, some gels can add up to 10.5 ohms to the circuit. Paddle pressure typically reduces impedance to 5% to 10% when compared to self-adherent patches without pressure. Geometric changes are probably responsible for this change in impedance. Similarly, there is clearly a small respiratory variation in impedance.

The distribution of current within the body and the heart is affected by size and location of electrodes. The goal is to achieve the most uniform distribution of current possible within the heart. This assures effective stimulation of all excitable tissue without causing damage by overdosing a portion of the heart. Outcome studies[32] of ventricular fibrillation in humans have shown no difference between anterior and anterior-posterior paddle placement. However, in atrial fibrillation, anterior-posterior placement is more effective.[33] The use of larger electrodes predictably lowers resistance somewhat but also increases current threshold. Any difference in therapeutic ratio would be too subtle to measure in humans.

These concepts of current and impedance are important. Even though the therapeutic ratio is large, the delivered current dose is usually unknown, making overdose easy. The deleterious effects of overdose are evident in animal studies[34] and studies of single-cell preparations.[29]

Programmed defibrillators

Automatic pacer-defibrillators[35] have existed since the early 1980s but have not been widely used. These instruments were designed to recognize asystole or ventricular arrhythmias requiring defibrillation and to provide the appropriate therapy without the intervention of a physician. Recognition of arrhythmias under adverse conditions of field resuscitation was difficult, and the protocols used for pacing or defibrillation were not the most successful. More recently, new devices that recognize ventricular arrhythmias and recommend defibrillation have been approved for use by paramedics, who are not otherwise permitted by local regulation to defibrillate in the field.

New waveforms

In the early 1970s, Mirowski, et al.[36] introduced automatic implantable cardioverter-defibrillators (AICDs) for the treatment of patients with otherwise intractable ventricular arrhythmias. Since that time, there has been renewed interest in other waveforms that might reduce the energy required for defibrillation. The lower thresholds obtained with myocardial patches or endocardial electrodes make more complicated electronic circuits practical in order to extend battery life. Knowledge gained from the development of AICDs suggests that the underdamped oscillator waveform may be nearly ideal by virtue of its small reverse polarity component. It should be noted that the presence of myocardial patch electrodes interferes significantly with external defibrillation.[37] In this case, defibrillation thresholds are approximately doubled.

New electrodes

Traditionally, anterior paddles used for adults are 8 cm in diameter, and a larger 10 to 12 cm paddle is used for posterior placement. One advantage of paddles is that they are applied with force, which reduces impedance. If repeated defibrillation is necessary or if surgical drapes might prevent ready access to the chest, preapplied adhesive electrodes, such as R2 electrodes,* are very convenient. The small increase in impedance is acceptable because more rapid defibrillation can be accomplished.[38] Newly developed adhesive pad electrodes† allow monitoring, pacing, or defibrillation through the same electrodes. The one disadvantage is that they may be less comfortable during external pacing. Gelled pads for use with regular paddles offer some convenience compared with paste or gel and avoid arching or short circuiting across the chest by leakage of conductive material between the paddles.

Appendix: Underdamped harmonic oscillator waveform

For readers who are interested this appendix presents the derivation of the equation for the defibrillator circuit. From Fig. 31-7, the sum of voltages around a closed circuit is zero:

$$V_C + V_L + VR = 0 \qquad (1)$$

Current is rate of change of charge on the capacitor:

$$i = -\frac{dq}{dt}$$

The equations for circuit components in terms of charge are as follows:

$$V_C = \frac{q}{C}$$

$$V_R = -iR = R\frac{dq}{dt}$$

$$V_L = -L\frac{di}{dt} = L\frac{d^2q}{dt^2}$$

---

* Zenex, Inc., Chicago, Ill.
† Such as those from ZMI, Inc., Woburn, Mass.

Substituting into equation 1 gives

$$\frac{d^2q}{dt^2} + \frac{R}{L}\frac{dq}{dt} + \frac{q}{LC} = 0 \tag{2}$$

This equation is identical to the archetypical equation of motion known in physics as the damped harmonic oscillator, applies at least to a first approximation to many systems, including the arterial pressure waveform as seen on a monitor. More detailed derivations are available in physics and mathematics texts.

It is usual practice to define the damping factor as $\beta = R/2L$ and the characteristic angular frequency as $\omega_o = (1/LC)^{1/2}$. The solution has the form $\sim e^{rt}$, where substitution into equation 2 gives

$$r^2 + 2\beta r + \omega_o^2 = 0$$

This is a quadratic equation with roots $r = -\beta \pm (\beta^2 - \omega_o^2)^{1/2}$. If the two roots are unequal, the general solution to equation 2 is

$$q = c_1 e^{r_1 t} + c_2 e^{r_2 t}, \quad r_1 \neq r_2$$

The constants c_1 and c_2 are determined from initial conditions. If $\beta^2 - \omega_o^2 = 0$, then $r_1 = r_2 = r$ and the system is critically damped. Then an additional term must be included to obtain two linearly independent solutions:

$$q = (c_1 + c_2 t)e^{rt} = (c_1 + c_2 t)e^{-\beta t}$$

The critically damped case produces the most rapid decay to rest at equilibrium.

For the underdamped situation where $\omega_1^2 = \omega_o^2 - \beta^2 > 0$, the solution can be rewritten:

$$q = Ae^{-\beta t}\cos(\omega_1 t - \delta)$$

where A and δ are constants. This equation represents oscillation within an exponentially decaying envelope.

For the overdamped situation, $\omega_2^2 = \beta^2 - \omega_o^2 > 0$, and

$$q = e^{-\beta t}(c_1 e^{\omega_2 t} + c_2 e^{-\omega_2 t})$$

The decay is longer than with the critically damped case.

With the component values shown in Fig. 31-7, critical damping occurs at 160 ohms patient impedance. At 50 ohms patient impedance, the solution is underdamped and the frequency of oscillation $\omega_1 = 750$ radians/sec or 8.3 ms/cycle. This compares with the actual result in Fig. 31-8.

Energy delivered to the patient is the sum over time of power. Power = VI and with voltage and current related as:

$$V = IR$$

then the energy, E, is:

$$E = \int I^2 R \, dt.$$

At constant energy and approximately constant shock duration, delivered current varies as $1/\sqrt{R}$. Compare this result with Fig. 31-10.

REFERENCES

1. Heller MB, Kaplan RM, Peterson J, et al: Comparison of performance of five transcutaneous pacing devices, *Ann Emerg Med* 16:166/493, 1987 (abstract).
2. Zoll PM: Resuscitation of the heart in ventricular standstill by external electric stimulation, *N Engl J Med* 247:768-771, 1952.
3. Abelman WH: Paul Zoll and electrical stimulation of the heart, *Clin Cardiol* 9:131-135, 1986.
4. Zoll PM, Frank HA, Zarsky LN, et al: Long term electric stimulation of the heart for Stokes-Adams disease, *Anesth Analg* 41:367-376, 1962.
5. Furman S, Robinson G: Use of an intracardiac pacemaker in the correction of total heart block, *Surg Forum* 9:245-248, 1958.
6. Feldman MD, McKay RS, Gervino EV, et al: Noninvasive transthoracic pacing tachycardia stress test: hemodynamic responses, *Circulation* 72(suppl) III-20, 1985 (abstract).
7. Feldman MD, Zoll PM, Aroesty JM, et al: Hemodynamic responses to noninvasive external cardiac pacing, *Am J Med* 84:395-400, 1988.
8. Belgard AH, Zoll PM, Zoll RZ: External noninvasive cardiac stimulation. United States Patent 4,349,030, 1982.
9. Falk RH, Zoll PM, Zoll RH: Safety and efficacy of noninvasive cardiac pacing, *N Eng J Med* 309:1166-1168, 1983.
10. Williams CR, Geddes LA, Bourland JD, et al: Analysis of the current-density distribution from a tapered, gelled-pad external cardiac pacing electrode, *Med Instrum* 21:329-334, 1987.
11. Wiggers CJ, Wégria R: Ventricular fibrillation due to single, localized induction and condenser shocks applied during the vulnerable phase of ventricular systole, *Am J Physiol* 128:500, 1940.
12. Zoll RH, Zoll PM, Belgard AH: *Noninvasive cardiac stimulation.* In Feruglio GA, editor: *Cardiac pacing: electrophysiology and pacemaker technology.* Padua, 1983, Piccin Medical Books, pp 593-595.
13. Voorhees WD 3d, Foster KS, Geddes LA, et al: Safety factor for precordial pacing: minimum current thresholds for pacing and for ventricular fibrillation by vulnerable-period stimulation, *PACE* 7:356-360, 1984.
14. Clinton JE, Zoll PM, Zoll R et al: Emergency noninvasive external cardiac pacing. *J Emerg Med* 2:155-162, 1985.
15. Estes NA 3d, Deering TF, Manolis AS, et al: External cardiac programmed stimulation for noninvasive termination of sustained supraventricular and ventricular tachycardia, *Am J Cardiol* 63:177-183, 1989.
16. Feldman MD, Warren SE, Gervino EV, et al: Noninvasive external cardiac pacing for thallium-201 scintigraphy, *Am J Physiol Imaging* 3:172-177, 1988.
17. Béland MJ, Hesslein PS, Finlay CD, et al: Noninvasive transcutaneous cardiac pacing in children, poster presentation, Dallas AHA, 1986.
18. Kirschenbaum LP, Eisenkraft JB, Mitchell J, et al: Transthoracic pacing for the treatment of severe bradycardia during induction of anesthesia, *J Cardiothorac Anesth* 3:329-332, 1989.
19. Thompson IR, Dalton BC, Lappas DG, et al: Right bundle branch block and complete heart block caused by the Swan-Ganz catheter, *Anesthesiology* 51:359-362, 1979.
20. Buran MJ: Transcutaneous pacing as an alternative to prophylactic transvenous pacemaker insertion, *Crit Care Med* 15:623-624, 1987 (letter).
21. Beck CS, Pritchard WH, Feil HS: Ventricular fibrillation of long duration abolished by electric shock, *JAMA* 135:985-986, 1953.
22. Zoll PM, Linenthal AJ, Gibson W, et al: Termination of ventricular fibrillation in man by externally applied electric countershock, *N Eng J Med* 254:727-732, 1956.
23. Lown B: Cardioversion of arrhythmias, *Br Heart J* 29:469-487, 1964.
24. Edmark KW: Simultaneous voltage and current waveforms generated during internal and external direct-current pulse defibrillation, *Surg Forum* 14:262-264, 1963.

25. Zipes DP, Fischer J, King RM, et al: Termination of ventricular fibrillation in dogs by depolarizing a critical amount of myocardium, *Am J Cardiol* 36:37-44, 1975.

26. Witkowski FX, Penkoske PA, Plonsey R: Mechanisms of defibrillation in open-chest dogs with unipolar DC-coupled simultaneous activation and shock potential recordings, *Circulation* 82:244-260, 1990.

27. Chen P-S, Shibata N, Dixon EG, et al: Comparison of the defibrillation threshold and the upper limit of vulnerability, *Circulation* 73:1022-1028, 1986.

28. Sweeney RJ, Gill RM, Syeinberg MI, et al: Ventricular refractory period extension caused by defibrillation shocks, *Circulation* 82:965-972, 1990.

29. Jones JL, Lepeschkin E, Rush S, et al: Depolarization-induced arrhythmias following high-intensity electric field stimulation of cultured myocardial cells, *Med Instrum* 12:54, 1978 (abstract of Second Purdue Cardiac Defibrillation Conference).

30. Geddes LA, Tacker WA, Rosborough JP, et al: Electrical dose for ventricular defibrillation of large and small animals using precordial electrodes, *J Clin Invest* 53:310-319, 1974.

31. Adgey AA, Patton JN, Campbell NP, et al: Ventricular defibrillation: appropriate energy levels, *Circulation* 60:219-223, 1979.

32. Kerber RE, Martins JB, Kelly KJ, et al: Self-adhesive preapplied electrode pads for defibrillation and cardioversion, *J Am Coll Cardiol* 3:815-820, 1984.

33. Zoll RH, Zoll PM, Belgard AH: personal communication.

34. Warner ED, Dahl C, Ewy GA: Myocardial injury from transthoracic defibrillator countershock, *Arch Pathol* 99:55-59, 1975.

35. Aronson AL, Haggar B: The automatic defibrillator-pacemaker: clinical rationale and engineering design, *Med Instrum* 20:27-35, 1985.

36. Mirowski M, Mower MM, Staewen WS, et al: The development of the transvenous automatic defibrillator, *Arch Intern Med* 129:773-779, 1972.

37. Lerman BB, Deale OC: Effect of epicardial patch electrodes on transthoracic defibrillation, *Circulation* 81:1409-1414, 1990.

38. Zoll RH, Zoll PM, Belgard AH: New defibrillation electrodes, *Med Instrum* 2:56, 1978 (abstract).

Chapter 32

INFUSION PUMPS

Roxanne F. Zarmsky, M.D.
Autry J. Parker, M.D.
Raymond S. Sinatra, M.D., Ph.D.

Infusion devices
Controllers
Positive pressure pumps
Syringe pumps
Patient-controlled analgesia devices
Commercially available PCA infusion devices
    Abbott LifeCare PCA Infuser "PCA Classic"
    Abbott LifeCare PCA Plus 4100 and LifeCare PCA
     Plus II
    Abbott LifeCare Provider 5500
    Bard (Harvard) PCA Infuser
    Bard PCA I and PCA II
    Bard Ambulatory PCA
    Graseby Patient-Controlled Analgesia System (PCAS)
    IVAC PCA Infuser 310
    Pharmacia CADD PCA 5800
    Stratofuse PCA
    PCA Infusor System and Basal-Bolus Infusor System
    WalkMed 430 PCA and 440 PIC

The proliferation of high-technology infusion devices has greatly influenced the practice of anesthesia by allowing precise delivery intraoperatively and postoperatively of intravenous anesthetics, analgesics, and vasopressors. Box 32-1 lists the various uses for infusion devices. Intravenous anesthesia via continuous infusions of anesthetic agents has become very popular because of the availability of infusion devices that are simple to use and are accurate. The ability to infuse multiple potent vasoactive substances at constant and accurate rates has improved patient care

Adapted in part from *Patient-controlled analgesia systems*. In Sinatra RS, Hord A, Ginsberg B, et al, editors: *Acute pain: mechanisms and management*. St Louis, 1992, Mosby–Year Book.

both inside and outside of the operating room. Many critically ill patients come to the operating room with several infusions controlled by a variety of devices. Finally, patient-controlled self-administration of opioids is an effective means of postoperative pain control that involves the use of specialized infusion pumps. Therefore, it is important for the anesthesiologist to be familiar with the types of available infusion control devices and the potential problems that can arise with their use.

Box 32-1. Clinical uses of infusion devices

Vasoactive drugs

Vasopressors
Vasodilators
Inotropes

Antibiotic and other nonbolus medications
Continuous infusion medications

Heparin
Aminophylline
Intravenous anesthetics such as propofol and alfentanil
Narcotics
Muscle relaxants
Protamine
Antiarrhythmics
Local anesthetics (epidural)

Total parenteral nutrition
Fluid maintenance (especially for children and those on fluid-restricted diets)
Maintenance of catheter patency (KVO)

Table 32-1. Types of infusion devices

Pumps (generate pressure to regulate flow)	Controllers (use gravity to regulate flow)	Special needs (may be controllers or pumps)
Volumetric	Manually clamped	PCA
Peristaltic	Automated	Epidural
Cassette	In-line disposable	infusions
Elastomeric		Insulin
reservoir		Chemotherapy
Syringe		Implantable
Electronic gear		Gastrointestinal
or lead screw		alimentation
Nonelectronic		

INFUSION DEVICES

Infusion devices can be divided into two major groups: (1) controllers that regulate the rate of gravity-induced flow and (2) positive displacement pumps that have a pressure-generating mechanism to control flow independently of gravity. In addition to these two broad categories, infusion devices can be classified according to their use (i.e., PCA) or type of reservoir (i.e., syringe). Table 32-1 shows a listing of the different classes of infusion control devices that the anesthesiologist may encounter. The choice of device depends on the purpose of the infusion and the type of solution being infused. For example, accuracy of total volume infused (and thus total calories per day) of a total parenteral nutrition solution (TPN) is more important than minor variations in flow rate. However, with a vasoactive solution (i.e., sodium nitroprusside), the constancy of flow rate is the prime factor in determining the safety of the infusion.

CONTROLLERS

Electrically powered infusion controllers automatically regulate and monitor flow through a gravity-fed system. There are three potential advantages over a simple, manually clamped IV tubing system. First, clotting of catheters is minimized due to early warning via alarms that sense increased back pressure. Second, when electrically powered controllers are used properly, the incidence of accidental rapid infusions and dry IV lines is decreased. Third, controllers may also be preferable to positive displacement pumps in that the incidence and severity of infiltrations can be reduced because the driving force is only the small hydrostatic pressure gradient between the height of the solution in the container and that of the catheter lumen.[1]

Infusion controllers are either drop rate–calibrated (drops/min) or flow rate–calibrated (ml/hr), and conversion charts are required if viscous solutions are used. Most controllers use drop sensors that work as part of a feedback system with the flow regulating mechanism. Regulation of flow is achieved by a system that pinches or intermittently occludes and releases the tubing.

All automated controllers have a catheter occlusion alarm. Most devices also have displays that alert the user prior to an occlusion. This indicates that the controller is sensing increased back pressure and is adjusting the flow-control mechanism to maintain the set flow rate. Medical personnel can therefore intervene before the infusion is shut off, for example, by repositioning the patient's extremity. As the back pressure increases, the accuracy of the flow rate decreases before the occlusion alarm sounds.[1]

Units with remote drop sensors that attach to the drip chamber can detect an empty container and stop the infusion before air enters the IV tubing. Controllers without this feature will draw air into the IV tubing unless the user

Table 32-2. Characteristics of selected electronic controllers*

Manufacturer	Model	Cost	Set cost	Flow range	Accuracy	Weight (lb)
Abbott Labs, Abbott Park, Il.	LifeCare 1050	$2084	$1.75-$3.50 (standard Abbott sets)	Microdrip 5-250 ml/hr Macrodrip 20-400 ml/hr	±10% total system	10
Critikon, Inc., Tampa, Fla.	Rateminder III	$1650	Uses standard sets $0.75 rate-flow clip	1-125 drops/min	NA†	3.5 including batteries
Critikon, Inc., Tampa, Fla.	Rateminder IV	$1750	Uses standard sets $0.75 rate-flow clip	3-500 ml/hr	NA†	3.5 including batteries
IVAC Corp., San Diego, Calif.	262+	$1800	$2.50	5-299 ml/hr	NA†	13
IVY Medical, Inc., Minneapolis, Minn.	Commander 600	$1695	Standard sets	5-600 ml/hr	±2%	9

*Information provided by manufacturers; prices subject to change.
†Information not available.

sets the volume-to-be-infused control to slightly less than the size of the IV fluid container. A separate air-in-line detector feature is present in only a few controllers. Some infusion control devices are solely battery powered, whereas most are electrically operated with a variable (at least 4 hours) battery backup. All have self-test features and fluid resistant switches, and all can be attached to a standard IV pole.

Several problems can occur when controllers are employed. Many controllers permit free flow of solution when the IV set is removed from the machine without the infusion tubing being clamped first. This can have devastating consequences if a potent vasoactive substance is being infused. Setting the correct flow rate can be a complex task if the machine is calibrated in drops/min. Drop size depends on the viscosity and specific gravity of a solution. A fluid code selection chart or a fluid type conversion chart needs to be consulted to compensate for the differing physical properties of the solutions infused. This adds another step and an opportunity for human error, and flow rates could be very different from those desired. Also, many infusion devices use more than one type of IV set (20 drops/ml or 60 drops/ml), and if the wrong set is chosen, infusion rates can be in error by a factor of 3.[1]

In-line disposable flow controllers are attractive because of their low cost, ease of use, and transportability. However, the accuracy of these devices is questionable. The height of the bag above the patient greatly influences the rate of flow, and the accuracy at low rates of flow is unreliable. A study of the Dial-a-Flo*[2] revealed an error of ±20% when flow rates were greater than 20 ml/hr and errors ranging from ±68% at flow rates of 5 ml/hr. The

*Sorensen Research, Salt Lake City, Utah.

Emergency Care Research Institute (ECRI)[1] evaluated the performance under normal and extreme conditions of nine electronic controllers in 1985. All of the controllers delivered nonviscous solutions (i.e., saline, D5W) to within 5% of the set rate when using a range of common infusion rates. Therefore, for the adult patient receiving a nonviscous solution, infusion controllers are adequate as long as only trained personnel operate them. This is because of the risk of free flow of solution when the IV tubing is removed from the controller without first being clamped.

Table 32-2 lists five commercially available controllers. The Abbott LifeCare 1050, IVAC Model 262+, and the Ivy Commander 600 are all large, pole-mounted devices. The Critikon Rateminder III and IV are lightweight (3.5 lb), battery-powered devices that can be pole-mounted or carried. The Abbott LifeCare 1050 has the capability to program a piggyback infusion, and this is reflected in the unit's higher price ($2084). All five controllers listed use standard IV sets except the IVAC 262+. All are flow rate– calibrated (ml/hr) except for the Critikon Rateminder III, in which the flow is set in drops/min. A conversion chart is required to convert from drops/min to ml/hr. An empty container sensor is present in all five controllers listed. The highest flow rate possible is the 600 ml/hr achieved by the Ivy Commander 600.

POSITIVE PRESSURE PUMPS

The infusion pump differs from the controller by its use of positive pressure to regulate flow. This has three advantages over the use of gravity to regulate flow. At very low flow rates accuracy can be achieved with positive-pressure–generating infusion devices.[3] Minor occlusions associated with viscous solutions and certain IV systems can be overcome. Also, positive pressure is required to infuse

Power	Battery (hr at ml/hr)	System alarms	Miscellaneous features
95-140 V AC	NA†	Dose delivered empty container flow	Dual rate, automatic piggybacking, uses most standard Abbott IV sets
6 V DC (4 D alkaline batteries)	NA†	Occlusion, flow status (end of infusion), low battery, service check, empty container	Has drop sensor, rate clip flow regulator reduces chance of accidental free flow, uses any manufacturer's IV set that flows with gravity, compact and cordless, titration capability without flow
6 V DC (4 D alkaline batteries)	NA†	Same as Rateminder III	Same as Rateminder III but flow is in ml/hr
115 V AC	6	Empty container, closed clamp, low battery, occlusion, unattainable rate, flow status, mispositioned flow sensor, opened latch, internal malfunction	Capable of detecting most infiltrations
110 V AC	NA†	No flow, empty container, IV complete, battery status	—

Table 32-3. Selected pumps that can function as controllers or pumps*

Manufacturer	Model	Pump mechanism	Cost	Set cost	Flow range	Accuracy
Abbott Labs Abbott Park, Il.	LifeCare 5000 Plum	Piston diaphragm	$3675	$4.50-$10.00	1-999 ml/hr 0.1-99.9 ml/hr	±5% total system
IMED Corp. San Diego, Calif.	Gemini PC-1	Linear peristaltic	NA†	$7.75	0.1-999 ml/hr	±5%
IMED Corp., San Diego, Calif.	Gemini PC-2	Linear peristaltic	$4250	$7.75	1-999 ml/hr per channel	±5%
Siemens Life Support Systems, Schaumburg, Il.	Mini Med III	Piston cylinder	$4250	$3.50-$12.50	0.1-999 ml/hr per channel	±2% normal range, ±5% extremes

*Information provided by manufacturers; prices subject to change.
†Information not available.

through indwelling arterial catheters. The high pressure generated by the pump can lead to such complications as increased severity of infiltrations and delay in the detection of occlusions at low infusion rates. Pumps manufactured in the 1970s generated high operating pressures (40 to 100 psig, equivalent to 2068 to 5170 mm Hg), whereas newer pumps operate in the range of 4 to 20 psig (207 to 1034 mm Hg).[4] Some pumps also allow the user to select the occlusion pressure limit and thus determine the maximum pressure generated by the pump. If the pressure limit can be set as low as 0.5 to 1 psig, then the pump is essentially acting as a controller.[3] The pump may be best used as a controller when the consequences of an undetected infiltration are severe (i.e., with caustic chemotherapeutic agents). The positive pressure capability of these pump/controllers is useful when viscous solutions are infused and in other situations of high back pressure.

Table 32-3 lists the features of four of the pump/controllers that are currently on the market. The Abbott Life-Care 5000 Plum and the IMED Gemini pumps are large, pole-mounted devices that use wall outlet AC power, have rechargeable variable-duration batteries, and are programmable to rates up to 999 ml/hr. The Gemini PC-2 is essentially two full pumps in one, as reflected in its higher cost ($4250) and greater weight (18.5 lb). The Siemens Mini-Med III is a compact (2.5 lb) device that is syringe capable and can be powered by one 9 V battery for 2.5 hours at a flow rate of 375 ml/hr. This pump can also achieve flow rates up to 999 ml/hr and has three separate channels with automatic piggybacking capability.

Infusion pumps are classified according to their mechanism of operation, which is either peristaltic, cassette, or elastomeric reservoir (Table 32-1). *Peristaltic* systems propel fluid by compression of fluid-filled tubing using either rotary cams (rotary peristaltic) or fingerlike projections (linear peristaltic). The fluid is pumped toward the patient in a fashion similar to the way food is propelled along the gastrointestinal tract. Most peristaltic pumps use a reservoir to which the tubing is attached, and this reservoir determines the range of volumes that the pump can deliver. Because the flexible tubing is constantly massaged, it may become deformed and stretched, leading to inaccuracy in delivered volumes. The range of accuracy of most peristaltic pumps is ±5% to ±10%.[3] *Cassette* pump systems consist of an administration set with a measured chamber that fits inside the pump. These devices have a cycle during which the chamber is filled, followed by a delivery cycle during which the measured volume is infused. Because a measured volume of infusate is delivered with each cycle, these pumps are also described as volumetric. In 1984, ECRI[4] reported on the accuracy of various infusion pumps. The majority of the pumps had an accuracy range of ±2% to ±10%; however, error rates as high as 20% were occasionally seen. The *elastomeric reservoir* system uses an elastic balloon-like reservoir that exerts a constant pressure on the infusate. A downstream restrictor controls the flow rate. Because the internal pressure of the reservoir is low, high rates of flow may be difficult to achieve with accuracy, and rates may depend on the solution's viscosity and temperature.[3] An example of this type of pump can be

Weight (lb)	Power	Battery (hr at ml/hr)	System alarms	Miscellaneous features
13	115 V AC	6 at 125	Distal occlusion, proximal occlusion, air in line, pressure out of range	Programmable operating modes, multiple intermittent piggybacking, syringe capable, opaque fluid capable
9.5	90-130 V AC	4 at 125	Occluded fluid side, occluded patient side, check IV set, open door with flowstop, close door, air in line, partial occlusion fluid side	Dual rate piggybacking, rapid occlusion detection, set occlusion pressure to 0.5-10 psi, computer interface capable, universal set for pump/controller mode, taper mode for ramp up or down of TPN infusions, opaque fluid capable
18.5	90-130 V AC	4 at 125 each channel	Same as PC-1	Same as PC-1 but dual channel, no taper mode
2.5	110 V AC; 9 V DC	2.5 at 375	Occluded, air in line, infusion complete, flow error, empty bottle, cassette disengaged, circuit malfunction, low and depleted battery	3 channels with 3 separate lines, syringe capable, optional battery pack 6 hr at 375 ml/hr, automatic piggybacking, opaque fluid capable

found in the section entitled "Commercially available PCA infusion devices (Baxter PCA Infusor)."

Table 32-4 lists the features of 23 currently available positive displacement pumps. The cost of these devices is significantly higher than that of controllers, ranging from approximately $2000 to more than $6000, depending on the features of the pump. An important factor in determining the cost of using an infusion pump is the cost of the infusion set. Prices can range from as little as $2.50 to as much as $14.85 per set. Three of the pumps (Baxter Flo-Gard 6200 and 6300, and the Smith & Nephew Sigma 6000+) use standard IV sets, which reduces the cost per use even more because separate inventories of pump tubing need not be stocked. However, the Flo-Gard 6200 and 6300 are relatively expensive, costing $3719 for the single-channel 6200 model and $6694 for the dual-channel 6300 model. Frequency of pump use helps to determine whether these models are cost-effective in a given institution. The Smith & Nephew Sigma 6000+ is shown in Fig. 32-1.

Pump accuracy ranges listed are from ±2% to ±10% (Table 32-4). All of the pumps listed can infuse opaque fluids and have air-in-line and infusion-complete alarms. Variable-duration back-up rechargeable batteries are provided in most of the AC-powered models. Several models have variable occlusion pressure limits that may reduce the incidence of nuisance alarms if properly set. Titration capability allows the user to change the rate without first shutting off the infusion. This can be very useful when potent vasoactive drugs are being infused. Of the 23 pumps

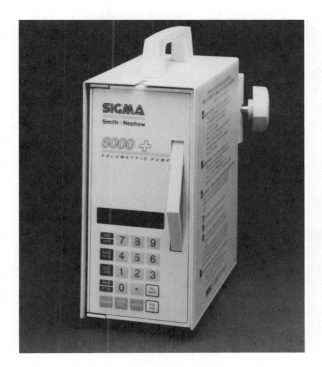

Fig. 32-1. Smith & Nephew Sigma 6000+ infusion pump. (Photo courtesy of Smith & Nephew Sigma, Medina, NY.)

listed, 10 have the capability to deliver flow in 0.1 ml/hr increments. However, four of these (Abbott LifeCare Micro, AVI 210A, Baxter Flo-Gard 8500 and IMED 965A Micro) have maximum flow rates of only 99.9 ml/hr. The AVI 210A is shown in Fig. 32-2. This pump and the AVI

Table 32-4. Characteristics of selected positive displacement pumps*

Manufacturer	Model	Pump mechanism	Cost	Set cost	Flow range (ml/hr)	Accuracy
Abbott Labs, Abbott Park, Ill.	LifeCare 3	Cassette: piston-actuated diaphragm	$2750	$4.50-$10.00	1-999	±5% total system
Abbott Labs, Abbott Park, Ill.	LifeCare 4	Cassette: piston-actuated diaphragm	$3045	$4.50-$10.00	1-999	±5% total system
Abbott Labs, Abbott Park, Ill.	LifeCare Micro	Cassette: piston-actuated diaphragm	$3045	$5.50-$11.00	0.1-99.9	±5% total system
Abbott Labs, Abbott Park, Ill.	LifeCare Hyperbaric	Cassette: piston-actuated diaphragm	$3360	$8.00-$11.00	10-800	±10% total system calibrated to ATM
Abbott Labs, Abbott Park, Ill.	LifeCare Omniflow 4000	Cassette: piston-actuated diaphragm	$5345	$10.25-$11.95	1.4-800	±4% total system
Abbott Labs, Abbott Park, Ill.	LifeCare Omniflow Therapist	Cassette: piston-actuated diaphragm	$7995	$10-$20	1.0-700	±4%
AVI Inc., St. Paul, Minn.	AVI 200A	Dual piston diaphragm cassette	$2235	$4.95	1-999	±2%
AVI Inc., St. Paul, Minn.	AVI 210A	Dual piston diaphragm cassette	$2395	$4.95	0.1-99.9	±2%
AVI Inc., St. Paul, Minn.	AVI 400A	Dual piston diaphragm cassette	$2500	$4.95	1-999	±2%
Baxter Healthcare Inc., Deerfield, Ill.	Flo-Gard 6200	Linear peristaltic	$3719	Uses standard sets	1-999	±5%
Baxter Healthcare Inc., Deerfield, Ill.	Flo-Gard 6300	Linear peristaltic	$6694	Uses standard sets	1-1999	±5%
Baxter Healthcare Inc., Deerfield, Ill.	Flo-Gard 8000	Piston actuated cassette diaphragm	$2779	$9.96-$12.80	1-999	±3%
Baxter Healthcare Inc., Deerfield, Ill.	Flo-Gard 8500	Piston actuated cassette diaphragm	$2909	$9.96-$12.80	0.1-99.9	±3%

*Information provided by manufacturers, prices subject to change.
†Information not available. Also have "air in-line" and "infusion complete" alarms.

Weight (lb)	Power	Battery (hr at ml/hr)	System alarms	Miscellaneous features
13	117 V AC	8 at 125	Occlusion pressure 10-20 psig, air in line, flow error, empty bottle, infusion complete, circuit malfunction, low battery, depleted battery	Can pump opaque fluids, cannot pump air because of siphon system
13	117 V AC	8 at 30	Same as LifeCare 3, except occlusion pressure variable	Can pump opaque fluid, differential pressure sensing, looks for 4, 8, or 12 psig change over normal operation to sense occlusion, titration feature, dual rate piggybacking, computer dataway
13	117 V AC	8 at 15	Same as LifeCare 3, except choice of 3 pressure limits	Can pump opaque fluid, uses microdrip or macrodrip IV sets
14.08	112-120 V AC	NA†	Dose complete, flow occlusion, battery low	Can pump opaque fluid, only device available for volumetric infusion in monoplace hyperbaric chambers
13.25	120 V AC	5 at 125	Occlusion pressure 1-12 psig, infusion complete, air in line, flow error, empty bottle, cassette disengaged, low battery, cassette malfunction	Can pump opaque fluid, 4 medications simultaneously and/or intermittently at different rates and volumes, takes bags, bottles or syringes, auto dilution, air in line elimination, auto 24-hr programming capability, needleless connections.
13.25	120 V AC	5 at 125	Cassette unlocked, faulty cassette, air in line, occlusion patient line, empty container, low battery	Same as Omniflow 4000 plus computer dataport communications, bar code readings, IV history storage, 48-hr battery backup, programmable and preprogrammable, multiple units for programming, programmable flush between medications
9.5	120 V AC	8 at 125	Occlusion pressure, 4 or 9 psi, air in line, empty bottle, door open, circuit malfunction, low battery, depleted battery	Opaque fluid capable, fluid delivery is continuous and nonpulsatile, upstream air detection and removal without violating fluid path integrity, user-selected occlusion pressure, titration capability
9.5	120 V AC	8 at 50	Same as AVI 200A	Same as AVI 200A but delivers in 0.1-ml increments
9.5	120 V AC	8 at 125	Same as AVI 200A	Same as 200A but with separate piggyback functions
14	115 V AC	6 at 125	Occlusion pressure 5-7 psi, air in line, flow error, door open, circuit malfunction, low battery, depleted battery, upstream and downstream occlusion	Opaque fluid capable, dual rate, automatic piggybacking, panel lockout, auto restart
17.5	115 V AC	6 at 125 one channel, 4 at 125 two channel	Same as FloGard 6200	Same as FloGard 6200 but with two channels
12	117-230 V AC ±10%	4 at 125	Occlusion pressure 1-10 psig, air in line, empty bottle, flow error, cassette disengaged, circuit malfunction, low battery, depleted battery	Opaque fluid capable, differential occlusion detection adjustable from 1-10 psig in 0.2 increments, dose volume feature that accommodates titration
12	117-230 V AC ±10%	4 at 125	Same as Flo-Gard 8000	Same as Flo-Gard 8000 but with 0.1-ml increments

Continued.

Table 32-4. Characteristics of selected positive displacement pumps—cont'd

Manufacturer	Model	Pump mechanism	Cost	Set cost	Flow range (ml/hr)	Accuracy
Baxter Healthcare Inc. Deerfield, Ill.	Flo-Gard VP	Peristaltic	$4250	$10.96-$14.85	0.1-999	±4%
Critikon Inc., Tampa, Fla.	Rateminder V	Cassette diaphragm	$2950	NA†	0.5-600	±2%
IMED Corp., San Diego, Calif.	965A Micro	Piston cylinder cassette	$3200	$8.10	0.1-99.9	±5%
IMED Corp., San Diego, Calif.	960A	Piston cylinder cassette	$3200	$6.75	1-999	±5%
IMED Corp., San Diego, Calif.	980C	Piston cylinder cassette	$3995	$6.75	1-2000	±5%
IVAC Corp., San Diego, Calif.	599	NA†	$2100	$2.50	1-999	NA†
IVAC Corp., San Diego, Calif.	570	NA†	$3400	$4.00	1-999 0.1-999.9	NA†
IVION Corp., Englewood Colo.	KIDS	NA†	$3895	NA†	0.1-999.9	±2%
Medical Technology Products Inc., Huntington, N.Y.	(MVP-1) 1000	Rotary peristaltic	$1,975	$4.35	0.1-499.9	±2%
Smith & Nephew Sigma, Medina, N.Y.	6000+	Linear peristaltic	$2995	Uses standard sets	0.1-999	±5%

200A and 400A (Fig. 32-3) allow free flow of fluid if a clamp is not closed before unloading the tubing from the pump.

Many pumps can infuse several drugs at once through separate channels, thus eliminating the need for a separate pump for each infusion that a patient is receiving. This reduces the amount of clutter around the bed and facilitates patient transportation and ambulation. The Baxter Flo-Gard 6300 has two separate channels and the Abbott Life-Care Omniflow 4000 and Omniflow Therapist (Fig. 32-4) have four separately controlled channels. However, the channels are merged into a single infusion line, so that drug compatibility must be considered. This function is different from a piggybacking feature present in several of the pumps in which more than one solution is infused through the same pumping mechanism. The Omniflow Therapist also is capable of being programmed to give intermittent flushes of up to four incompatible solutions being run through the same IV line. This feature is important in the critically-ill patient with limited IV access. Three of the pumps listed weigh less than the average 9.5-14.5 lbs. Of the other pumps, the Critikon Rateminder V operates only on battery power, but the IVAC 599 and the Medical Technology Products MVP-1 have line AC capability in addition to a battery mode. The compact design of the MVP-1 pump is shown in Fig. 32-5.

Weight (lb)	Power	Battery (hr at ml/hr)	System alarms	Miscellaneous features
13.5	115 V AC	5-hr rate not specified	Occlusion air, door open, check site, low battery	Infiltration detection, auto restart, variable occlusion pressure, time programming
7	6 V DC, 6 D alkaline batteries	2 months at 125	Occlusion pressure 2-8 psig, air, empty bottle, flow error, cassette disengaged, door open, circuit malfunction, depleted battery	Opaque fluid capable, compact and cordless, variable pressure settings of 2-8 psig, rate in decimals below 25 ml/hr, cassette valve eliminates free flow on cassette removal
14	120 V AC	10 at 50	Occlusion pressure 15-25 psig, air, flow error, door open, circuit malfunction, low battery, depleted battery	Opaque fluid capable, automatic priming, syringe adaptable, 0.1-ml increments
14	120 V AC	10 at 125	Same as 965A	Same as 965A but with 1-ml increments
14	90-130 V AC, 206-260 V AC	8 at 125	Occlusion pressure 8 or 18 psig, air, flow error, door open, circuit malfunction, low battery, depleted battery	Opaque fluid capable, dual rate sequential piggybacking, computer linking capable, high rate capability (2000 ml/hr), syringe adaptable, optional empty bottle detector, auto prime selectable, tamper proof mode
6	90-126 V AC	NA†	Occlusion, air, set out, low battery, open door, malfunction, discharge battery	Small and lightweight, dual rate capable
14.25	100-120 V AC	5 at 125	Occlusion, low battery, air, malfunction	Variable occlusion pressure, all range, computer interface, optional flow sensor, adjustable air-in-line setting (50-150 μl)
11	117 V AC	NA†	Occlusion on bottle and patient sides, air	Marketed for pediatric use
4.5	110-115 V AC 12 V DC adaptor	up to 6 hr	Occlusion pressure 8-12 psig, air, empty bottle, flow error, cassette disengaged, circuit malfunction, low battery, depleted battery	Opaque fluid capable, gravity prime, impact resistant case, nitro tubing available
10.2	105-135 V AC	6 at 125	Occlusion pressure 6-18 psig, air, empty, flow error, door open, circuit malfunction, low battery, depleted battery	Program for 12 different rate and volume schedules leading to gradual rate change, opaque fluid capable

SYRINGE PUMPS

Syringe pumps have become increasingly popular because of their convenience and lower cost per use. Often standard syringes already stocked by the hospital can be used in these pumps. Also, less medication waste occurs in drug preparation and priming the system. The electronic syringe pump uses either a motor-driven lead screw or has a gear mechanism to move the plunger into the syringe barrel. The rate of infusion is controlled by the speed of the motor driving the plunger into the syringe. The type of flow is pulsatile continuous delivery.[5] Non-electronic syringe pumps use mechanisms (i.e. springs) to apply a constant force to the plunger and deliver medication continu-

ously at a rate determined by the force applied as well as by external factors such as the viscosity of the solution. Electronic syringe pumps usually provide a greater accuracy (±2% to ±5%) than volumetric or peristaltic pumps and controllers.[3] A drawback to the syringe pump is the limitation of its reservoir size to 60 ml, which makes it inappropriate for large volume infusions. Some syringe pumps are capable of generating high pressures before the alarm signals excess pressure. If the IV line suddenly opens after a blockage, a large bolus of infusate may be released. Because of their decreased cross-sectional areas small syringes may develop higher pressures before the occlusion alarm is annunciated.[5]

Table 32-5 contains a listing of 15 currently available electronic syringe pumps. The Bard InfusO.R., the Baxter AS20GH and AS20G, the Graseby MS16A and the IVAC 710 can accept only one large size (50 or 60 ml) syringe. The Baxter AS20GH and AS20G and the MedFusion 2010 (Fig. 32-6) have multiple infusion modes available (μg/kg/min versus ml/hr), and a programmed bolus is possible. The Bard InfusO.R. (Fig. 32-7), a device powered only by battery, has multiple magnetic face plates available that provide a program to deliver a specific drug. The patient's weight and drug dose are selected (μg/kg/min) and the device delivers the medication at the appropriate ml/hr. It is especially easy to bolus with this pump because it has a separate bolus dial with listed bolus dosage possibilities provided on the face plate. A disadvantage of this pump is that it cannot be operated without an expensive, drug-specific face plate. Most of the syringe pumps listed are compact, lightweight devices weighing under 2 pounds. The Becton-Dickinson Program 2 (Fig. 32-8) is larger (9.2 lb) but is also a two-channel device capable of accommodating a wide range of syringe sizes. The IVAC 710 is only a one-channel pump but has the added feature of detecting back pressures in excess of 6 psig and annunciating an alarm should this occur. The Baxter AS5D pump has an adjustable occlusion pressure limit up to 15 ± 2 psig. The Kendall McGaw (Bard) 150XL and 300XL (Fig. 32-9) are battery-powered devices and less expensive than the other pumps listed, but these pumps are very simple and do not allow the extensive programming ability provided by most syringe pumps. The plunger is moved 5.5 inches per hour for the 150XL and 5.5 inches over a flexible time period for the 300XL; a calibration chart is provided to convert plunger distance moved to ml/hr.

The selection of a pump depends on several factors. If pumps of one design and manufacturer are already in use at an institution, the feasibility of changing to another design that requires extensive employee training must be considered. The intended use of a pump (i.e., large-volume infusion versus intermittent delivery of medication) will determine whether a syringe pump, positive-pressure

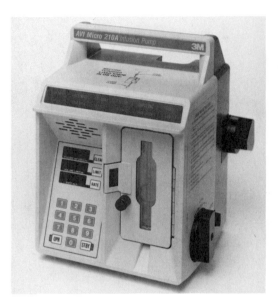

Fig. 32-2. AVI Micro 210A infusion pump. (Photo courtesy of AVI Inc., St. Paul, Minn.)

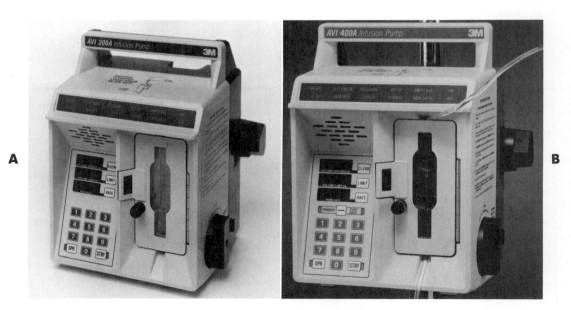

Fig. 32-3. A, AVI 200A pump and **B,** 400A infusion pump. (Photo courtesy of AVI Inc., St. Paul, Minn.)

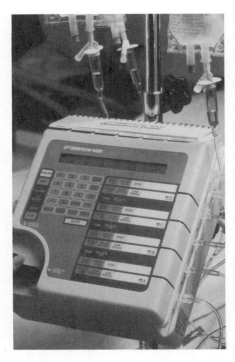

Fig. 32-4. Abbott LifeCare Omniflow 4000 infusion pump. (Photo courtesy of Abbott Labs, Abbott Park, Ill.)

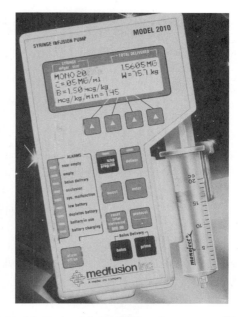

Fig. 32-6. Medfusion Model 2010 syringe pump. (Photo courtesy of Medfusion, Inc., Duluth, Ga.)

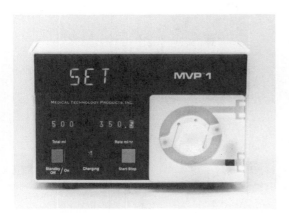

Fig. 32-5. Medical Technology Products MVP-1 infusion pump. (Photo courtesy of Medical Technology Products Inc., Huntington, NY.)

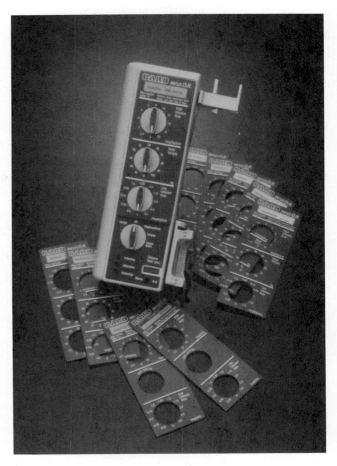

Fig. 32-7. Bard InfusO.R. syringe pump. (Photo courtesy of Bard, Medical Systems Division, North Reading, Mass.)

pump, or controller is appropriate. The available features, the cost of the pump, the cost of the infusion sets, and the safety and ease of use ultimately determine which pumps are purchased and used by an institution.

Infusion pumps are mechanical devices, and therefore they must undergo routine inspection and maintenance in order to assure their accuracy. Usually these checkout procedures are best performed by an institution's biomedical engineering staff or by the manufacturer under a mainte-

Table 32-5. Selected electronic non-PCA syringe pumps*

Manufacturer	Model	Cost	Set cost	Syringe size	Flow range
Bard Medical Systems Division North Reading, Mass.	Infus O.R. 6461500	$1,995	$2.95	60 ml	0-600 ml/h
Baxter Healthcare Corp., Hooksett, N.H.	AS2F	$1,345	Uses standard microvolume tubing	1-60 ml	0.02-88 ml/hr; 0.5-49.5 hr in 0.5-hr increments
Baxter Healthcare Corp., Hooksett, N.H.	AS5D	$1,765	Uses any microvolume tubing	20-60 ml	0.1-99.99 ml/hr; 0.001-9.999 ml/min
Baxter Healthcare Corp., Hooksett, N.H.	AS20A	$1795	Uses any microvolume tubing	1-60 ml	0.05-84.7 ml/hr (depends on mode and syringe size)
Baxter Healthcare Corp., Hooksett, N.H.	AS20GH	$2,195	Uses any high flow rate set	60 ml	Depends on programmed information
Baxter Healthcare Corp., Hooksett, N.H.	AS20G	$1,895	Uses any high flow rate set	60 ml	Depends on programmed information
Baxter Healthcare Corp.	AS20S	$1,785	Uses any microvolume tubing	1-60 ml	Depends on syringe selected
Becton Dickinson Infusion Systems, Lincoln. Park, N.J.	360 infuser	$695	S2.95	3-60 ml	1.5-360 ml/hr 10-60 min
Becton Dickinson Infusion Systems, Lincoln Park, N.J.	Program 2	$2,895	$2.95	5-60 ml	0.1-99.9 ml/hr each channel dependent on syringe size
Becton Dickinson Infusion Systems, Lincoln Park, N.J.	Rate Infuser II	$1,750	$2.95	1-60 ml	0.1-99.9 ml/hr
Graseby Medical Ltd., Millersville Md.	MS16A	$995	$2.00	60 ml	0.02-33 ml/hr
IVAC Corp., San Diego, Calif.	710	$1,700	$1.50	50 ml	0.1-99.9 ml/hr

*Information provided by manufacturers: prices subject to change.
†Information not available.
‡These pumps carry the brand name Bard.

Accuracy	Weight	Power	Battery	System alarms	Miscellaneous features
±3%	2 lb	Battery only	4 C alkaline batteries	End of syringe, occlusion, low battery, internal fault	Multiple face plates for different drugs, program weight and desired dose (μg/kg/min) and pump calculates rate
±4%	19.3 oz	105-125 V AC; DC	Internal rechargeable NiCad	System, near empty, runaway	Also available in infusion time settings 0.5-24.75 hr with 0.25-hr increments
±3%	7.5 lb	105-125 V AC; DC	Internal rechargeable lead acid	System, excess force, runaway, low battery, bad battery, battery power only	Excess force adjustable 15±2 lb
±3%	24 oz	105-125 V AC; DC	Internal rechargeable NiCad	System, high pressure, low battery, bad battery, charging, volume limit	Continuous intermittent, or standby modes
±3%	27 oz	105-125 V AC; DC	Internal rechargeable NiCad	System, low battery, bad battery, volume limit, charging, high pressure	Multiple infusion modes; body weight (kg), drug concentration (mg/ml), dose (μg/kg/min), continuous (ml/hr) (μg/hr)
±3%	27 oz	105-125 V AC; DC	Internal rechargeable NiCad	System, high pressure, low battery, bad battery, volume limit, charging	Multiple infusion modes, body weight (kg), drug concentration (mg/ml), dose (μg/min) (μg/kg/min), continuous rate (ml/hr)
±3%	24 oz	105-125 V AC; DC	Internal rechargeable NiCad	System, high pressure, low battery, bad battery, volume limit, charging	—
±3%	2 lb with batteries	Battery only	4 C alkaline batteries (400 hr)	System occlusion, end of infusion, low battery, syringe displaced	Primarily for intermittent medication delivery up to 1-hr infusion length
±3%	9.5 lb	105-125 V AC	Internal chargeable lead acid	System, invalid program, occlusion, syringe tampering, low volume, time limit, 2-minute pause, low or bad battery	2 independent channels, 0.1 ml/hr minimum on all syringe sizes, includes IV pole clamp
±3%-±5%	2 lb, 10 oz with batteries	Battery only	4 C alkaline batteries (265 hr)	System, occlusion, low volume, low battery, syringe tamper, incorrect setting, wait state	Includes IV pole clamp
±5%	0.4 lb with battery	Battery only	9V battery	Occlusion, completion of infusion, low battery	Designed for ambulatory use
NA†	7 lb	95-135 V AC	Lead acid	Empty syringe, occlusion, low battery, syringe clamp, zero rate	Detects pressure in excess of 6 psig

Continued.

Table 32-5. Selected electronic non-PCA syringe pumps—cont'd

Manufacturer	Model	Cost	Set cost	Syringe size	Flow range
Kendall McGaw Labs, Inc. Irvine, Calif.	150 XL Mini Infuser‡	$695	$3.25	5-60 ml	Flat rate 5.5 inches/hr
Kendall McGaw Labs, Inc. Irvine, Calif.	300 XL Mini Infuser‡	$795	$3.25	5-60 ml	Flexible rate, 5.5 inches over 7.5-120 minutes
MedFusion Inc., Duluth, Ga.	1001	$1,695	Any tubing	1-60 ml	0.1-99.9 ml/hr
MedFusion Inc., Duluth, Ga.	2001	$2,125	Any tubing	1-60 ml	0.01-99.99 ml/hr
MedFusion Inc., Duluth Ga.	2010	$2,375	Any tubing	1-60 ml	0.1-378.0 ml/hr dependent on syringe

‡These pumps carry the brand name Bard.

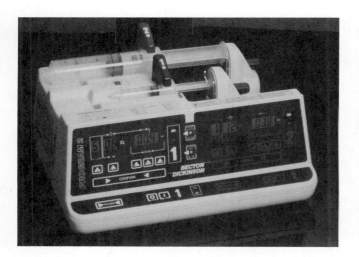

Fig. 32-8. Becton-Dickinson Program 2 syringe pump. (Photo courtesy of Becton-Dickinson Infusion Systems, Lincoln Park, N.J.)

nance contract. ECRI[6] has published the following recommendations for routine six-monthly pump maintenance:

1. Examine the physical condition of the unit and correct problems. The instrument should be clean and the markings legible. Check operation of moveable parts.
2. Inspect fuses and circuit breakers.
3. Check chassis grounding resistance by using an ohm meter to measure the resistance between the grounding pin on the plug and the bare metal on the chassis. This value should not exceed 0.1 ohm.

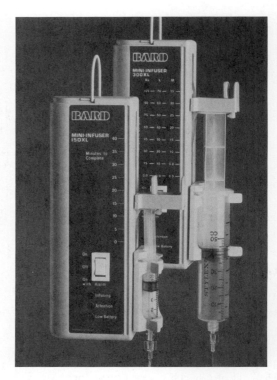

Fig. 32-9. Kendall McGaw (Bard Mini-Infuser) 150XL and 300XL syringe pumps. (Photo courtesy of Kendall McGaw Lab, Irvine, Calif.)

Accuracy	Weight	Power	Battery	System alarms	Miscellaneous features
±3%	1 lb, 12 oz with batteries	Battery only	4 C alkaline batteries	Occlusion, end of infusion, low battery	
±3%	1 lb, 12 oz with batteries	Battery only	4 C alkaline batteries	Occlusion, end of infusion, low battery	
±3%	5 lb	120 V AC	NiCad (not rechargeable)	System, near empty, empty, low battery, depleted battery, occlusion, volume limit	Battery for backup only
±3%	2.5 lb	120 V AC (adaptor)	Rechargeable battery backup, type not specified, 10 hr at 5 ml/hr with 60-ml syringe	System, near empty, empty, volume limit, occlusion, low battery, depleted battery, over delivery, under delivery, program error	Multiple programming modes: continuous, volume/time, intermittent: manual or automatic
±3%	2.5 lb	120 V AC	Rechargeable battery backup, type not specified, 10 hr at 5 ml/hr with 60 ml syringe	Same as 2001	Multiple programming modes: continuous volume/time, body weight mode, mass mode, bolus capability

4. Check the maximum leakage current by measuring the leakage current between the chassis and the ground in all wiring configurations while the unit is connected to the AC power outlet (grounded, ungrounded, unit on, unit off). When the unit is ungrounded, leakage current should be less than 100 μA and no more than a few microamperes when grounded.
5. Check rate accuracy by measuring at two or more points typical of the pump's clinical usage. A graduated cylinder and a stopwatch are needed to perform this test. The percent error should be less than 10%.
6. Test the alarms.
7. Test battery condition by running the pump at a high rate for 1 hour and then check flow accuracy using the battery as the power source.

PATIENT-CONTROLLED ANALGESIA DEVICES

Potent opioid analgesics continue to be the mainstay in the treatment of moderate to severe postoperative pain and are traditionally administered on an as-needed basis via intramuscular, oral, or intravenous routes. The standard protocols that have evolved, although emphasizing patient safety, all too often provide inadequate analgesia. To achieve optimal analgesic benefit, several principles must be followed: (1) Therapeutic plasma levels and adequate central nervous system (CNS) delivery must be achieved in order to assure sufficient occupancy and activation of opiate receptors. (2) therapeutic concentrations exhibit wide variability for each opioid and for different individuals; (3) the dose-response curve is very steep (i.e., small changes in plasma concentration may be all that separate inadequate from clinically adequate analgesia[7] and (4) the therapeutic window is relatively narrow (i.e., underdosing and overdosing can easily occur). The introduction of new drug delivery systems, far more than any other development, has made possible the application of the above principles.

Plasma and CNS concentrations are most uniform when opioids are administered by either continuous infusion or as multiple small doses.[8] Unfortunately, the high workload of contemporary surgical floors does not lend itself to the repeated administration of small doses. Instead, patients are given a relatively large intramuscular bolus of analgesic drug, usually every 4 hours. This dosing regimen all too often leads to a well described "pain cycle"[9] in which pain therapy is dependent on nursing variables (i.e., response to the patient's complaint, "screening," preparation of the syringe, and administration of drug) and the patient's characteristics (i.e., absorption from administration site, pharmacokinetics, and pharmacodynamics). To accommodate significant variability in pain perception, and minimum effective analgesic concentrations (MEAC) between individuals, a patient-interactive system is necessary. Patient-controlled analgesia is an interactive form of therapy that permits patients to treat pain by self-administering small doses of intravenous and epidural analgesics. Through the use of microprocessor technology, patients are allowed to control the rate of drug administration on the basis of the degree of pain relief needed. This control allows patients to compensate for differences in individual pharmacodynamics and pharmacokinetics, changes in pain stimulus intensity, and inappropriate "screening" by house staff.[7,9]

A sizeable number of PCA or "demand" analgesia systems have been developed (Tables 32-6 and 32-7). These systems have several modes of operation and incorporate many unique features. The feature that most of the modern PCA systems have in common is a microprocessor that allows the patient to interact (within preset dose limits and lockout intervals) with an infusion pump connected to the intravenous line. Patients usually activate the pump by pressing a remote activation button connected to the apparatus. Each push of the button is termed an *analgesic demand,* and successful pump activation results in the delivery of an *incremental,* or *bolus* dose. The size of the incremental dose ranges from 0.5 to 2.5 ml (first-generation devices) and 0.1 to 5 ml (second-generation devices) and is administered over 10 to 30 seconds. The industry standard regarding accuracy of incremental dose delivery is ± 0.5% of the programmed dose.[10] Depending on the technology employed, the incremental dose may be delivered according to drug concentration (mg/ml or μg/ml), volume of solution (ml), or both. Many PCA devices store in memory the number of attempts (demands) as well as the total number of incremental boluses delivered during the previous 12 to 24 hours of therapy. With appropriate education of the patient and adequate size of the bolus, the ratio of demands versus incremental boluses delivered should approach 1.0.[8] Some PCA infusors provide audible (beep, chirp) or visual (increasing cumulative dose display) cues in association with the successful delivery of an incremental bolus. This technology offers important dosing reinforcement for elderly and confused patients. Other devices designed to chirp with every analgesic demand offer the potential advantage of a "placebo effect." A lockout interval is engaged at the time the incremental dose is delivered, thereby assuring that another dose cannot be administered within a preset time limit. This dose delay represents the most important safety mechanism associated with PCA. It is designed to protect the patient from excessive button pushing (secondary to patient confusion or overly concerned visitors) and potential overdosage. The lockout interval in effect limits the number of incremental boluses that a patient can self-administer over a period of time; thus sedation and sleep usually ensue before the patient is able to administer a dose large enough to cause severe overdosage. A second safety mechanism that helps to minimize the risk of overdose is the maximum dose limit. Depending on the manufacturer, either a 1- or 4-hour lim-

itation in cumulative PCA dose can be set. The 1-hour maximum dosage has the advantage of warning if a pump runaway occurs. A pump runaway is a situation in which the pump continues to deliver drug beyond the dose programmed into the device.[11] The maximum dose limit may be eliminated for patients who have a high degree of opioid tolerance and for persons recovering from extremely painful procedures.

Incremental bolus size, delivery rate, and lockout interval are clinician-programmed functions of most PCA systems. Patients control only the frequency at which the boluses are given. The size of the incremental bolus should be large enough to make the *steady-state error* (patient's pain) as small as possible but not so large as to make the feedback system unstable.[12,13] Thus the choice of the size of the incremental bolus and the lockout interval depends mainly upon the kinetics of the particular drug employed.

Several PCA delivery options that have been approved by the Food and Drug Administration include incremental bolus on demand, incremental bolus on demand plus continuous (basal) infusion, and continuous infusion (Fig. 32-10). The most popular and simplest mode of patient-controlled administration is incremental bolus dose on demand. This dosing option is completely dependent on patient control and responds via preprogrammed dose and lockout interval. One major drawback to this system is that patients may awaken in severe pain because they cannot activate the system during periods of sleep.

Bolus dose on demand plus continuous infusion is usually employed when short-acting opioids such as fentanyl are prescribed; however, the addition of a basal infusion has also been advocated when longer acting analgesics are administered.[14] The demand plus continuous infusion mode provides a background (usually subtherapeutic) plasma concentration on top of which patient demands permit titration to an individualized MEAC.[15] The addition of a continuous infusion offers the theoretical advantage of allowing the patient to sleep without experiencing marked reductions in plasma opioid levels, thereby maintaining a concentration that is close to effective upon awakening. It also allows the bolus dose to be made smaller while increasing the interval between successive demands. A variation of the demand plus continuous infusion mode is the demand plus tail dose option offered by the Pharmacia Prominject PCA infuser.[15,16] A third continuous infusion option, not yet commercially available, is the patient-adjusted infusion system. This system uses a microprocessor to sense the number of demands made by the patient over a set time interval and then increases or decreases the infusion rate accordingly. One potential drawback of this system is that if a patient "revs up" the system to potential overdose levels, the time before the machine "senses" the delay may be prolonged, thereby increasing the likelihood of a severe overdose.[17] Another proposed option, similar to the adjustable infusion, is a patient-adjusted infusion plus incremental bolus doses on demand.

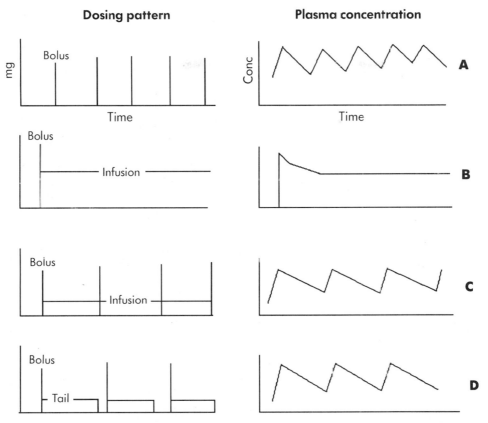

Fig. 32-10. Dosing patterns and plasma concentrations achieved with a variety of infusion options. The addition of either a basal infusion or a tail dose slows the decline in plasma concentration and lengthens the interval between demand boluses. **A,** Bolus dose on demand (PCA); **B,** continuous therapeutic infusion; **C,** bolus dose on demand plus basal infusion (PCA and BI); **D,** bolus dose on demand plus tail dose.

This option would also utilize microprocessor technology to "sense" the need of the patient by the number of demands made for medication. It would have the advantage of a faster response to increased pain needs but would also suffer from the same potential drawback as the adjustable infusion system.

In addition to the delivery modes discussed above, most modern pumps can be used in a continuous mode, which basically converts the pump from a PCA device to a simple positive displacement pump. This option allows the pump to be used for both epidural and subcutaneous infusions, or where the physician wishes fully to control systemic analgesic delivery. Using the systemic route, the simplest infusion regimen consists of a loading dose (to fill the volume in which the drug is initially distributed) followed by a constant infusion (to replace drug eliminated from the body). Infusion regimens ideally should be based on the drug's pharmacokinetics so that a desired drug concentration is achieved and maintained. Complex, pharmacokinetic-based regimes utilizing computer software are presently being developed, and these will facilitate the titration of the opioid to a plasma concentration specified by the physician and patient together.[17,18]

Many practical issues must be addressed when a patient-controlled analgesia system is considered. Mode of delivery, safety, availability of trained personnel, and adequacy of patient monitoring must all be considered. Box 32-2 outlines some important differences in the design and function among modern PCA infusion devices.

The power supply of a PCA system is an important consideration. If a system is primarily AC powered, back-up battery run time is the key specification to be addressed, especially when patients are transported off the floor for diagnostic testing. Ideally the back-up battery should provide power for 4 to 6 hours following AC disconnection, and the PCA prescription should be retained if the back-up battery charge is lost. Battery-powered PCA devices should retain power for at least 24 hours of operation at maximum current drain.

All PCA systems must have protection against accidental purging because of the large amount of drug that could potentially be infused into the patient. Nevertheless, the amount of drug available within the pump usually represents a compromise between potential safety in case of accidental overdose and the frequency with which the system must be refilled manually. Because modern PCA devices

Table 32-6. Specifications of selected PCA infusion devices

Device	Maker	Cost*	Specifications	Reservoir	Pump mechanism	Dosing modes	Flow rates
Lifecare PCA Classic	Abbott	$3450	14 lb, 8.25″ × 13.25″ × 6″ 120V AC internal rechargeable lead acid battery (8 hr) (pole-mounted)	Abbott 30-ml syringe, vial injector	Lead screw	PCA, bolus	1.0 ml/14 sec
Lifecare PCA Plus 4100	Abbott	$3750	14 lb, 8.25″ × 13.25″ × 6″ 120V AC internal rechargeable lead acid battery (8 hr) (pole-mounted)	Abbott 30-ml syringe, vial injector	Lead screw	PCA, bolus, CBI, CBI+, bolus	1.0 ml/14 sec continuous 0.5-10 ml dose
Lifecare PCA Plus II	Abbott	$3900	14 lb, 8.25″ × 13.25″ × 6″ 120V AC internal rechargeable lead acid battery (8 hr) (pole-mounted)	Abbott 30-ml syringe, vial injector	Lead screw	PCA, bolus, CBI, CBI+, bolus	1.0 ml/14 sec continuous 0.1-10 ml dose
Bard Harvard PCA	Bard	$3550	10 lb, 12.5″ × 10″ × 4.5″ 110/120V AC+ internal rechargeable lead acid battery (3 hr) (pole-mounted)	Standard 60-ml syringe, 50-ml prefilled syringe	Lead screw	PCA, CBI, PCA+ CBI	Bolus: 150 ml/hr CBI 0 to 9.9 ml/hr continuous 0.1-99.9 ml/hr
Bard Ambulatory PCA	Bard	$3095	11 oz; 4.75″ × 3.26″ × 1.2″ primary 9 V lithium, backup 3 V lithium (ambulatory)	100-ml or 250-ml reservoir	Linear peristaltic	PCA, CBI, PCA+ CBI	Bolus: 0-9.9 ml CBI: 0 to 20 ml/hr
PCA I	Bard	$3195	4.2 lb, 13.0″ × 6.3″ × 2.8″ four D-size alkaline batteries (pole-mounted)	Standard 60-ml syringe	Lead screw	PCA, CBI, PCA+ CBI	Bolus: 0-9.9 ml at 150 ml/hr CBI: 0-9.9 ml/hr
PCA II	Bard	$3795	4.2 lb, 13.0″ × 6.3″ × 2.8″ four D-size alkaline batteries or 110/120 V AC (pole-mounted)	Standard 60-ml syringe	Lead screw	PCA, CBI, PCA+ CBI	0.1-150 ml/hr depending on cartridge

Device	Manufacturer	Price*	Size/Power	Reservoir	Mechanism	Modes	Rate
IVAC PCA Infuser 310	IVAC	$3210	6 lb; 6.3" × 12" × 3" Four D-size alkaline batteries (pole-mounted)	Standard 20-, 30-, or 60-ml syringe	Lead screw	CBI, CBI+ bolus	1.0-60 ml/hr
Basal Bolus Infusor	Baxter	$40	3 oz; 8" × 1.5" chamber plus wristwatch style administrator, no battery (ambulatory)	60-ml balloon reservoir	Balloon internal pressure	CBI+ bolus	CBI:0.5 ml/hr bolus: 0.5 or 2.0 ml/hr
PCA Infusor	Baxter	$37	3 oz; 8" × 1.5" chamber plus wristwatch administrator, no battery (ambulatory)	60-ml balloon reservoir	Balloon internal pressure	PCA bolus only	2 ml/hr or 5 ml/hr preset
Graseby PCA	Graseby Medical	$3495	6 lb; 14.4" × 5" × 3.2" 110 V AC internal rechargeable battery (8 hr) (pole-mounted)	Standard 60-ml syringe or 30-ml prefilled	Lead screw	PCA, CBI, PCA+ CBI, loading	CBI: 0-20 ml/hr bolus: 10 μg/ml-99.5 mg
Provider	Abbott	$3000	14 oz; 5.2" × 3.4" × 1.3" 9 V lithium battery (ambulatory)	No captive reservoir, uses 250-500 ml bags	Eccentric rotor peristaltic	PCA, CBI, PCA+ CBI, Intermittent	CBI: 0.1-250 ml/hr
Stratofuse PCA Infuser	Strato Medical	$3900	3.8 lb; 14" × 3.31" × 7.06" 110/130 V AC modified to DC, internal rechargeable NiCad cells (6 hr) (pole-mounted)	Baxter 30-ml prefilled glass syringe or standard 50/60-ml syringe	Direct belt drive	PCA, CBI, PCA+ CBI	Bolus: 0.1-5.0 ml CBI: 0.1-10.0 ml/hr
Walkmed 430 PCA	Medfusion	$2695	12.75 oz; 1.8" × 4" × 4.5" 9 V alkaline battery (165 hr) (ambulatory)	Disposable 65-, 150- and 250-ml bags	Linear peristaltic	PCA, CBI, PCA+ CBI	Bolus: 0-1999 ml/hr CBI: 0.1-30.0 ml/hr
WalkMed 440 PIC	Medfusion	$3095	12.75 oz; 1.8" × 4" × 4.5" 9 V alkaline battery (165 hr) (ambulatory)	Disposable 65-, 150- and 250-ml bags	Linear peristaltic	PCA, CBI, Intermittent	Bolus: 0-1999 ml/hr CBI: 0.1-30.0 ml/hr
CADD PCA 5800	Pharmacia Deltec	$2995	15 oz; 1.1" × 3.5" × 6.3" 9 V alkaline battery (24 hr at 20 ml/hr) (ambulatory)	50- or 100-ml cassette reservoir with remote adapter	Linear peristaltic	PCA CBI PCA+ CBI	Bolus: 0-6 ml CBI: 0-20 ml/hr

*Prices and specifications are subject to change by the manufacturer.

Table 32-7. Special characteristics of selected PCA devices

Pump	Special features	Pros	Cons
Lifecare PCA Classic	Locked cover prevents access to programming controls and syringe Backlit LCD screen	Very easy to program Rugged and reliable	Large, heavy device Bolus mode only Requires Lifecare prefilled syringes
Lifecare PCA Plus 4100	Program: mg or ml Printer capability Key security access Backlit LCD screen	Prompts facilitate programming, continuous display of cumulative dose	Large, heavy device Requires Lifecare prefilled syringes
Lifecare PCA Plus II	Program: mg or ml Printer capability Key security access Backlit LCD screen	Prompts facilitate programming, continuous display of cumulative dose	Large, heavy device Expensive Requires Lifecare prefilled syringes
Bard PCA (Harvard)	Programmable in ml only Key and code security access Display: attempts versus injections and times Printer capability	Easy to program	Large, heavy device Short battery life Keyed access code may be discovered by the patient
Bard Ambulatory PCA	Program: mg or ml Display: TD, attempts versus injects Printer capability Key and code security access	Small size Backup battery Can be used for epidural infusions	Requires Bard tubing and reservoir sets Very fragile Key-Lock mechanism
PCA I	Dials for programming Backlit LCD screen Lockable pole mount Printer capability	Uses standard syringes Simple to program	Limited versatility in selecting operating parameters
PCA II	Backlit screen Lockable pole mount Printer capability Customization cartridge	Uses standard syringes Upgradable	Detachable 110/120 V AC cable connector is very fragile
IVAC PCA	Backlit screen Menu driven program 24-hr memory	Can use a variety of syringes 25-60 ml Dosing history saved for 99 hr	Programming in mg only
Basal Bolus Infusor	Tamper evident design Wristwatch dosing device	Simple Small No power source Disposable	Preset dose based on concentration Expensive Partial dose can be given within "lockout" Lockout interval 15 or 60 minutes only
PCA Infusor	Tamper evident design Wristwatch dosing device	Simple Small No power source Disposable	Preset dose based on concentration Expensive Partial dose can be given within "lockout" Lockout interval 2 or 5 min only
Graseby PCA	Program: mg or ml Display: TD Printer capability Key acess	Loading dose can be delivered over 5-15 minutes Uses standard syringes Unique remote	Not lockable to pole Small display screen
Provider	Program: ml or mg Optional reservoir "lock box"	Small size Lithium battery offers prolonged duration Can be used for epidural infusions	Requires expensive Abbott pump-tubing sets "Lockbox" is essential when infusing narcotics
Stratofuse PCA Infuser	Program: ml only On-board printer Key access	On-board printer Clinician controlled dosing capability	Can be programmed only in ml Expensive
Walkmed 430 PCA	Program: mg or ml Display: 24-hr history Optional access lock	Small size	9 V alkaline battery runs down quickly Lock levels are confusing
WalkMed 440 PIC	Program: mg or ml Display: 24-hr history Optional access lock	Small size	Same as the 430 PCA
CADD PCA 5800	Program: ml or mg Display: total dose, attempts, injects, key and code access	Small size Easy bolus	Lock levels plus code may be confusing

ards when prepared by either the nursing or pain service staff. The cost of preparation by the pharmacy, although initially more expensive, decreases as the number of syringes filled increases. Drug purchase expenses plus nursing or pharmacy preparation time must therefore be considered in the overall cost. Devices utilizing dedicated prefilled syringes are simple to set up and have less potential for errors in filling and risk of contamination, although the significant cost of the specialized administration sets ($7.00 per 30 mg Abbott morphine syringe) is usually passed on to the patient.

The advantages of prefilled syringes over hospital-filled syringes involve many variables, and the ultimate choice is dependent on the particular characteristics of the hospital. Usually, smaller pain services in community-based hospitals require a limited number of pumps and have lower PCA drug requirements. These smaller services may be best served by the purchase of prefilled syringes. Pain services requiring a large number of syringes may realize significant cost savings by having them prepared daily by a dedicated pharmacist. One advantage associated with the purchase of prefilled syringes and dedicated tubing sets is that a small surcharge added to the cost of these supplies will permit deferred purchase of the PCA device. Other options available for pump acquisition include outright purchase and leasing from either the manufacturer or medical supply companies. Features that should be considered prior to the purchase or lease of a PCA pump are presented in Box 32-3.

PCA pumps are positive displacement pumps that can be divided into two broad categories on the basis of their pumping mechanisms: peristaltic pumps and syringe

are designed to fail in a noninfusion mode (preventing a pump runaway) and incorporate antisiphon and backflow valves, overdosage related to pump malfunction is less likely. Although pumps are tested by the manufacturer prior to shipping, calibration and flow-rate checks should be performed upon delivery and every 6 months thereafter by the hospital's biomedical engineering staff.[11] In this regard, Bard MedSystems provides a miniinfusion calibrator to check the accuracy of delivery volumes.

The purchase of administration sets, drug reservoirs, prefilled syringes, and disposable batteries represents another important consideration in the evaluation of different PCA systems because these supplies will in time cost considerably more than the infusion pump itself. Devices utilizing standard syringes and IV tubing may appear to be more cost-effective but require a large time commitment, and they pose potential overdose and contamination haz-

pumps. Peristaltic pumps occlude and release specialized tubing sets in a distally migrating periodic pattern that propels boluses of fluid at a rate that is controlled by the microprocessor. These pumps may be rotary or linear, but all produce an intermittent flow pattern. With demand growing for smaller ambulatory PCA units, peristaltic pumps are becoming more prevalent.

As previously described, syringe-driven pumps deliver flow by means of a turning lead screw mechanism that forces the plunger into the barrel of a syringe reservoir. Many of the larger PCA pumps employ rotating lead screws, which provide accurate delivery while preventing free flow when the syringe or syringe-cartridge is being changed. Because drug delivery is limited to the volume of drug within the syringe (25 to 60 ml), the frequency of syringe changes may be excessive unless the drug is formulated in a concentrated solution.

PCA pumps may also be characterized as either nonambulatory (pole-mounted) or ambulatory devices. Ambulatory devices are small, lightweight, and battery powered. These devices are fragile, but they offer the following advantages: (1) A relatively large amount of drug may be stored in cassettes or pouches (enough drug may be loaded to satisfy the patient's entire postsurgical analgesic requirement; (2) the device is easily carried by the patient (in a belt or sling), therefore minimizing the need for an IV pole; and (3) the small size of the pump facilitates transport and storage. A potential disadvantage of ambulatory PCA devices is that in some hospital settings their small size may encourage tampering and theft.

Nonambulatory, or pole-mounted, pumps are usually larger and heavier than typical ambulatory devices and cannot be carried by the patient. These infusion pumps will permit effective ambulation provided that they are mounted on a freely movable IV pole. Nonambulatory pumps typically require a 110-V AC power supply and utilize drug-filled syringes that are secured within a locked chamber. Major advantages associated with nonambulatory pumps are: (1) Built-in rechargeable batteries eliminate costs associated with disposable batteries; and (2) the devices are far more robust and less likely to be damaged, tampered with, or stolen than are ambulatory pumps. The section that follows describes a number of commercially marketed pole-mounted and ambulatory PCA pumps. These devices have been evaluated with respect to security and ease of use. All were able to meet or exceed the industry standard for accuracy of delivery, alarm sensitivity, and electrical safety.[10]

COMMERCIALLY AVAILABLE PCA INFUSION DEVICES
Abbott LifeCare PCA Infuser "PCA Classic"

The LifeCare PCA Infuser* is a first-generation, FDA-approved device that was developed and successfully mar-

*Abbott Laboratories, North Chicago, Ill.

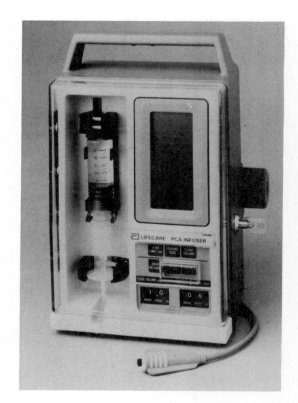

Fig. 32-11. Abbott LifeCare PCA Infuser "PCA Classic." (Photo courtesy of Abbott Labs, Abbott Park, Ill.)

keted in the United States (Fig. 32-11). Although the design is almost 8 years old, its ruggedness, reliability, and ease of use have ensured its continued popularity. The LifeCare Infuser is a full-size device that combines microprocessor and stepping motor technology and permits demand doses of opioids to be administered from specialized disposable syringe-cartridges. A locked security door prevents unauthorized access to both the drug cartridge and the thumbwheels that control dose and lockout interval. A liquid crystal display (LCD) indicates the total dose administered, the number of demand doses, and alarm messages. Minimum demand dose volume is 0.5 ml; the 4-hour maximum dose volume is 30 ml. The device is powered by 110-V AC and has an 8 hour back-up battery. Available prefilled 30-ml cartridges include morphine 1 mg/ml, morphine 5 mg/ml, and meperidine 10 mg/ml. Unfilled cartridges are also available for preparation by the pharmacy. A specialized connection tubing set that incorporates a one-way check valve must be used for proper Infuser function.

Abbott LifeCare PCA Plus 4100 and LifeCare PCA Plus II

The Abbott LifeCare Plus 4100 and the LifeCare PCA Plus II* are full-size devices representative of "state of the art" second-generation PCA infusers (Fig. 32-12). The

*Abbott Laboratories, North Chicago, Ill.

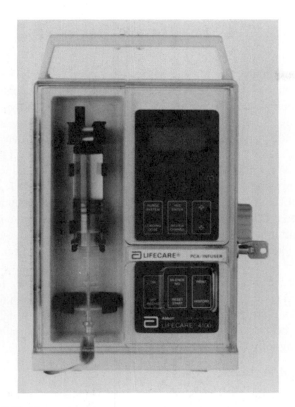

Fig. 32-12.   Abbott LifeCare PCA Plus 4100. (Photo courtesy of Abbott Labs, Abbott Park, Ill.)

basic mechanism of their operation and that of other PCA devices is illustrated in Fig. 32-13. The PCA Plus devices incorporate powerful microprocessors and LCD and light emitting diode (LED) features. The operator is guided by a self-prompting LCD, which facilitates programming and understanding of various alarms. To initiate the use of the PCA Plus devices, the user places the specialized drug cartridge into a spring-loaded connector, purges the syringe, and then selects the drug to be used from a display menu (either morphine 1 mg/ml, morphine 5 mg/ml, meperidine 10 mg/ml, or other drug). The user must then decide on one of three modes of therapy: (a) PCA only (patient activated demand), (b) continuous mode (continuous "basal" infusion), and (c) combined PCA plus continuous mode (patient activated demands plus continuous infusion). The PCA demand dose (0.5 ml minimum with PCA Plus, 0.1 ml minimum with PCA Plus II), lockout interval (5 to 99 minutes), and 4-hour maximum dose (30 mg morphine, 300 mg meperidine) limits are then set. The Plus II permits both milligram-based, and microgram-based dosing. Both infusers continually display cumulative dose administered, offer 1-hour and 24-hour patient history (mg delivered, attempts, doses) and can provide a 12-hour hard copy of PCA dosing via an optional printer. Each is powered by 110-V AC and contains an 8-hour back-up battery. Drug cartridges and

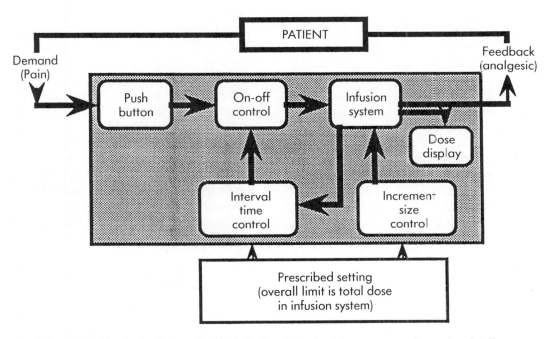

Fig. 32-13.   The basic design of a PCA device. The physician programs the mode of delivery (i.e., incremental bolus, incremental bolus plus infusion) as well as the prescription (i.e., drug, dose size, interval between doses, maximum dose). The patient then interacts with the device using a control button.

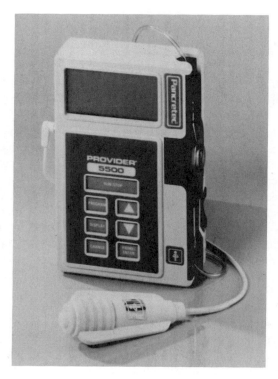

Fig. 32-14. Abbott LifeCare Provider 5500. (Photo courtesy of Abbott Labs, Abbott Park, Ill.)

specialized tubing sets are identical to those utilized by the LifeCare PCA "Classic" infuser.

Abbott LifeCare Provider 5500

The Abbott LifeCare Provider 5500* is a versatile ambulatory infuser that utilizes a disposable 9-V extended-duration lithium battery and can accommodate a 500-ml external reservoir bag (Fig. 32-14). An optional reservoir lock box is available for use with opioid solutions. The pump unit weighs only 14 ounces, has a maximum delivery rate of 250 ml/hr, and is FDA-approved for both intravenous and epidural administration. It is programmable in mg or ml and has four modes of operation: PCA, basal, PCA plus basal, and intermittent dosing. The Provider employs a unique microcomputer-controlled eccentric-rotor pump that is built into the disposable tubing set. This pumping mechanism insures precise dosing and overcomes the high resistance to flow of epidural catheters. The expense of these specialized pump and tubing sets should be factored into the overall cost of operation.

Bard (Harvard) PCA Infuser

The Bard (Harvard) Infuser,† a large, first-generation, FDA approved PCA device, has been marketed since 1985. This device represented the first modern PCA pump

*Abbott Laboratories, North Chicago, Ill.
†Bard MedSystems Division, C.R. Bard, Inc., North Reading, Mass.

offering flexibility in dosing, including PCA bolus, continuous infusion, and PCA bolus plus continuous infusion. The infuser is microprocessor controlled and utilizes a lead screw-stepper motor mechanism to empty a self-contained 60-ml syringe. A three-digit code typed into the control panel enables the operator to gain access to the programming prompts. Programming is relatively straightforward; an alphanumeric LCD control panel provides guidance. The LCD reviews the patient's history, including total dose administered, injections, and attempted injections. The pump can deliver a minimum PCA bolus of 0.1 ml and has a maximum flow rate of 99.9 ml/hr in continuous mode. It lacks the ability to be programmed in mg/ml concentrations. The syringe chamber has a tamper-proof cover and key access, and the device itself is locked to a specialized IV pole. The infuser is powered by 110-V AC source and has a 3-hour battery backup. An optional printer for hard copy of patient information is available. Although the device utilizes standard 60-ml syringes that are filled by the hospital, a prefilled 50-ml syringe containing morphine 1 mg/ml is available from the manufacturer.

Bard PCA I and PCA II

The Bard PCA I and PCA II infusers* are moderately sized pole-mounted, lead screw-driven syringe pumps that run on battery or 110-V AC power (Fig. 32-15). The PCA I can be programmed in three modes: PCA, continuous basal infusion, and PCA plus continuous basal infusion, by way of three dials mounted on the face plate. PCA dose, delay (lockout interval), and basal infusion rate are restricted to the values displayed on the face plate. Its LCD is backlit and provides patient history, cumulative dose, injections, and attempted injections. The PCA I utilizes four disposable (D size) alkaline batteries that provide power for 30 days.

PCA II is an updated "state of the art" contemporary of the PCA I. This device, expected to gain FDA approval in 1992, offers a number of advances, including simplified menu-driven programming, increased flexibility, and upgradability. The device may be powered by D size alkaline batteries or 110-V AC and can be programmed in milligrams or milliliters, and in three different infusion modes. The AC power cord can be detached from the pump in order to facilitate patient ambulation. The PCA II will employ snap-in type of microprocessor cartridges designed to provide customized menus, dosing options, and future upgrade capability; all of these features should minimize obsolescence.

Bard Ambulatory PCA

The Bard Ambulatory PCA,* a battery operated, linear peristaltic action, ambulatory infusion pump, is one of the smallest units presently on the market (Fig. 32-16).

*Bard MedSystems Division, C.R. Bard, Inc., North Reading, Mass.

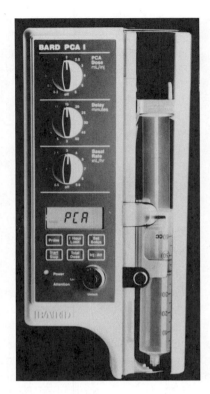

Fig. 32-15. Bard PCA I infuser. (Photo courtesy of Bard, Medical Systems Division, North Reading, Mass.)

Weighing only 11 ounces, it is FDA-approved for both intravenous and epidural applications. Like larger models offered by Bard, the device is microprocessor-controlled, menu-driven, and programmable in three modes (PCA, PCA plus continuous basal infusion, and continuous infusion). Access to programming is via a three-digit security code and prescriptions may be entered in milliliters or milligrams. PCA bolus size ranges from 0 to 9.9 ml, and maximum continuous infusion rate is 20 ml/hr. An LCD provides patient history of total milliliters delivered, injections, and attempted injections. The pump has a tamper-proof cover with key access to the self-contained drug reservoir. Reservoir pouches of 100 and 250 ml are presently available, and a 500-ml bag designed for continuous epidural infusions will soon be released. The device utilizes 9-V alkaline and lithium batteries for pump operation and a 3-V lithium back-up battery that maintains the program if the primary batteries should fail. An optional printer is also available.

Graseby Patient-Controlled Analgesia System (PCAS)

The Graseby PCAS* is a medium-sized, pole-mounted device that utilizes lead-screw driven pump technology and uses standard 60-ml syringes. It can be programmed in mass units (10μg to 99.5 mg/hr) but not in milliliters and

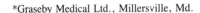

*Graseby Medical Ltd., Millersville, Md.

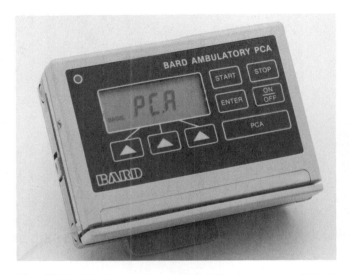

Fig. 32-16. Bard Ambulatory PCA. (Photo courtesy of Bard, Medical Systems Division, North Reading, Mass.)

has the added feature of programming the size and length of time over which a loading dose may be given. Dosing options include PCA bolus doses and a "background" continuous infusion of up to 20 ml/hr. The PCAS employs a unique air-driven demand button that is less likely to be mistaken for a nurse call button and poses no electrical hazard to the patient. The device is powered by 110-V AC and contains an 8-hour battery backup. Its LCD gives the patient's history of injections and attempted injections and a constant display of total drug given. An optional printer can be attached to the unit to provide a hard copy of the PCA history.

IVAC PCA Infuser 310

The IVAC PCA Infuser 310* is an updated version of the Becton-Dickinson PCA infuser. It is a medium-sized, pole-mounted, lead screw-driven, syringe pump. The device offers great flexibility in syringe choice, and its locking chamber can accommodate standard 20-, 30-, and 60-ml plastic syringes. The LCD guides the operator through the programming procedure with step-by-step alphanumeric prompts. The device stores in memory a 24-hour history of PCA use. This history is maintained for up to 99 hours after the pump is turned off. The IVAC PCA is programmable in milligrams per milliliter, and drug may be infused via three different dosing options: PCA, continuous mode, and PCA plus continuous mode. The pump unit weighs 6 lb, has a maximum flow rate of 60 ml/hr, and can run for 400 hours on four D-size alkaline batteries.

Pharmacia CADD PCA 5800

The Pharmacia CADD PCA 5800† is a battery-powered, linear-peristaltic driven, ambulatory pump that uses cassette

*IVAC Corporation, San Diego, Calif.
†Pharmacia Deltec Inc., St. Paul, Minn.

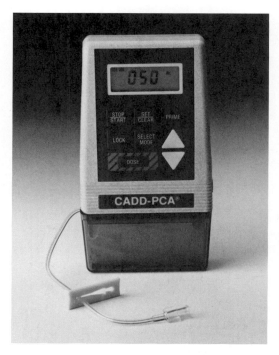

Fig. 32-17. Pharmacia Deltec CADD PCA 5800. (Photo courtesy of Pharmacia Deltec Inc., St. Paul, Minn.)

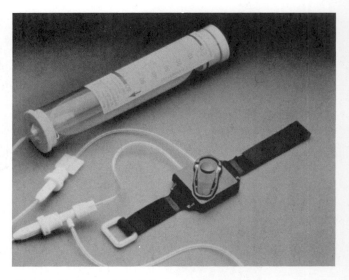

Fig. 32-18. Baxter PCA Infusor system. (Photo courtesy of Baxter Healthcare Inc., Deerfield, Ill.)

reservoirs or can be adapted to use a remote reservoir (Fig. 32-17). The pump unit weighs only 15 ounces and is powered by a 9-V alkaline or lithium battery. It is programmable in milliliters or milligrams and has three modes of operation: PCA, basal, and PCA plus basal. It has a maximum delivery rate of 20 ml/hr in continuous mode. In addition, a clinician-activated bolus can be instituted within any mode. The device utilizes three different lock levels and a three-digit security code to access dosing prompts and history. The different lock levels make the device more difficult to program than pumps utilizing menu-driven prompts; however, they provide safety and greater flexibility in patient dosing, which is ideal for home PCA therapy. For example, in lock level 1 the patient can adjust the continuous rate and patient activated dose within limits set by the clinician.

Stratofuse PCA

The Stratofuse PCA* is a medium-sized, pole-mounted, lead screw action, syringe pump that uses standard 60-ml syringes or prefilled 30-ml glass syringes. Programming is simple and direct: the LCD control panel guides the operator with setup, operation, and history. Dosage is programmed in milliliters only. The device permits three modes of operation: PCA bolus, continuous infusion, and clinician-controlled bolus. The PCA mode can be used in conjunction with clinician boluses and continuous infu-

sions. The minimum incremental dose volume is 0.1 ml, and the maximum continuous rate is 10 ml/hr. The device contains a rechargeable battery with approximately 4 hours of operating life and requires specialized Baxter administration sets. Most notably the Stratofuse PCA has an onboard printer, which yields hardcopy of the patient's drug history with corresponding times. Prefilled 30-ml glass syringes containing morphine 1 mg/ml are available from Baxter.

PCA Infusor System and Basal-Bolus Infusor System

The PCA Infusor and the more recently developed Basal-Bolus Infusor* represent a fundamentally different approach to PCA technology (Fig. 32-18). The units are totally disposable and thus do not require a large capital expenditure.[19] These systems are self-powered through a balloon reservoir and have no programmability. With the PCA Infusor, patients activate a 0.5-ml bolus via a wristwatch type of control module. The amount of medication available to the patient is controlled by the concentration of the drug in the system and the rate of infusion. The lockout interval, which is the time required to fill the 0.5-ml reservoir, cannot be changed and can be partially overridden. A patient who activates the demand button within the lockout period will receive the amount of medication that has accumulated in the 0.5-ml reservoir. The Basal Bolus Infusor has the same mechanism of action but adds continuous basal infusion (Fig. 32-19). Although these devices are inexpensive (ranging from $30 to $40 each), the fact that they can be used on one patient only suggests that long-term costs per patient treated may be greater than that of a typical infusion pump.

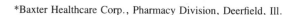

*Baxter Healthcare Corp., Pharmacy Division, Deerfield, Ill.

*Baxter Healthcare Corp. I.V. Systems Division, Deerfield, Ill.

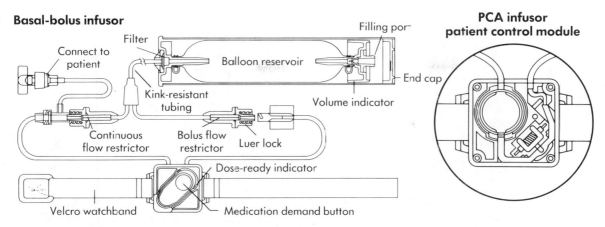

Basal-bolus infusor

**PCA infusor
patient control module**

Connect to patient — Filter — Balloon reservoir — Filling port — End cap — Volume indicator — Kink-resistant tubing — Continuous flow restrictor — Bolus flow restrictor — Luer lock — Dose-ready indicator — Velcro watchband — Medication demand button

Fig. 32-19. A schematic of the Baxter Basal-Bolus infusor. (Diagram courtesy of Baxter Healthcare Inc., Deerfield, Ill.)

The WalkMed 430 PCA and 440 PIC

The WalkMed 430 PCA and 440 PIC* devices are battery-operated, peristaltic-action, ambulatory PCA pumps that utilize disposable reservoirs. The pump requires a 9-V alkaline battery, and the reservoir bags range in size from 65 to 250 ml. The units weigh only 12.75 ounces and are programmable in milligrams or milliliters. Both units have a maximum flow rate of 30 ml/hr in continuous mode. The WalkMed devices employ a number of visual and audible alarms, including a highly effective occlusion alarm. The 430 has two modes of operation: PCA and continuous. The 440 also has an intermittent mode. Access to programming is similar to that of the CADD-PCA and employs two lock levels and a three digit code.

The development of new drug delivery systems has provided marked improvements in pain management by allowing our present knowledge of pharmacology, psychology, physiology, and pathophysiology to be incorporated into management regimens. Patient-controlled analgesia systems have, over the last 10 years, evolved from their limited role in clinical research to become powerful tools for the control of postoperative and chronic pain. Continued refinement of PCA technology will further improve analgesic efficacy, patient safety, and cost effectiveness.

*Medfusion, Inc., Duluth, Ga.

REFERENCES

1. Emergency Care Research Institute: Infusion controllers, *Health Devices* 14:219-257, 1985.
2. Rithhalia SV, Rozkovec A: Evaluation of a simple device for regulating intravenous infusions, *Intensive Care Med* 5:41-43, 1979.
3. Kwan, JW: High-technology i.v. infusion devices, *Am J Hosp Pharm* 46:320-325, 1989.
4. Emergency Care Research Institute: Infusion pumps, *Health Devices* 13:31-62, 1984.
5. Emergency Care Research Institute: Syringe infusion pumps, *Health Devices* 16:3-30, 1987.
6. Emergency Care Research Institute: Inspection and preventive maintenance of infusion pumps, *Health Devices* 4:217-221, 1975.
7. Austin KL, Stapleton JV, Mather LE: Relationships between blood meperidine concentration and analgesic response, *Anesthesiology* 53:460-466, 1980.
8. Hull CJ: *The pharmacokinetics of opioid analgesia, with special reference to PCA*. In Harmer M, Rosen M, Vickers MD, editors: *Patient controlled analgesia*, Oxford, 1984, Blackwell Scientific, pp 8-17.
9. Graves DA, Foster TS, Batenhorst RL, et al: Patient-controlled analgesia, *Ann Intern Med* 99:360-366, 1983.
10. Emergency Care Research Institute: Patient controlled analgesia infusion pumps, *Health Devices* 17:137-167, 1988.
11. Kreitzer JM, Kirshenbaum LA, Eisenkraft JB: Safety of PCA devices, *Anesthesiology* 70:881, 1989 (letter).
12. Harmer M, Rosen M, Vickers MD: Patient controlled analgesia. Proceedings of the first international workshop on patient controlled analgesia 1:11-12, 1985.
13. Jacobs OL, Bullingham RE: *Modelling, estimation and control for demand analgesia*. In Harmer M, Rosen M, Vickers MD, editors: *Patient controlled analgesia*, Oxford, 1984, Blackwell Scientific, pp 57-72.
14. Sinatra RS, Chung KS, Silverman DG, et al: An evaluation of morphine and oxymorphone administered via PCA or PCA plus basal infusion in postcesarean patients, *Anesthesiology* 71:502-507, 1989.
15. Tamsen A, Hartvig P, Dahlstrom B, et al: Patient-controlled analgesic therapy in the early postoperative period, *Acta Anaesthesiol Scand* Suppl 74:157-160, 1982.
16. Tamsen A: *The Prominject*. In Harmer M, Rosen M, Vickers MD, editors: *Patient controlled analgesia*, Oxford, 1984, Blackwell Scientific, pp 92-93.
17. Hill HF: *Pharmacokinetic tailoring of computer-controlled alfentanil infusions*. In Krobeth PD, Smith RB, Juhl RP, editors: *Pharmacokinetics and pharmacodynamics, vol 2, Current problems, potential solutions*, Cincinnati, 1988, Harvey Whitney.
18. Hill HF, Jacobson RC, Coda BA, et al: A computer-based system for controlling plasma opioid concentration according to patient need for analgesia, *Clin Pharmacokinet* 20:319-330, 1991.
19. Wermeling DP, Foster TS, Rapp RP, et al: Evaluation of a disposable nonelectronic PCA device for postoperative pain, *Clin Pharm* 6:307-314, 1987.

Chapter 33

FUTURE DIRECTIONS IN ANESTHESIA APPARATUS

Leslie Rendell-Baker, M.D.

The change in intensive care unit (ICU) ventilators from the mechanical Engström of 1955 to the modern, entirely electronic, Puritan Bennett 7200, point the way for a similar change in anesthesia apparatus, the basic design of which has not changed in 30 years.

Milestones along the way are listed below:

1976: The microprocessor-controlled prototype Boston Anesthesia System included electronic gas-flow control, jet vaporizer, machine monitoring, and message/alarm system.

1986: The Engström Elsa was in production; this followed the same basic design as the Boston apparatus.

1982-1988: Dräger (Lubeck) designs for electronic apparatus demonstrated that digital measurement improved the accuracy necessary for precise control of closed system anesthesia.

1989: The prototype microprocessor-controlled apparatus of Sykes, et al. further explored electronic control methods.

1989: The Prototype Utah Anesthesia Workstation of Westenskow, et al. demonstrated effective servo loop control of an anesthesia apparatus via a Macintosh Plus computer.

1990: The Dutch PhysioFlex production microprocessor ventilator-closed system anesthesia apparatus effectively culminates these developments. This apparatus will require certain safety features for safe use. International Standards Organization (ISO) and European Community (CEN) safety standards are currently being developed.

PRESENT-DAY DESIGNS

The basic design of present-day anesthesia apparatus has changed little since the 1930s, when Richard Salt, with encouragement from Professor Robert Macintosh, introduced the rotameter flowmeter into anesthesia practice[1-4] and later in 1957 when Cyprane* introduced the

*Yorkshire, U.K.

674

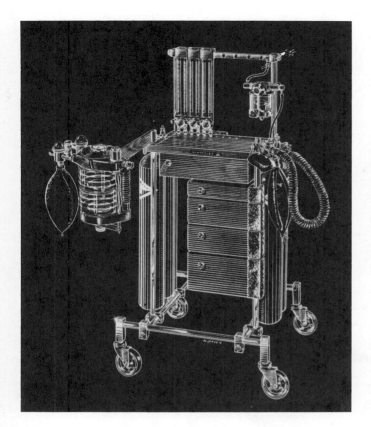

Fig. 33-1. The Fraser Sweatman Quantiflex Anesthesia Machine of 1964 displayed the essentials of a present-day apparatus: rotameter flowmeters, a temperature-compensated variable bypass Fluotec vaporizer, and large-capacity carbon dioxide absorption canister. Although there is a total absence of current electronic monitoring equipment, it is otherwise essentially the same as the latest machine of the 1990s (shown in Fig. 33-4). (From Fraser Sweatman Inc. advertisement in *Anesthesiology*, 21:1, Jan-Feb 1964.)

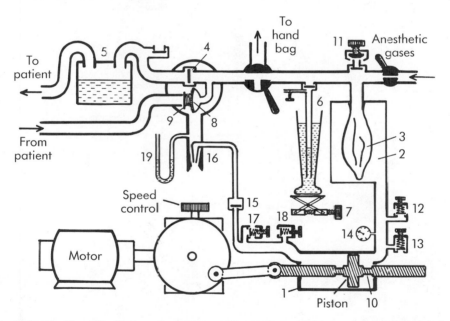

Fig. 33-2. The Engström Universal ventilator of the 1950s was driven and controlled entirely by mechanical means. The large piston in the reciprocating pump (*1*) provided the force necessary to deliver the gases from the reservoir bag (*3*) to the patient's lungs. The tidal volume was determined by the quantity of gas in the bag (*3*) and the respiratory rate by the speed control. The safety valve (*6*) controlled the maximum pressure exerted. (*2*) Rigid plastic pressure chamber; (*4*) one-way valve; (*5*) humidifier; (*6*) water manometer (with one-way valve and slow leak) indicating positive pressure and acting as a safety valve; (*7*) safety blow-off control; (*8*) rubber diaphragm; (*9*) expiratory valve; (*10*) pressure release groove; (*11*) air inlet control; (*12*) valve limiting positive pressure in pressure chamber (*2*); (*13*) valve limiting negative pressure in pressure chamber (*2*); (*14*) manometer; (*15*) one-way valve; (*16*) injector; (*17*) control for adjusting negative pressure applied to patient during the expiratory phase; (*18*) air-inlet valve to cylinder; (*19*) water manometer indicating pressure in the patient circuit during the expiratory phase. (Illustration from Mushin WW, Rendell-Baker L, Thompson PW: *Automatic ventilation of the lungs,* ed 1, Oxford, 1965, Blackwell, Fig. 51, p 126.)

temperature-compensated Fluotec vaporizer. The currently used circle carbon dioxide absorption breathing system introduced by Brian Sword[5] in 1926 has essentially not changed since it was improved by James Elam and his colleagues in 1958. These components fitted together formed an anesthesia machine of the 1960s era (see Fig. 33-1) and are still recognizable as the basis of present-day apparatus. The main difference is that there was no present-day monitoring equipment.

It is instructive to compare the great changes that have taken place in the design of ICU ventilators with those that have been made in the design of the anesthesia apparatus. When the entirely mechanically driven and controlled Engström ventilator of the 1950s (Fig. 33-2) is compared with the all-electronic Puritan Bennett 7200ae ventilator of today (Fig. 33-3), the extent of the electronic revolution is clear. By comparison, the basic design of anesthesia apparatus has changed little during this time; only the monitoring devices show the influence of electronics (Fig. 33-4). The gas flows are still indicated by rotameter or ball flowmeters with an accuracy of ±10%. The volatile agents are still delivered from temperature-compensated variable-bypass vaporizers similar to those of the 1957 Fluotec, which had an accuracy of ±15% at fresh-gas flow rates of 4 to 10 L/min.

These cumbersome flowmeters and vaporizers are usually mounted on the back of the apparatus. This makes it necessary for the user to turn at least 90° from the patient to check the apparatus. Such an arrangement is not acceptable in an aircraft, where the pilot must be able simultaneously to observe the instruments and the glide path into the airport while landing the aircraft.

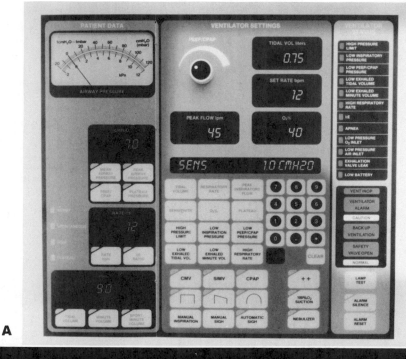

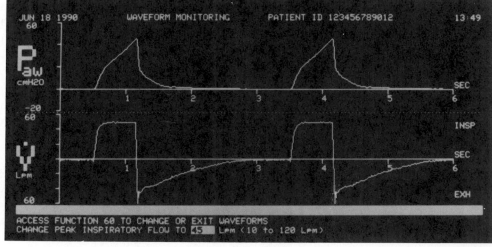

Fig. 33-3. For legend see opposite page.

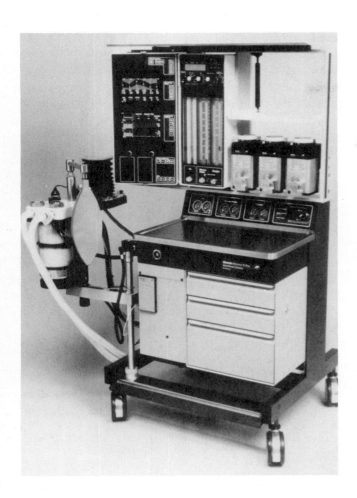

Fig. 33-4. The Ohmeda Modulus CD (Central Display) Anesthesia Apparatus of 1991 has flowmeters, vaporizers, and an absorber similar to those of the Quantiflex apparatus from the mid 1960s. However, a complete panel of electronic monitoring devices and an electronically controlled ventilator have been added. A convenient space has been left on the upper-right portion of the apparatus for additional monitoring equipment. (Illustration courtesy Ohmeda, a Division of BOC Healthcare Inc., Madison, Wis.)

Fig. 33-3. A, The 1990 Puritan Bennett 7200ae ventilator with graphic display. The control panel is color-coded and divided into several sections. On the left is the green Patient Data section, which displays the airway pressure, the *I:E* ratio, respiratory rate, and the tidal and minute volumes. The central, blue section displays the setting of the ventilator and the alarm status. The setting keys are arranged from the top down in a logical order, to set tidal volume, respiratory rate, peak inspiratory flow, sensitivity, oxygen percentage, and plateau pressure. These are followed by the alarm settings. The three choices for the breathing pattern are next: CMV, SIMV, and CPAP, with a choice of three different wave forms: square wave, descending ramp wave, and sine wave. On the right-hand panel are the Ventilator Status Indicators. *NORMAL-green* indicates normal function, *CAUTION-yellow* indicates an error condition corrected. *VENTILATOR ALARM-red* indicates an uncorrected error in the ventilator operation or patient setting. The alarm indicators above indicate the nature of the problem. This ventilator is supplied with a display panel that can display menu options for the operator or display messages requiring the operator's attention. When the power is turned on, the ventilator checks both the electronics and the microprocessor to determine that they are functioning properly. It then checks for leaks in the patient breathing system before indicating it is ready for duty. **B,** The display panel can be used to show pressure, flow, or volume loops, thus permitting analysis of the ventilator's function and the patient's respiratory status. (Illustrations courtesy of Puritan Bennett.)

FUTURE DESIGNS OF APPARATUS

Boston Anesthesia System

The prototype Boston Anesthesia System,[6] introduced in 1976, was the first to herald future developments (Fig. 33-5). In their design, Cooper, et al.[6] sought to exploit the benefit of electronics and incorporated good human factors engineering to simplify the user's task. On this apparatus, the flows of the gases and the concentration of vapors were indicated by illuminated bar graphs on the display panel (Fig. 33-6). The gas flow settings were changed by "increment/decrement" switches located below each illuminated bar graph. The gas flow was controlled by opening solenoid controlled orifices of known resistance in an 8-orifice flow-control unit. The gases were supplied at a constant pressure of 50 psig so that each calibrated orifice delivered a known flow of gas. Each orifice delivered twice the flow of the one below it in the sequence. The smallest orifice delivered a flow rate of 49 ml/min. The maximum flow rate with all orifices open was 12.7 L/min. In this system there were no moving parts to get out of calibration and no

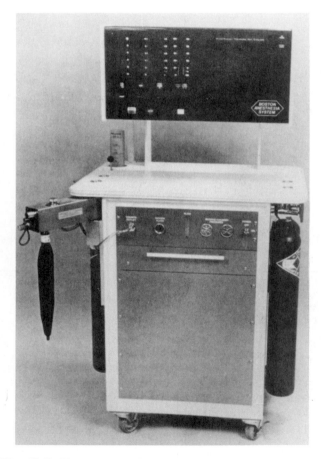

Fig. 33-5. The prototype Boston Anesthesia System of 1976 used electronic controls for gas and vapor delivery. All functions were controlled by a microprocessor. (Illustration from Cooper JB, Newbower RS, Moore JW, et al: A new anesthesia delivery system, *Anesthesiology* 49: 310-318, 1978.)

needle valves that might wear. A small rotameter flowmeter was placed in the center of the front panel of the cabinet to reassure the skeptical user of the total gas flowing.

For vaporizing potent volatile anesthetics, this machine utilized a device similar to a Bosch automotive fuel injector. This device controlled a solenoid-operated valve that delivered pulses of liquid anesthetic of precise volume into the circuit. The pulse frequency controlled the concentration of vapor delivered to the circuit. The apparatus was controlled by an INTEL 880 microprocessor (Fig. 33-7), which interpreted the commands from the control console and displayed these settings along with the actual measured values. It also displayed alarms if any unsafe or inappropriate conditions resulted from errors by either the apparatus or the user. The flat control panel could be detached from the base and mounted in any convenient location.

Although the Boston Anesthesia System represented a major step forward with its centralized alarms and messages, it was still left to the user to take the necessary corrective action. There was no feedback control mechanism to correct a problem before it developed. A rechargeable battery provided back-up power, because the flow of gases and anesthetic vapor were completely dependent on an available power supply. The emergency oxygen flush control was mechanical and could be used to provide life-support oxygen if all power supplies failed.

Engström Elsa

Although the principles of the Boston Anesthesia System were demonstrated in detail to all anesthesia equipment manufacturers in the United States, none of them adopted any of its design features in their own apparatus. However, Professor O.P. Norlander[7] of Stockholm was extremely impressed with the design and eventually persuaded the Engström Company to develop an apparatus based on the Boston design. This appeared in 1986 and was given the name Engström Elsa (Fig. 33-8). Unlike the original Boston design, the Engström design retained needle valves to control the gas flow, so that in the event that the electrical power failed, the gas flow could still be controlled. Each dot on the scale around the control knobs represented approximately 3 L/min of gas flow. In this design, the needle valve controls the flow and a hot wire anemometer measures the flow, which is then displayed on the control panel as a bar graph (Fig. 33-9). Alarm levels can be set for the airway pressure, minute volume, anesthetic agent, carbon dioxide, and oxygen. The apparatus is not provided with a battery back-up power source.

The upper panel (Fig. 33-8) has the monitor displays for fresh-gas flow, expired minute volume or tidal volume, airway pressure, inspired or fresh gas oxygen concentration, inspired or end-tidal carbon dioxide, and fresh gas or inspired anesthetic concentration. There is also a window for display of messages and alarms. All the key compo-

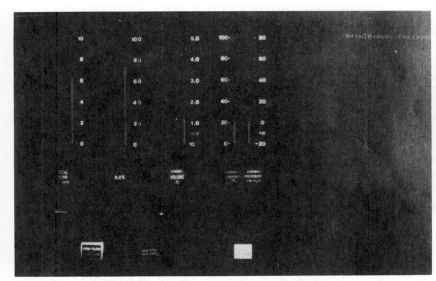

Fig. 33-6. The Boston Anesthesia System's electronic display and control panel. The electronic bar graphs are color-coded; reading from left to right they indicate total gas flow in L/min (white), percentage nitrous oxide (blue), percentage of enflurane being delivered (red), the expired oxygen percentage, and the airway pressure in cm H_2O. On the right side of the panel, messages are displayed drawing attention to possible problems with the patient or apparatus. (Illustration from Cooper JB, Newbower RS, Moore JW, et al: A new anesthesia delivery system, *Anesthesiology* 49:310-318, 1978.)

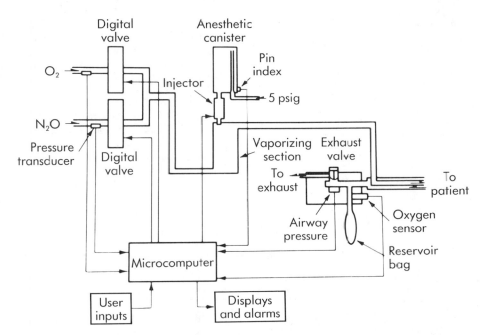

Fig. 33-7. Diagram of the Boston Anesthesia System illustrating how the electronic digital valves and various sensors are connected to the microprocessor. (Illustration from Cooper JB, Newbower RS, Moore JW, et al: A new anesthesia delivery system, *Anesthesiology* 49:310-318, 1978.)

nents of the breathing system are incorporated into an easily detachable "patient cassette," which may be autoclaved. The Engström Elsa's design did not incorporate any servo-controlled feedback loop controls to assist the user's tasks.

Liquid anesthetic agents in their original bottles (Fig. 33-10) are attached to the back of the apparatus by specially keyed caps that prevent misconnection of the agents. These caps are also fitted with electronic sensors that indicate on the front panel the level of liquid in the bottle. When the vaporizer control knob is turned on, driving gas

at a constant pressure enters the bottle, which delivers the agent to a vaporizing chamber that is maintained at a constant temperature. Delivery of vapor from the chamber is controlled by a magnetic valve that pulsates to permit the pressure of the driving gas to deliver known quantities of anesthetic vapor into the fresh gas supply (Fig. 33-11). The faster the pulsation rate, the more vapor that is delivered. The concentration of the volatile agent can be monitored at any of these points within the breathing system as desired. This mechanism is again based upon the same principle as that used in the Bosch fuel injection systems.

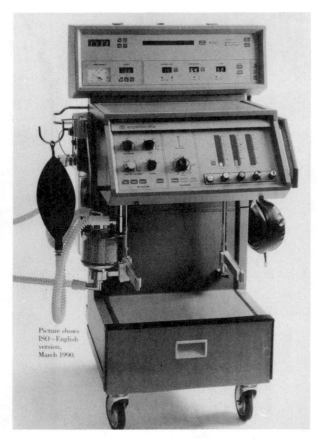

Fig. 33-8. The Engström Elsa microprocessor-controlled electronic anesthesia apparatus of 1986. (Illustration courtesy of the Gambro Engström Company, Bromma, Sweden.)

Fig. 33-9. Engström Elsa control panel. On the right are the control knobs for the gases, *(3)* air, *(4)* nitrous oxide, and *(5)* oxygen, above which are the electronic bar graphs showing the flows measured by the hot wire anemometers. Above the bar graphs are the alarm controls for high and low carbon dioxide and oxygen levels. In the center of the panel are controls for the vaporizers: *(8)* selects either halothane, enflurane, or isoflurane; *(9)* controls the percentage vapor concentration in the fresh-gas flow; and *(10)* shows the level of agent in the bottle. At the top of the panel are the alarm controls for high and low levels of the anesthetic agent. On the left are the ventilator controls; *(15)* tidal volume; *(16)* respiratory rate, and *(12)* I:E ratio. *(14)* PEEP or inspiratory assistance; and *(13)* selects either CMV, EMMV, or spontaneous respiration. Above these are the alarm controls for the high and low airway pressure and minute volume. (Illustration from Engström Elsa user's instruction manual, courtesy of Gambro Engström AB, Bromma, Sweden.)

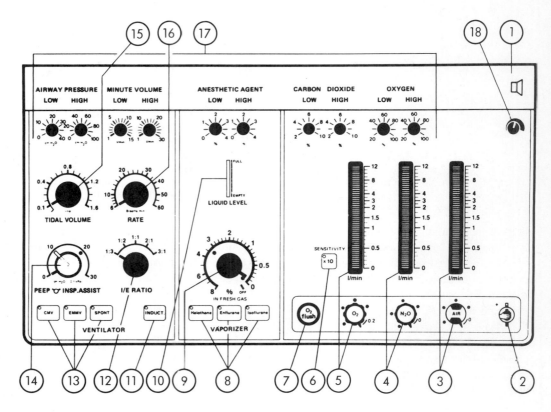

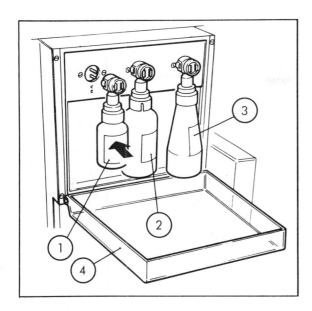

Fig. 33-10. Liquid volatile anesthetic agents in their original bottles attached to the back of the Engström Elsa. Screw-on indexed caps prevent erroneous connection. *1*, *2* and *3* are agent specific bottles containing isoflurane, halothane and enflurane, respectively. *4* is a hinged protective cover for the three bottles of agents. (Illustration from Engström Elsa user's instruction manual, courtesy of Gambro Engström AB, Bromma, Sweden.)

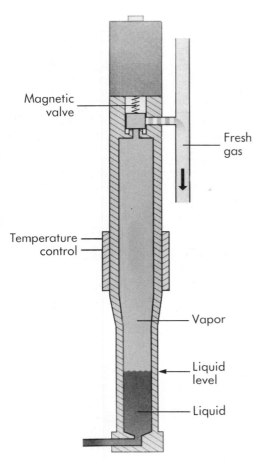

Fig. 33-11. Engström Elsa vaporizer mechanism. Liquid anesthetic is forced into the heated vaporizing chamber by the pressure of the driving gas. The normally closed magnetic valve opens in a pulsatile fashion, permitting measured quantities of 100% concentration of anesthetic vapor to pass into the fresh gas stream. The quantity of vapor released into the breathing system is determined by the pulsation frequency. (Illustration from Engström Elsa user's instruction manual, courtesy of Gambro Engström AB, Bromma, Sweden.)

The Elsa was specifically designed to facilitate closed circuit anesthesia with volatile agents. Reviewing their 2 years of experience with six of these machines, Alexander, et al.[8] stated that, "Once familiarization was achieved, the machines proved easy to operate and are particularly satisfactory when used with low fresh gas flows." After 1½ to 2 years' use without routine service, the flowmeter and vaporizer outputs and monitor readings of their machines were checked (see Table 33-1). They noted some variability in the vaporizer's output of enflurane and found that the readings of the vapor monitors were not within the manufacturer's stated ±5% accuracy after 2 years without routine service.

THE DRÄGER AS3 ELECTRONIC ANESTHESIA APPARATUS, 1988

The Dräger AS3 Electronic Anesthesia apparatus of 1988 (Fig. 33-12), a third-generation prototype microprocessor-controlled anesthesia workstation, uses digital quantification of fresh-gas flow, vaporization of volatile anesthetics, and the minute volume ventilation provided by the ventilator. The digital technology increases the overall accuracy of the metering systems from the conventional ±25% to 30% to ±4% to 8%[9-13] (Fig. 33-13).

Measurement of gas flow

For greater accuracy in measurement of gas delivery, a digitally controlled volumetric gas measuring system is used (Fig. 33-14). In this system, a known volume is filled to a preset pressure, and that volume of gas is then released into the system, which is at a lower pressure. The frequency of these gas pulses determines the flow rate, which is independently monitored by a hot wire anemometer.

Table 33-1. Summary of measurements made to validate the performance of six Engström Elsa anesthesia machines after 18–24 months' regular use without routine service

Variable	Average difference from test equipment (%)	Range of differences (%) (six machines)	Manufacturer's claimed accuracy (%)
Fresh gas flow N_2O/O_2 400-1000 ml/min	−19	−11 to −28	±10
Fresh gas flow N_2O/O_2 1.5-10 L/min	± 7	+8 to −10	±10
Tidal volume	+ 5	+2 to +9	±7
Expired minute volume	+ 6	0 to +11	±7
Vaporizer at 2% settings			
Halothane	± 8	+10 to −10	±5
Enflurane	±25	+10 to −55	±5
Isoflurane	± 9	+10 to −20	±5
Vapor monitor			
Halothane	+12	0 to +22	±5
Enflurane	+18	+6 to +32	±5
Isoflurane	+17	+6 to +33	±5
Oxygen monitor	± 1.3	+4 to −2	±2

From Alexander JP, et al: The Engström Elsa anaesthetic machine, *Anaesthesia* 45: 746-750, 1990.

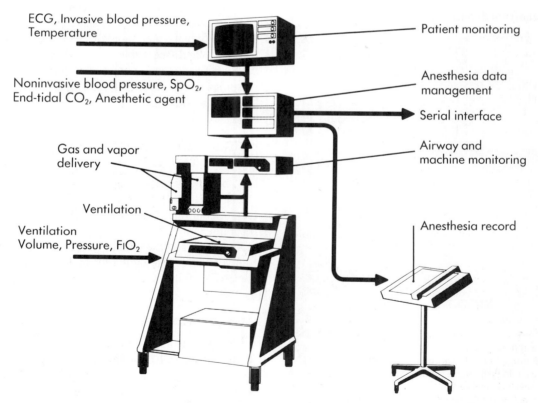

Fig. 33-12. Dräger Anesthesia Workplace, 1988. (Illustration courtesy Westenskow DR, Wallroth CF: Regelkreise für Anaesthesia-Atemsysteme Beit, *Anaesth Intensivther Notfallmed* 35: 137-151, 1990.)

Overall accuracy of metering
and ventilation systems

	Conventional	Analog servoloop	Digital volumetric
Gas	± 24%	± 14%	± 4%
Liquid	± 32%	± 14%	± 8%
Ventilation	± 29%	± 21%	± 7%
Summary	± 25% to 30%	± 15% to 20%	± 4% to ± 8%
Classification for quantitative anesthesia	Unacceptable	Marginal	Desirable

Fig. 33-13. Dräger Anesthesia Workplace, 1988. Overall accuracy of metering and ventilation systems.

Vaporization of volatile agents

A micropump (Fig. 33-15) is employed to deliver a fixed volume of liquid anesthetic agent at a variable frequency into a heated mixing chamber, where it is mixed with a measured flow of gas (Fig. 33-16). The micropump is fail-safe in that it cannot fail in the open position. The concentration of the resultant vapor is monitored independently by an infrared analyzer. The pulse rate of the micropump is controlled by a closed-loop servo mechanism to achieve and maintain the agents' preset end-tidal concentration.[9]

A digitally controlled ventilator

The ventilator is digitally controlled to provide more accurate gas delivery (Fig. 33-17). A cylinder with a defined volume is filled with the gas mixture. The displacement of the piston within the cylinder is measured with a linear displacement transducer, which provides an accurate control of volume. As in Frumin and Lee's 1956 Auto-Anestheton,[14,15] the minute ventilation delivered by the ventilator is varied by a closed-loop servo mechanism to maintain the preset end-tidal carbon dioxide level.

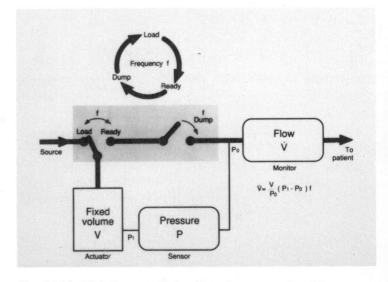

Fig. 33-14. Digitally controlled volumetric gas metering (Illustration courtesy of Wallroth CF, Jaklitsch R, Wied HA: *Technical realization of quantitative metering and ventilation*. In Van Akern K, Frankenberger H, Koneeny E, et al, editors: *Quantitative anaesthesia, low flow and closed circuit*, New York, 1989, Springer-Verlag, p 98.)

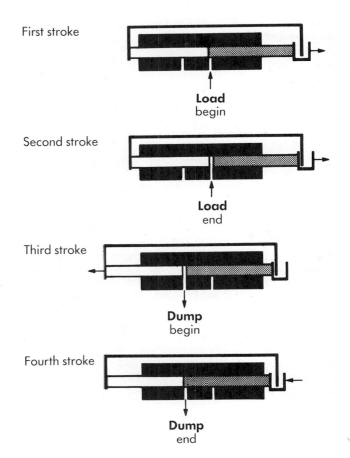

Fig. 33-15. Micropump for delivering fixed volumes of liquid anesthetic agent to the mixing chamber. On the first stroke, the free-moving piston moves to the right and loading begins. On the second stroke, both pistons and agent start to move to the left. On the third stroke, dumping of the agent commences as the free-moving piston is driven to the left. Finally, on the fourth stroke, both pistons are transferred to the loading position. In the event of a power failure, no liquid agent is delivered. (Illustration from Wallroth CF, Jaklitsch R, Wied HA: *Technical realization of quantitative metering and ventilation*. In Van Ackern K, Frankenberger H, Koneeny E, et al, editors: *Quantitative anaesthesia, low flow and closed circuit*, New York, 1989, Springer-Verlag, p 102.)

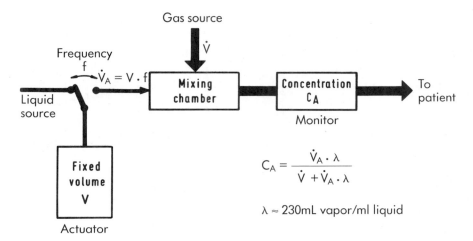

$$C_A = \frac{\dot{V}_A \cdot \lambda}{\dot{V} + \dot{V}_A \cdot \lambda}$$

$\lambda \approx 230\text{mL vapor/ml liquid}$

Fig. 33-16. Digitally controlled volumetric anesthetic agent metering system. A fixed volume of liquid anesthetic from the micropump is added to a known volume of gas mixture delivered to the mixing chamber. The final concentration is checked by the independent infrared monitor. (Illustration courtesy of Wallroth CF, Jaklitsch R, Wied HA: *Technical realization of quantitative metering and ventilation.* In Van Ackern, K, Frankenberger H, Koneeny E, et al, editors: *Quantitative anaesthesia, low flow and closed circuit,* New York, 1989, Springer-Verlag, p. 101.)

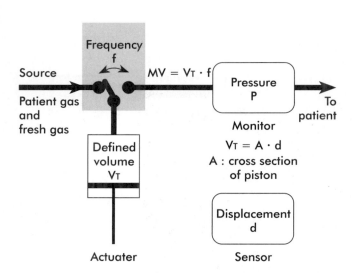

Fig. 33-17. Digitally controlled ventilation. To minimize the effect of system compliance and fresh-gas flows on the volume delivered, a defined volume is filled with gas mixture. The displacement of the piston is measured by the displacement transducer, and this displacement, multiplied by the cross-sectional area of the piston, gives the filling volume. After filling, the control valve changes and the defined volume is delivered to the patient at a pressure (*P*) indicated by the monitor. (Illustration courtesy of Wallroth CF, Jaklitsch R, Wied HA: *Technical realization of quantitative metering and ventilation.* In Van Ackern, K, Frankenberger H, Koneeny E, et al, editors: *Quantitative anaesthesia, low flow and closed circuit,* New York, 1989, Springer-Verlag, p 104.)

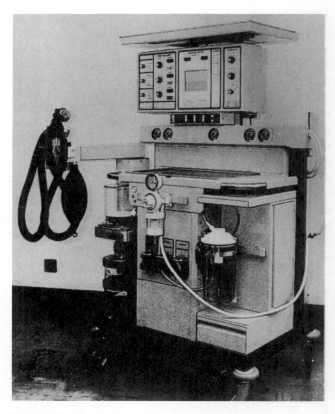

Fig. 33-18. The Oxford microprocessor-controlled anaesthetic machine of 1989 was built in the Nuffield Department of Anaesthetics, Oxford, U.K., in cooperation with the Penlon Company The base of the unit contains the gas supplies, gas mixing, vaporizers, gas analysis, breathing system, and ventilator modules plus suction. (Illustrations from Sykes MK, Sugg BR, Hahn CE et al: A new microprocessor-controlled anaesthetic machine, *Br J Anaesth* 62: 447, 1989.)

THE OXFORD MICROPROCESSOR-CONTROLLED ANAESTHETIC MACHINE, 1989

The Oxford microprocessor-controlled machine (Fig. 33-18) design utilizes the power of five microprocessors to simplify the mechanical components of the fresh gas delivery and vaporizer components of the machine.[16] Figure 33-19 shows the arrangement of the mechanical components. Figure 33-20 shows the relationship between the controls and the monitoring for each machine function.

Gas flow control and mixing

Supplies of oxygen, air, and nitrous oxide at 300 kPa (43 psig) are fed to microprocessor-controlled solenoid-operated valves. Pulses of gas released from these valves pass through chokes to the mixing chambers. These chambers are maintained at a constant pressure of 100 cm H_2O by variable-orifice valves that incorporate transducers to indicate the gas flow (Fig. 33-21).[17,18] As a known volume of gas is released with each pulse, the gas mixture and flow can be varied by the microprocessor by varying the pulse rate for each individual gas (Figs. 33-22 and 33-23).

Vaporizers

Gas from the second constant back-pressure valve is divided into bypass flow and vaporizer flow (Fig. 33-24). The latter is controlled by a solenoid valve and is released fully saturated in pulses from the Copper Kettle type of vaporizer. Because both the vaporizer temperature and the vapor pressure curve of the agent are known, the flow of gas through the vaporizer is controlled by a microprocessor to produce the desired concentration of agent in the final mixture. An interferometer measures the gas and vapor in the fresh gas.[19] The oxygen concentration in the inspiratory limb of the breathing system is measured by a paramagnetic analyzer. An infrared analyzer monitors the carbon dioxide level in the circuit at the patient Y piece. Inspired and expired gas volumes are measured by turbine flowmeters, and airway pressure is sensed by a pressure transducer close to the inspiratory unidirectional valve.

All functions of the machine are programmed and controlled by a microprocessor, that receives its instructions from the settings on the manual control. The measured values are displayed on the control panel, enabling the user to compare them with the set values. The microprocessors also compare these parameters and alert the user to any discrepancy. The base unit contains the gas supplies, gas mixing, vaporizing, gas analysis, the breathing system and ventilator modules, and suction.

Controls

The control panel can be moved sideways and rotated in order to position it close to the patient's head and facing the user (Figs. 33-18 and 33-25). Controls on the left side of the control panel are for selecting the gas mixture, breathing system, and volatile agent together with oxygen concentration, total fresh-gas flow, and vapor concentration. In each case the measured values are displayed digitally to the right of the controls. On the right side are the ventilator controls for frequency, tidal volume, *I:E* ratio, and on/off. In the center section are the breathing system monitors for inspired oxygen concentration and minute volume, together with a screen displaying a tidal volume bar graph, with both analog and digital displays of airway pressure or carbon dioxide concentration plus malfunction messages.

Any of the following breathing systems can be selected electronically: circle system, with or without carbon dioxide absorption; Mapleson A or D systems; and PEEP. The machine is designed to deliver a minimum oxygen flow of 1 L/min and a minimum fresh-gas flow of 3 L/min, except with the carbon dioxide absorption system, when a "low flow option" permits a total fresh-gas flow of 2 L/min.

THE UTAH ANESTHESIA WORKSTATION

Loeb, et al.[20] designed the prototype Utah Anesthesia Workstation to demonstrate the feasibility of computer-assisted anesthesia apparatus (Fig. 33-26). A Macintosh Plus computer is used to control a standard Dräger Narkomed anesthesia machine to which have been added electronic sensors and analyzers, electronic gas flow controls (Fig. 33-27), and an Ohmeda 7000 ventilator. A large computer screen provides a central display for system data and controls. To help the user, the amount of information is limited and preprocessed. Alarms identify the cause of the problem rather than merely indicating that a signal has exceeded its threshold (see Fig. 33-28).

Information is displayed on the screen, and the system is controlled by using the track ball controller to point to on-screen images (Fig. 33-29). Below the display are three control-mode buttons. In "Manual," the machine is operated in the normal fashion, with the system's monitoring and electronic control functions inoperative. This mode is used at the beginning of anesthesia, before the patient is tracheally intubated. After intubation, mechanical ventilation is begun and the apparatus is changed to either "Autopilot" or "Electronic Control," activating monitoring and electronic control of the flow of oxygen and nitrous oxide and the quantity of anesthetic vapor delivered from the Verni-Trol vaporizer. In "Electronic Control," the flows are set by the anesthesiologist. In "Autopilot," fresh-gas flow, oxygen concentration, and the anesthetic vapor concentration in the fresh gas are set by the user, with the computer calculating the flow that must be delivered to achieve these set points.

Monitors

The sensors and analyzers send signals to the computer preprocessor. The latter detects each breath on the basis of

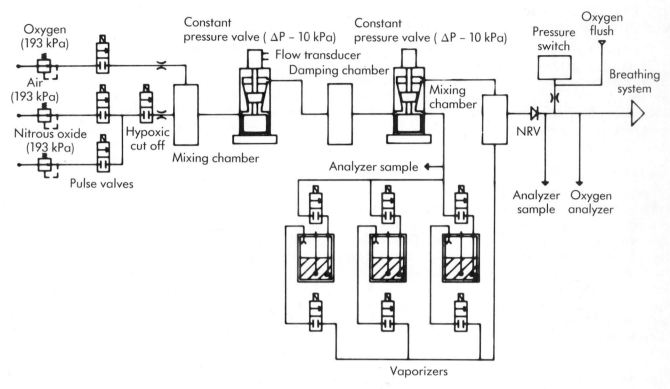

Fig. 33-19. Arrangement of the mechanical components of the fresh gas and vaporizer units of the Oxford machine. 1 kPa = 7.5 mm Hg, so that 10 kPa = 75 mm Hg and 193 kPa = 1448 mm Hg. *NRV*, nonreturn valve. (Illustration from Sykes MK, Sugg BR, Hahn CE, et al: A new microprocessor-controlled anaesthesia machine, *Br J Anaesth* 62: 446, 1989.)

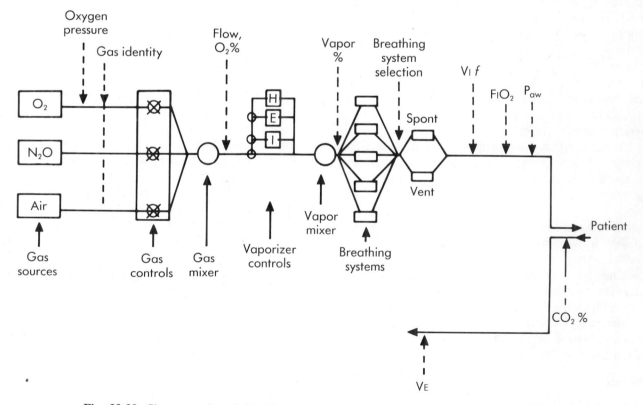

Fig. 33-20. Shown are the relationships between the controls (*solid arrows*), and the monitors (*dotted arrows*) monitoring the machine's function. V_I, Inspired volume; V_E, expired volume; *f*, frequency; P_{aw}, airway pressure. (Illustration from Sykes MK, Sugg BR, Hahn CE, et al: A new microprocessor-controlled anaesthesia machine, *Br J Anaesth* 62: 445-455, 1989.)

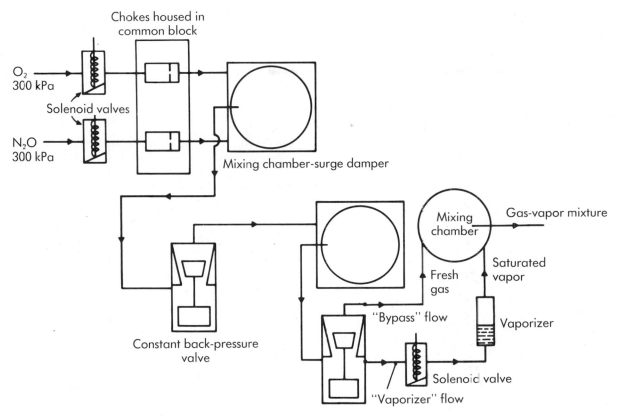

Fig. 33-21. Schematic of the system for gas mixing, flow stabilizing, and vaporizer systems. (From Hahn CE, Palayiwa E, Sugg BR, et al: A microprocessor-controlled anaesthetic vaporizer, *Br J Anaesth* 58:1161-1166, 1986.)

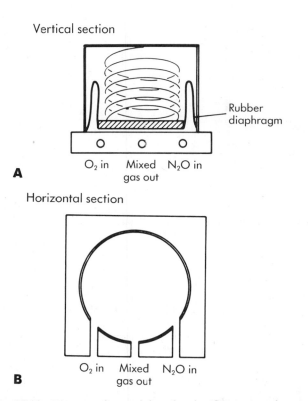

Fig. 33-22. Diagram of gas-mixing chamber/flow surger damper in **A**, vertical and **B**, horizontal sections.

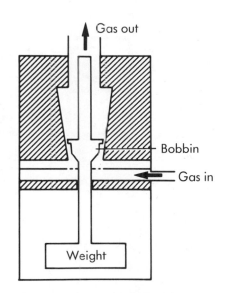

Fig. 33-23. Diagram of constant back-pressure valve with flow-rate transducer. (Note the similarity to Heidbrink flowmeters of the 1930s in Macintosh R, Mushin W, and Epstein H, *Physics for the anaesthetist*, 2nd edition, Oxford, 1958, Blackwell, Fig. 219, p 209.)

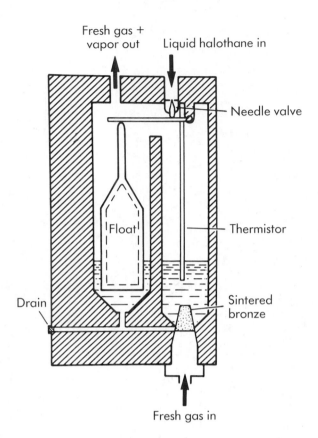

Fresh gas + vapor out | Liquid halothane in
Needle valve
Float
Thermistor
Drain
Sintered bronze
Fresh gas in

Fig. 33-24. Schematic of the Copper Kettle type of vaporizer. To avoid problems with the nitrous oxide dissolving in the halothane, the vaporizer contains only 10 ml of the agent in the vaporizing chamber. When the level of the liquid falls, the float also falls and the needle valve opens and admits more agent to the vaporizer. The thermistor informs the microprocessor of the temperature within the vaporizer so that the microprocessor can control the gas flow through the vaporizer to maintain a steady concentration of the agent in the final gas mixture. (Illustration from Hahn CE, Palayiwa E, Sugg BR, et al: A microprocessor-controlled anaesthetic vaporizer, *Br J Anaesth* 58:1163, 1986.)

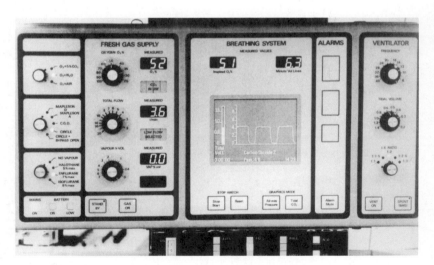

Fig. 33-25. The Oxford microprocessor-controlled anaesthetic machine. The control panel is divided into three main sections. The left section controls the fresh gas mixture, the breathing systems, and the volatile agents, together with the controls for the oxygen concentration, total fresh-gas flow, and the anesthetic vapor concentration. The measured values in the fresh gas for oxygen concentration, total gas flow, and vapor concentration are displayed digitally to the right of these controls. The right-hand section has the controls for the ventilator. The center panel has the breathing system monitors and alarms and an electroluminescent screen, which displays the tidal volume and airway pressures or carbon dioxide concentration, together with any messages concerning malfunction. (Illustration from Sykes MK, Suggs BR, Hahn CE, et al: A new microprocessor-controlled anaesthetic machine, *Br J Anaesth* 62:445-455, 1989.)

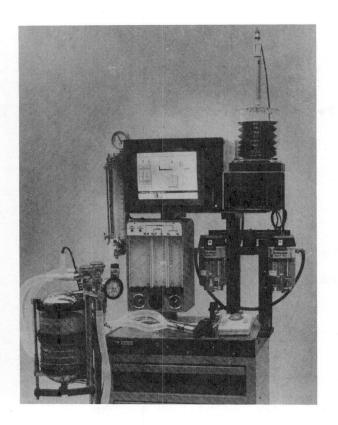

Fig. 33-26. The Utah Anesthesia Workstation, 1989. (Illustration from Loeb RG, Brunner JX, Westenskow DR, et al., *Anesthesiology* 70:999-1007, 1989.

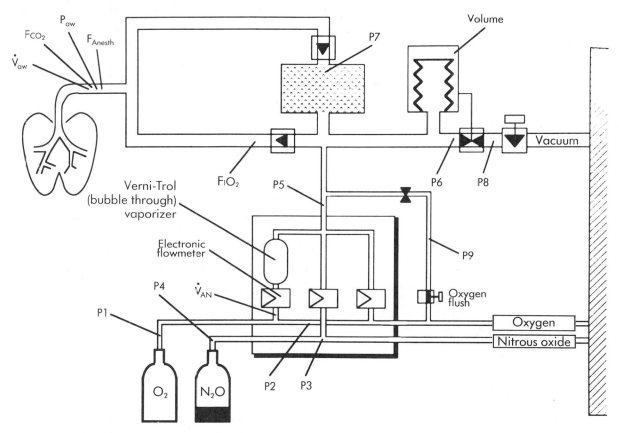

Fig. 33-27. Utah Anesthesia Workstation. Location of sensors on the anesthesia apparatus and breathing system. *P1 through P9*, Pressure sensors; $\dot{V}_{aw}$, measures gas flow at the airway: $\dot{V}_{an}$, measures oxygen flow into the Verni-Trol vaporizer: *FiO₂, Fanesth, FCO₂*, measure concentrations of oxygen, halogenated anesthetic, and carbon dioxide, respectively. *Volume* senses the position of the ventilator bellows. (Illustration courtesy of Loeb RG, Brunner JX, Westenskow Dr, et al: The Utah Anesthesia Workstation, *Anesthesiology* 70:999-1007, 1989.)

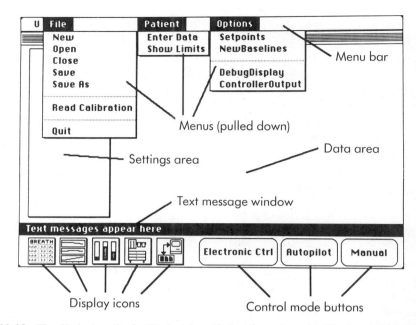

Fig. 33-28. The Utah Anesthesia Workstation display format on the Macintosh Plus computer screen. The control mode buttons are used to select the operating mode. In "Manual" the machine is operated normally and there is no electronic monitoring. During "Electronic Control" and "Autopilot" the machine is controlled electronically and electronic monitoring is active. (Illustration courtesy of Loeb RG, Brunner JX, Westenskow DR, et al: The Utah Anesthesia Workstation, *Anesthesiology* 70:999-1007, 1989.)

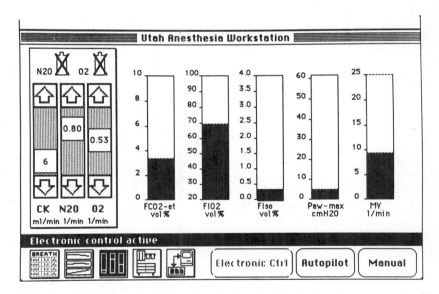

Fig. 33-29. The Utah Anesthesia Workstation display. In this display, the apparatus is operating under "Electronic Control". On the left, the gas flow settings indicate flows of 6 ml/min through the vaporizer, 0.80 L/min nitrous oxide, and 0.53 L/min oxygen. The crossed out nitrous oxide and oxygen cylinders indicate that these cylinders are closed. The bar graphs indicate expired carbon dioxide of 3.5 volumes percent, inspired oxygen 70%, inspired isoflurane 0.3%, maximum airway pressure of 10 cm H_2O, and a minute volume of 9 L/min. (Illustration courtesy of Loeb RG, Brunner JX, Westenskow DR, et al: The Utah Anesthesia Workstation, *Anesthesiology* 70:999-1007, 1989.)

the carbon dioxide concentration and the flow through the pneumotachometer and then reports the duration of inspiration, the peak pressure, the end-tidal carbon dioxide, and so on. The computer evaluates these data and can detect any unexpected events. Should an event be detected, the display alerts the user by flashing a written message and indicating the location of the failure on a diagram (Fig. 33-30). Should more than one event occur simultaneously, all of the affected areas on the schematic flash, but the text of only the most important priority is displayed. The current program enables the computer to detect and diagnose 26 system problems, and when tested had an accuracy of 94%. This system collects 17 signals and summarizes them on a breath-by-breath basis. The data are then analyzed to detect patterns, and these are compared with the model-based threshold values when necessary. The advantage of this integrated approach is that problems can be detected which otherwise might be missed. Although this present apparatus provided limited computer-assisted control, future versions will include a "sophisticated self-tuning interlinked controller" for anesthetic concentration, oxygen concentration, and fresh-gas flow.[20,21]

The PhysioFlex Rotterdam ventilator, 1989

Designed from the start as a closed system,[22,23] analogous to a lung function spirometer, the PhysioFlex (Fig. 33-31) is a combined ventilator-anesthesia apparatus that bears little resemblance to a customary anesthesia machine. For example, it has no flowmeters and provides no indication of the fresh-gas flow rates. It simplifies the operator's task by making extensive use of servo feedback systems.[24] Once the operator has set the parameters, the

machine's computer performs the necessary calculations and carries out minute-to-minute adjustments to ensure that the parameters are met (Fig. 33-32). A blower circulates the gases around the system at a rate of 70 L/min, providing optimal gas mixing. There is an absorber to remove the carbon dioxide and a charcoal absorber to remove the volatile agent at the end of the anesthesia. A paramagnetic oxygen analyzer displays the oxygen concentration in the system continuously, and an infrared multigas analyzer samples from the Y piece, returning the sampled gas to the system. Volatile anesthetic is aspirated from the agent bottle and injected from a syringe by a computer-controlled injection pump. All gases are admitted to the system through computer-controlled valves. For mechanical ventilation, the customary bag-in-a-box arrangement is replaced by four membrane chambers positioned in parallel, one or more of which is employed depending on the tidal volume required. Although designed as a closed system for use with controlled ventilation, a simple knob converts it to spontaneous or manually controlled ventilation. Much of the patient's breathing system is enclosed within the apparatus, making cleaning and sterilization an apparent problem. It is therefore essential to use a fresh, disposable bacterial filter for each patient.

In use

When the apparatus is switched on, it performs an automatic system check of the gas supply, leakage, oxygen analyzer calibration, infrared analyzer test with calibration gas, and the computer itself. It also displays a checklist of six items that the user must verify have been checked before the computer is ready to start (Fig. 33-33). The user then enters the patient's body weight, age, and sex; and

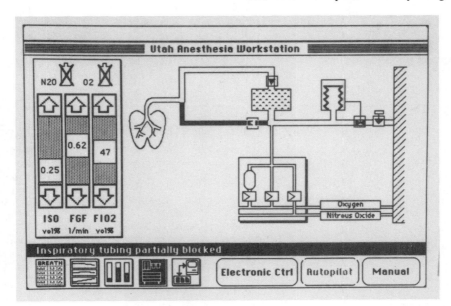

Fig. 33-30. Utah Anesthesia Workstation. The user is alerted by the computer monitor message saying, "inspiratory tubing partially blocked," and the diagram indicating where the blockage has occurred. (Illustration courtesy of Loeb RG, Brunner JX, Westenskow DR, et al: The Utah Anesthesia Workstation, *Anesthesiology* 70:999-1007, 1989.)

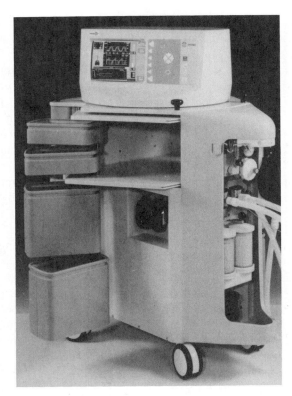

Fig. 33-31. The PhysioFlex Rotterdam Ventilator (1989). The control console, with its touch button controls and display panel on top of the apparatus, may be rotated to permit the machine to be placed either on the user's left-hand or right-hand side, as desired. The bottles of volatile anesthetic agents are seen in the small recess, where they are attached directly to the apparatus for delivery of the liquid agent to the vaporizer. The breathing hose and carbon dioxide absorbers are seen on the right. Mobile equipment trays and bins are attached to the apparatus on the left. (Illustration courtesy of Physio BV, Amsterdam, The Netherlands.)

the computer displays on the screen the proposed tidal volume and respiratory rate based on the Radford Tables[25] (Fig. 33-34). If these values are satisfactory the user presses the "OK" button on the console. If not, different parameters may be entered. The computer then selects only the appropriate number of ventilatory chambers to provide the required tidal exchange. This minimizes the system's internal compression volume, making possible ventilation of infants. The *I:E* ratio and the shape of the inspiratory and expiratory curves with PEEP or with negative end-expiratory pressure (NEEP) can be displayed on the screen before being applied. The oxygen percentage with nitrous oxide or air in the gas mixture is then chosen. When satisfied with the machine's settings, the user initiates the set-up procedure whereby the system is flushed with 95% oxygen and the oxygen analyzer is calibrated. The carrier gas, either nitrous oxide or air, is then injected until the reservoir bags in the membrane chambers are completely filled. The oxygen concentration in the breathing system is thus diluted to the preselected value. The computer then calculates the volume of the system. At the same time, the syringe is filled with the chosen volatile anesthetic. The system is now ready and requests permission to start. When the system is in use, all gas concentrations are automatically maintained at the preset values and the ventilation provided is the preselected pattern that had been previewed on the screen.

Vaporizer

A computer-controlled step motor drives the vaporizer syringe, which injects the liquid directly into the breathing system. There, the gas flow of 70 L/min causes its immediate evaporation. The system is feedback servocontrolled to achieve the chosen end-tidal concentration. To reach a

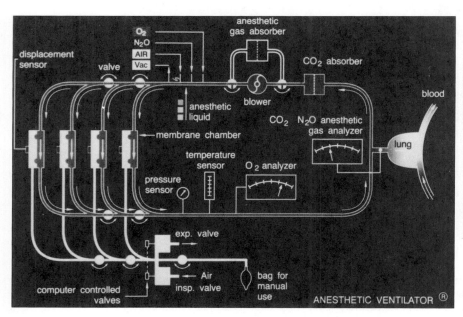

Fig. 33-32. Functional diagram of the PhysioFlex Rotterdam Ventilator. The gas mixture in this closed system is circulated by a blower because there are no unidirectional valves. The tidal exchange is produced by compression of one or more of the membrane chambers. The activated charcoal adsorber is used to remove the volatile anesthetic agent to terminate the anesthesia. (Illustration courtesy of Physio BV, Amsterdam, The Netherlands.)

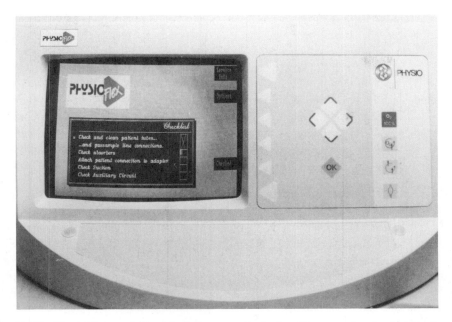

Fig. 33-33. PhysioFlex machine. Monitor screen displaying 6 items to be checked by the user before the computer will activate the apparatus. The PhysioFlex color monitor has 15 keys, 6 of which are soft keys, whereby the user controls the apparatus. The apparatus displays menus from which the user may choose that which best suits the patient. (Illustration courtesy of Physio BV, Amsterdam, The Netherlands.)

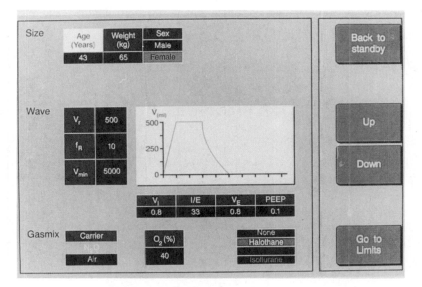

Fig. 33-34. PhysioFlex machine. The anesthesiologist has entered the patient's statistics: A 43-year-old female weighing 65 kg. The anesthesiologist has chosen to use 40% oxygen with nitrous oxide and halothane. The apparatus suggested a tidal exchange of 500 ml with a frequency of 10 breaths per minute, making a minute ventilation of 5 L. (Illustration courtesy of Physio BV, Amsterdam, The Netherlands.)

steady state of anesthesia rapidly, a priming dose of the volatile agent is injected at the start. Based on Lowe and Ernst's recommendation,[26] this priming dose is calculated by the computer on the basis of the patient's body weight and the system's volume. The system then provides an optimum computer-controlled wash-in and prevents an overshoot of the desired end-tidal concentration. To lower the concentration of volatile anesthetic, the computer switches in the activated charcoal filter, which is normally in a bypass position. At the end of the anesthetic, the step motor automatically returns the remainder of the liquid volatile anesthetic to the reservoir bottle.

The monitor and control panel

The control panel (Fig. 33-35) may be rotated to provide the user with the best possible visibility. In this feedback control system, the function of the apparatus is varied by the computer in order to produce the preset desired conditions. Oxygen uptake and the end-tidal carbon dioxide concentration are presented in trend curves on the color monitor, together with most of the ventilatory parameters presented in real-time curves. The inspiratory and end-tidal volatile anesthetic concentrations are also displayed, together with a bar graph showing the exact composition of the gas mixture in the system.

Alarms

The chosen limits for the functions are monitored by the computer, and the system warns and alarms with different sound levels depending on the amount of deviation from the preset level. Each alarm or warning is accompanied by a message in red on the screen. The warnings cannot be switched off, and the alarm sound can be silenced for only 1 minute. Esophageal intubation is recognized by the ab-

sence of carbon dioxide on the capnogram. A circuit disconnection is detected by the absence of the plateau pressure in the system. If occlusion of the sample line is sensed, the injection of volatile anesthetic into the system is interrupted. In the event of a power failure, a battery supplies 30 minutes of back-up power to operate the system.

This apparatus represents a complete break from traditional designs in that it does not attempt to reproduce electronically such features of a traditional anesthesia machine as flowmeters for the gases. On the other hand, it displays on its color screen many parameters not normally available to the anesthesiologist in the OR. In addition, the system's feedback control enables it to make the necessary minor adjustments to keep the respiratory parameters, the gas mixture, the volatile agent, and many other features within the preset limits. It thus relieves the anesthesiologist of the need to constantly adjust the controls of the apparatus. Like the cruise control on a modern automobile, it probably provides a much smoother management than can be achieved by even the most careful human attention. Furthermore, because it is a totally closed system, it brings to fruition in modern times the intention of Dennis Jackson who, in 1915, designed the first nitrous oxide–oxygen circle absorption system to provide economy together with accurate control of the depth of anesthesia.[27]

Human factors in design of anesthesia apparatus

As pointed out earlier (see Chapter 18), the design of anesthesia apparatus lags markedly behind the design of aircraft cockpits from the point of view of human engineering. The American National Standard on Minimum Performance and Safety Requirements for Anesthesia Apparatus (Z79.8, published in 1979) required that "flowmeters, gauges, controls and other displays that should be

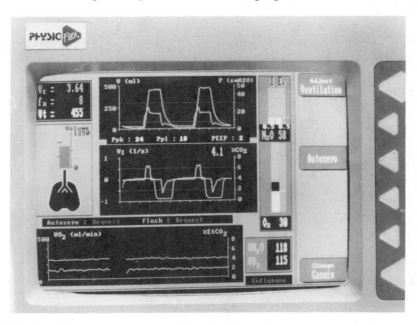

Fig. 33-35. PhysioFlex monitor and control panel. (Illustration courtesy of Physio BV, Amsterdam, The Netherlands.)

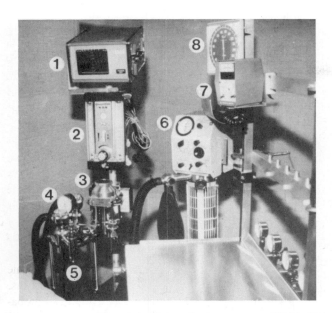

Fig. 33-36. The "line of sight" anesthesia apparatus (1976). Designed by Chalmers M. Goodyear and Leslie Rendell-Baker, M.D., and built by the Harris-Lake Co. for The Mount Sinai Hospital in New York. The machine's gauges and controls face a user seated at the patient's head. *1*, ECG; *2*, flowmeters; *3*, vaporizer; *4*, breathing system pressure gauge; *5*, carbon dioxide absorber; *6*, ventilator controls; *7*, oxygen analyzer; *8*, sphygmomanometer. (Copyright 1976, L. Rendell-Baker, M.D.)

checked most frequently should be grouped together and should be placed in the optimum visual zone as close as possible to the operator's line of sight when viewing the patient." There is little evidence, however, that this has been followed in the intervening period. An apparatus (Fig. 33-36) built in 1976 and widely exhibited at that time clearly demonstrated that the ECG, flowmeters, vaporizer, and ventilator controls could be placed so that they faced the user when the patient was being observed. In spite of this practical demonstration, present designs show little tendency to follow this lead.

The design for a future electronic anesthesia workstation that incorporates good human factors in its design and uses current available technology is shown in Fig. 33-37. The patient monitor (*1*) together with the monitor and controls for the apparatus (*3*) can be placed near the side of the patient's head, where they can be easily seen by the user at all times. In this design, the usual position for these devices is occupied by the automatic anesthesia chart recorder (*10*) and its controls (11).

FUTURE TRENDS

Studies of airline pilots and operators of other complex systems have shown that when faced with stressful situations, an excessive amount of information, and numerous alarms sounding, the tendency is to switch off this excess input and to "fly by the seat of their pants," ignoring the instrumentation. Airplanes are now designed to present the pilot with only the most essential information in a "heads up" display so that the pilot can concentrate on the task at hand. The bulk of the information is handled by the computers. If future anesthesia workstation designers are to follow this lead, computers will be used to monitor the myriad of details of minute-to-minute control, clearly alerting the operator when either the apparatus or the patient deviates from the desired parameters. Westenskow and colleagues' Utah Anesthesia Workstation and the PysioFlex designs clearly show how the computer can be used to spare the operator from the minute-to-minute task of monitoring the function of the apparatus. The several models of the Puritan Bennett 7200 ventilator have clearly demonstrated how easily a machine's function can be modified in response to changing needs merely by changing the circuit boards.

It is most likely that future volatile anesthetic agents will be even more expensive than those currently available. This will make closed circuit methods more desirable to help contain anesthesia costs.

Safety features

An electronic anesthesia apparatus cannot be used safely without a back-up battery power supply. This should provide power for 1 to 2 hours in the event that the main power supply fails. Some essential monitoring should also be available on reserve power. Finally, a reserve supply of oxygen must be available to be used with manual ventilation in the event that all power supplies, including the reserve battery supply, are lost.

Safety standards

The International Standards Organization* Technical Committee 121, and the European Community Standards Committee† CEN/TC215/WG1 are writing safety standards for anesthesia workstations that will be applied when the European Community's central authority assumes control of medical equipment safety in Europe in 1992. Manufacturers in the United States will clearly be impacted because they supply anesthesia and ventilator equipment to Europe. It seems likely that the European standard, mandatory in Europe, will also greatly influence what equipment is available in the United States market in the future.

In reviewing the apparatus described here, along with the recently published papers it is clear that all the essential systems necessary to assemble a modern electronic servo-controlled anesthesia workstation are available to present-day designers. In Europe the two advanced electronic anesthesia workstations—the Engström Elsa and the PhysioFlex Rotterdam—are already commercially avail-

*For information on US or ISO standards, contact Beth Kilburn Moran, ASTM, 1916 Race St., Philadelphia, Pa. 19103-1187, USA.
†For CEN standards, contact Dr. Carl F. Wallroth, PE, Drägerwerk A.G., Moislinger Allee, 53-55 P.O. Box 1339, D-2400 Lubeck 1, Germany.

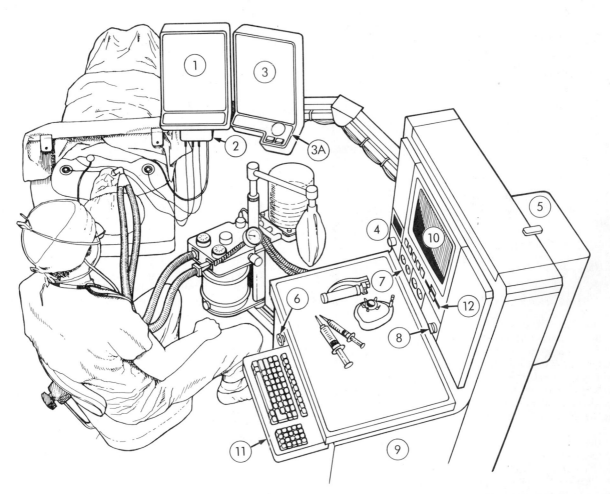

Fig. 33-37. Good human factors design of future anesthesia workstation: Presently available components have been arranged so that the patient monitor (*1*) and the apparatus controls and monitor (*3*) can be placed close to the patient's head. The patient monitor (*1*) may have analog and digital displays of the ECG, pulse rate, noninvasive blood pressure, arterial and other pressure readings, pulse oximeter and body temperature, inspired and expired oxygen and carbon dioxide, and anesthetic agents. The minute volume, tidal volume, respiratory frequency, and airway pressure are also displayed. The patient connections to the monitor enter at (*2*). Panel 3 displays the information concerning the function of the anesthesia apparatus, which the computer monitors to aid the user in its control. The computer controls the flow and delivery of gases and anesthetic vapors. The anesthesiologist controls the system with the track ball controller (*3A*), which controls the menus displayed on the screen, enabling the user to choose the one desired. If the computer detects a malfunction, a visual and audible alarm, together with a message on the screen, will simplify the user's task and speed the correct response. *4,* This monitor shows the total gas flow and also controls the emergency oxygen supply in the event that all power supplies are lost; *5,* contains the bottles of volatile anesthetic agents from which the agent is delivered by the pump to the vaporizer; *6,* the emergency oxygen flush control; *7,* the pipeline pressure and cylinder pressure gauges; *8,* the on/off control for gases and electrical power; *9,* within the cabinet are the electronic gas flowmeters, the micropump-operated vaporizer, the ventilator, and back-up battery power with trickle charger; *10,* displays the anesthesia chart, which is automatically recorded on a floppy disk inserted at (*12*) for later preparation of hard-copy printout in the PACU; (*11*), keyboard for additions to be made to the patient record. This proposed design brings together features of the present-day Ohmeda anesthesia delivery system and ventilator, the volatile anesthetic bottle attachment and vaporizer of the Engström Elsa apparatus, the control keyboard of the North American Dräger, and present automatic record-keeping systems. What sets this design apart from the others is that it has been arranged according to good human factors engineering, with the apparatus display panels arranged alongside the patient, who, after all, should be the prime focus of attention. (Copyright 1991, L. Rendell-Baker, M.D.)

able and will undoubtedly "break the ice" for the acceptance of the designs that will certainly follow in Europe.

When will this electronic feedback-controlled anesthesia delivery system appear on the United States' market? All major manufacturers have prototype equipment in advanced stages of development, and this will no doubt be put into production when they believe that there is sufficient demand from clinicians.In the past, however, anesthesiologists have tended to prefer 30-year-old equipment designs. This has restricted the implementation of changes, which may have to wait for a new generation of anesthesiologists who are more comfortable with computer technology.

REFERENCES

1. Foregger R: The rotameter in anesthesia, *Anesthesiology* 7:549-556, 1946.
2. Macintosh RR, Epstein HG: 50 Jahre rotameter for narkoseapparat, *Der Anaesthetist* 10:213-214, 1961.
3. Magill IW: Anaesthetic flowmeters, *Lancet* ii:776, 1941.
4. Trost AH: Anaesthetic flowmeters, *Lancet* i:92, 1942.
5. Sword BC: The closed circle method of administration of gas anesthesia, *Anesth Analg* 9:198, 1930.
6. Cooper JB, Newbower RS, Moore JW, et al: A new anesthesia delivery system, *Anesthesiology* 49:310-318, 1978.
7. Norlander OP, Hahn CEW, Palayiwa E, et al: A new integrated system for anesthesia. Abstract #99. Presented at the seventh European Congress in Anesthesiology, Vienna, 1986.
8. Alexander JP, Watters CH, Dodds WJ, et al: The Engström Elsa anaesthetic machine, *Anaesthesia* 45:746-750, 1990.
9. Westenskow DR, Wallroth CF: Closed loop control for anesthesia breathing systems, *J Clin Monit* 6:249-256, 1990.
10. Wallroth CF: Design of anesthesia equipment for quantitative anesthesia. Proceedings of the Closed Circuit and Low Flow Anesthesia Systems Society's third international symposium, Washington, DC, May 1988, p 33.
11. Wallroth CF: Technical conceptions for an anesthesia system with electronic metering of gases and vapors, *Acta Anaesthesiol Belg* 34:279-294, 1984.
12. Wallroth CF, Jaklitsch R, Wied HA: Technical realization of quantitative metering and ventilation. In Van Akern K, Frankenberger H, Koneeny E, et al, editors: *Quantitative anaesthesia*, New York, 1989, Springer-Verlag.
13. Westenskow DR, Walroth CF: Regelkreise für Anesthesia-Atemsysteme Beit, *Anaesth Intensivther Notfallmed* 35:137-151, 1990.
14. Frumin MJ, Lee ASJ: A physiologically oriented artificial respirator which produces N_2O-O_2 anesthesia in man, *J Lab Clin Med* 49:617, 1957.
15. Frumin MJ: Clinical use of a physiological respirator producing N_2O-O_2 amnesia-analgesia, *Anesthesiology* 18:290, 1957.
16. Sykes MK, Sugg BR, Hahn CE, et al: A new microprocessor-controlled anaesthetic machine, *Br J Anaesth* 62:445-455, 1989.
17. Palayiwa E, Hahn CE, Sugg BR, et al: A microprocessor-controlled gas mixing device, *Br J Anaesth* 58:1041-1047, 1986.
18. Hahn CE, Palayiwa E, Sugg BR, et al: A microprocessor-controlled anesthetic vaporizer, *Br J Anaesth* 58:1161-1166, 1986.
19. Sugg BR, Palayiwa E, Davies WL, et al: An automatic interferometer for the analysis of anaesthetic gas mixtures, *Br J Anaesth* 61:484-491, 1988.
20. Loeb RG, Brunner JX, Westernskow DR, et al: The Utah Anesthesia Workstation, *Anesthesiology* 70:999-1007, 1989.
21. Westenskow DR, Loughlen PL: *Quantitative anesthesia with the help of closed loop control*. In Van Akern K, Frankenberger H, Koneeny E, et al, editors: *Quantitative anesthesia*, New York, 1989, Springer-Verlag, p 115.
22. Versichelen L, Rolly G: Mass-spectrometric evaluation of some recently introduced low flow, closed circuit systems, *Acta Anas Belgica* 41:225-237, 1990.
23. Verkaaik A, Erdmann W, Grogono AW, et al: A new totally closed circle anesthesia ventilator, *The Circular* 6: October 1989.
24. Erdmann W, Schipper-Veeger A, Verkaaik A, et al: Closing the loop from sensor to therapy: implementation for respiratory closed-circuit systems, *Eur J Anaesthesiol* 6:67, 1989 (abstract).
25. Radford EP: Ventilation standards for use in artificial ventilation, *J Appl Physiol* 7:451, 1955.
26. Lowe HJ, Ernst EA: *The quantitative practice of anesthesia: use of the closed circuit*, Baltimore, 1981, Williams & Wilkins.
27. Jackson DE: New method for production of general analgesia and anesthesia with description of the apparatus used, *J Lab Clin Med* 1:1, 1915.

INDEX